ELECTRONIC PDR®

NP91

PDR on CD-ROM. Send me the PDR on CD-ROM system I have checked below for 30-day preview. If not completely satisfied, I may return the system for a full refund.

CHECK SYSTEM OF YOUR CHOICE:
☐ Item #1M1. Expanded PDR on CD-ROM containing all 5 PDR volumes and The Merck Manual ($895).
☐ Item #1P1. Expanded PDR on CD-ROM containing all 5 PDR volumes ($595).

CHECK TYPE OF DISKETTE DRIVE IN YOUR COMPUTER:
☐ 5¼ inch ☐ 3½ inch CD-ROM drive required.

CHECK METHOD OF PAYMENT:
☐ Payment enclosed (shipping and handling are free).
☐ Bill me or charge my credit card prior to shipment. (Add $3.95 shipping and handling.)
☐ My purchase order is enclosed. (Add $3.95 shipping and handling.)

PDR DRUG INTERACTIONS AND SIDE EFFECTS DISKETTES. Send me the PDR Drug Interactions and Side Effects DISKETTES in the format checked below. If, after 10 days, I decide that they do not fit my needs, I may return them for a full refund.

CHECK SYSTEM OF YOUR CHOICE:
☐ Item #2A1. Complete DISKETTES System
(Includes Drug Interactions and Side Effects *plus* Indications Index) ($219).
☐ Item #2B1. Interactions and Side Effects only ($159).
☐ Item #2C1. Indications only ($79).

CHECK FORMAT: ☐ 360K 5¼″ diskettes ☐ High-density 5¼″ diskettes
☐ 720K 3½″ diskettes ☐ High-density 3½″ diskettes

CHECK METHOD OF PAYMENT:
☐ Payment enclosed (shipping and handling are free).
☐ Bill me or charge my credit card. (Add $3.95 shipping and handling.)
☐ Purchase order enclosed. (Add $3.95 shipping and handling.)

FOR CREDIT CARD ORDERS, please fill in account information below.

Charge my ☐ VISA ☐ MasterCard
(Add $3.95 shipping and handling.)

Account # ________________ Exp. Date ________
MO. YR.

Signature ________________

Your charge will not be processed until your order is shipped.
Residents of NJ, IL, IA, CA, VA and KY please add sales tax.
Purchase of reference materials for professional use may be tax deductible.

Name ________________

Institution ________________

Address ________________

City ________________ State ________ Zip ________

Occupation ________________

Detach along dotted line and mail in an envelope to:
Physicians' Desk Reference,
P.O. Box 824, Mahwah, NJ 07430

Put the Power of PDR on your personal computer! Fill out and return the special order form above. For faster service order by fax: (201) 529-4077.
(Letterhead or purchase order preferred.) ***Do not mail a confirmation order in addition to this fax.***

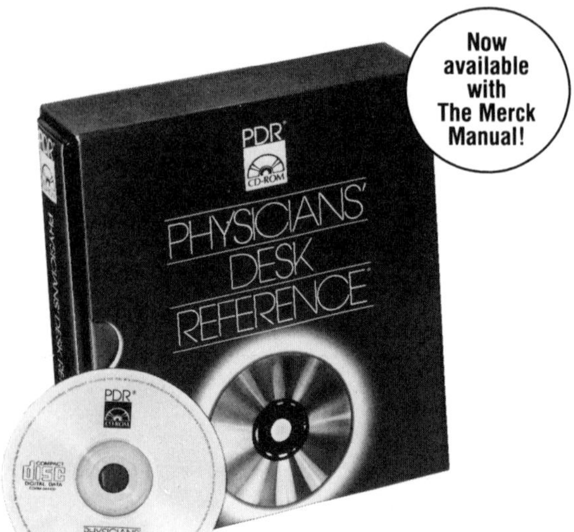

Fast, fail-safe access to the complete text of all 5 PDR® volumes in one integrated program!

PDR® on CD-ROM

The complete contents of all five PDR volumes—plus The Merck Manual—on one CD-ROM disk! United under a single index for quickest access possible. Find the exact text you need in seconds! Compare drugs on a special split screen. Put the power of today's technology—and the vital information of a *complete drug reference library*—to work for you as never before! Choose the PDR on CD-ROM system you want on the order card above.

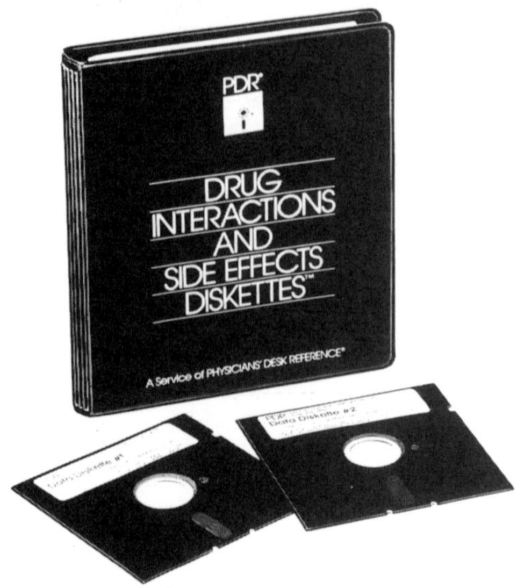

PDR DRUG INTERACTIONS AND SIDE EFFECTS DISKETTES™

Let PDR 1991 Drug Interactions and Side Effects DISKETTES check for interactions of up to 20 drugs at a time—or automatically screen out the source of a side effect. Search 5,000 brand and generic listings found in the PDR,® PDR For Nonprescription Drugs,® and PDR For Ophthalmology.® Check 2,500 side effects as quickly as you can name the reaction...and... find approved alternatives for more than 2,000 indications whenever you pinpoint a problem prescription through the optional Indications Index feature. Select the system and format you need on the order card above.

PDR®

12 EDITION

1991

PHYSICIANS' DESK REFERENCE

CONSUMERS' GUIDE TO NONPRESCRIPTION DRUGS

The same reference that doctors use...now in a paperback version for the general reader!

Publisher • EDWARD R. BARNHART

Director of Sales: KEVIN D. MILLER

Account Managers: CHAD E. ALCORN
CHARLIE J. MEITNER
JOANNE C. TERZIDES

Marketing and Circulation Director:
ROBIN B. BARTLETT

Assistant Circulation Director:
ANNETTE G. VERNON

Fulfillment Manager: ANITA H. MOORE

Professional Relations Manager:
ANNA E. BARBAGALLO

Marketing Administrator: DAWN TERRANOVA

Customer Support Coordinator:
ANNEMARIE LUTOSTANSKI

Senior Research Analyst: PATRICIA DeSIMONE

Publication Manager: ALICE S. MACNOW

Director of Production: MARJORIE A. DUFFY

Manager of Production Services:
ELIZABETH H. CARUSO

Format Editor: MILDRED M. SCHUMACHER

Index Editor: ADELE L. DOWD

Medical Consultant:
LOUIS V. NAPOLITANO, M.D.

Art Associate: JOAN AKERLIND

Director, PDR Development:
DAVID W. SIFTON

Database Manager: MUKESH MEHTA, R.Ph.

Database Coordinator: BEVERLY A. PFOHL

Administrative Assistants: SONIA C. RYAN
HELENE WATTMAN

Officers of Medical Economics Data, a division of Medical Economics Inc.: President and Chief Executive Officer: Norman R. Snesil; Senior Vice President and Chief Financial Officer: Joseph T. Deithorn; Senior Vice President and Group Publisher: Edward R. Barnhart; Senior Vice President, Business Development: Stephen J. Sorkenn; Vice President of Circulation: Scott I. Rockman; Vice President, Information Services: Edward J. Zecchini.

ISBN 0-87489-721-1

Foreword to the Twelfth Edition

PHYSICIANS' DESK REFERENCE For NONPRESCRIPTION DRUGS® is the over-the-counter—drug companion volume to Physicians' Desk Reference. It is organized in a similar manner with a Manufacturers' Index, Product Name Index, Product Category Index, Active Ingredients Index—all color coded for quick reference. Descriptive labeling appears in the Product Information Section and Diagnostics, Devices and Medical Aids Section.

The transferring of some drug ingredients and dosage forms from prescription to over-the-counter status is continuing. This trend has broadened the range of effective products available to health conscious consumers for self-medication. Improved labeling helps to ensure appropriate use of these products. Manufacturers of nonprescription drug products have included inactive ingredients as well as active ingredients to alert those who may have sensitivity to certain ingredients.

The PHYSICIANS' DESK REFERENCE For NONPRESCRIPTION DRUGS® is published annually by Medical Economics Data, a division of Medical Economics Company Inc., with the cooperation of the manufacturers whose products are described in the Product Information and Diagnostics, Devices and Medical Aids Sections. Its purpose is to make available essential information on nonprescription products.

The function of the Publisher is the compilation, organization, and distribution of this information. Each product description has been prepared by the manufacturer, and edited and approved by the manufacturer's medical department, medical director, and/or medical consultant. In organizing and presenting the material in PHYSICIANS' DESK REFERENCE For NONPRESCRIPTION DRUGS®, the Publisher does not warrant or guarantee any of the products described herein or perform any independent analysis in connection with any of the product information contained herein. PHYSICIANS' DESK REFERENCE For NONPRESCRIPTION DRUGS® does not assume, and expressly disclaims, any obligation to obtain and include information other than that provided to it by the manufacturer. In making this material available it should be understood that the Publisher is not advocating the use of any product described herein. Besides the information given here, additional information on any product may be obtained through the manufacturer.

EDWARD R. BARNHART
Publisher

HOW TO USE THIS EDITION

If you want to find . . .	And you already know . . .	Here's where to look . . .
the brand name of a product	the manufacturer's name	White Section: Manufacturers' Index
	its generic name	Yellow Section: Active Ingredients Index*
the manufacturer's name	the product's brand name	Pink Section: Product Name Index*
	the product's generic name	Yellow Section: Active Ingredients Index*
essential product information, such as: active ingredients indications actions warnings drug interaction precautions symptoms & treatment of oral overdosage dosage & administration how supplied	the product's brand name	Pink Section: Product Name Index*
	the product's generic name:	Yellow Section: Active ingredients Index*
a product with a particular chemical action	the chemical action	Yellow Section: Active Ingredients Index*
a product with a particular active ingredient	the active ingredient	Yellow Section: Active Ingredients Index*
a similar acting product	the product classification	Blue Section: Product Category Index*
generic name of a brand name product	the product's brand name	Pink Section: Product Name Index. Generic name will be found under "Active Ingredients" in Product Information Section.

* *In the Pink, Blue and Yellow Sections, the page numbers following the product name refer to the pages in the Product Identification Section where the product is pictured and the Product Information Section where the drug is comprehensively described.*

Contents

SECTION 1

Manufacturers' Index

The manufacturers whose names appear in this index have provided information concerning their products in either the Product Information Section, Product Identification Section, or the Diagnostics, Devices and Medical Aids Section.

Included in this index are the names and addresses of manufacturers, individuals or departments to whom you may address inquiries, a partial list of products as well as emergency telephone numbers wherever available.

The symbol ◆ indicates that the product is shown in the Product Identification Section.

(◆ Shown in Product Identification Section)

AU PHARMACEUTICALS, INC. 508
P.O. Box 476
Grand Saline, TX 75140
Address inquiries to:
Michael Vick (800) 232-2246
For Medical Emergencies Contact:
Rita Gates, PhD (214) 340-1503
OTC Products Available
Aurum - The Gold Lotion
Feminine Gold
Gold Plus - The Gold Lotion
Theragold - The Gold Lotion
Therapeutic Gold - The Gold Lotion

AYERST LABORATORIES 509
Division of American Home Products Corporation
685 Third Avenue
New York, NY 10017-4071
For information for Ayerst's consumer products, see product listings under Whitehall Laboratories.
Please turn to Whitehall Laboratories, page 745.

BAKER CUMMINS DERMATOLOGICALS, INC. 509
8800 NW 36th Street
Miami, FL 33178
Address inquiries to:
(305) 590-2282
For Medical Emergencies Contact:
Medical Dept. (305) 590-2451
(305) 590-2218
(305) 590-2254
OTC Products Available
Aqua-A Cream
Aquaderm Combination Treatment/Moisturizer (SPF 15 Formula)
Aquaderm Cream
Aquaderm Lotion
P & S Liquid
P & S Plus Tar Gel
P & S Shampoo
Ultra Mide 25
X-Seb Shampoo
X-Seb Plus Conditioning Shampoo
X-Seb T Shampoo
X-Seb T Plus Conditioning Shampoo

BAUSCH & LOMB PERSONAL PRODUCTS DIVISION 404, 511
1400 North Goodman Street
Rochester, NY 14692-0450
OTC Products Available
◆Allergy Drops
◆Dry Eye Therapy Lubricating Eye Drops
◆Duolube Eye Ointment
◆Eye Wash
◆Moisture Drops

BEACH PHARMACEUTICALS 512
Division of Beach Products, Inc.
Executive Office
5220 S. Manhattan Ave.
Tampa, FL 33611 (813) 839-6565
Manufacturing and Distribution
Main St. at Perimeter Rd.
Conestee, SC 29605
Toll Free 1-(800) 845-8210
Address inquiries to:
Victor De Oreo, R Ph, V.P., Sales
(803) 277-7282
Richard Stephen Jenkins, Exec. V.P.
(813) 839-6565
OTC Products Available
Beelith Tablets

BECTON DICKINSON CONSUMER PRODUCTS 512
One Becton Drive
Franklin Lakes, NJ 07417-1883
Address inquiries to:
Consumer Service (201) 848-6574
OTC Products Available
B-D Glucose Tablets

BEIERSDORF INC. 404, 512
P.O. Box 5529
Norwalk, CT 06856-5529
Address inquiries to:
Medical Division (203) 853-8008
OTC Products Available
◆Aquaphor Healing Ointment
◆Basis Facial Cleanser (Normal to Dry Skin)
◆Basis Soap-Combination Skin
◆Basis Soap-Extra Dry Skin
◆Basis Soap-Normal to Dry Skin
◆Basis Soap-Sensitive Skin
◆Eucerin Cleansing Lotion (Fragrance-free)
◆Eucerin Dry Skin Care Cleansing Bar (Fragrance-free)
◆Eucerin Dry Skin Care Creme (Fragrance-free)
◆Eucerin Dry Skin Care Lotion (Fragrace-free)
◆Nivea Bath Silk Bath Oil
◆Nivea Bath Silk Bath & Shower Gel (Extra-Dry Skin)
◆Nivea Bath Silk Bath & Shower Gel (Normal-to-Dry Skin)
◆Nivea Moisturizing Creme
◆Nivea Moisturizing Lotion (Extra Enriched)
◆Nivea Moisturizing Lotion (Original Formula)
◆Nivea Moisturizing Oil
◆Nivea Skin Oil
◆Nivea Sun After Sun Lotion
◆Nivea Sun SPF 15
◆Nivea Visage Facial Nourishing Creme
◆Nivea Visage Facial Nourishing Lotion

BENSON PHARMACAL COMPANY 516
Division of American Victor Co., Inc.
431 Hempstead Avenue
West Hempstead, NY 11552
Address inquiries to:
Sami M. Moukaddem, RPh
(516) 486-5560
OTC Products Available
Altocaps-400 Capsules
Combi-Cap Capsules
Roygel 25 mg Capsules
Roygel 50 mg Capsules
Roygel 100 mg Capsules
Roygel Ultima Capsules
Toco-A-Benson Capsules
Vit "A" Capsules

BLAINE COMPANY, INC. 516
2700 Dixie Highway
Fort Mitchell, KY 41017
Address inquiries to:
Mr. Alex M. Blaine (606) 341-9437
OTC Products Available
Mag-Ox 400
Uro-Mag

BLOCK DRUG COMPANY, INC. 516
257 Cornelison Avenue
Jersey City, NJ 07302
Address inquiries to:
Steve Gattanella (201) 434-3000
For Medical Emergencies Contact:
James Gingold (201) 434-3000
OTC Products Available
Arthritis Strength BC Powder
BC Powder
BC Cold Powder Multi-Symptom Formula
BC Cold Powder Non-Drowsy Formula
Nytol Tablets
Promise Toothpaste
Mint Gel Sensodyne
Mint Sensodyne Toothpaste
Original Sensodyne Toothpaste
Tegrin for Psoriasis Lotion, Cream & Soap
Tegrin Medicated Shampoo

BOEHRINGER INGELHEIM PHARMACEUTICALS, INC. 519
90 East Ridge
P.O. Box 368
Ridgefield, CT 06877
Address inquiries to:
Medical Services Dept.
(203) 798-9988
OTC Products Available
Dulcolax Suppositories
Dulcolax Tablets
Nōstril Nasal Decongestant
Nōstrilla Long Acting Nasal Decongestant

BOIRON 404, 520
1208 Amosland Road
Norwood, PA 19074
Address inquiries to:
Gina M. Casey
Assistant to the President
(800) 258-8823
For Medical Emergencies Contact:
Mark Land
Technical Services Department
(800) 258-8823
OTC Products Available
◆Oscillococcinum

BRISTOL LABORATORIES 521
A Bristol-Myers Squibb Company
2400 W. Lloyd Expressway
Evansville, IN 47721
(812) 429-5000
Naldecon X-line is now being distributed by Apothecon.
OTC Products Available
Naldecon CX Adult Liquid
Naldecon DX Adult Liquid
Naldecon DX Children's Syrup
Naldecon DX Pediatric Drops
Naldecon EX Children's Syrup
Naldecon EX Pediatric Drops
Naldecon Senior DX Cough/Cold Liquid
Naldecon Senior EX Cough/Cold Liquid

BRISTOL-MYERS PRODUCTS 404, 524
(A Bristol-Myers Squibb Company)
345 Park Avenue
New York, NY 10154
Address Inquiries to:
Bristol-Myers Products Division
Consumer Affairs Department
US Highway 202/206 North
P.O. Box 1279
Somerville, NJ 08876
In Emergencies Call:
(800) 468-7746
Address Inquiries on KERI, FOSTEX and PRESUN to:
Westwood-Squibb Pharmaceuticals
Consumer Affairs Department
100 Forest Avenue
Buffalo, NY 14213
In Emergencies Call:
(716) 887-3773
OTC Products Available
◆Alpha Keri Moisture Rich Body Oil
Alpha Keri Moisture Rich Cleansing Bar
Alpha Keri Moisturizing Body Powder
Alpha Keri Moisturizing Spray Mist
Alpha Keri Shower & Bath Gelee
Ammens Medicated Powder
B.Q. Cold Tablets
BAN Antiperspirant Cream Deodorant
BAN Antiperspirant Deodorant Spray
BAN Basic Non-Aerosol Antiperspirant Spray
BAN Roll-On Antiperspirant Deodorant
BAN Solid Antiperspirant Deodorant
◆Arthritis Strength Bufferin Analgesic Caplets
◆Extra Strength Bufferin Analgesic Tablets
◆Bufferin Analgesic Tablets and Caplets
◆Allergy-Sinus Comtrex Multi-Symptom Allergy/Sinus Formula Tablets & Caplets
Cough Formula Comtrex
◆Comtrex Multi-Symptom Cold Reliever Tablets/Caplets/Liqui-Gels/Liquid
◆Congespirin For Children Aspirin Free Chewable Cold Tablets
◆Datril Extra-Strength Analgesic Tablets & Caplets
◆Aspirin Free Excedrin Analgesic Caplets
◆Excedrin Extra-Strength Analgesic Tablets & Caplets
◆Excedrin P.M. Analgesic/Sleeping Aid Tablets, Caplets and Liquid
◆Sinus Excedrin Analgesic, Decongestant Tablets & Caplets

(◆ Shown in Product Identification Section)

◆4-Way Cold Tablets
◆4-Way Fast Acting Nasal Spray (regular & mentholated) & Metered Spray Pump (regular)
◆4-Way Long Lasting Nasal Spray & Metered Spray Pump
Fostex 10% Benzoyl Peroxide Bar
Fostex 5% Benzoyl Peroxide (Vanish) Gel
Fostex 10% Benzoyl Peroxide (Vanish) Gel
Fostex 10% Benzoyl Peroxide Wash
Fostex Medicated Cleansing Bar
Fostex Medicated Cleansing Cream
Keri Creme
Keri Facial Soap
◆Keri Lotion - Fresh Herbal Scent
◆Keri Lotion - Original Formula
◆Keri Lotion - Silky Smooth Formula
Minit-Rub Analgesic Ointment
Mum Antiperspirant Cream Deodorant
◆No Doz Fast Acting Alertness Aid Tablets
No Doz Maximum Strength Caplets
◆Nuprin Ibuprofen/Analgesic Tablets & Caplets
◆Pazo Hemorrhoid Ointment & Suppositories
PreSun 15 Facial Stick Sunscreen
PreSun 15 Facial Sunscreen
PreSun 15 Lip Protector Sunscreen
PreSun for Kids
PreSun for Kids Spray Mist
PreSun 8, 15 and 39 Creamy Sunscreens
◆PreSun 15 and 29 Sensitive Skin Sunscreen
PreSun 23 Spray Mist
◆Therapeutic Mineral Ice, Pain Relieving Gel
◆Therapeutic Mineral Ice Exercise Formula, Pain Relieving Gel
Tickle Roll-On Antiperspirant/Deodorant

BURROUGHS WELLCOME COMPANY **406, 538**
3030 Cornwallis Road
Research Triangle Park, NC 27709
(800) 722-9292
For Medical or Drug Information:
Contact Drug Information Service
Business hours only
(8:15 AM to 4:15 PM EST)
(800) 443-6763
For 24-hour Medical Emergency Information, call (800) 443-6763
For Sales Information:
Contact Sales Distribution Department
Address Other Inquiries to:
Consumer Products Division
OTC Products Available
Actidil Syrup
◆Actidil Tablets
◆Actifed Capsules
◆Actifed Plus Caplets
◆Actifed Plus Tablets
◆Actifed Syrup
◆Actifed Tablets
◆Actifed 12-Hour Capsules
Ammonia Aromatic, Vaporole
Borofax Ointment
◆Empirin Aspirin
◆Filteray Broad Spectrum Sunscreen Lotion
Lubafax Surgical Lubricant, Sterile
◆Marezine Tablets
◆Neosporin Cream
◆Neosporin Ointment
◆Neosporin Maximum Strength Ointment
◆Nix Creme Rinse
◆Polysporin Ointment
◆Polysporin Powder
◆Polysporin Spray
◆Sudafed Children's Liquid
◆Sudafed Cough Syrup
◆Sudafed Plus Liquid
◆Sudafed Plus Tablets
◆Sudafed Sinus Caplets
◆Sudafed Sinus Tablets
◆Sudafed Tablets, 30 mg
◆Sudafed Tablets, Adult Strength, 60 mg
◆Sudafed 12 Hour Capsules
Wellcome Lanoline

CAMPBELL LABORATORIES INC. **546**
Address Inquiries to:
Richard C. Zahn, President
P.O. Box 812, FDR Station
New York, NY 10150-0812
(212) 688-7684
OTC Products Available
Herpecin-L Cold Sore Lip Balm

CHATTEM INC., CONSUMER PRODUCTS DIVISION **546**
Division of Chattem, Inc.
1715 West 38th Street
Chattanooga, TN 37409
Address Inquiries to:
David Robb (615) 821-4571
For Medical Emergencies Contact:
Walter Ludwig (615) 821-4571
OTC Products Available
Black-Draught Granulated
Black-Draught Lax-Senna Tablets
Black-Draught Syrup
Blis-To-Sol Liquid
Blis-To-Sol Powder
Flex-all 454 Pain Relieving Gel
Norwich Extra-Strength Aspirin
Norwich Regular Strength Aspirin
Nullo Deodorant Tablets
Pamprin Multi-Symptom Extra-Strength Pain Relief Formula Tablets
Pamprin Maximum Cramp Relief Formula Tablets, Caplets & Capsules
Pamprin-IB
Prēmsyn PMS Capsules & Caplets
Soltice Quick-Rub

CHURCH & DWIGHT CO., INC. **548**
469 North Harrison Street
Princeton, NJ 08540
Address inquiries to:
Mr. Stephen Lajoie (609) 683-5900
For Medical Emergencies Contact:
Mr. Stephen Lajoie (609) 683-5900
OTC Products Available
Arm & Hammer Pure Baking Soda
OTIX Drops Ear Wax Removal Aid

CIBA CONSUMER PHARMACEUTICALS **407, 548**
Division of CIBA-GEIGY Corporation
Raritan Plaza III
Edison, NJ 08837
Address inquiries to:
(201) 906-6000
For Medical Emergencies Contact:
(201) 277-5000
OTC Products Available
◆Acutrim 16 Hour Steady Control Appetite Suppressant
◆Acutrim Late Day Strength Appetite Suppressant
◆Acutrim II Maximum Strength Appetite Suppressant
◆Doan's - Extra-Strength Analgesic
◆Doan's - Regular Strength Analgesic
◆Eucalyptamint 100% All Natural Ointment
Fiberall Chewable Tablets, Lemon Creme Flavor
◆Fiberall Fiber Wafers - Fruit & Nut
◆Fiberall Fiber Wafers - Oatmeal Raisin
◆Fiberall Powder Natural Flavor
◆Fiberall Powder Orange Flavor
◆Nupercainal Cream and Ointment
◆Nupercainal Pain Relief Cream
◆Nupercainal Suppositories
◆Otrivin Nasal Spray & Nasal Drops
◆Otrivin Pediatric Nasal Drops
◆Privine Nasal Solution
◆Privine Nasal Spray
◆Q-vel Muscle Relaxant Pain Reliever
◆Slow Fe Tablets
◆Sunkist Children's Chewable Multivitamins - Complete
◆Sunkist Children's Chewable Multivitamins - Plus Extra C
◆Sunkist Children's Chewable Multivitamins - Plus Iron
◆Sunkist Children's Chewable Multivitamins - Regular
◆Sunkist Vitamin C - Chewable
◆Sunkist Vitamin C - Easy to Swallow

COLGATE-PALMOLIVE COMPANY **408, 554**
A Delaware Corporation
300 Park Avenue
New York, NY 10022
Address inquiries to:
Consumers:
Consumer Affairs
300 Park Avenue
New York, NY 10022
(212) 310-2000
Physicians:
Medical Director
909 River Road
Piscataway, NJ 08854
(201) 878-7500
For Medical Emergencies Contact:
9 AM to 5 PM (201) 878-7500
5 PM to 9 AM (201) 547-2500
OTC Products Available
Colgate Dental Cream
◆Colgate Junior Fluoride Gel Toothpaste
◆Colgate MFP Fluoride Gel
◆Colgate MFP Fluoride Toothpaste
◆Colgate Mouthwash Tartar Control Formula
◆Colgate Tartar Control Formula
◆Colgate Tartar Control Gel
Colgate Toothbrushes
Curad Bandages
Dermassage Dish Liquid
◆Fluorigard Anti-Cavity Fluoride Rinse
Mersene Denture Cleanser
Ultra Brite Toothpaste

COLUMBIA LABORATORIES, INC. **409, 555**
4000 Hollywood Boulevard
Hollywood, FL 33021
Address inquiries to:
Professional Services Department
(305) 964-6666
For Medical Emergencies Contact
(800) 749-1919
OTC Products Available
◆Diasorb Liquid
◆Diasorb Tablets
◆Legatrin
◆Replens
Vaporizer in a Bottle Nasal Decongestant

COMBE, INC. **409, 556**
1101 Westchester Avenue
White Plains, NY 10604
Address inquiries to:
Theresa C. Infantino (914) 694-5454
For Medical Emergencies Contact:
Mark K. Taylor (914) 694-5454
OTC Products Available
◆Gynecort 5 Creme
◆Lanabiotic Ointment
◆Lanacane Creme
◆Lanacane Spray
◆Lanacort 5 Creme and Ointment
◆Odor-Eaters Spray Powder
◆Vagisil Creme
◆Vagisil Feminine Powder

COPLEY PHARMACEUTICAL INC. **558**
25 John Road
Canton, MA 02021
Address inquiries to:
Copley Pharmaceutical Inc.
(617) 821-6111
For Medical Emergencies Contact:
Dr. Antoon (617) 821-6111
OTC Products Available
Hydrocortisone 0.5% Aerosol
Lice•Enz Foam
Saliv-Aid Oral Lubricant
Simethicone Drops
Tolnaftate 1% Liquid Aerosol
Tolnaftate 1% Powder Aerosol

FISONS CONSUMER HEALTH **409, 558**
Fisons Corporation
P.O. Box 1212
Rochester, NY 14603

(◆ Shown in Product Identification Section)

Address inquiries to:
Product Service Department
P.O. Box 1212
Rochester, NY 14603
(716) 475-9000
FAX (716) 274-5304
For Medical Emergencies Contact
Fisons Corporation
(716) 475-9000
OTC Products Available
Allerest Children's Chewable Tablets
Allerest Eye Drops
Allerest Headache Strength Tablets
Allerest 12 Hour Caplets
Allerest 12 Hour Nasal Spray
◆Allerest Maximum Strength Tablets
◆Allerest No Drowsiness Tablets
Allerest Sinus Pain Formula
◆Americaine Hemorrhoidal Ointment
◆Americaine Topical Anesthetic First Aid Ointment
◆Americaine Topical Anesthetic Spray
Bacid Capsules
◆CaldeCORT Anti-Itch Hydrocortisone Cream
◆CaldeCORT Anti-Itch Hydrocortisone Spray
◆CaldeCORT Light Cream
◆Caldesene Medicated Ointment
◆Caldesene Medicated Powder
Cholan HMB
◆Cruex Antifungal Cream
◆Cruex Antifungal Powder
◆Cruex Antifungal Spray Powder
Delsym Cough Formula
Desenex Antifungal Cream
Desenex Antifungal Foam
◆Desenex Antifungal Ointment
◆Desenex Antifungal Powder
◆Desenex Antifungal Spray Powder
◆Desenex Foot & Sneaker Deodorant Spray
Desenex Soap
Emul-O-Balm
Isoclor Liquid
Isoclor Tablets
◆Isoclor Timesule Capsules
Kondremul
Neo-Cultol
Sinarest 12 Hour Nasal Spray
Sinarest No Drowsiness Tablets
Sinarest Tablets & Extra Strength Tablets
◆Ting Antifungal Cream
◆Ting Antifungal Powder
◆Ting Antifungal Spray Liquid
◆Ting Antifungal Spray Powder
Vaponefrin
Vitron-C and Vitron-C Plus

FLEMING & COMPANY **563**
1600 Fenpark Dr.
Fenton, MO 63026
Address inquiries to:
John J. Roth, M.D. (314) 343-8200
For Medical Emergencies Contact:
John R. Roth, M.D. (314) 343-8200
OTC Products Available
Chlor-3 Condiment
Impregon Concentrate
Magonate Tablets and Liquid
Marblen Suspension Peach/Apricot
Marblen Suspension Unflavored
Marblen Tablets
Nephrox Suspension
Nicotinex Elixir
Ocean Nasal Mist
Ocean-A/S Nasal Spray
Ocean-Plus Mist
Purge Concentrate

FLEX AID, INC. **410, 564**
a Division of NDL Products, Inc.
P.O. Box 1917
Pompano Beach, FL 33061
Address inquiries to:
Customer Service Department
(305) 942-4560
OTC Products Available
Flex Aid Elastic Athletic Supporters
◆Flex Aid Elastic Braces
◆Flex Aid Elastic Splint Wrist Brace
◆Flex Aid Elastic Support Hosiery
◆Flex Aid Neoprene Supports
◆Flex Aid Neoprene Knee Support
Flex Aid Pouch Style Arm Slings

G&W LABORATORIES, INC. **410, 564**
111 Coolidge Street
South Plainfield, NJ 07080
Address inquiries to:
Joel Zacklin (201) 753-2000
OTC Products Available
◆G&W Glycerin Suppositories, Adult and Pediatric

GLENBROOK LABORATORIES **410, 564**
Division of Sterling Drug Inc.
90 Park Avenue
New York, NY 10016
Address inquiries to:
Medical Director (212) 907-2764
OTC Products Available
◆Children's Bayer Chewable Aspirin
◆Genuine Bayer Aspirin Tablets & Caplets
◆Maximum Bayer Aspirin Tablets & Caplets
◆Bayer Plus Aspirin Tablets
◆Therapy Bayer Aspirin Caplets
◆8 Hour Bayer Timed-Release Aspirin
◆Haley's M-O, Regular & Flavored
◆Midol 200 Cramp Relief Formula
◆Maximum Strength Midol Multi-Symptom Menstrual Formula
◆Maximum Strength Midol PMS Premenstrual Syndrome Formula
◆Regular Strength Midol Multi-Symptom Menstrual Formula
◆Children's Panadol Chewable Tablets, Liquid, Infants' Drops
◆Junior Strength Panadol
◆Maximum Strength Panadol Tablets and Caplets
◆Phillips' LaxCaps
◆Concentrated Phillips' Milk of Magnesia
◆Phillips' Milk of Magnesia Liquid
◆Phillips' Milk of Magnesia Tablets
◆Stri-Dex Dual Textured Maximum Strength Pads
Stri-Dex Dual Textured Maximum Strength Big Pads
◆Stri-Dex Dual Textured Regular Strength Pads
Stri-Dex Dual Textured Regular Strength Big Pads
◆Vanquish Analgesic Caplets

HERALD PHARMACAL, INC. **574**
6503 Warwick Road
Richmond, VA 23225
Address inquiries to:
Henry H. Kamps
(804) 745-3400
For Medical Emergencies Contact:
Henry H. Kamps
(804) 745-3400
OTC Products Available
Aqua Glycolic Lotion
Aqua Glycolic Shampoo
Aqua Glyde Cleanser
Aquaray 20 Sunscreen
Cam Lotion

HOECHST-ROUSSEL PHARMACEUTICALS INC. **574**
Routes 202-206
P.O. Box 2500
Somerville, NJ 08876-1258
Address medical inquiries to:
Scientific Services Dept.
(800) 445-4774
(8:30 AM-5:00 PM EST)
For medical emergency information only, after hours and on weekends, call: (201) 231-2000
OTC Products Available
Festal II Digestive Aid

ICN PHARMACEUTICALS, INC. **411, 574**
ICN Plaza
3300 Hyland Avenue
Costa Mesa, CA 92626
Address inquiries to:
Professional Service Department
(800) 556-1937
In CA (800) 331-2331
(714) 545-0100
For Medical Emergencies Contact:
Medical Department
(800) 548-5100
OTC Products Available
◆Fototar Cream
◆Insta-Glucose

INTER-CAL CORPORATION **575**
421 Miller Valley Road
Prescott, AZ 86301
Address inquiries to:
Gerald W. Elders (602) 445-8063
OTC Products Available
Ester-C Tablets

JACKSON-MITCHELL PHARMACEUTICALS, INC. **576**
1485 East Valley Road, Suite C
P.O. Box 5425
Santa Barbara, CA 93108
Address inquiries to:
Carol Jackson (805) 565-1538
For Medical Emergencies Contact:
Carol Jackson (805) 565-1538
Branch Offices
Turlock, CA 95380
P.O. Box 934 (209) 667-2019
OTC Products Available
Meyenberg Evaporated Goat Milk - 12 fl. oz.
Meyenberg Powdered Goat Milk - 4 oz. & 14 oz.

JOHNSON & JOHNSON CONSUMER PRODUCTS, INC. **411, 577**
Grandview Road
Skillman, NJ 08558
Address inquiries to:
(800) 526-3967
For Medical Emergencies Contact:
(800) 526-3967
OTC Products Available
JOHNSON'S Baby Sunblock Cream (SPF 15)
JOHNSON'S Baby Sunblock Lotion (SPF 15)
JOHNSON'S Baby Sunblock Lotion (SPF 30+)
◆JOHNSON'S Medicated Diaper Rash Ointment
K-Y Brand Lubricating Jelly
PURPOSE Dual Treatment Moisturizer (SPF 12)
PURPOSE Soap
SUNDOWN Sunblock Combi Pack, Ultra Protection (SPF 15)
SUNDOWN Sunblock Cream, Ultra Protection (SPF 15)
SUNDOWN Sunblock Stick, Ultra Protection (SPF 15)
SUNDOWN Sunblock Stick, Ultra Protection (SPF 30+)
SUNDOWN Sunscreen Lotions
Maximal Protection (SPF 8)
Ultra Protection Sunblock (SPF 15)
Ultra Protection Sunblock (SPF 20)
Ultra Protection Sunblock (SPF 25)
Ultra Protection Sunblock (SPF 30+)

JOHNSON & JOHNSON • MERCK CONSUMER PHARMACEUTICALS COMPANY **412, 577**
Camp Hill Road
Fort Washington, PA 19034
Address inquiries to:
Consumer Affairs Department
(215) 233-7000
For Medical Emergencies Contact:
(215) 233-7000
OTC Products Available
◆ALternaGEL Liquid
◆Dialose Capsules
◆Dialose Plus Capsules
◆Effer-Syllium Natural Fiber Bulking Agent
Ferancee Chewable Tablets
◆Ferancee-HP Tablets

(◆ Shown in Product Identification Section)

◆Kasof Capsules
◆Mylanta Liquid
◆Mylanta Tablets
◆Mylanta-Double Strength Liquid
◆Mylanta-Double Strength Tablets
◆Mylicon Drops
◆Mylicon Tablets
◆Mylicon-80 Tablets
◆Mylicon-125 Tablets
◆Orexin Softab Tablets
◆Probec-T Tablets
◆The Stuart Formula Tablets
◆Stuartinic Tablets

KREMERS URBAN COMPANY 581
See SCHWARZ PHARMA

LACTAID INC. 413, 581
P.O. Box 111
Old Egg Harbor Road and Delancy Avenue
Pleasantville, NJ 08232-0111
Address inquiries to:
Alan E. Kligerman (609) 645-5100
(800) 257-8650
Also (800) 522-8243
Canada (800) 387-5711
OTC Products Available
◆Beano Drops
◆Lactaid Caplets
◆Lactaid Drops

LAVOPTIK COMPANY, INC. 583, 773
661 Western Avenue North
St. Paul, MN 55103
Address inquiries to:
661 Western Avenue North
St. Paul, MN 55103 (612) 489-1351
For Medical Emergencies Contact:
B. C. Brainard (612) 489-1351
OTC Products Available
Lavoptik Eye Cup
Lavoptik Eye Wash

LEDERLE LABORATORIES 413, 583
Division of American Cyanamid Co.
One Cyanamid Plaza
Wayne, NJ 07470
Address inquiries on medical matters to:
Professional Services Dept.
Lederle Laboratories
Pearl River, NY 10965
8 AM to 4:30 PM EST
(914) 735-2815
All other inquiries and after hours emergencies
(914) 732-5000
Distribution Centers
ATLANTA
Contact EASTERN (Philadelphia) Distribution Center
CHICAGO
Bulk Address
1100 East Business Center Drive
Mt. Prospect, IL 60056
Mail Address
P.O. Box 7614
Mt. Prospect, IL 60056-7614
(800) 533-3753
(708) 827-8871
DALLAS
Bulk Address
7611 Carpenter Freeway
Dallas, TX 75247
Mail Address
P.O. Box 655731
Dallas, TX 75247 (800) 533-3753
(214) 631-2130
LOS ANGELES
Bulk Address
2300 S. Eastern Ave.
Los Angeles, CA 90040
Mail Address
T.A. Box 2202
Los Angeles, CA 90051
(800) 533-3753
(213) 726-1016
EASTERN (Philadelphia)
Bulk Address
202 Precision Drive
P.O. Box 99
Horsham, PA 19044
Mail Address
P.O. Box 93
Horsham, PA 19044 (800) 533-3753
(215) 672-5400
OTC Products Available
Acetaminophen Capsules, Tablets, Elixir, Liquid
Aureomycin Ointment 3%
◆Caltrate 600
◆Caltrate 600 + Iron
◆Caltrate 600 + Vitamin D
◆Caltrate, Jr.
◆Centrum
◆Centrum, Jr. (Children's Chewable) + Extra C
◆Centrum, Jr. (Children's Chewable) + Extra Calcium
◆Centrum, Jr. (Children's Chewable) + Iron
◆Centrum Liquid
◆Centrum Silver
Docusate Sodium (DSS) USP Capsules, Syrup
Docusate Sodium (DSS) w/Casanthranol Capsules, Syrup
◆Ferro-Sequels
Ferrous Gluconate Iron Supplement
Ferrous Sulfate
◆FiberCon
Filibon Prenatal Vitamin Tablets
Gevrabon Liquid
Gevral Protein Powder
Gevral T Tablets
Gevral Tablets
Guaifenesin w/D-Methorphan Hydrobromide Syrup
Guaifenesin Syrup
Incremin w/Iron Syrup
Lederplex Capsules and Liquid
Neoloid Emulsified Castor Oil
Peritinic Tablets
Pseudoephedrine HCl Syrup & Tablets
Quinine Capsules
Stresscaps Capsules
◆Stresstabs
◆Stresstabs + Iron, Advanced Formula
◆Stresstabs + Zinc
Triprolidine HCl with Pseudoephedrine HCl Syrup & Tablets
◆Zincon Dandruff Shampoo

LIFESCAN INC. 773
1051 South Milpitas Blvd.
Milpitas, CA 95035
For the name of your local representative, call toll-free:
In the US: (800) 227-8862
In Canada: (800) 663-5521
OTC Products Available
One Touch Blood Glucose Monitoring System

LUYTIES PHARMACAL COMPANY 590
P. O. Box 8080
St. Louis, MO 63156
Address Inquiries to:
Customer Service (800) 325-8080
OTC Products Available
Yellolax

MACSIL, INC. 590
1326 Frankford Avenue
Philadelphia, PA 19125
(215) 739-7300
OTC Products Available
Balmex Baby Powder
Balmex Emollient Lotion
Balmex Ointment

MARION MERRELL DOW INC. 414, 591
Consumer Products Division
10123 Alliance Road
Mail: P.O. Box 429553
Cincinnati, OH 45242-9553
Address inquiries to:
Professional Information Department
Business hours only
(9:00 AM to 4:30 PM EST)
(800) 552-3656
For Medical Emergency Information Only after hours or on weekends
(513) 948-9111
OTC Products Available
◆Cēpacol Anesthetic Lozenges (Troches)
◆Cēpacol/Cēpacol Mint Mouthwash/Gargle
◆Cēpacol Dry Throat Lozenges, Cherry Flavor
◆Cēpacol Dry Throat Lozenges, Honey-Lemon Flavor
◆Cēpacol Dry Throat Lozenges, Menthol-Eucalyptus Flavor
◆Cēpacol Dry Throat Lozenges, Original Flavor
◆CĒPASTAT Cherry Flavor Sore Throat Lozenges
◆CĒPASTAT Extra Strength Sore Throat Lozenges
◆CITRUCEL Orange Flavor
◆CITRUCEL Regular Flavor
◆Debrox Drops
◆Gaviscon Antacid Tablets
◆Gaviscon-2 Antacid Tablets
◆Gaviscon Extra Strength Relief Formula Liquid Antacid
◆Gaviscon Extra Strength Relief Formula Antacid Tablets
◆Gaviscon Liquid Antacid
◆Gly-Oxide Liquid
◆Novahistine DMX
◆Novahistine Elixir
◆Os-Cal 500 Chewable Tablets
◆Os-Cal 500 Tablets
◆Os-Cal 250+D Tablets
◆Os-Cal 500+D Tablets
◆Os-Cal Fortified Tablets
◆Os-Cal Plus Tablets
Simron Capsules
Simron Plus Capsules
Singlet Tablets
◆Throat Discs Throat Lozenges

MARLYN HEALTH CARE 598
6324 Ferris Square
San Diego, CA 92121
(800) 462-7596
OTC Products Available
4-Hair
4-Nails
Hep-Forte Capsules
Marlyn Formula 50
Marlyn Formula 50 Mega Forte
Marlyn PMS
Osteo Fem
Pro-Skin-E (Face Capsule)
Pro-Skin Nutribloxx

McNEIL CONSUMER PRODUCTS CO. 415, 599
Division of McNeil-PPC, Inc.
Camp Hill Road
Fort Washington, PA 19034
(215) 233-7000
Address inquiries to:
Consumer Affairs Department
Fort Washington, PA 19034
Manufacturing Divisions
Fort Washington, PA 19034
Southwest Manufacturing Plant
4001 N. I-35
Round Rock, TX 78664
OTC Products Available
◆Imodium A-D Caplets and Liquid
◆Medipren ibuprofen Caplets and Tablets
◆PediaCare Allergy Relief Formula Liquid
◆PediaCare Cough-Cold Formula Liquid and Chewable Tablets
◆PediaCare Infants' Oral Decongestant Drops
◆PediaCare Night Rest Cough-Cold Formula Liquid
◆Sine-Aid Maximum Strength Sinus Headache Caplets
◆Sine-Aid Maximum Strength Sinus Headache Tablets

(◆ **Shown in Product Identification Section**)

◆Tylenol acetaminophen Children's Chewable Tablets & Elixir
◆Tylenol Allergy Sinus Medication Caplets and Gelcaps, Maximum Strength
◆Children's Tylenol Cold Liquid Formula and Chewable Tablets
◆Tylenol Cold & Flu Hot Medication, Packets
◆Tylenol Cold Medication Caplets and Tablets
◆Tylenol Cold Medication, Effervescent Tablets
◆Tylenol Cold Medication No Drowsiness Formula Caplets
◆Tylenol Cold Night Time Medication Liquid
Tylenol, Extra-Strength, acetaminophen Adult Liquid Pain Reliever
◆Tylenol, Extra-Strength, acetaminophen Caplets, Gelcaps, Tablets
◆Tylenol, Infants' Drops
◆Tylenol, Junior Strength, acetaminophen Coated Caplets, Grape Chewable Tablets
◆Tylenol, Maximum Strength, Sinus Medication Tablets, Caplets and Gelcaps
◆Tylenol, Regular Strength, acetaminophen Tablets and Caplets

MEAD JOHNSON NUTRITIONALS 417, 611
A Bristol-Myers Squibb Company
2400 W. Lloyd Expressway
Evansville, IN 47721
(812) 429-5000
Address inquiries to:
Scientific Information Section
Medical Department
OTC Products Available
Casec
Ce-Vi-Sol
Criticare HN
Enfamil Infant Formula
Enfamil With Iron Infant Formula
Enfamil Infant Formula Nursette
Fer-In-Sol
HIST 1
HIST 2
HOM 1
HOM 2
Isocal
Isocal HCN
Isocal HN
LYS 1
LYS 2
Lofenalac Iron Fortified Low Phenylalanine Diet Powder
Lonalac
Low Methionine Diet Powder (Product 3200K)
Low PHE-TYR Diet Powder (Product 3200AB)
MCT Oil
MSUD Diet Powder
MSUD 1
MSUD 2
Moducal Dietary Carbohydrate
Mono- and Disaccharide-Free Diet Powder (Product 3232A)
Nutramigen Hypoallergenic Protein Hydrolysate Formula
OS 1
OS 2
PKU 1
PKU 2
PKU 3
Phenyl-Free Phenylalanine-Free Diet Powder
◆Poly-Vi-Sol Vitamins, Chewable Tablets and Drops (without Iron)
◆Poly-Vi-Sol Vitamins, Circus Shapes Chewable (without Iron)
◆Poly-Vi-Sol Vitamins with Iron, Chewable Tablets and Circus Shapes Chewable
◆Poly-Vi-Sol Vitamins with Iron, Drops
Portagen
Pregestimil Iron Fortified Protein Hydrolysate Formula with Medium Chain Triglycerides
ProSobee Soy Isolate Formula
ProSobee Soy Isolate Formula Nursette
Protein-Free Diet Powder (Product 80056)
◆Ricelyte, Rice-Based Oral Electrolyte Maintenance Solution
Special Metabolic Diets
Special Metabolic Modules
Sustacal HC
Sustacal Liquid, Powder, Pudding
Sustacal with Fiber
Sustagen
TYR 1
TYR 2
◆Tempra, Acetaminophen
TraumaCal
Trind
Trind-DM
◆Tri-Vi-Sol Vitamin Drops
◆Tri-Vi-Sol Vitamin Drops with Iron
UCD 1
UCD 2
Ultracal

MEAD JOHNSON PHARMACEUTICALS 417, 614
A Bristol-Myers Squibb Company
2400 W. Lloyd Expressway
Evansville, IN 47721-0001
(812) 429-5000
Address Inquiries to:
Scientific Information Section
Medical Department
OTC Products Available
◆Colace
◆Peri-Colace

MENLEY & JAMES LABORATORIES 417, 615
A Division of WKW, Inc.
Commonwealth Corporate Center
100 Tournament Drive, Suite 110
Horsham, PA 19044
Address inquiries to:
Consumer Affairs Department
(800) 321-1834
OTC Products Available
◆A.R.M. Allergy Relief Medicine Caplets
◆Acnomel Cream
◆Aqua Care Cream
◆Aqua Care Lotion
AsthmaHaler Mist Epinephrine Bitartrate Bronchodilator
AsthmaNefrin Solution "A" Bronchodilator
◆Benzedrex Inhaler
◆Congestac Caplets
◆FemIron Multi-Vitamins and Iron
◆Hold Cough Suppressant Lozenge
◆Liquiprin Children's Elixir
◆Liquiprin Infants' Drops
◆Ornex Caplets
S.T.37 Antiseptic Solution
◆Serutan Toasted Granules
Thermotabs
Troph-Iron Liquid
Trophite Liquid

MILES INC. CONSUMER HEALTHCARE DIVISION 418, 620
1127 Myrtle Street
Elkhart, IN 46514
Address inquiries to:
Manager, Consumer Affairs Dept.
(219) 264-8955
OTC Products Available
◆Alka-Mints Chewable Antacid
◆Alka-Seltzer Advanced Formula Antacid & Non-Aspirin Pain Reliever
◆Alka-Seltzer Effervescent Antacid
◆Alka-Seltzer Effervescent Antacid and Pain Reliever
◆Alka-Seltzer Extra Strength Effervescent Antacid and Pain Reliever
◆Alka-Seltzer (Flavored) Effervescent Antacid and Pain Reliever
◆Alka-Seltzer Plus Cold Medicine
◆Alka-Seltzer Plus Night-Time Cold Medicine
◆Alka Seltzer Plus Sinus Allergy Medicine
◆Bactine Antiseptic/Anesthetic First Aid Spray
◆Bactine First Aid Antibiotic Ointment
◆Bactine Hydrocortisone Anti-Itch Cream
◆Biocal 500 mg Tablet Calcium Supplement
◆Bugs Bunny Children's Chewable Vitamins + Minerals with Iron and Calcium (Sugar Free)
◆Bugs Bunny Children's Chewable Vitamins (Sugar Free)
◆Bugs Bunny With Extra C Children's Chewable Vitamins (Sugar Free)
◆Bugs Bunny Plus Iron Children's Chewable Vitamins (Sugar Free)
◆Domeboro Astringent Solution Effervescent Tablets
◆Domeboro Astringent Solution Powder Packets
◆Flintstones Children's Chewable Vitamins
◆Flintstones Children's Chewable Vitamins With Extra C
◆Flintstones Children's Chewable Vitamins Plus Iron
◆Flintstones Complete With Calcium, Iron & Minerals Children's Chewable Vitamins
◆Miles Nervine Nighttime Sleep-Aid
◆One-A-Day Essential Vitamins
◆One-A-Day Maximum Formula Vitamins and Minerals
◆One-A-Day Plus Extra C Vitamins
◆Stressgard Stress Formula Vitamins
◆Within Women's Formula Multivitamin with Calcium, Extra Iron and Zinc

MORE DIRECT HEALTH PRODUCTS 628
6351-E Yarrow Drive
Carlsbad, CA 92009
Address inquiries to:
(619) 438-1935
For Medical Emergencies Contact:
(619) 438-1935
OTC Products Available
CigArrest Tablets

MURO PHARMACEUTICAL, INC. 628
890 East Street
Tewksbury, MA 01876-9987
Address inquiries to:
Professional Service Dept.
(800) 225-0974
(508) 851-5981
OTC Products Available
Bromfed Syrup
Guaifed Syrup
Salinex Nasal Mist and Drops

NATURE'S BOUNTY, INC. 419, 629
90 Orville Drive
Bohemia, NY 11716
Address inquiries to:
Professional Service Department
(516) 567-9500
(800) 645-5412
OTC Products Available
ABC to Z
Acidophilus
B-Complex and B-12
B-Complex +C (Long Acting) Tablets
B-6 50 mg., 100 mg., 200 mg.
B-12 & B-12 Sublingual Tablets
B-50 Tablets
B-100 Tablets-Ultra B Complex
Beta-Carotene Capsules
Bounty Bears (Children's Chewables)
C-500 mg., C-1000 mg., C-1500 mg. & Time Release Formulas
Chromium Picolinate 200 mcg.
E-Oil
◆Ener-B Vitamin B_{12} Nasal Gel Dietary Supplement
Garlic Oil 15 gr. & 77 gr.
KLB6 Capsules
l-Lysine 500 mg. Tablets
Lecithin 1200 mg. Capsules
M-KYA
Nature's Bounty 1 Tablets
Nature's Bounty Slim Quick

(◆ Shown in Product Identification Section)

◆Pepto-Bismol Liquid & Tablets
◆Maximum Strength Pepto-Bismol Liquid

REED & CARNRICK **422, 651**
1 New England Avenue
Piscataway, NJ 08854
Address Inquiries to:
Professional Service Dept.
(201) 981-0070
For Medical Emergencies Contact:
Medical Director (201) 434-3000
OTC Products Available
Alphosyl Lotion
◆Phazyme Drops
Phazyme Tablets
◆Phazyme-125 Softgels Maximum Strength
◆Phazyme-95 Tablets
proctoFoam/non-steroid
◆R&C Lice Treatment Kit
◆R&C Shampoo
◆R&C Spray III
Trichotine Liquid, Vaginal Douche
Trichotine Powder, Vaginal Douche

THE REESE CHEMICAL COMPANY **423, 653**
10617 Frank Avenue
Cleveland, OH 44106
Address inquiries to:
George W. Reese, III
(216) 231-6441
OTC Products Available
Bi-Zet Throat Lozenges
Cold Control+ Caplets
◆Colicon Drops
Dentapaine Gel
Dermatox Skin Lotion
Kao-Paverin w/Paregoric Liquid
Keep Alert Caplets
Licide Lice Control Shampoo
Licide Lice Control Spray
Podactin Anti-Fungal Cream
Red Hearts Vitamin Tonic Tablets
◆Reese's Pinworm Medicine
Sinadrin Tablets
◆Sleep-ettes-D Tablets
Theracof Cough & Cold Liquid
Tri-Biozene Ointment

REQUA, INC. **653**
Box 4008
1 Seneca Place
Greenwich, CT 06830
Address inquiries to:
Geoffrey Geils (203) 869-2445
(800) 321-1085
OTC Products Available
Charcoaid
Charcoal Tablets
Charcocaps

RHONE-POULENC RORER PHARMACEUTICALS INC. **423, 654**
Consumer Pharmaceutical Products
a division of
Rhone-Poulenc Rorer Pharmaceuticals Inc.
500 Virginia Drive
Fort Washington, PA 19034
For Medical Emergencies/ Product Information Contact:
Medical Services
(215) 628-6627
(215) 628-6065
For Reports of Adverse Drug Experiences Contact:
Product Surveillance (215) 956-5136
For Quality Assurance Questions Contact:
John Chiles
Complaint Coordinator
(215) 628-6416
For Regulatory Questions Contact:
Margaret Masters
Assoc. Director, Regulatory Control
(215) 628-6085
For Product Information Contact:
Medical Services
(215) 628-6627
(215) 628-6065
OTC Products Available
◆Ascriptin A/D Caplets
◆Regular Strength Ascriptin Tablets
◆Extra Strength Maalox Plus Suspension
◆Maalox Plus Tablets
◆Perdiem Fiber Granules
◆Perdiem Granules

RICHARDSON-VICKS INC. **424, 656**
One Far Mill Crossing
Shelton, CT 06484
Address inquiries to:
Medical Director
Vicks Research Center
(203) 925-7888
For Medical Emergencies Contact:
(301) 328-2425
OTC Products Available
◆Children's Chloraseptic Lozenges
◆Chloraseptic Liquid, Cherry, Menthol or Cool Mint
◆Chloraseptic Liquid - Nitrogen Propelled Spray
◆Chloraseptic Lozenges, Cherry and Cool Mint
◆Chloraseptic Lozenges, Menthol
◆Clearasil Adult Care Medicated Blemish Cream
Clearasil Adult Care Medicated Blemish Stick
Clearasil Antibacterial Soap
Clearasil 10% Benzoyl Peroxide Acne Medication Vanishing Lotion
◆Clearasil Double Textured Pads - Regular and Maximum Strength
◆Clearasil 10% Benzoyl Peroxide Maximum Strength Acne Medication Cream, Tinted
◆Clearasil 10% Benzoyl Peroxide Maximum Strength Acne Medication Cream, Vanishing
◆Dramamine Chewable Tablets
◆Dramamine Liquid
◆Dramamine Tablets
Head & Chest Cold Medicine
◆Icy Hot Balm
◆Icy Hot Cream
◆Icy Hot Stick
◆Percogesic Analgesic Tablets
Vicks Children's Cough Syrup
◆Vicks Children's NyQuil
Vicks Cough Silencers Cough Drops
◆Vicks Daycare Daytime Cold Medicine Caplets
◆Vicks Daycare Daytime Cold Medicine Liquid
Vicks Formula 44 Cough Control Discs
◆Vicks Formula 44 Cough Medicine
◆Vicks Formula 44D Decongestant Cough Medicine
◆Vicks Formula 44M Multi-Symptom Cough Medicine
Vicks Inhaler
◆Vicks NyQuil Nighttime Colds Medicine-Original & Cherry Flavor
Vicks Oracin Cherry Flavor Cooling Throat Lozenges
Vicks Oracin Cooling Throat Lozenges
◆Vicks Pediatric Formula 44 Cough Medicine
◆Vicks Pediatric Formula 44 Cough & Cold Medicine
◆Vicks Pediatric Formula 44 Cough & Congestion Medicine
◆Vicks Sinex Decongestant Nasal Spray
◆Vicks Sinex Decongestant Nasal Ultra Fine Mist
◆Vicks Sinex Long-Acting Decongestant Nasal Spray
◆Vicks Sinex Long-Acting Decongestant Nasal Ultra Fine Mist
Vicks Throat Drops
  Cherry Flavor
  Ice Blue
  Lemon Flavor
  Regular Flavor
Vicks Throat Lozenges
◆Vicks Vaporub
Vicks Vaposteam
Vicks Vatronol Nose Drops
Victors Menthol-Eucalyptus Vapor Cough Drops
  Cherry Flavor
  Regular

ORAL HEALTH PRODUCTS
Benzodent Analgesic Denture Ointment
Fixodent Denture Adhesive Cream
Complete Denture Cleanser and Toothpaste in One
Extra Hold Fasteeth for Lowers Denture Adhesive Powder
Fasteeth Denture Adhesive Powder
Kleenite Denture Cleanser

ROBERTS PHARMACEUTICAL CORPORATION **425, 667**
6-G Industrial Way West
Eatonton, NJ 07724
Address inquiries to:
Customer Service Department
(800) 828-2088
For Medical Emergencies Contact:
Medical Services Department
(201) 389-1182
OTC Products Available
Alkets Tablets
Cheracol Cough Syrup
◆Cheracol D Cough Formula
Cheracol Nasal Spray Pump
◆Cheracol Plus Head Cold/Cough Formula
Cheracol Sore Throat Spray
Citrocarbonate Antacid
Clocream Skin Protectant Cream
Diostate D Tablets
◆Haltran Tablets
Lipomul Oral Liquid
Orthoxicol Cough Syrup
◆P-A-C Analgesic Tablets
◆Pyrroxate Capsules
◆Sigtab Tablets
Super D Perles
Zymacap Capsules

A. H. ROBINS COMPANY, INC. CONSUMER PRODUCTS DIVISION **425, 670**
Subsidiary of AMERICAN HOME PRODUCTS CORPORATION
3800 Cutshaw Avenue
Richmond, VA 23230
Address inquiries to:
The Medical Department
(804) 257-2000
For Medical Emergencies Contact:
Medical Department (804) 257-2000
(day or night)
If no answer, call answering service
(804) 257-7788
OTC Products Available
Allbee with C Caplets
Allbee C-800 Plus Iron Tablets
Allbee C-800 Tablets
◆Chap Stick Lip Balm
◆Chap Stick Petroleum Jelly Plus
◆Chap Stick Petroleum Jelly Plus with Sunblock 15
◆Chap Stick Sunblock 15 Lip Balm
Cough Calmers Lozenges
Dimacol Caplets
◆Dimetane Decongestant Caplets
◆Dimetane Decongestant Elixir
◆Dimetane Elixir
◆Dimetane Extentabs 8 mg
◆Dimetane Extentabs 12 mg
◆Dimetane Tablets
◆Dimetapp Elixir
◆Dimetapp DM Elixir
◆Dimetapp Extentabs
◆Dimetapp Plus Caplets
◆Dimetapp Tablets
◆Donnagel
◆Robitussin
◆Robitussin Cough Calmers
◆Robitussin Night Relief
◆Robitussin Pediatric
◆Robitussin-CF
◆Robitussin-DM
◆Robitussin-PE
Z-Bec Tablets

(◆ Shown in Product Identification Section)

ROSS LABORATORIES 426, 679
Division of Abbott Laboratories USA
P.O. Box 1317
Columbus, OH 43216-1317
Address Inquiries to:
Medical Director (614) 227-3333
OTC Products Available
◆Clear Eyes Lubricating Eye Redness Reliever
◆Ear Drops by Murine—(See Murine Ear Wax Removal System/Murine Ear Drops)
◆Murine Ear Drops
◆Murine Ear Wax Removal System
◆Murine Eye Lubricant
◆Murine Plus Lubricating Eye Redness Reliever
Pedialyte Oral Electrolyte Maintenance Solution
Rehydralyte Oral Electrolyte Rehydration Solution
Ross Pediatric Nutritional Products
Alimentum Protien Hydrolysate Formula With Iron
Isomil Soy Protein Formula With Iron
Isomil SF Sucrose-Free Soy Protein Formula With Iron
PediaSure Liquid Nutrition for Children
RCF Ross Carbohydrate Free Low-Iron Soy Protein Formula Base
Similac Low-Iron Infant Formula
Similac PM 60/40 Low-Iron Infant Formula
Similac Special Care With Iron 24 Premature Infant Formula
Similac With Iron Infant Formula
◆Selsun Blue Dandruff Shampoo
◆Selsun Blue Dandruff Shampoo-Extra Medicated
◆Selsun Blue Extra Conditioning Dandruff Shampoo
◆Tronolane Anesthetic Cream for Hemorrhoids
◆Tronolane Anesthetic Suppositories for Hemorrhoids

RUSS PHARMACEUTICALS, INC. 427, 682
22 Inverness Center Parkway
Birmingham, AL 35242
P.O. Box 380188
Birmingham, AL 35238-0188
Address inquiries to:
(205) 995-5000
For Medical Emergencies Contact:
Judy Davis (205) 995-5000
Branch Offices
151 Passaic Street, Suite B-1
Rochelle Park, NJ 07622
(201) 368-1196
550 North Brand Blvd., Seventh Floor
Glendale, CA 91203 (818) 546-5029
Fuller Square Building, Suite 346
8100 Burlington Pike
Florence, KY 41042
(606) 485-6306
OTC Products Available
Amesec
◆Corticaine
◆Vicon Plus
◆Vicon-C
◆Vi-Zac

RYDELLE LABORATORIES 427, 683
Division of S.C. Johnson & Son, Inc.
1525 Howe Street
Racine, WI 53403
Address inquiries to:
Carol Hansen
Consumer Affairs Director
(414) 631-4000
For Medical Emergencies Contact:
Marvin G. Parker, M.D., F.A.C.P.
(414) 631-2111
OTC Products Available
◆Aveeno Anti-Itch Concentrated Lotion
◆Aveeno Anti-Itch Cream
◆Aveeno Bath Oilated
◆Aveeno Bath Regular
◆Aveeno Cleansing Bar for Acne
◆Aveeno Cleansing Bar for Dry Skin
◆Aveeno Cleansing Bar for Normal to Oily Skin
◆Aveeno Moisturizing Lotion
◆Aveeno Shower and Bath Oil
◆Rhulicream
◆Rhuligel
◆Rhulispray

SANDOZ PHARMACEUTICALS/ CONSUMER DIVISION 427, 684
59 Route 10
East Hanover NJ 07936
Address Medical Inquiries To:
Medical Department
Sandoz Pharmaceuticals Corporation
East Hanover, NJ 07936
(201) 503-7500
Other Inquiries To:
(201) 503-7500
FAX (201) 503-8265
OTC Products Available
Acid Mantle Creme
◆BiCozene Creme
Cama Arthritis Pain Reliever
◆Dorcol Children's Cough Syrup
◆Dorcol Children's Decongestant Liquid
◆Dorcol Children's Fever & Pain Reducer
◆Dorcol Children's Liquid Cold Formula
◆Ex-Lax Chocolated Laxative
◆Ex-Lax Pills, Unflavored
◆Extra Gentle Ex-Lax
◆Gas-X Tablets
◆Extra Strength Gas-X Tablets
◆Gentle Nature Natural Vegetable Laxative
◆TheraFlu Flu and Cold Medicine
Thera-Flu Flu, Cold and Cough Medicine
Triaminic Allergy Tablets
Triaminic Chewables
◆Triaminic Cold Tablets
◆Triaminic Expectorant
◆Triaminic Nite Light
◆Triaminic Syrup
◆Triaminic-12 Tablets
◆Triaminic-DM Syrup
◆Triaminicin Tablets
◆Triaminicol Multi-Symptom Cold Tablets
◆Triaminicol Multi-Symptom Relief
Ursinus Inlay-Tabs

SCHERING CORPORATION
See SCHERING-PLOUGH HEALTHCARE PRODUCTS, INC.

SCHERING-PLOUGH HEALTHCARE PRODUCTS, INC. 428, 692
110 Allen Road
Liberty Corner, NJ 07938
Address inquiries to:
Regulatory Affairs (908) 604-1960
For Medical Emergencies Contact:
Clinical Department
(901) 320-2421
OTC Products Available
◆A and D Ointment
◆Afrin Cherry Scented Nasal Spray 0.05%
◆Afrin Children's Strength Nose Drops 0.025%
◆Afrin Menthol Nasal Spray, 0.05%
◆Afrin Nasal Spray 0.05% and Nasal Spray Pump
◆Afrin Nose Drops 0.05%
◆Afrin Saline Mist
◆Afrin Tablets
◆Aftate for Athlete's Foot
◆Aftate for Jock Itch
Aspergum
◆Chlor-Trimeton Allergy Syrup, Tablets & Long-Acting Repetabs Tablets
◆Chlor-Trimeton Decongestant Tablets
◆Chlor-Trimeton Long Acting Decongestant Repetabs Tablets
◆Chlor-Trimeton Maximum Strength Timed Release Allergy Tablets
◆Chlor-Trimeton Sinus Caplets
Cod Liver Oil Concentrate Capsules
Cod Liver Oil Concentrate Tablets
Cod Liver Oil Concentrate Tablets w/Vitamin C
◆Complex 15 Hand & Body Moisturizing Cream
◆Complex 15 Hand & Body Moisturizing Lotion
◆Complex 15 Moisturizing Face Cream
◆Coppertone Sunblock Lotion SPF 15
◆Coppertone Sunblock Lotion SPF 25
◆Coppertone Sunblock Lotion SPF 30
◆Coppertone Sunblock Lotion SPF 45
◆Coppertone Sunscreen Lotion SPF 6
◆Coppertone Sunscreen Lotion SPF 8
◆Coricidin 'D' Decongestant Tablets
◆Coricidin Demilets Tablets for Children
◆Coricidin Tablets
◆Correctol Laxative Tablets
Cushion Grip Denture Adhesive
Demazin Nasal Decongestant/ Antihistamine Repetabs Tablets & Syrup
Dermolate Anti-Itch Cream
◆Di-Gel Antacid/Anti-Gas
Disophrol Chronotab Sustained-Action Tablets
Disophrol Tablets
◆Drixoral Antihistamine/Nasal Decongestant Syrup
◆Drixoral Non-Drowsy Formula
◆Drixoral Plus Extended-Release Tablets
◆Drixoral Sinus
◆Drixoral Sustained-Action Tablets
◆Duration 12 Hour Mentholated Nasal Spray
◆Duration 12 Hour Nasal Spray
◆Duration 12 Hour Nasal Spray Pump
◆Emko Because Contraceptor Vaginal Contraceptive Foam
◆Emko Vaginal Contraceptive Foam
◆Feen-A-Mint Gum
◆Feen-A-Mint Laxative Pills and Chocolated Mint Tablets
◆Gyne-Lotrimin Vaginal Cream Antifungal
◆Gyne-Lotrimin Vaginal Inserts
◆Lotrimin AF Antifungal Cream, Lotion and Solution
Mol-Iron Tablets
Mol-Iron w/Vitamin C Tablets
Muskol Insect Repellent Aerosol Liquid
Muskol Insect Repellent Lotion
Muskol Insect Repellent Pump Spray
Muskol Insect Repellent Roll-on
◆OcuClear Eye Drops (See PDR For Ophthalmology)
◆Regutol Stool Softener
◆Shade Oil-Free Gel SPF 15
Shade Oil-Free Gel SPF 25
◆Shade Sunblock Lotion SPF 15
Shade Sunblock Lotion SPF 30
Shade Sunblock Lotion SPF 45
Shade Sunblock Stick SPF 30
◆Solarcaine
St. Joseph Adult Aspirin (325 mg.)
◆St. Joseph Adult Chewable Aspirin (81 mg.)
St. Joseph Anti-Diarrheal for Children
◆St. Joseph Aspirin-Free Fever Reducer for Children Chewable Tablets, Liquid & Infant Drops
St. Joseph Cold Tablets for Children
◆St. Joseph Cough Suppressant for Children
◆St. Joseph Nighttime Cold Medicine
Stay Trim Diet Gum
Stay Trim Diet Mints
◆Tinactin Aerosol Liquid 1%
◆Tinactin Aerosol Powder 1%
◆Tinactin Antifungal Cream, Solution & Powder 1%
◆Tinactin Jock Itch Cream 1%
◆Tinactin Jock Itch Spray Powder 1%
◆Water Babies by Coppertone Sunblock Cream SPF 25
◆Water Babies by Coppertone Sunblock Lotion SPF 15
◆Water Babies by Coppertone Sunblock Lotion SPF 30
◆Water Babies by Coppertone Sunblock Lotion SPF 45
◆Water Babies Little Licks SPF 30 Sunblock Lip Balm

(◆ Shown in Product Identification Section)

SCHWARZ PHARMA 431, 707
Kremers Urban Company
P.O. Box 2038
Milwaukee, WI 53201
Address inquiries to:
Technical Services Department
(414) 354-4300
(800) 558-5114
For Medical Emergencies Contact:
(414) 354-4300
(800) 558-5114
OTC Products Available
Calciferol Drops
Fedahist Decongestant Syrup
Fedahist Expectorant Pediatric Drops
Fedahist Expectorant Syrup
Fedahist Tablets
Gemnisyn Tablets
Kudrox Suspension
◆Lactrase Capsules
Milkinol

SLIM•FAST FOODS COMPANY 431, 707
919 Third Avenue
New York, NY 10022
Address inquiries to:
Consumer Services (212) 688-4420
OTC Products Available
Slim•Fast
◆Ultra Slim•Fast

SMITHKLINE BEECHAM CONSUMER BRANDS 431, 708
Unit of SmithKline Beecham, Inc.
P.O. Box 1467
Pittsburgh, PA 15230
Address inquiries to:
Professional Services Department
(800) BEECHAM
(412) 928-1050
OTC Products Available
◆A-200 Pediculicide Shampoo & Gel
◆Clear by Design Medicated Acne Gel
◆Clear By Design Medicated Cleansing Pads
◆Contac Allergy 12 Hour Capsules
◆Contac Continuous Action Decongestant/Antihistamine Capsules
◆Contac Cough Formula
◆Contac Cough & Sore Throat Formula
◆Contac Jr. Children's Cold Medicine
◆Contac Maximum Strength Continuous Action Decongestant/Antihistamine Caplets
◆Contac Nighttime Cold Medicine
◆Contac Severe Cold and Flu Formula Caplets
◆Contac Sinus Caplets Maximum Strength Non-Drowsy Formula
◆Contac Sinus Tablets Maximum Strength Non-Drowsy Formula
◆Ecotrin Enteric Coated Aspirin Maximum Strength Tablets and Caplets
◆Ecotrin Enteric Coated Aspirin Regular Strength Tablets and Caplets
Esotérica Medicated Fade Cream
◆Feosol Capsules
◆Feosol Elixir
◆Feosol Tablets
Geritol Complete Tablets
Geritol Extend Tablets and Caplets
Geritol Liquid - High Potency Iron & Vitamin Tonic
Massengill Baby Powder Soft Cloth Towelette and Unscented Soft Cloth Towelette
Massengill Disposable Douche
Massengill Liquid Concentrate
◆Massengill Medicated Disposable Douche
Massengill Medicated Liquid Concentrate
Massengill Medicated Soft Cloth Towelette
Massengill Powder
◆Nature's Remedy Natural Vegetable Laxative
◆N'ICE Medicated Sugarless Sore Throat and Cough Lozenges
N'ICE Sore Throat Spray
◆N'ICE Sugarless Vitamin C Drops
◆Oxy Clean Lathering Facial Scrub
◆Oxy Clean Medicated Cleanser
◆Oxy Clean Medicated Pads - Regular, Sensitive Skin, and Maximum Strength
◆Oxy Clean Medicated Soap
◆Oxy Night Watch Nighttime Acne Medication-Maximum Strength and Sensitive Skin Formulas
◆Oxy 10 Daily Face Wash Antibacterial Skin Wash
◆Oxy-5 and Oxy-10 Tinted and Vanishing Formulas with Sorboxyl
◆Sine-Off Maximum Strength Allergy/Sinus Formula Caplets
◆Sine-Off Maximum Strength No Drowsiness Formula Caplets
◆Sine-Off Sinus Medicine Tablets-Aspirin Formula
◆Sominex Caplets and Tablets
Sominex Liquid
◆Sominex Pain Relief Formula
◆Sucrets (Original Mint and Mentholated Mint)
◆Sucrets Children's Cherry Flavored Sore Throat Lozenges
◆Sucrets Cold Formula
◆Sucrets Cough Control Formula
◆Sucrets Maximum Strength Wintergreen and Sucrets Wild Cherry (Regular Strength) Sore Throat Lozenges
◆Sucrets Maximum Strength Sprays
◆Teldrin Timed-Release Allergy Capsules, 12 mg.
◆Tums Antacid Tablets
◆Tums E-X Antacid Tablets
◆Tums Liquid Extra-Strength Antacid
◆Tums Liquid Extra-Strength Antacid with Simethicone
Vivarin Stimulant Tablets

SMITHKLINE CONSUMER PRODUCTS
See MENLEY & JAMES LABORATORIES and SMITHKLINE BEECHAM CONSUMER BRANDS.

E. R. SQUIBB & SONS, INC. 433, 727
Apothecon®
A Bristol-Myers Squibb Company
P.O. Box 4000
Princeton, NJ 08543-4000
(609) 987-6800
Address Inquiries to:
Bristol-Myers Squibb Pharmaceutical Group
Drug Information
1 Squibb Drive
Cranbury, NJ 08512 (609) 243-6303
Distribution Centers
ATLANTA, GEORGIA
P.O. Box 16503
Atlanta, GA 30321
FAX: (404) 968-2684
All Customers Call
(800) 241-5364
CHICAGO, ILLINOIS
P.O. Box 788
Arlington Heights, IL 60006-0788
FAX: (312) 439-4960
State of IL Customers Call
(800) 942-0674
All Others Call (800) 323-0665
IRVING, TEXAS
Mail or telephone orders and customer service inquiries should be directed to Atlanta, GA (see above)
All customers call
(800) 241-5364
LOS ANGELES, CALIFORNIA
P.O. Box 19618
Irvine, CA 92713-9618
State of CA Customers Call
(800) 422-4254
State of HI Customers Call
(714) 727-7200
All Others Call (800) 854-3050
SEATTLE, WASHINGTON
Mail or telephone orders and customer service inquiries should be directed to Los Angeles (see above)
States of AK and MT Customers Call
(714) 727-7200
State of CA Customers Call
(800) 422-4254
All Others Call (800) 854-3050
NEW YORK AREA
CN 5250
Princeton, NJ 08543-5250
State of NJ Customers Call
(800) 352-4865
All Others Call (800) 631-5244

Theragran line is now being distributed by Apothecon.
OTC Products Available
◆Theragran Liquid
◆Theragran Stress Formula
◆Theragran Tablets
◆Theragran-M Tablets

STANDARD HOMEOPATHIC COMPANY 728
210 West 131st Street
Box 61067
Los Angeles, CA 90061
OTC Products Available
Hyland's Bed Wetting Tablets
Hyland's Calms Forté Tablets
Hyland's Colic Tablets
Hyland's Cough Syrup with Honey
Hyland's C-Plus Cold Tablets
Hyland's Teething Tablets
Hyland's Vitamin C for Children

STELLAR PHARMACAL CORPORATION 434, 729
1990 N.W. 44th Street
Pompano Beach, FL 33064-8712
Address inquiries to:
Scott L. Davidson (305) 972-6060
Customer Service & Order Department
(800) 845-7827
OTC Products Available
◆Star-Otic Ear Solution

STUART PHARMACEUTICALS 434, 729
a business unit of ICI Americas Inc.
Wilmington, DE 19897 USA
Address inquiries to:
Yvonne A. Graham, Manager
Professional Services
(302) 886-2231
For Medical Emergencies:
After hours & on weekends
(302) 886-3000
OTC Products Available
◆HIBICLENS Antimicrobial Skin Ckeanser
HIBISTAT Germicidal Hand Rinse
HIBISTAT Towelette
◆STUART PRENATAL Tablets

SYNTEX LABORATORIES, INC. 732
3401 Hillview Avenue
P.O. Box 10850
Palo Alto, CA 94304
Direct General/Sales/Order inquiries for U.S. Marketed products to:
Marketing Information Department
Specify product (415) 855-5050
Direct Medical inquiries on U.S. marketed products to:
Medical Services Department
General Medical Inquiries
(415) 855-5545
Adverse Reactions Inquiries
(415) 852-1386

OTC Products Available
Carmol 20 Cream
Carmol 10 Lotion

TEC LABORATORIES, INC. 434, 732
P.O. Box 1958
Albany, OR 97321
Address inquiries to:
P.O. Box 1958
Albany, OR 97321
(503) 926-4577
For Medical Emergencies Contact:
Dr. Robert Smith (503) 926-4577
OTC Products Available
Sting-X Tractor
Tec Labs 10 Hour Insect Repellent
◆Tecnu Poison Oak-N-Ivy Cleaner

THOMPSON MEDICAL COMPANY, INC. 434, 732
222 Lakeview Avenue
West Palm Beach, FL 33401
Address inquiries to:
Medical Services (212) 751-9090
OTC Products Available
Appedrine, Maximum Strength Tablets
Aqua-Ban, Maximum Strength Plus Tablets
Aqua-Ban Tablets
Arthritis Hot
Aspercreme Creme & Lotion Analgesic Rub
Control Capsules
◆Cortizone-5 Creme & Ointment
Dexatrim Capsules
Dexatrim Maximum Strength Caffeine-Free Caplets
Dexatrim Maximum Strength Caffeine-Free Capsules
◆Dexatrim Maximum Strength Plus Vitamin C/Caffeine-free Caplets
◆Dexatrim Maximum Strength Plus Vitamin C/Caffeine-free Capsules
Dexatrim Maximum Strength Pre-Meal Caplets
Diar Aid Tablets
Encare Vaginal Contraceptive Suppositories
End Lice
Ibuprin
◆NP-27 Cream, Solution, Spray Powder & Powder Antifungal
Prolamine Maximum Strength Capsules
◆Sleepinal Night-time Sleep Aid Capsules
Sportscreme Analgesic Rub
Tempo Antacid with Antigas Action
Tribiotic Plus

TRITON CONSUMER PRODUCTS, INC. 734
561 West Golf Road
Arlington Heights, IL 60005
Address inquiries to:
Karen Shrader (800) 942-2009
For Medical Emergencies Contact
(800) 942-2009
OTC Products Available
MG 217 Psoriasis Ointment and Lotion
MG 217 Psoriasis Shampoo and Conditioner
ProTech First-Aid Stik
Skeeter Stik Insect Bite Medication
Skeeter Stop 100 Insect Repellent
Tick Away Insect Repellent

UAS LABORATORIES 735
9201 Penn Avenue South #10
Minneapolis, MN 55431
Address inquiries to:
Dr. S. K. Dash (612) 881-1915
(800) 422-3371
OTC Products Available
DDS-Acidophilus

THE UPJOHN COMPANY 434, 735
7000 Portage Road
Kalamazoo, MI 49001
For Medical and Pharmaceutical Information, Including Emergencies:
(616) 329-8244
(616) 323-6615
Pharmaceutical Sales Areas and Distribution Centers
Atlanta (Chamblee)
GA 30341-2626 (404) 451-4822
Boston (Wellesley)
MA 02181 (617) 431-7970
Buffalo (Amherst)
NY 14221 (716) 632-5942
Chicago (Oak Brook Terrace)
IL 60181 (708) 574-3300
Cincinnati, OH 45202
(513) 723-1010
Dallas (Irving)
TX 75062 (214) 256-0022
Denver, CO 80216 (303) 399-3113
Hartford (Enfield)
CT 06082 (203) 741-3421
Honolulu, HI 96818 (808) 422-2777
Kalamazoo, MI 49001
(616) 323-4000
Kansas City, MO 64131
(816) 361-2286
Los Angeles, CA 90038
(213) 463-8101
Memphis, TN 38119 (901) 685-8192
Minneapolis (Bloomington), MN 55437
(612) 921-8484
New York (Uniondale)
NY 11553 (516) 745-6100
Orlando, FL 32809 (407) 859-4591
Philadelphia (Berwyn)
PA 19312 (215) 993-0100
Pittsburgh (Bridgeville)
PA 15017 (412) 257-0200
Portland, OR 97232 (503) 232-2133
St. Louis, MO 63141 (314) 872-8626
San Francisco (Foster City)
CA 94404 (415) 377-0203
Shreveport, LA 71129
(318) 688-3700
Washington, DC 20011
(202) 882-6163
OTC Products Available
Baciguent Antibiotic Ointment
◆Cortaid Cream with Aloe
◆Cortaid Lotion
◆Cortaid Ointment with Aloe
◆Cortaid Spray
Cortef Feminine Itch Cream
◆Doxidan Capsules
◆Kaopectate Concentrated Anti-Diarrheal, Peppermint Flavor
◆Kaopectate Concentrated Anti-Diarrheal, Regular Flavor
◆Kaopectate Children's Chewable Tablets
◆Kaopectate Maximum Strength Caplets
◆Motrin IB Caplets and Tablets
Myciguent Antibiotic Cream
Myciguent Antibiotic Ointment
◆Mycitracin Plus Pain Reliever
◆Mycitracin Triple Antibiotic Ointment
Phenolax Wafers
Progaine Shampoo
◆Surfak Capsules
◆Unicap Softgel Capsules & Tablets
Unicap Jr Chewable Tablets
◆Unicap M Tablets
Unicap Plus Iron Vitamin Formula Tablets
◆Unicap Sr. Tablets
◆Unicap T Tablets

WAKUNAGA OF AMERICA CO., LTD. 435, 739
Subsidiary of Wakunaga Pharmaceutical Co., Ltd.
23501 Madero
Mission Viejo, CA 92691
Address inquires to:
(714) 855-2776
OTC Products Available
◆Kyolic
Kyo-Dophilus, Capsules: Acidophilus, Bifidus, S. Faecalis
Kyo-Green, Powder: Barley & Wheat Grass, Chlorella, Brown Rice, Kelp
Kyolic Formula 106 Capsules: Aged Garlic Extract Powder (300 mg) & Vitamin E
Kyolic Super Formula 104 Capsules: Aged Garlic Extract Powder (300 mg)
Kyolic Super Formula 105 Capsules: Aged Garlic Extract Powder (200 mg)
Kyolic Super Formula 100 Capsules & Tablets: Aged Garlic Extract Powder (300 mg)
Kyolic Super Formula 100 Tablets: Aged Garlic Extract Powder (270 mg)
◆ Kyolic-Aged Garlic Extract Flavor & Odor Modified Enriched with Vitamins B_1 and B_{12}
Kyolic-Aged Garlic Extract Flavor & Odor Modified Plain
Kyolic-Aged Garlic Extract Liquid Enriched with Vitamin B, & Vitamin B_{12}
Kyolic-Aged Garlic Extract Liquid Plain
◆ Kyolic-Formula 101 Capsules: Aged Garlic Extract (270 mg)
Kyolic-Formula 103 Capsules: Aged Garlic Extract Powder (220 mg)
Kyolic-Formula 101 Tablets: Aged Garlic Extract Powder (270 mg)
Kyolic-Super Formula 104, Aged Garlic Extract Powder (300 mg) with Lecithin
Kyolic-Super Formula 103, Capsules: Aged Garlic Extract Powder (220 mg) with Vitamin C, Astragalus, Calcium
Kyolic-Super Formula 105, Capsules: Aged Garlic Extract Powder (250 mg) with Selenium, Vitamins A & E
Kyolic-Super Formula 106, Capsules: Aged Garlic Extract Powder (300 mg) with Vitamin E, Cayenne Pepper, Hawthorn Berry
◆ Kyolic-Super Formula 101 Garlic Plus Tablets & Capsules: Aged Garlic Extract Powder (270 mg) with Brewer's Yeast, Kelp & Algin
Kyolic-Super Formula 102, Tablets & Capsules: Aged Garlic Extract Powder (350 mg) with Enzyme Complex

WALKER, CORP & CO., INC. 435, 739
203 E. Hampton Place
Syracuse, NY 13206
Address inquiries to:
P.O. Box 1320
Syracuse, NY 13201 (315) 463-4511
For Medical Emergencies Contact:
George J. Eschenfelder
(315) 492-0947
OTC Products Available
◆Evac-U-Gen Mild Laxative

WALKER PHARMACAL COMPANY 740
4200 Laclede
St. Louis, MO 63108
Address Inquiries to:
Customer Service (314) 533-9600
OTC Products Available
HIKE Antiseptic Ointment
PRID Salve

WALLACE LABORATORIES 435, 740
Half Acre Road
Cranbury, NJ 08512
Address inquiries to:
Wallace Laboratories
Div. of Carter-Wallace, Inc.
P.O. Box 1001
Cranbury, NJ 08512 (609) 655-6000
For Medical Emergencies:
(609) 799-1167
OTC Products Available
◆Maltsupex Liquid, Powder & Tablets
◆Ryna Liquid
◆Ryna-C Liquid
◆Ryna-CX Liquid
◆Syllact Powder

WARNER-LAMBERT COMPANY 435, 742
Consumer Health Products Group
201 Tabor Road
Morris Plains, NJ 07950
See also Parke-Davis

(◆ Shown in Product Identification Section)

Address Inquiries to:
Robert Kirpitch (201) 540-3204
For Medical Emergencies Call:
(201) 540-2000
OTC Products Available
Bromo-Seltzer
Corn Husker's Lotion
Efferdent Extra Strength Denture Cleanser
◆Professional Strength Efferdent
◆Halls Cough Formula
◆Halls Mentho-Lyptus Cough Suppressant Tablets
◆Halls Plus Cough Suppressant Tablets
◆Halls Vitamin C Drops
Listerex Lotion
◆Listerine Antiseptic
◆Listerine Antiseptic Lozenges Regular Strength
◆Listerine Maximum Strength Antiseptic Lozenges
◆Listermint with Fluoride
◆Lubriderm Cream
◆Lubriderm Lotion
◆Lubriderm Skin Conditioning Oil
◆Rolaids
◆Rolaids (Calcium Rich/Sodium Free)
◆Extra Strength Rolaids
Super Anahist Tablets

WESTWOOD-SQUIBB PHARMACEUTICALS INC. 436, 744
100 Forest Avenue
Buffalo, NY 14213
(716) 887-3400
Address inquiries to:
Consumer Affairs Department
(716) 887-3773
OTC Products Available
Balnetar
Estar Gel
Fostril Lotion
◆Lac-Hydrin Five
Lowila Cake
◆Moisturel Cream
◆Moisturel Lotion
◆Moisturel Sensitive Skin Cleanser
Pernox Lotion
Pernox Medicated Scrub
Pernox Shampoo
Sebucare Lotion
◆Sebulex Antiseborrheic Treatment Shampoo
Sebulex Shampoo with Conditioners
Sebulon Dandruff Shampoo
◆Sebutone and Sebutone Cream Antiseborrheic Tar Shampoos

WHITEHALL LABORATORIES INC. 436, 745, 775
Division of American Home Products Corporation
685 Third Avenue
New York, NY 10017
Address Professional Inquiries to:
(800) 343-0856
Address Consumer Inquiries to:
(212) 878-5503
OTC Products Available
◆Advil Ibuprofen Caplets and Tablets
◆Anacin Coated Analgesic Caplets
◆Anacin Coated Analgesic Tablets
Anacin Maximum Strength Analgesic Coated Tablets
Anacin-3 Children's Acetaminophen Chewable Tablets, Alcohol-Free Liquid and Infants' Drops
◆Anacin-3 Maximum Strength Acetaminophen Film Coated Caplets
◆Anacin-3 Maximum Strength Acetaminophen Film Coated Tablets
Anacin-3 Regular Strength Acetaminophen Film Coated Tablets
◆Anbesol Baby Teething Gel Anesthetic
◆Anbesol Gel Antiseptic-Anesthetic
◆Anbesol Gel Antiseptic-Anesthetic - Maximum Strength
◆Anbesol Liquid Antiseptic-Anesthetic
◆Anbesol Liquid Antiseptic-Anesthetic - Maximum Strength
Arthritis Pain Formula Aspirin-Free by the Makers of Anacin Analgesic Tablets
Arthritis Pain Formula by the Makers of Anacin Analgesic Tablets and Caplets
Bisodol Antacid Powder
Bisodol Antacid Tablets
Bronitin Asthma Tablets
Bronitin Mist
◆Clearblue Easy
◆Clearplan Easy
Clusivol Syrup
◆CoAdvil
Compound W Gel
Compound W Solution
Denalan Denture Cleanser
◆Denorex Medicated Shampoo and Conditioner
◆Denorex Medicated Shampoo, Extra Strength
◆Denorex Medicated Shampoo, Extra Strength With Conditioners
◆Denorex Medicated Shampoo, Regular & Mountain Fresh Herbal Scent
Dermoplast Anesthetic Pain Relief Lotion
Dermoplast Anesthetic Pain Relief Spray
◆Dristan Decongestant/Antihistamine/ Analgesic Coated Caplets
◆Dristan Decongestant/Antihistamine/ Analgesic Coated Tablets
◆Dristan Advanced Formula Decongestant/Antihistamine/ Analgesic Tablets
Dristan Inhaler
◆Dristan Long Lasting Menthol Nasal Spray
◆Dristan Long Lasting Nasal Spray, Regular
◆Maximum Strength Dristan Decongestant/Analgesic Coated Caplets
Dristan Nasal Spray, Menthol
◆Dristan Nasal Spray, Regular and Regular with Metered Dose Pump
Dristan Room Vaporizer
Dristan-AF Decongestant/Antihistamine/ Analgesic Tablets
Dry and Clear Acne Medicated Lotion & Double Strength Cream
Enzactin Cream
Fiber Guard
Freezone Solution
Heather Feminine Deodorant Spray
Heet Analgesic Liniment
Heet Analgesic Spray
InfraRub Analgesic Cream
Kerodex Cream 51 (for dry or oily work)
Kerodex Cream 71 (for wet work)
Larylgan Throat Spray
Medicated Cleansing Pads by the Makers of Preparation H Hemorrhoidal Remedies
Momentum Muscular Backache Formula
Outgro Solution
Oxipor VHC Lotion for Psoriasis
◆Posture 600 mg
◆Posture-D 600 mg
◆Preparation H Hemorrhoidal Cream
◆Preparation H Hemorrhoidal Ointment
◆Preparation H Hemorrhoidal Suppositories
◆Primatene Mist
Primatene Mist Suspension
◆Primatene Tablets-M Formula
◆Primatene Tablets-P Formula
◆Primatene Tablets-Regular Formula
Quiet World Nighttime Pain Formula
Riopan Antacid Chew Tablets
Riopan Antacid Chew Tablets in Rollpacks
◆Riopan Antacid Suspension
Riopan Antacid Swallow Tablets
Riopan Plus Chew Tablets
Riopan Plus Chew Tablets in Rollpacks
◆Riopan Plus 2 Chew Tablets
◆Riopan Plus Suspension
◆Riopan Plus 2 Suspension
◆Semicid Vaginal Contraceptive Inserts
Sleep-eze 3 Tablets
Today Personal Lubricant
◆Today Vaginal Contraceptive Sponge
Trendar Ibuprofen Tablets
Viro-Med Tablets
Youth Garde Moisturizer Plus PABA

WINTHROP CONSUMER PRODUCTS 437, 757
Division of Sterling Drug Inc.
90 Park Avenue
New York, NY 10016
Address inquiries to:
Winthrop Consumer Products
For Medical Emergencies Contact:
Medical Department (212) 907-3027
OTC Products Available
◆Bronkaid Mist
Bronkaid Mist Suspension
◆Bronkaid Tablets
◆Campho-Phenique Cold Sore Gel
◆Campho-Phenique Liquid
◆Campho-Phenique Triple Antibiotic Ointment Plus Pain Reliever
Fergon Elixir
◆Fergon Tablets
NTZ Long Acting Nasal Spray & Drops 0.05%
◆NāSal Moisturizing Nasal Spray
◆NāSal Moisturizing Nose Drops
Neo-Synephrine 12 Hour Adult Nose Drops
Neo-Synephrine 12 Hour Nasal Spray
◆Neo-Synephrine 12 Hour Nasal Spray Pump
Neo-Synephrine 12 Hour Vapor Nasal Spray
Neo-Synephrine Jelly
Neo-Synephrine Nasal Spray (Mentholated)
◆Neo-Synephrine Nasal Sprays
◆Neo-Synephrine Nose Drops
◆pHisoDerm Cleansing Bar
◆pHisoDerm For Baby
◆pHisoDerm Skin Cleanser and Conditioner - Regular and Oily
◆pHisoPUFF
WinGel Liquid & Tablets

WINTHROP PHARMACEUTICALS 761
90 Park Avenue
New York, NY 10016
Address Medical Inquiries to:
Professional Services Department
(800) 446-6267
All Other Information:
Main Office
90 Park Avenue
New York, NY 10016
(212) 907-2000
OTC Products Available
Anti-Rust Tablets
Breonsin Capsules
Bronkolixir
Bronkotabs Tablets
Drisdol
Measurin Caplets
pHisoDerm (see Winthrop Consumer Products)
Pontocaine Cream
Pontocaine Ointment
Zephiran Chloride Aqueous Solution
Zephiran Chloride Concentrate Solution
Zephiran Chloride Spray
Zephiran Chloride Tinted Tincture
Zephiran Towelettes

WYETH-AYERST LABORATORIES 438, 764
Division of American Home Products Corporation
P.O. Box 8299
Philadelphia, PA 19101
Address inquiries to:
Professional Service (215) 688-4400
For EMERGENCY Medical Information
Day or night call (215) 688-4400

WYETH-AYERST DISTRIBUTION CENTERS

Atlanta, GA—P.O. Box 1773
Paoli, PA 19301-1773
(800) 666-7248
Freight address:
221 Armour Drive NE
Atlanta, GA 30324
Mail DEA order forms to:
P.O. Box 4365
Atlanta, GA 30302

Boston MA—P.O. Box 1773
Paoli, PA 19301-1773
(800) 666-7248
Freight address:
7 Connector Road
Andover, MA 01810
Mail DEA order forms to:
P.O. Box 1776
Andover, MA 01810

Chamblee, GA—P.O. Box 1773
Paoli, PA 19301-1773
(800) 666-7248
Freight address:
3600 American Drive
Chamblee, GA 30341

Chicago, IL—P.O. Box 1773
Paoli, PA 19301-1773
(800) 666-7248
Freight address:
745 N. Gary Avenue
Carol Stream, IL 60188
Mail DEA order forms to:
P.O. Box 140
Wheaton, IL 60189-0140

Dallas, TX—P.O. Box 1773
Paoli, PA 19301-1773
(800) 666-7248
Freight address:
11240 Petal Street
Dallas, TX 75238
Mail DEA order forms to:
P.O. Box 650231
Dallas, TX 75265-0231

Foster City, CA—P.O. Box 1773
Paoli, PA 19301-1773
(800) 666-7248
Freight address:
1147 Chess Drive
Foster City, CA 94404

Hawaii—P.O. Box 1773
Paoli, PA 19301-1773
(800) 666-7248
Mail DEA order forms to:
96-1185 Waihona, Street, Unit C1
Pearl City, HI 96782

Kansas City, MO—P.O. Box 1773
Paoli, PA 19301-1773
(800) 666-7248
Freight address:
1340 Taney Street
North Kansas City, MO 64116
Mail DEA order forms to:
P.O. Box 7588
North Kansas City, MO 64116

Los Angeles, CA—P.O. Box 1773
Paoli, PA 19301-1773
(800) 666-7248
Freight address:
6530 Altura Blvd.
Buena Park, CA 90622
Mail DEA order forms to:
P.O. Box 5000
Buena Park, CA 90622-5000

Philadelphia, PA—P.O. Box 1773
Paoli, PA 19301-1773
(800) 666-7248
Freight address:
31 Morehall Road
Frazer, PA 19355
Mail DEA order forms to:
P.O. Box 61
Paoli, PA 19301

Seattle, WA—P.O. Box 1773
Paoli, PA 19301-1773
(800) 666-7248
Freight address:
19255 80th Ave. South
Kent, WA 98032
Mail DEA order forms to:
P.O. Box 5609
Kent, WA 98064-5609

South Plainfield, NJ—P.O. Box 1773
Paoli, PA 19301-1773
(800) 666-7248
Freight address:
4000 Hadley Road
South Plainfield, NJ 07080

OTC Products Available

◆Aludrox Oral Suspension
◆Amphojel Suspension
◆Amphojel Suspension without Flavor
◆Amphojel Tablets
◆Basaljel Capsules
◆Basaljel Suspension
◆Basaljel Tablets
◆Cerose-DM
◆Collyrium for Fresh Eyes
◆Collyrium Fresh
◆Nursoy, Soy Protein Isolate Formula for Infants, Concentrated Liquid, Ready-to-Feed, and Powder
◆SMA Iron Fortified Infant Formula, Concentrated, Ready-to-Feed and Powder
◆SMA lo-iron Infant Formula, Concentrated, Ready-to-Feed, and Powder
◆Wyanoids Relief Factor Hemorrhoidal Suppositories

ZILA PHARMACEUTICALS, INC. **439, 768**
777 East Thomas Road
Phoenix, AZ 85014-5454
Address inquiries to:
Ed Pomerantz,
Vice President, Marketing
(602) 957-7887

OTC Products Available

ZilaBrace Oral Analgesic Gel
◆Zilactin Medicated Gel
Zilactol Medicated Liquid
ZilaDent Oral Analgesic Gel

(◆ **Shown in Product Identification Section)**

SECTION 2

Product Name Index

In this section only described products are listed in alphabetical sequence by brand name or generic name. They have page numbers to assist you in locating the descriptions. For additional information on other products, you may wish to contact the manufacturer directly. The symbol ◆ indicates the product is shown in the Product Identification Section.

A

B

C

D

(◆ Shown in Product Identification Section)

E

F

G

(◆ Shown in Product Identification Section)

N

O

P

Q

R

S

T

U

SECTION 3

Product Category Index

Products described in the Product Information (White) Section are listed according to their classifications. The headings and subheadings have been determined by the OTC Review process of the U.S. Food and Drug Administration. Classification of products have been determined by the Publisher with the cooperation of individual manufacturers. In cases where there were differences of opinion or where the manufacturer had no opinion, the Publisher made the final decision.

A

AMEBICIDES & TRICHOMONACIDES (see under ANTIPARASITICS)

AMINO ACID PREPARATIONS

ANALGESICS

ACETAMINOPHEN

ACETAMINOPHEN & COMBINATIONS

DECONGESTANTS

ORAL & COMBINATIONS

TOPICAL

LONG-ACTING

M

W

SECTION 4

Active Ingredients Index

In this section the products described in the Product Information (White) Section are listed under their chemical (generic) name according to their principal ingredient(s). Products have been included under specific headings by the Publisher with the cooperation of individual manufacturers.

A

H

I

U

V

VITAMIN B_{12}

VITAMIN B_{12}, NASAL DELIVERY

VITAMIN C

VITAMIN D

VITAMIN D_2

VITAMIN E

SECTION 5

Product Identification Section

This section is designed to help you identify products and their packaging.

Participating manufacturers have included selected products in full color. Where capsules and tablets are included they are shown in actual size. Packages generally are reduced in size.

For more information on products included, refer to the description in the PRODUCT INFORMATION SECTION or check directly with the manufacturer.

While every effort has been made to reproduce products faithfully, this section should be considered only as a quick-reference identification aid.

INDEX BY MANUFACTURER

ADRIA

Original Flavor

Cherry Flavor

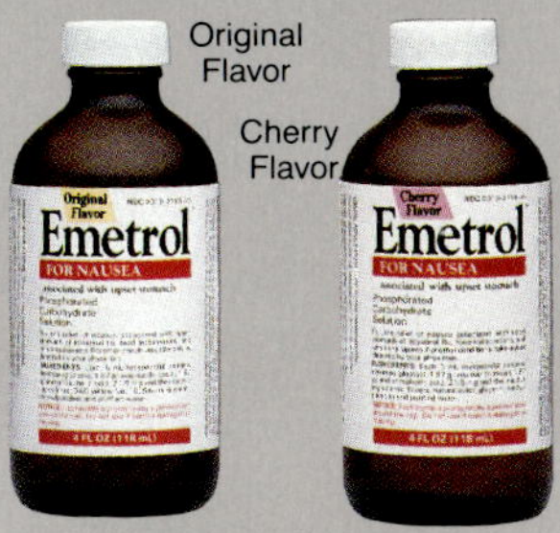

EMETROL®
(phosphorated carbohydrate solution)

Allergan

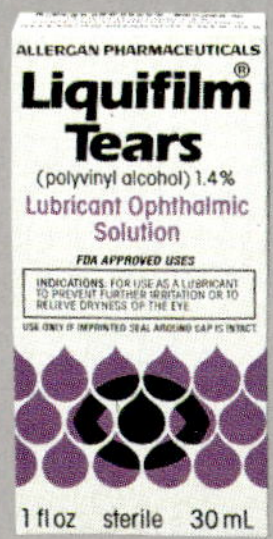

1 fl oz

Also available: ½ fl oz

LIQUIFILM TEARS®
Lubricant Ophthalmic Solution

Allergan

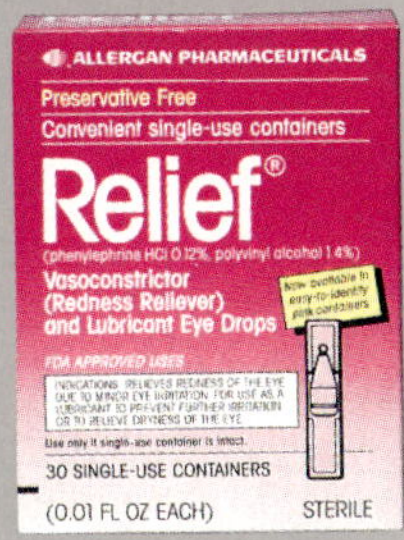

30 single-use containers
(0.01 fl oz each)

RELIEF®
Vasoconstrictor (Redness Reliever) and Lubricant Eye Drops

B. F. Ascher & Co., Inc.

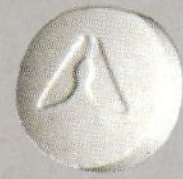

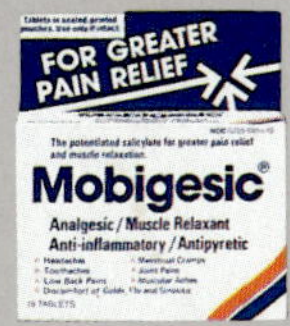

Available: 18's, 50's & 100's

MOBIGESIC®
ANALGESIC TABLETS

Adria

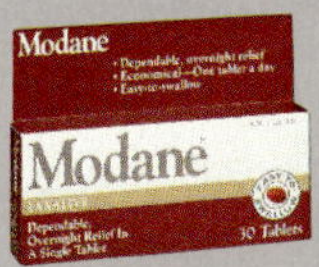

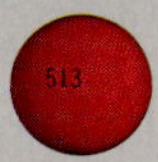

MODANE®
(phenolphthalein)

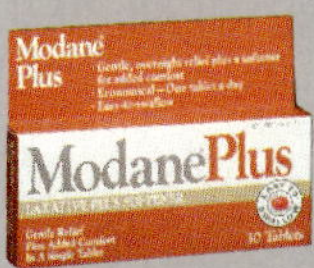

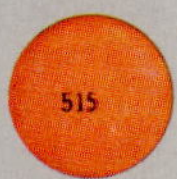

MODANE® PLUS
(phenolphthalein and docusate sodium)

Allergan

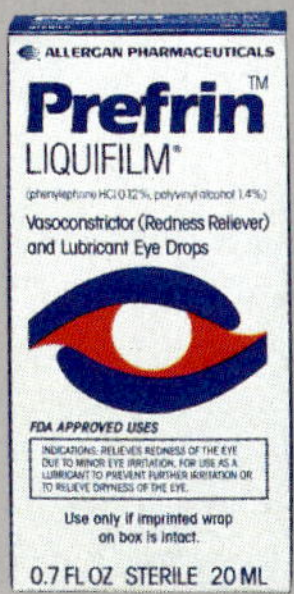

0.7 fl oz

PREFRIN™ LIQUIFILM®
Vasoconstrictor (Redness Reliever) and Lubricant Eye Drops
(phenylephrine HCl 0.12%, polyvinyl alcohol 1.4%)

Allergan

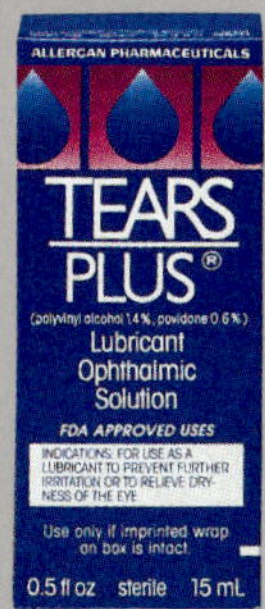

½ fl oz

Also available: 1 fl oz

TEARS PLUS®
Lubricant Ophthalmic Solution

B. F. Ascher & Co., Inc.

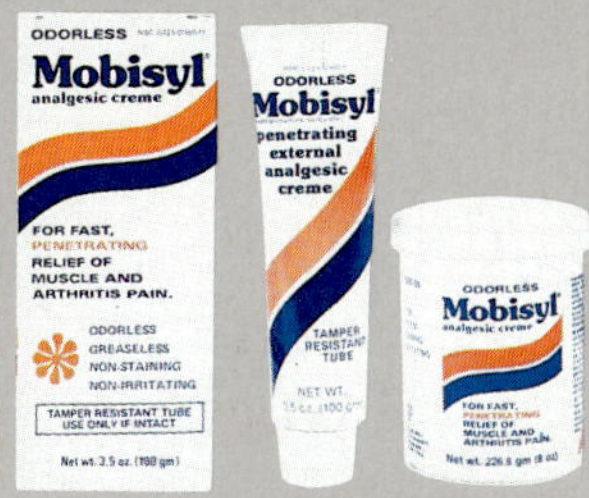

Also Available: 1.25 oz

MOBISYL®
ANALGESIC CREME

ALLERGAN

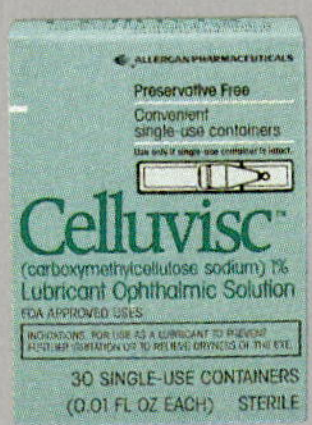

30 single-use containers
(0.01 fl oz each)

CELLUVISC®
Lubricant Ophthalmic Solution

Allergan

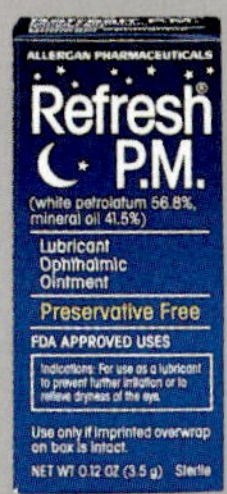

0.12 oz (3.5 g)

Preservative-free
Nighttime treatment for dry eyes.

REFRESH® P.M.
Lubricant Ophthalmic Ointment

ASCHER

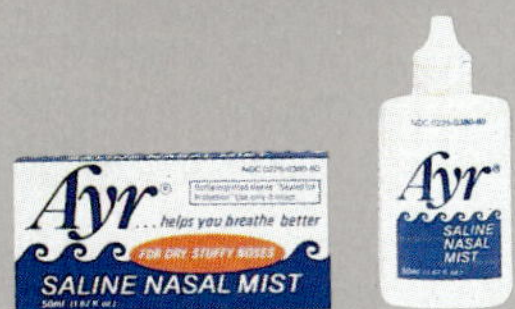

AYR® SALINE NASAL MIST

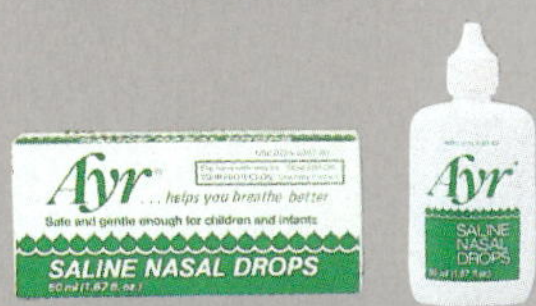

AYR® SALINE NASAL DROPS

B. F. Ascher & Co., Inc.

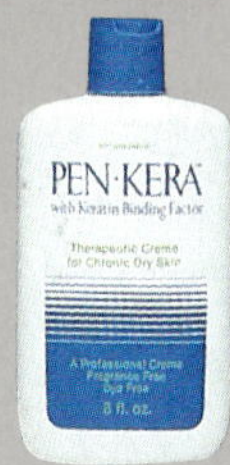

Available in 8 oz bottle

PEN•KERA®

Therapeutic Creme for Chronic Dry Skin

Allergan

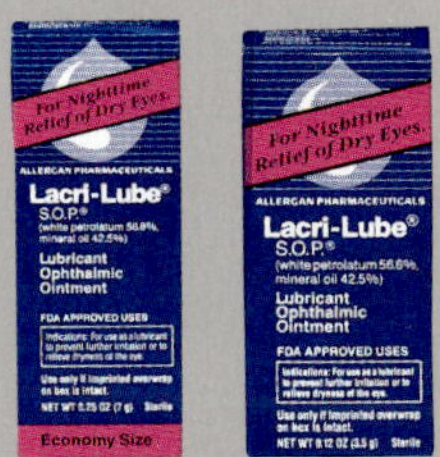

7 g 3.5 g

Also available:
0.7 g unit dose (24 pack)

LACRI-LUBE® S.O.P.®
Lubricant Ophthalmic Ointment

Allergan

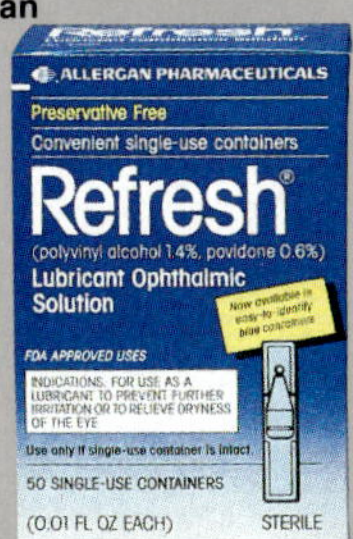

50 single-use containers
(0.01 fl oz each)

Also available:
30 single-use containers

REFRESH®
Lubricant Ophthalmic Solution

B. F. Ascher & Co., Inc.

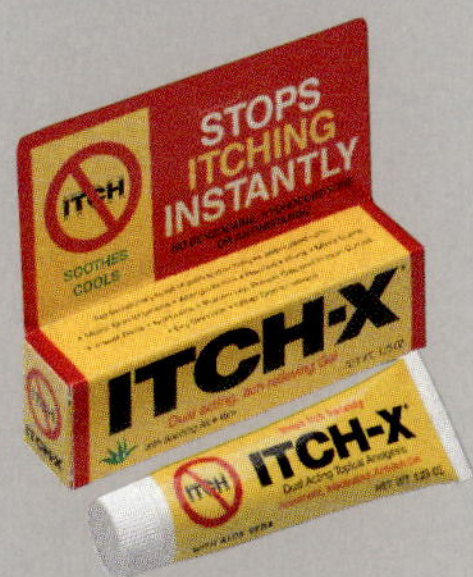

Available in 1.25 oz tube

ITCH-X® GEL
(benzyl alcohol 10% & pramoxine hydrochloride 1%)

B. F. Ascher & Co., Inc.

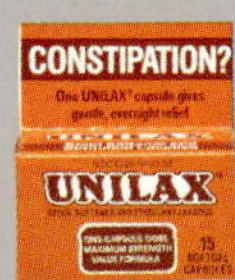

Available in 15's & 60's

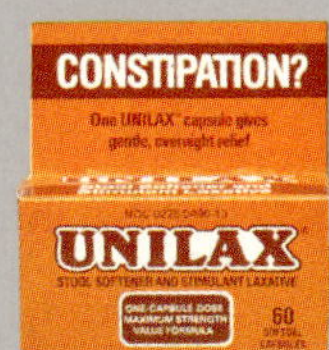

UNILAX®
Softgel Capsules

ASTRA

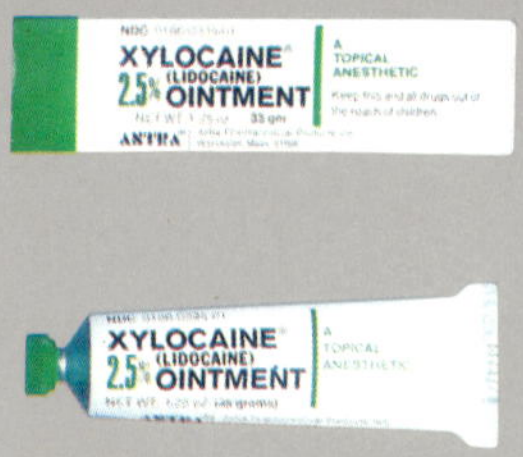

Available in 35g Tube

XYLOCAINE® 2.5% OINTMENT
(lidocaine)

Bausch & Lomb

4 fl. oz.

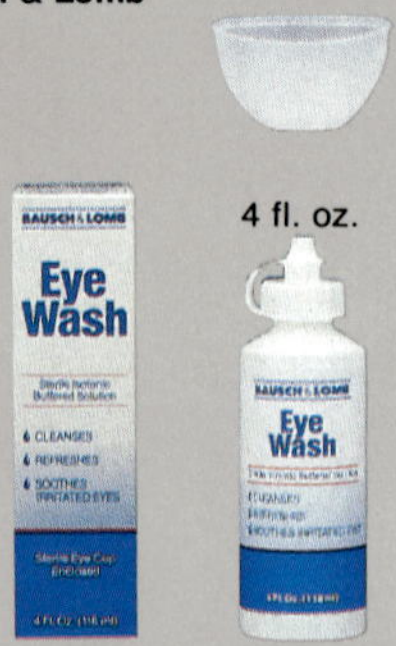

EYE WASH
Cleanses, Refreshes and Soothes Irritated Eyes

Beiersdorf

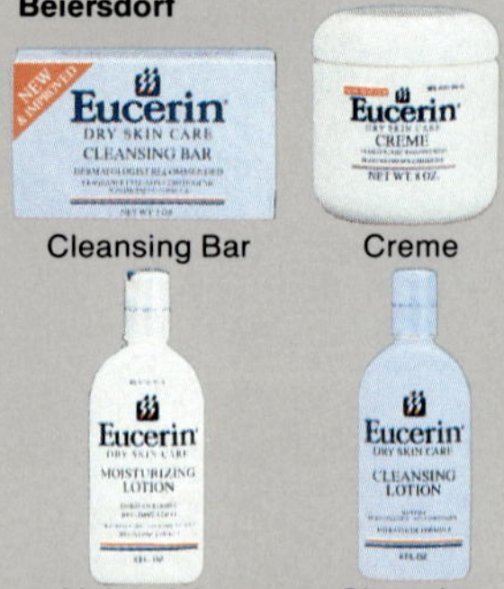

Cleansing Bar
Creme
Moisturizing
Cleansing

EUCERIN®
Fragrance-Free Dry Skin Care

BOIRON

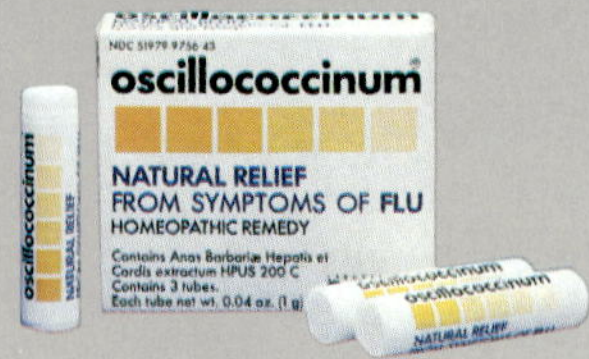

OSCILLOCOCCINUM®
Homeopathic remedy for relief of flu-like symptoms

BAUSCH & LOMB

0.5 fl. oz.

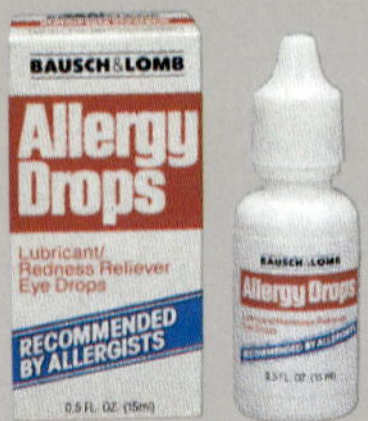

ALLERGY DROPS
Lubricant/Redness Reliever Eye Drops

Bausch & Lomb

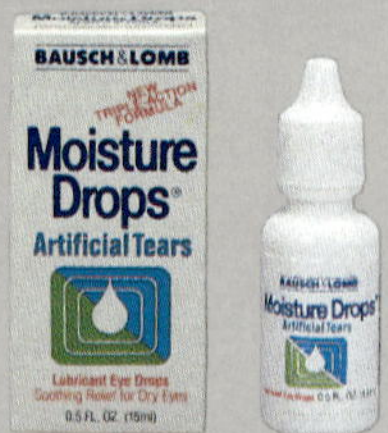

0.5 and 1.0 oz. sizes
MOISTURE DROPS®
ARTIFICIAL TEARS

Lubricant Eye Drops
Soothing Relief for Dry Eyes

Beiersdorf

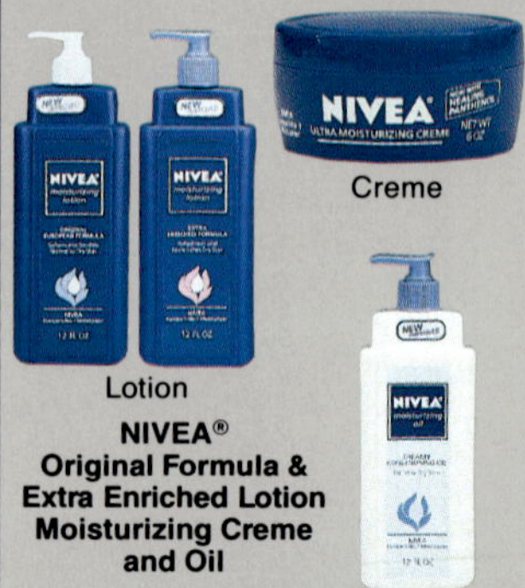

Creme
Lotion
Oil

NIVEA®
Original Formula & Extra Enriched Lotion Moisturizing Creme and Oil

For Very Dry Skin

Bristol-Myers Products

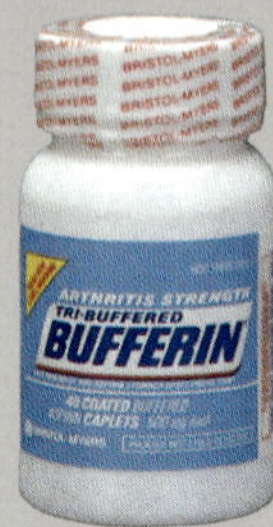

Bottles of 40 and 100 coated caplets

ARTHRITIS STRENGTH BUFFERIN® CAPLET
(buffered aspirin)

Bausch & Lomb

Sterile Single-Use Container

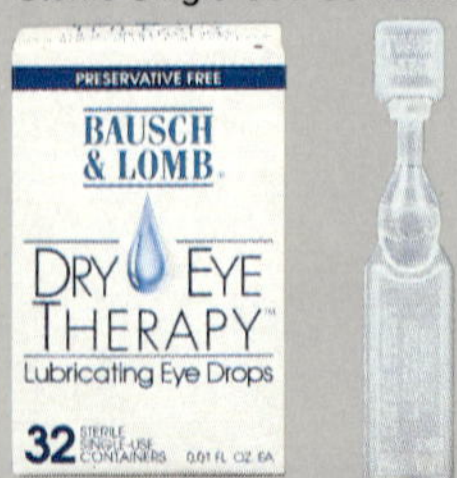

Preservative Free
32 Sterile Single-Use Containers
0.01 fl. oz. Each

DRY EYE THERAPY™
Lubricating Eye Drops

BEIERSDORF

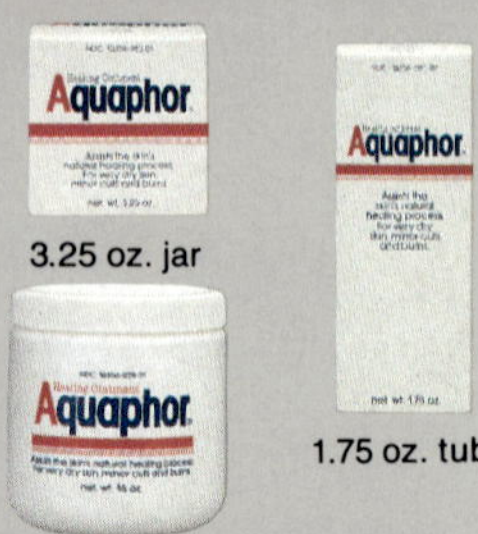

3.25 oz. jar
1.75 oz. tube
16 oz. jar

AQUAPHOR®
Healing Ointment
For dry skin, minor cuts and burns

Beiersdorf

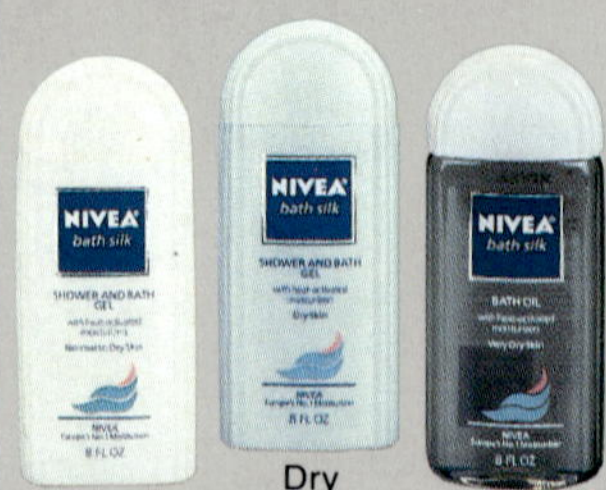

Normal to Dry Skin
Dry Skin
Very Dry Skin

NIVEA®
Bath Silk Shower & Bath Gel Bath Oil

Bristol-Myers Products

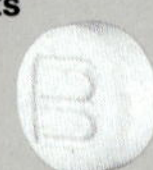

Bottles of 12, 30, 36, 50, 60, 100, 200, 275 and 1000 and vials of 10

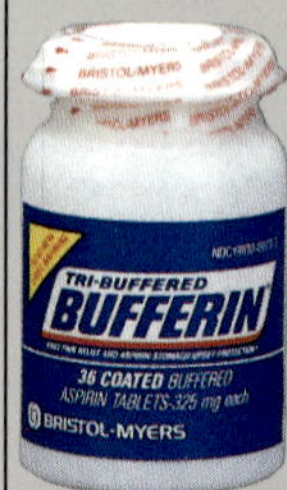

Hospital/Institutional packs of 150 x 2 tablets in foil packets

BUFFERIN® TABLET
(buffered aspirin)

Bausch & Lomb

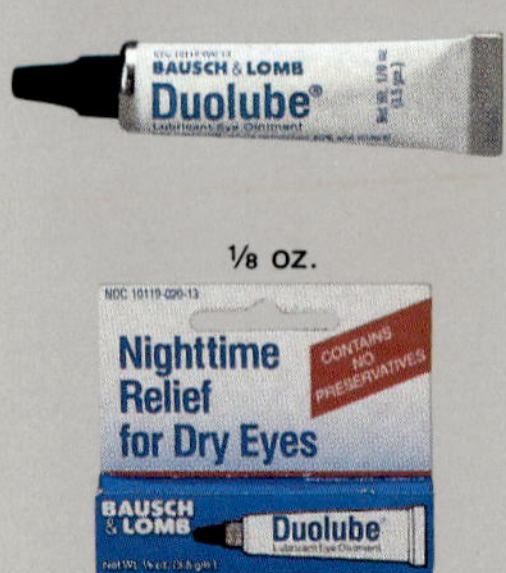

⅛ oz.

DUOLUBE®
Lubricant Eye Ointment
Nighttime Relief for Dry Eyes

Beiersdorf

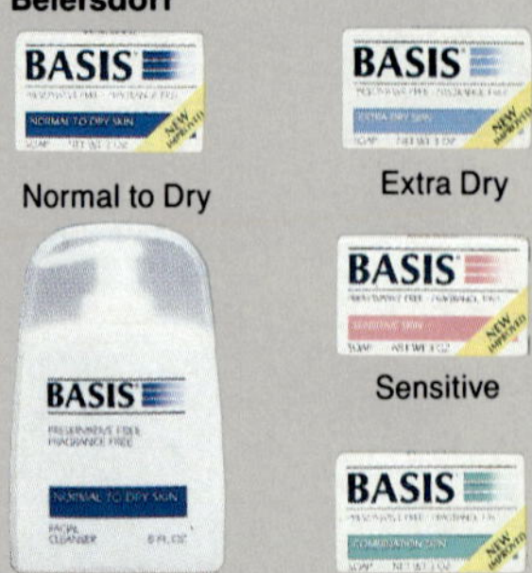

Normal to Dry
Extra Dry
Sensitive
Facial Cleanser
Combination

BASIS®
Soap & Facial Cleanser
Cleans and Softens the Skin

Beiersdorf

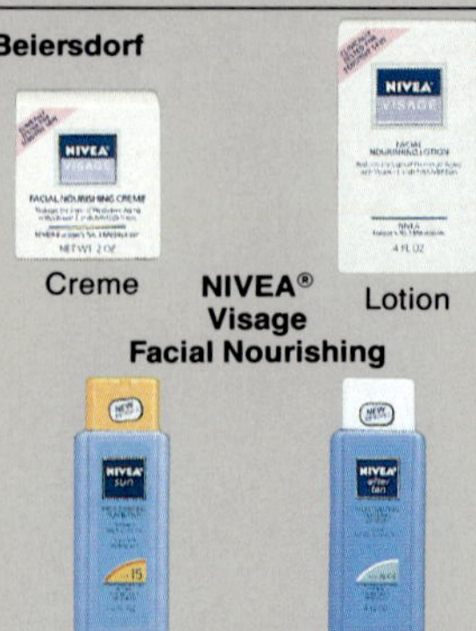

Creme
Lotion

NIVEA®
Visage
Facial Nourishing

Sun
After Tan

NIVEA®
Sun Block and Cooling Lotion

Bristol-Myers Products

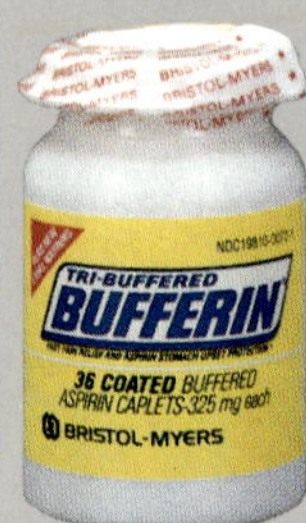

Bottles of 30, 36, 50, 60 and 100 coated caplets

BUFFERIN® CAPLET
(buffered aspirin)

Bristol-Myers Products

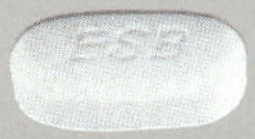
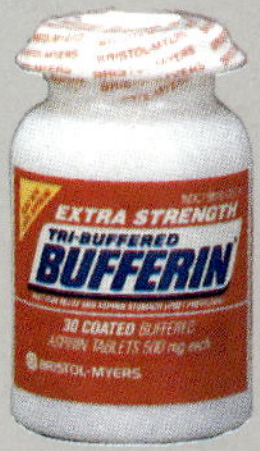

Bottles of 30, 50, 60 and 100 coated tablets

EXTRA STRENGTH BUFFERIN® TABLET
(buffered aspirin)

Bristol-Myers Products

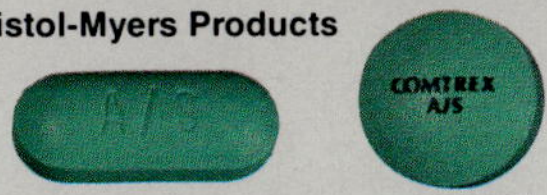

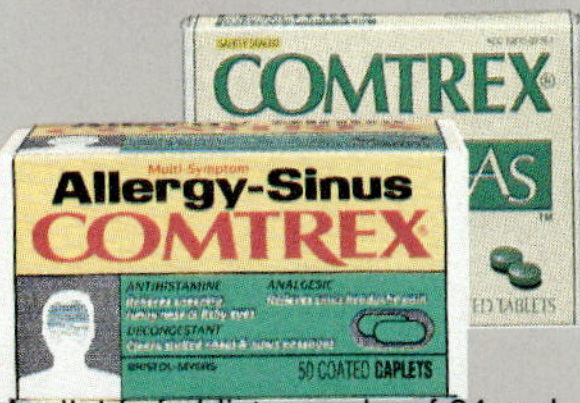

Available in blister packs of 24 and bottles of 50 tablets

COMTREX® A/S MULTI-SYMPTOM CAPLETS AND TABLETS ALLERGY-SINUS FORMULA
(acetaminophen, pseudoephedrine, chlorpheniramine)

Bristol-Myers Products

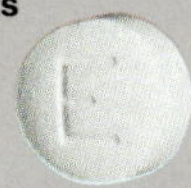
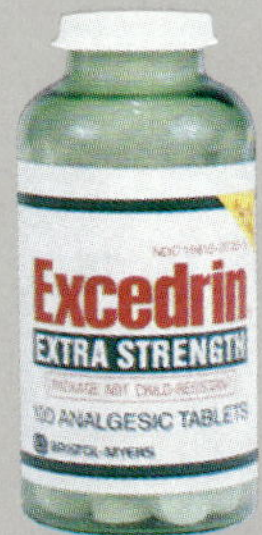

Bottles of 12, 30, 60, 100, 165, 225 and 275 metal tins of 12 and vials of 10

EXCEDRIN® TABLETS
Aspirin/Acetaminophen/Caffeine

Bristol-Myers Products

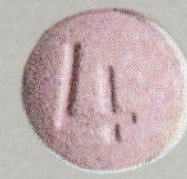
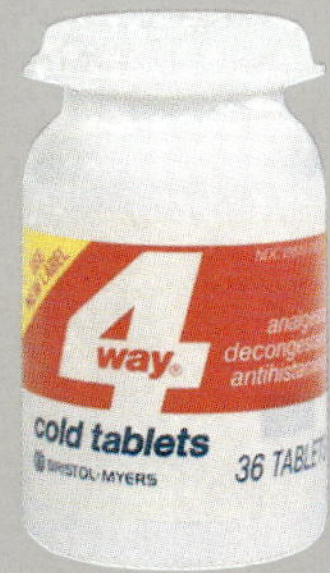

Bottles of 36 and 60

4-WAY® COLD TABLETS

Bristol-Myers Products

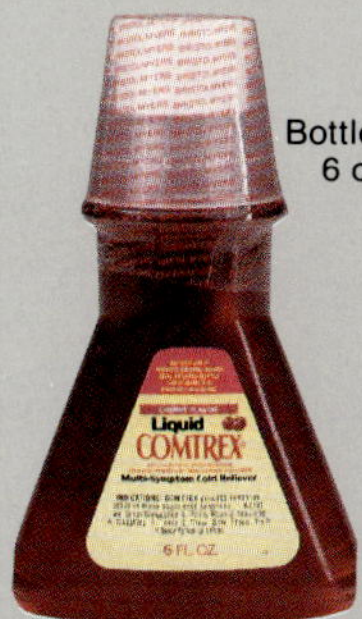

Bottles of 6 oz.

COMTREX® LIQUID

Bristol-Myers Products

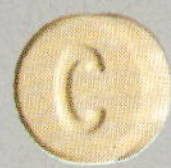
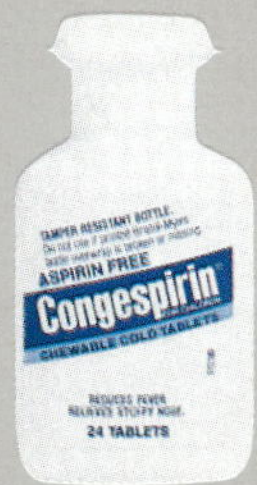

Bottles of 24

ASPIRIN FREE CONGESPIRIN®
(acetaminophen 81 mg., phenylephrine 1.25 mg.)

Bristol-Myers Products

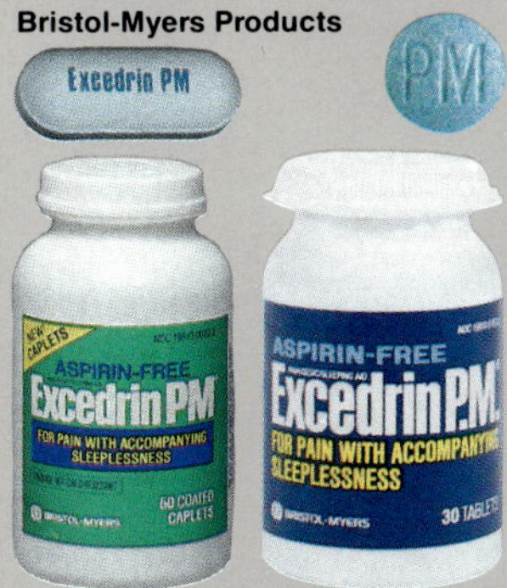

Bottles of 10, 30, 50 and 80 and vials of 10

EXCEDRIN P.M.®

Bristol-Myers Products

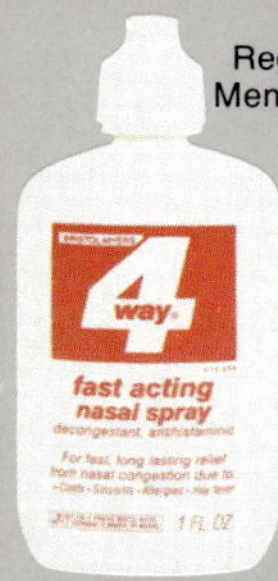

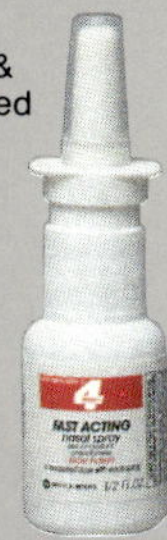

Regular & Mentholated

Atomizers of ½ and 1 oz.

Available in ½ oz. metered spray pump

4-WAY® FAST ACTING NASAL SPRAY

Bristol-Myers Products

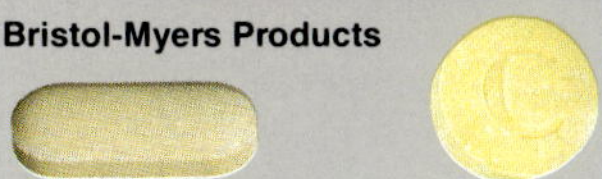
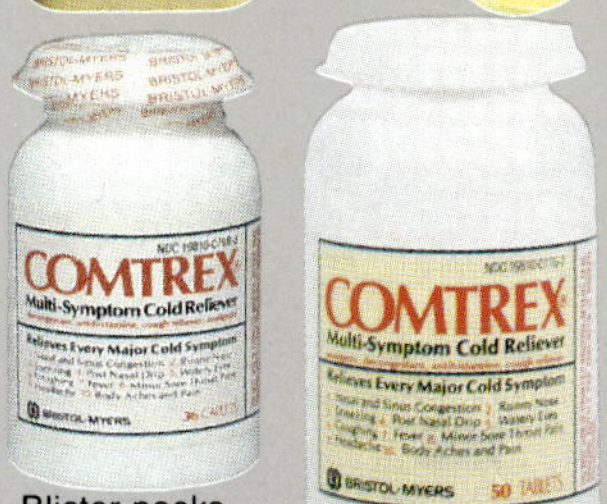

Blister packs of 24 and bottles of 50
COMTREX® CAPLETS

Blister packs of 24, bottles of 50, vials of 10
COMTREX® TABLETS

Bristol-Myers Products

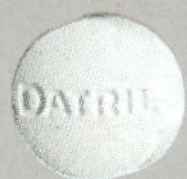
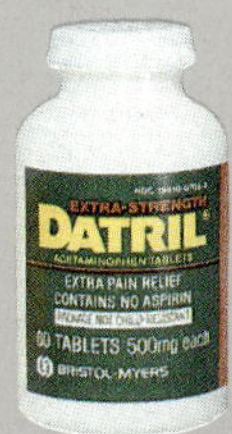

Bottles of 30, 60 and 100 tablets and vials of 10

EXTRA STRENGTH DATRIL® TABLETS
(acetaminophen)

Bristol-Myers Products

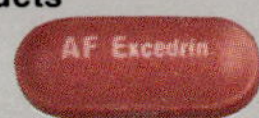

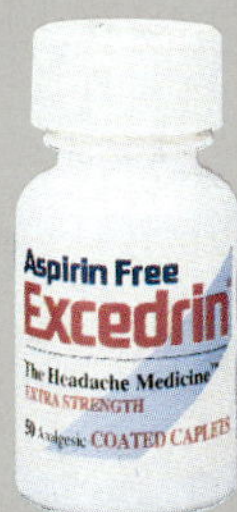

Bottles of 24, 50 and 100

ASPIRIN FREE EXCEDRIN® CAPLETS
(acetaminophen/caffeine)

Bristol-Myers Products

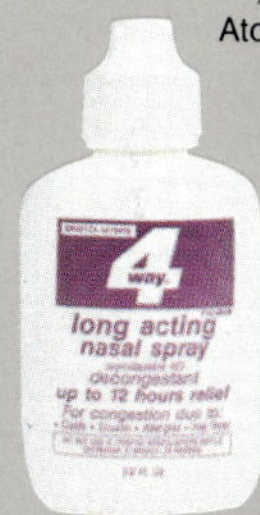

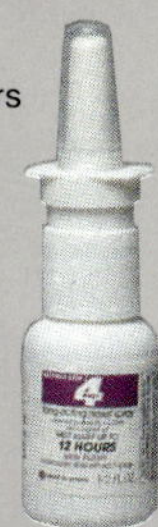

½ oz. Atomizers

Available in ½ oz. metered spray pump

4-WAY® LONG ACTING NASAL SPRAY
(oxymetazoline hydrochloride 0.05%)

Bristol-Myers Products

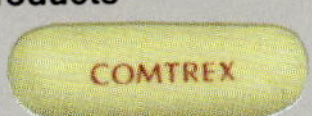

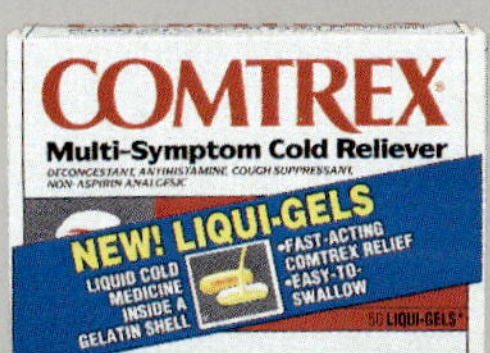

Blister packs of 24 and 50

COMTREX® LIQUI-GELS

Bristol-Myers Products

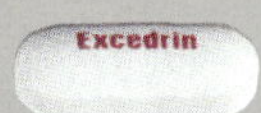

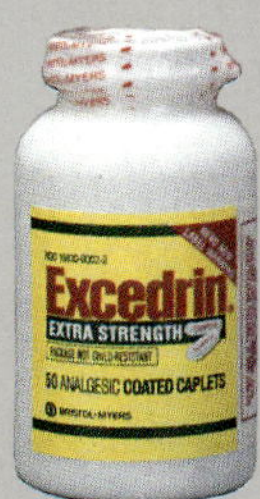

Bottles of 24, 50 and 100

EXCEDRIN® CAPLETS
Aspirin/Acetaminophen/Caffeine

Bristol-Myers Products

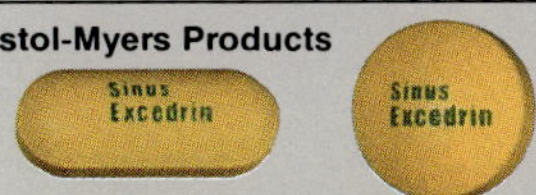

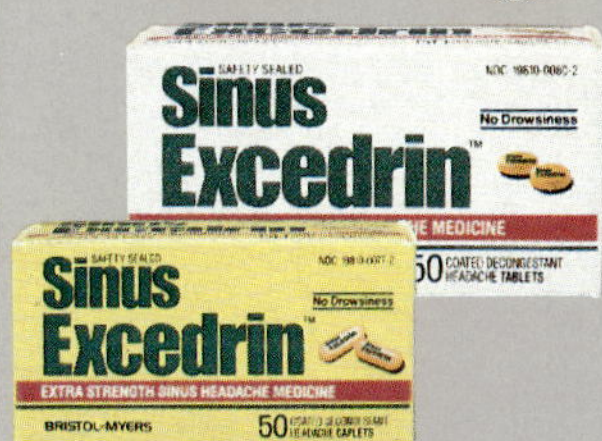

Available in blister packs of 24 and bottles of 50 caplets and tablets

SINUS EXCEDRIN® CAPLETS & TABLETS
(acetaminophen, pseudoephedrine)

Bristol-Myers Products

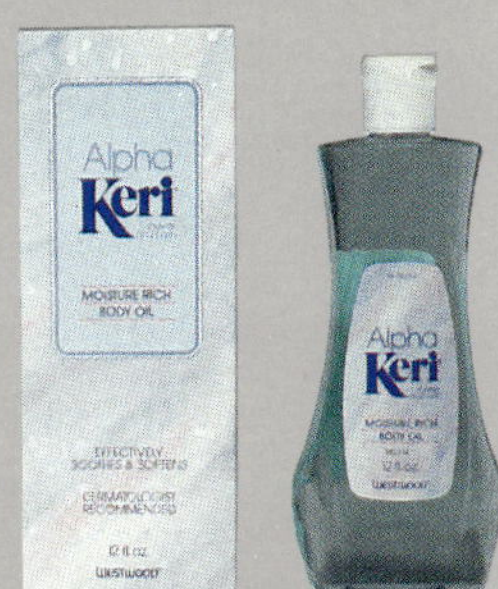

4, 8, 12 and 16 oz.

ALPHA KERI® Shower and Bath Products

Bristol-Myers Products

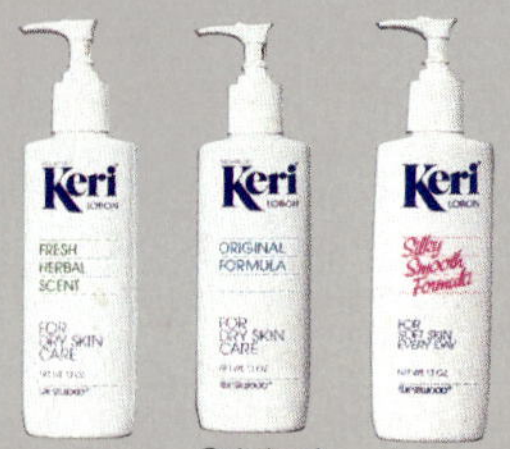

Fresh Herbal Scent
Original Formula
Silky Smooth Formula

6.5, 13 and 20 oz.

KERI® LOTION
For Dry Skin Care

Bristol-Myers Products

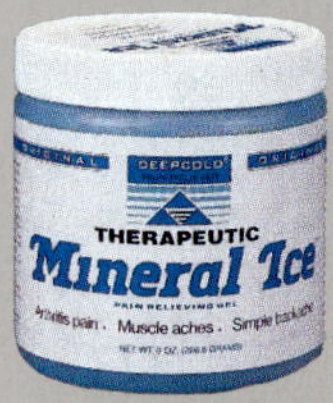

Available in:
3.5 oz., 8 oz. and 16 oz.

THERAPEUTIC
MINERAL ICE™
Pain Relieving Gel

Burroughs Wellcome

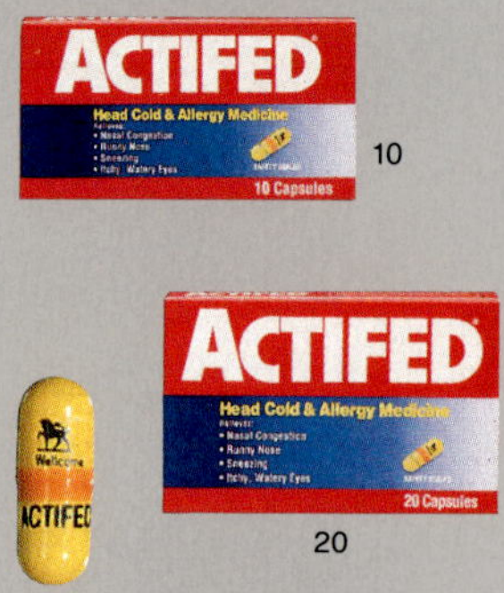

10

20

ACTIFED® CAPSULES

Burroughs Wellcome

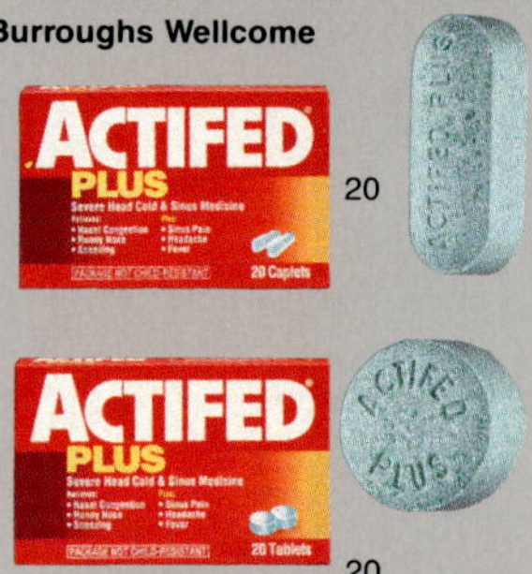

20

20

Also available in 40s

ACTIFED® PLUS
CAPLETS & TABLETS

Bristol-Myers Products

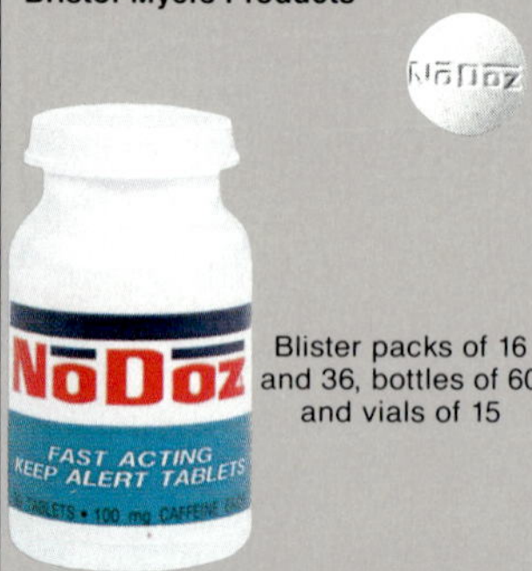

Blister packs of 16 and 36, bottles of 60 and vials of 15

NO-DOZ® TABLETS
(caffeine)

Bristol-Myers Products

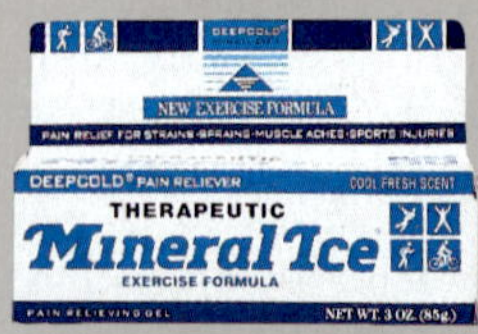

Tubes of 3.5 oz.

THERAPEUTIC
MINERAL ICE®
EXERCISE FORMULA

Pain Relieving Gel

Burroughs Wellcome

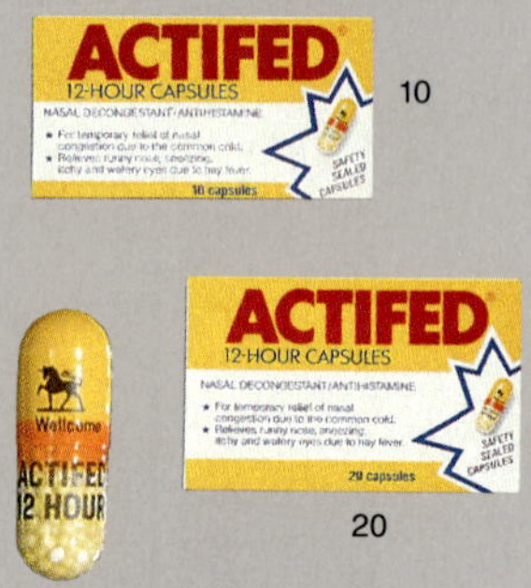

10

20

ACTIFED® 12-HOUR CAPSULES

Burroughs Wellcome

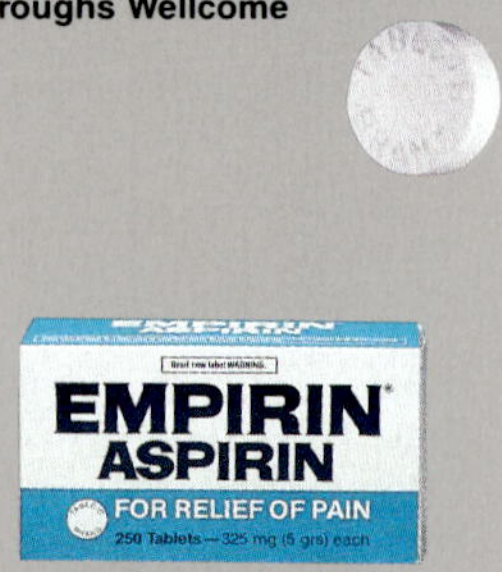

250

Also available in 50s and 100s

EMPIRIN® ASPIRIN TABLETS

Bristol-Myers Products

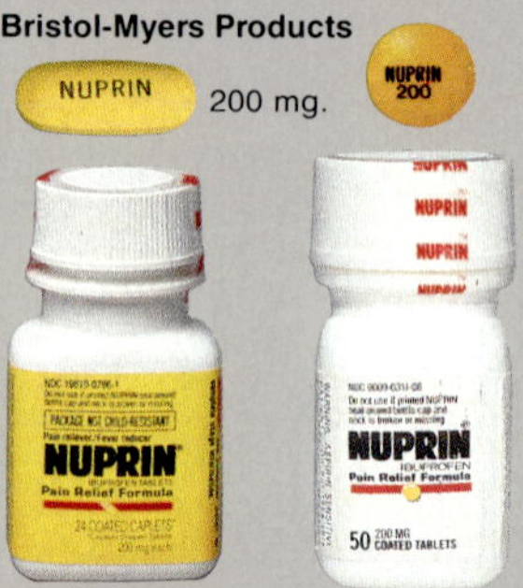

200 mg.

Bottles of 24, 50 and 100 caplets

Bottles of 24, 50, 100, 150 and 225 and vials of 10

NUPRIN® CAPLET & TABLET
(ibuprofen)

Bristol-Myers Products

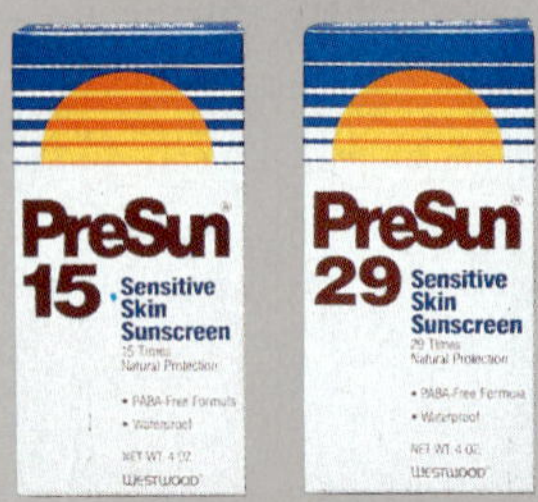

Sensitive Skin Sunscreen 15

Sensitive Skin Sunscreen 29

4 oz.

PRESUN®
Creamy, Lotion, Facial, Sensitive Skin and Stick Formulas

Burroughs Wellcome

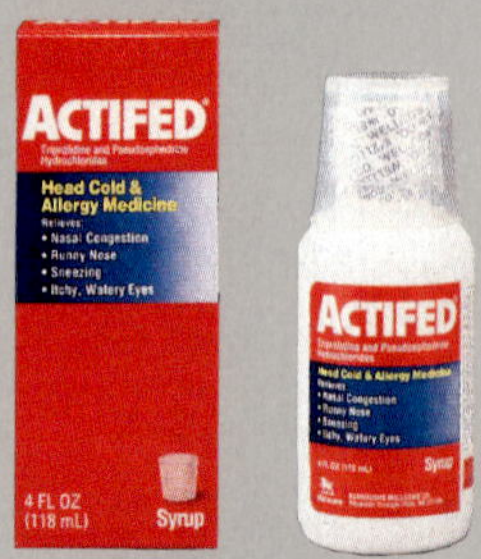

4 fl. oz.

Also available in pints

ACTIFED® SYRUP

Burroughs Wellcome

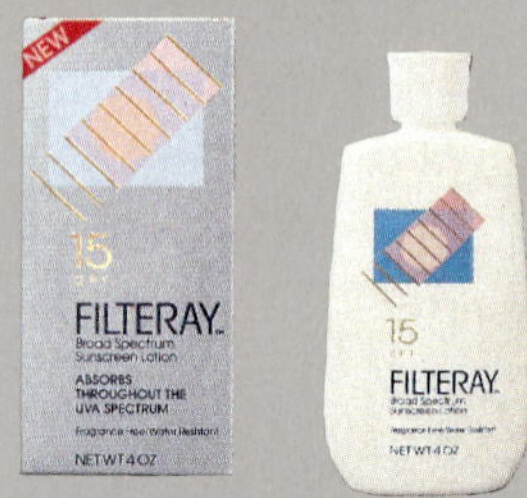

4 oz.

FILTERAY®
BROAD SPECTRUM
SUNSCREEN LOTION

Bristol-Myers Products

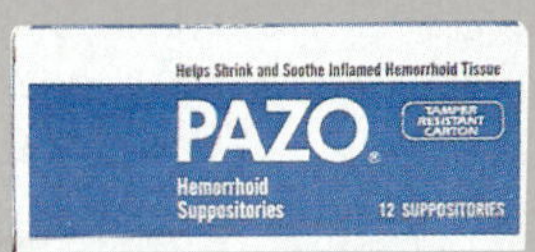

Boxes of 12 and 24 suppositories

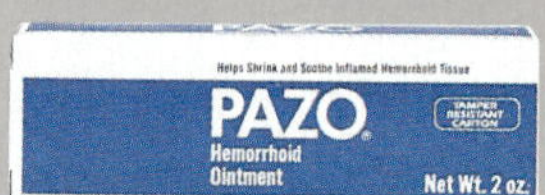

Tubes of 1 and 2 oz.

PAZO®
Hemorrhoid Ointment and Suppositories

BURROUGHS WELLCOME

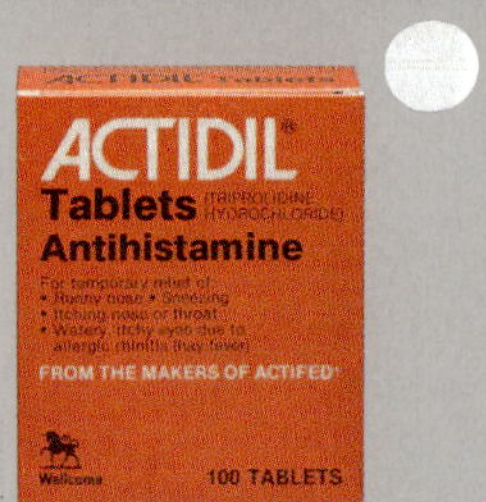

100
Syrup available in pints

ACTIDIL®
TABLETS & SYRUP

Burroughs Wellcome

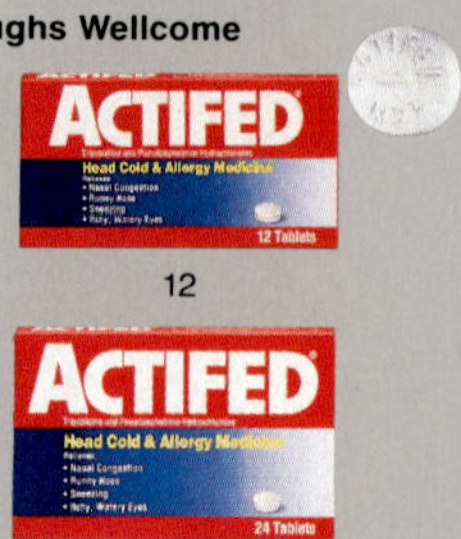

12

24

Also available in 48s and in bottles of 100

ACTIFED®
TABLETS

Burroughs Wellcome

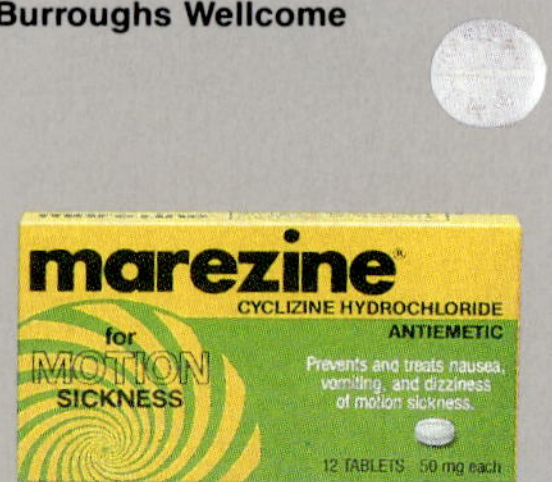

12

Also available in 100s

MAREZINE® TABLETS

Burroughs Wellcome

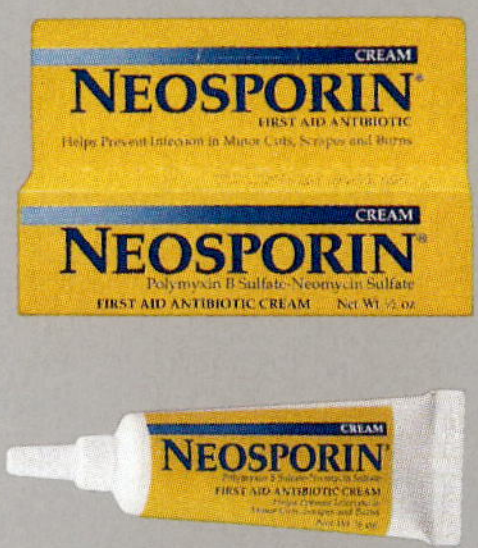

Available in ½ oz. tubes

NEOSPORIN® FIRST AID ANTIBIOTIC CREAM

Burroughs Wellcome

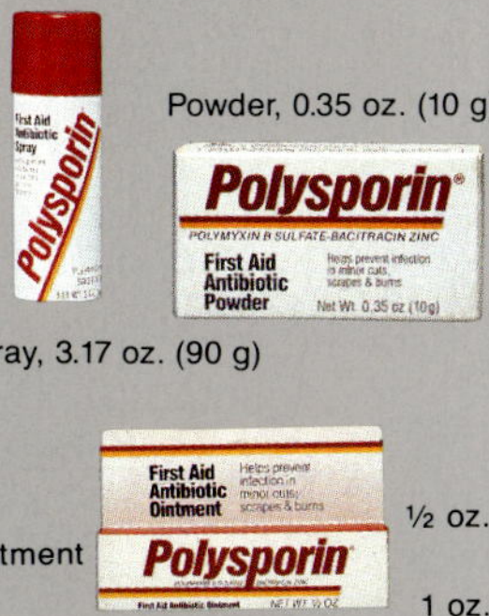

Powder, 0.35 oz. (10 g)

Spray, 3.17 oz. (90 g)

Ointment ½ oz. 1 oz.

POLYSPORIN® FIRST AID ANTIBIOTIC SPRAY, POWDER & OINTMENT

Burroughs Wellcome

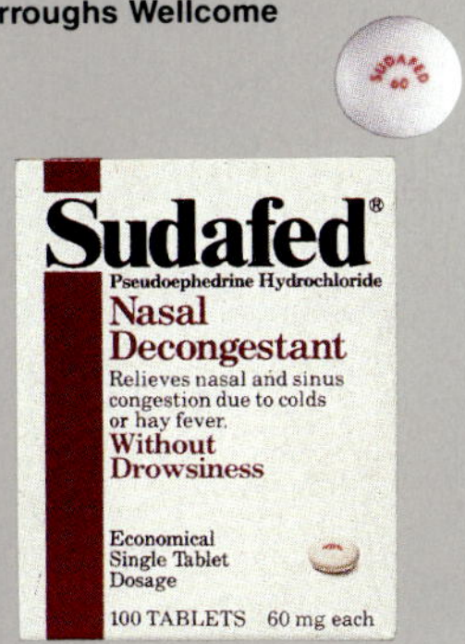

100

SUDAFED® 60 mg TABLETS

CIBA CONSUMER

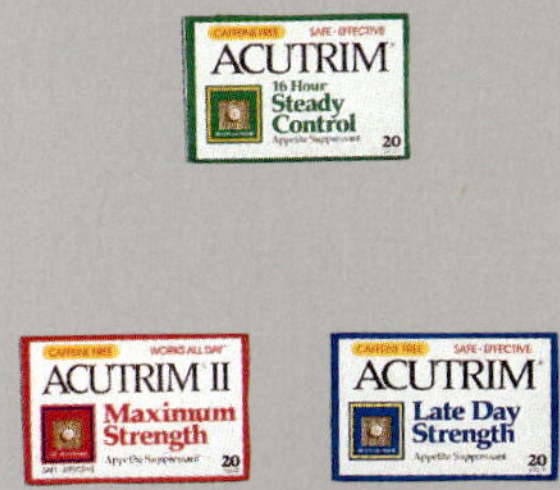

ACUTRIM® Appetite Suppressants

Caffeine Free/Works All Day

Burroughs Wellcome

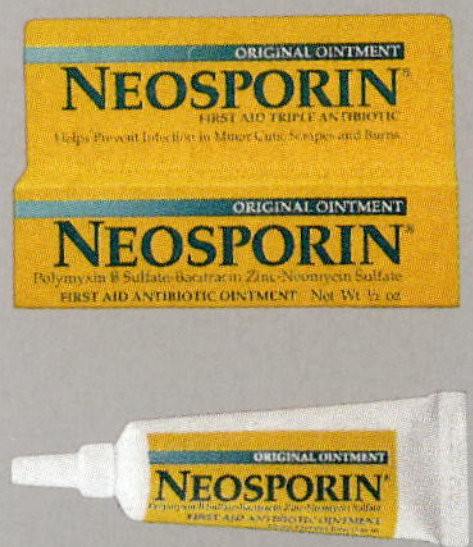

Available in ½ and 1 oz. tubes

NEOSPORIN® FIRST AID ANTIBIOTIC OINTMENT

Burroughs Wellcome

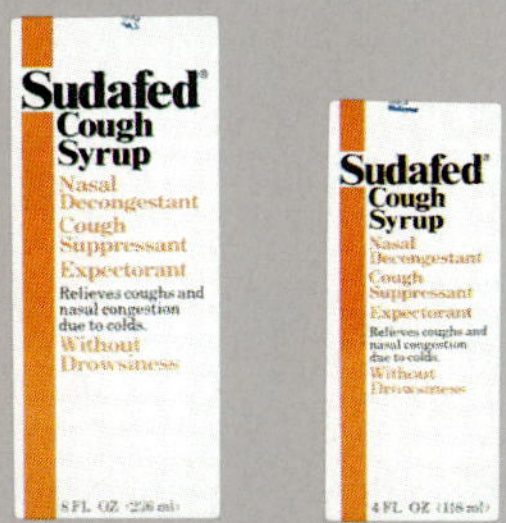

8 fl. oz. 4 fl. oz.

SUDAFED® COUGH SYRUP

Burroughs Wellcome

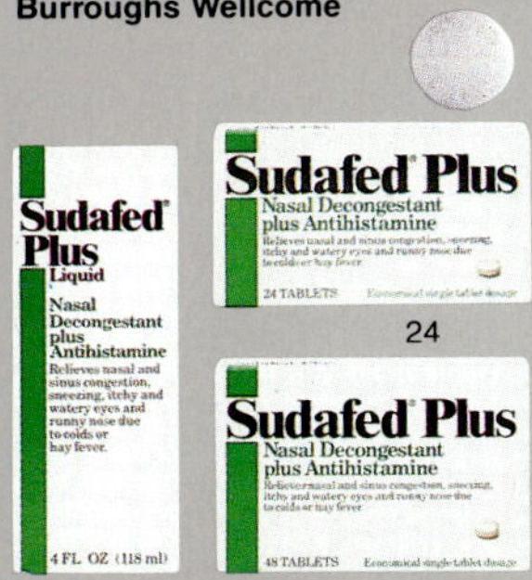

24

4 fl. oz. 48

SUDAFED® PLUS LIQUID & TABLETS

Ciba Consumer

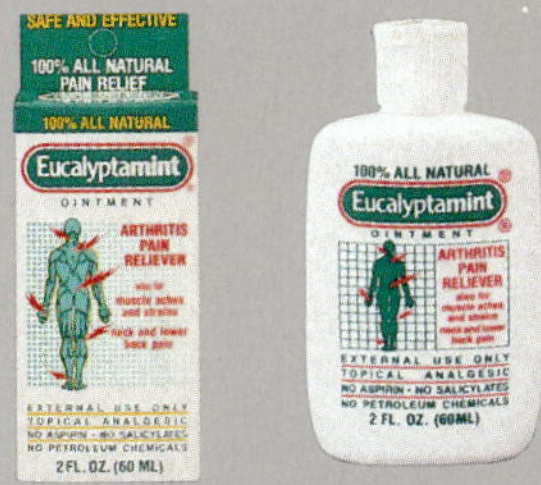

Available in 2 oz & 4 oz bottles

EUCALYPTAMINT® 100% All Natural External Analgesic Ointment

Burroughs Wellcome

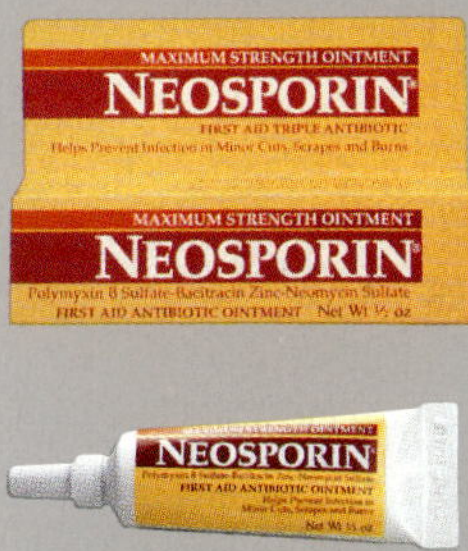

Available in ½ oz. tubes

MAXIMUM STRENGTH NEOSPORIN® FIRST AID ANTIBIOTIC OINTMENT

Burroughs Wellcome

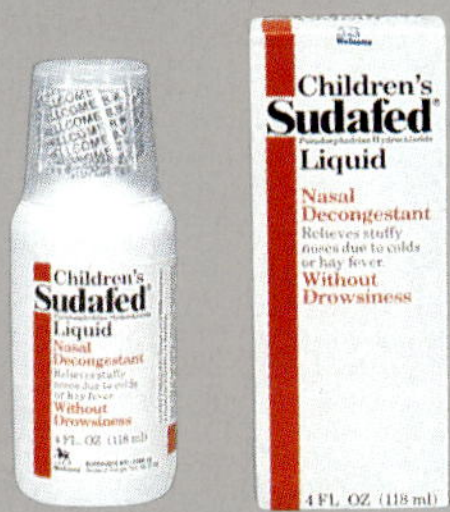

4 fl. oz.

CHILDREN'S SUDAFED® LIQUID

Burroughs Wellcome

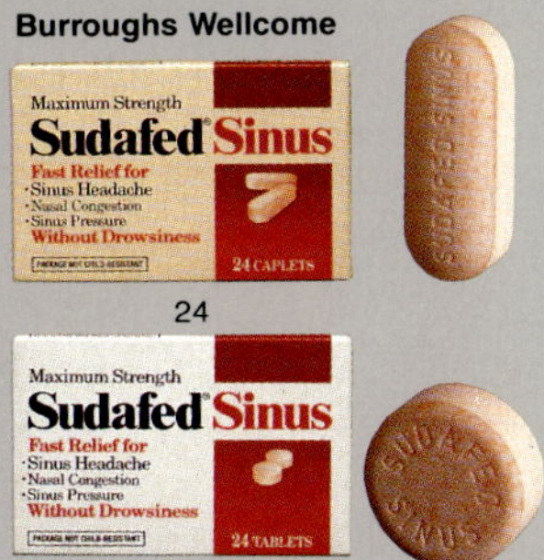

24

24

Also available in 48s

SUDAFED® SINUS CAPLETS & TABLETS

CIBA Consumer

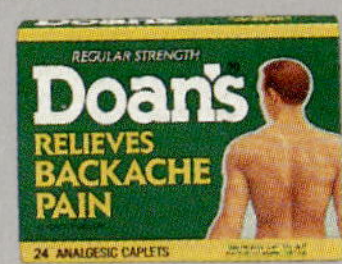

REGULAR STRENGTH DOAN'S®

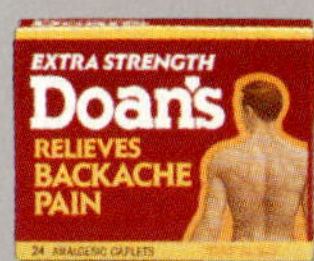

EXTRA STRENGTH DOAN'S®

DOAN'S® Backache Analgesic Relieves back pain

Available in packages of 24 & 48

Burroughs Wellcome

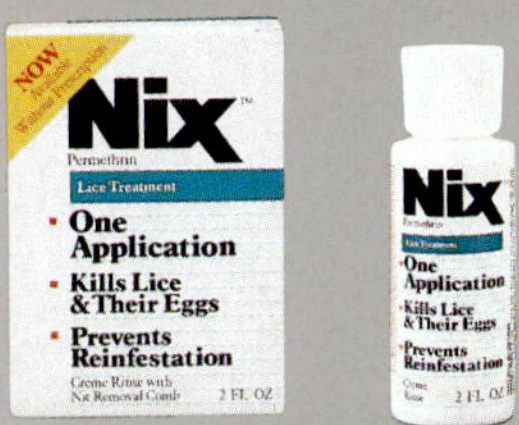

2 fl. oz.

Also available: 2-bottle family pack

NIX™ LICE TREATMENT CREME RINSE

Burroughs Wellcome

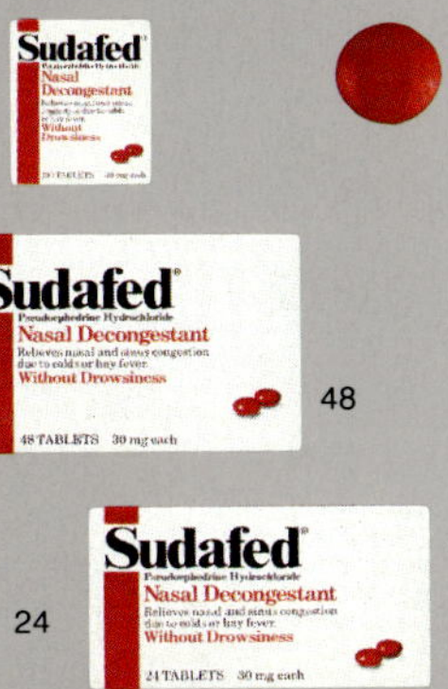

100

48

24

SUDAFED® 30 mg TABLETS

Burroughs Wellcome

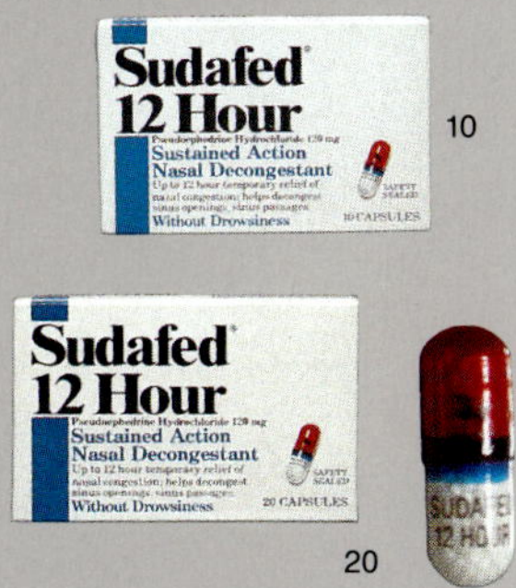

10

20

Also available in 40s

SUDAFED® 12 HOUR CAPSULES

CIBA Consumer

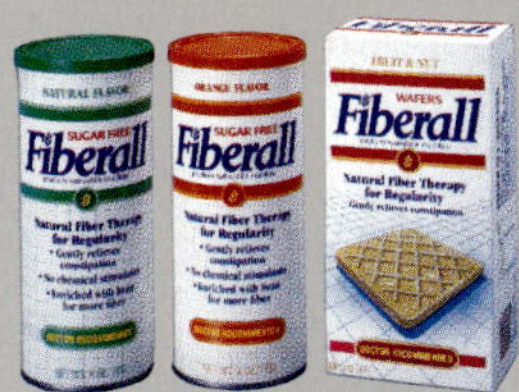

FIBERALL Natural Fiber Therapy for Regularity

Available in:
Powders: 10 and 15 oz. Natural, Orange
Wafers: 14 Fruit & Nut, Oatmeal Raisin
Tablets: 18

CIBA Consumer

Available in 2 oz and 1 oz tubes

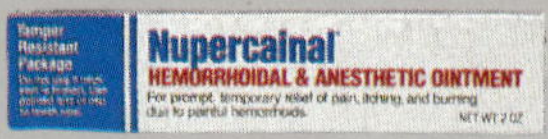

Prompt, temporary relief of pain, itching, and burning due to hemorrhoids.

NUPERCAINAL®
Hemorrhoidal & Anesthetic Ointment

CIBA Consumer

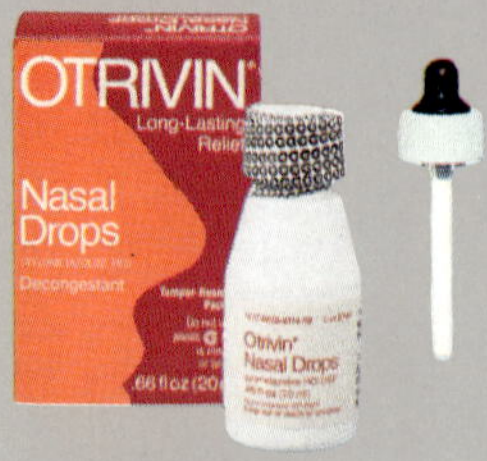

.66 fl oz

OTRIVIN®
Nasal Decongestant Drops

CIBA Consumer

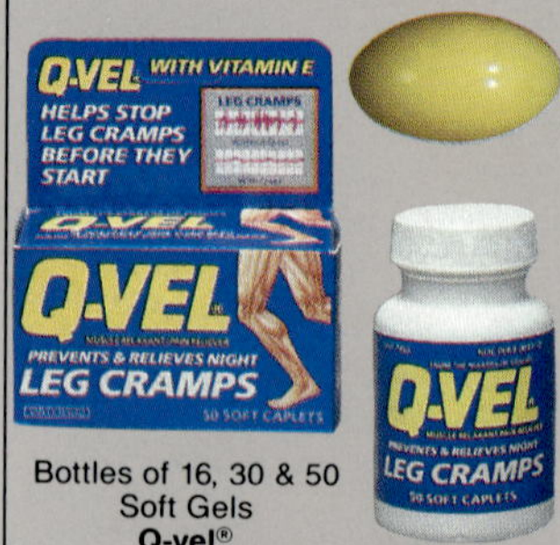

Bottles of 16, 30 & 50 Soft Gels
Q-vel®
Muscle Relaxant
Pain Reliever

CIBA Consumer

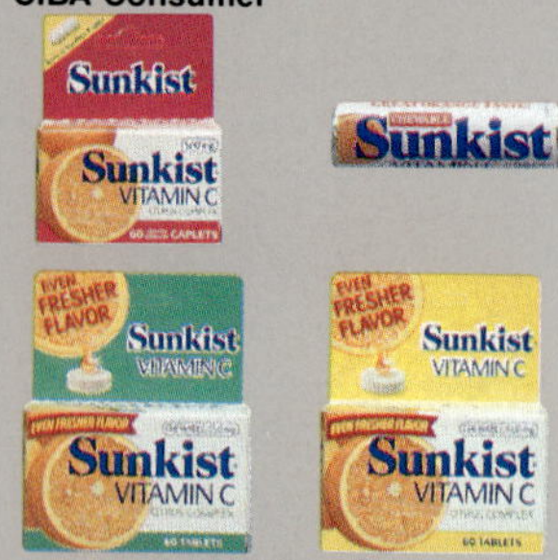

SUNKIST®
Vitamin C Citrus Complex
250 & 500 mg chewable tablets;
500 mg easy to swallow caplets;
60 mg chewable tablets
(11-tablet roll)

CIBA Consumer

Available in boxes of 12 and 24 suppositories

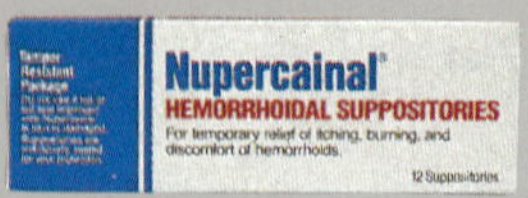

Temporary relief of itching, burning, and discomfort of hemorrhoids.

NUPERCAINAL®
Hemorrhoidal Suppositories

CIBA Consumer

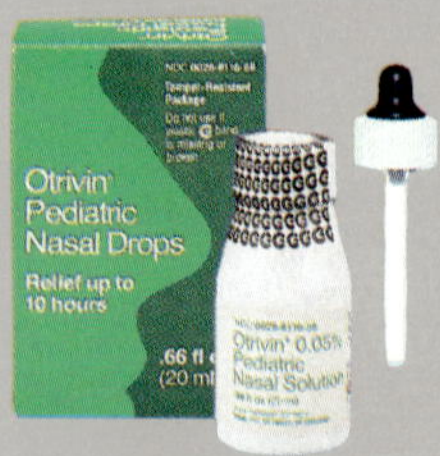

.66 fl oz

OTRIVIN®
Pediatric
Nasal Decongestant Drops

CIBA Consumer

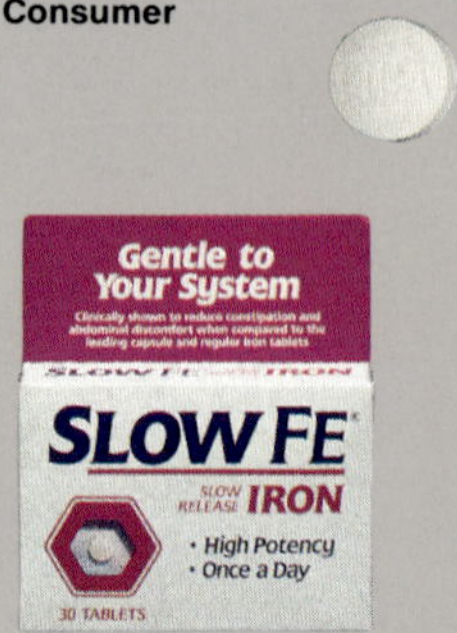

Available in packages of 30, 60 & 100 tablets
SLOW FE®
Slow Release Iron

COLGATE-PALMOLIVE

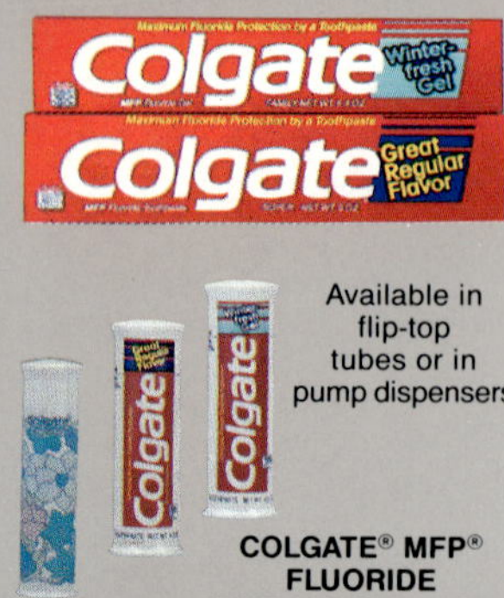

Available in flip-top tubes or in pump dispensers

COLGATE® MFP®
FLUORIDE
TOOTHPASTE & GEL

CIBA Consumer

1½ oz

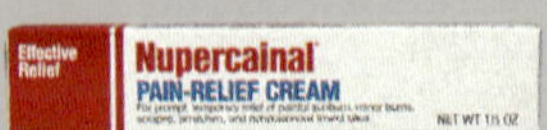

Prompt, temporary relief of painful sunburn, minor burns, scrapes, scratches, and nonpoisonous insect bites.

NUPERCAINAL®
Pain-Relief Cream

CIBA Consumer

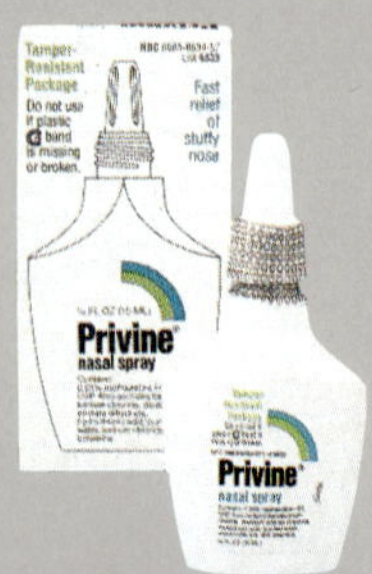

½ fl oz

PRIVINE®
Nasal Decongestant Spray

CIBA Consumer

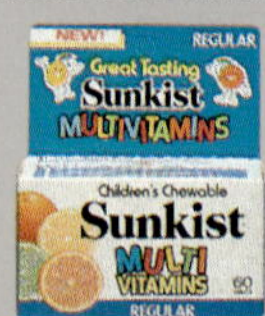

Regular

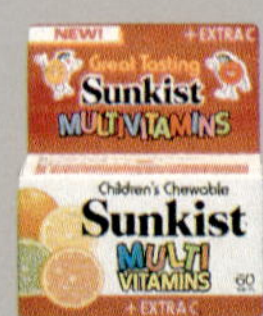

+Extra C

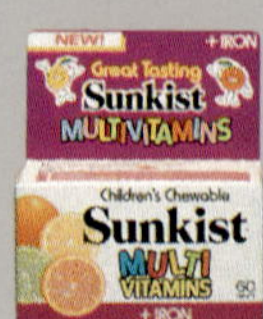

+Iron

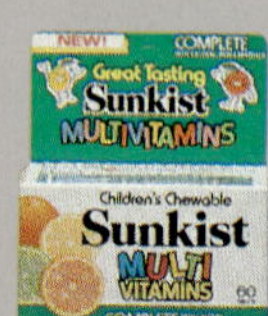

Complete

SUNKIST®
Children's Multivitamins

Colgate-Palmolive

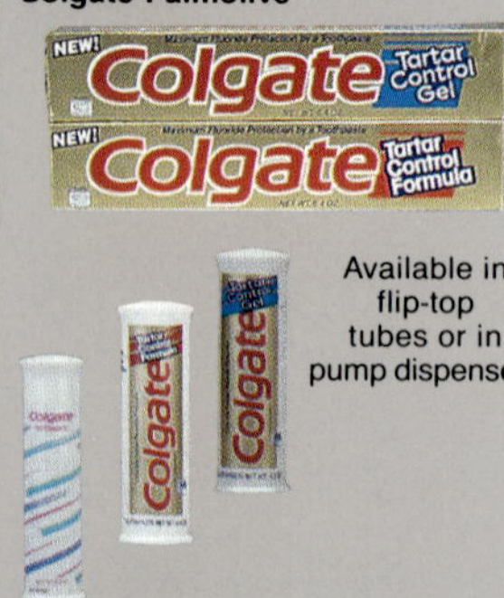

Available in flip-top tubes or in pump dispensers

COLGATE®
TARTAR CONTROL
FORMULA & GEL

CIBA Consumer

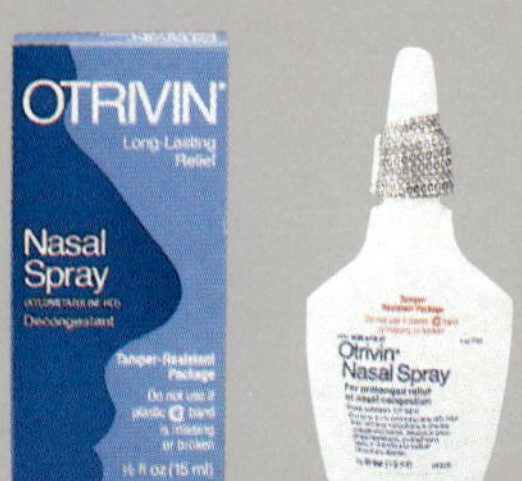

½ fl oz

OTRIVIN®
Nasal Decongestant Spray

CIBA Consumer

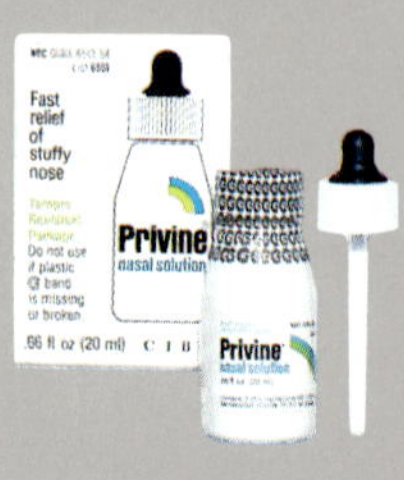

.66 fl oz

PRIVINE®
Nasal Decongestant Solution

Colgate-Palmolive

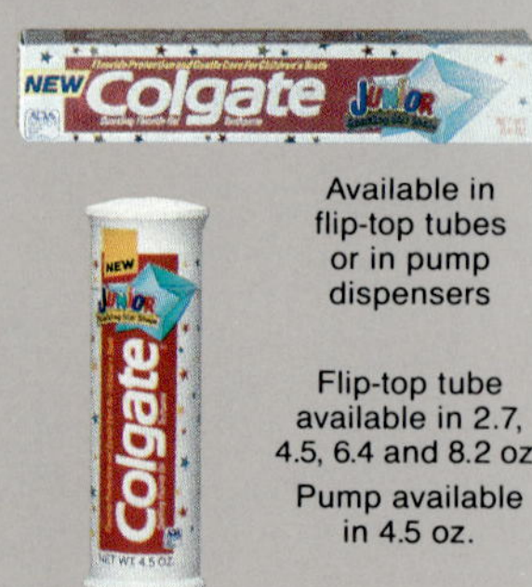

Available in flip-top tubes or in pump dispensers

Flip-top tube available in 2.7, 4.5, 6.4 and 8.2 oz.

Pump available in 4.5 oz.

COLGATE® JUNIOR
Fluoride Gel Toothpaste

Colgate-Palmolive

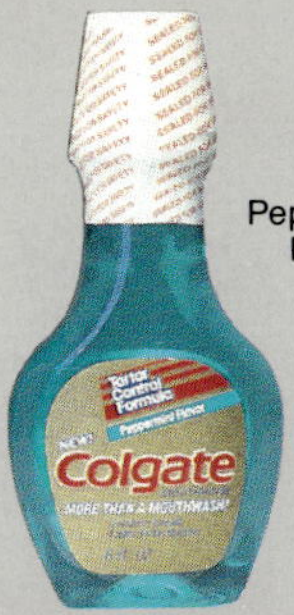

Peppermint Flavor

COLGATE® MOUTHWASH
Tartar Control Formula

Columbia

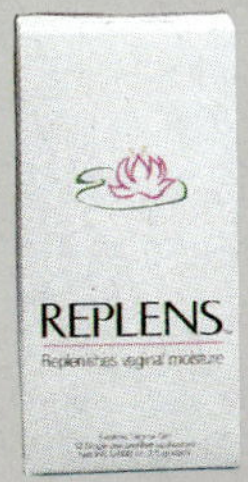

Available in Boxes of 3 and 12 Single-Use Applicators

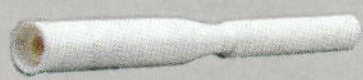

REPLENS®
Vaginal Moisturizer

Combe

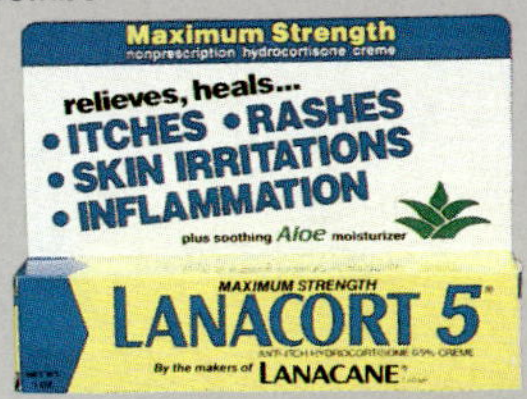

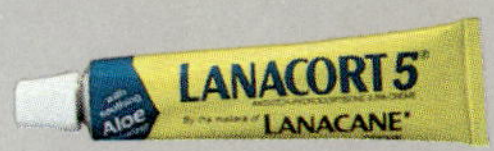

½ or 1 oz. creme—½ oz. ointment

LANACORT 5®
Anti-Itch Hydrocortisone 0.5%
Creme or Ointment

FISONS

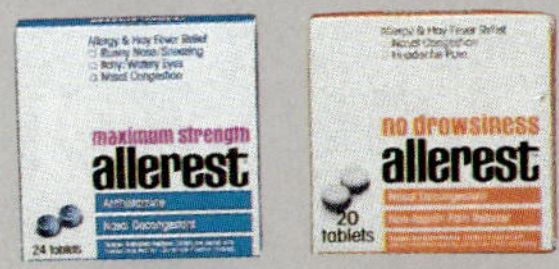

24 tablets
MAXIMUM STRENGTH ALLEREST® TABLETS

20 tablets
NO DROWSINESS ALLEREST® TABLETS

Allergy & Hay Fever Relief

Colgate-Palmolive

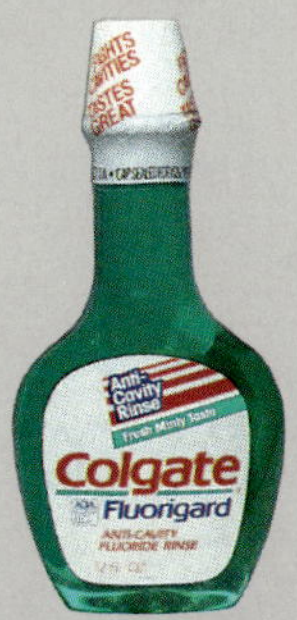

FLUORIGARD™
Anti-Cavity Fluoride Rinse

COMBE

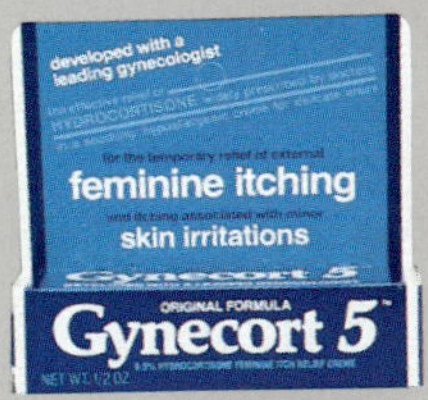

½ oz.

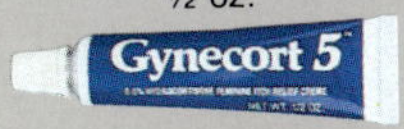

GYNECORT 5™
(0.5% Hydrocortisone)
Feminine Itch Relief Creme

Combe

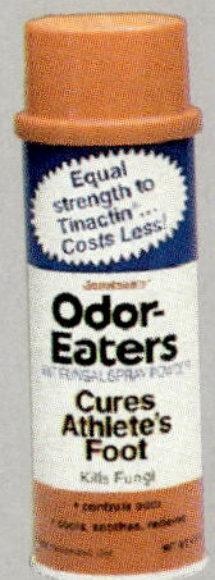

Available in 3 oz. Container

ODOR-EATERS
Antifungal Spray Powder
Cures Athlete's Foot

Fisons

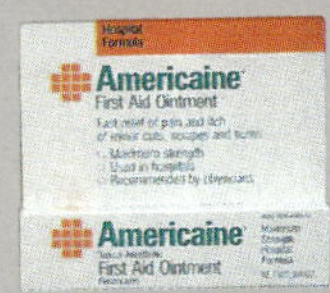

Ointment
¾ oz.

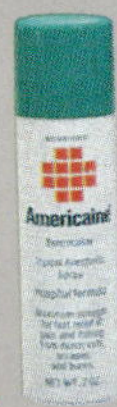

Spray
2 oz.

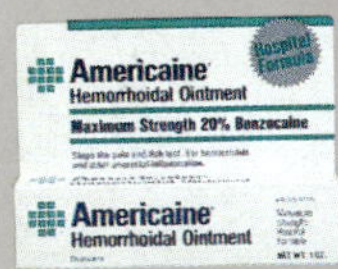

Hemorrhoidal Ointment
1 oz.

AMERICAINE®
(benzocaine)

COLUMBIA

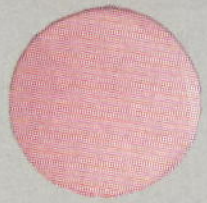

Tablets

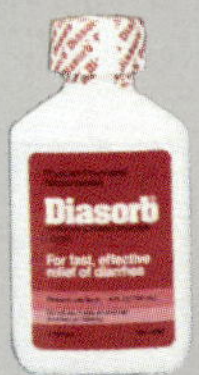

Liquid

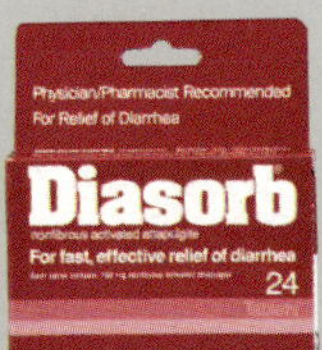

DIASORB®
Nonfibrous Activated Attapulgite
ANTI-DIARRHEAL

Combe

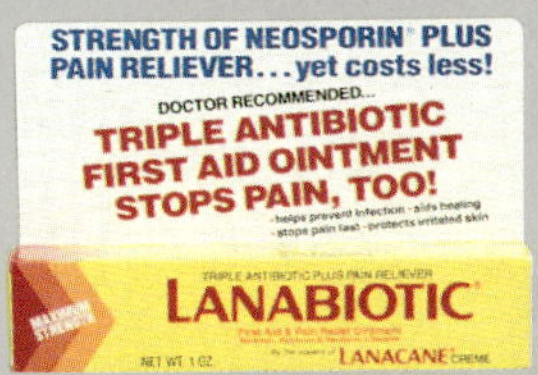

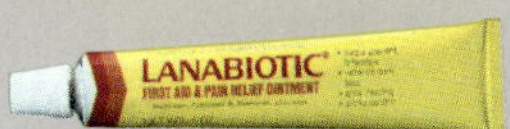

½ oz. or 1 oz. Tubes

LANABIOTIC® Ointment
Triple Antibiotic Plus
Pain Reliever
First Aid Ointment

Combe

VAGISIL®
FEMININE POWDER
Available in
7 oz. or 11 oz.
Container

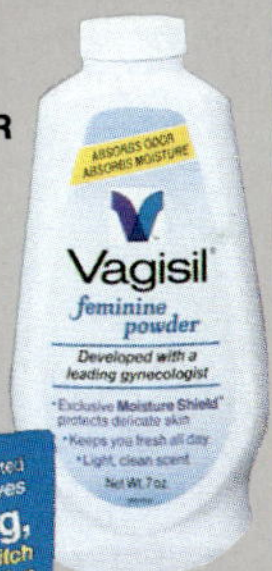

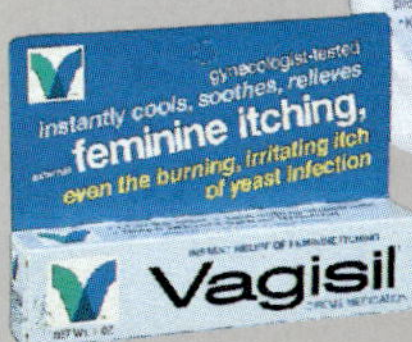

VAGISIL® CREME MEDICATION
Available in 1 oz. or 2 oz. Tubes

Fisons

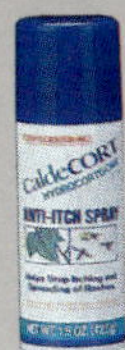

1.5 oz.

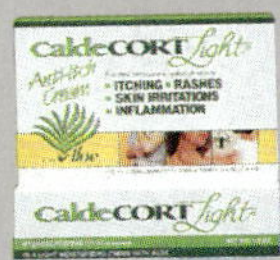

½ oz.

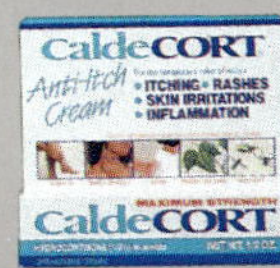

½ oz.

CaldeCORT Light™
CaldeCORT® CREAM and SPRAY
(hydrocortisone acetate, 0.5%)

Columbia

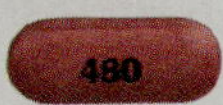

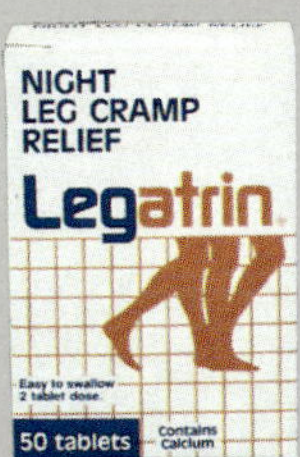

Available in Packages of 30 and 50 Tablets

LEGATRIN®
Night leg cramp relief

Combe

LANACANE®
SPRAY MEDICATION
Available in
4 oz. Container

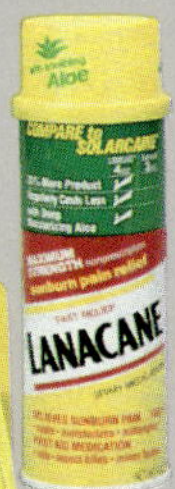

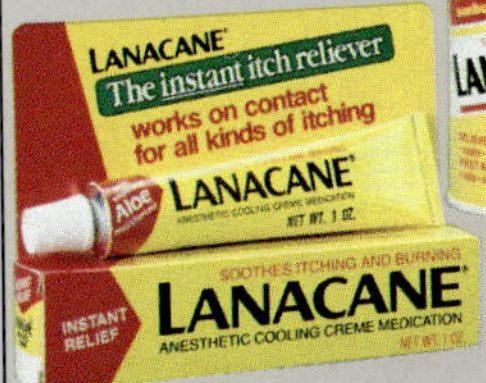

LANACANE®
MEDICATED CREME
Available in 1 oz.
and 2 oz. Tubes

Copley Pharmaceutical

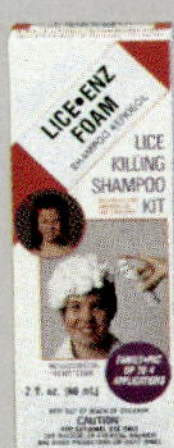

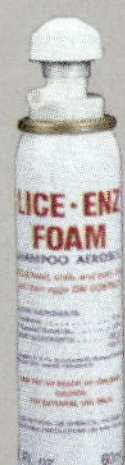

LICE • ENZ FOAM
Pediculicide Mousse
Easy to use—child friendly

Fisons

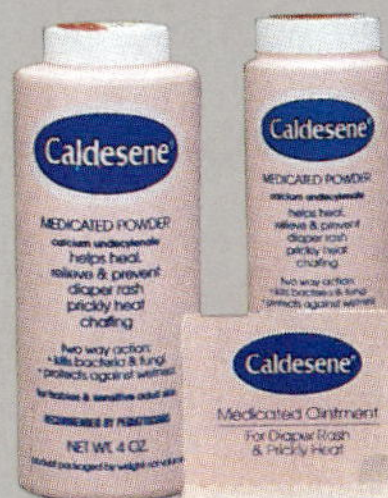

2 oz.

4 oz.

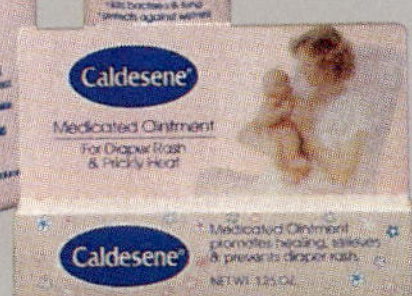

1.25 oz.

CALDESENE®
MEDICATED POWDER and OINTMENT

Fisons

Spray Powder

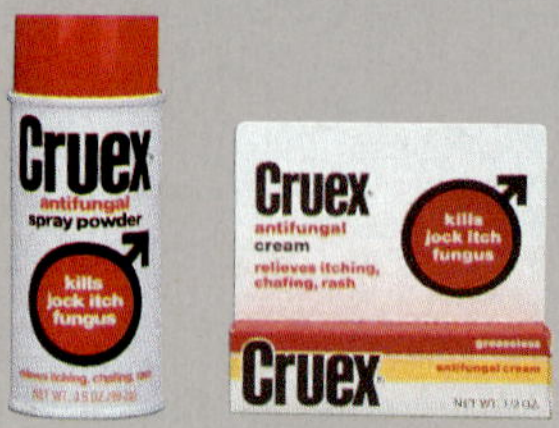

Cream

CRUEX®
Antifungal Spray Powder & Cream
Relieves Itching, Chafing, Rash

Fisons

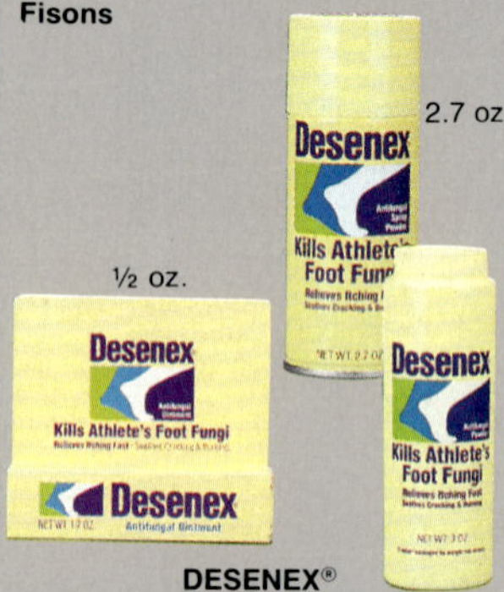

2.7 oz.

½ oz.

DESENEX®
Spray Powder, Powder, Cream & Ointment
Relieves Symptoms of Athlete's Foot

Fisons

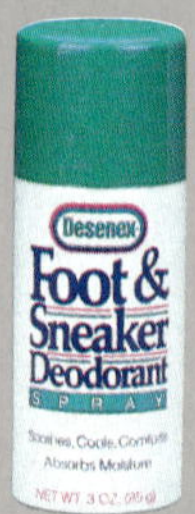

3 oz.

DESENEX®
FOOT & SNEAKER DEODORANT
Soothes, Cools, Comforts & Absorbs Moisture

Fisons

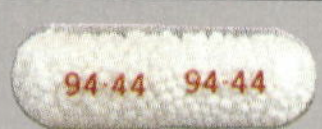

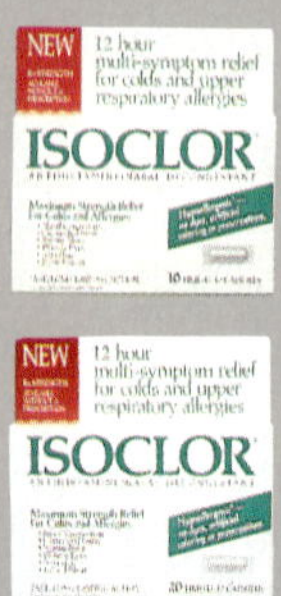

10's

20's

ISOCLOR® TIMESULE® CAPSULES
Nasal Decongestant/Antihistamine

Fisons

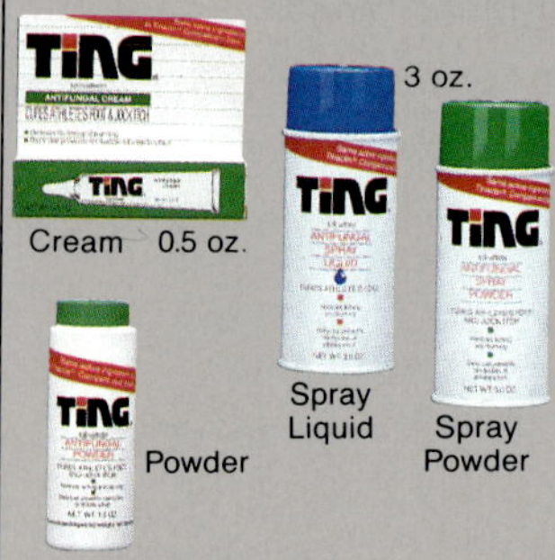

3 oz.

Cream 0.5 oz.

Powder

Spray Liquid

Spray Powder

TING®
For Athlete's Foot & Jock Itch

FLEXAID

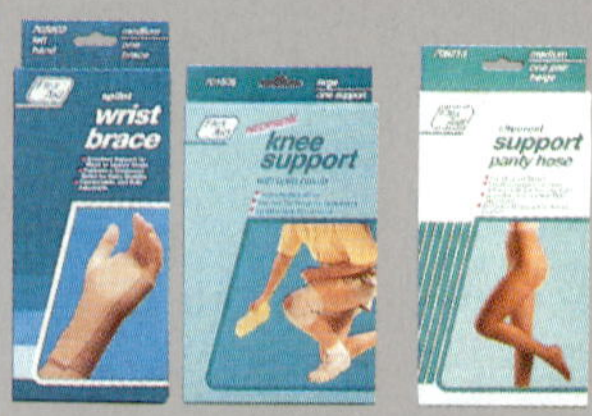

FLEXAID™

Elastic and Neoprene Supports, Braces and Hosiery

G & W LABORATORIES

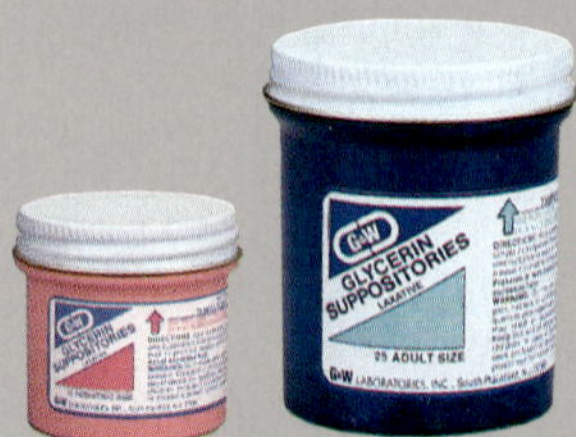

Jars of 12 & 25

Jars of 12, 25, 50 & 100

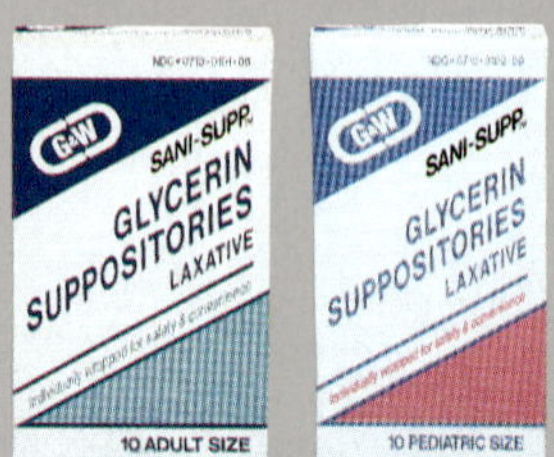

Adult Boxes of Foil Wrapped 10, 25, 50

Pediatric Boxes of Foil Wrapped 10, 25

GLYCERIN SUPPOSITORIES
Laxative

GLENBROOK

Division of Sterling Drug Inc.

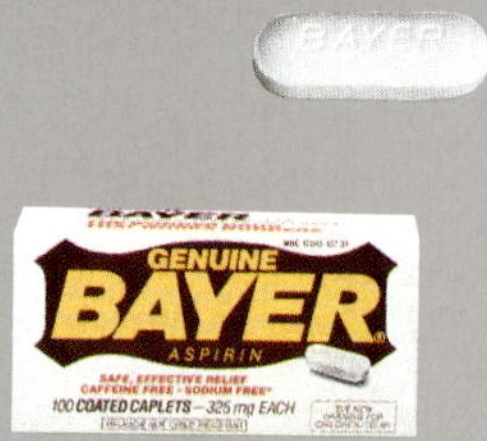

Caplets available in bottles of 50, 100 and 200

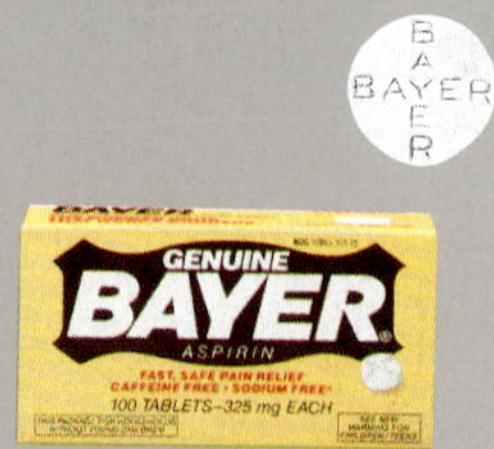

Available in packs of 12 tablets and bottles of 24, 50, 100, 200, 300 and 365

GENUINE BAYER® ASPIRIN
Toleraid® Micro-Thin Coating
Sodium Free • Caffeine Free

Glenbrook

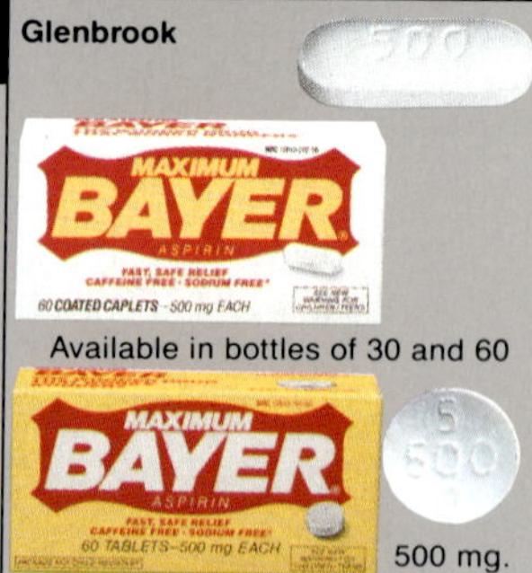

Available in bottles of 30 and 60

500 mg.

Available in boxes of 30, 60 and 100 tablets

MAXIMUM BAYER® ASPIRIN
Toleraid® Micro-Thin Coating
Sodium Free • Caffeine Free

Glenbrook

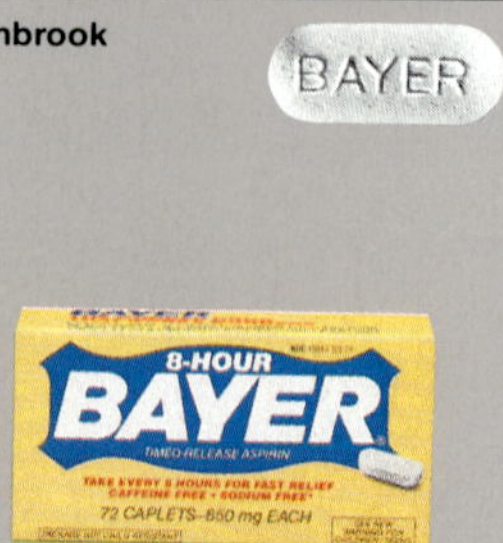

Available in bottles of 30, 72, and 125 caplets

8-HOUR BAYER®
TIMED-RELEASE ASPIRIN
Sodium Free • Caffeine Free

Glenbrook

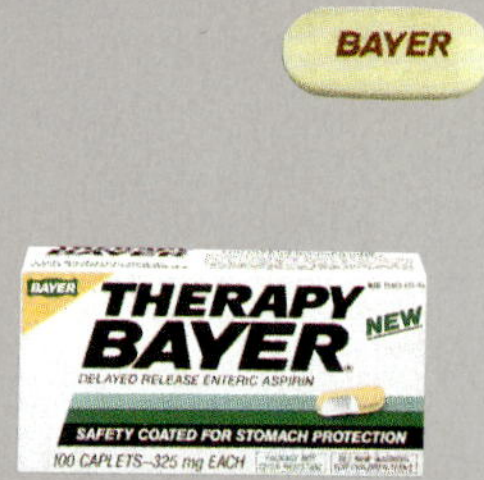

Available in bottles of 50 and 100 caplets

THERAPY BAYER®
Delayed Release Enteric Aspirin
Sodium Free • Caffeine Free

Glenbrook

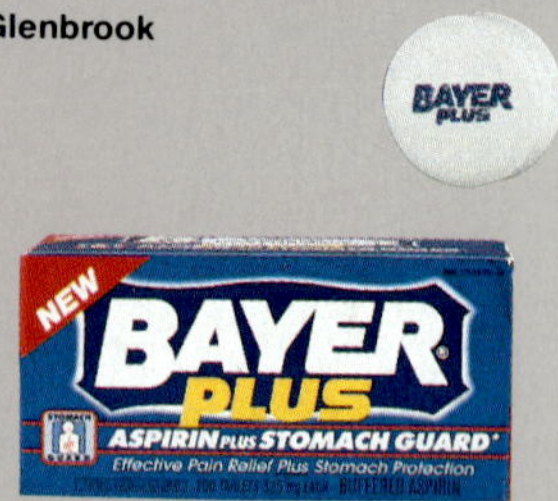

Available in bottles of 24, 50 and 100

BAYER® PLUS
Stomach Guard™
Effective Pain Relief Plus Stomach Protection. Coated For Easy Swallowing.

Glenbrook

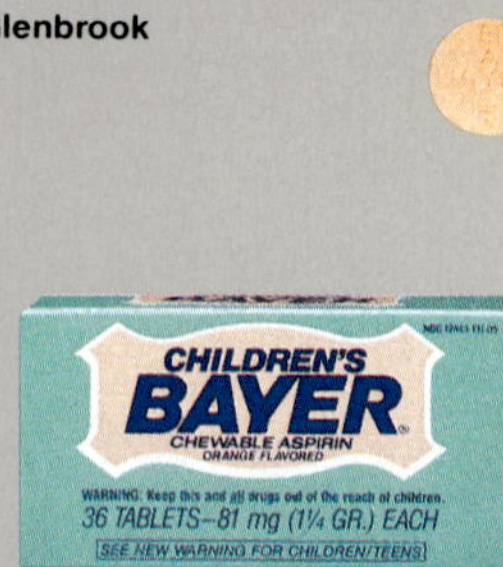

Available in bottle of 36 tablets

BAYER® CHILDREN'S CHEWABLE ASPIRIN

Glenbrook

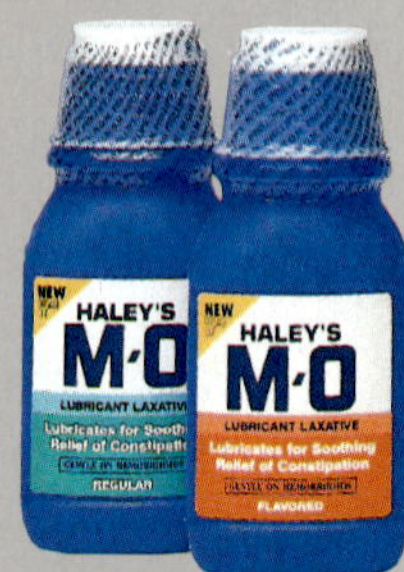

Available in regular and flavored 12 oz. and 26 oz. plastic bottles

HALEY'S M-O®

Glenbrook

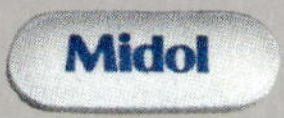

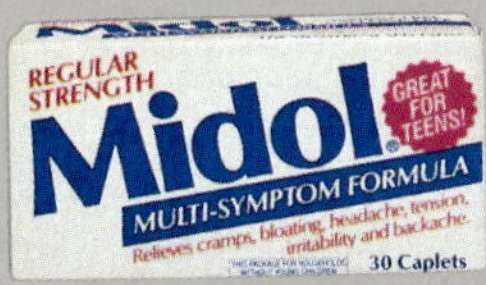

Available in packages of 12, 30 and 60 caplets®

MIDOL®

Glenbrook

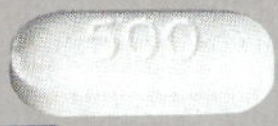

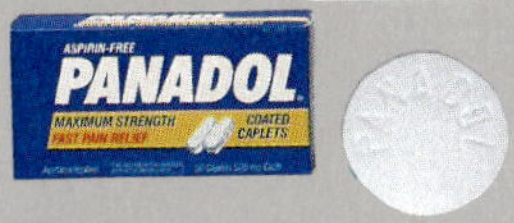

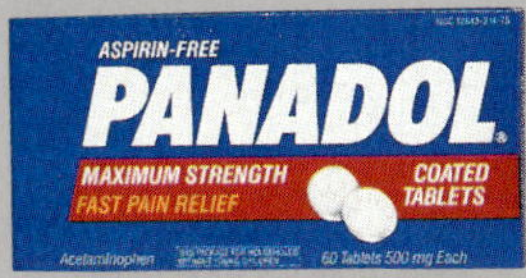

MAXIMUM STRENGTH PANADOL®
Coated Caplets and Tablets
Acetaminophen

Glenbrook

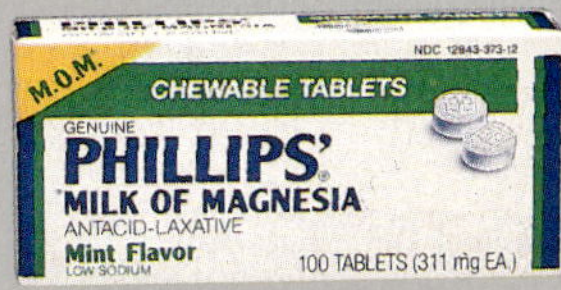

PHILLIPS'® MILK OF MAGNESIA TABLETS
Available in mint flavored chewable tablets in blister packed 24 and bottles of 100 and 200

ICN

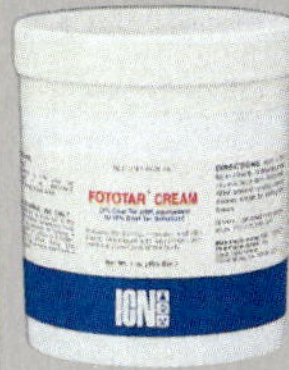

1 lb. jar

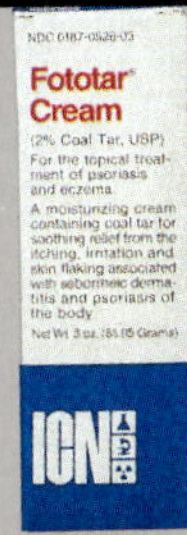

3 oz. tube

FOTOTAR® CREAM
(2% Coal Tar USP, equivalent to 10% Coal Tar Solution)

Glenbrook

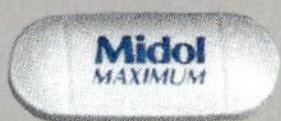

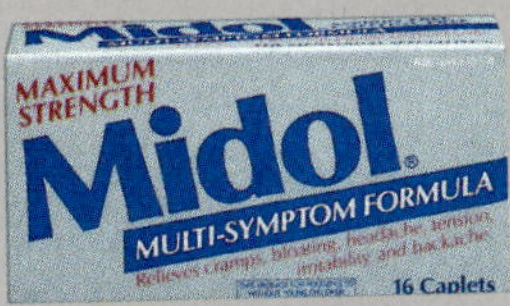

Available in packages of 8, 16 and 32 caplets®

MIDOL®
MAXIMUM STRENGTH

Glenbrook

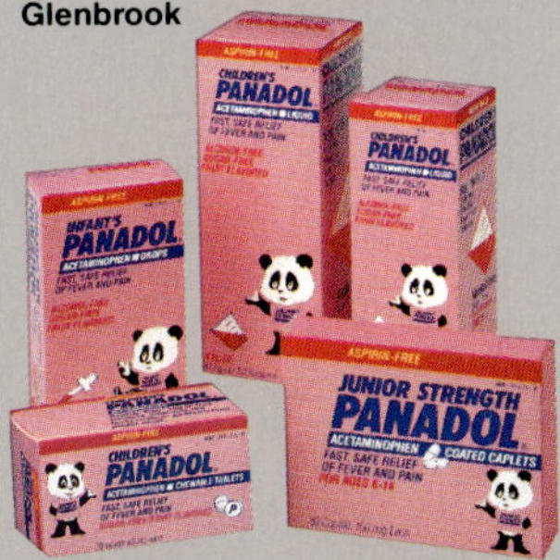

CHILDREN'S PANADOL®
Chewable Tablets, Caplets, Liquid and Drops
Acetaminophen

Glenbrook

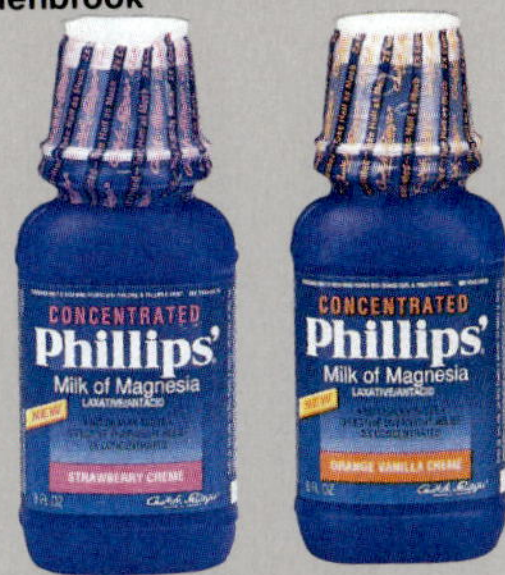

Available in Strawberry Creme and Orange Vanilla Creme 8 oz. plastic bottles

Concentrated
PHILLIPS'® MILK OF MAGNESIA

ICN

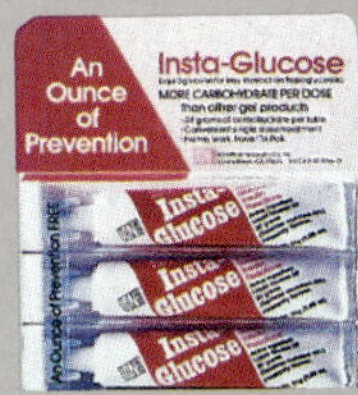

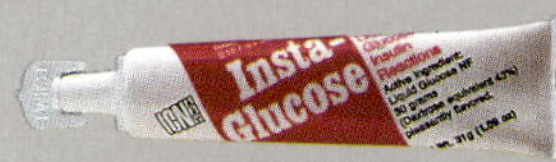

INSTA-GLUCOSE
For treatment of insulin reaction/hypoglycemia

Glenbrook

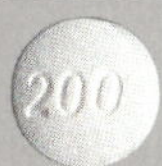

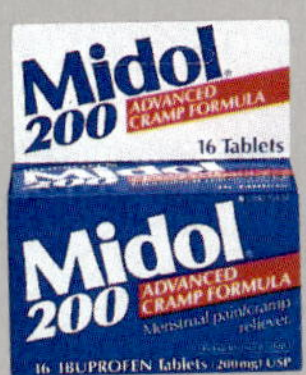

Available in packages of 16 and 32 coated tablets

MIDOL® 200

Glenbrook

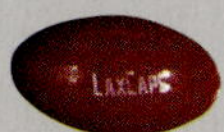

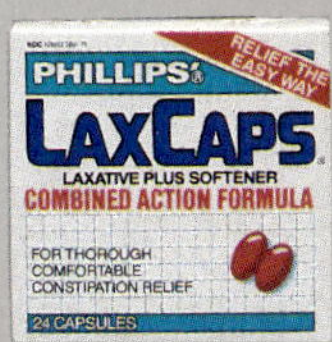

Available in 8 and 24 capsules

LAXCAPS®
Laxative Plus Softener
Combined Action Formula

Glenbrook

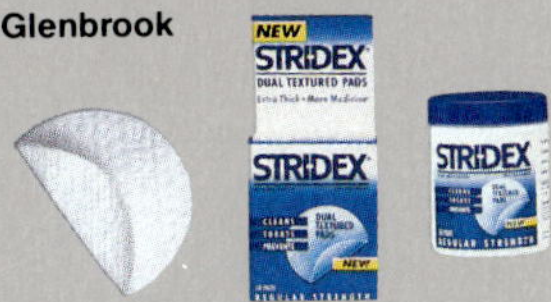

Regular Strength Pads

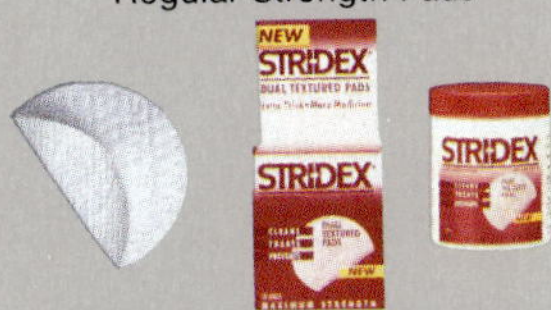

Maximum Strength Pads
New Dual Textured Pads in containers of 32 and 50 pads
STRI-DEX®

JOHNSON & JOHNSON

Consumer Products Inc.

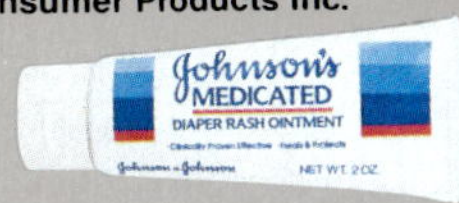

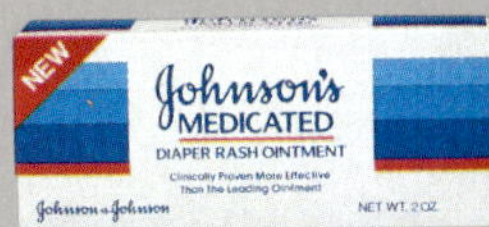

Available in 2 oz. Tubes

JOHNSON'S MEDICATED DIAPER RASH OINTMENT

Glenbrook

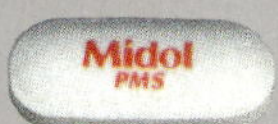

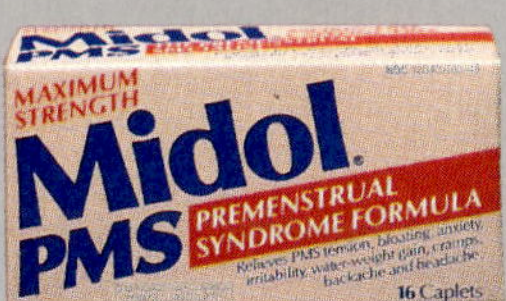

Available in bottles of 8, 16 and 32 caplets

MIDOL® PMS
MAXIMUM STRENGTH

Glenbrook

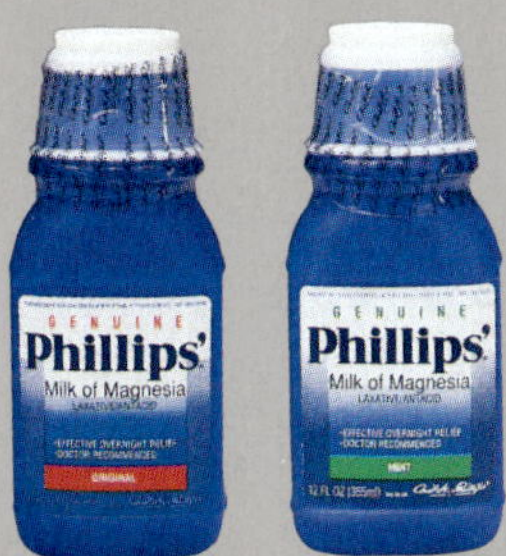

Available in regular and mint flavor 4 oz., 12 oz., 26 oz. plastic bottles

PHILLIPS'® MILK OF MAGNESIA

Glenbrook

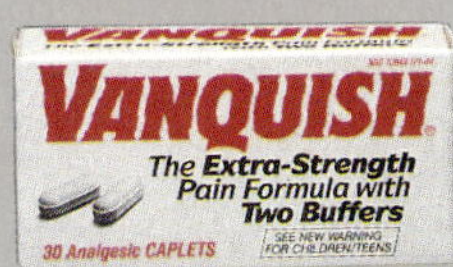

Available in packages of 30, 60 and 100 caplets

VANQUISH®
Extra-Strength Pain Formula with Two Buffers

While every effort has been made to reproduce products faithfully, this section is to be considered a Quick-Reference identification aid.

J&J-MERCK

12 oz

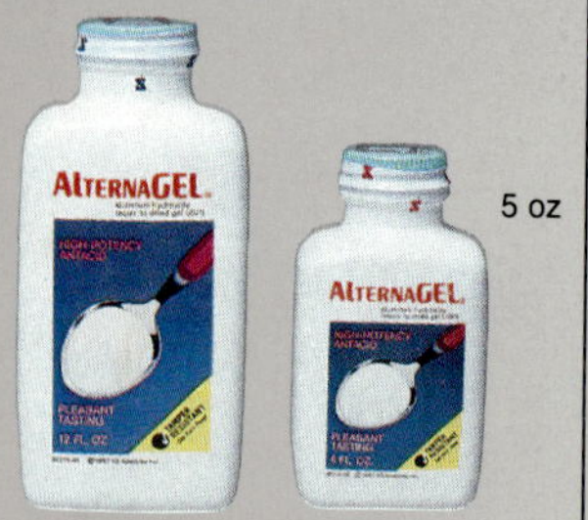

5 oz

ALternaGEL®
High Potency Aluminum Hydroxide Antacid

J&J-Merck

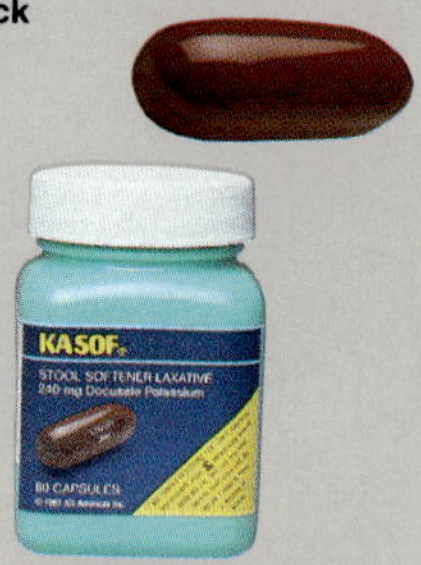

Bottles of 30 and 60 capsules

KASOF®
(docusate potassium, 240 mg)

High Strength Stool Softener

J&J-Merck

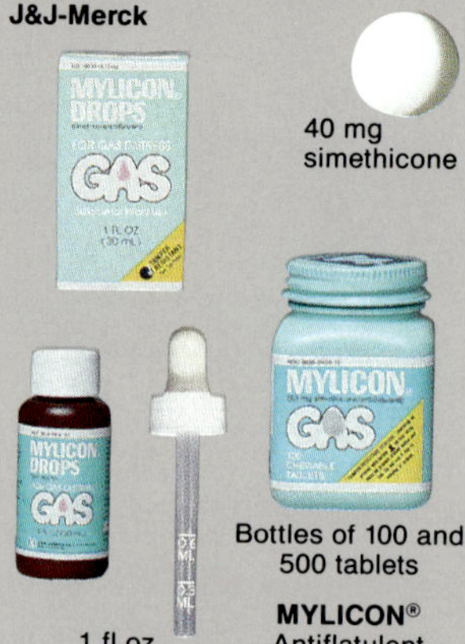

40 mg simethicone

Bottles of 100 and 500 tablets

1 fl oz

MYLICON®
Antiflatulent

J&J-Merck

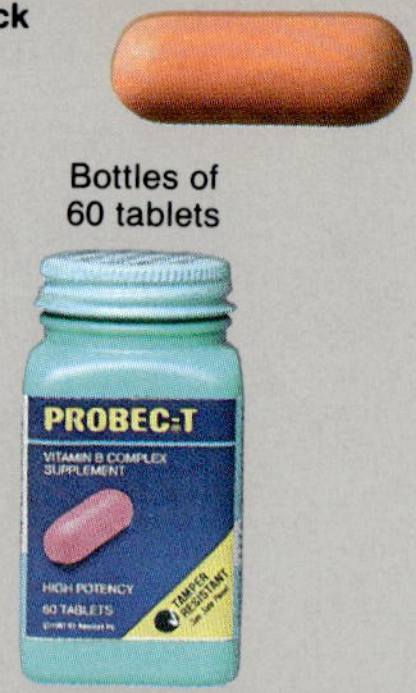

Bottles of 60 tablets

PROBEC®-T
High potency B complex supplement with 600 mg of vitamin C

J&J-Merck

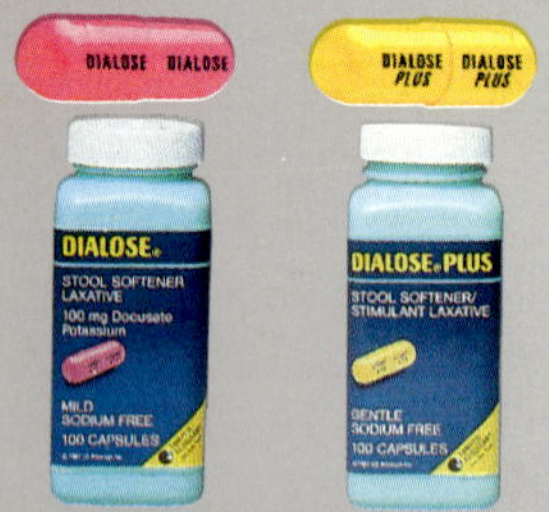

Stool Softeners

Bottles of 36 and 100 capsules

Bottles of 36, 100 and 500 capsules

DIALOSE®
(docusate potassium, 100 mg)

DIALOSE® PLUS
(docusate potassium, 100 mg and casanthranol, 30 mg)

J&J-Merck

Sodium Free

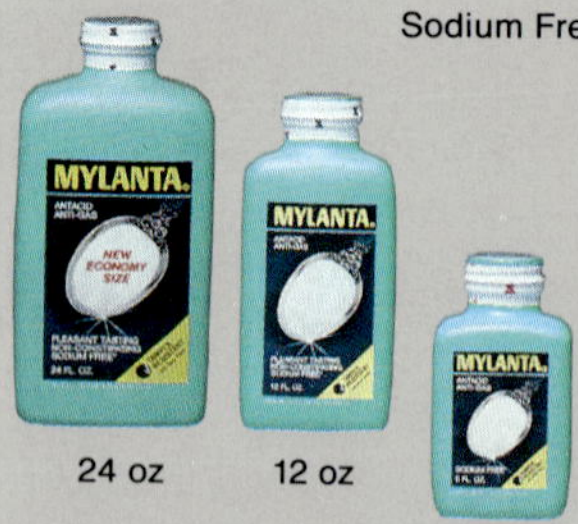

24 oz 12 oz 5 oz

MYLANTA® LIQUID
Antacid/Anti-Gas

(magnesium and aluminum hydroxides with simethicone)

J&J-Merck

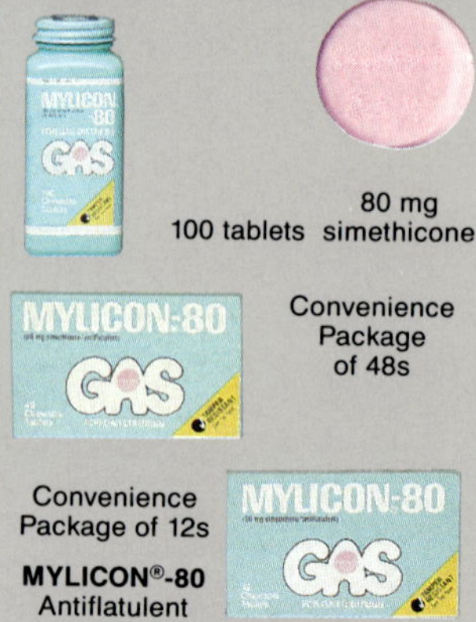

100 tablets

80 mg simethicone

Convenience Package of 48s

Convenience Package of 12s

MYLICON®-80
Antiflatulent

J&J-Merck

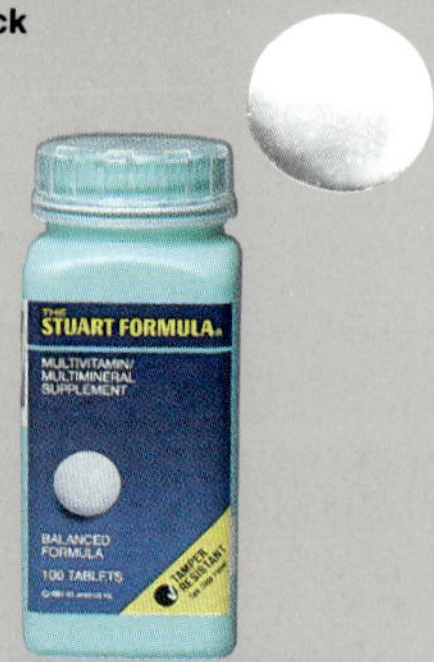

Bottles of 100 and 250 tablets

STUART FORMULA® TABLETS
Multivitamin/Multimineral Supplement

J&J-Merck

Available in 9 oz and 16 oz bottles

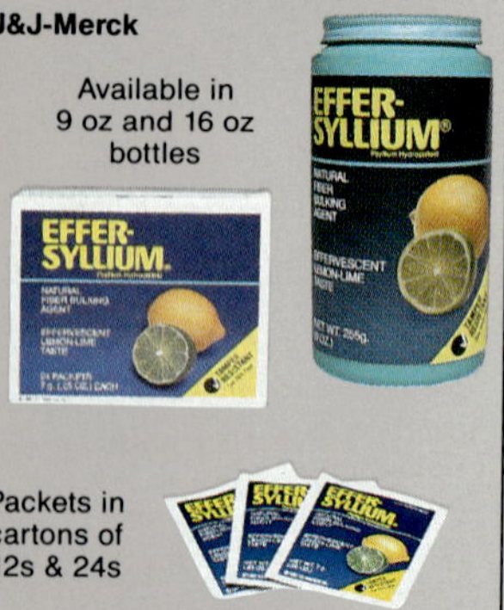

Packets in cartons of 12s & 24s

EFFER-SYLLIUM®
Natural Fiber Bulking Agent

J&J-Merck

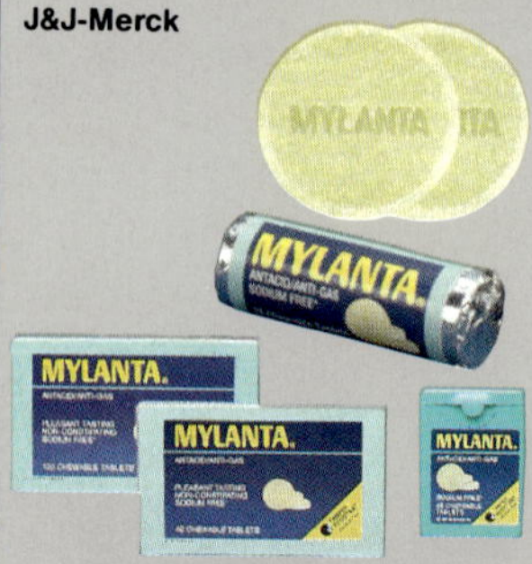

Available in boxes of 40 and 100, bottles of 180, flip-top Convenience Packs of 48 and 12 tablet rolls

MYLANTA® TABLETS
Antacid/Anti-Gas

J&J-Merck

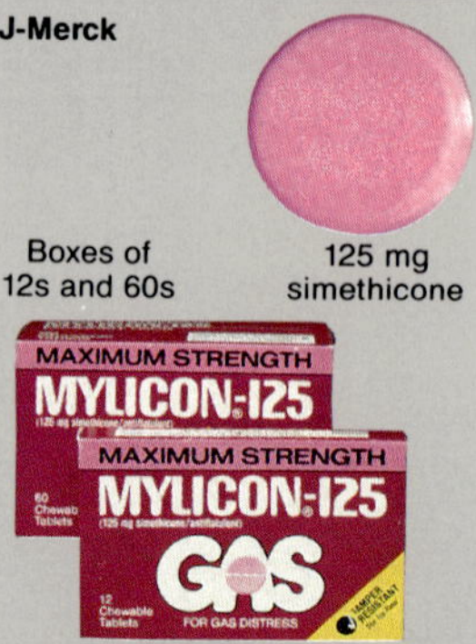

Boxes of 12s and 60s

125 mg simethicone

MAXIMUM STRENGTH MYLICON®-125
Antiflatulent

J&J-Merck

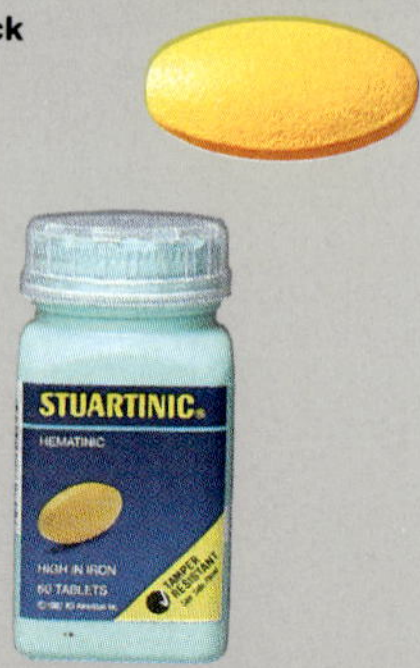

Bottles of 60 tablets

STUARTINIC®
Hematinic

J&J-Merck

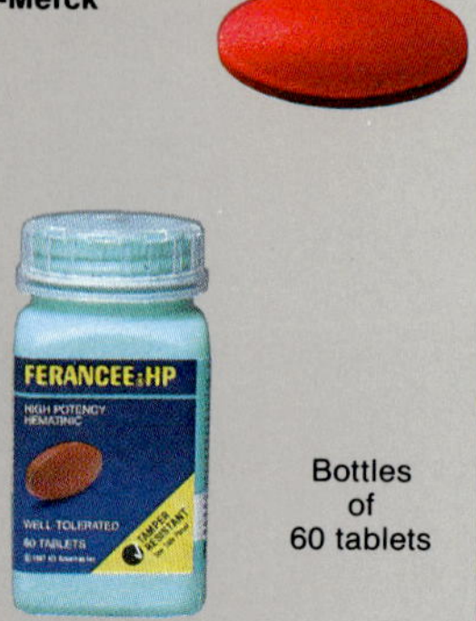

Bottles of 60 tablets

FERANCEE®-HP
High Potency Hematinic

J&J-Merck

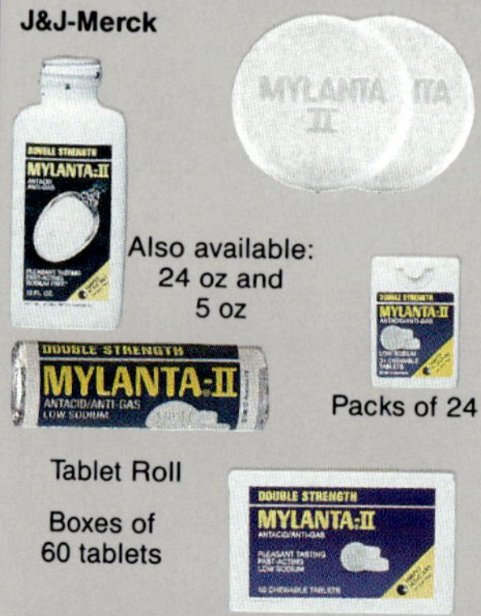

Also available: 24 oz and 5 oz

Tablet Roll

Packs of 24

Boxes of 60 tablets

MYLANTA®-II LIQUID and TABLETS
Double Strength Antacid/Anti-Gas

J&J-Merck

Bottles of 100 tablets

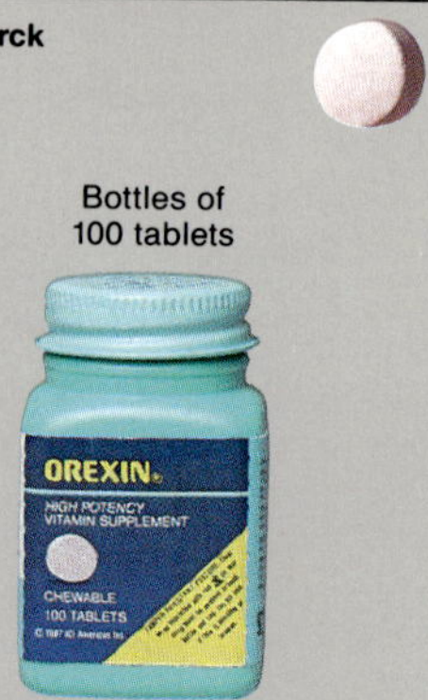

OREXIN®
Therapeutic Vitamin Supplement

For more detailed information on products illustrated in this section, consult the Product Information Section or manufacturers may be contacted directly.

LACTAID INC.

After JAN. 1, 1991
Marketed by AKPharma Inc.

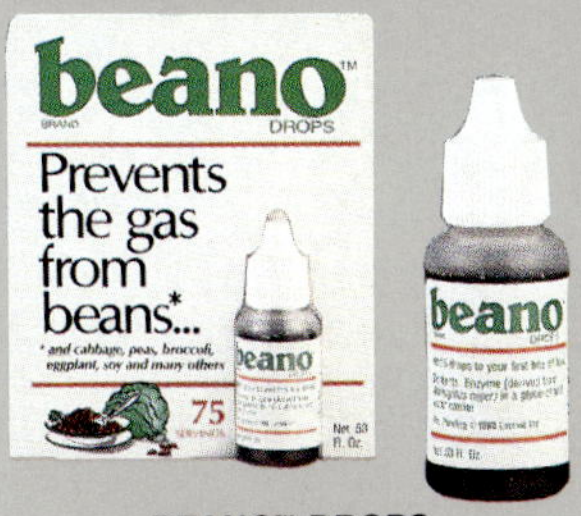

BEANO™ DROPS
(enzyme from Aspergillus niger in a glycerol and water carrier)
(Shown smaller than actual size)

Lederle

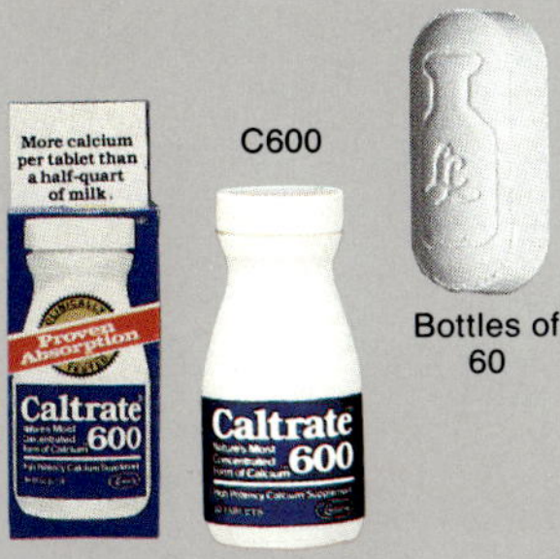

C600

Bottles of 60

CALTRATE® 600
High Potency Calcium Supplement

Lederle

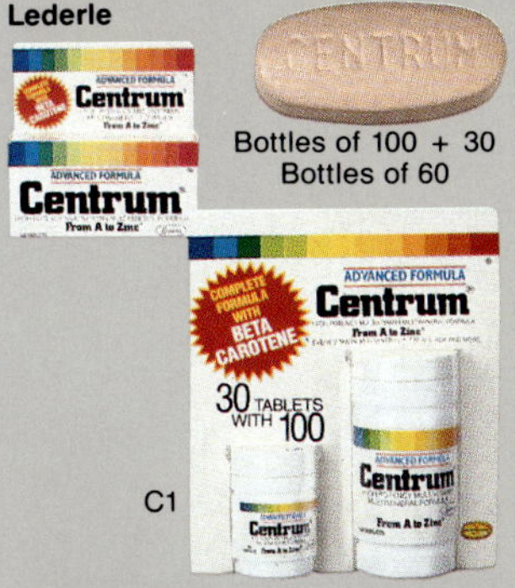

Bottles of 100 + 30
Bottles of 60

C1

Advanced Formula CENTRUM®
High Potency Multivitamin/ Multimineral Formula

Lederle

CS11

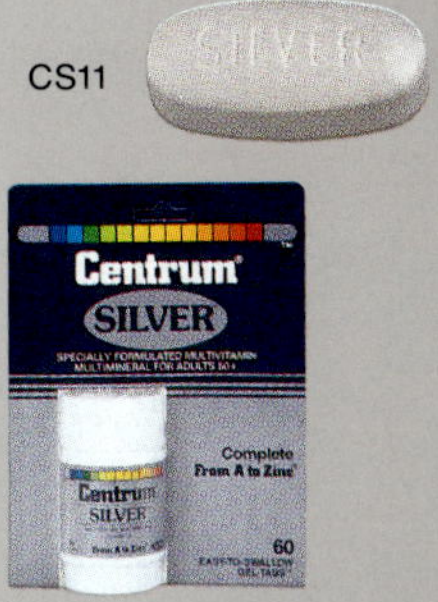

CENTRUM® SILVER™
Specially Formulated Multivitamin/multimineral

For adults 50+

Lactaid Inc.

After JAN. 1, 1991
Marketed by McNeil Consumer Products

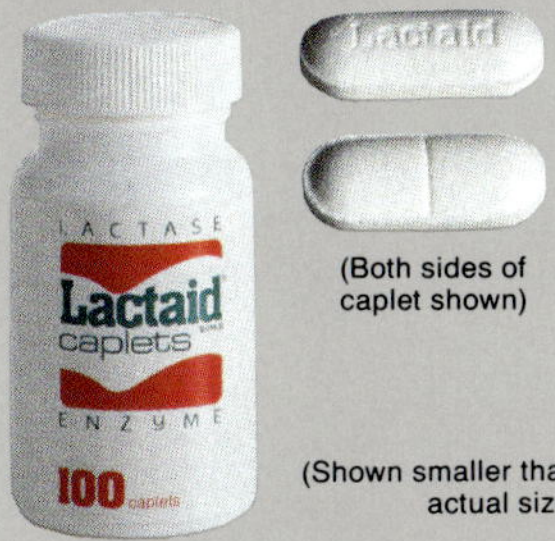

(Both sides of caplet shown)

(Shown smaller than actual size)

LACTAID® CAPLETS
(lactase enzyme caplets)

Lederle

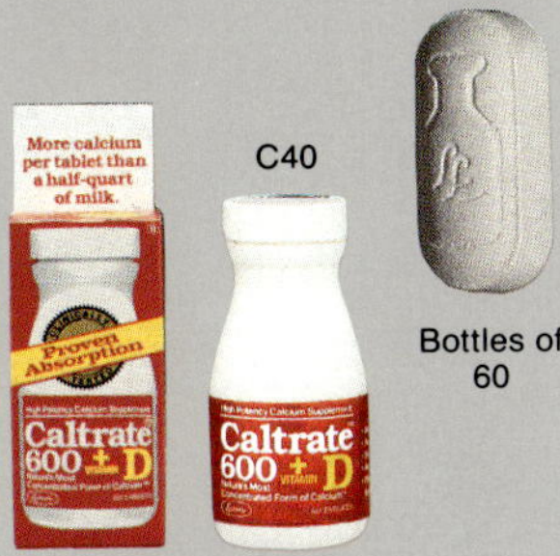

C40

Bottles of 60

CALTRATE® 600+D
High Potency Calcium Supplement

Lederle

C2

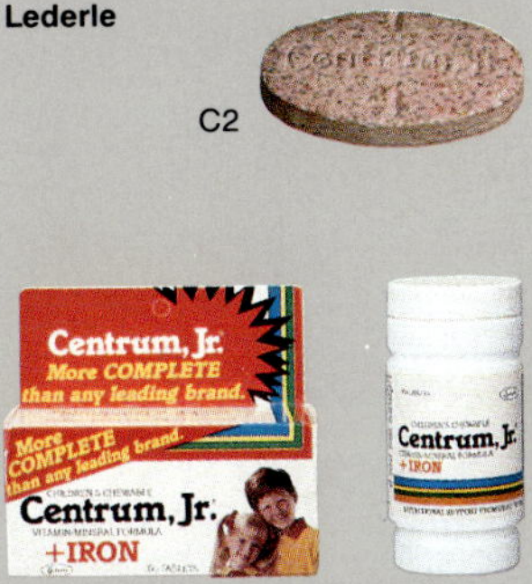

60 tablets

CENTRUM, JR.® + Iron
Children's Chewable Vitamin/Mineral Formula

Lederle

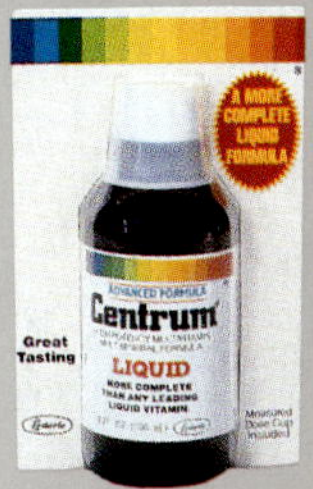

CENTRUM® LIQUID
High Potency Multivitamin/Multimineral Formula

Lactaid Inc.

(Shown smaller than actual size)

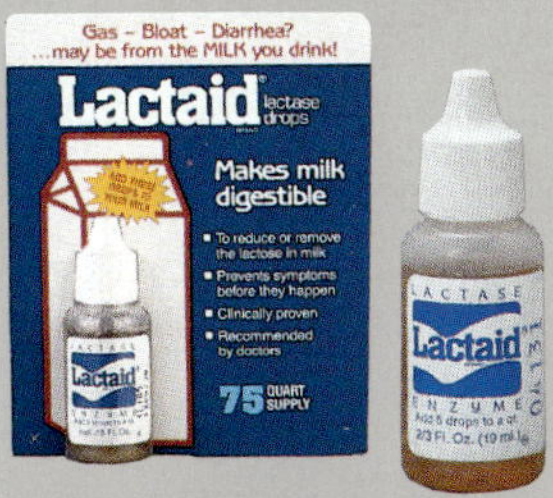

LACTAID®
(lactase enzyme)

Lederle

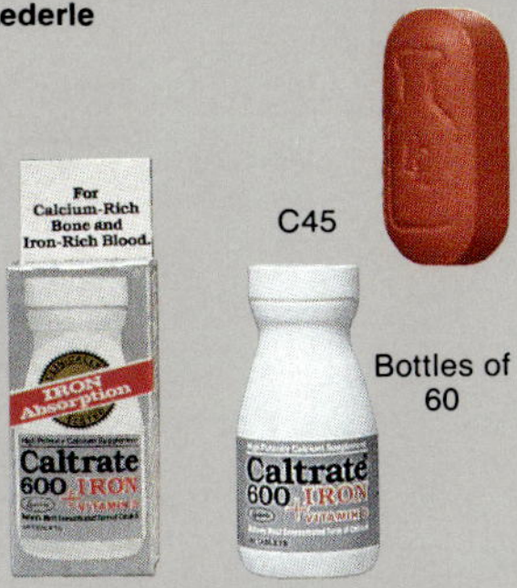

C45

Bottles of 60

CALTRATE® 600+IRON+ VITAMIN D
High Potency Calcium Supplement

Lederle

C39

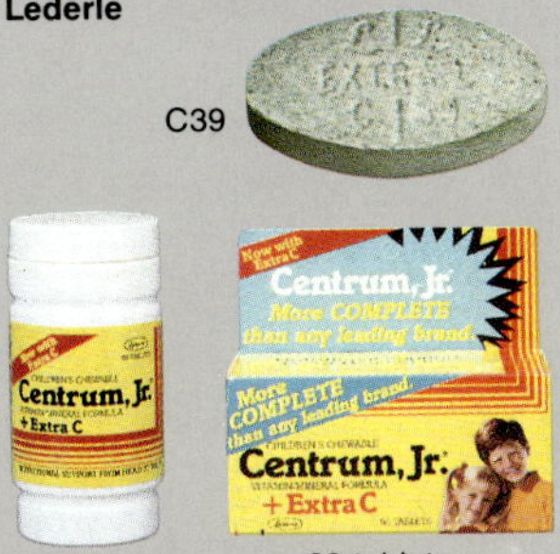

60 tablets

CENTRUM, JR.® + Extra C
Children's Chewable Vitamin/Mineral Formula

Lederle

F66

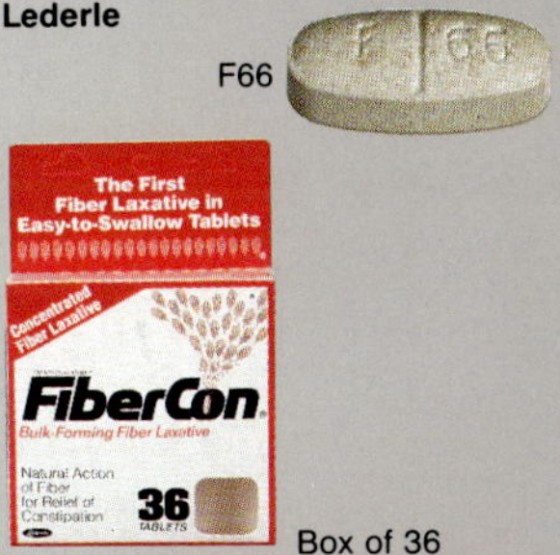

Box of 36

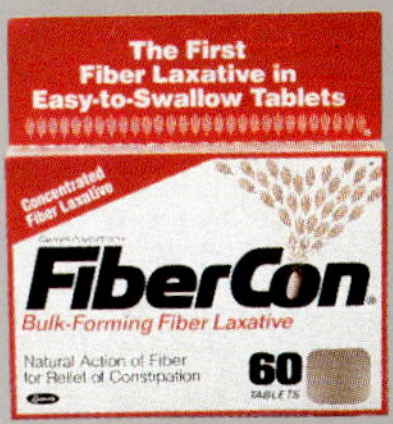

Box of 60

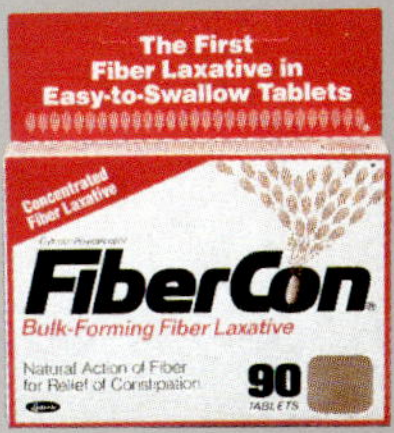

Box of 90

Also available in bottles of 500 and unit dose

FIBERCON®
Calcium Polycarbophil
Bulk-Forming Fiber Laxative

LEDERLE

LEDERMARK®
Product Identification Code

Many Lederle tablets and capsules bear an identification code, and these codes are listed with each product pictured. A current listing appears in the Product Information Section of the 1991 Physicians' Desk Reference.

Lederle

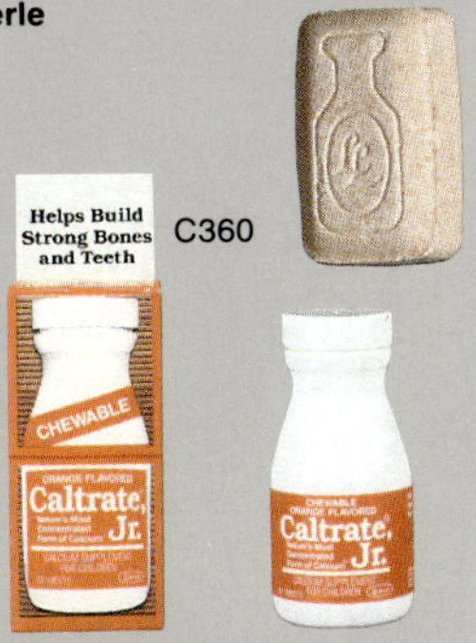

C360

CALTRATE® JR.
Chewable Calcium Supplement For Children

Lederle

C60

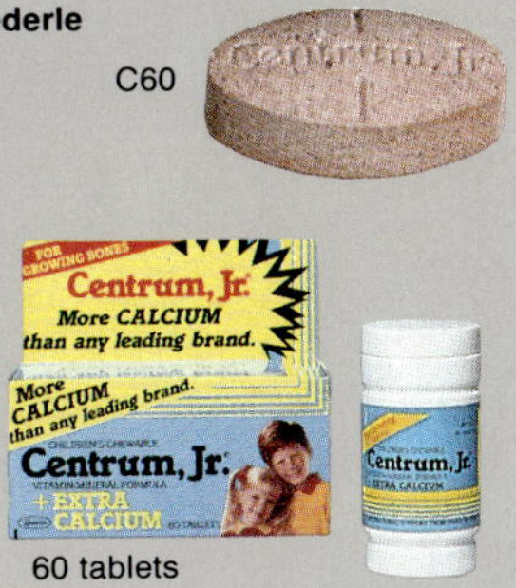

60 tablets

CENTRUM, JR® + Extra Calcium
Children's Chewable Vitamin/Mineral Formula

Lederle

F2

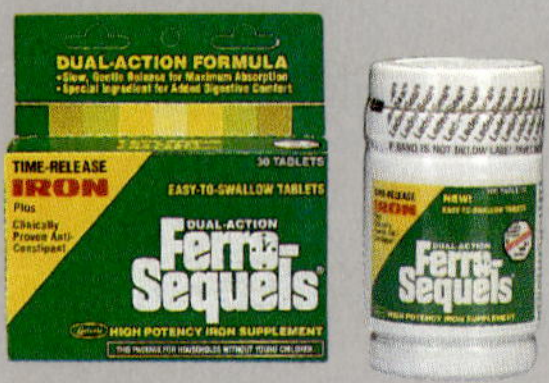

Available in blister packs of 30 and bottles of 30 and 100

FERRO-SEQUELS®
High Potency Iron Supplement with Proven Anti-Constipant

Lederle

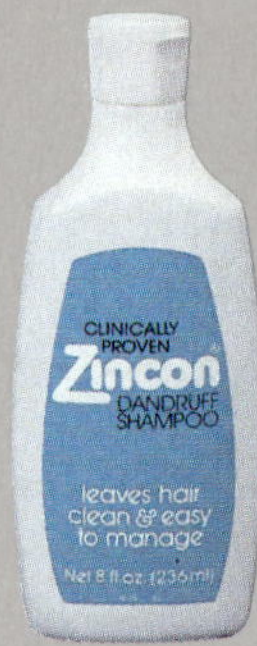

Bottles of 4 fl. oz. and 8 fl. oz.

ZINCON®
Pyrithione Zinc 1%
Dandruff Shampoo

Marion Merrell Dow

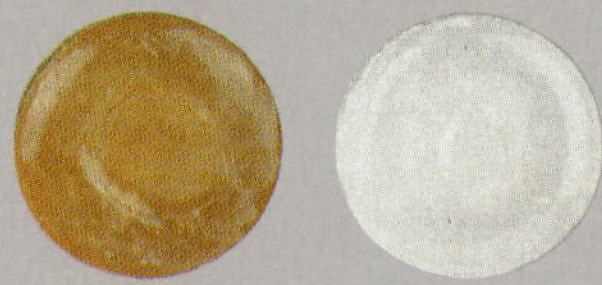

18 lozenges per package

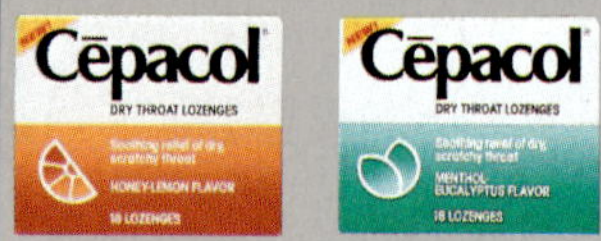

Honey-Lemon Menthol-Eucalyptus

CĒPACOL®
DRY THROAT LOZENGES

Marion Merrell Dow

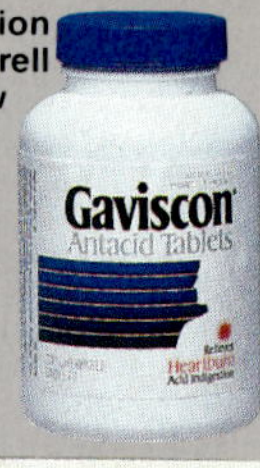

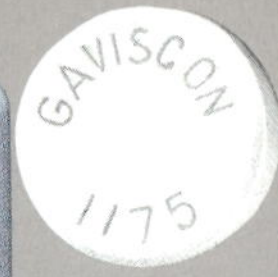

100-tablet bottle

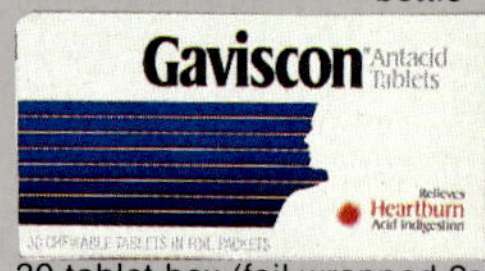

30-tablet box (foil-wrapped 2s)

GAVISCON®
Antacid Tablets

Lederle

S1

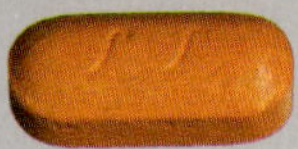

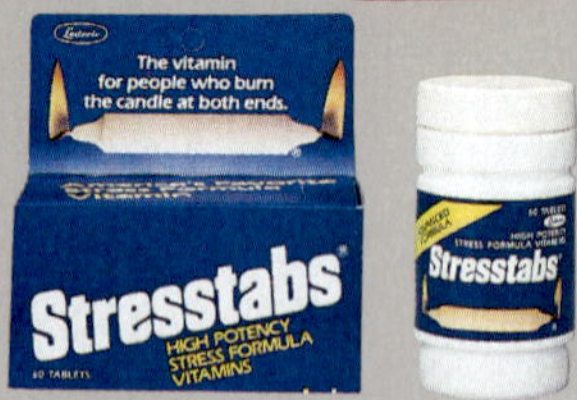

Bottles of 30 and 60

Advanced Formula STRESSTABS®

High Potency Stress Formula Vitamins

MARION MERRELL DOW

Consumer Products

Cēpacol Gold

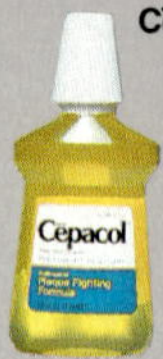

Available in 4, 12, 18, 24 and 32 fl. oz. bottles

Cēpacol Mint

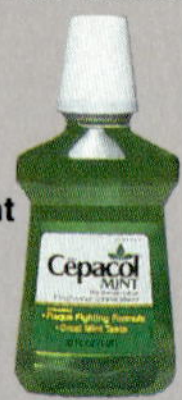

CĒPACOL®
Mouthwash/Gargle

Marion Merrell Dow

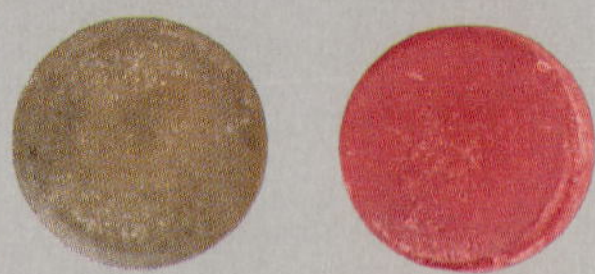

18 lozenges per package

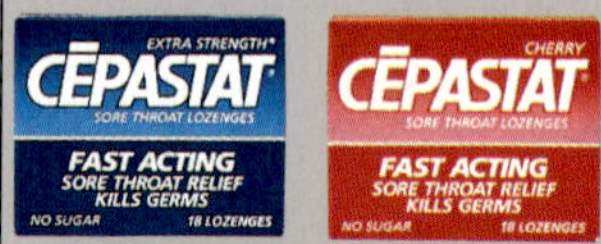

Extra Strength Cherry

CĒPASTAT®
SORE THROAT LOZENGES

Marion Merrell Dow

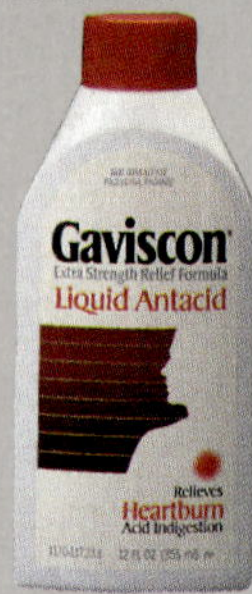

12 fl. oz.

GAVISCON®
Extra Strength Relief Formula Liquid Antacid

Lederle

S2

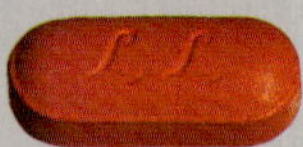

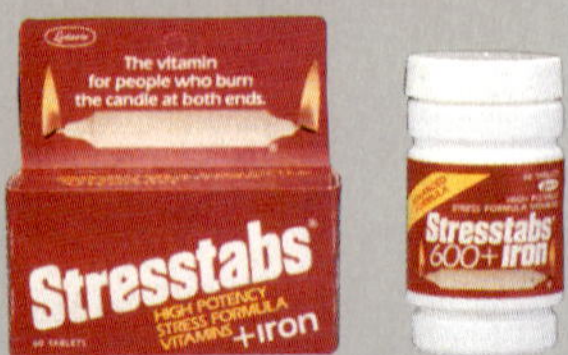

Bottles of 30 and 60

Advanced Formula STRESSTABS®
with IRON

High Potency Stress Formula Vitamins

Marion Merrell Dow

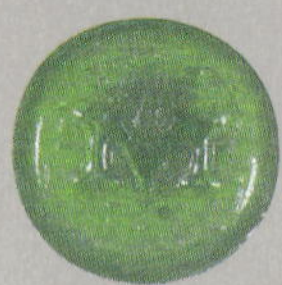

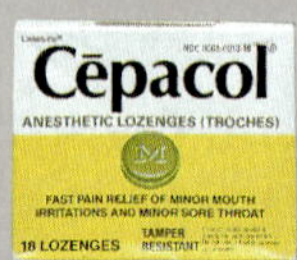

18 lozenges per package

CĒPACOL® ANESTHETIC LOZENGES (Troches)

Marion Merrell Dow

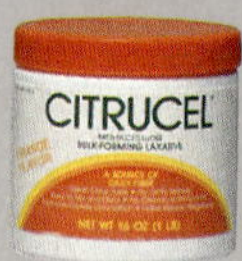

CITRUCEL
Orange
Available in 16 oz. and 30 oz. containers

CITRUCEL
Regular
Available in 7 oz. and 10 oz. containers

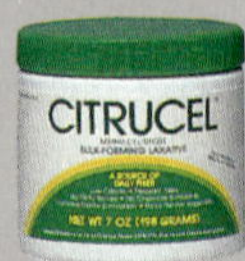

CITRUCEL®
Therapeutic Fiber for Regularity

Marion Merrell Dow

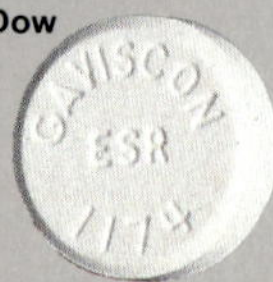

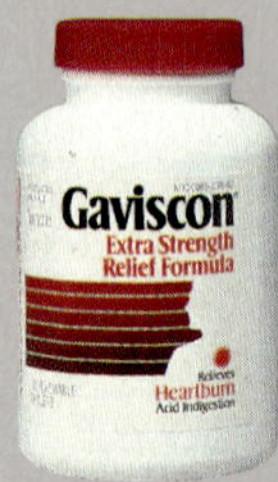

100-tablet bottle

GAVISCON®
Extra Strength Relief Formula Antacid Tablets

Lederle

S3

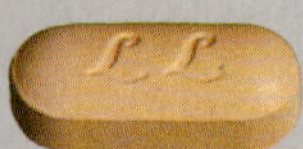

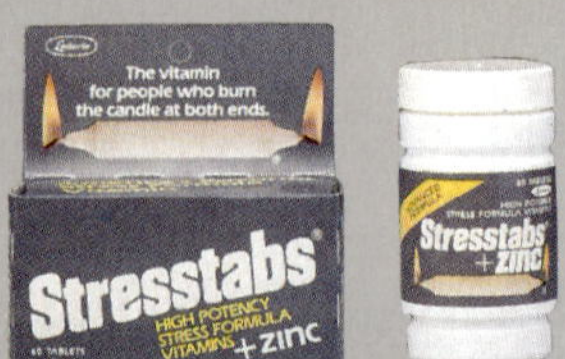

Bottles of 30 and 60

Advanced Formula STRESSTABS®
with ZINC

High Potency Stress Formula Vitamins

Marion Merrell Dow

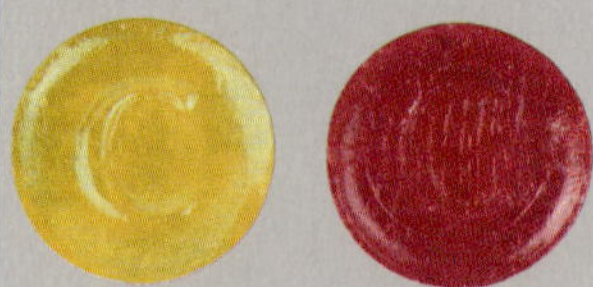

18 lozenges per package

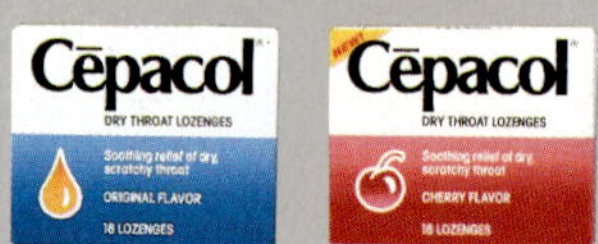

Original Flavor Cherry

CĒPACOL®
DRY THROAT LOZENGES

Marion Merrell Dow

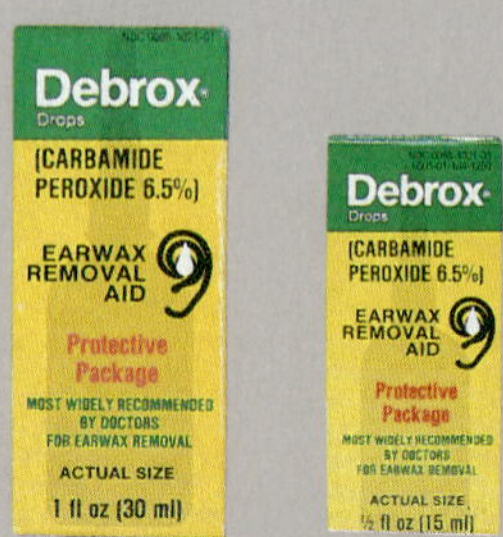

1 fl. oz. ½ fl. oz.

DEBROX®
Drops

Marion Merrell Dow

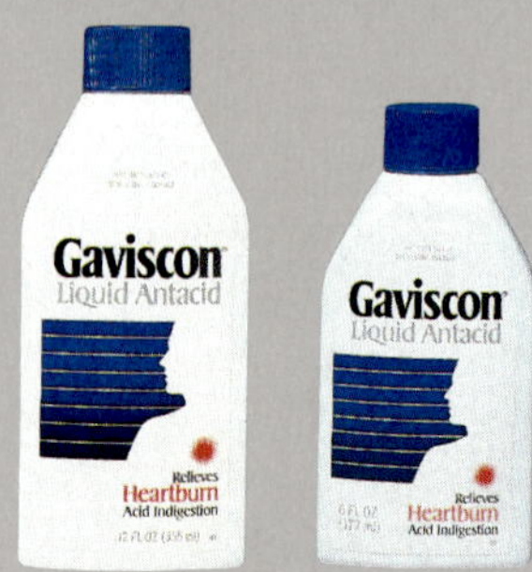

12 fl. oz. 6 fl. oz.

GAVISCON®
Liquid Antacid

Marion Merrell Dow

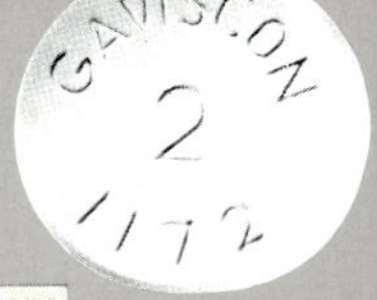

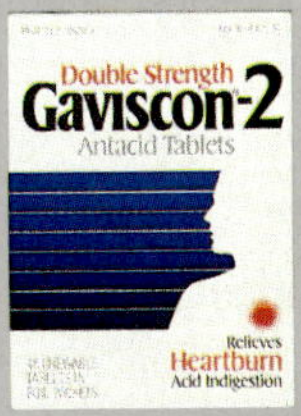

Box of 48 foil-wrapped tablets

GAVISCON®-2 Antacid Tablets

Marion Merrell Dow

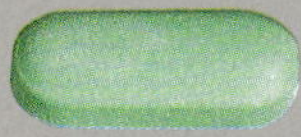

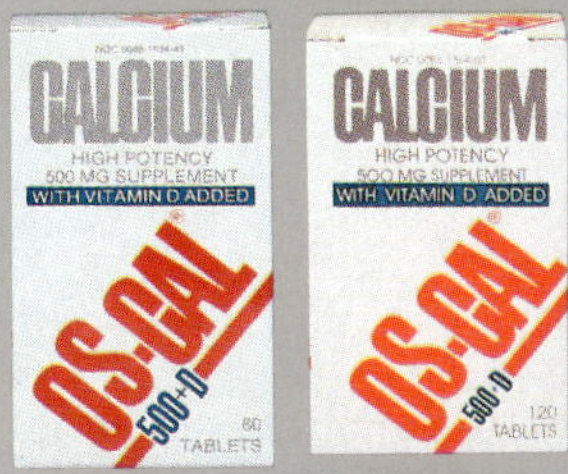

Bottle of 60 tablets

OS-CAL® 500+D Tablets
(calcium with vitamin D)

Marion Merrell Dow

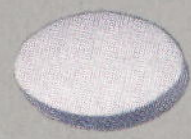

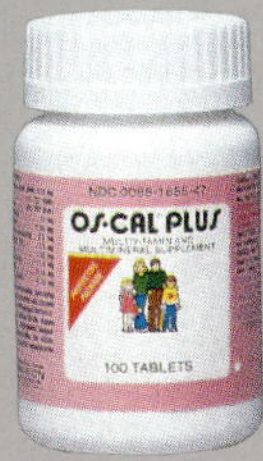

Bottle of 100 tablets

OS-CAL® PLUS Multivitamin and Multimineral Supplement

McNeil Consumer

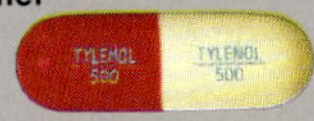

500 mg.

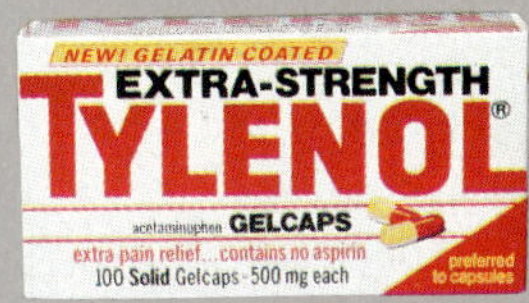

Gelcaps available in tamper-resistant bottles of 24, 50, 100 and 150.

EXTRA-STRENGTH TYLENOL®
acetaminophen
GELCAPS®

Marion Merrell Dow

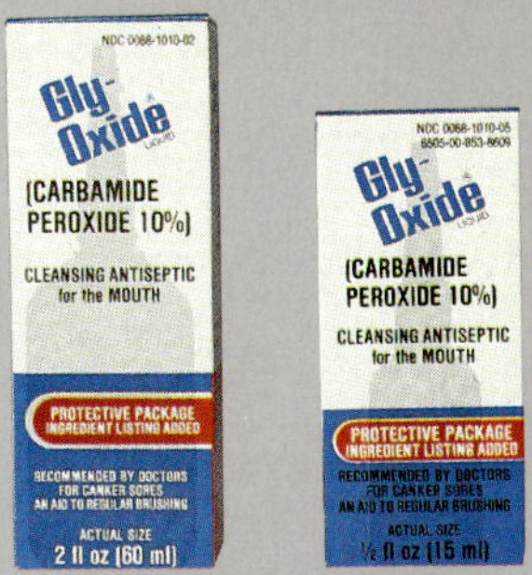

2 fl. oz. ½ fl. oz.

GLY-OXIDE® Liquid

Marion Merrell Dow

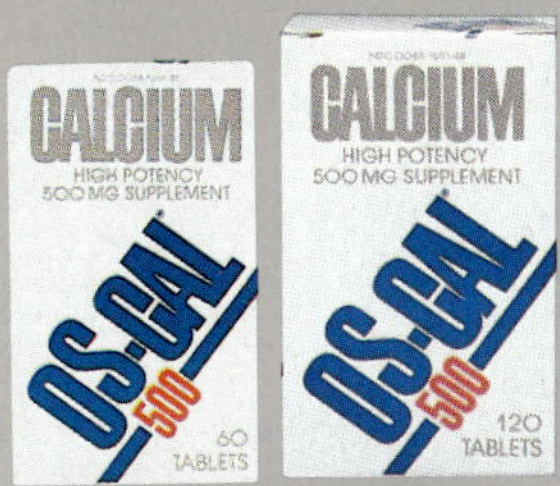

Bottles of 60 and 120 tablets

OS-CAL® 500 Tablets

Marion Merrell Dow

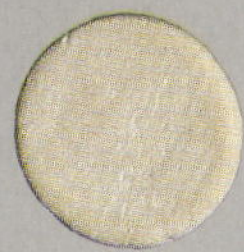

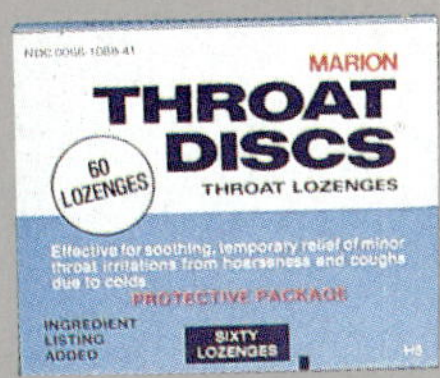

Box of 60 lozenges

THROAT DISCS® Throat Lozenges

McNeil Consumer

500 mg.

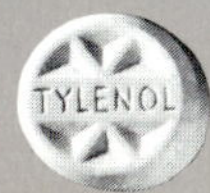

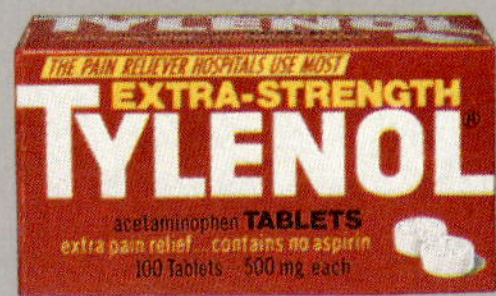

Tablets available in tamper-resistant vials of 10 and bottles of 30, 60, 100 and 200. Liquid: 8 fl. oz.

EXTRA-STRENGTH TYLENOL®
acetaminophen
Tablets & Liquid

Marion Merrell Dow

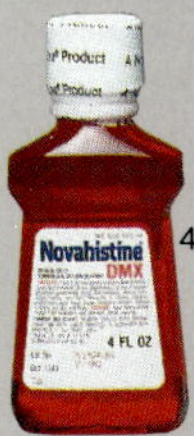

Novahistine DMX
Cough/Cold Formula & Decongestant

4 fl. oz.

4 fl. oz.

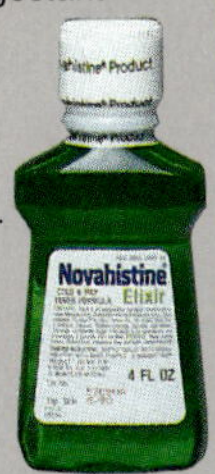

Novahistine Elixir
Cold & Hay Fever Formula

NOVAHISTINE® DMX & ELIXIR Cough/Cold Products

Marion Merrell Dow

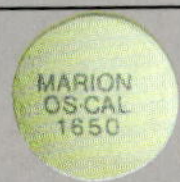

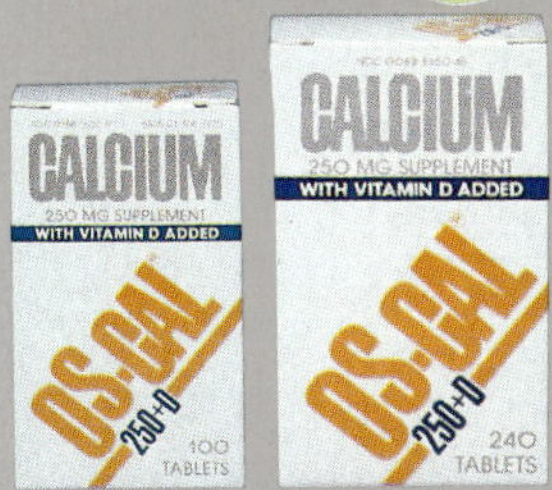

Bottles of 100 and 240 tablets

OS-CAL® 250+D Tablets
(calcium with vitamin D)

McNEIL CONSUMER

325 mg.

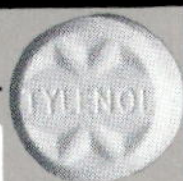

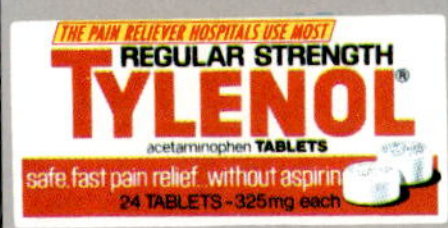

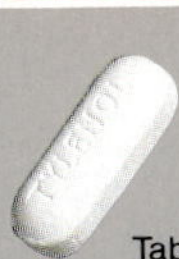

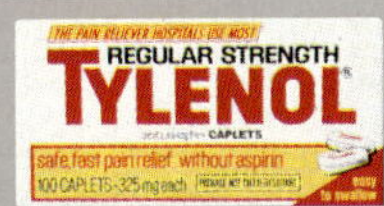

Tablets and Caplets Available in 24's, 50's, 100's and 200's.

REGULAR STRENGTH TYLENOL®
acetaminophen Tablets and Caplets

McNeil Consumer

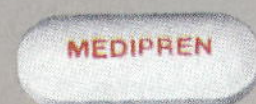

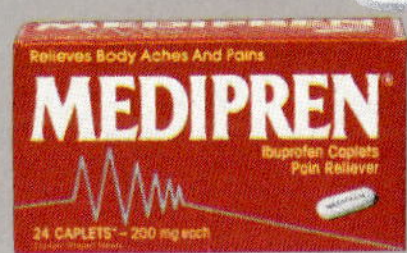

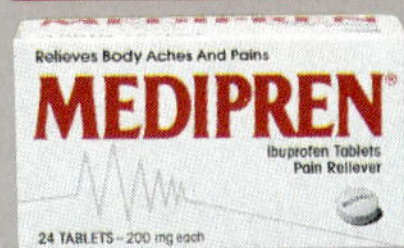

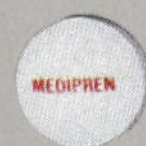

Caplets and Tablets available in bottles of 24 and 50. Caplets also available in bottles of 125.

MEDIPREN®
ibuprofen

Marion Merrell Dow

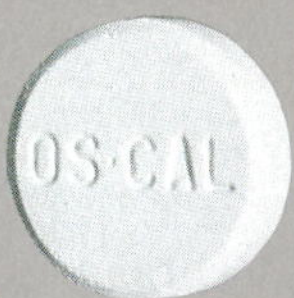

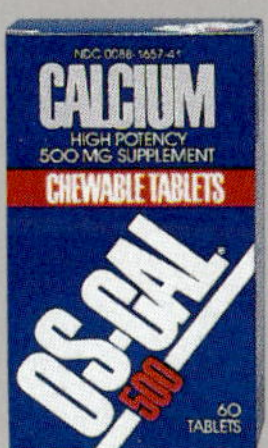

Bottle of 60 tablets

OS-CAL® 500 Chewable Tablets

Marion Merrell Dow

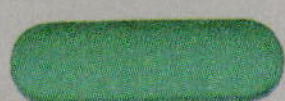

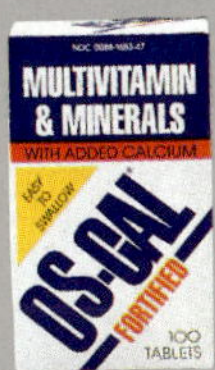

Bottle of 100 tablets

OS-CAL® Fortified Multivitamin and Minerals With Added Calcium

---

McNeil Consumer

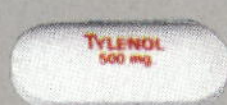

500 mg.

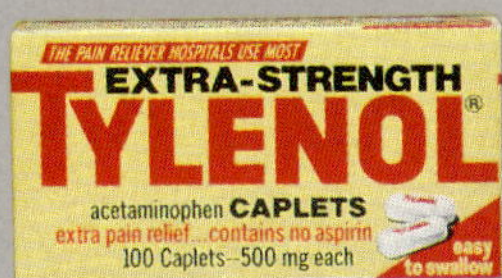

Caplets available in tamper-resistant vials of 10 and bottles of 24, 50, 100, 175 and 250.

EXTRA-STRENGTH TYLENOL®
acetaminophen
Caplets

McNeil Consumer

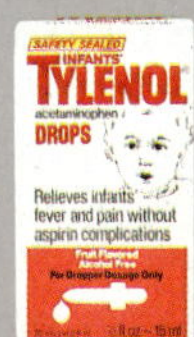

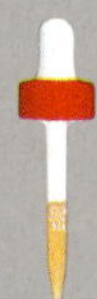

Available in ½ and 1 fl. oz. bottle with child-resistant safety cap and calibrated dropper.

INFANTS' TYLENOL®
acetaminophen
Alcohol Free Drops

McNeil Consumer

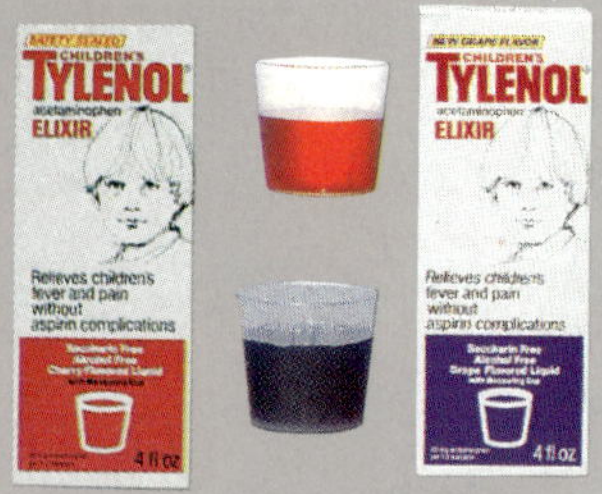

Available in cherry and grape flavors in 2 and 4 fl. oz. bottles with child-resistant safety cap and convenient dosage cup.

CHILDREN'S TYLENOL®
acetaminophen
Alcohol Free Elixir

McNeil Consumer

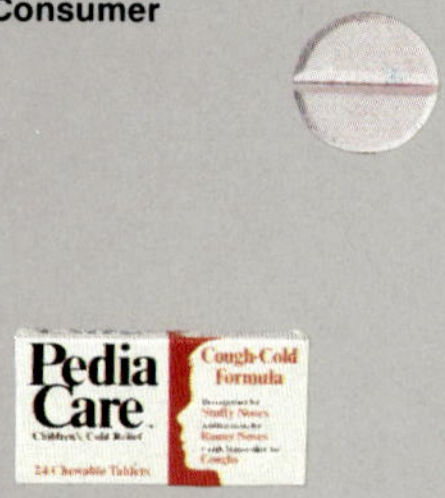

Bottles of 24 chewable tablets.

McNeil Consumer

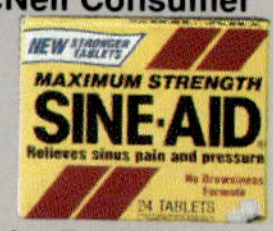

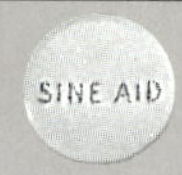

SINE-AID®

Available in blister packs of 24 and bottles of 50 and 100 tablets.

No Drowsiness Formula

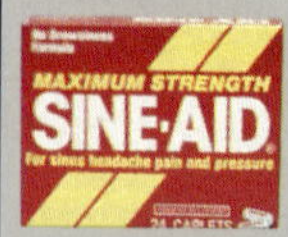

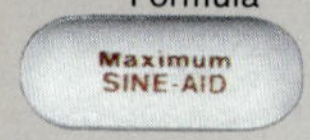

Available in blister packs of 24 and bottles of 50 caplets.

MAXIMUM-STRENGTH SINE-AID®
Relieves sinus headache and pressure

McNeil Consumer

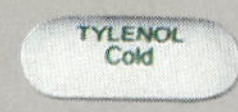

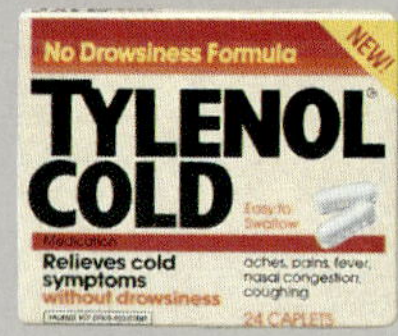

Available in blister-packs of 24 and bottles of 50.

TYLENOL® COLD Medication
No Drowsiness Formula Caplets

McNeil Consumer

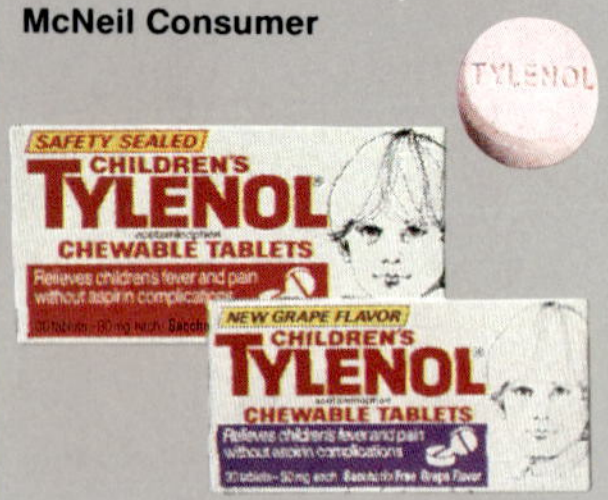

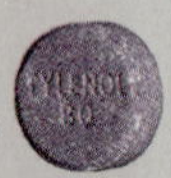

Fruit flavor: available in bottles of 30 with child-resistant safety cap and blister-packs of 48.
Grape flavor: available in bottles of 30 with child-resistant safety cap.

CHILDREN'S TYLENOL®
acetaminophen
80 mg. Chewable Tablets

McNeil Consumer

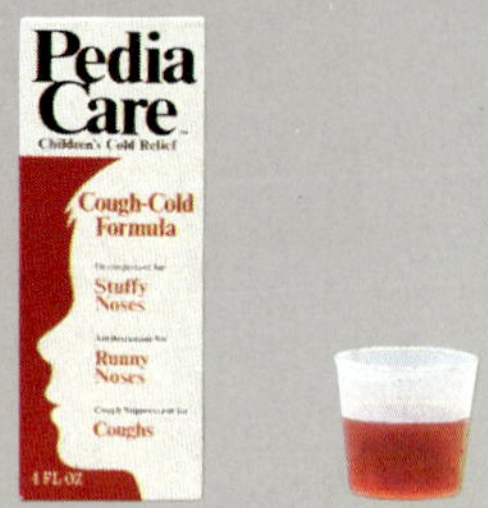

4 fl. oz. bottle with convenient dosage cup.

Both with child-resistant safety cap.

PEDIACARE®
Cough-Cold Formula

McNeil Consumer

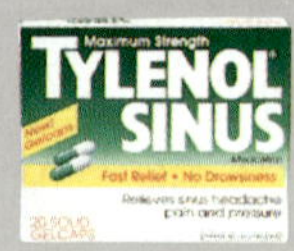

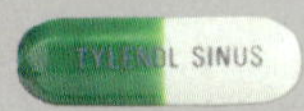

Blister pack of 20's & bottles of 40's

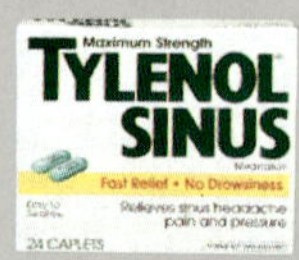

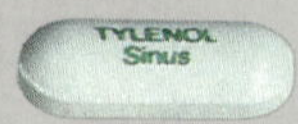

Blister pack of 24's & bottles of 50's

Also available in tablet form.

MAXIMUM-STRENGTH TYLENOL® SINUS MEDICATION

McNeil Consumer

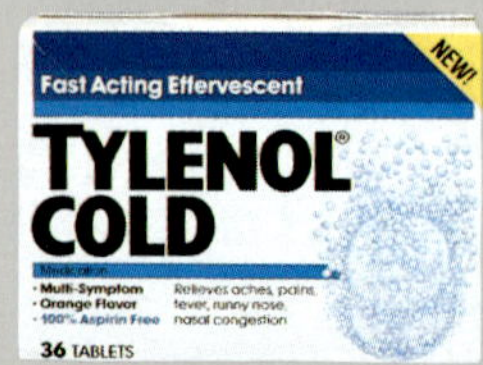

Available in cartons of 20 & 36 effervescent tablets

TYLENOL® COLD MEDICATION
Effervescent Formula

McNeil Consumer

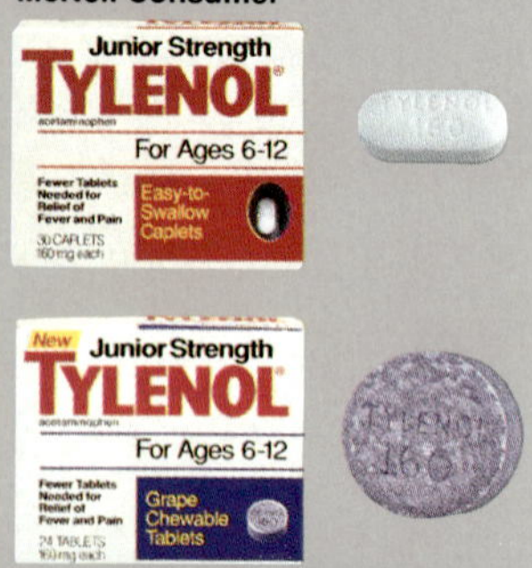

JUNIOR STRENGTH TYLENOL®
160 mg. acetaminophen
Swallowable Caplets: Blister pack of 30
Chewable Tablets: Blister pack of 24

McNeil Consumer

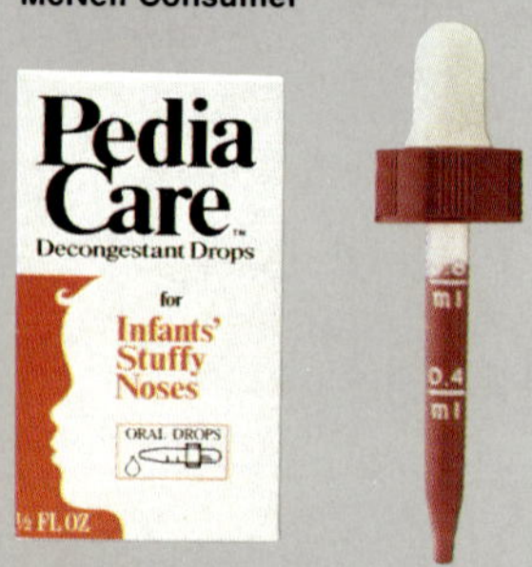

Available in ½ fl. oz. bottle with child-resistant safety cap and calibrated dropper.

PEDIACARE®
Oral Decongestant Drops

McNeil Consumer

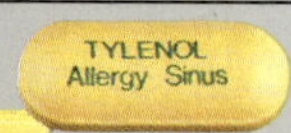

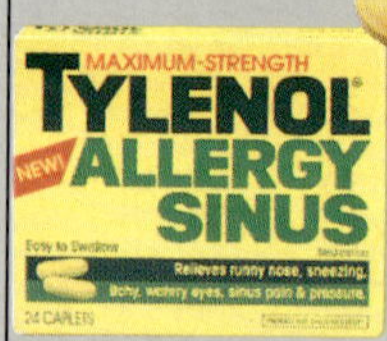

Blister pack of 24's & bottles of 50's

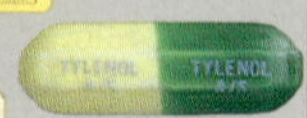

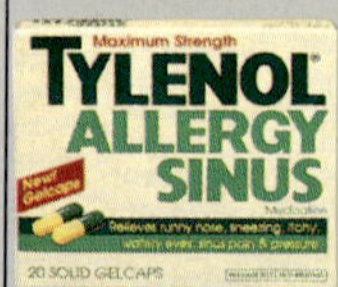

Blister pack of 20's & bottles of 40's

MAXIMUM-STRENGTH TYLENOL® ALLERGY SINUS MEDICATION

McNeil Consumer

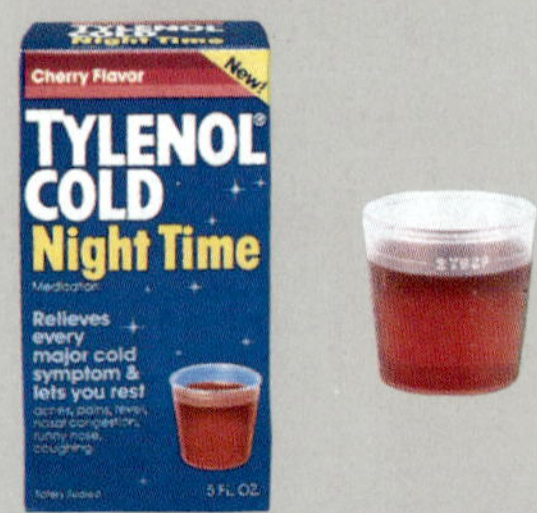

Available in 5 fl. oz. bottle with child-resistant safety cap and convenient dosage cup enclosed.

TYLENOL® COLD NIGHT TIME
Medication Liquid

McNeil Consumer

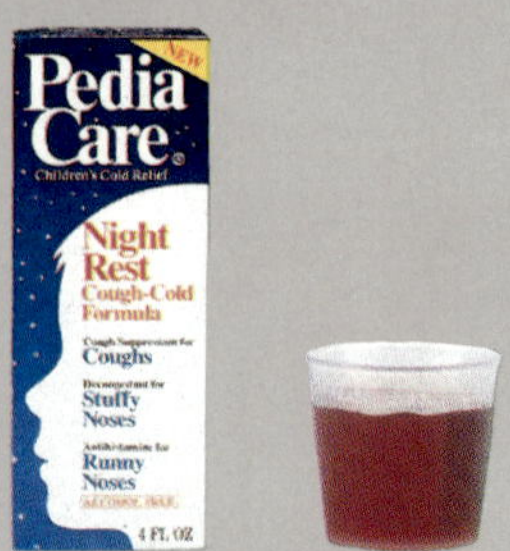

Available in 4 fl. oz. bottle with child-resistant safety cap and convenient dosage cup.

PEDIACARE® NIGHTREST
Cough-Cold Formula

McNeil Consumer

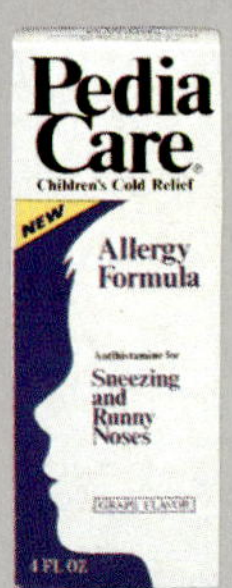

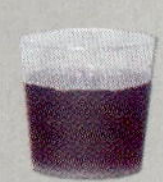

Available in 4 fl. oz. bottle with child-resistant safety cap and convenient dosage cup.

PEDIACARE®
Allergy Formula

McNeil Consumer

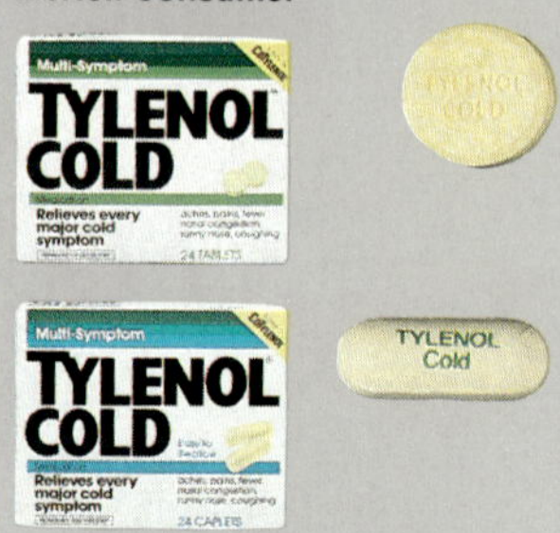

Available in blister-packs of 24 and bottles of 50.

TYLENOL® COLD Medication
Tablets and Caplets

McNeil Consumer

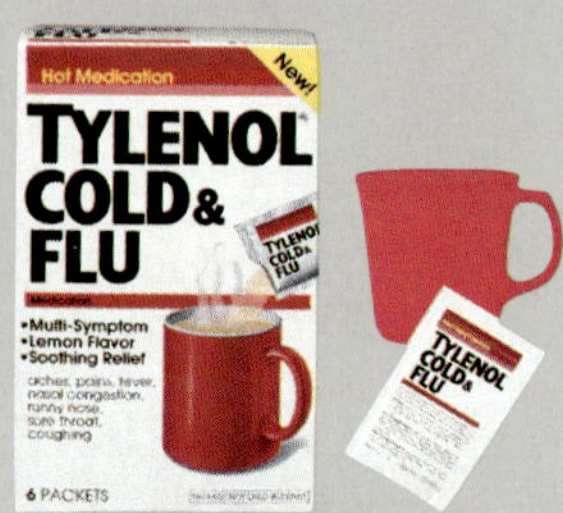

Available in cartons of 6 or 12 individual packets

TYLENOL® COLD & FLU
Hot Liquid Medication

McNeil Consumer

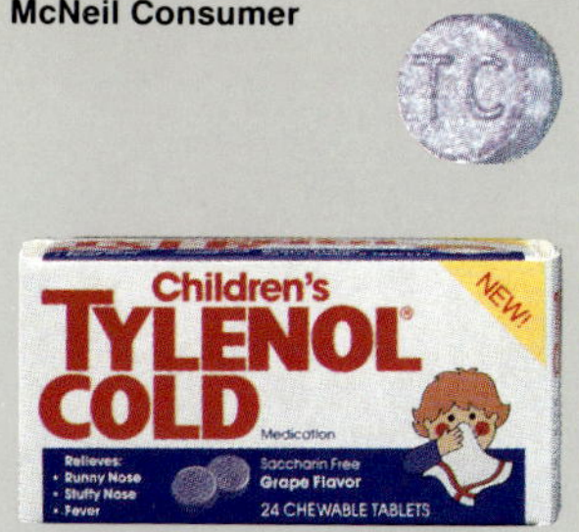

Available in bottles of 24 chewable tablets with child-resistant safety cap.

CHILDREN'S TYLENOL® COLD
Chewable Cold Tablets

Mead Johnson Nutritionals

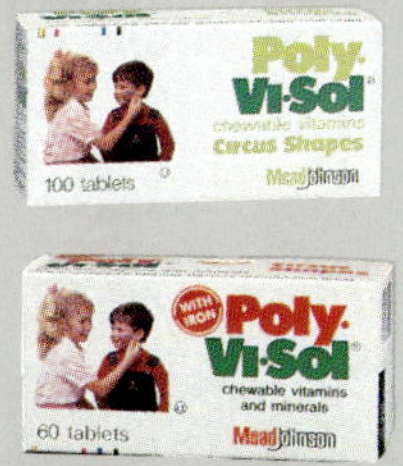

Available in bottles of 60 and 100 tablets

POLY-VI-SOL® CIRCUS SHAPES CHEWABLE VITAMINS
with and without iron

MEAD JOHNSON PHARM.

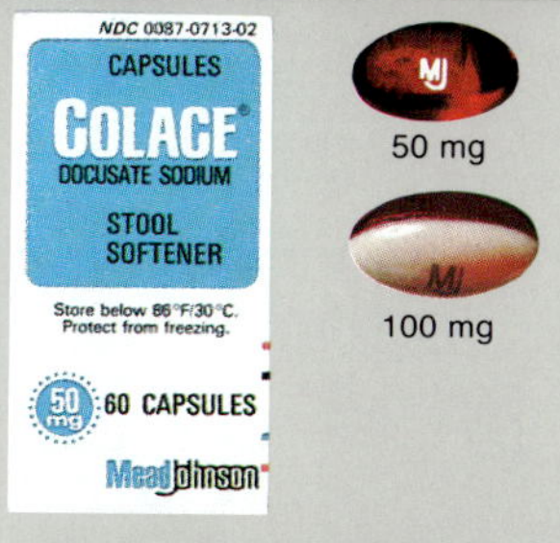

Bottles of 30, 60, 250 and 1000 Stool Softener

†COLACE®
(docusate sodium)

Menley & James

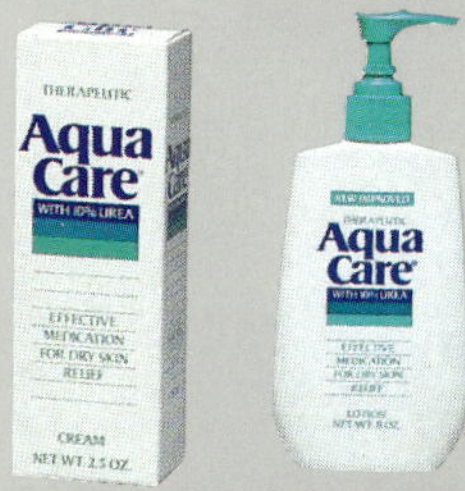

2.5 oz. tube

8 oz. and 16 oz. bottles

AQUA CARE® CREAM AND LOTION with 10% Urea

McNeil Consumer

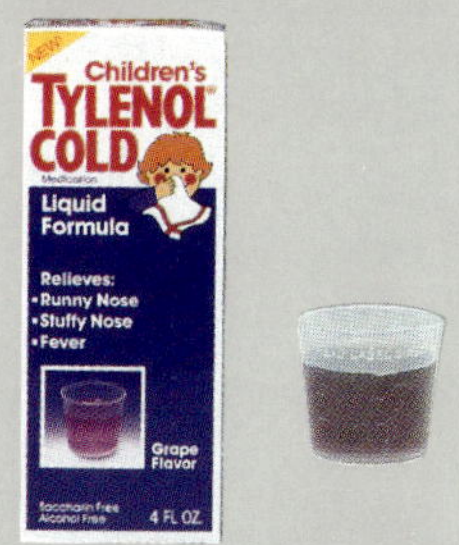

Available in 4 fl. oz. bottle with child-resistant safety cap and convenient dosage cup.

CHILDREN'S TYLENOL® COLD
Liquid Cold Formula

Mead Johnson Nutritionals

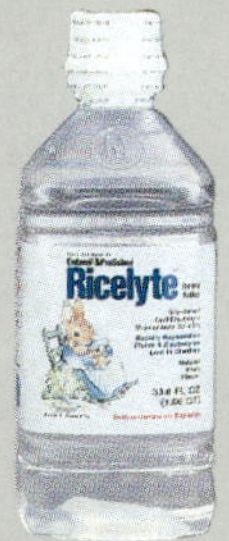

RICELYTE™
Rice-Based Oral Electrolyte Maintenance Solution

Mead Johnson Pharmaceuticals

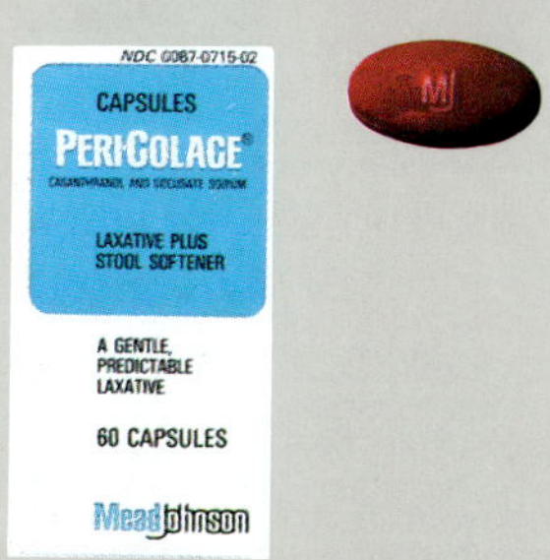

Bottles of 30, 60, 250 and 1000 Laxative and Stool Softener

†PERI-COLACE®
(casanthranol and docusate sodium)

Menley & James

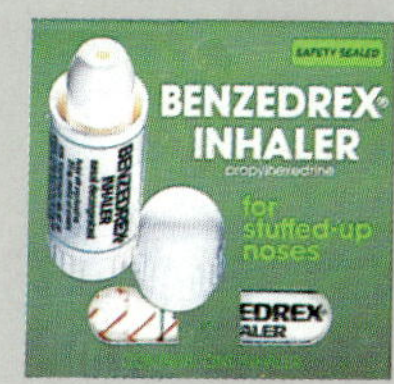

1 inhaler per package

BENZEDREX® INHALER
(propylhexedrine)

McNeil Consumer

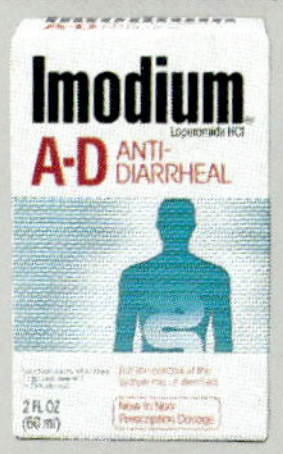

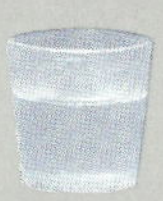

Available in 2, 3 and 4 fl. oz. bottles with a convenient dosage cup, and caplets in 6's and 12's.

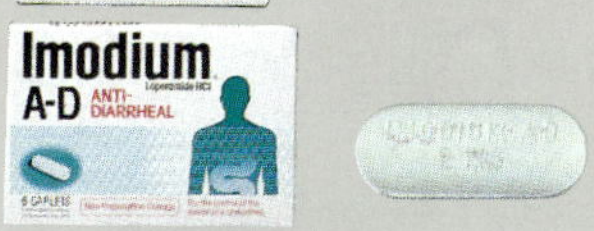

IMODIUM® A-D
loperamide HCl
ANTI-DIARRHEAL

Mead Johnson Nutritionals

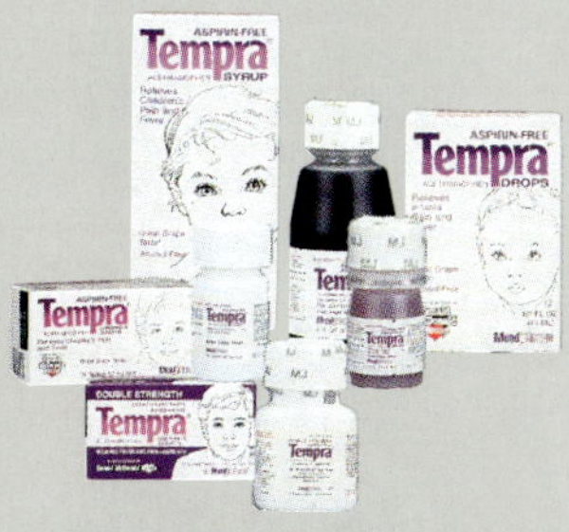

Alcohol-free
Aspirin-free
TEMPRA®
Acetaminophen for children

MENLEY & JAMES

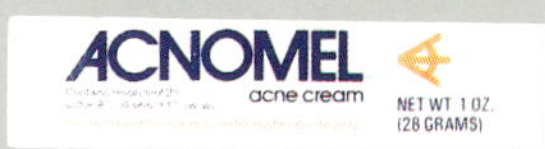

1 oz. tube

ACNOMEL® ACNE CREAM
(resorcinol, sulfur, alcohol)

Menley & James

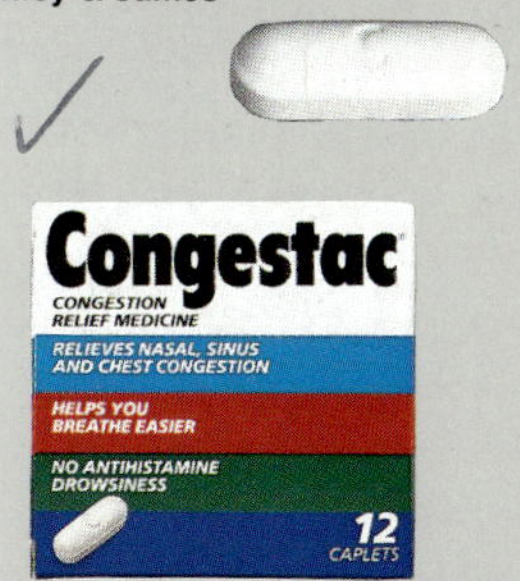

Packages of 12 and 24 caplets

CONGESTAC®
Congestion Relief Medicine
Decongestant/Expectorant

MEAD JOHNSON

Nutritionals

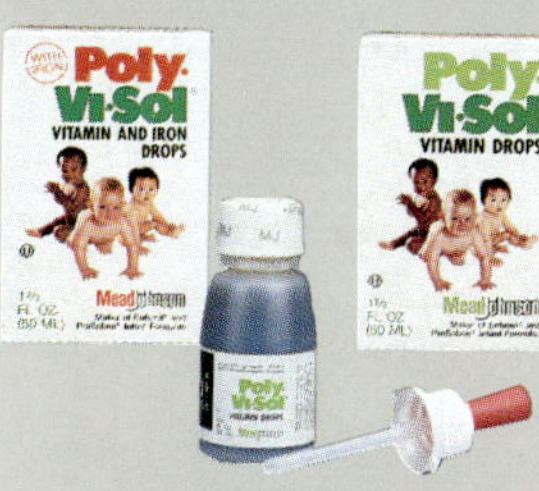

POLY-VI-SOL®
VITAMIN DROPS
with and without iron

Mead Johnson Nutritionals

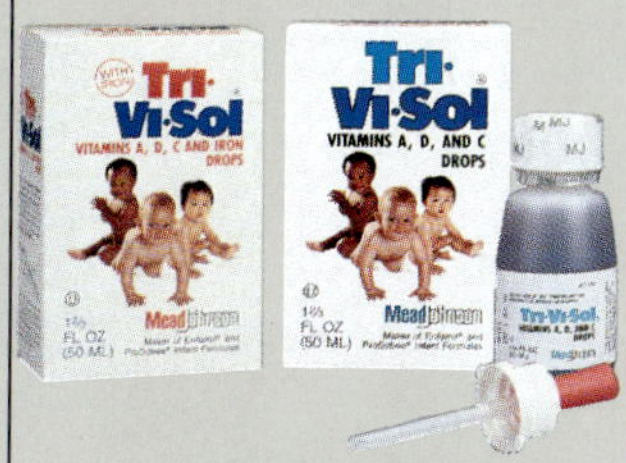

TRI-VI-SOL®
VITAMIN DROPS
with and without iron

Menley & James

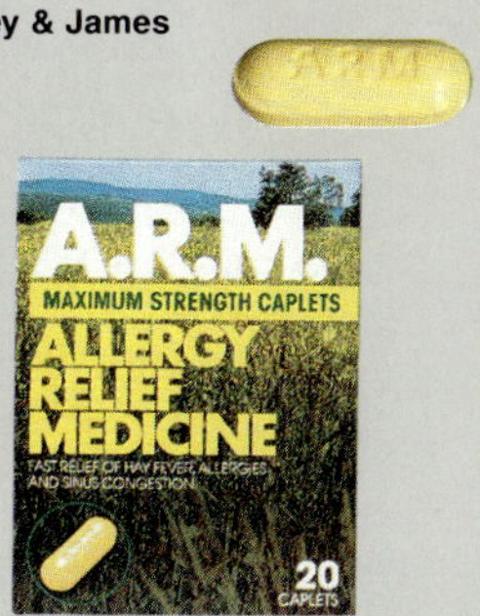

Packages of 20 and 40 caplets

A.R.M.® ALLERGY RELIEF MEDICINE
(chlorpheniramine maleate, phenylpropanolamine HCl)

Menley & James

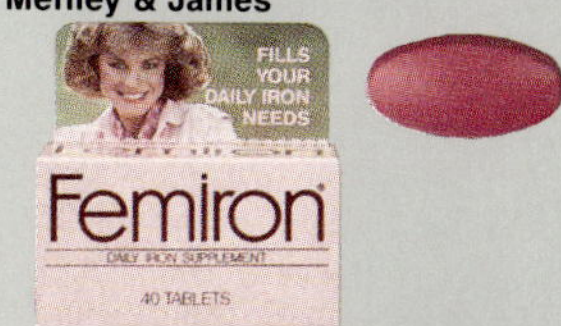

FEMIRON® REGULAR
Bottles of 40 and 120

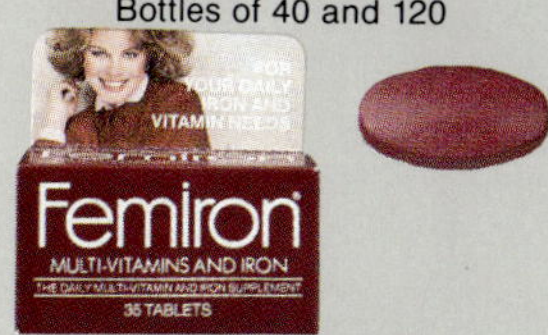

FEMIRON® WITH VITAMINS
Bottles of 35, 60 and 90

Menley & James

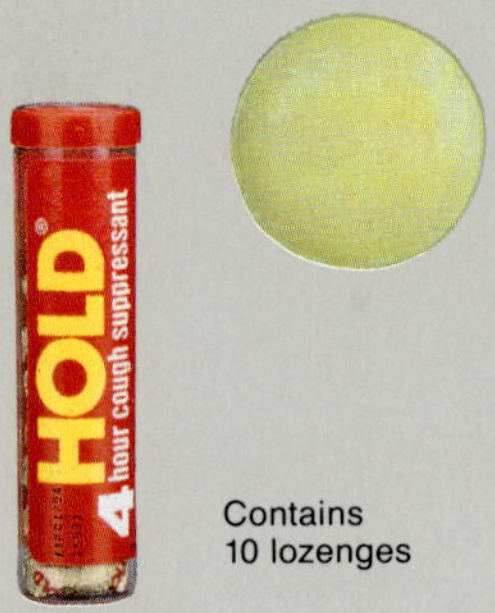

Contains 10 lozenges

HOLD®
Cough Suppressant
Lozenges with Dextromethorphan

MILES INC.

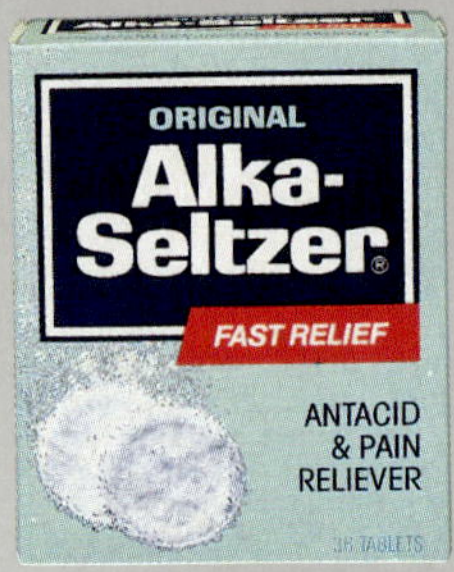

**ALKA-SELTZER®
EFFERVESCENT
ANTACID & PAIN RELIEVER**

Miles Inc.
Consumer Healthcare Division

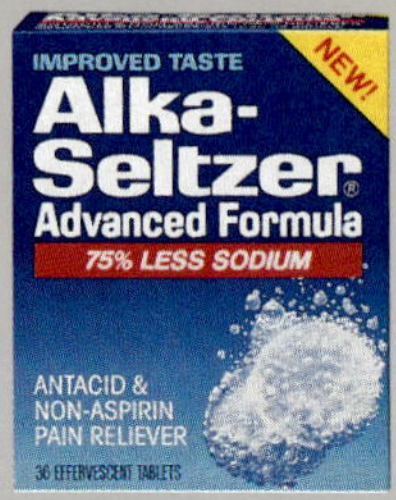

**ALKA-SELTZER®
ADVANCED FORMULA**

Miles Inc.
Consumer Healthcare Division

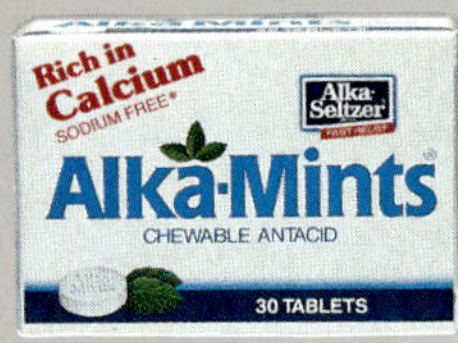

**ALKA-MINTS® CHEWABLE
ANTACID**
(Calcium Carbonate 850 mg)

Menley & James

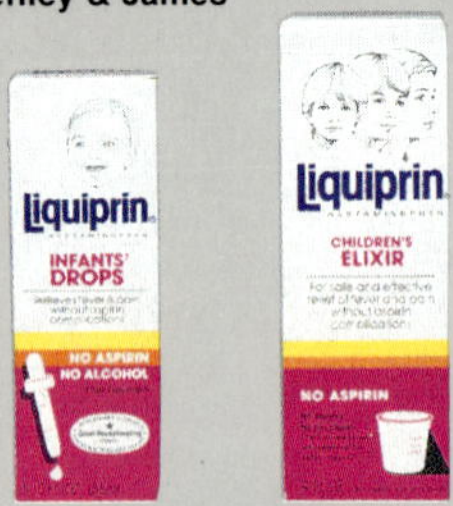

1.16 fl. oz. 4 fl. oz.
Fruit Flavored Drops and
Cherry Elixir
Alcohol Free
Child Resistant Safety Cap

LIQUIPRIN®
Acetaminophen

Miles Inc.
Consumer Healthcare Division

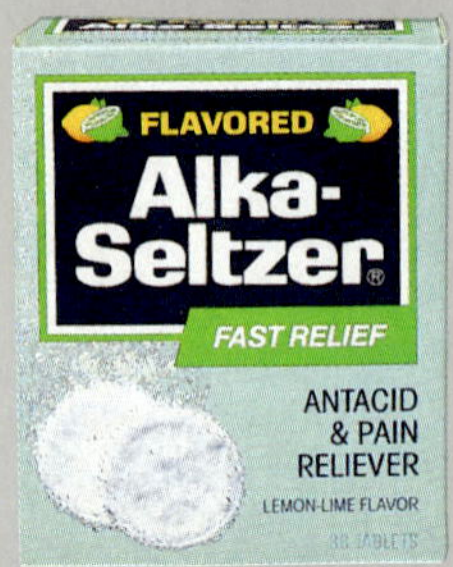

**ALKA-SELTZER®
FLAVORED EFFERVESCENT
ANTACID & PAIN RELIEVER**

Miles Inc.
Consumer Healthcare Division

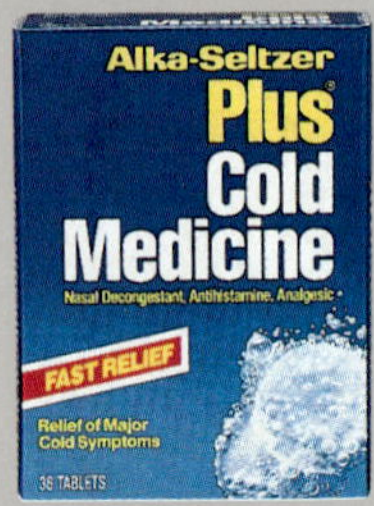

**ALKA-SELTZER PLUS®
COLD MEDICINE**

Miles Inc.
Consumer Healthcare Division

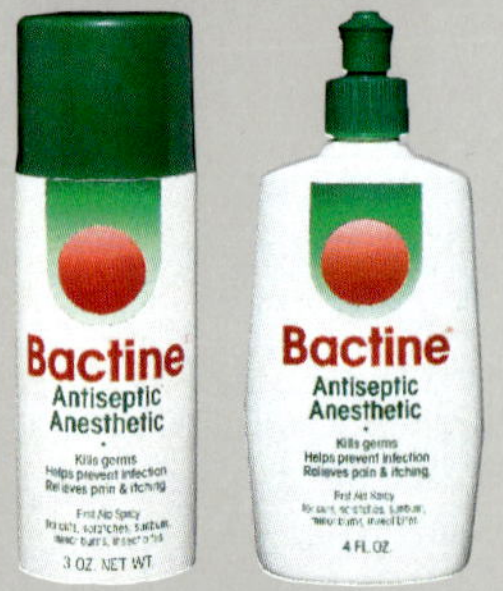

**BACTINE®
ANTISEPTIC • ANESTHETIC
FIRST AID SPRAY**
Aerosol and Liquid

Menley & James

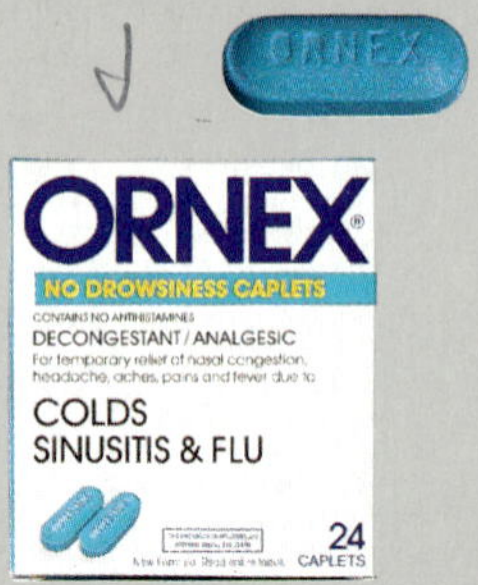

Packages of 24 and
48 caplets

ORNEX® CAPLETS
Decongestant/Analgesic

Miles Inc.
Consumer Healthcare Division

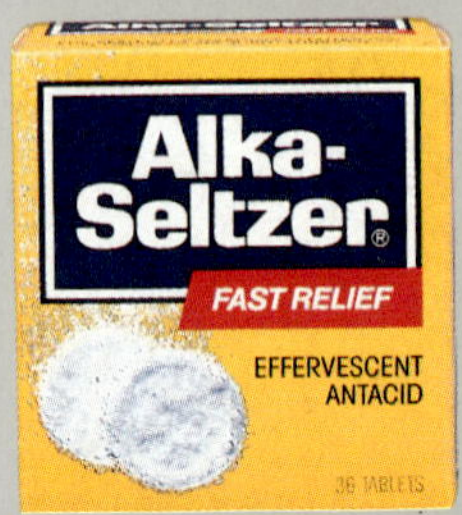

**ALKA-SELTZER®
EFFERVESCENT ANTACID**

Miles Inc.
Consumer Healthcare Division

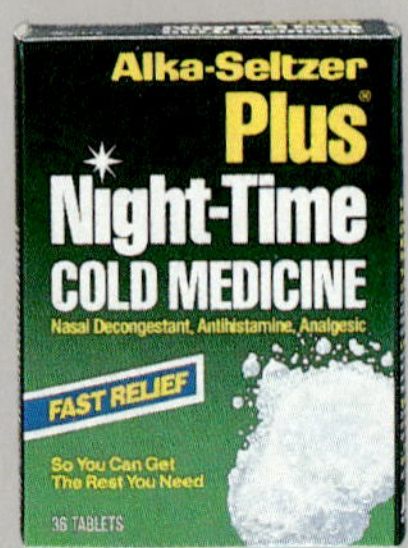

**ALKA-SELTZER PLUS®
NIGHT-TIME
COLD MEDICINE**

Miles Inc.
Consumer Healthcare Division

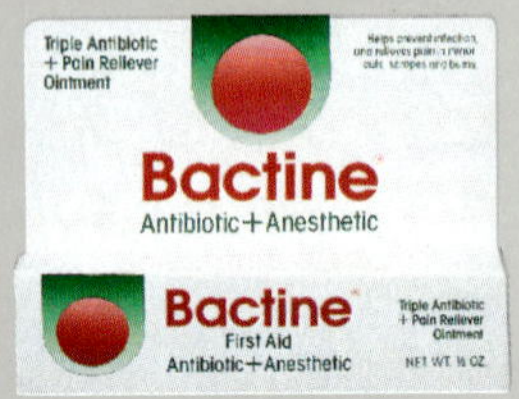

**BACTINE®
FIRST AID
ANTIBIOTIC OINTMENT**

Menley & James

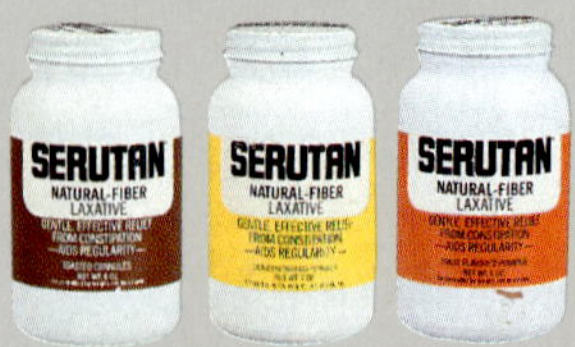

Toasted Granules Concentrated Powder Fruit Flavored

**SERUTAN®
Natural Fiber
Therapy For Regularity (psyllium)**

Available in:
Toasted Granules—6 and 18 oz.
Regular Powder—7, 14 and 21 oz.
Fruit Flavored Powder—6, 12 and 18 oz.

Miles Inc.
Consumer Healthcare Division

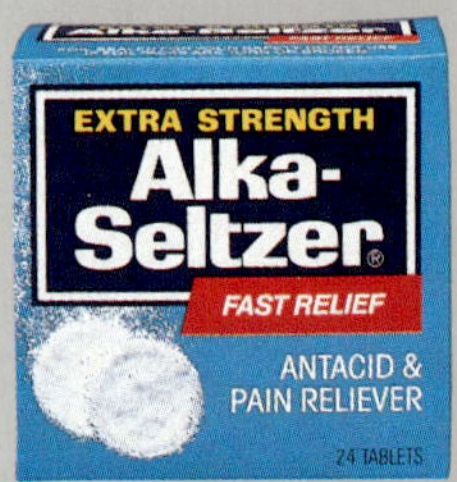

**ALKA-SELTZER®
EXTRA STRENGTH
EFFERVESCENT ANTACID &
PAIN RELIEVER**

Miles Inc.
Consumer Healthcare Division

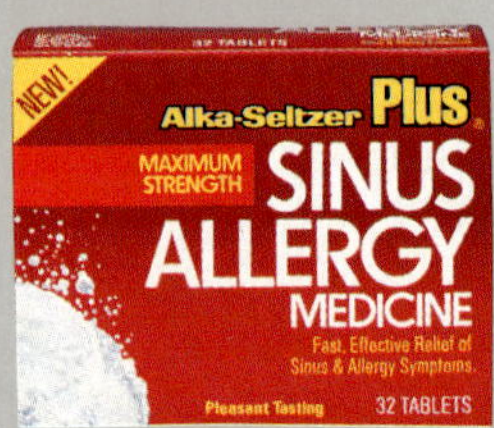

**ALKA-SELTZER PLUS®
SINUS ALLERGY
MEDICINE**

Miles Inc.
Consumer Healthcare Division

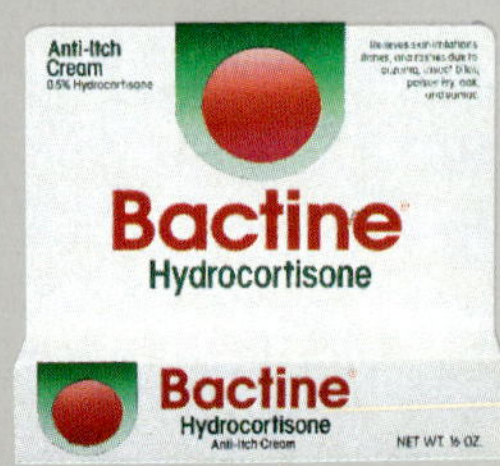

**BACTINE®
HYDROCORTISONE (0.5%)
SKIN CARE CREAM**

Miles Inc.
Consumer Healthcare Division

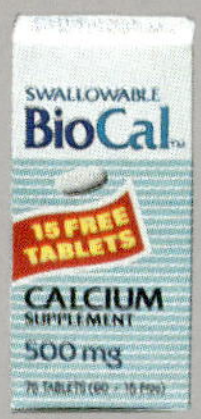

500 mg

BIOCAL™
CALCIUM SUPPLEMENT
(Calcium Carbonate)

Miles Inc.
Consumer Healthcare Division

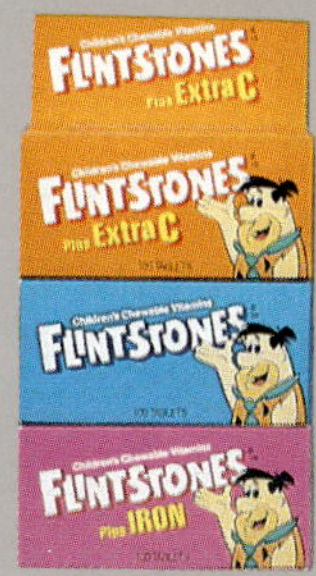

FLINTSTONES® BRAND
CHILDREN'S CHEWABLE VITAMINS
WITH EXTRA C, REGULAR,
AND PLUS IRON

Miles Inc.
Consumer Healthcare Division

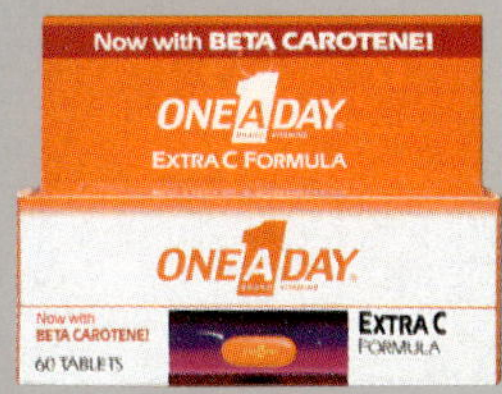

ONE A DAY® BRAND PLUS EXTRA C
VITAMINS
11 essential vitamins
with high potency
300 mg Vitamin C

NATURE'S BOUNTY

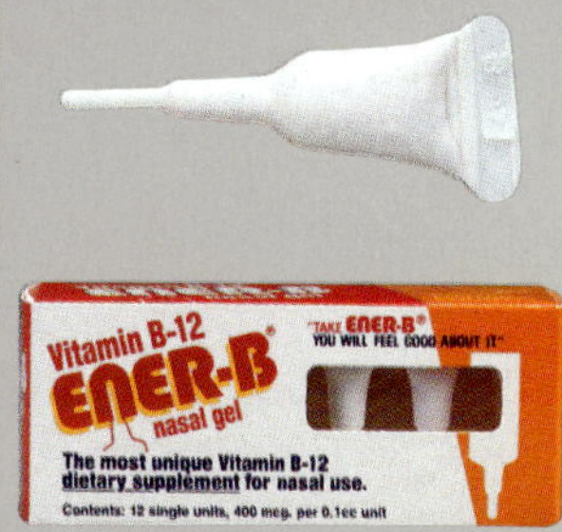

ENER-B®
Vitamin B-12 Nasal Gel

Miles Inc.
Consumer Healthcare Division

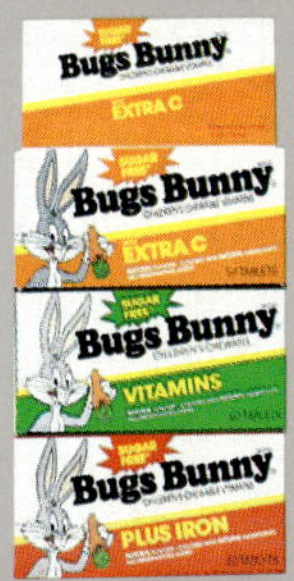

BUGS BUNNY® BRAND SUGAR FREE
CHILDREN'S CHEWABLE VITAMINS
WITH EXTRA C, REGULAR,
AND PLUS IRON

Miles Inc.
Consumer Healthcare Division

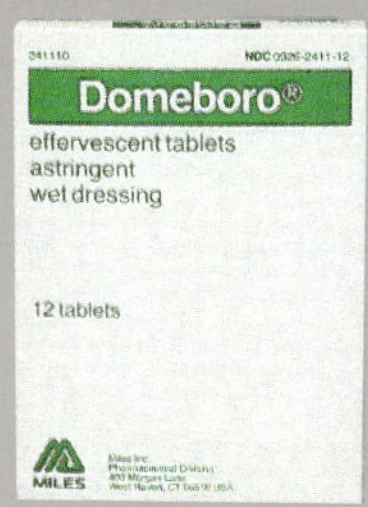

DOMEBORO®
ASTRINGENT SOLUTION

Miles Inc.
Consumer Healthcare Division

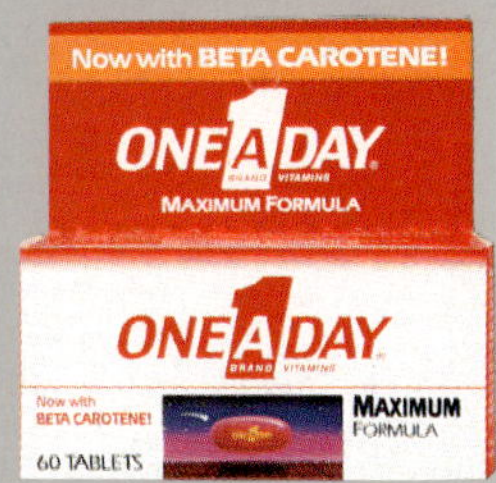

ONE A DAY® BRAND
MAXIMUM FORMULA
THE MOST COMPLETE
ONE A DAY® BRAND

NEUTRIN DRUG

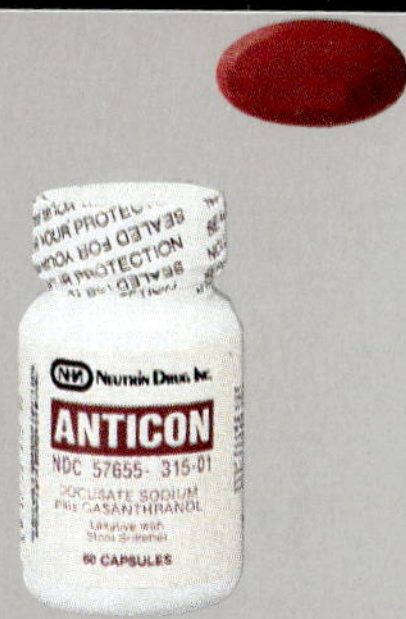

ANTICON
Laxative and Stool
Softener

Miles Inc.
Consumer Healthcare Division

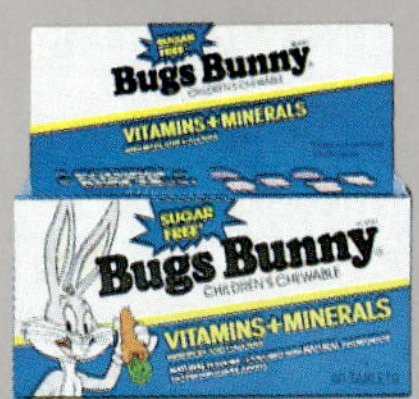

BUGS BUNNY® BRAND SUGAR FREE
CHILDREN'S CHEWABLE
VITAMINS + MINERALS

Miles Inc.
Consumer Healthcare Division

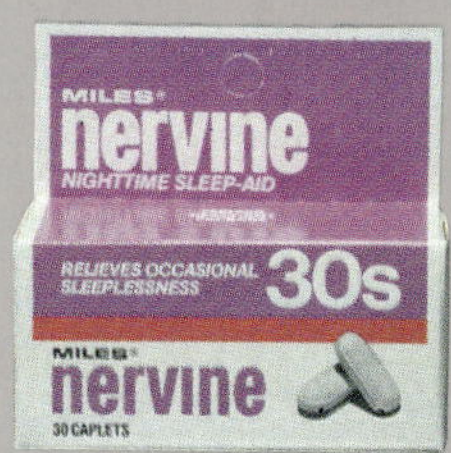

MILES® NERVINE
NIGHTTIME SLEEP-AID
(Diphenhydramine HCl 25 mg)

Miles Inc.
Consumer Healthcare Division

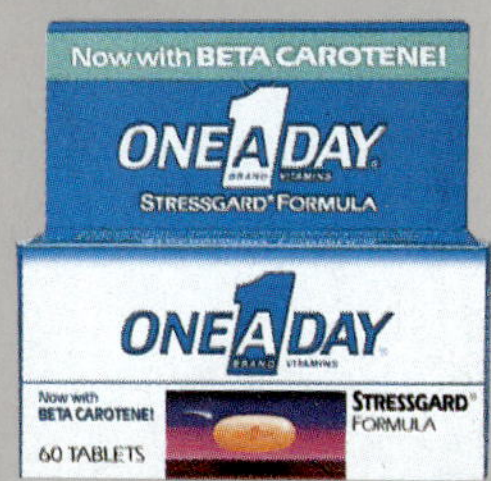

STRESSGARD®
STRESS FORMULA VITAMINS

NEUTROGENA

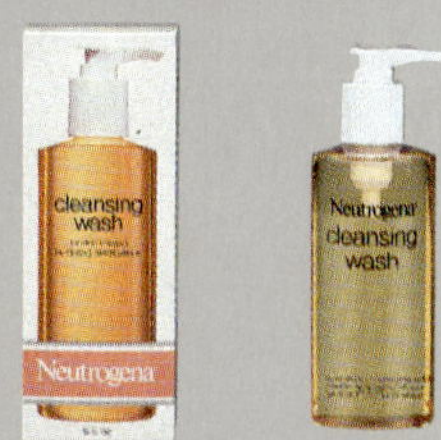

6 fl. oz.

NEUTROGENA® CLEANSING WASH

Especially formulated for
skin irritated by
drying medications

Miles Inc.
Consumer Healthcare Division

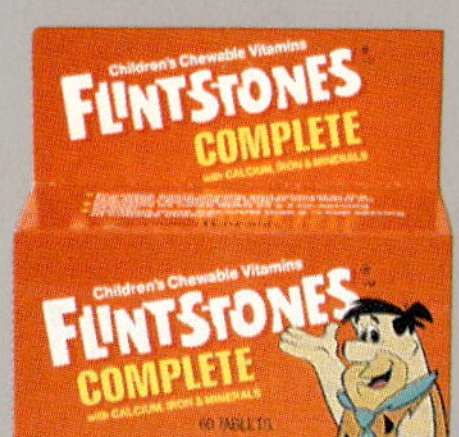

FLINTSTONES® BRAND COMPLETE
CHILDREN'S CHEWABLE VITAMINS
WITH IRON, CALCIUM & MINERALS

Miles Inc.
Consumer Healthcare Division

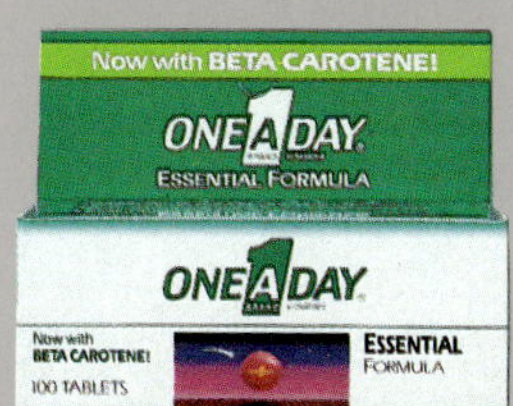

ONE A DAY® BRAND
ESSENTIAL VITAMINS

Miles Inc.
Consumer Healthcare Division

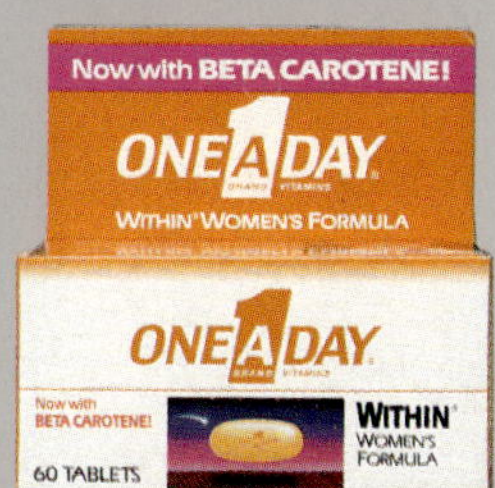

ONE-A-DAY® WITHIN®
Advanced Multivitamin
For Women With Calcium &
Extra Iron

Neutrogena

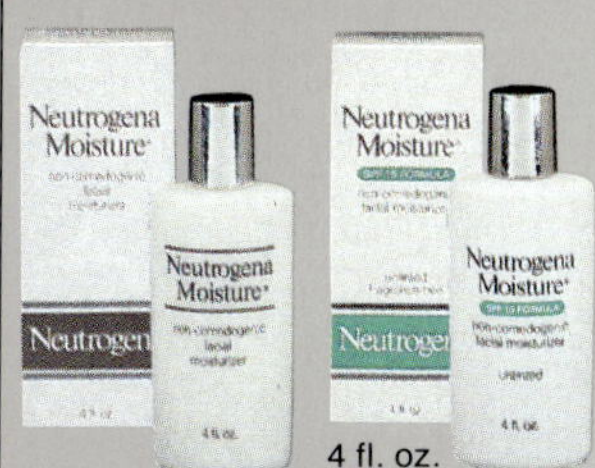

4 fl. oz.

NEUTROGENA MOISTURE®
and
NEUTROGENA MOISTURE®
SPF 15 Formula Untinted*

Non-Comedogenic
Facial Moisturizer
*Also available in Sheer Tint

Neutrogena

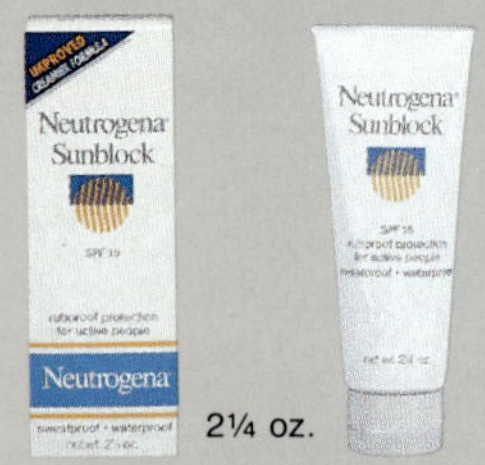

2¼ oz.

NEUTROGENA® SUNBLOCK SPF 15

Ideal for the Active Patient

Rubproof—Sweatproof Waterproof—Paba-free

ORTHO

Ortho—Advanced Care Prods.

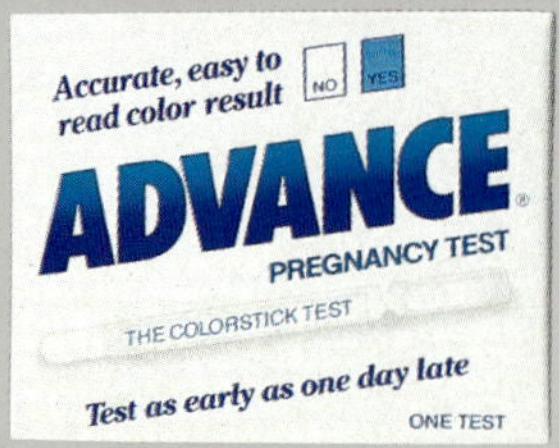

Test as early as one day late
ADVANCE®
Pregnancy Test

Ortho—Advanced Care Prods.

Available in Single and Double Kits

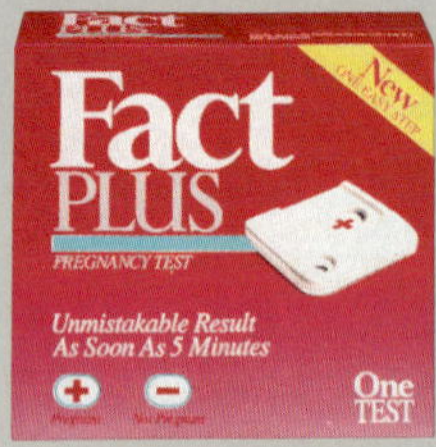

One Step Unmistakable +/– Result
FACT PLUS®
Pregnancy Test

PARKE-DAVIS

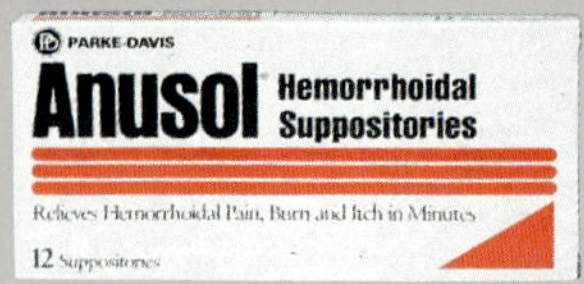

Available in boxes of 12, 24 and 48

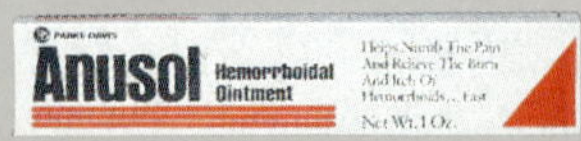

Available in 1 Oz. and 2 Oz. Tubes

ANUSOL®
Suppositories and Ointment

NUMARK

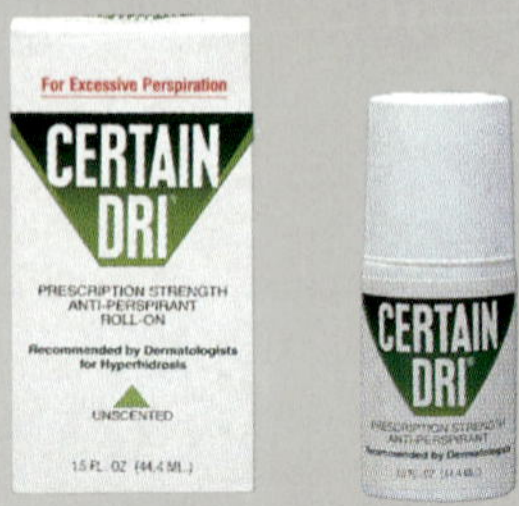

CERTAIN DRI®
Anti-Perspirant Roll-On

For Excessive Perspiration

Ortho—Advanced Care Prods.

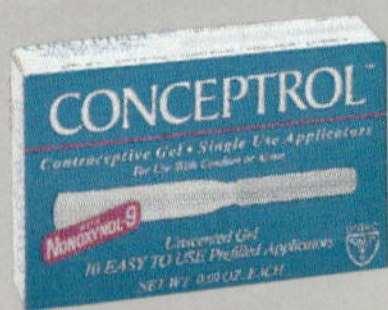

CONCEPTROL®
Contraceptive Gel
Single Use Contraceptive
[nonoxynol-9, 8.34% (150 mg)]

For use with condom or alone.

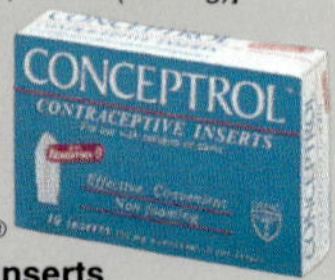

CONCEPTROL®
Contraceptive Inserts
[nonoxynol-9, 4% (100 mg)]

Ortho—Advanced Care Prods.

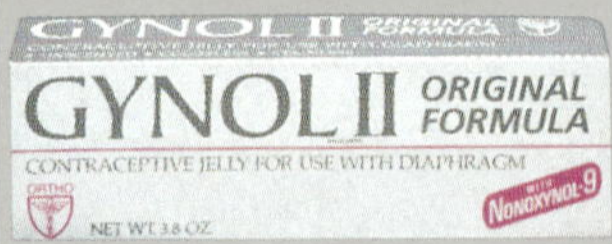

GYNOL II® ORIGINAL FORMULA
Contraceptive Jelly
[nonoxynol-9, 2% (100 mg)]

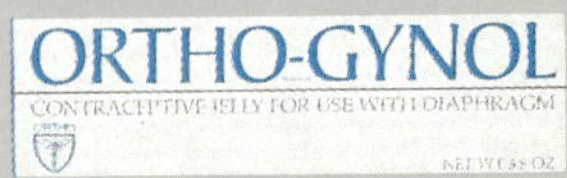

ORTHO-GYNOL®
Contraceptive Jelly
(diisobutylphenoxypolyethoxyethanol, 1%)

Parke-Davis

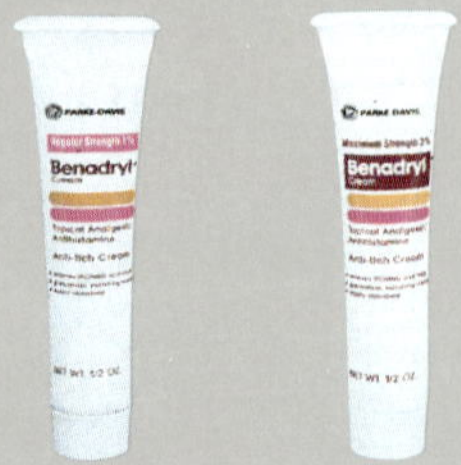

Regular Strength — Maximum Strength

BENADRYL®
Cream
Topical Antihistamine

OHM LABORATORIES

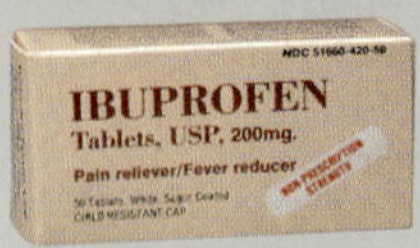

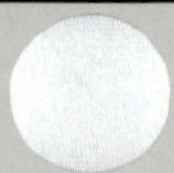

200 mg.

200 mg.

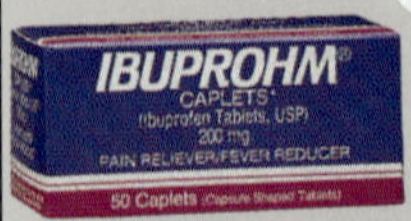

Tablets and Caplets available in bottles of 24, 50 and 100

IBUPROFEN TABLETS
IBUPROHM CAPLETS

Ortho—Advanced Care Prods.

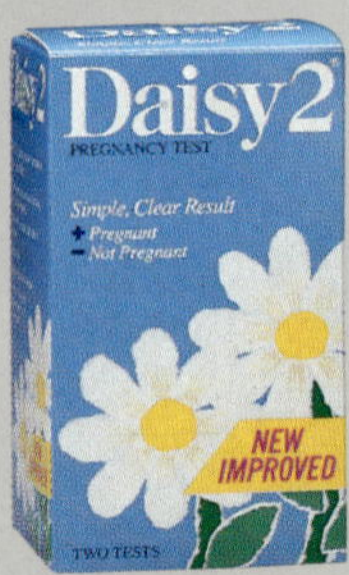

Two complete tests in each kit.

DAISY 2®
Pregnancy Test

Ortho—Advanced Care Prods.

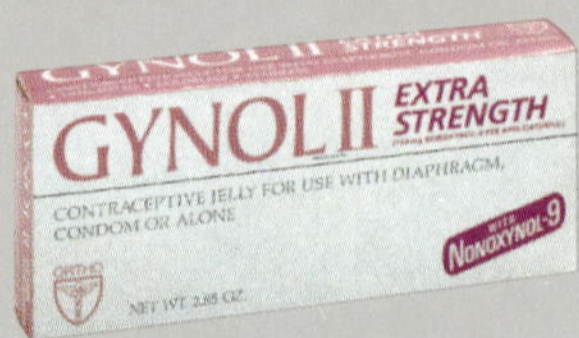

Contraceptive Jelly.
For use with condom, diaphragm or alone.

GYNOL II™
Extra Strength
[nonoxynol 9, 3% (150 mg)]

Parke-Davis

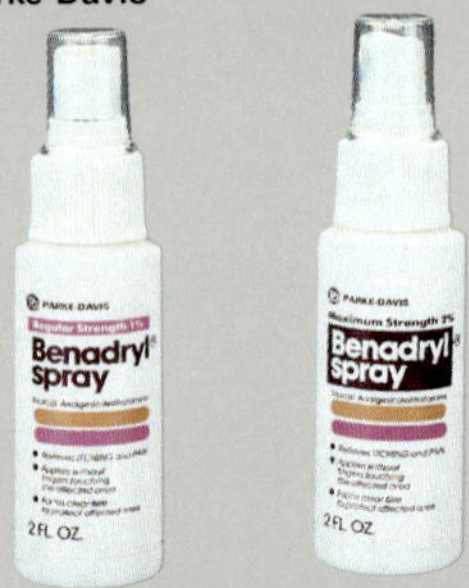

Regular Strength — Maximum Strength

BENADRYL®
Spray
Topical Antihistamine

While every effort has been made to reproduce products faithfully, this section is to be considered a Quick-Reference identification aid.

Ortho—Advanced Care Prods.

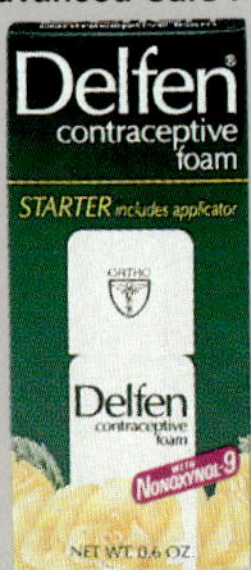

Starter (0.60 oz. vial w/applicator package)
Refill (1.40 oz. vial only packages)

DELFEN® Contraceptive Foam
[nonoxynol-9, 12.5% (100 mg)]

Ortho—Advanced Care Prods.

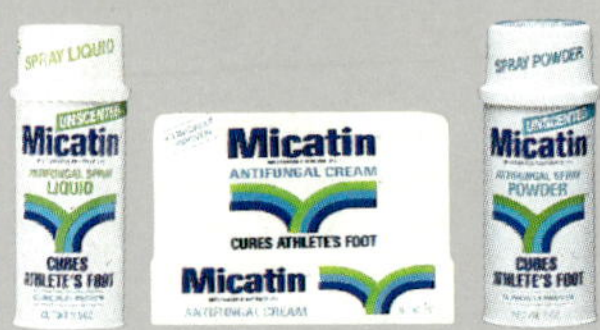

Spray Liquid (3.5 oz.) — Cream (½ oz. and 1 oz.) — Spray Powder and Spray Deodorant (3.0 oz.)

MICATIN® Antifungal
For Athlete's Foot
(miconazole nitrate, 2%)

Parke-Davis

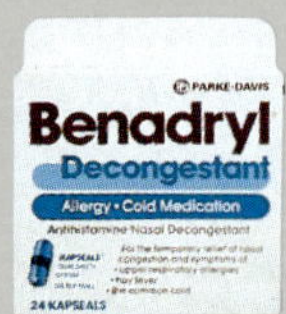

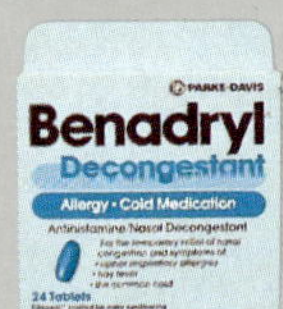

Available in boxes of 24

BENADRYL®
Decongestant

Parke-Davis

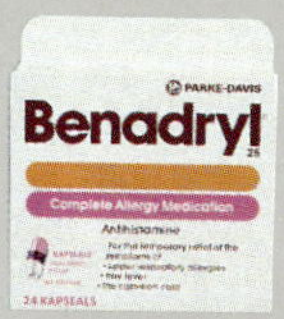

Kapseals available in boxes of 24 and 48

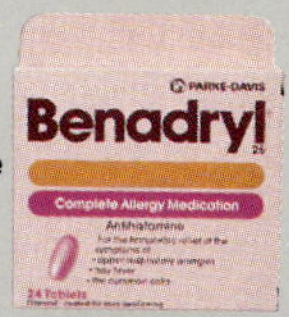

Tablets available in boxes of 24 and bottles of 100

BENADRYL® 25

Parke-Davis

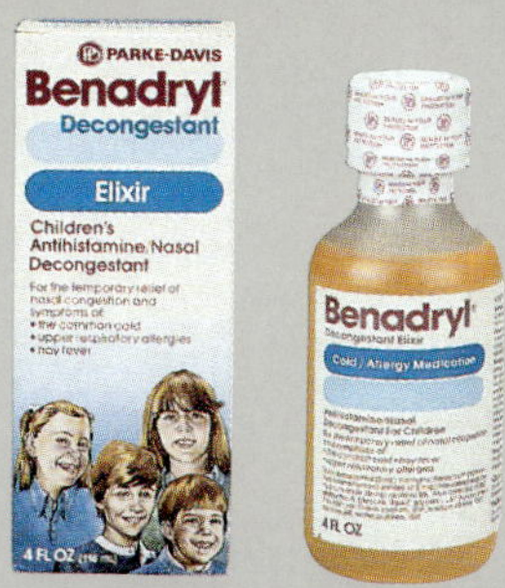

Available in 4 Oz. Bottles

BENADRYL®
Decongestant Elixir

Parke-Davis

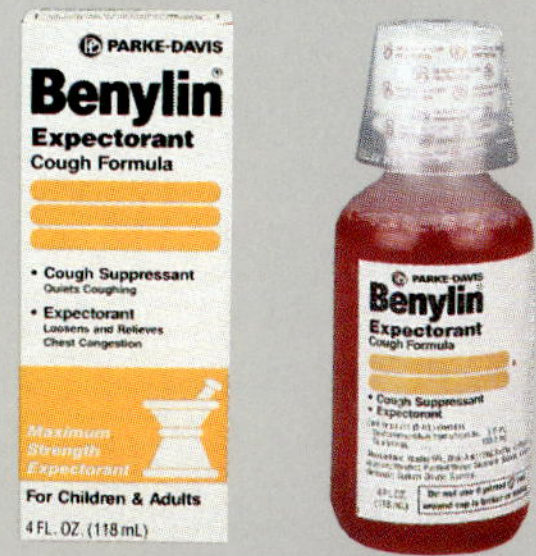

Available in 4 Oz. and 8 Oz. Bottles

BENYLIN® EXPECTORANT

Parke-Davis

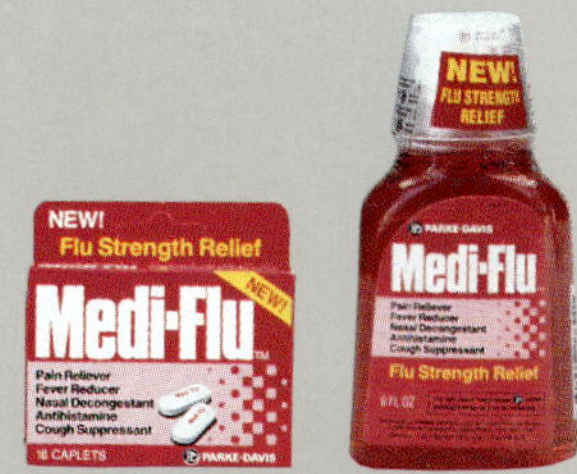

16 Caplets 6 Fl. Oz.

FLU STRENGTH RELIEF™
MEDI-FLU™

Parke-Davis

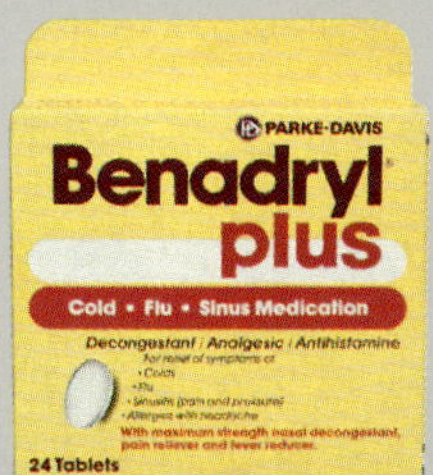

Available in boxes of 24 and 48

BENADRYL® PLUS
Decongestant/Analgesic/
Antihistamine

Parke-Davis

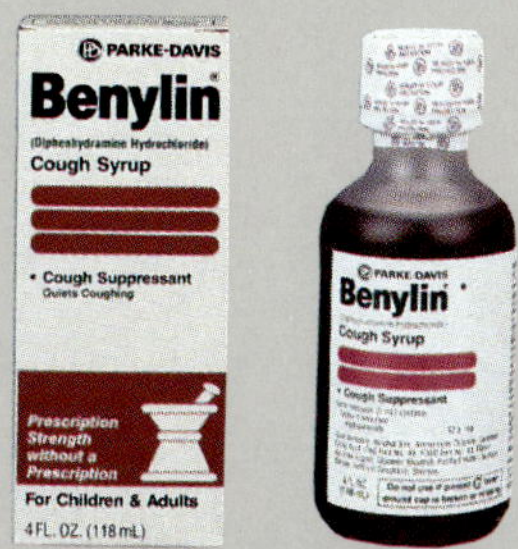

Available in 4 Oz. and 8 Oz. Bottles

BENYLIN®
Cough Syrup

Parke-Davis

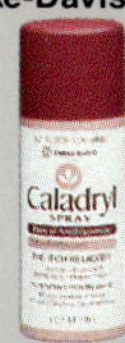

Spray

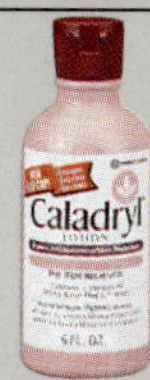

Lotion

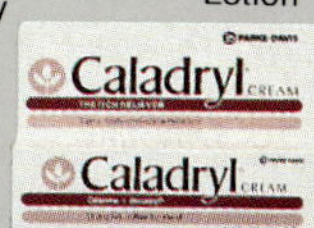

Cream

For relief from itching due to:
Poison Ivy, Insect Bites, Poison Oak,
Skin Irritation

CALADRYL®
Topical Antihistamine/Skin Protectant

Parke-Davis

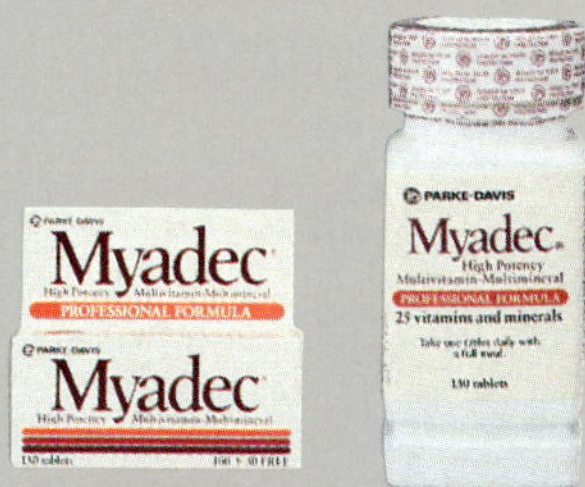

Available in bottles of 130 Tablets

MYADEC®
Multivitamin-Multimineral
Supplement

Parke-Davis

Honey-Lemon Flavor

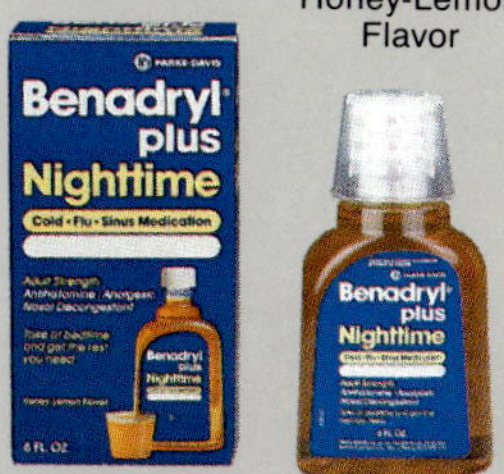

Available in 6 Fl. Oz. and 10 Fl. Oz. Bottles

BENADRYL® PLUS
NIGHTTIME

Parke-Davis

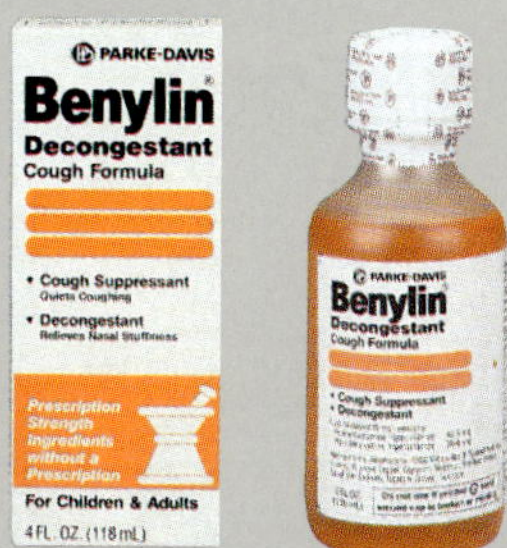

Available in 4 Oz. Bottles

BENYLIN®
Decongestant Cough Formula

Parke-Davis

1 test kit

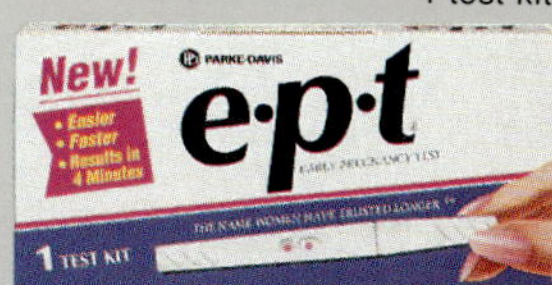

e·p·t® Simple to do.
Easy to read.
Accurate results in 4 minutes.

e·p·t®
STICK TEST
Early Pregnancy Test

Parke-Davis

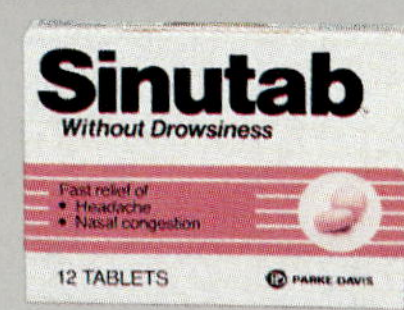

Easy-to-open package
(Non-child resistant)

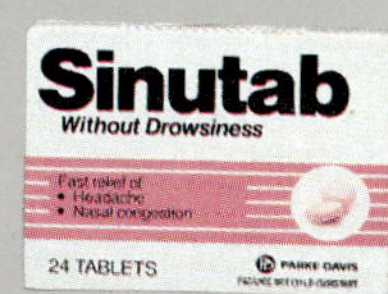

Child-resistant package
REGULAR SINUTAB®

Parke-Davis

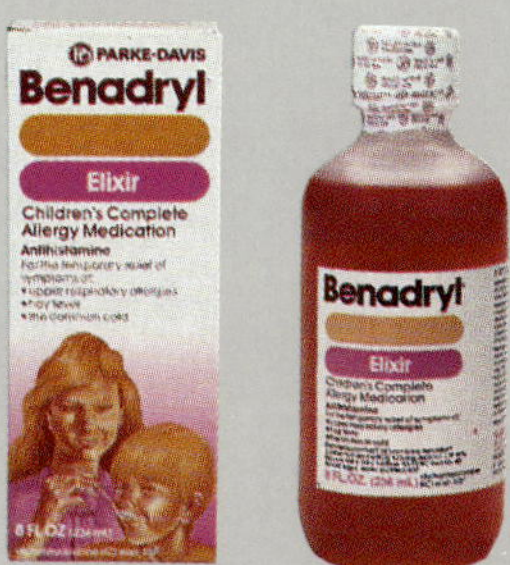

Available in 4 Oz. and 8 Oz. Bottles

BENADRYL®
Elixir

Parke-Davis

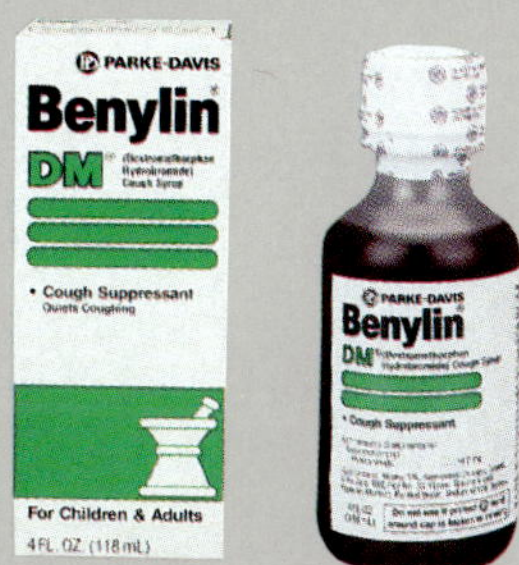

Available in 4 Oz. Bottles

BENYLIN DM®
Cough Syrup

Parke-Davis

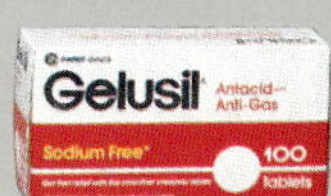

100 tablets
Also available:
50 tablets

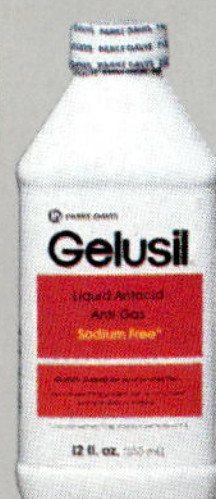

GELUSIL®
Antacid-Anti-gas
Sodium Free

12 Fl. Oz.

Parke-Davis

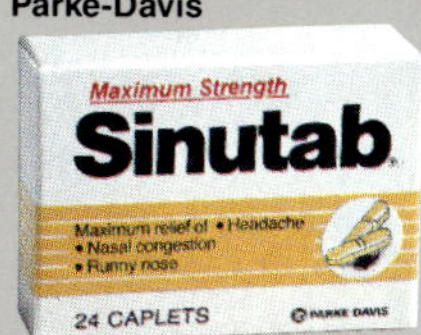

Caplets

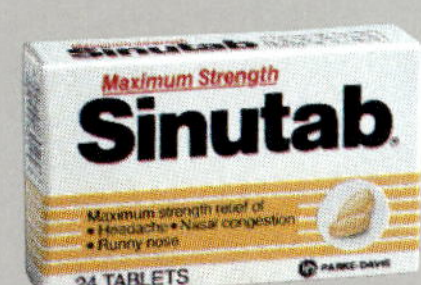

Tablets

MAXIMUM STRENGTH
SINUTAB®

Parke-Davis

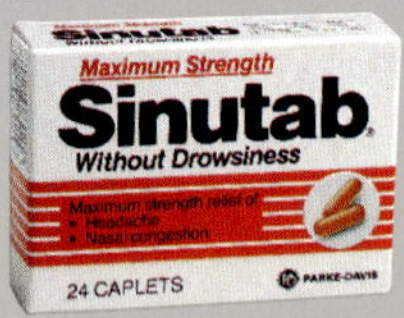

Caplets

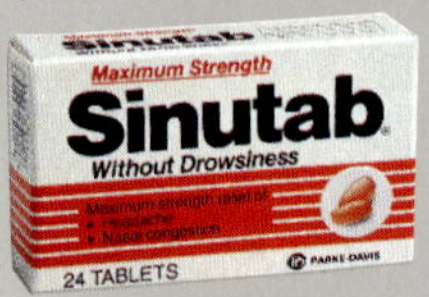

Tablets

MAXIMUM STRENGTH SINUTAB® Without Drowsiness

PFIZER

Consumer Health Care

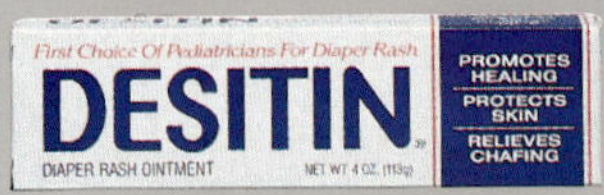

DESITIN® Diaper Rash Ointment

Procter & Gamble

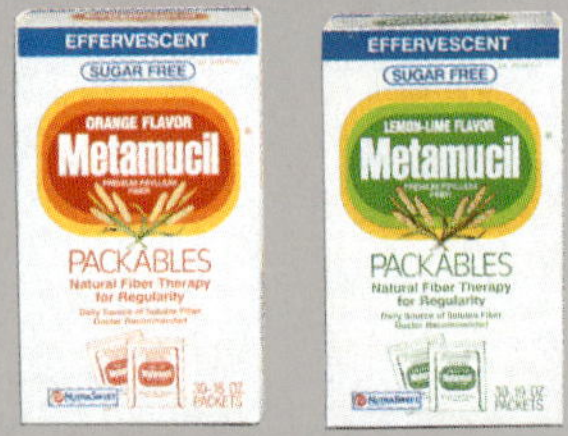

EFFERVESCENT SUGAR FREE METAMUCIL® Natural Therapeutic Fiber for Regularity

Procter & Gamble

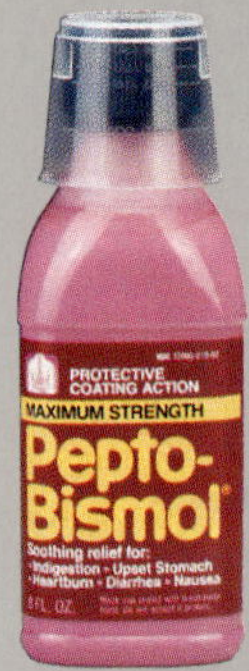

Liquid available in 4 oz., 8 oz. and 12 oz. plastic bottles

PEPTO-BISMOL® MAXIMUM STRENGTH LIQUID

Parke-Davis

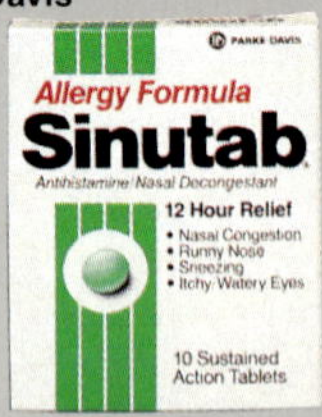

10 Sustained Action Tablets

12 Hour Relief of Nasal Congestion, Runny Nose, Sneezing, Itchy/Watery Eyes

ALLERGY FORMULA SINUTAB®

Consumer Health Care

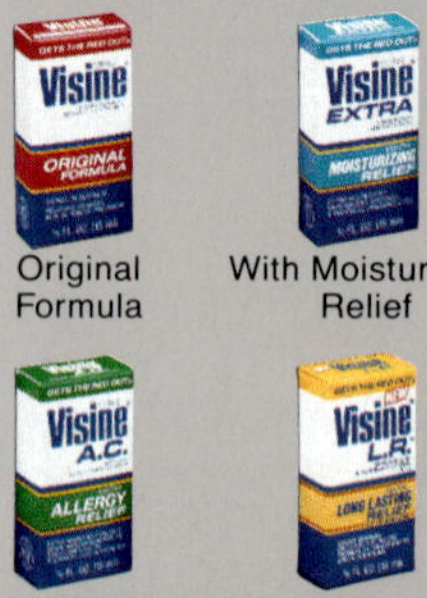

Original Formula

With Moisturizing Relief

With Allergy Relief

With Long Lasting Relief

VISINE® Redness Reliever Eye Drops

Procter & Gamble

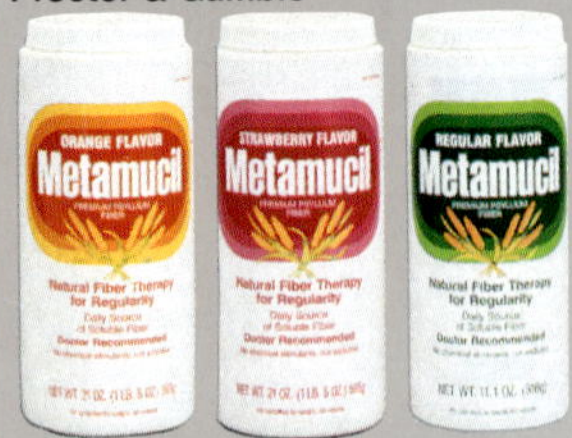

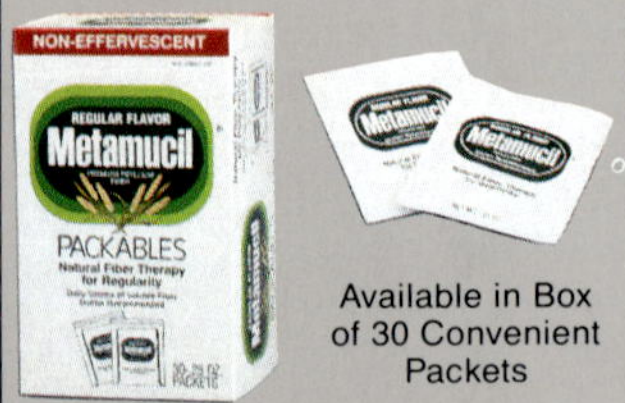

Available in Box of 30 Convenient Packets

METAMUCIL®

Natural Therapeutic Fiber for Regularity

Procter & Gamble

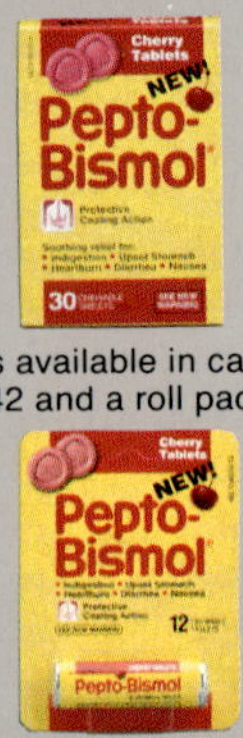

Tablets available in cartons of 30 & 42 and a roll pack of 12

PEPTO-BISMOL® CHERRY TABLETS

Parke-Davis

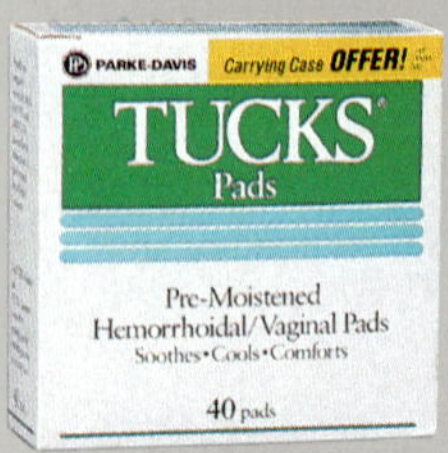

40 pads

Also available in 100 pad packages

TUCKS® Pre-Moistened Pads

PROCTER & GAMBLE

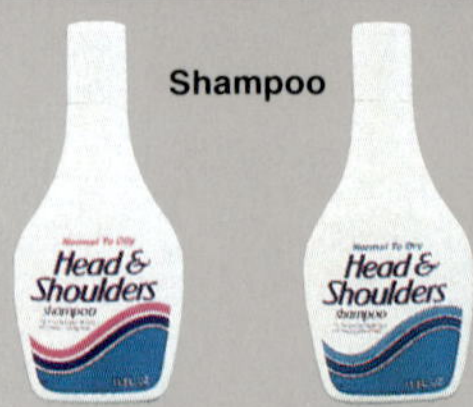

Shampoo

Normal to Oily

Normal to Dry

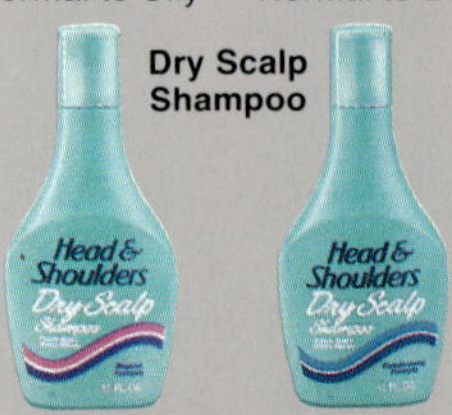

Dry Scalp Shampoo

Regular Formula

Conditioning Formula

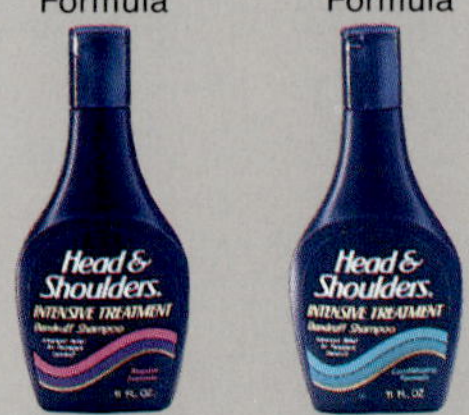

Regular Formula

Conditioning Formula

Intensive Treatment Dandruff Shampoo

HEAD & SHOULDERS®

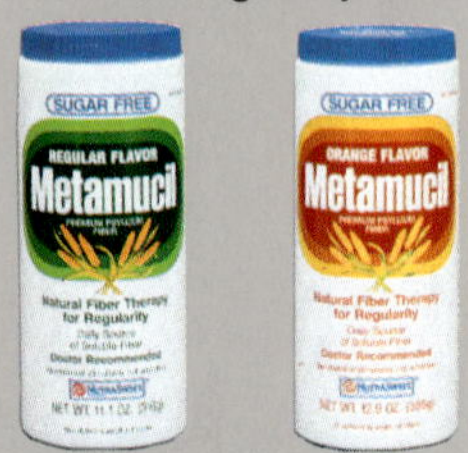

SUGAR FREE METAMUCIL®

Natural Therapeutic Fiber for Regularity

REED & CARNRICK

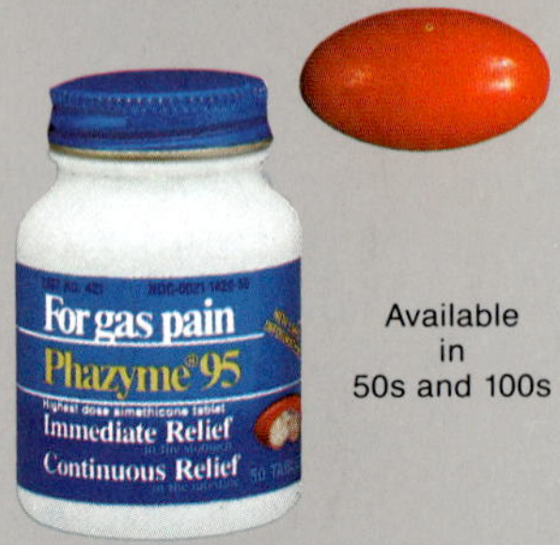

Available in 50s and 100s

PHAZYME® 95
An antiflatulent to alleviate or relieve symptoms of gas.

Parke-Davis

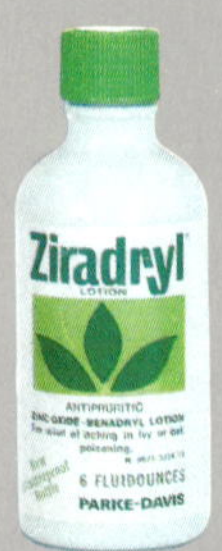

6 Fl. Oz.

ZIRADRYL® LOTION

Procter & Gamble

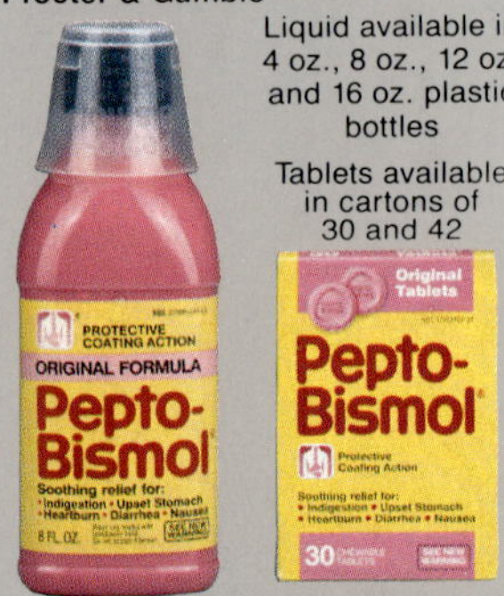

Liquid available in 4 oz., 8 oz., 12 oz. and 16 oz. plastic bottles

Tablets available in cartons of 30 and 42

PEPTO-BISMOL® ORIGINAL FORMULA LIQUID AND ORIGINAL TABLETS

Reed & Carnrick

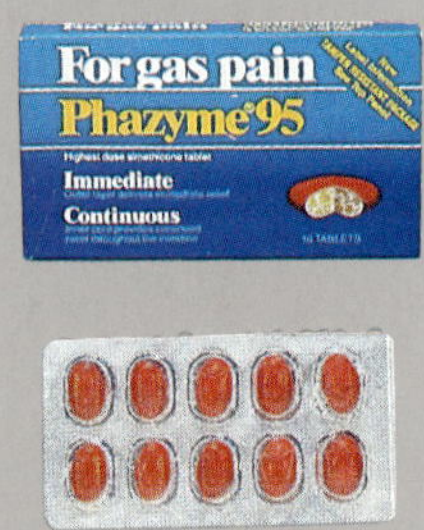

PHAZYME® 95 Consumer 10 Packs

An antiflatulent to alleviate or relieve symptoms of gas.

Reed & Carnrick

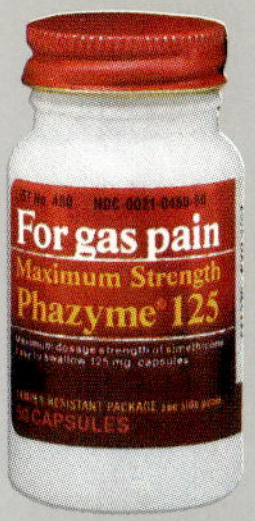

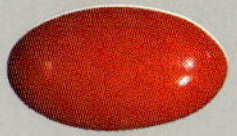

Available in 50s

MAXIMUM STRENGTH PHAZYME® 125

An antiflatulent to alleviate or relieve symptoms of gas. Softgel capsule for ease of swallowing.

Reed & Carnrick

Available in 2 and 4 fl. oz. sizes

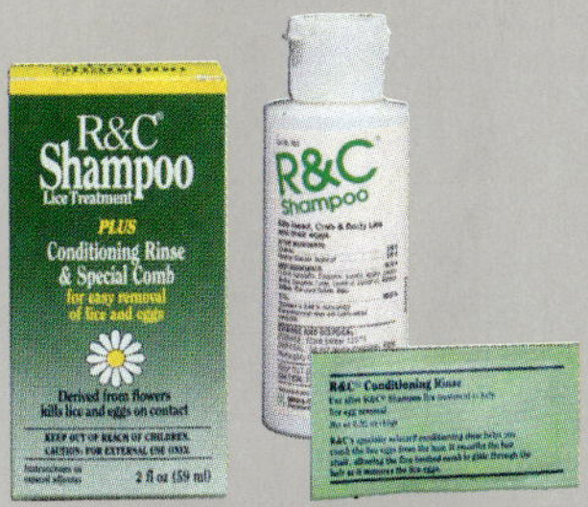

R&C SHAMPOO®

Kills head, crab and body lice and their eggs. Effective nit comb and R&C Conditioning Rinse Packet included.

Reese

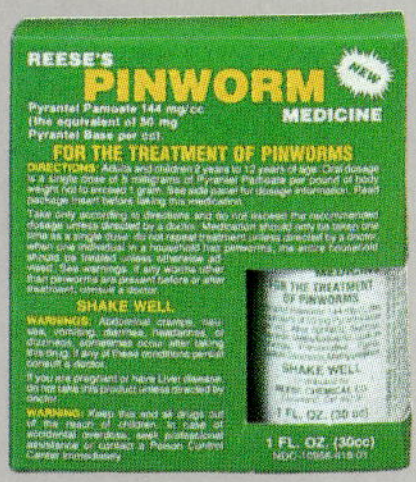

REESE'S PINWORM MEDICINE

With English and Spanish directions

Rhône-Poulenc Rorer Consumer Div.

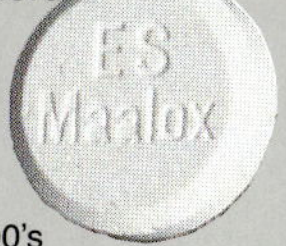

Tablets: 24's, 50's, 100's

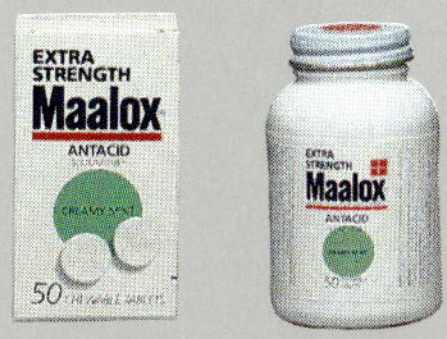

EXTRA STRENGTH MAALOX®

(dried aluminum hydroxide gel 400 mg and magnesium hydroxide 400 mg)

Reed & Carnrick

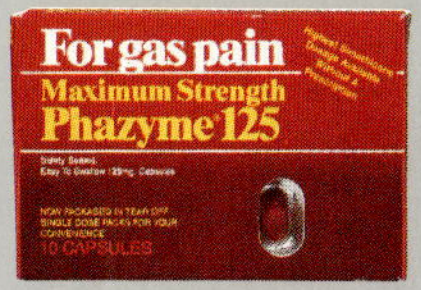

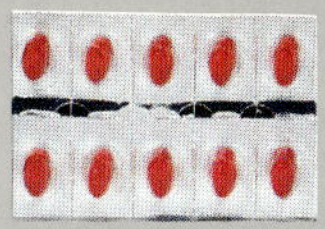

MAXIMUM STRENGTH PHAZYME® 125 Consumer 10 Packs

An antiflatulent to alleviate or relieve symptoms of gas.

Reed & Carnrick

Available in 5 and 10 oz. sizes

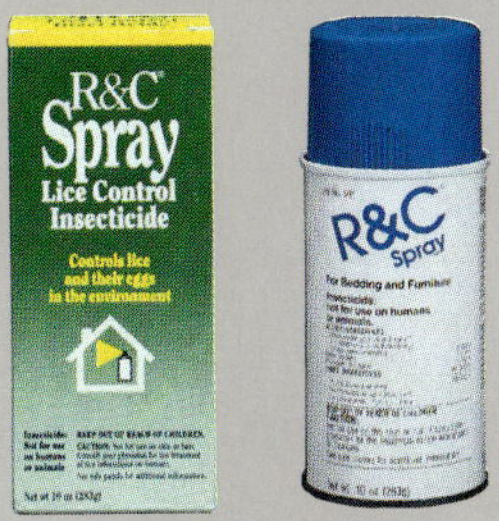

R&C SPRAY®

Controls lice and their eggs in the home. Insecticide: not for use on humans or animals.

Reese

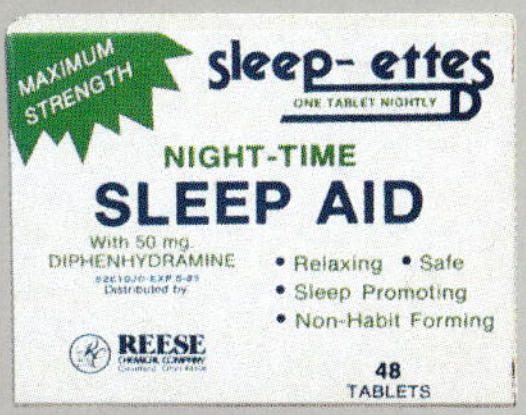

24's and 48's

SLEEP-ETTES-D

Maximum Strength with 50 mg. Diphenhydramine

Rhône-Poulenc Rorer Consumer Div.

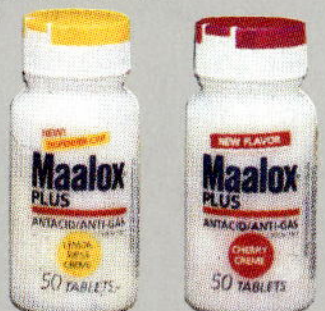

Lemon and Cherry Tablets 50's, 100's

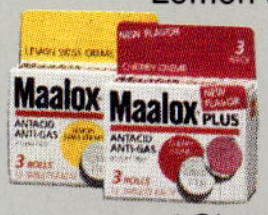

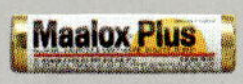

Lemon and Cherry 3 roll pack

Single Roll Lemon only

MAALOX® PLUS

(magnesium hydroxide 200 mg, dried aluminum hydroxide gel 200 mg, and simethicone 25 mg)

Reed & Carnrick

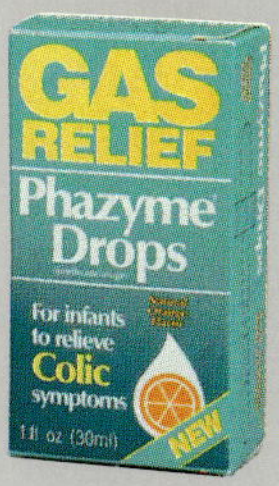

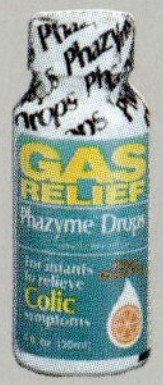

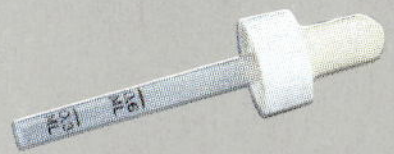

Available in 1 oz. Bottles

PHAYZME® DROPS

A liquid antiflatulent suitable for relieving infant colic symptoms and for those who prefer liquid dosage forms

Reed & Carnrick

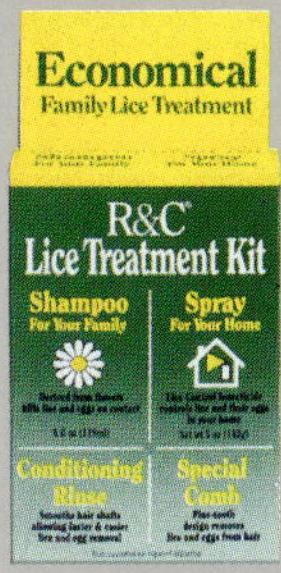

R&C LICE TREATMENT KIT

Contains 4 oz. R&C SHAMPOO, 5 oz. R&C SPRAY, R&C Conditioning Rinse Packet and nit comb.

REESE CHEMICAL CO.

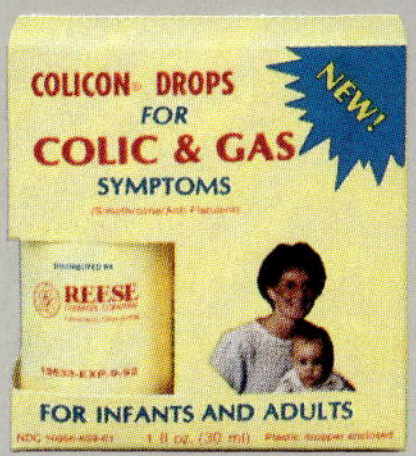

1 fl. oz. w/dropper

COLICON® DROPS

With English and Spanish directions

RHÔNE-POULENC RORER

Consumer Div.

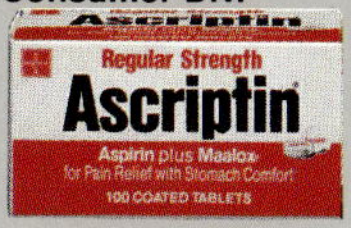

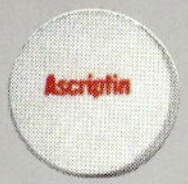

bottles of 50, 100, 225 & 500 tablets

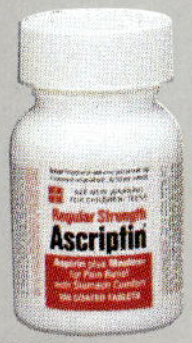

REGULAR STRENGTH ASCRIPTIN®

(Aspirin [325 mg] and Maalox [magnesium hydroxide 50 mg, dried aluminum hydroxide gel 50 mg], buffered with calcium carbonate)

Rhône-Poulenc Rorer Consumer Div.

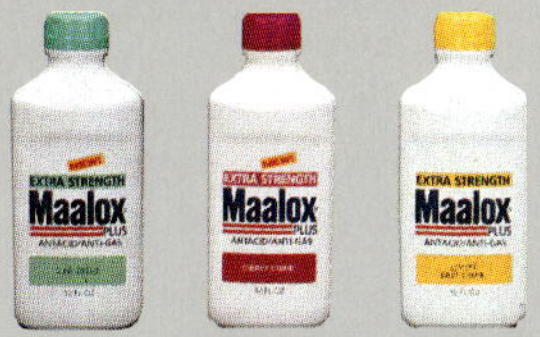

Mint | Cherry | Lemon

12 oz. Suspension

Lemon 26 oz.

EXTRA STRENGTH MAALOX® PLUS

(magnesium hydroxide 450 mg, aluminum hydroxide 500 mg, and simethicone 40 mg)

Rhône-Poulenc Rorer Consumer Div.

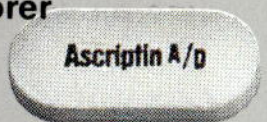

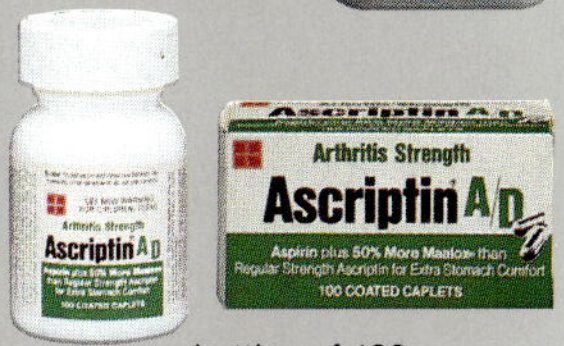

bottles of 100, 225 & 500 caplets

FOR ARTHRITIS PAIN ASCRIPTIN® A/D

(Aspirin [325 mg] and Maalox [magnesium hydroxide 75 mg, dried aluminum hydroxide gel 75 mg], buffered with calcium carbonate)

Rhône-Poulenc Rorer Consumer Div.

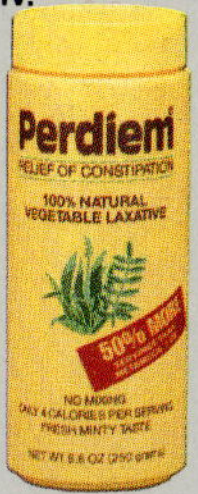

Granules 100 gm. and 250 gm.

PERDIEM®

100% Natural Vegetable Laxative

82 percent psyllium (Plantago Hydrocolloid)
18 percent senna (Cassia Pod Concentrate)

Rhône-Poulenc Rorer Consumer Div.

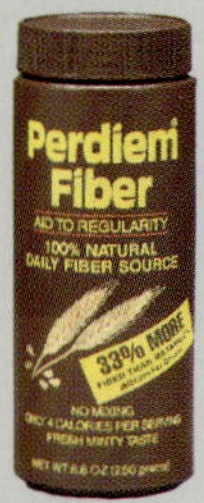

Granules
100 gm. and 250 gm.

PERDIEM® FIBER
100% Natural Daily Fiber Source
100% Psyllium (Plantago Hydrocolloid)

Richardson-Vicks Inc.

Bottles of 6 oz. and 10 oz. and packets of 20 Caplets

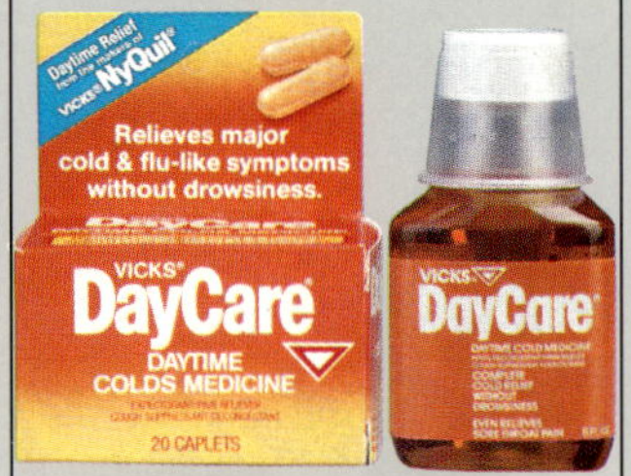

VICKS® DAYCARE®
Daytime Colds Medicine
(acetaminophen, pseudoephedrine hydrochloride, dextromethorphan hydrobromide, guaifenesin)

Richardson-Vicks Inc.

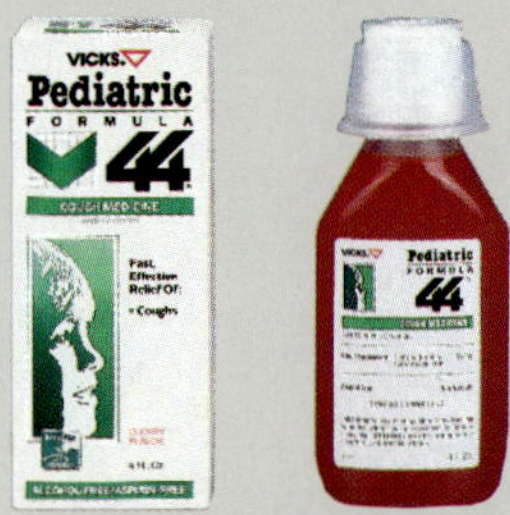

Available in 4 oz.

VICKS®
PEDIATRIC FORMULA 44®
Cough Medicine
(dextromethorphan hydrobromide)

Richardson-Vicks Inc.

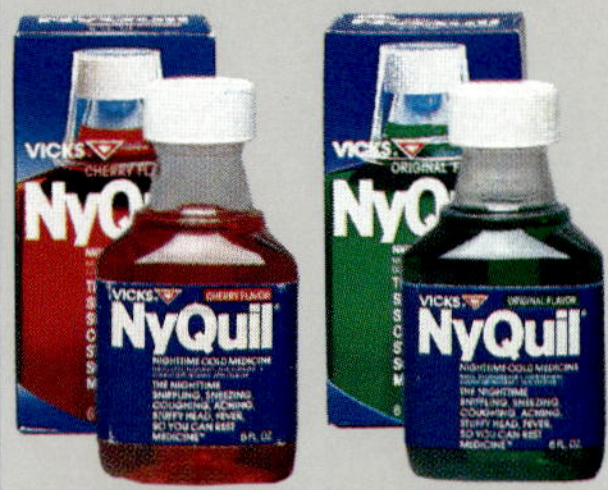

Original Flavor: 6 oz., 10 oz., 14 oz.
Cherry Flavor: 6 oz., 10 oz., 14 oz.

VICKS® NYQUIL®
NIGHTTIME COLDS MEDICINE
(acetaminophen, doxylamine succinate, pseudoephedrine hydrochloride, dextromethorphan hydrobromide)

RICHARDSON-VICKS INC.

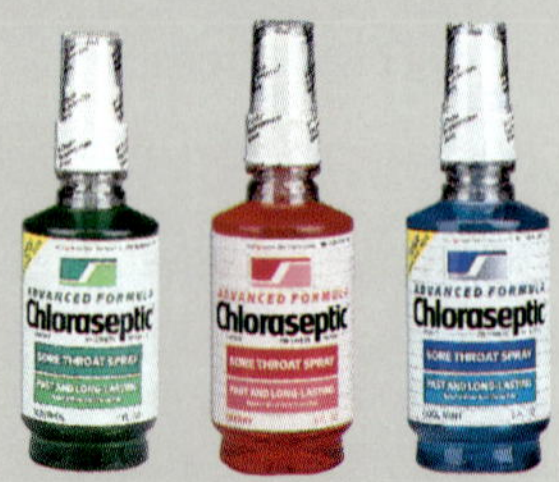

Available: Menthol, Cherry and Cool Mint in 6 oz. spray. Menthol and Cherry in 12 oz. gargle and 1.5 oz. aerosol spray.

CHLORASEPTIC® LIQUID

Richardson-Vicks Inc.

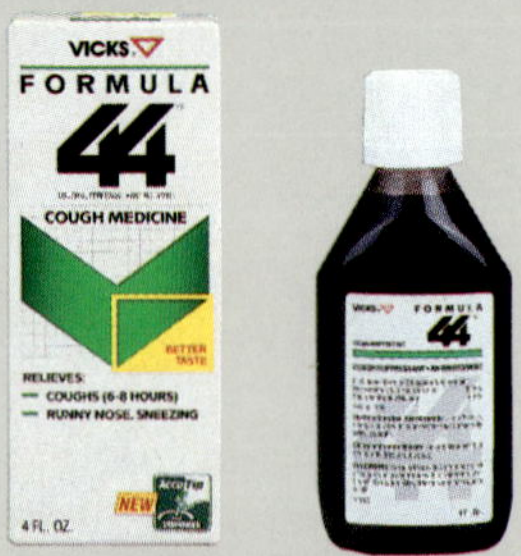

Available in 4 oz. and 8 oz.

VICKS® FORMULA 44®
Cough Medicine
(dextromethorphan hydrobromide, chlorpheniramine maleate)

Richardson-Vicks Inc.

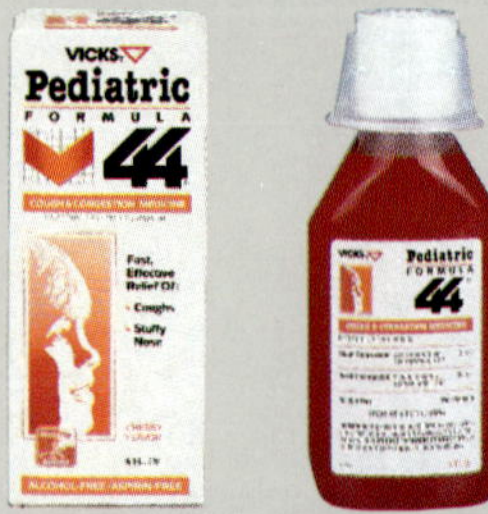

Available in 4 oz.

VICKS®
PEDIATRIC FORMULA 44®
Cough & Congestion Medicine
(dextromethorphan hydrobromide, pseudoephedrine hydrochloride)

Richardson-Vicks Inc.

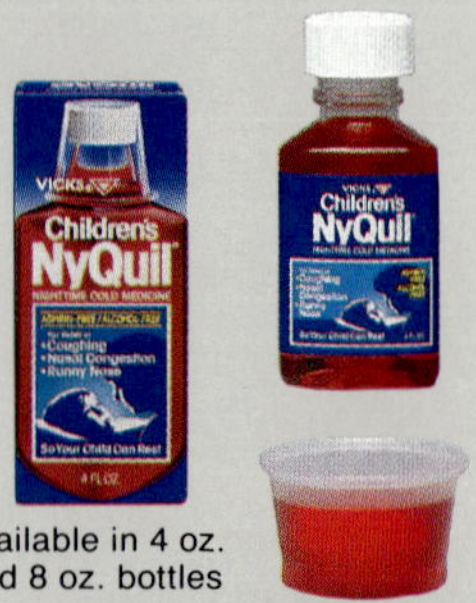

Available in 4 oz. and 8 oz. bottles

VICKS® CHILDREN'S NYQUIL®
(chlorpheniramine maleate, pseudoephedrine HCl, dextromethorphan hydrobromide)

Richardson-Vicks Inc.

Children's Grape

Cool Mint

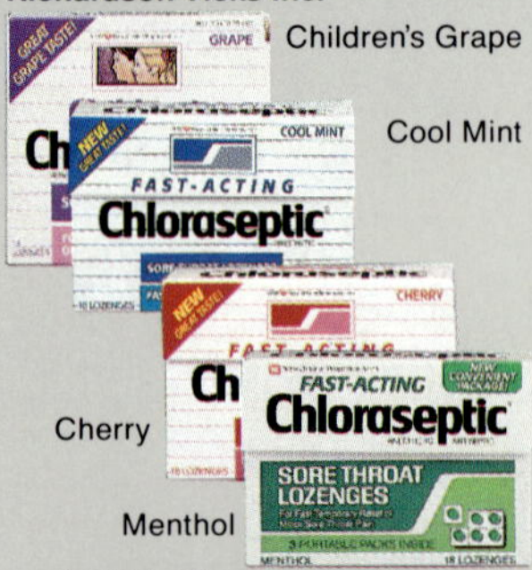

Cherry

Menthol

Available: Cherry and Cool Mint in cartons of 18 and 36; Menthol and Children's Grape in cartons of 18.

CHLORASEPTIC® LOZENGES

Richardson-Vicks Inc.

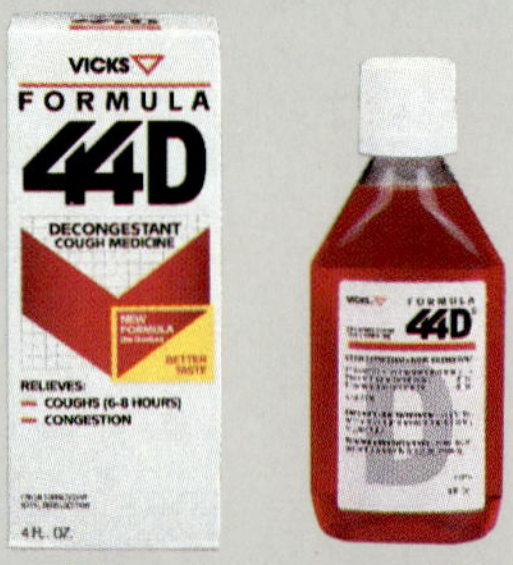

Available in 4 oz., 8 oz. and 12 oz.

VICKS® FORMULA 44D®
Decongestant Cough Medicine
(dextromethorphan hydrobromide, pseudoephedrine hydrochloride)

Richardson-Vicks Inc.

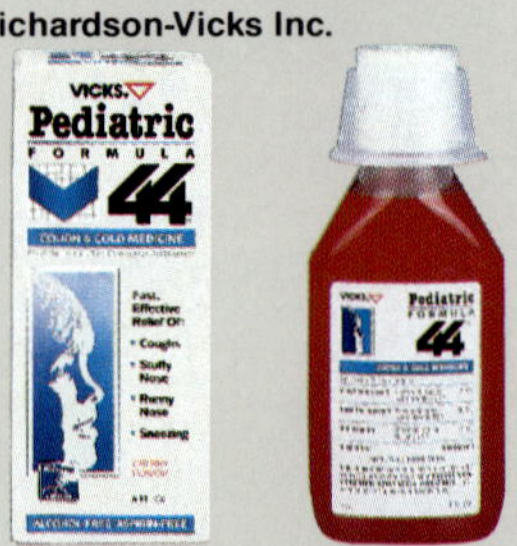

Available in 4 oz.

VICKS®
PEDIATRIC FORMULA 44®
Cough & Cold Medicine
(dextromethorphan hydrobromide, pseudoephedrine hydrochloride, chlorpheniramine maleate)

Richardson-Vicks Inc.

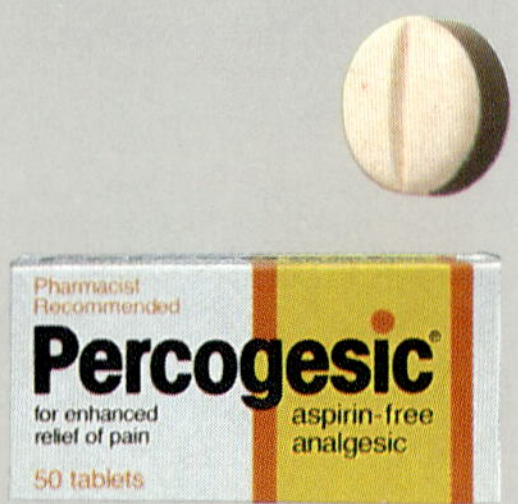

Available in bottles of 24, 50 and 90

PERCOGESIC®
analgesic
(acetaminophen and phenyltoloxamine citrate)

Richardson-Vicks Inc.

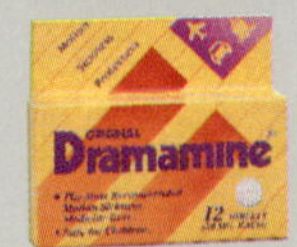

DRAMAMINE®
(dimenhydrinate)
Tablets 12s, 36s & 100s

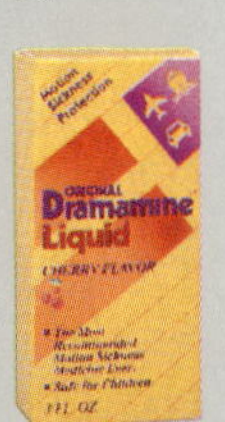

DRAMAMINE® LIQUID
(dimenhydrinate syrup USP)
Liquid 3 fl. oz.

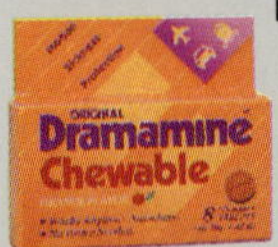

DRAMAMINE® CHEWABLE
(dimenhydrinate)
Tablets 8s & 24s

Richardson-Vicks Inc.

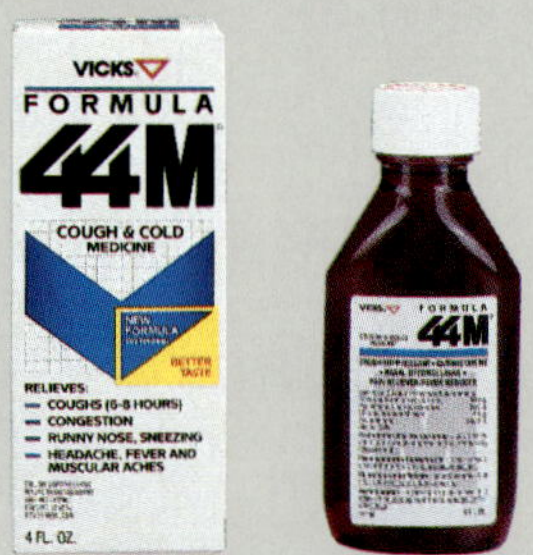

Available in 4 oz. and 8 oz.

VICKS® FORMULA 44M®
(dextromethorphan hydrobromide, pseudoephedrine hydrochloride, chlorpheniramine maleate, acetaminophen)

Richardson-Vicks Inc.

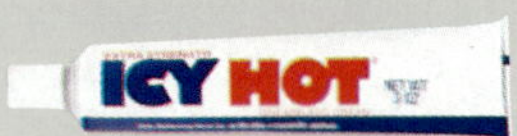

Rub, greaseless,
1¼-oz and 3-oz tubes

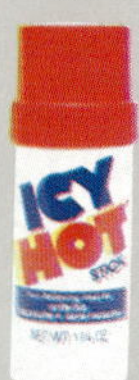

Stick, 1¾ oz

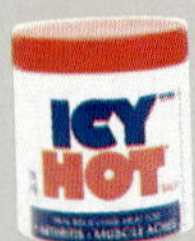

Balm, 3½-oz

ICY HOT®
Analgesic Balm, Rub and Stick for Pain from Arthritis and Muscle Aches

Richardson-Vicks Inc.

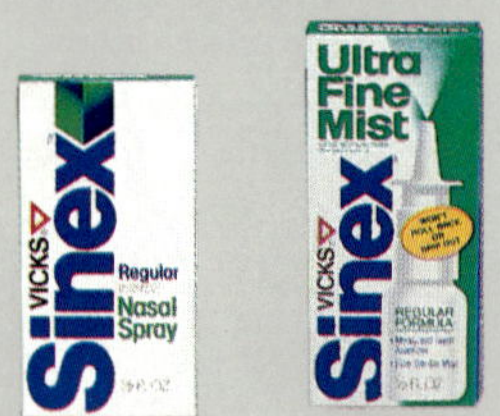

Sinex®

Sinex®
Ultra Fine Mist

Available in ½ oz., 1 oz. squeeze bottles and ½ oz. measured dose atomizer.

VICKS® SINEX® ULTRA FINE MIST
Decongestant Nasal Spray
(phenylephrine hydrochloride, cetylpyridinium chloride)

Richardson-Vicks Inc.

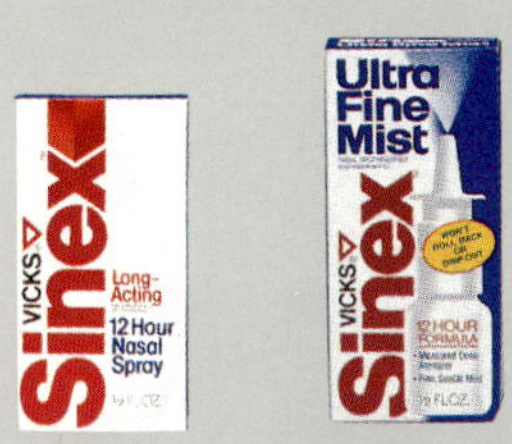

Sinex®
Long-Acting

Sinex® Ultra Fine
Mist 12 Hour

Available in ½ oz., 1 oz. squeeze bottles and ½ oz. measured dose atomizer.

VICKS® SINEX® LONG-ACTING
Decongestant Nasal Spray
(oxymetazoline hydrochloride)

Richardson-Vicks Inc.

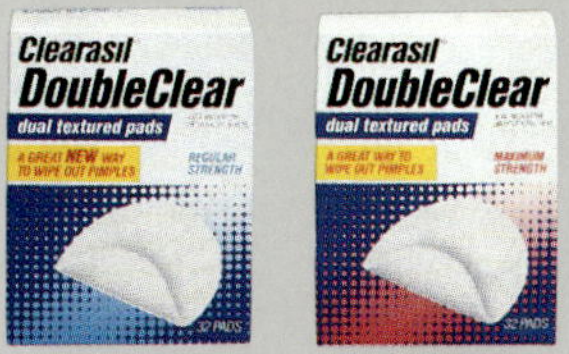

Regular Strength (1.25% salicylic acid)

Maximum Strength (2.0% salicylic acid)

32 pads

CLEARASIL®
Double Clear Dual Textured
Medicated Pads

Roberts Pharmaceutical

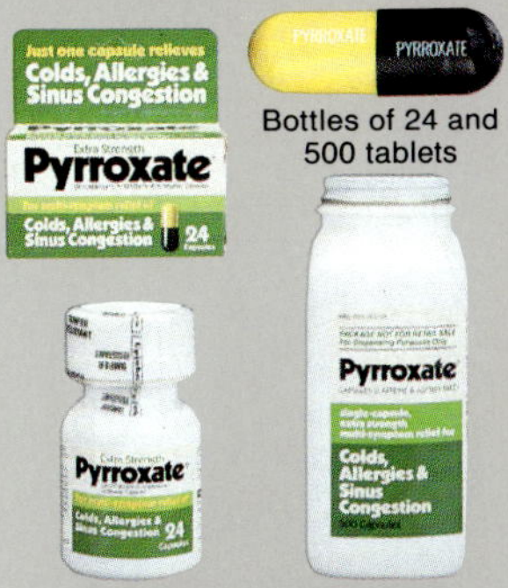

Bottles of 24 and 500 tablets

PYRROXATE® Capsules
Nasal Decongestant/Antihistamine/ Analgesic

A. H. Robins

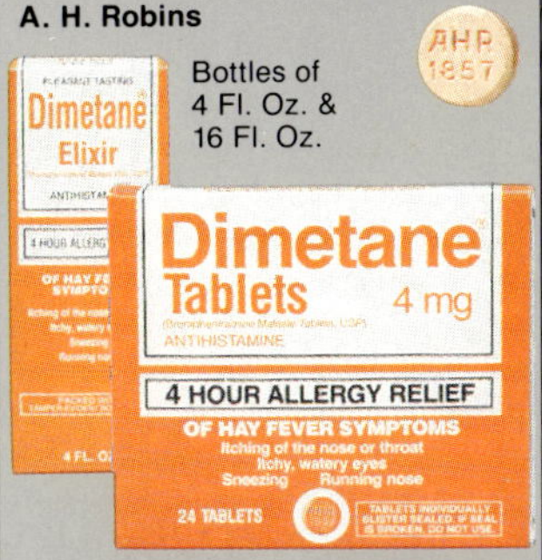

Bottles of 4 Fl. Oz. & 16 Fl. Oz.

Consumer cartons of 24 and bottles of 100 and 500

DIMETANE® ELIXIR AND TABLETS
(Brompheniramine Maleate)

Richardson-Vicks Inc.

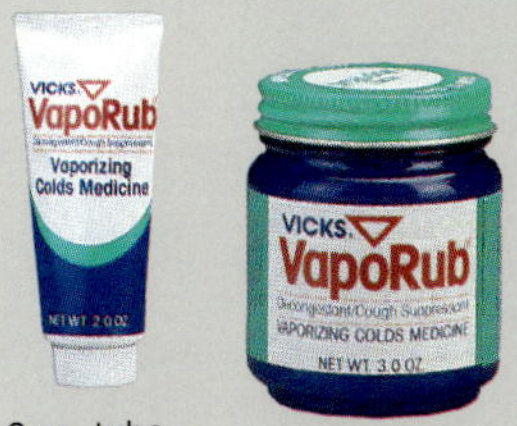

2 oz. tube

1.5 oz., 3.0 oz., 6 oz. jar

VICKS® VAPORUB®
Decongestant Cough Suppressant
(menthol, camphor, eucalyptus oil)

ROBERTS

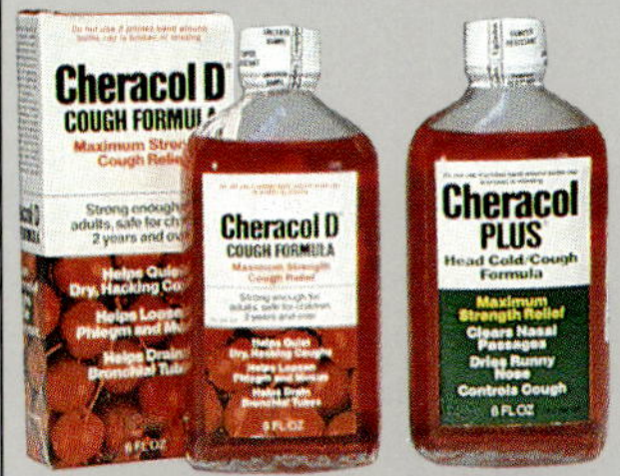

2 oz, 4 oz, 6 oz

4 oz, 6 oz

CHERACOL D®
Cough Formula

CHERACOL PLUS®
Head Cold/Cough Formula

Roberts Pharmaceutical

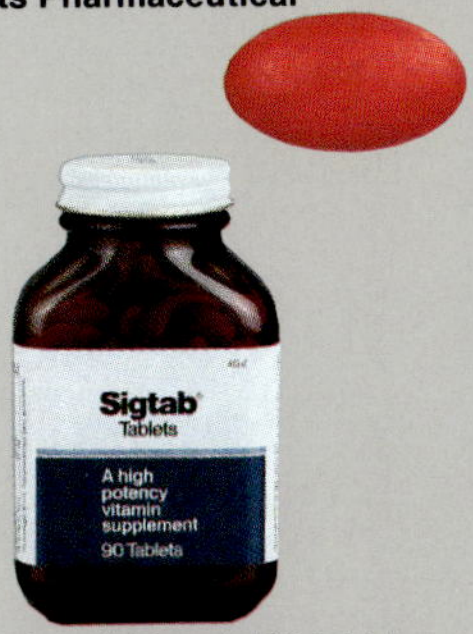

Bottles of 90 and 500 tablets

SIGTAB® Tablets
High potency vitamin supplement

A. H. Robins

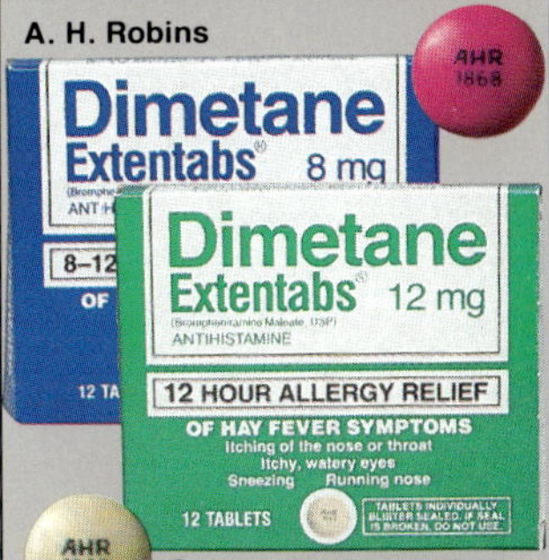

Consumer cartons of 12 and bottles of 100

DIMETANE EXTENTABS®
8 mg & 12 mg TABLETS
(Brompheniramine Maleate, USP)

Richardson-Vicks Inc.
Also Available: Clearasil® Acne Treatment Vanishing Lotion

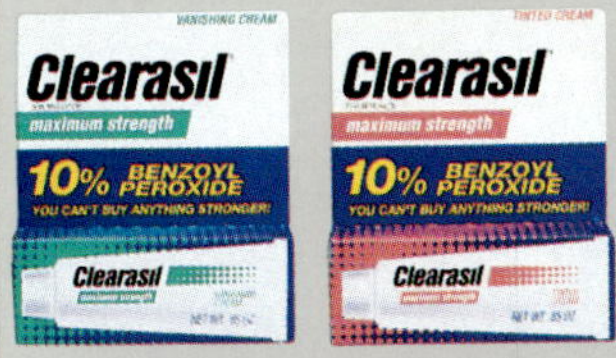

Vanishing

Tinted

Both available in .65 and 1.0 oz. sizes

CLEARASIL®
Acne Treatment Cream
(10% benzoyl peroxide)

Roberts Pharmaceutical

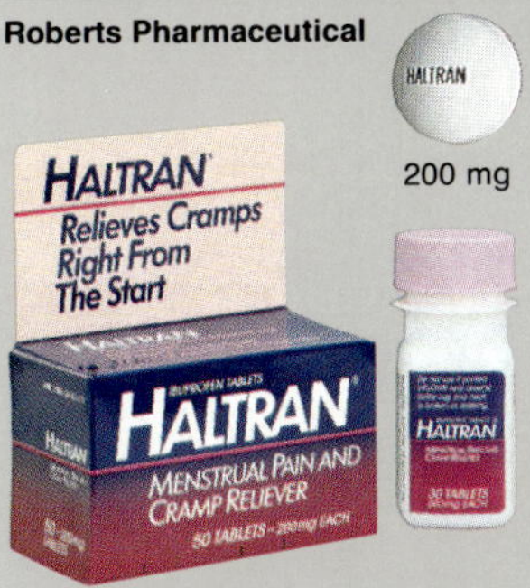

200 mg

Bottles of 30

HALTRAN® Tablets
(ibuprofen tablets, USP)

A. H. ROBINS

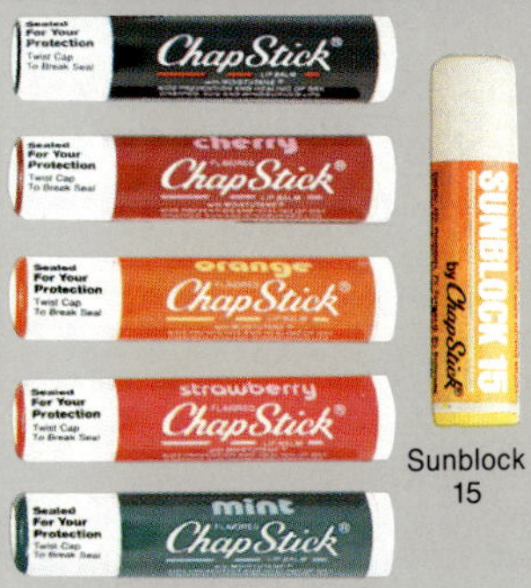

Sunblock 15

CHAP STICK®

Lip Balm

A. H. Robins

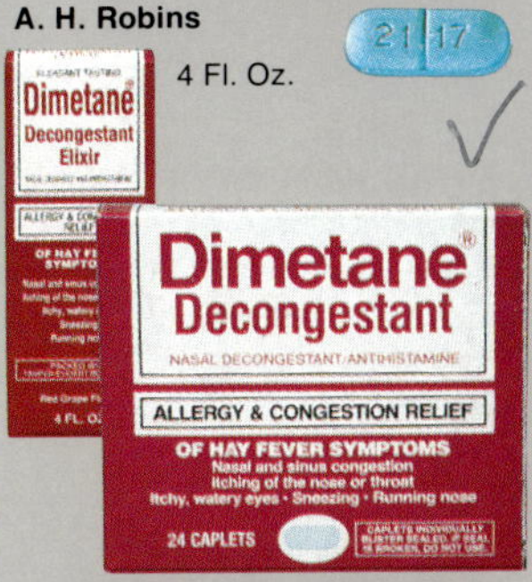

4 Fl. Oz.

Consumer cartons of 24 and 48

DIMETANE®
DECONGESTANT ELIXIR
AND CAPLETS

Richardson-Vicks Inc.

Also Available:
Clearasil Medicated Blemish Stick

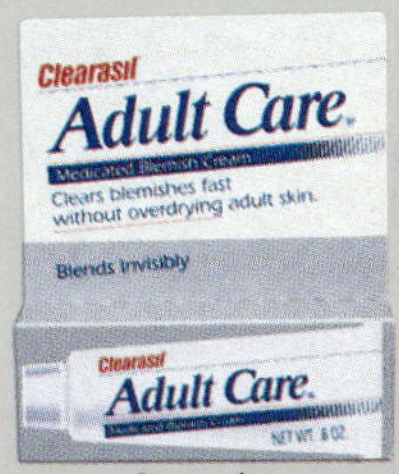

.6 oz. size

CLEARASIL® ADULT CARE®
(sulfur, resorcinol)

Roberts Pharmaceutical

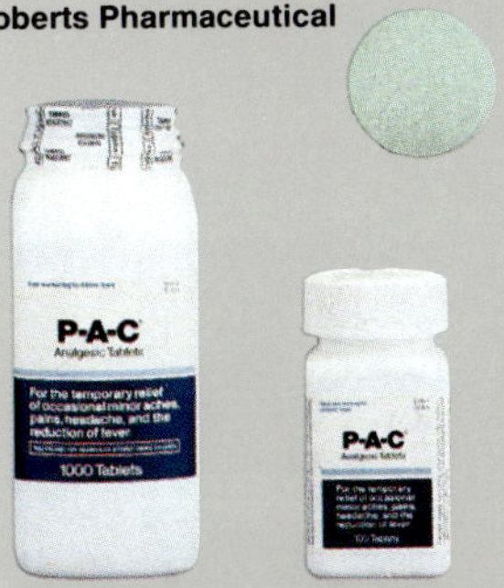

1,000 tablets

100 tablets

P-A-C®
Analgesic Tablets

A. H. Robins

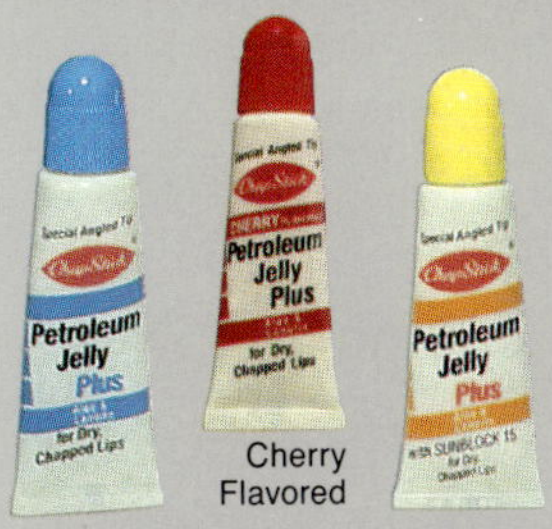

Cherry Flavored

for Dry, Chapped Lips

for Dry, Chapped Lips with SUNBLOCK 15

CHAP STICK® Petroleum Jelly Plus

A. H. Robins

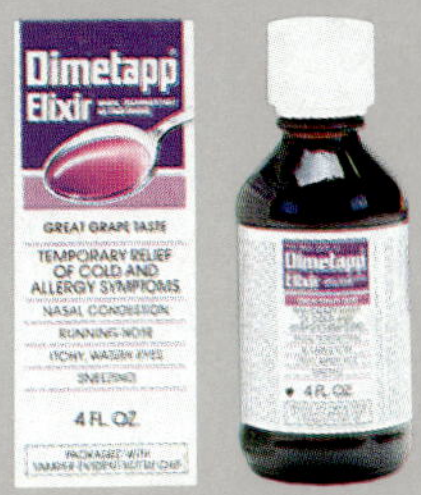

Available in bottles of 4 Fl. Oz., 8 Fl. Oz., 16 Fl. Oz. and 128 Fl. Oz.

DIMETAPP® ELIXIR

A. H. Robins

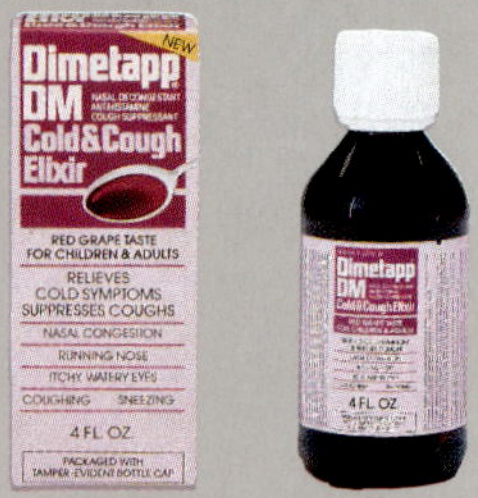

Available in bottles of 4 Fl. Oz. and 8 Fl. Oz.

DIMETAPP® DM COLD & COUGH ELIXIR
(Brompheniramine Maleate, Phenylpropanolamine HCl, Dextromethorphan Hydrobromide)

A. H. Robins

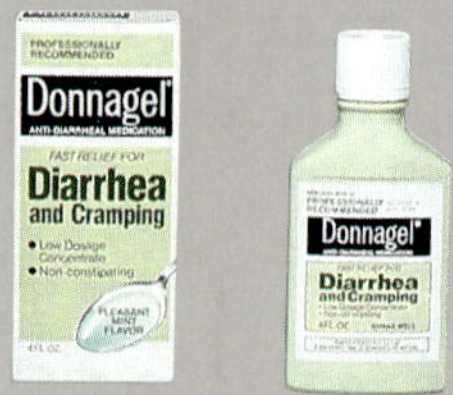

Available in bottles of 4 Fl. Oz., 8 Fl. Oz. and 16 Fl. Oz.

DONNAGEL®

A. H. Robins

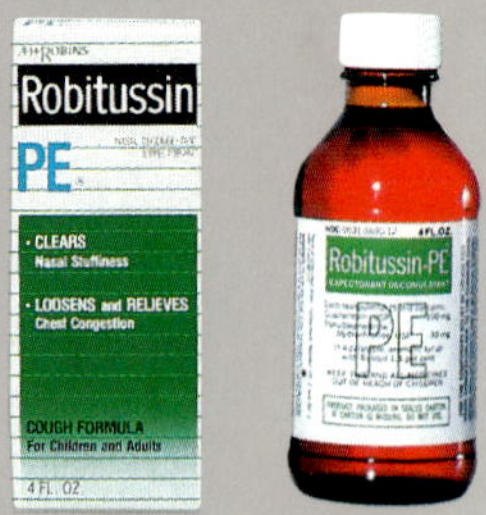

Available in bottles of 4 Fl. Oz., 8 Fl. Oz. and 16 Fl. Oz.

ROBITUSSIN-PE® SYRUP

ROSS

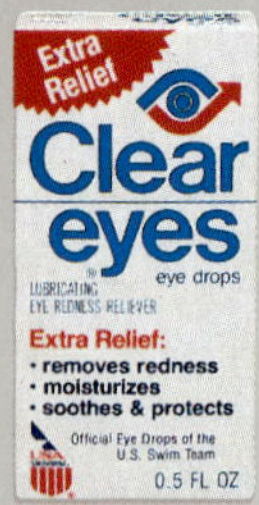

CLEAR EYES® Lubricating Eye Redness Reliever

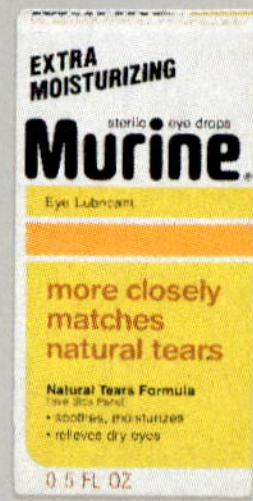

MURINE® EYE LUBRICANT More Closely Matches Natural Tears

A. H. Robins

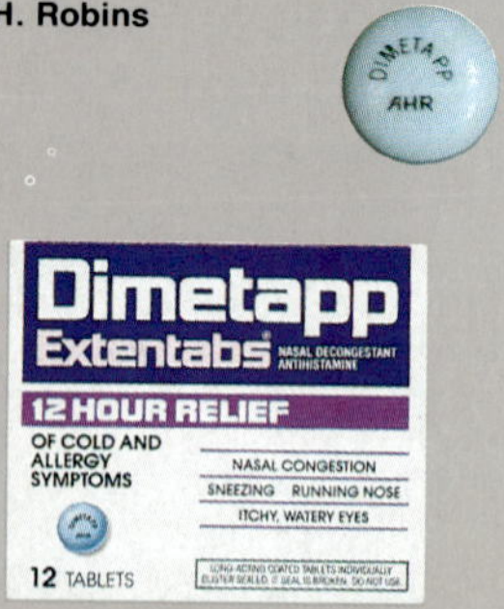

Available in consumer cartons of 12, 24 and 48 and bottles of 100 and 500

DIMETAPP EXTENTABS®

A. H. Robins

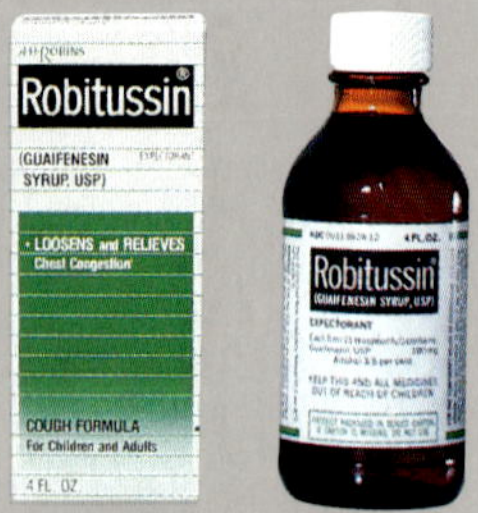

Available in bottles of 4 Fl. Oz., 8 Fl. Oz., 16 Fl. Oz. and 128 Fl. Oz.

ROBITUSSIN® SYRUP
(Guaifenesin Syrup, USP)

A. H. Robins

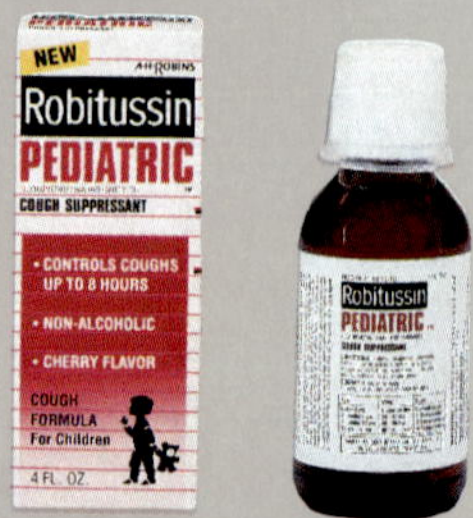

Available in bottles of 4 Fl. Oz. and 8 Fl. Oz.

ROBITUSSIN PEDIATRIC™ COUGH SUPPRESSANT
(Dextromethorphan Hydrobromide)

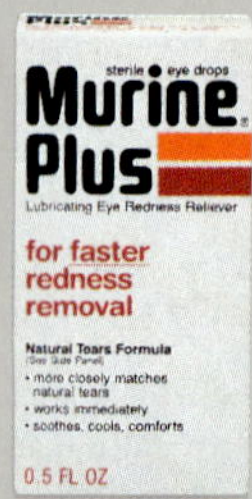

MURINE® PLUS Lubricating Eye Redness Reliever

Available in: 0.5 and 1.0 Fl. Oz.

A. H. Robins

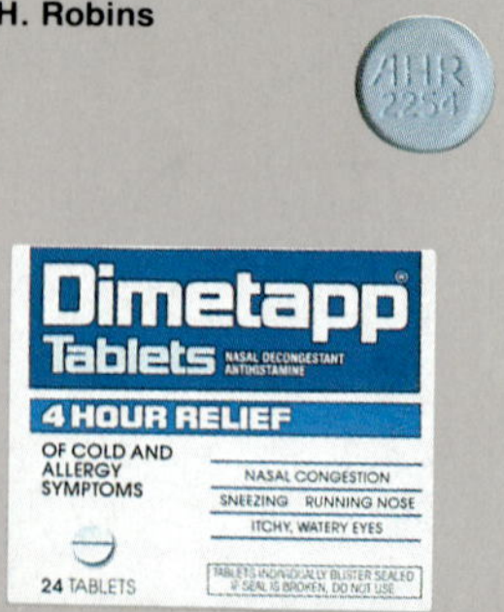

Available in consumer cartons of 24

DIMETAPP® TABLETS

A. H. Robins

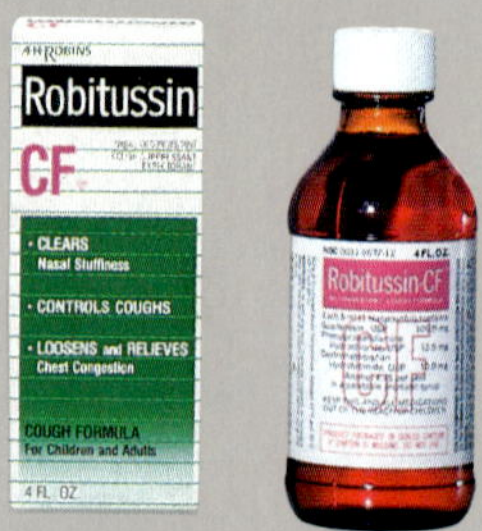

Available in bottles of 4 Fl. Oz., 8 Fl. Oz. and 16 Fl. Oz.

ROBITUSSIN-CF® SYRUP

A. H. Robins

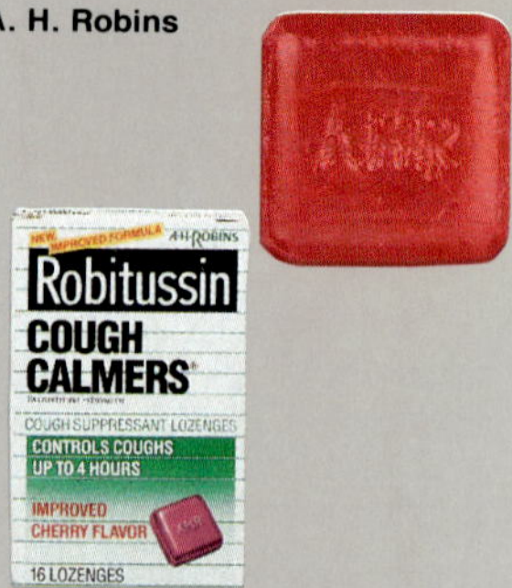

Available in consumer cartons of 16 lozenges

ROBITUSSIN COUGH CALMERS®
(Dextromethorphan Hydrobromide)

Ross

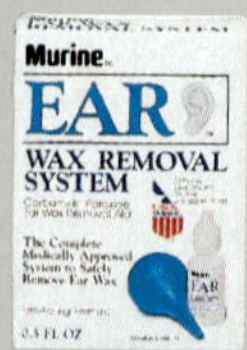

0.5 Fl. Oz.

MURINE® EAR WAX REMOVAL SYSTEM

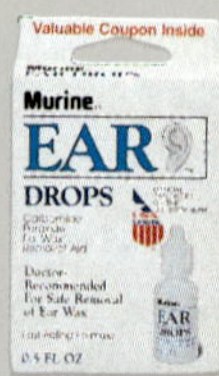

0.5 Fl. Oz.

MURINE® EAR DROPS

A. H. Robins

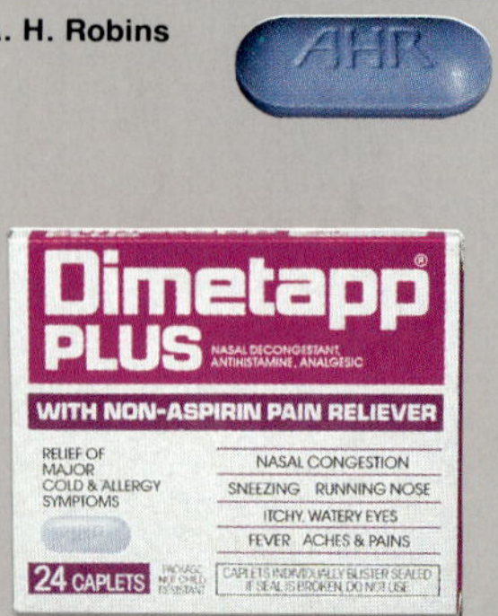

Available in consumer cartons of 24 and bottles of 48

DIMETAPP® PLUS CAPLETS

A. H. Robins

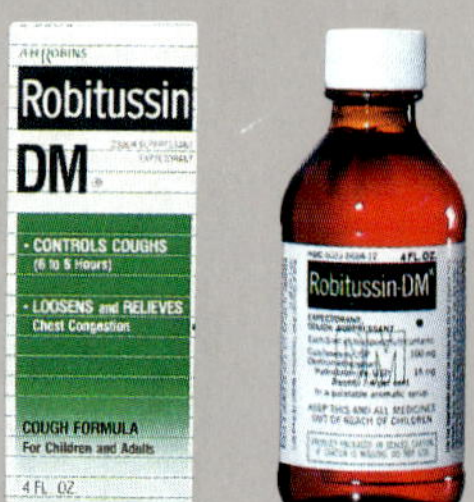

Available in bottles of 4 Fl. Oz., 8 Fl. Oz., 16 Fl. Oz. and 128 Fl. Oz.

ROBITUSSIN-DM® SYRUP

A. H. Robins

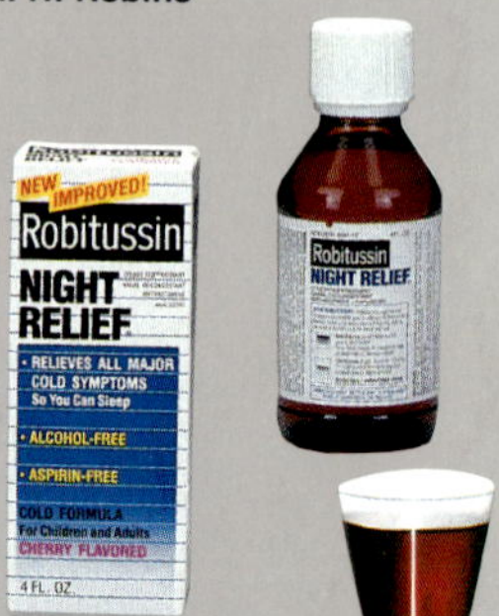

Available in bottles of 4 Fl. Oz. and 8 Fl. Oz. with convenient dosage cup.

ROBITUSSIN NIGHT RELIEF®

For more detailed information on products illustrated in this section, consult the Product Information Section or manufacturers may be contacted directly.

Ross 4 Fl. Oz.

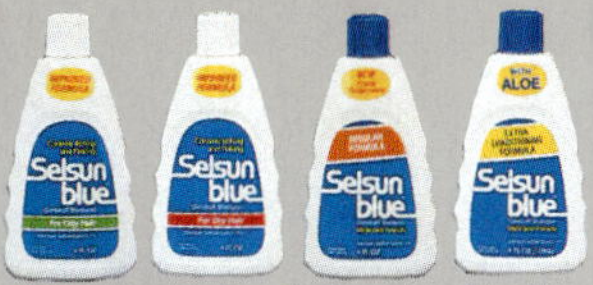

For Oily Hair | For Dry Hair | For Regular Hair | For All Hair Types

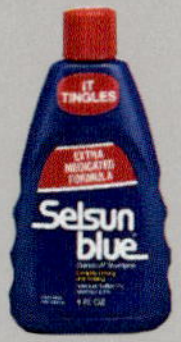

Extra Medicated
For All Hair Types

SELSUN BLUE® Dandruff Shampoo

Also available in 7 and 11 Fl. Oz.

Russ Pharmaceuticals

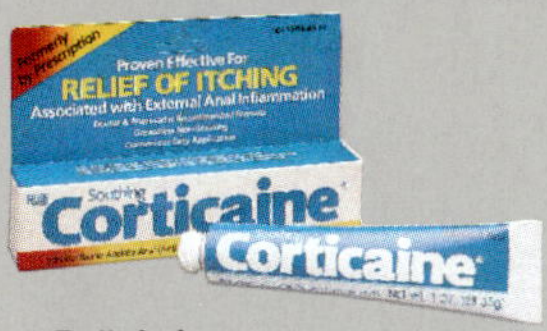

Relief of itching

CORTICAINE®
(hydrocortisone acetate)

Rydelle

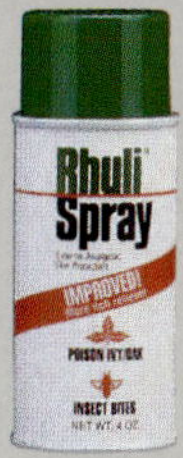

4 oz.

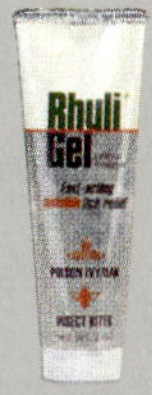

2 oz.

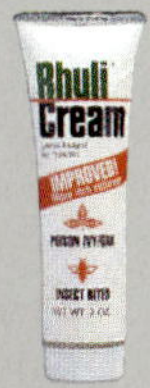

2 oz.

RHULI®
SPRAY, GEL & CREAM
Fast, Cooling Relief of Itching

Sandoz Consumer Division

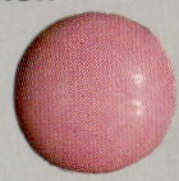

24's

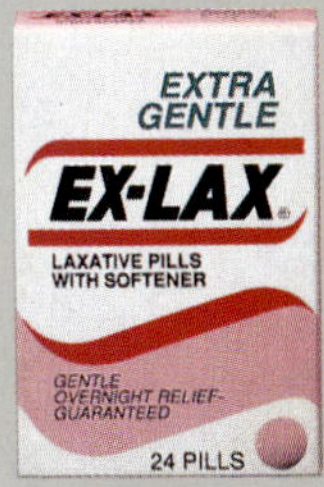

EXTRA GENTLE EX-LAX®

Ross

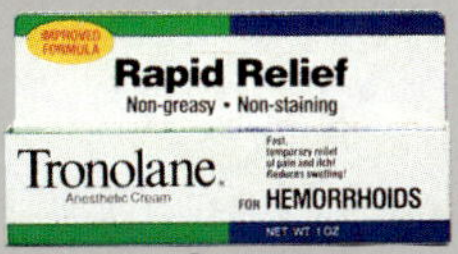

Cream
1 Oz. and 2 Oz. Tubes

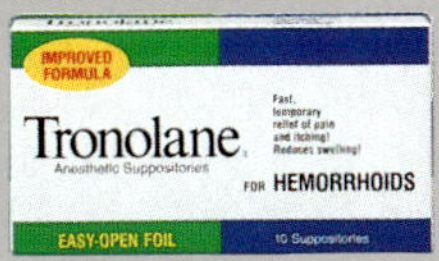

Suppositories
10's and 20's

TRONOLANE®
Anesthetic Cream and Suppositories for Hemorrhoids

RYDELLE

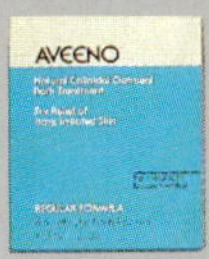

Regular

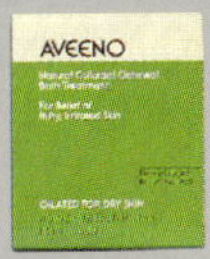

For Dry Skin

AVEENO® BATH

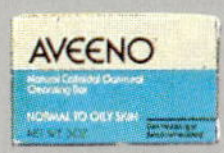

Normal to Oily Skin

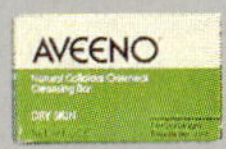

Dry Skin

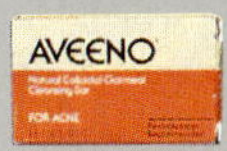

For Acne

AVEENO® BAR

SANDOZ

Consumer Division

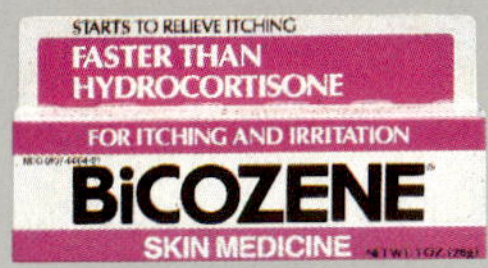

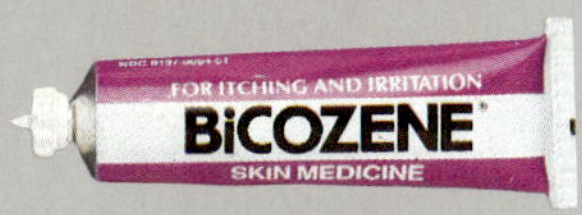

1 oz. (28.4 g.)

BICOZENE® CREME

Sandoz Consumer Division

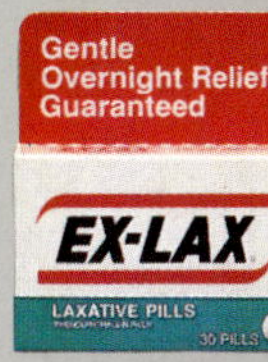

8's, 30's, 60's

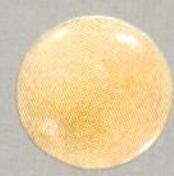

Pill

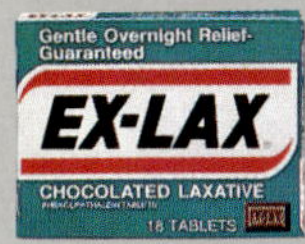

6's, 18's, 48's and 72's

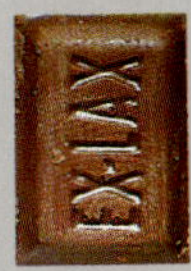

Chocolated Tablet

EX-LAX®

Russ Pharmaceuticals

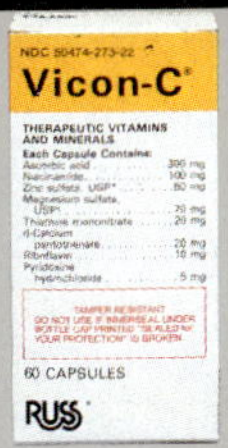

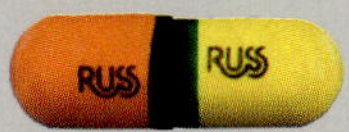

VICON-C

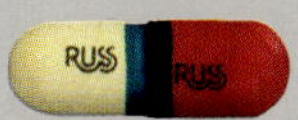

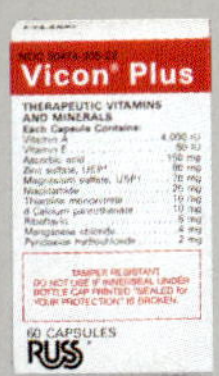

VICON PLUS

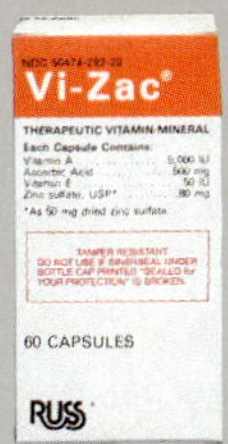

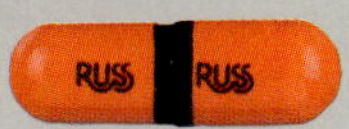

VI-ZAC

(Therapeutic Vitamins and Minerals)

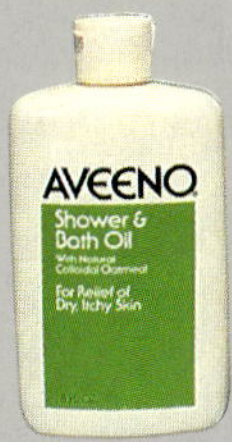

Shower and Bath Oil

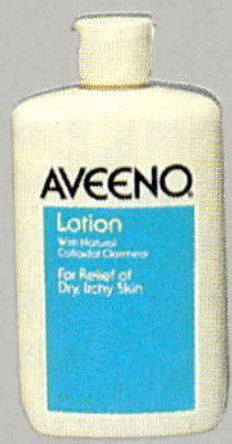

Lotion

AVEENO®
With Natural Colloidal Oatmeal
For the Relief of Dry, Itchy Skin

Rydelle

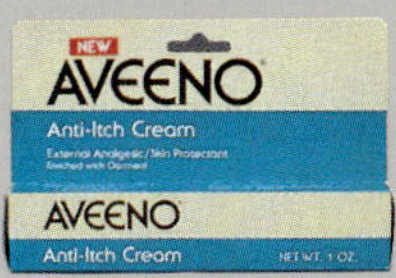

Cream

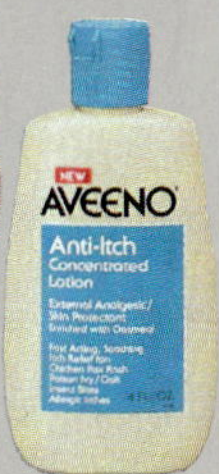

Concentrated Lotion

AVEENO®
ANTI-ITCH
External Analgesic/Skin Protectant
Enriched with Oatmeal

Sandoz Consumer Division

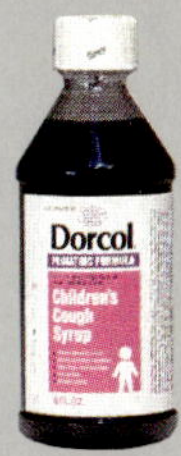

4 oz., 8 oz.

DORCOL®
Children's Cough Syrup

4 oz.

DORCOL®
Children's Liquid Cold Formula

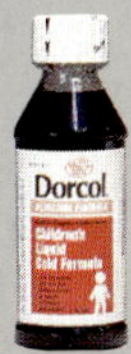

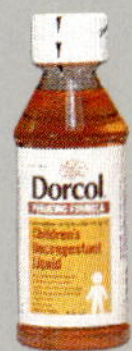

4 oz.

DORCOL®
Children's Decongestant Liquid

4 oz.

DORCOL®
Children's Fever & Pain Reducer

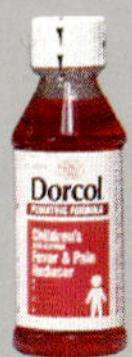

DORCOL®
PEDIATRIC FORMULAS

Sandoz Consumer Division

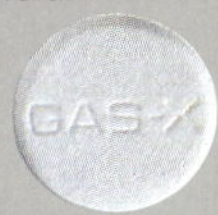

12's, 36's

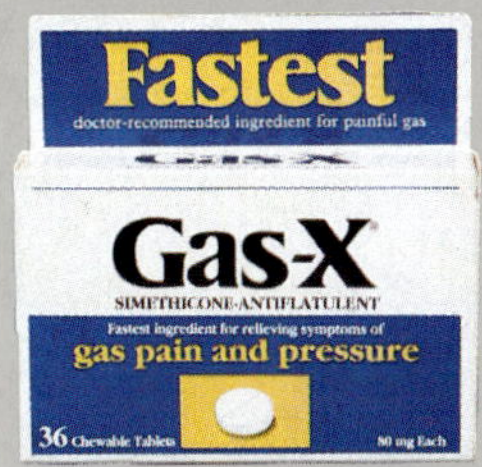

GAS-X®
(80 mg. simethicone)

Sandoz Consumer Division

18 tablets
48 tablets

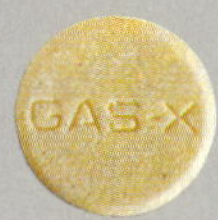

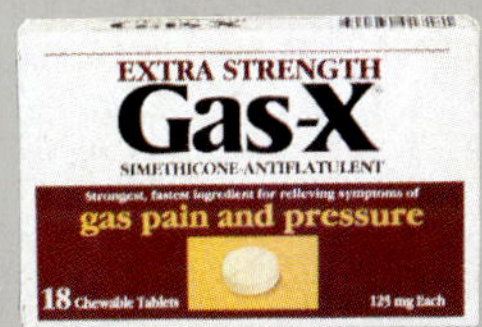

EXTRA-STRENGTH GAS-X®
(125 mg. simethicone)

Sandoz Consumer Division

16's

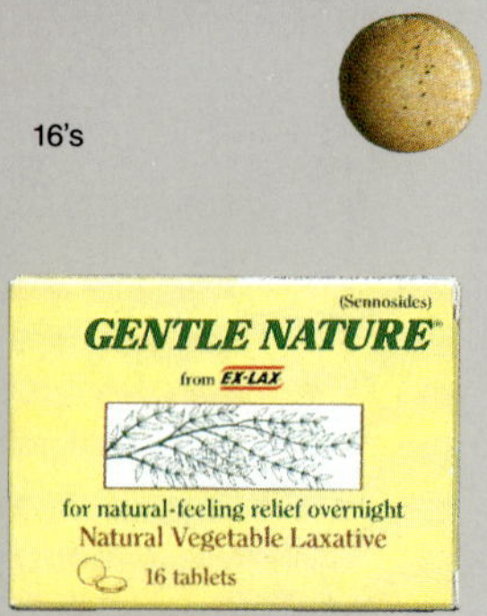

GENTLE NATURE®
(20 mg. sennosides)

Sandoz Consumer Division

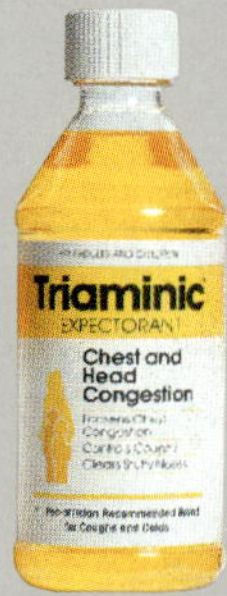

4 oz., 8 oz.

TRIAMINIC®
EXPECTORANT

SCHERING-PLOUGH
HealthCare

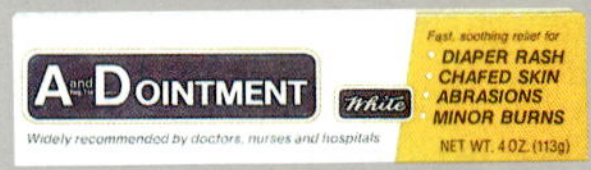

WMJ

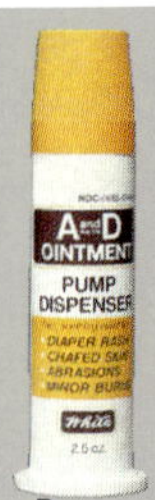

Pump
Dispenser

A and D[Reg. ™] Ointment

Schering-Plough HealthCare

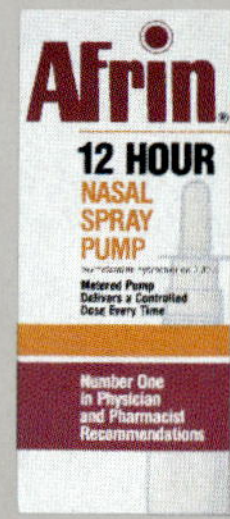

Safety Sealed

AFRIN® NASAL SPRAY PUMP
(oxymetazoline hydrochloride 0.05%)

Sandoz Consumer Division

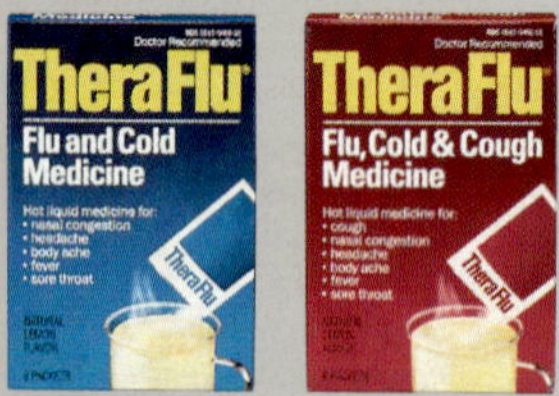

6's and 12's

THERA FLU®
Flu and Cold
Medicine

THERA FLU®
Flu, Cold &
Cough Medicine

Sandoz Consumer Division

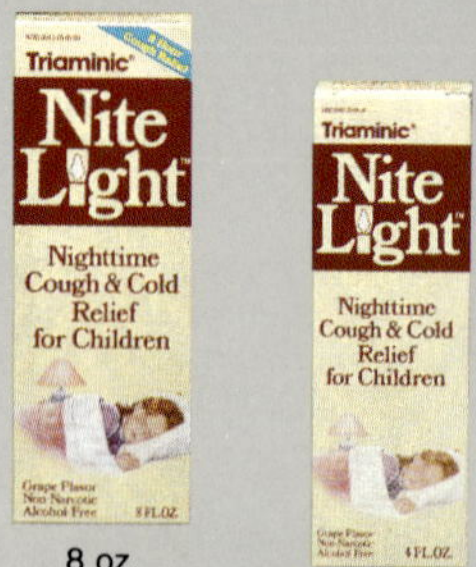

8 oz.

4 oz.

TRIAMINIC®
NITE LIGHT™
Nighttime Cough & Cold
Relief for Children

Schering-Plough HealthCare

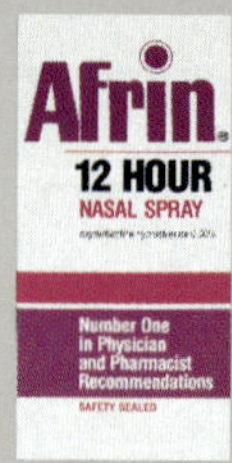

Safety Sealed

AFRIN®
NASAL SPRAY
0.05%

(oxymetazoline hydrochloride, USP)

Schering-Plough HealthCare

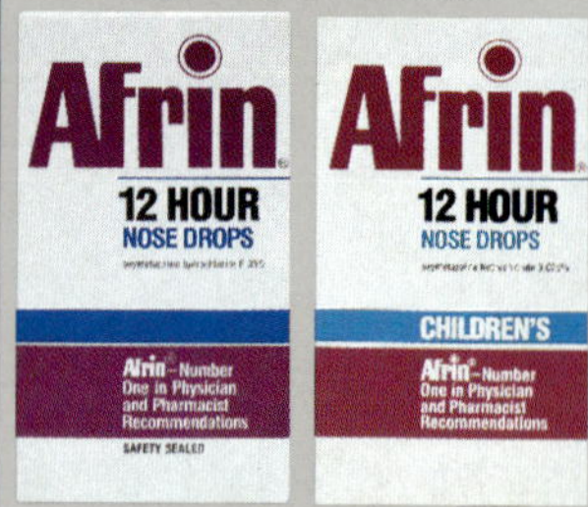

Safety Sealed

Nose Drops
0.05%

Children's Strength
Nose Drops
0.025%

AFRIN® NOSE DROPS
(oxymetazoline hydrochloride)

Sandoz Consumer Division

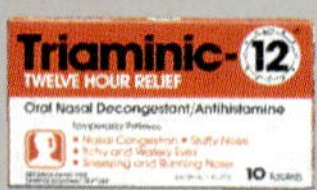

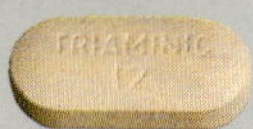

TRIAMINIC-12®
Tablets
(Sustained Release)

10's, 20's

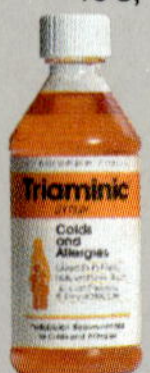

24's

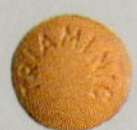

TRIAMINIC®
Cold Tablets

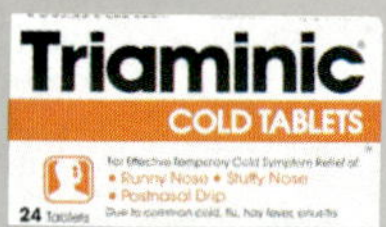

4 oz., 8 oz.
TRIAMINIC®
Cold Syrup

TRIAMINIC®

Sandoz Consumer Division

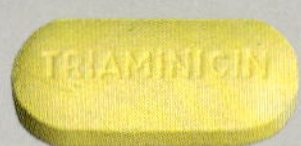

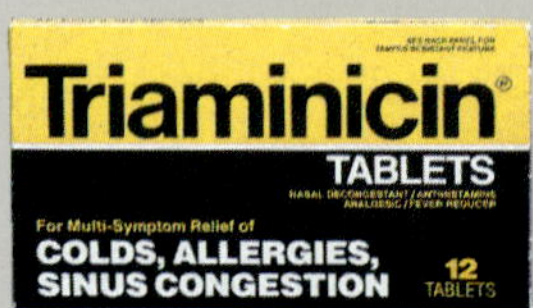

12's, 24's, 48's, 100's

TRIAMINICIN®
TABLETS

Schering-Plough HealthCare

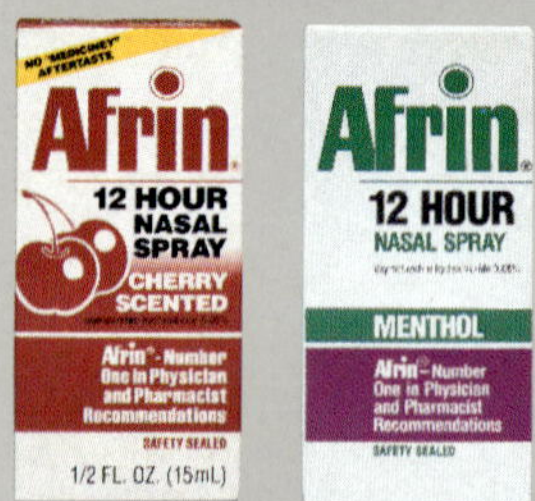

Safety Sealed

AFRIN®
CHERRY SCENTED
NASAL SPRAY
0.05%

AFRIN®
MENTHOL
NASAL SPRAY
0.05%

(oxymetazoline hydrochloride, USP)

Schering-Plough HealthCare

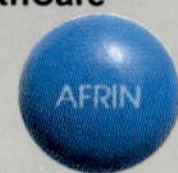

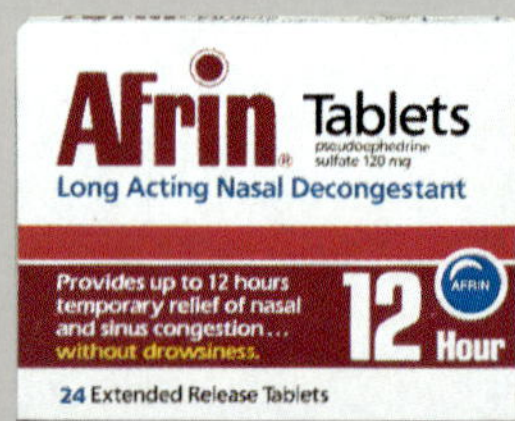

AFRIN®
EXTENDED RELEASE
TABLETS

(pseudoephedrine sulfate)

Sandoz Consumer Division

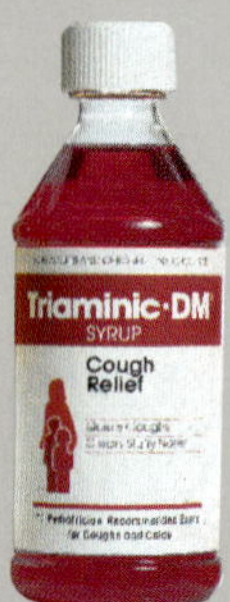

4 oz., 8 oz.

TRIAMINIC-DM®
COUGH FORMULA

Sandoz Consumer Division

4 oz., 8 oz.

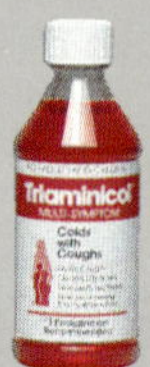

TRIAMINICOL®
MULTI-SYMPTOM
RELIEF

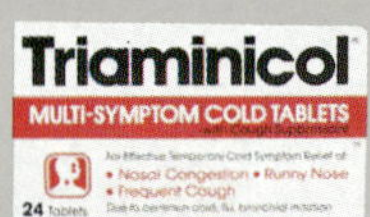

24's

TRIAMINICOL®
MULTI-SYMPTOM COLD TABLETS

Schering-Plough HealthCare

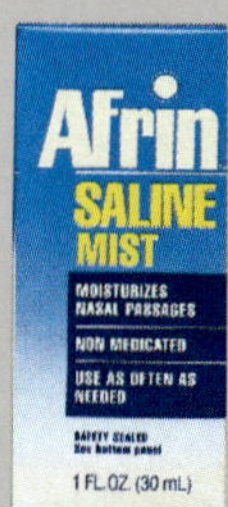

AFRIN®
SALINE MIST
(oxymetazoline hydrochloride, USP)

Schering-Plough HealthCare

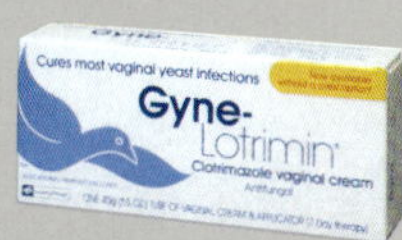

Cream

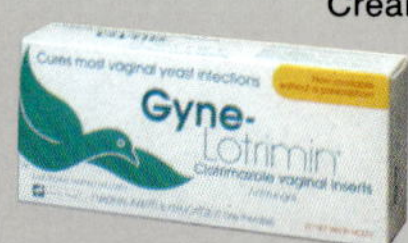

Inserts

GYNE-LOTRIMIN®
Clotrimazole Vaginal
Antifungal

Schering-Plough HealthCare

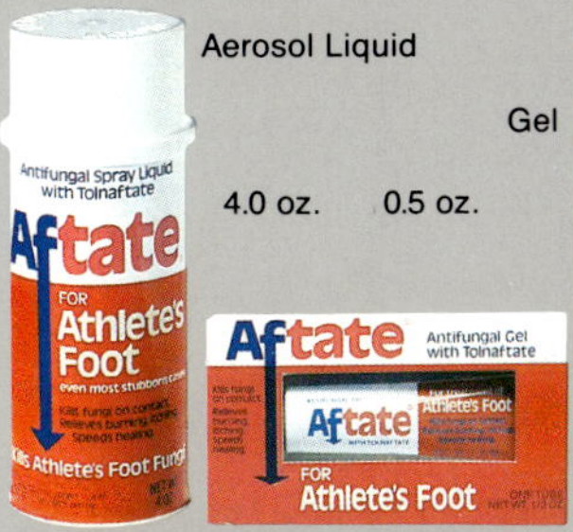

Aerosol Liquid

Gel

4.0 oz. 0.5 oz.

Also available in 3.5 oz. spray powder and 2.25 oz. shaker powder.

AFTATE® FOR ATHLETE'S FOOT

(tolnaftate 1%)

Schering-Plough HealthCare

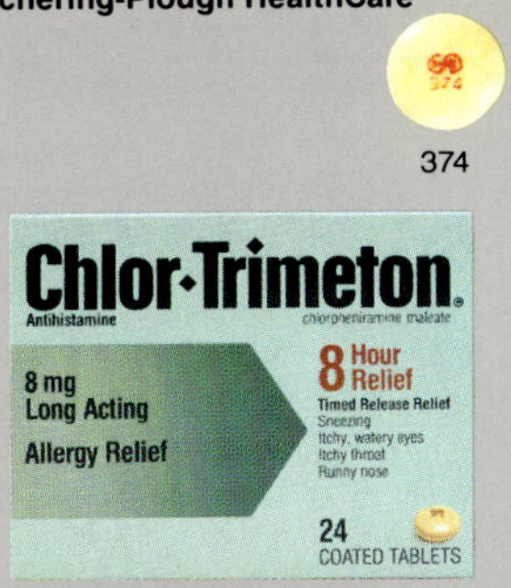

374

CHLOR-TRIMETON® LONG ACTING ALLERGY REPETABS® TABLETS

(8 mg chlorpheniramine maleate)

Schering-Plough HealthCare

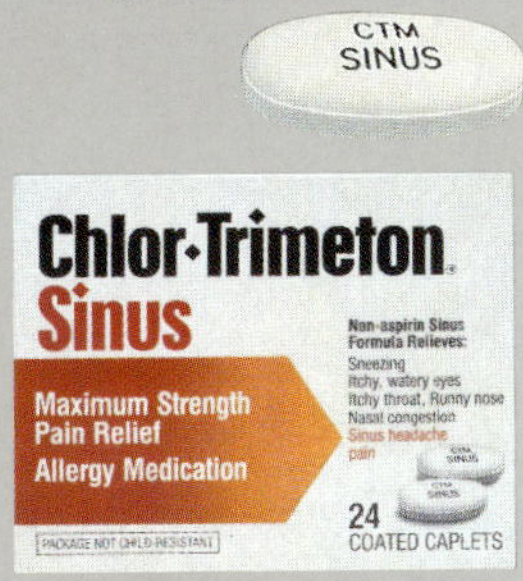

CHLOR-TRIMETON® SINUS CAPLETS

(2 mg chlorpheniramine maleate, 12.5 mg phenylpropanolamine HCl, and 500 mg acetaminophen)

Schering-Plough HealthCare

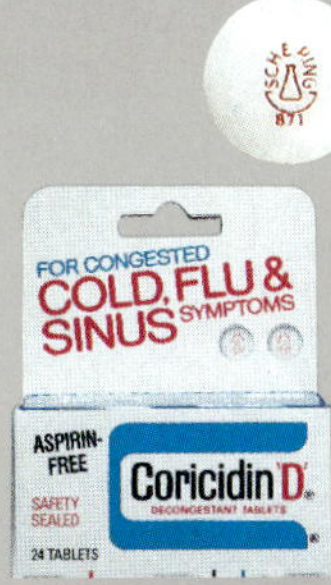

871 or 307

CORICIDIN 'D'® DECONGESTANT TABLETS

(2 mg chlorpheniramine maleate, 12.5 mg phenylpropanolamine HCl, and 325 mg acetaminophen)

Schering-Plough HealthCare

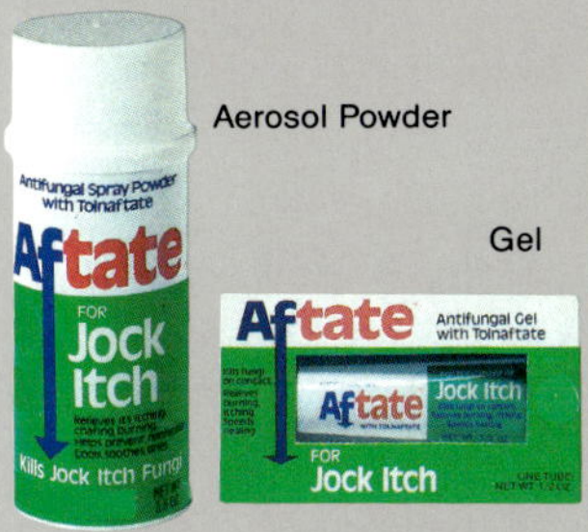

Aerosol Powder

Gel

3.5 oz. 0.5 oz.

Also available in 1.5 oz. shaker powder.

AFTATE® FOR JOCK ITCH

(tolnaftate 1%)

Schering-Plough HealthCare

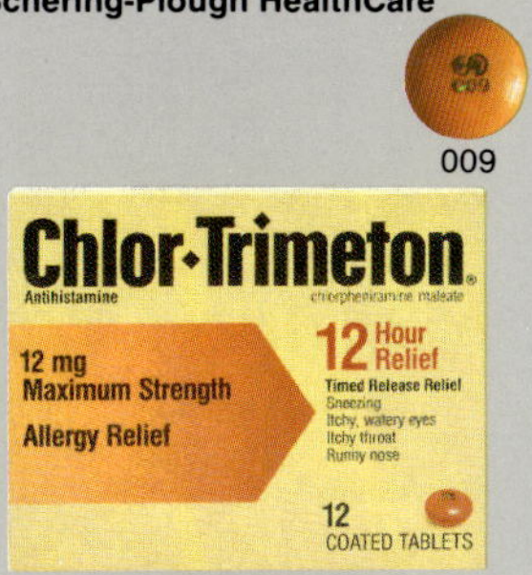

009

CHLOR-TRIMETON® MAXIMUM STRENGTH TIMED RELEASE ALLERGY TABLETS

(12 mg chlorpheniramine maleate)

Schering-Plough HealthCare

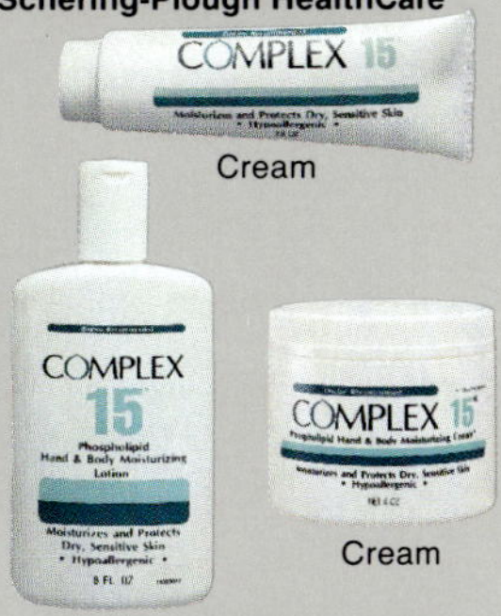

Cream

Cream

Lotion

COMPLEX 15® HAND AND BODY MOISTURIZING CREAM

Schering-Plough HealthCare

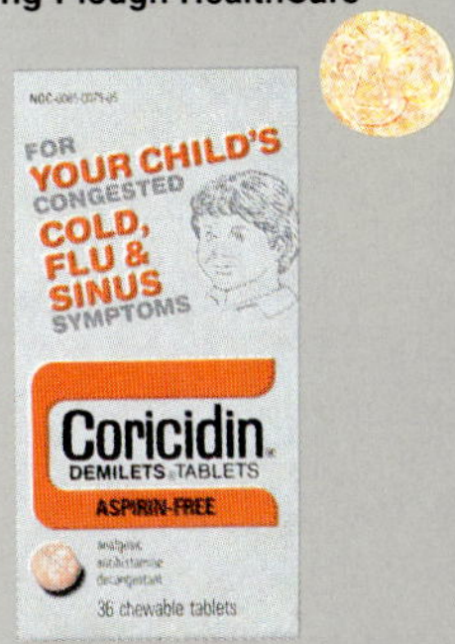

CORICIDIN® DEMILETS® TABLETS

(1.0 mg chlorpheniramine maleate, 80 mg acetaminophen, 6.25 mg phenylpropanolamine HCl)

Schering-Plough HealthCare

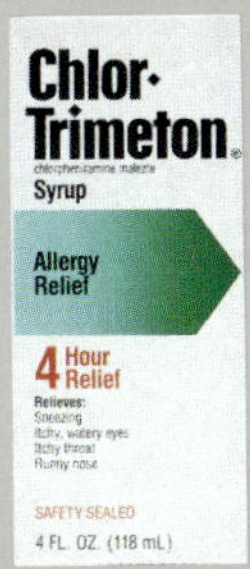

CHLOR-TRIMETON® ALLERGY SYRUP

(2 mg chlorpheniramine maleate)

Schering-Plough HealthCare

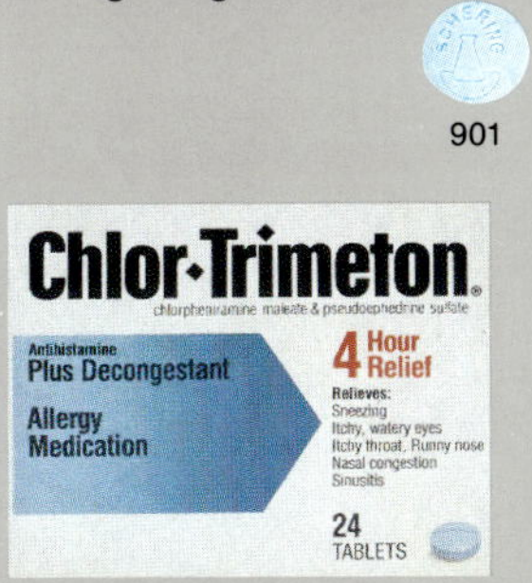

901

CHLOR-TRIMETON® DECONGESTANT TABLETS

(4 mg chlorpheniramine maleate and 60 mg pseudoephedrine sulfate)

Schering-Plough HealthCare

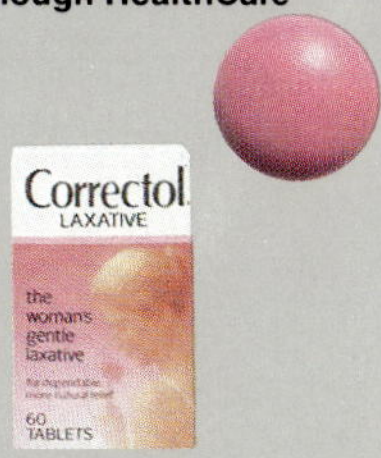

Available in 15, 30, 60 and 90 tablet sizes.

CORRECTOL® LAXATIVE

(Tablet contains 100 mg. docusate sodium and 65 mg. yellow phenolphthalein.)

Schering-Plough HealthCare

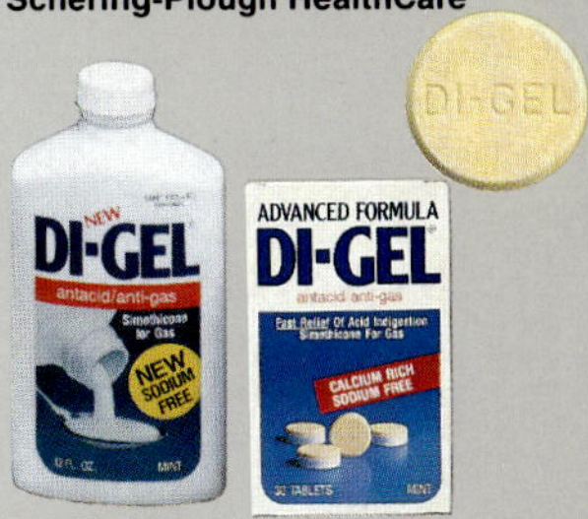

Liquid Tablets

Mint and Lemon/Orange flavors, 6 fl. oz. and 12 fl. oz. liquid plus 30 and 90 tablet sizes.
Now also available in 3-roll pack and 60 tablet bottle (Mint only).

DI-GEL®

Schering-Plough HealthCare

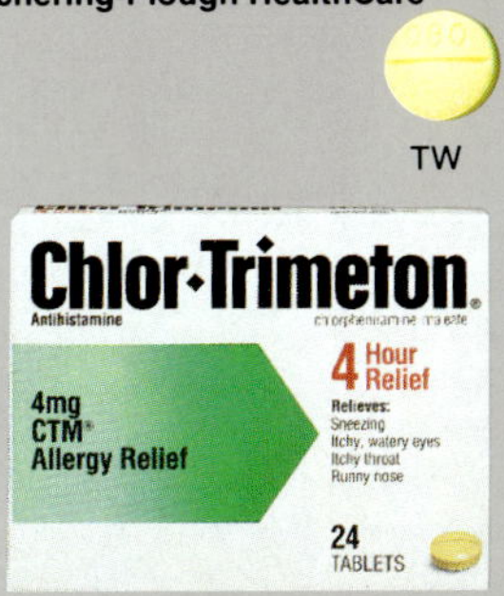

TW

CHLOR-TRIMETON® ALLERGY TABLETS

(4 mg chlorpheniramine maleate)

Schering-Plough HealthCare

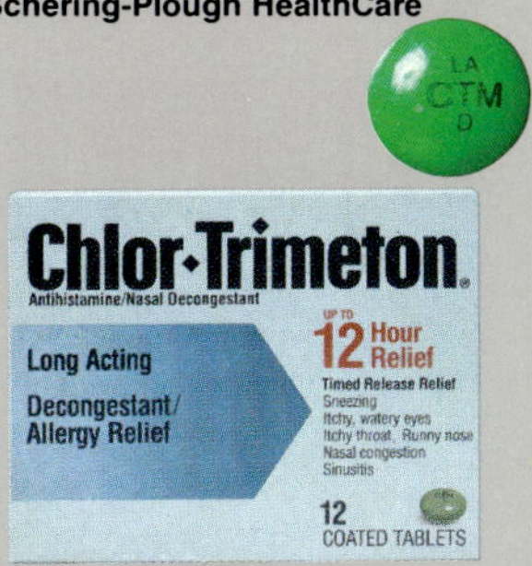

LONG ACTING CHLOR-TRIMETON® DECONGESTANT REPETABS®

(8 mg chlorpheniramine maleate and 120 mg pseudoephedrine sulfate)

Schering-Plough HealthCare

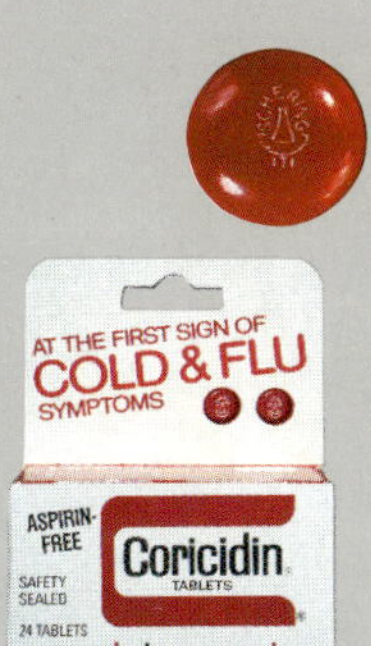

PKD or SN or 171 or 522

CORICIDIN® TABLETS

(2 mg chlorpheniramine maleate and 325 mg acetaminophen)

Schering-Plough HealthCare

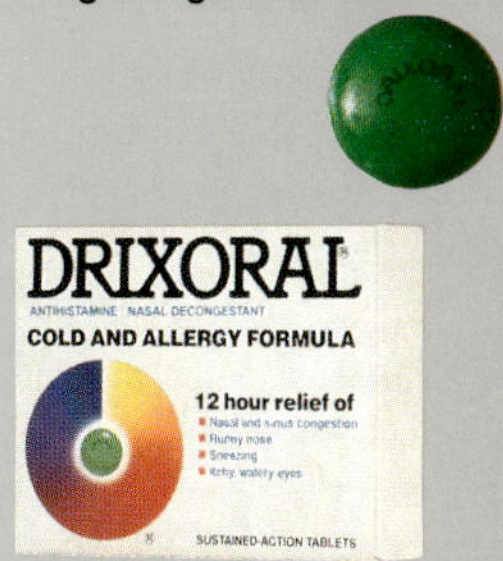

DRIXORAL® SUSTAINED-ACTION TABLETS

(6 mg dexbrompheniramine maleate and 120 mg pseudoephedrine sulfate)

Schering-Plough HealthCare

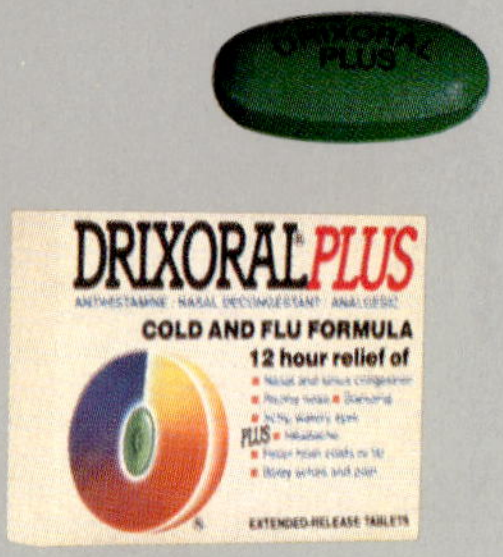

DRIXORAL® PLUS EXTENDED-RELEASE TABLETS
(60 mg pseudoephedrine sulfate, 3 mg dexbrompheniramine maleate and 500 mg acetaminophen)

Schering-Plough HealthCare

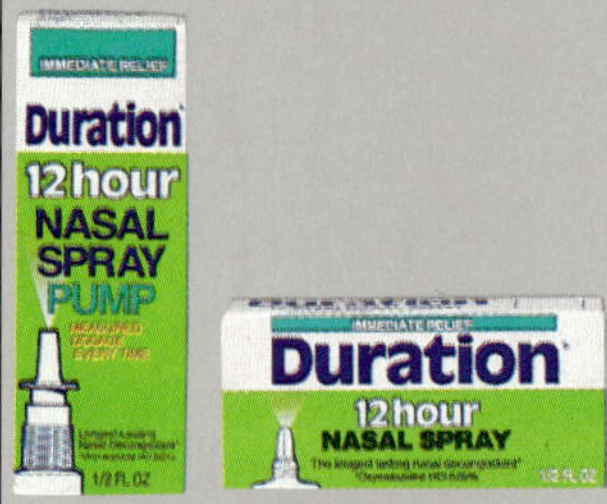

Available in ½ oz., 1 oz.; ½ oz. measured dosage pump spray; and ½ oz. mentholated.
(oxymetazoline HCl)

DURATION® NASAL SPRAY

Schering-Plough HealthCare

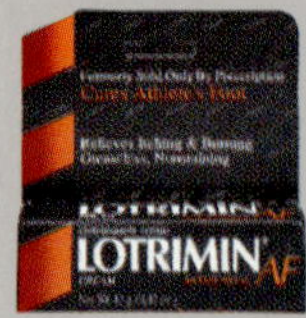

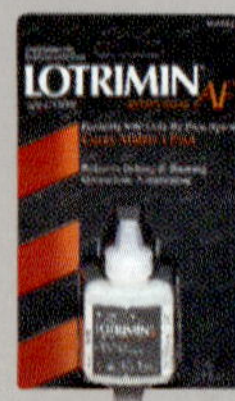

LOTRIMIN® AF
(1% clotrimazole)
For athlete's foot

Schering-Plough HealthCare

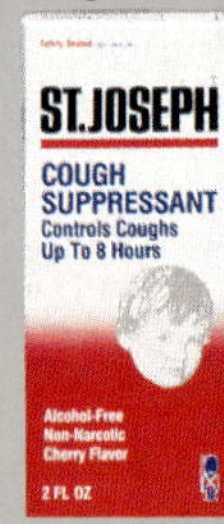

Available in 2 fl. oz. and 4 fl. oz. sizes.

ST. JOSEPH® COUGH SUPPRESSANT FOR CHILDREN
(dextromethorphan hydrobromide)

Schering-Plough HealthCare

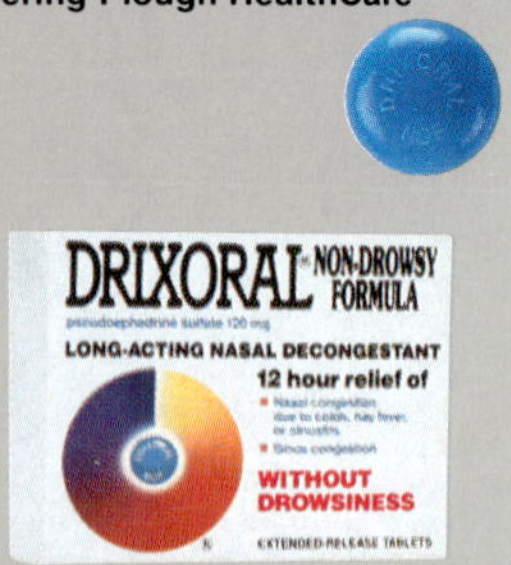

DRIXORAL® NON-DROWSY FORMULA EXTENDED-RELEASE TABLETS
(120 mg pseudoephedrine sulfate)

Schering-Plough HealthCare

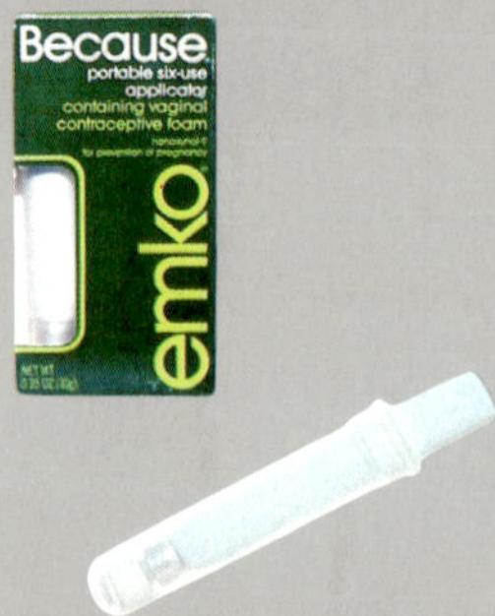

BECAUSE® CONTRACEPTOR®
(nonoxynol-9)

Schering-Plough HealthCare

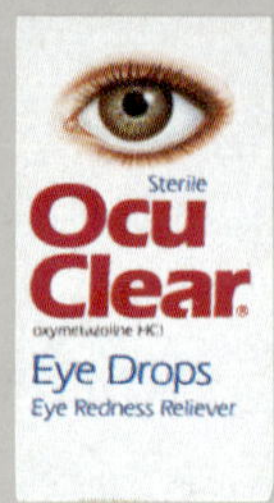

Safety Sealed

OCUCLEAR® EYE DROPS

(oxymetazoline HCl 0.025%)

Schering-Plough HealthCare

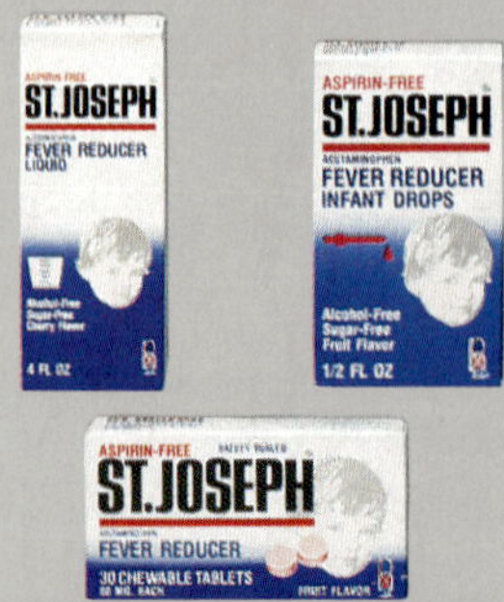

ST. JOSEPH® ASPIRIN-FREE Fever Reducers Alcohol-Free, Sugar-Free Infant Drops—Liquid and Tablets

Schering-Plough HealthCare

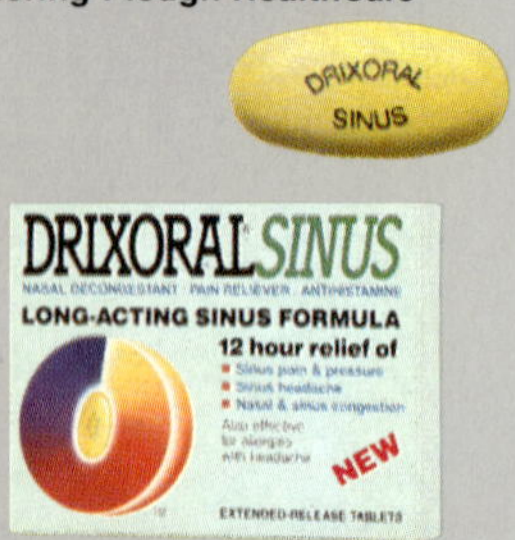

DRIXORAL® SINUS
(60 mg pseudoephedrine sulfate, 3 mg dexbrompheniramine maleate, 500 mg acetaminophen)

Schering-Plough HealthCare

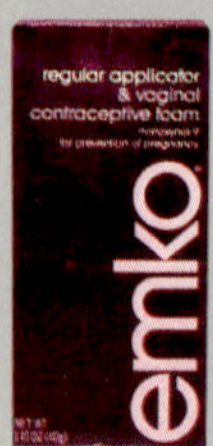

EMKO® CONTRACEPTIVE FOAM

(nonoxynol-9)

Schering-Plough HealthCare

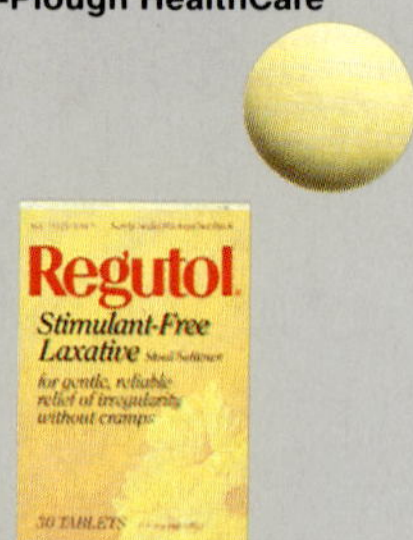

Available in 30, 60 and 90 tablet sizes.

REGUTOL® STOOL SOFTENER
(100 mg. docusate sodium per tablet)

Schering-Plough HealthCare

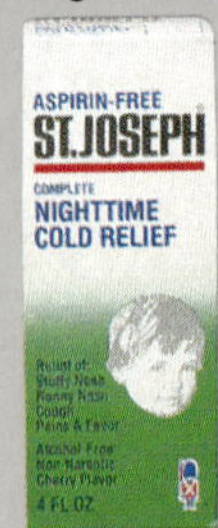

4 fl. oz. bottle

Each 5 cc (average teaspoon) contains: Chlorpheniramine maleate 1 mg., pseudoephedrine hydrochloride 15 mg., acetaminophen 160 mg., dextromethorphan hydrobromide 5 mg.

ST. JOSEPH® NIGHTTIME COLD RELIEF

Schering-Plough HealthCare

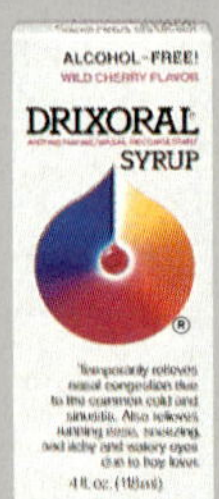

Safety Sealed

DRIXORAL® SYRUP
(2 mg brompheniramine maleate and 30 mg pseudoephedrine sulfate)

Schering-Plough HealthCare

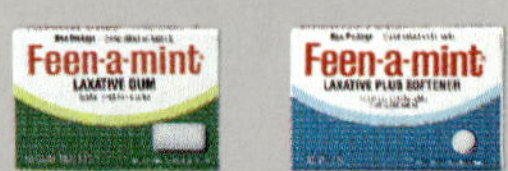

Laxative Gum

Laxative plus Softener

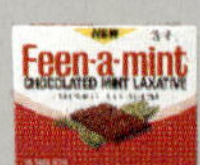

Chocolated Mint Laxative

FEEN-A-MINT® LAXATIVE

Gum contains: 97.2 mg. phenolphthalein.
Pills contain: 100 mg. docusate sodium and 65 mg. phenolphthalein.
Chocolate contains: 65 mg. phenolphthalein.

Schering-Plough HealthCare

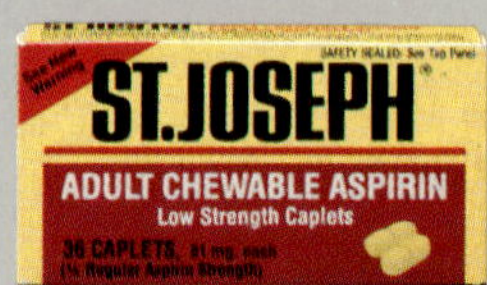

36 caplets

ST. JOSEPH® ADULT CHEWABLE ASPIRIN Low Strength Caplets

Each caplet contains 81 mg. of aspirin

Schering-Plough HealthCare

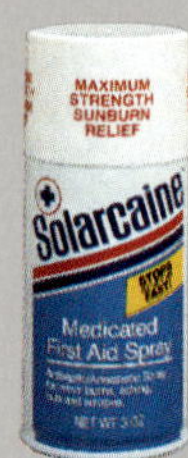

3 oz.
Also available in regular lotion, aloe aerosol, aloegel, aloe mist and aloe cream

SOLARCAINE® FIRST AID PRODUCTS
For sunburns, minor burns, cuts and scrapes

Schering-Plough HealthCare

4 fl. oz.

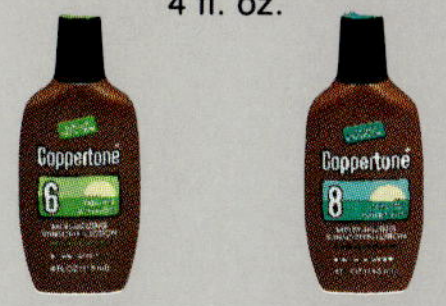

SPF 6 SPF 8

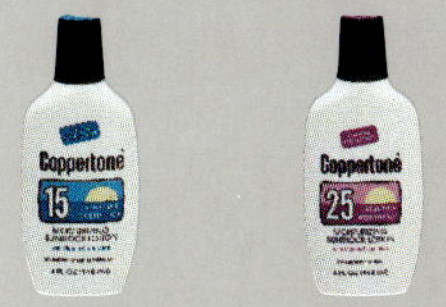

SPF 15 SPF 25

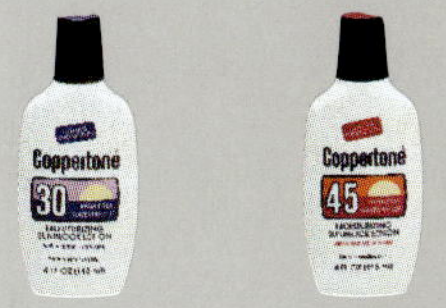

SPF 30 SPF 45

New PABA-free ingredients:
SPF 6–15: Ethylhexyl p-methoxycinnamate, oxbenzone
SPF 25, 30: Ethylhexyl p-methoxycinnamate, 2-ethylhexyl salicylate, homosalate, oxybenzone
SPF 45: Ethylhexyl p-methoxycinnamate, 2-ethylhexyl salicylate, octocrylene, oxybenzone.

COPPERTONE® WATERPROOF SUNSCREENS

Schering-Plough HealthCare

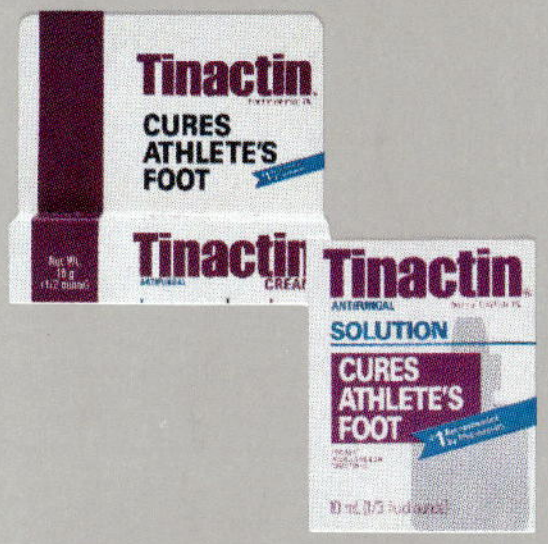

TINACTIN®
CREAM AND SOLUTION
(tolnaftate 1%)

SCHWARZ PHARMA

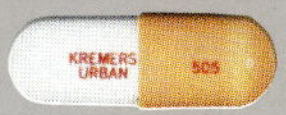

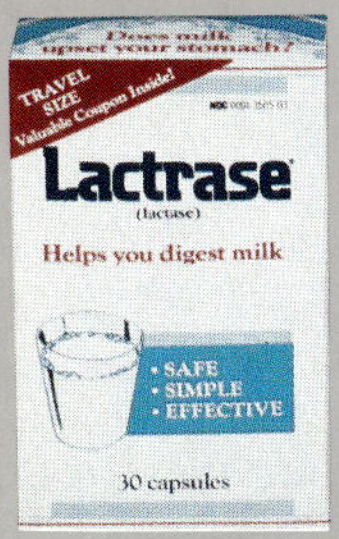

Available in cartons of 10 and 30 and bottles of 100

LACTRASE® Capsules
(lactase) 250 mg

SmithKline Beecham Consumer Brands

60 Pads

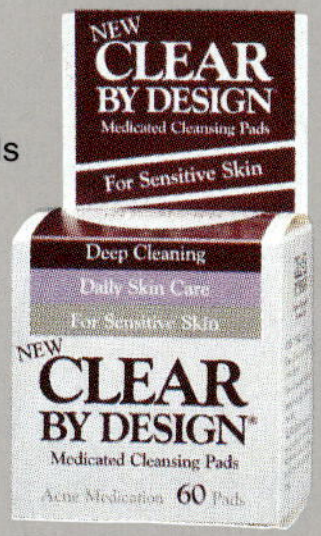

CLEAR BY DESIGN®
Medicated
Cleansing Pads

Schering-Plough HealthCare

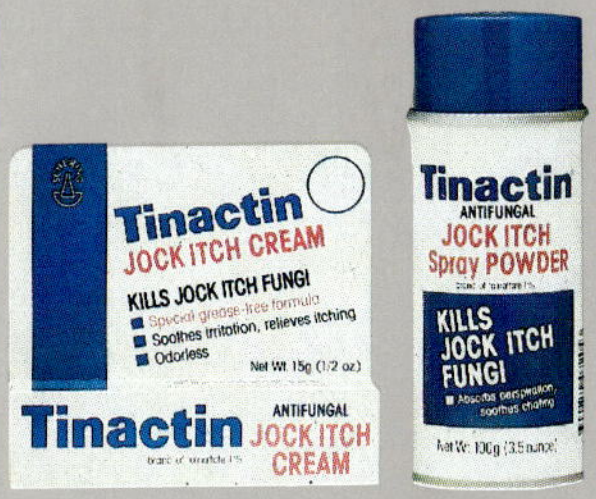

TINACTIN® JOCK ITCH
CREAM AND SPRAY POWDER
(tolnaftate 1%)

SLIM•FAST FOODS

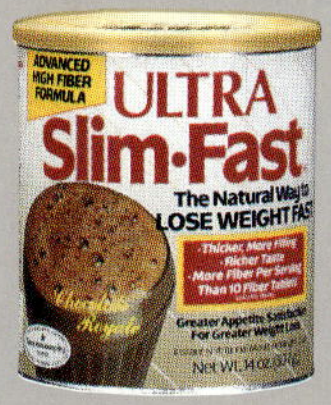

Available in Chocolate Royale, French Vanilla, Strawberry Supreme, Mocha and Fruit Juice mix

ULTRA SLIM•FAST®

SmithKline Beecham Consumer Brands

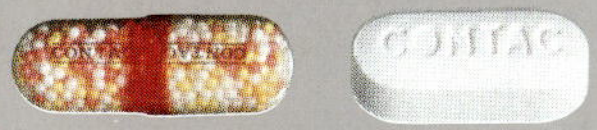

Packages of 10, 20 and 40 capsules and caplets

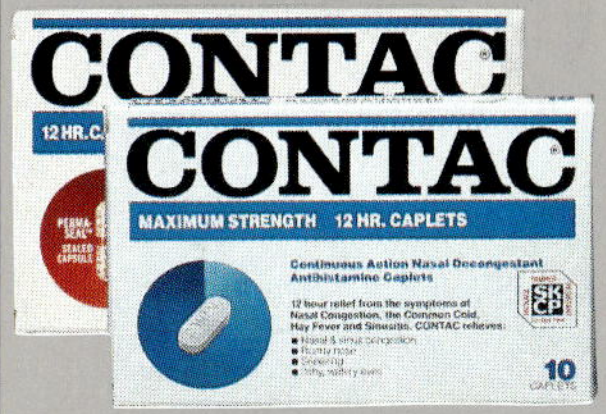

CONTAC®
CONTINUOUS ACTION NASAL DECONGESTANT ANTIHISTAMINE CAPLETS & CAPSULES

Schering-Plough HealthCare

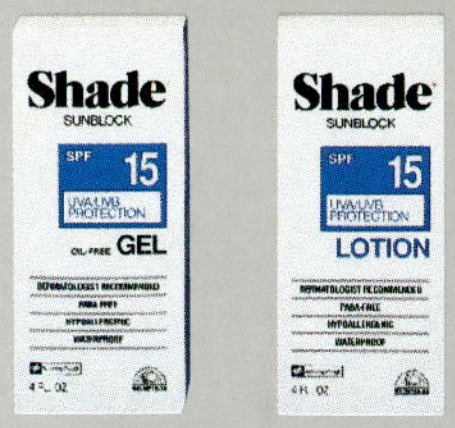

4 fl. oz.

Also available in SPF 30 and 45 Lotions, SPF 25 Gel and SPF 30 Stick

SHADE®
WATERPROOF SUNBLOCKS

Schering-Plough HealthCare

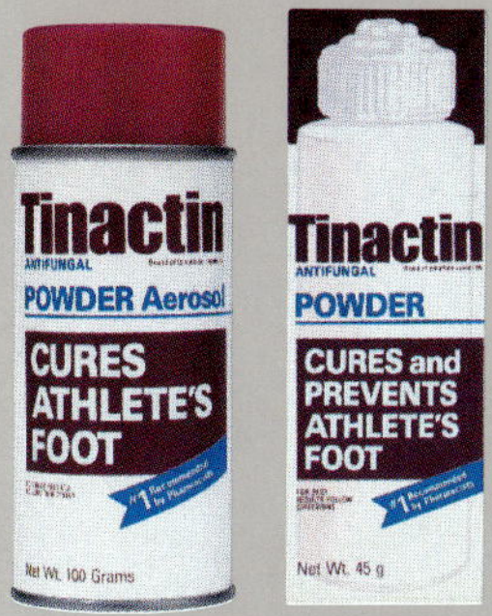

TINACTIN® POWDER AEROSOL AND POWDER
(tolnaftate 1%)

SMITHKLINE BEECHAM

Consumer Brands

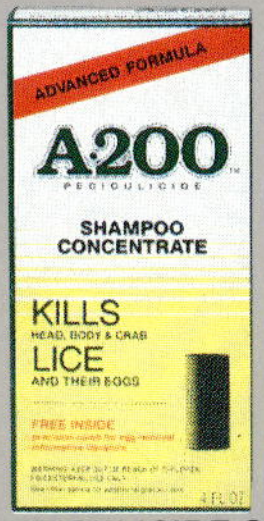

4 fl. oz.

A-200® PEDICULICIDE SHAMPOO

Also available:
A-200® Pediculicide Shampoo, 2 fl. oz.
A-200® Pediculicide Gel, 1 oz.

SmithKline Beecham Consumer Brands

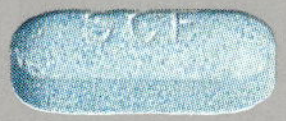

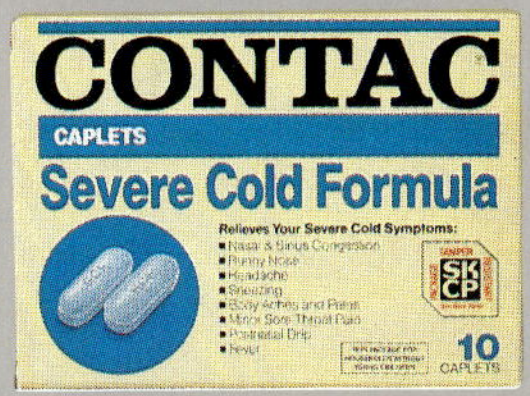

Packages of 10, 20 and 40 caplets

CONTAC®
SEVERE COLD FORMULA

Schering-Plough HealthCare

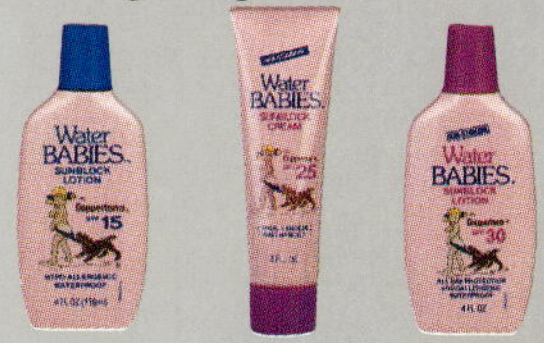

SPF 15 SPF 25 SPF 30
4 fl. oz. 3 fl. oz. 4 fl. oz.

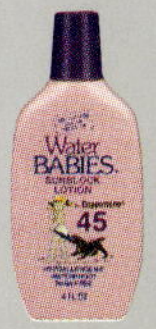

SPF 45
4 fl. oz.

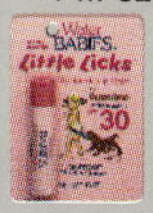

SPF 30

WATER BABIES®
SUNBLOCKS

Schering-Plough HealthCare

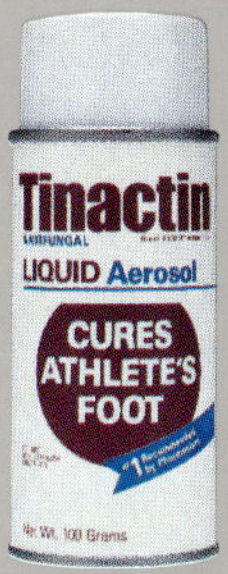

TINACTIN®
LIQUID AEROSOL
(tolnaftate 1%)

SmithKline Beecham Consumer Brands

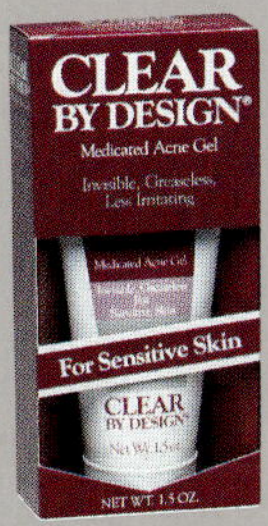

1.5 oz. tube

CLEAR BY DESIGN®
Medicated Acne Gel
(benzoyl peroxide 2.5%)

SmithKline Beecham Consumer Brands

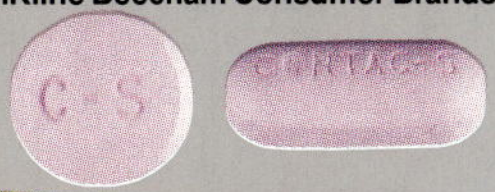

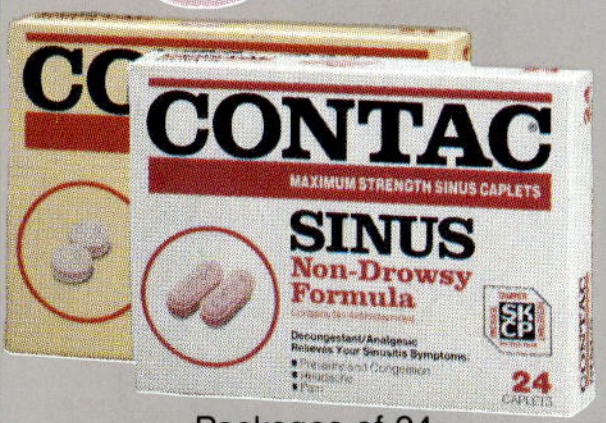

Packages of 24

CONTAC®
MAXIMUM STRENGTH SINUS TABLETS AND CAPLETS NON-DROWSY FORMULA

SmithKline Beecham Consumer Brands

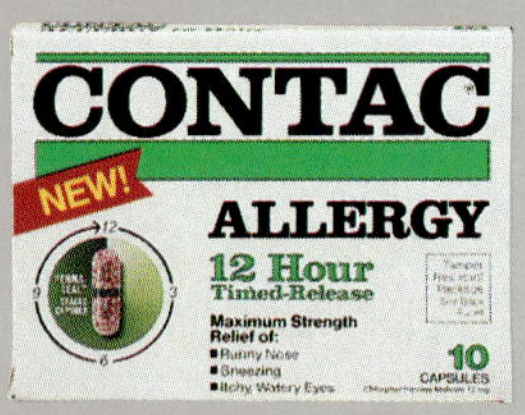

Packages of 10 and 20 Capsules

CONTAC®
Allergy 12 Hour Capsules

SmithKline Beecham Consumer Brands

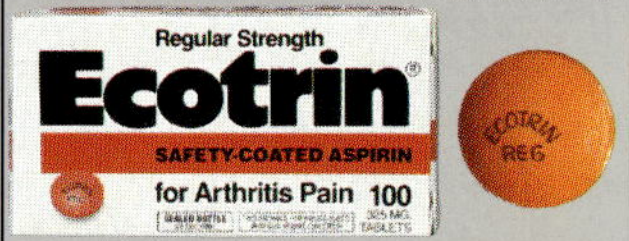

In 100, 250 and 1000 tablet bottles

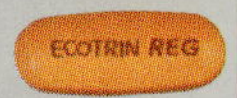

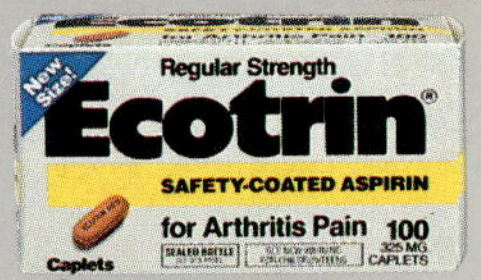

Caplets in bottles of 100

REGULAR STRENGTH ECOTRIN® TABLETS AND CAPLETS
Duentric® coated 5 gr. aspirin

SmithKline Beecham Consumer Brands

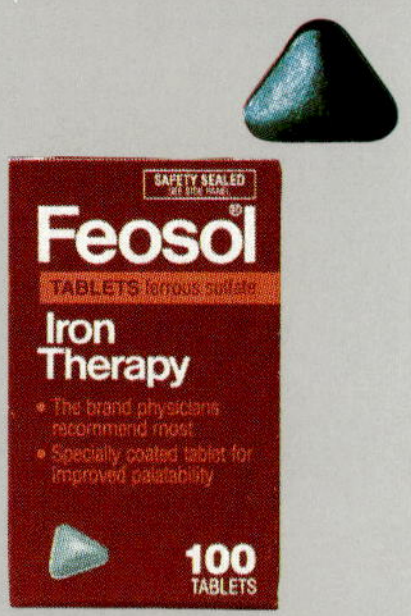

In 100 and 1000 tablet bottles

FEOSOL® TABLETS
(ferrous sulfate USP)

SmithKline Beecham Consumer Brands

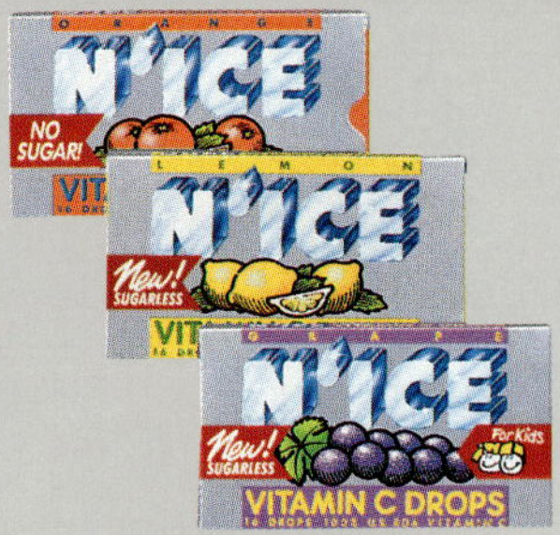

Available in Orange, Lemon, Children's Grape in 16 count packages

N'ICE®
Vitamin C Drops

SmithKline Beecham Consumer Brands

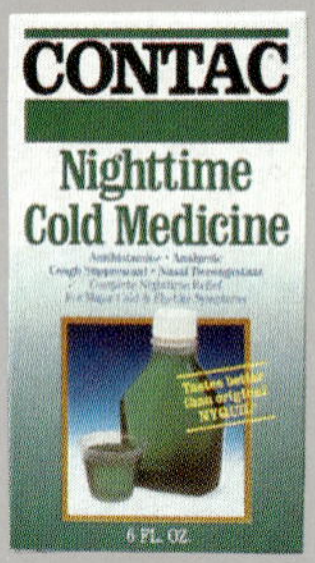

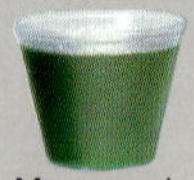

Measured dose cup

CONTAC® NIGHTTIME COLD MEDICINE

SmithKline Beecham Consumer Brands

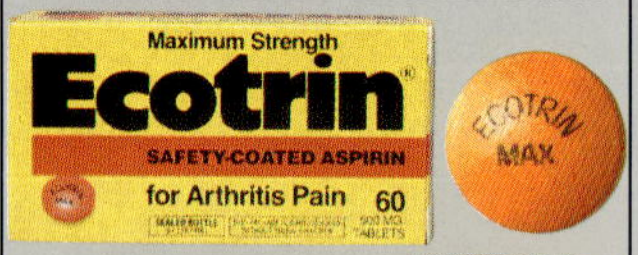

In 60 and 150 tablet bottles

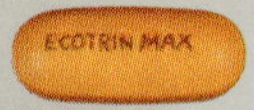

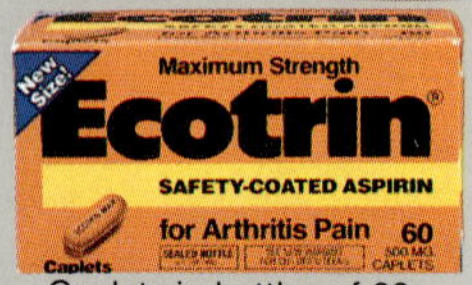

Caplets in bottles of 60

MAXIMUM STRENGTH ECOTRIN® TABLETS AND CAPLETS
Duentric® coated 7.7 gr. aspirin

SmithKline Beecham Consumer Brands

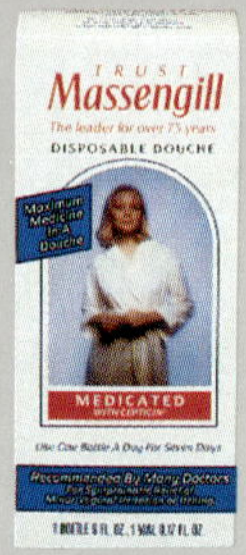

Available in single or twin packs

MASSENGILL® Medicated
Disposable Douche
With Povidone-iodine

SmithKline Beecham Consumer Brands

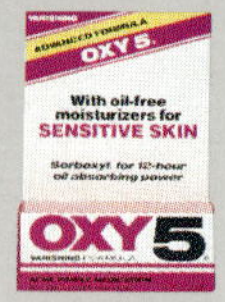

OXY® 5
Vanishing

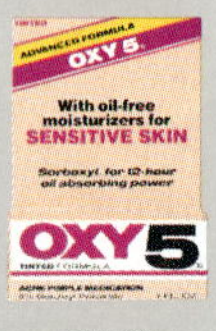

OXY® 5
Tinted

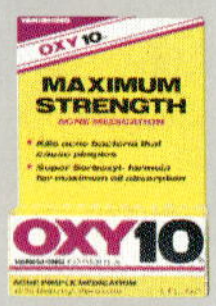

OXY® 10
Vanishing

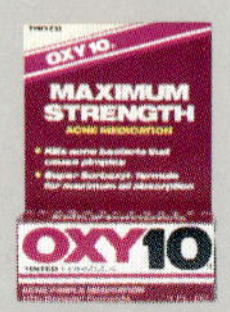

OXY® 10
Tinted

SmithKline Beecham Consumer Brands

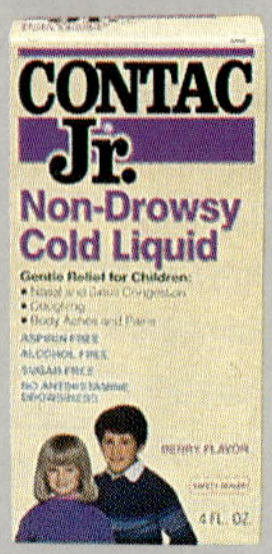

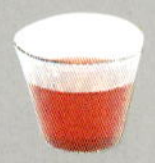

Includes dose-by-weight cup

CONTAC JR.® COLD MEDICINE FOR CHILDREN

SmithKline Beecham Consumer Brands

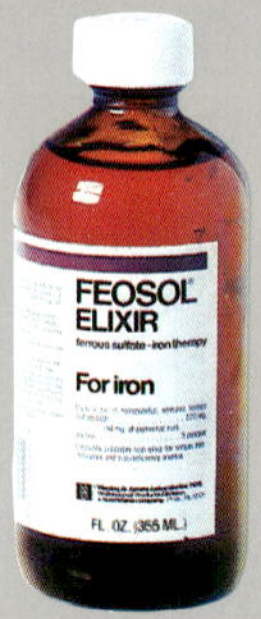

16 oz. bottle
FEOSOL® ELIXIR
(ferrous sulfate USP)

SmithKline Beecham Consumer Brands

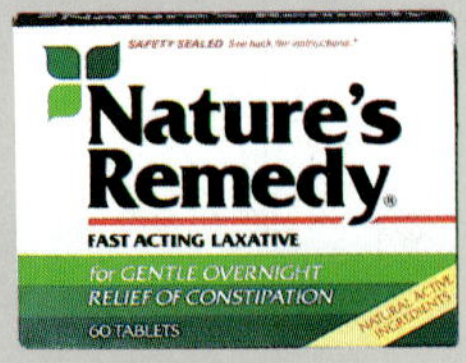

60 tablets

NATURE'S REMEDY®

Also available:
Box 12s and 30s

SmithKline Beecham Consumer Brands

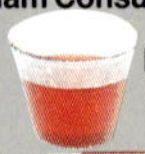

Measured dose cup

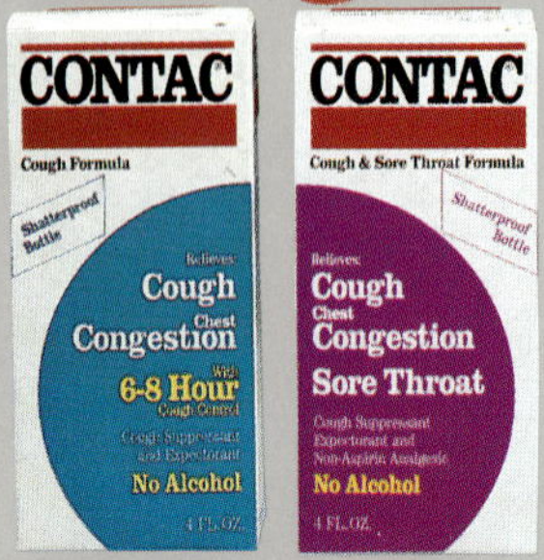

CONTAC® COUGH AND COUGH & SORE THROAT FORMULA

SmithKline Beecham Consumer Brands

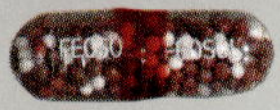

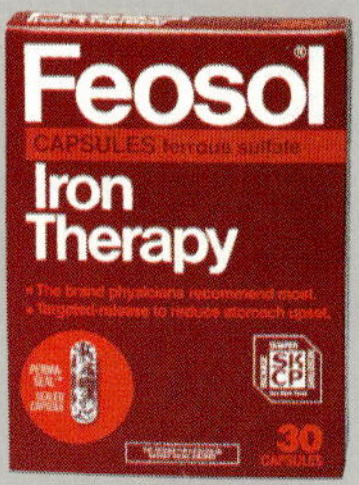

Packages of 30 and 60 capsules and bottles of 500

FEOSOL® CAPSULES
(ferrous sulfate USP)

SmithKline Beecham Consumer Brands

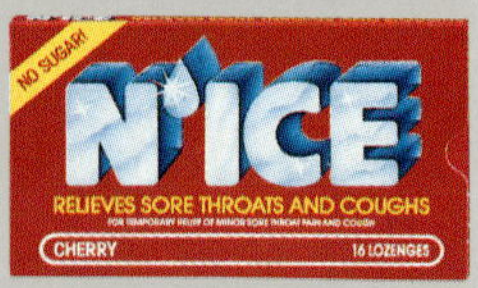

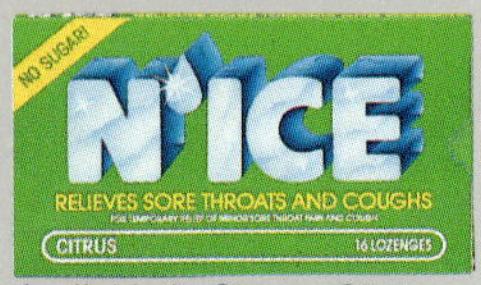

Available in Cherry, Citrus, Menthol Eucalyptus, Menthol Mint, Children's Berry

N'ICE®
Sore Throat Lozenges

SmithKline Beecham Consumer Brands

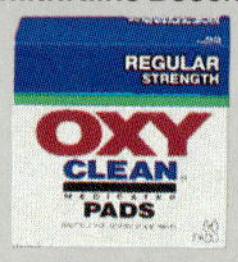

Regular Strength

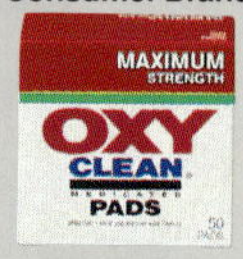

Maximum Strength

Sensitive Skin

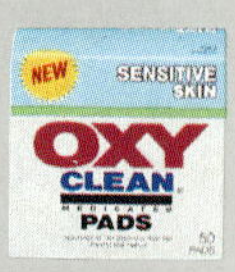

50 pads
Also available: 90 pads

OXY CLEAN® MEDICATED PADS

SmithKline Beecham Consumer Brands

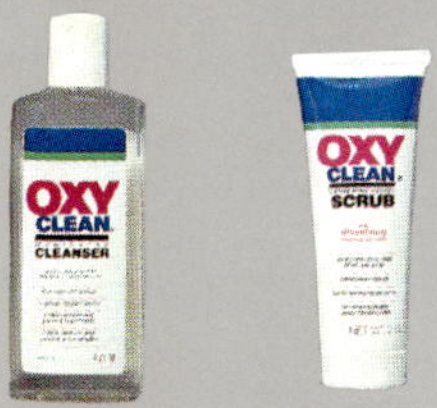

Medicated Cleanser 4 fl. oz.

Lathering Facial Scrub 2.65 oz.

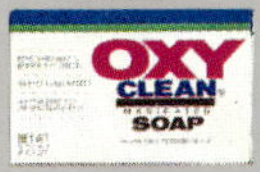

Medicated Soap 3.25 oz.

OXY CLEAN®

SmithKline Beecham Consumer Brands

24 caplet package

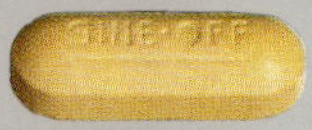

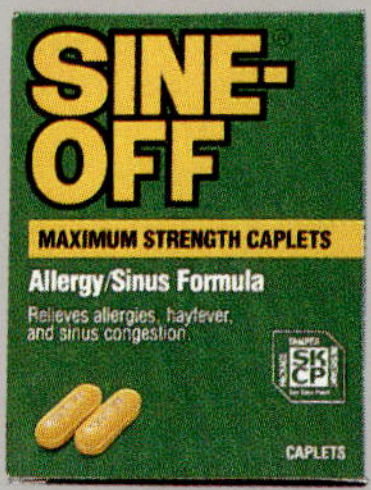

SINE-OFF®
MAXIMUM STRENGTH ALLERGY/ SINUS FORMULA CAPLETS

SmithKline Beecham Consumer Brands

Cherry Mint

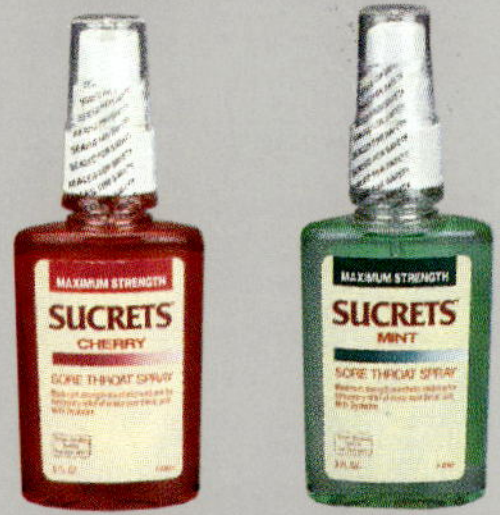

Available in 3 oz and 6 oz Bottles

SUCRETS®
Maximum

SmithKline Beecham Consumer Brands

Available in Extra Strength and Extra Strength with Simethicone

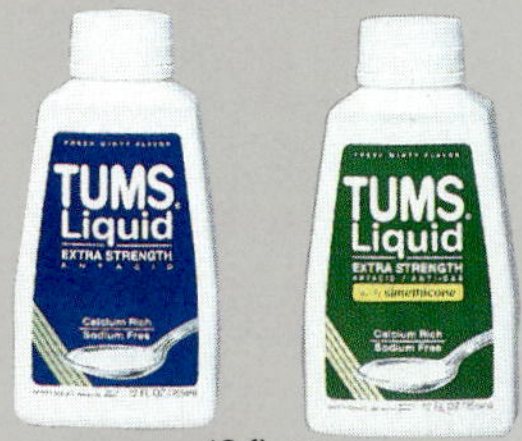

12 fl. oz.

TUMS® LIQUID
Extra Strength Antacid
(calcium carbonate)

SmithKline Beecham Consumer Brands

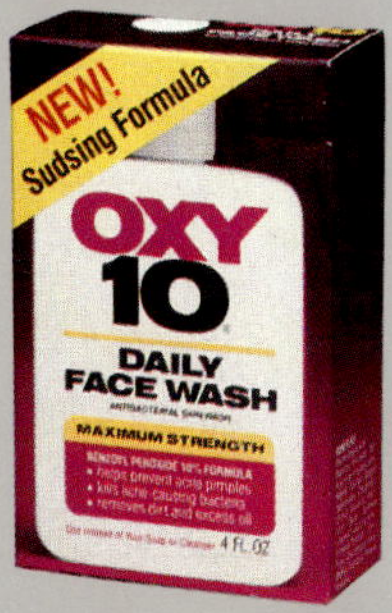

OXY 10® DAILY FACE WASH

SmithKline Beecham Consumer Brands

24 caplet package

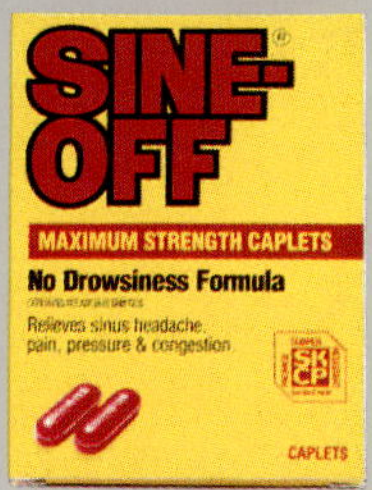

SINE-OFF®
MAXIMUM STRENGTH
NO DROWSINESS FORMULA CAPLETS

SmithKline Beecham Consumer Brands

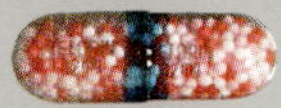

Packages of 12, 24 and 48 capsules

12 mg.

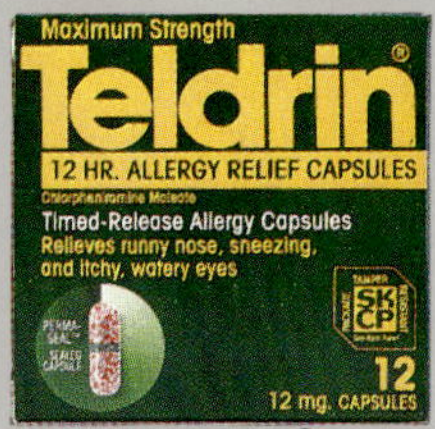

TELDRIN®
TIMED-RELEASE CAPSULES
(chlorpheniramine maleate)

SQUIBB

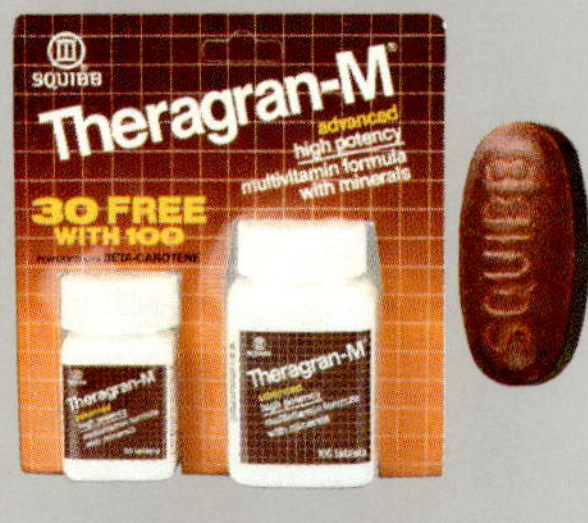

ADVANCED FORMULA THERAGRAN-M®
High Potency Multivitamin Formula with Minerals

SmithKline Beecham Consumer Brands

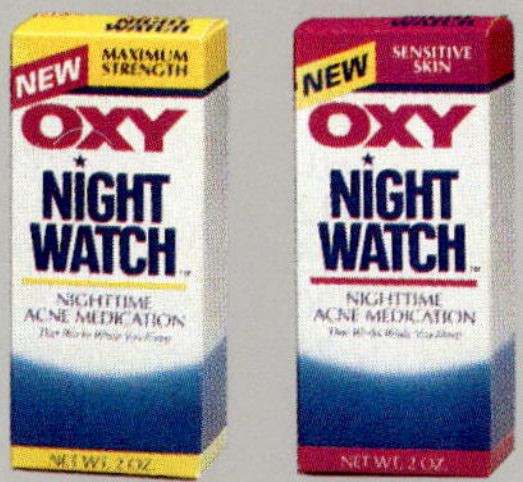

Maximum Strength

Sensitive Skin

OXY NIGHT WATCH™

SmithKline Beecham Consumer Brands

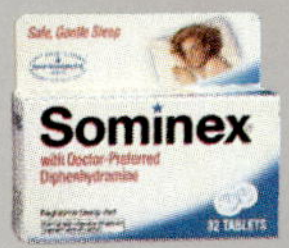

Boxes of 16, 32 and 72 Tablets

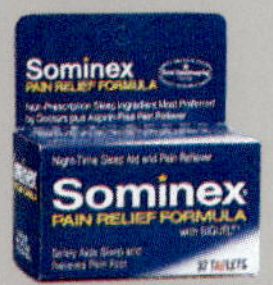

Boxes of 16 and 32 Tablets

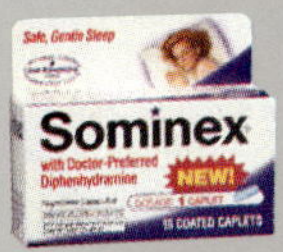

Boxes of 8, 16 and 32 Caplets

SOMINEX®
Night-Time Sleep Aids

SmithKline Beecham Consumer Brands

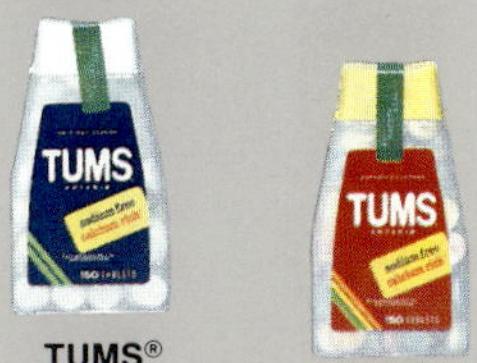

TUMS®
Peppermint

TUMS®
Assorted Flavors

E. R. Squibb & Sons

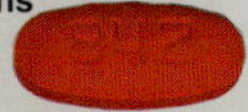

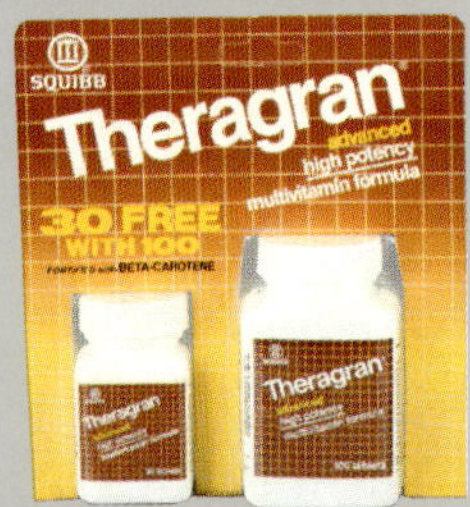

ADVANCED FORMULA THERAGRAN®
High Potency Multivitamin Formula

SmithKline Beecham Consumer Brands

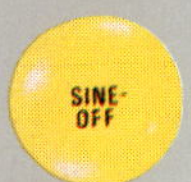

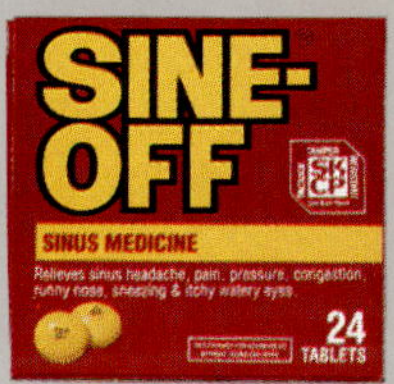

Packages of 24, 48, and 100 tablets

SINE-OFF® REGULAR STRENGTH ASPIRIN FORMULA

SmithKline Beecham Consumer Brands

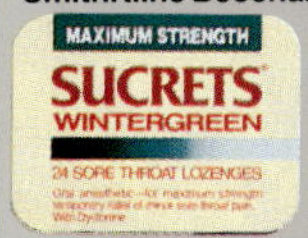

Maximum Strength

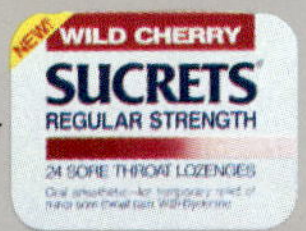

Regular

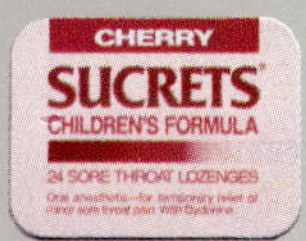

Children's Formula

SUCRETS®
Sore Throat Lozenges

SmithKline Beecham Consumer Brands

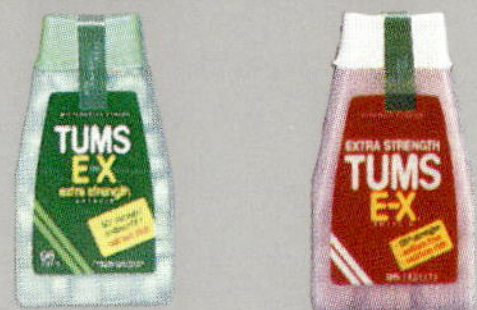

TUMS E-X®
Wintergreen

TUMS E-X®
Cherry

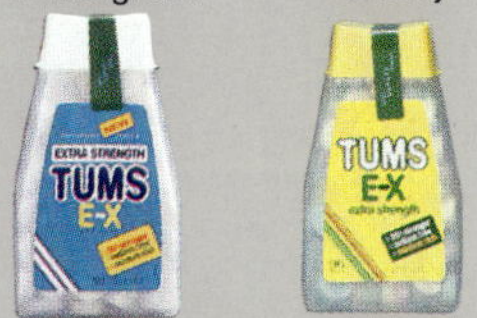

TUMS E-X®
Peppermint

TUMS E-X®
Assorted Flavors

E. R. Squibb & Sons

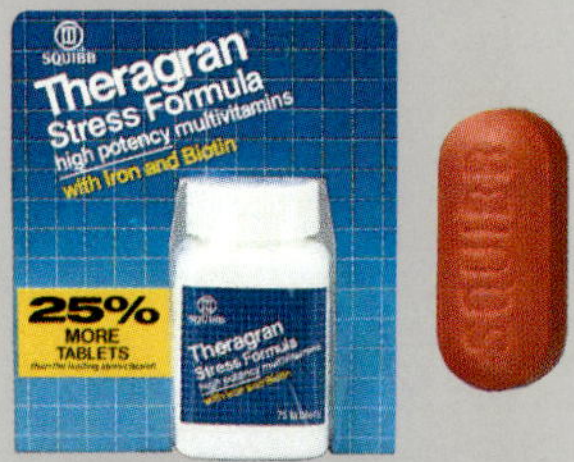

THERAGRAN® STRESS FORMULA
High Potency Multivitamin Formula with Iron and Biotin

E. R. Squibb & Sons

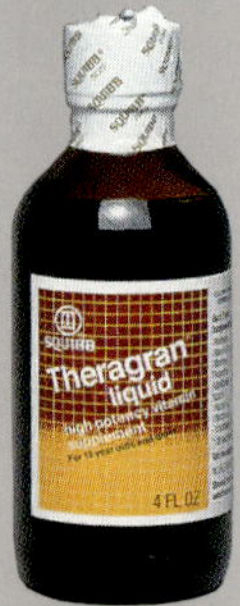

THERAGRAN® LIQUID
High Potency Liquid
Vitamin Supplement

TEC LABORATORIES

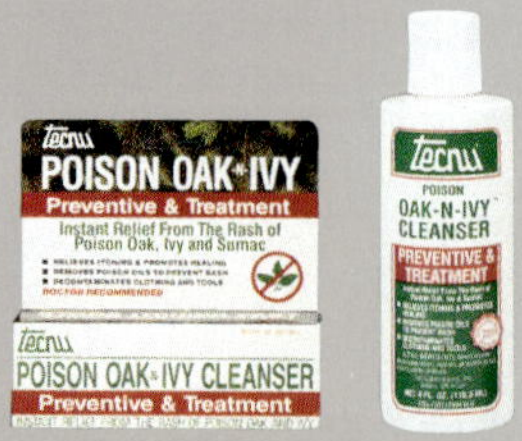

tecnu®
POISON OAK -N- IVY CLEANSER
Preventive & Treatment
Instant Relief from the Rash of
Poison Oak and Ivy

Thompson Medical Company, Inc.

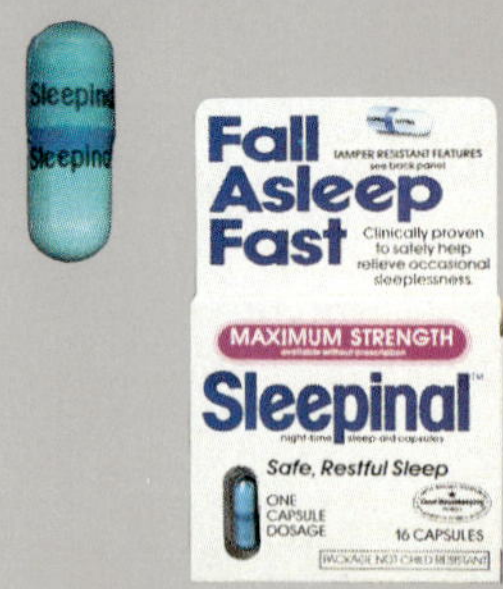

Available in 16, 32 capsule sizes

SLEEPINAL™
(diphenhydramine HCl 50 mg.)

Upjohn

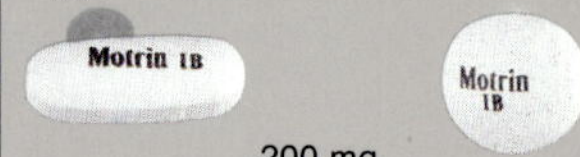

200 mg

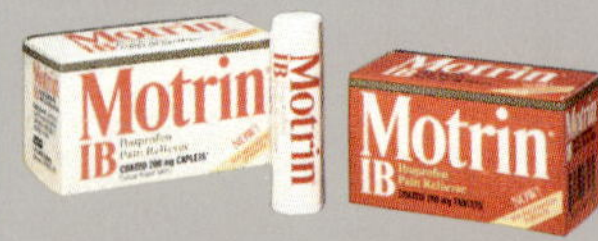

MOTRIN® IB
Caplets and Tablets
(ibuprofen, USP)
Bottles of 24, 50, 100 and 165;
Convenience pack (vial) of 8

STELLAR

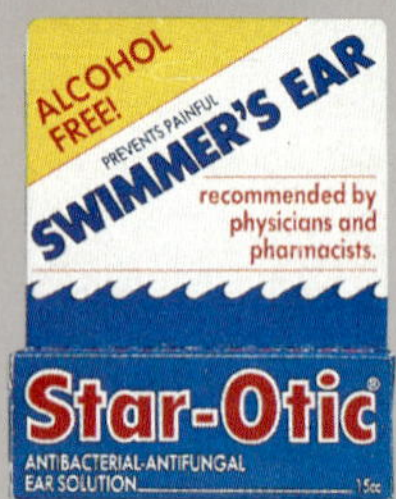

Prevent Swimmer's Ear

STAR-OTIC®
Antibacterial • Antifungal

THOMPSON MEDICAL

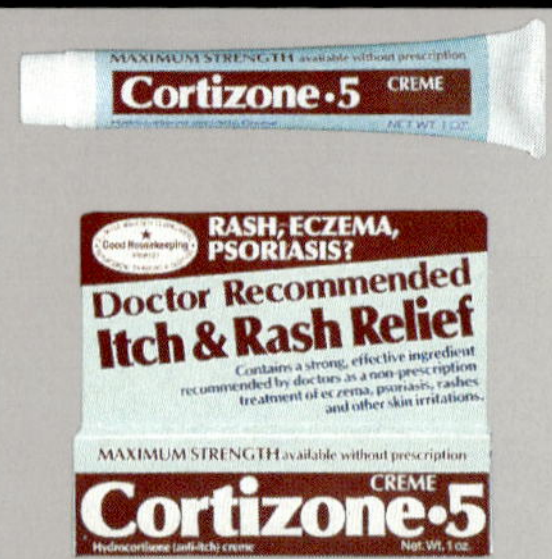

Available in ½, 1, 2 oz. creme;
1 oz. ointment

CORTIZONE-5
(hydrocortisone 0.5%)

UPJOHN

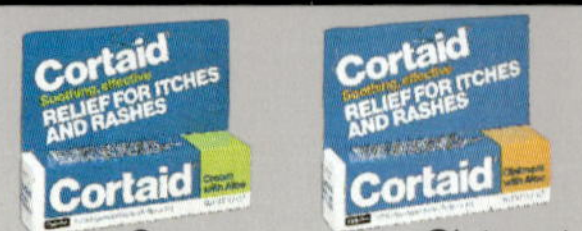

Cream with Aloe ½ oz, 1 oz

Ointment with Aloe ½ oz, 1 oz

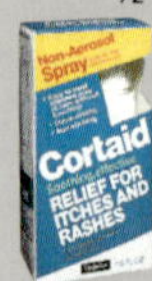

Spray 1.5 oz

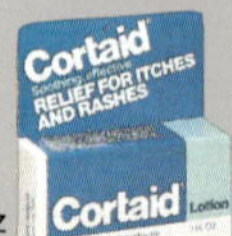

Lotion 1 oz

CORTAID®
Cream & Ointment with Aloe; Lotion
(hydrocortisone acetate)
Spray (hydrocortisone)

Upjohn

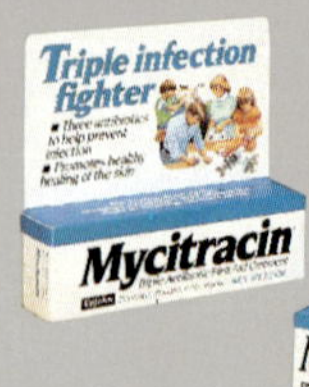

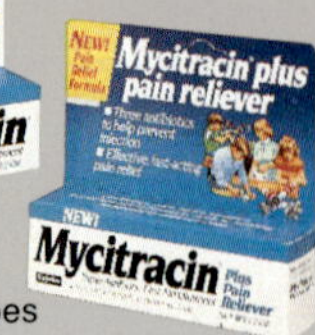

½ oz & 1 oz tubes

MYCITRACIN®
Triple Antibiotic Ointment
(bacitracin-polymyxin-neomycin)

MYCITRACIN® Plus Pain Reliever
(bacitracin-polymyxin-neomycin-lidocaine
topical ointment)

STUART

4 oz 8 oz

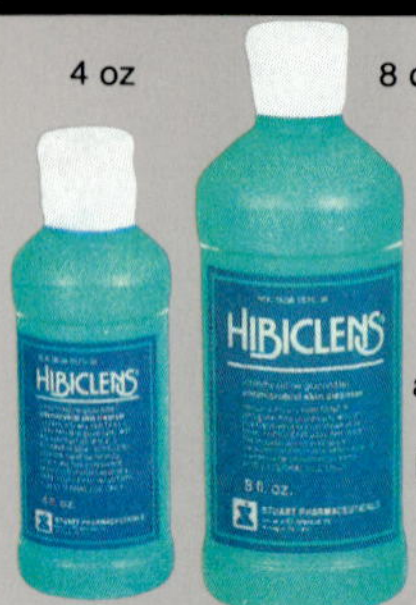

Also bottles of 16 oz, 32 oz and 1 gal; 15 ml packettes

HIBICLENS®
(chlorhexidine gluconate)
Antiseptic Antimicrobial
Skin Cleanser

Thompson Medical Company, Inc.

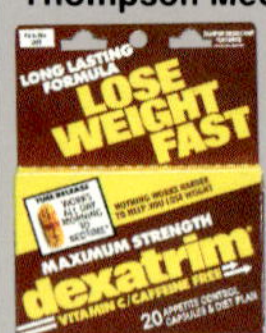

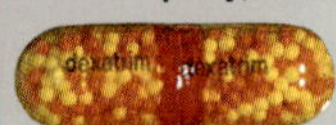

Available in
10, 20 and 40
capsule sizes

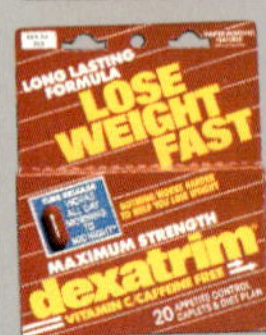

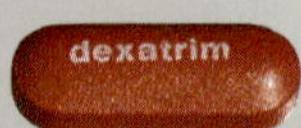

Available in
10, 20 and 40
caplet sizes

MAXIMUM STRENGTH DEXATRIM®
Capsules & Caplets
Plus Vitamin C

Upjohn

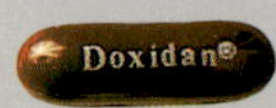

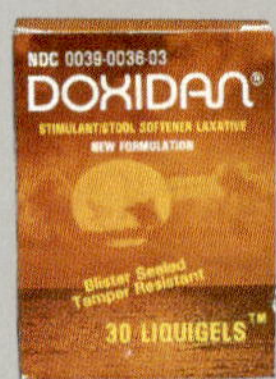

Packages of
10, 30, 100
and 1,000

Stimulant/Stool Softener Laxative

DOXIDAN® Capsules
(docusate calcium and
phenolphthalein)

Upjohn

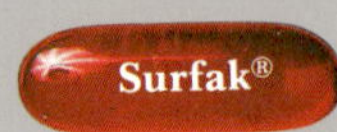

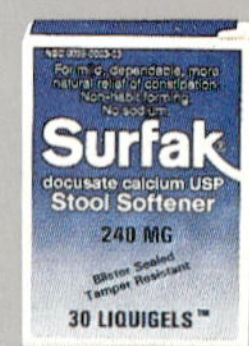

Packages of 7, 30,
100 and 500

Stool Softener

SURFAK® Capsules
(docusate calcium)

Stuart

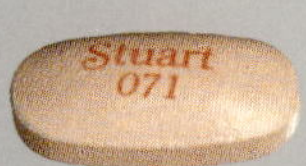

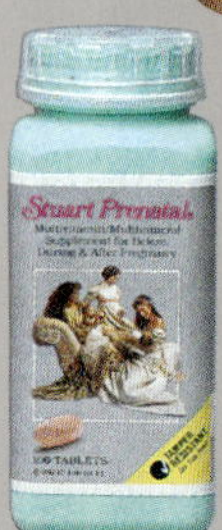

Bottles of
100 tablets

STUART PRENATAL® TABLETS
Multivitamin/Multimineral Supplement
for pregnant or lactating women

Thompson Medical Company, Inc.

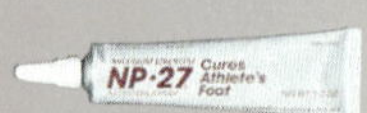

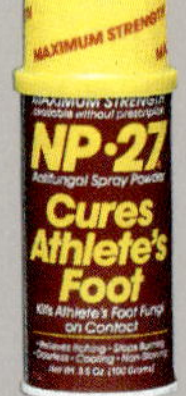

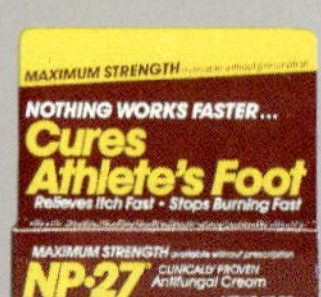

Available in ½, 1 oz. cream; ½ oz.
solution; 3.5 oz. spray powder

NP-27®
(tolnaftate 1%)

Upjohn

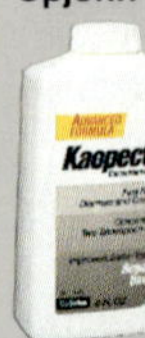

Regular Flavor Liquid

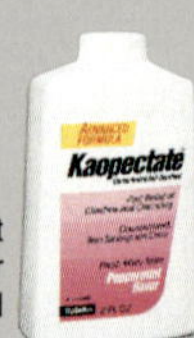

Peppermint Flavor Liquid

3.8, 12, 16 oz. 8, 12 oz.

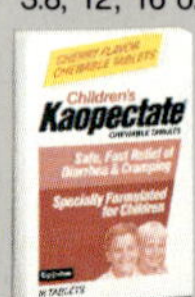

Children's Cherry Flavor Chewable Tablets

16's

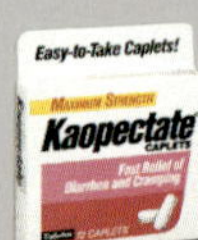

Maximum Strength Caplets

12's, 20's

KAOPECTATE® Anti-Diarrheal

Upjohn

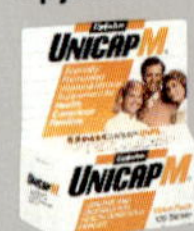

UNICAP M® Tablets
Bottle of 120

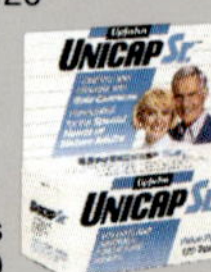

UNICAP Sr.® Tablets
Bottle of 120

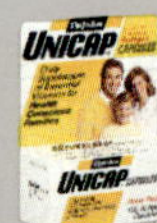

UNICAP® Capsules
Bottle of 120
Softgel Capsules

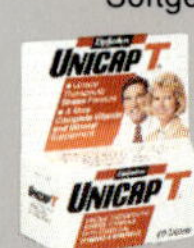

UNICAP T® Tablets
Stress Formula
Bottle of 60

Multivitamin Supplement

WAKUNAGA

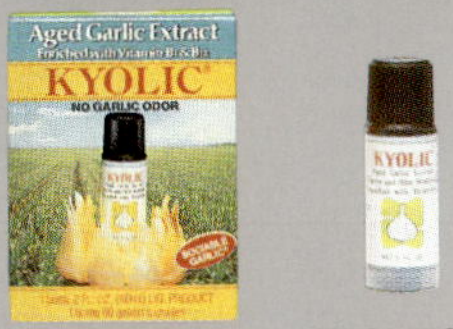

KYOLIC®
Aged Garlic Extract
with B_1, B_{12}

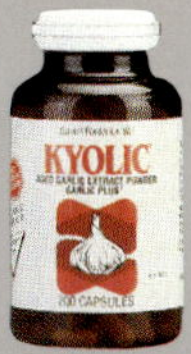

KYOLIC®
Aged Garlic Extract
Super Formula
101-Capsules

Wallace

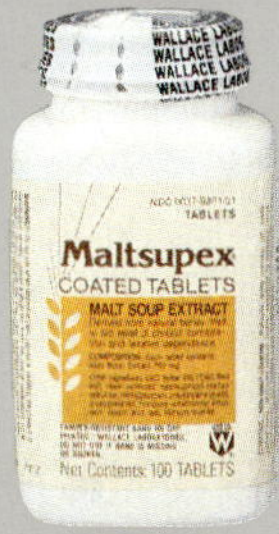

100 tablets

MALTSUPEX® TABLETS
(malt soup extract)

Wallace

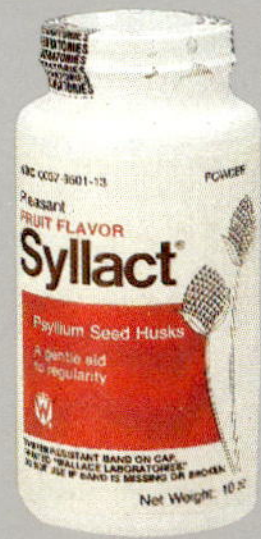

SYLLACT™
(powdered psyllium seed husks)

Warner-Lambert Co.

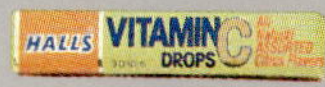

Assorted Citrus

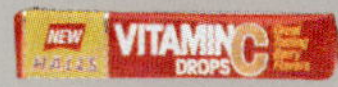

Assorted Berry

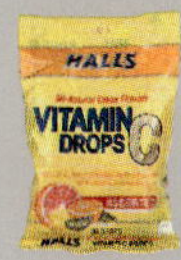

HALLS® VITAMIN C DROPS

WALKER, CORP & CO.

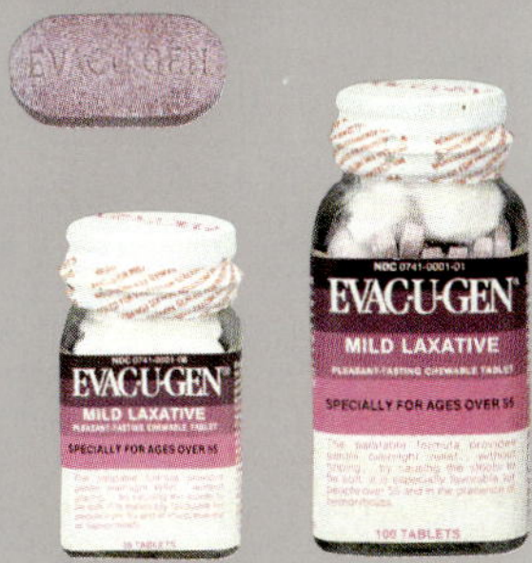

35 Tablets 100 Tablets

EVAC-U-GEN®
Mild Laxative

Wallace

1 pint
(473 ml)

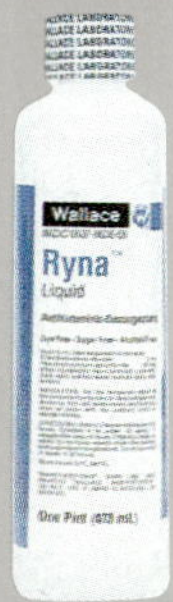

Also available: 4 fl oz (118 ml)

RYNA™ LIQUID
(antihistamine-decongestant)

WARNER-LAMBERT CO.

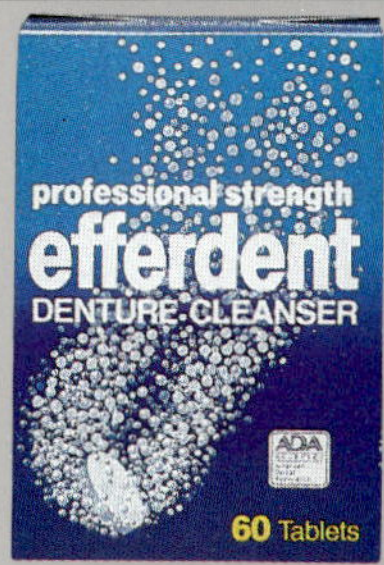

PROFESSIONAL STRENGTH EFFERDENT®

Denture Cleanser

Warner-Lambert Co.

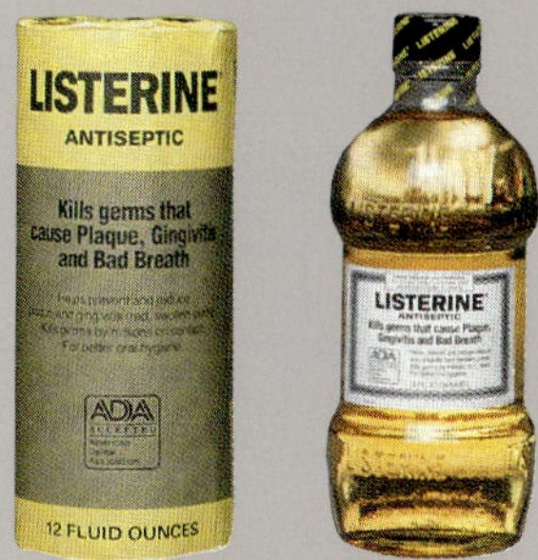

LISTERINE® ANTISEPTIC

WALLACE

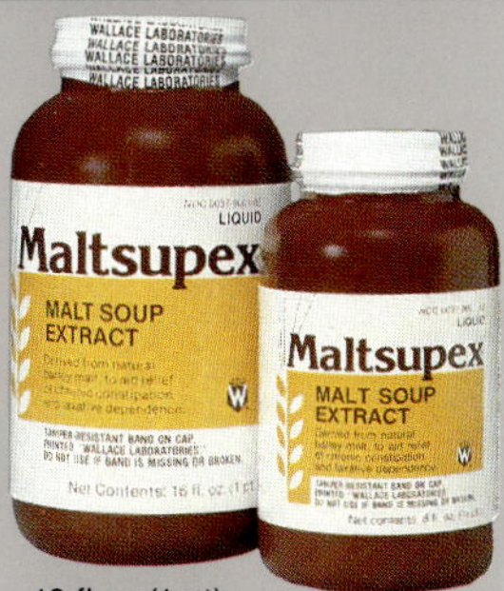

16 fl oz (1 pt) 8 fl oz (½ pt)

MALTSUPEX® LIQUID
(malt soup extract)

Wallace

1 pint
(473 ml)

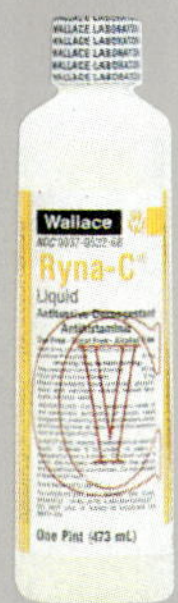

Also available: 4 fl oz (118 ml)

RYNA-C® LIQUID
(antitussive-antihistamine-decongestant)

Warner-Lambert Co.

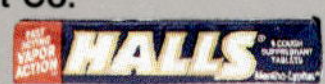

Mentho-Lyptus

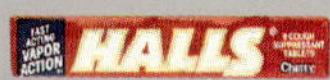

Cherry

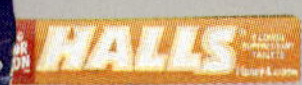

Honey-Lemon

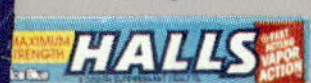

Ice Blue

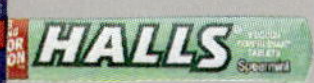

Spearmint

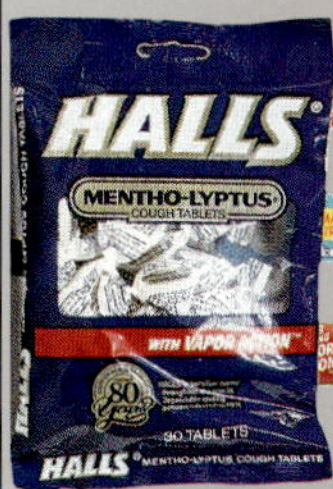

HALLS® MENTHO-LYPTUS
Cough Suppressant Tablets

Warner-Lambert Co.

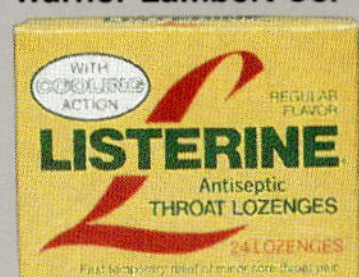

24
Lozenges

LISTERINE®
Antiseptic Throat Lozenges

24
Lozenges

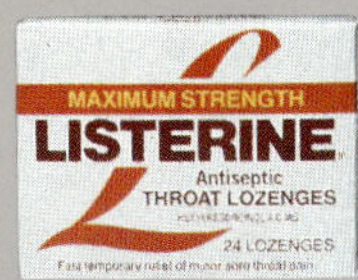

MAXIMUM STRENGTH LISTERINE®
Antiseptic Throat Lozenges

Wallace

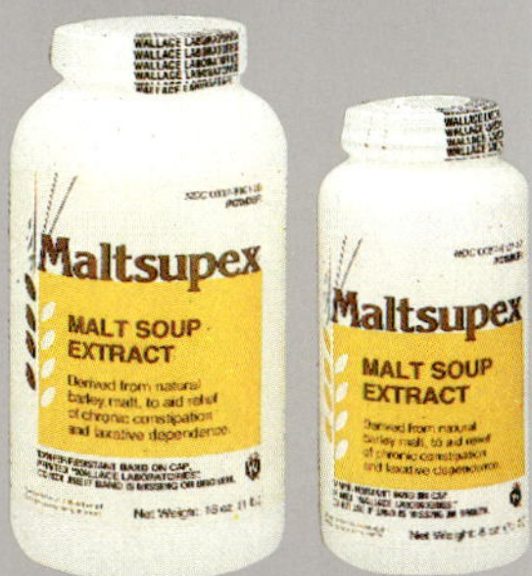

16 oz (1 lb) 8 oz (½ lb)

MALTSUPEX® POWDER
(malt soup extract)

Wallace

1 pint
(473 ml)

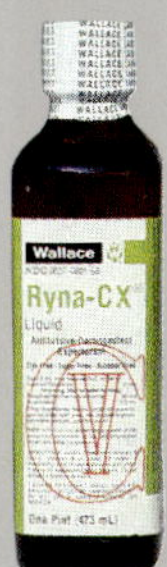

Also available: 4 fl oz (118 ml)

RYNA-CX® LIQUID
(antitussive-decongestant-expectorant)

Warner-Lambert Co.

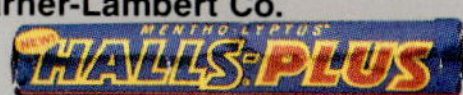

Mentho-Lyptus

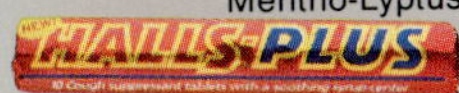

Cherry

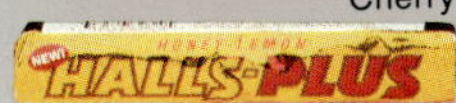

Honey-Lemon

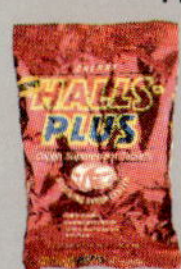

HALLS® PLUS
Cough Suppressant Tablets

Soothing Syrup Center

Warner-Lambert Co.

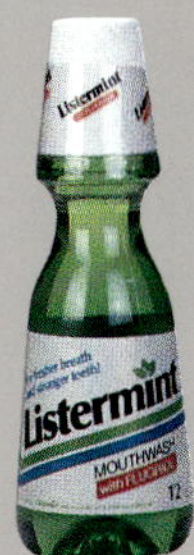

LISTERMINT™ with FLUORIDE
Anticavity Dental Rinse &
Mouthwash

Warner-Lambert Co.

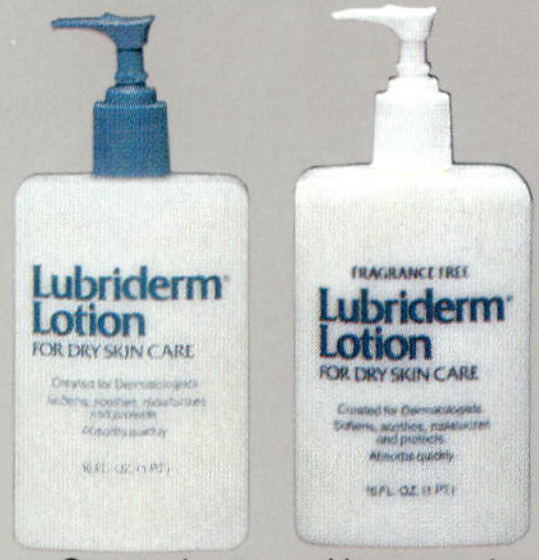

Scented Unscented

LUBRIDERM® LOTION

For Dry Skin Care

Warner-Lambert Co.

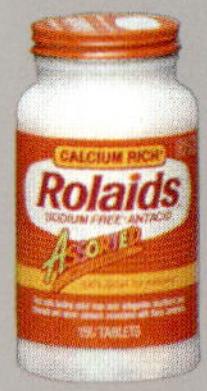

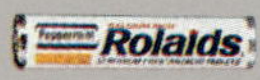

Peppermint

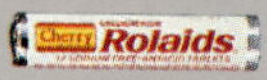

Cherry

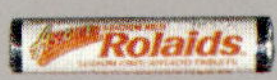

Assorted Fruit

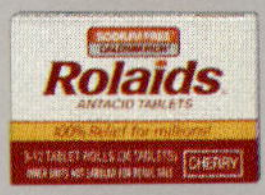

CALCIUM RICH SODIUM FREE ROLAIDS®

Calcium Rich, Sodium Free Relief from Heartburn, Sour Stomach or Acid Indigestion and Upset Stomach Associated with these Symptoms

Westwood-Squibb

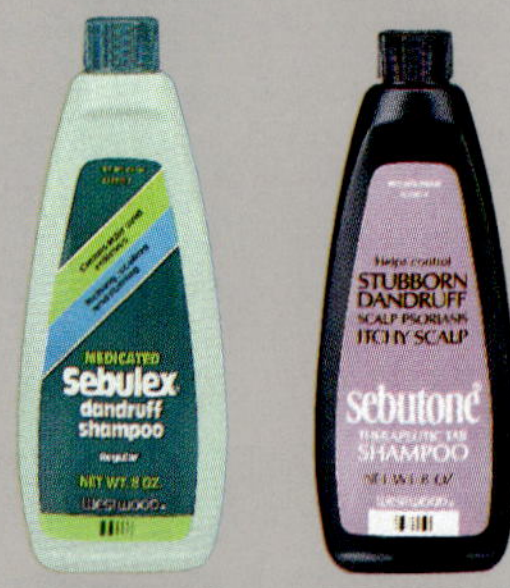

SEBULEX® **SEBUTONE®**
Medicated Dandruff Shampoos

Whitehall

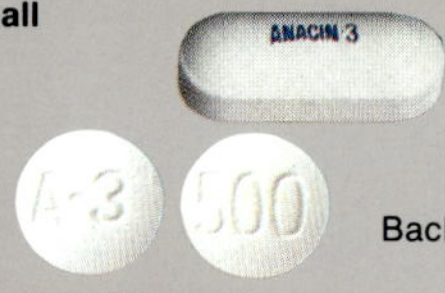

Front Back

500 mg.

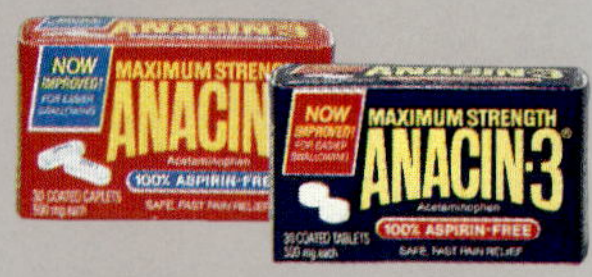

Coated Tablets: Tins of 12, Bottles of 30, 60 and 100. Coated Caplets: Bottles of 30, 60 and 100.

MAXIMUM STRENGTH ANACIN-3®
Acetaminophen Tablets and Caplets

Warner-Lambert Co.

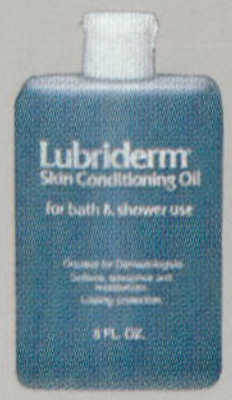

8 fl. oz.

LUBRIDERM® SKIN CONDITIONING OIL

For Dry Skin Care

Warner-Lambert Co.

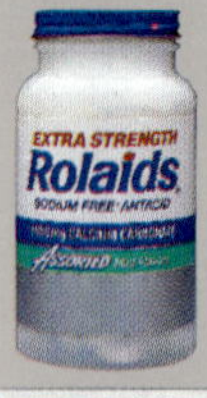

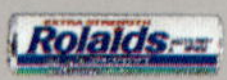

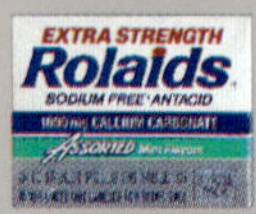

EXTRA STRENGTH ROLAIDS®

Extra Strength Calcium, Sodium Free Relief from Heartburn, Sour Stomach or Acid Indigestion and Upset Stomach Associated with these Symptoms

WHITEHALL

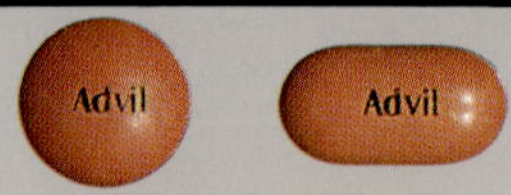

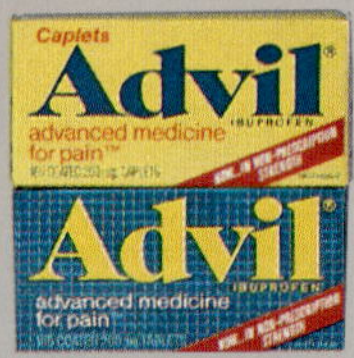

Coated Tablets in Bottles of 24, 50, 100, 165 and 250. Coated Caplets in Bottles of 24, 50, 100, 165 and 250.
ADVIL®
Ibuprofen Tablets and Caplets, USP

Whitehall

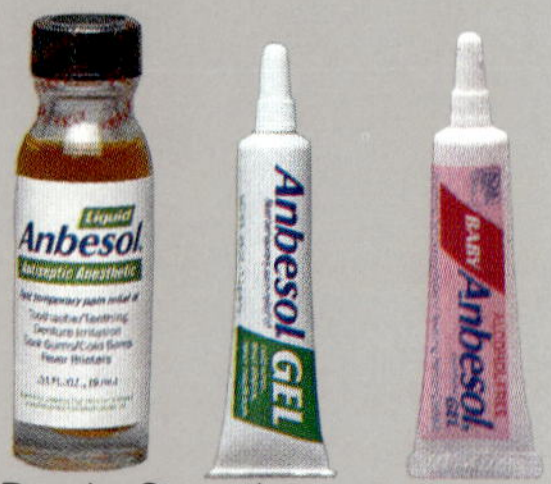

Regular Strength
Liquid .31 oz. and .74 oz. Gel .25 oz. Baby Teething Gel .25 oz.

ANBESOL®

Warner-Lambert Co.

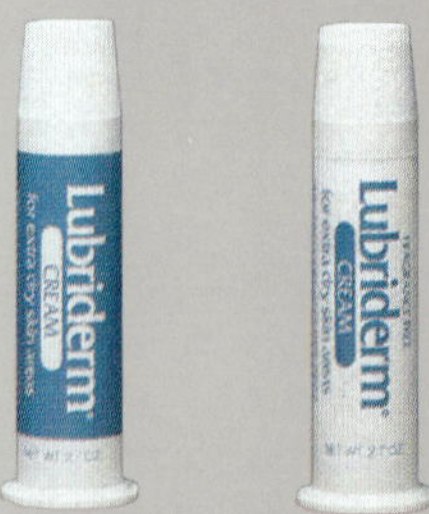

Scented Unscented

LUBRIDERM® CREAM

For Extra Dry Skin Areas

WESTWOOD-SQUIBB

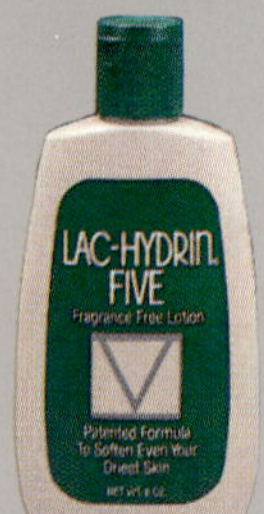

8 oz.

LAC-HYDRIN® FIVE
Fragrance Free Lotion

Patented—Softens Even Your Driest Skin

Whitehall

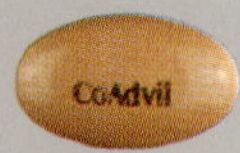

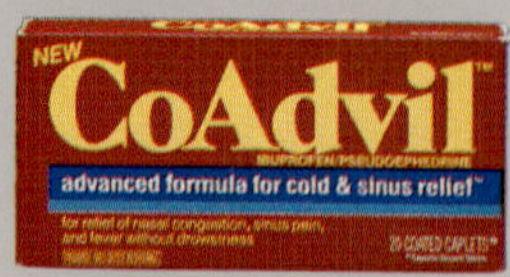

Coated Caplets in Packages of 20 and Bottles of 48 and 100.

CoADVIL™
Ibuprofen/Pseudoephedrine Caplets

Whitehall

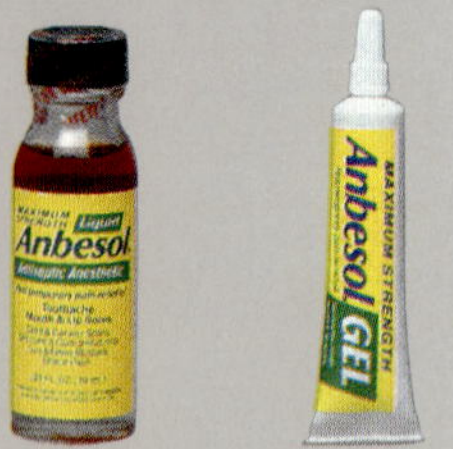

Liquid .31 oz. Gel .25 oz.

MAXIMUM STRENGTH ANBESOL®
Anesthetic for Oral Topical Pain Relief

Warner-Lambert Co.

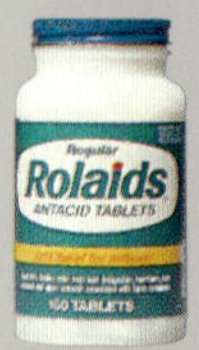

Spearmint

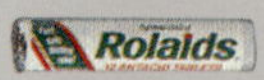

Wintergreen

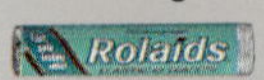

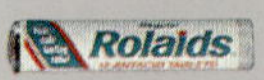

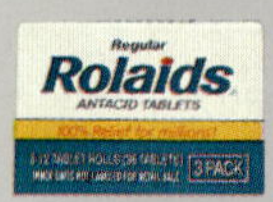

Regular

ROLAIDS®

Fast, Safe, Lasting Relief from Heartburn, Sour Stomach or Acid Indigestion and Upset Stomach Associated with these Symptoms

Westwood-Squibb

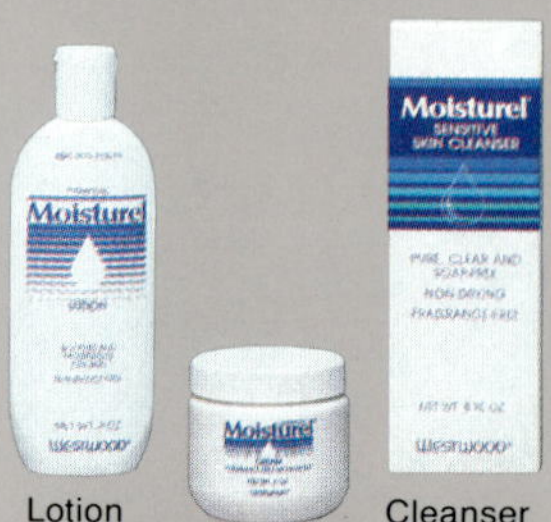

Lotion Cream Cleanser

Fragrance-Free MOISTUREL®

Whitehall

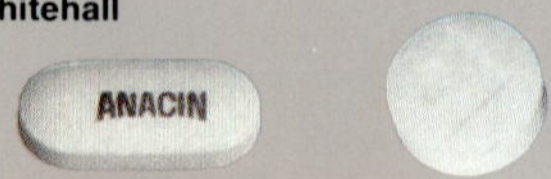

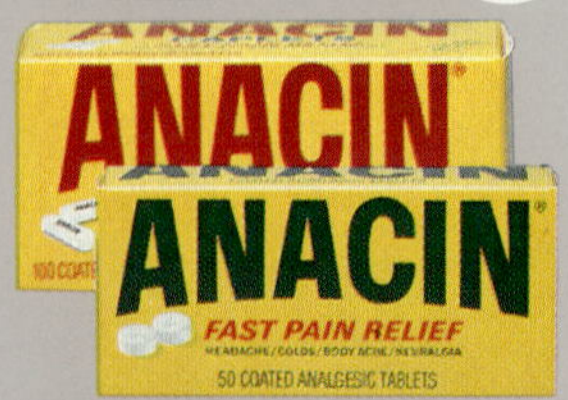

Coated Tablets in Tins of 12 and Bottles of 30, 50, 100, 200 and 300. Coated Caplets in Bottles of 30, 50 and 100.

ANACIN®
Analgesic Tablets and Caplets

Whitehall

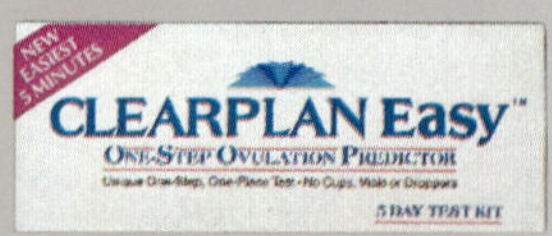

CLEARPLAN EASY™
One-Step Ovulation Predictor

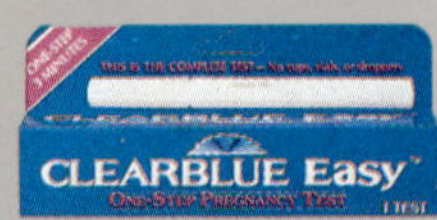

CLEARBLUE EASY™
One-Step Pregnancy Test

Whitehall

(Shown smaller than actual size)

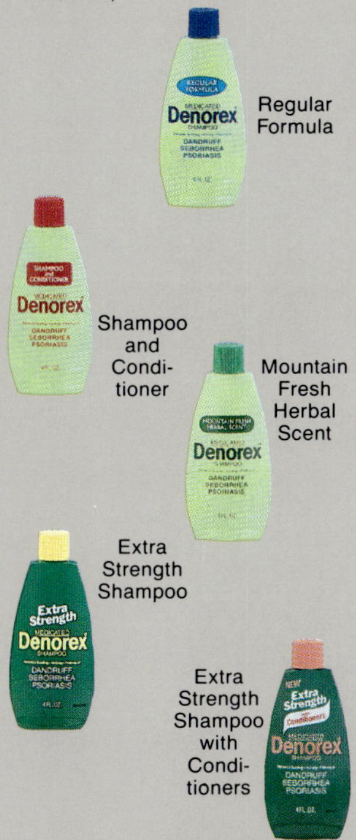

Regular Formula

Shampoo and Conditioner

Mountain Fresh Herbal Scent

Extra Strength Shampoo

Extra Strength Shampoo with Conditioners

DENOREX®
Medicated Shampoo

Whitehall

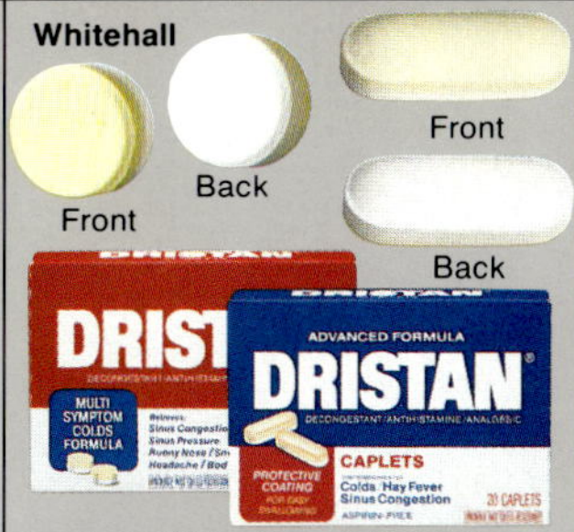

Front Back Front Back

Coated Tablets: Tins of 12, Packages of 24, and Bottles of 48 and 100. Coated Caplets: Packages of 20 and 40.

DRISTAN®
COATED TABLETS AND CAPLETS
Decongestant/Antihistamine/ Analgesic

Whitehall

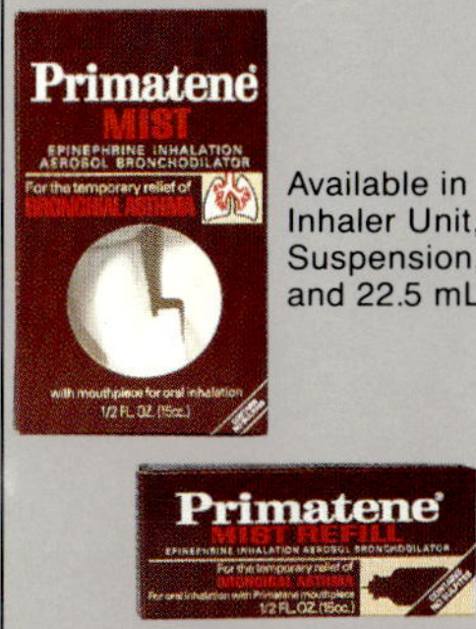

Available in 15 mL Inhaler Unit, 10 mL Suspension, 15 mL and 22.5 mL Refills.

PRIMATENE® MIST

Asthma Remedy

Whitehall

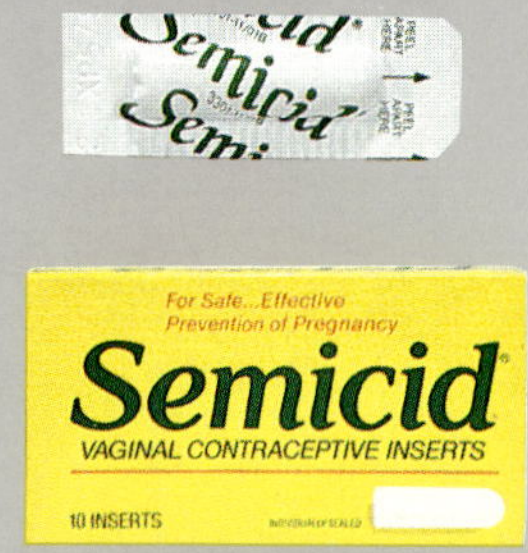

Available in Packages of 10 and 20.

SEMICID®
Vaginal Contraceptive Inserts

Whitehall

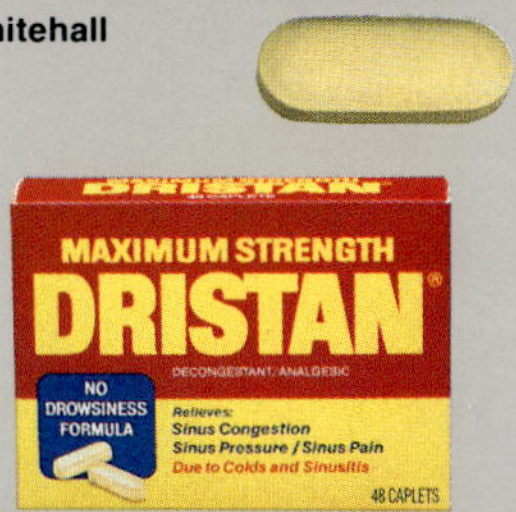

Coated Caplets: Packages of 24, 48 and Bottles of 100.

MAXIMUM STRENGTH DRISTAN®
(acetaminophen 500 mg., pseudoephedrine HCl 30 mg.)

Whitehall

Regular Front Back

P Formula Front Back

M Formula Front Back

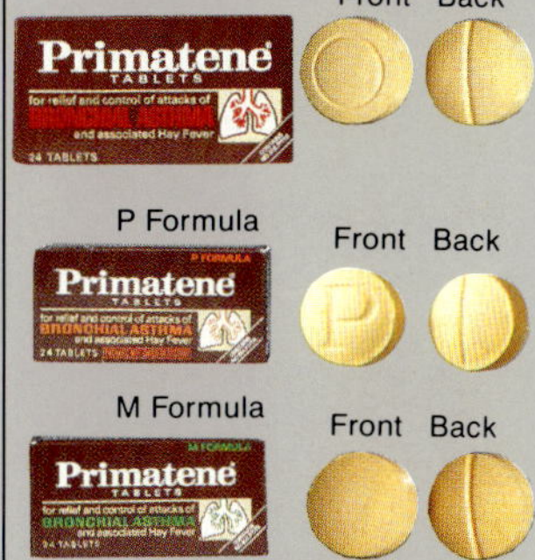

PRIMATENE® TABLETS
Asthma Remedy

Whitehall

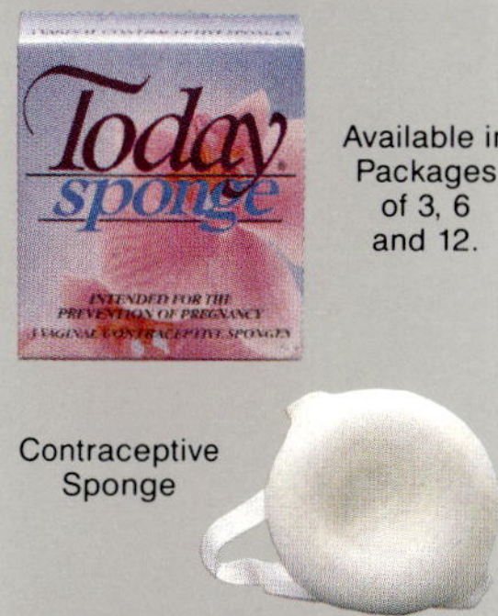

Available in Packages of 3, 6 and 12.

Contraceptive Sponge

TODAY®
Vaginal Contraceptive Sponge

Whitehall

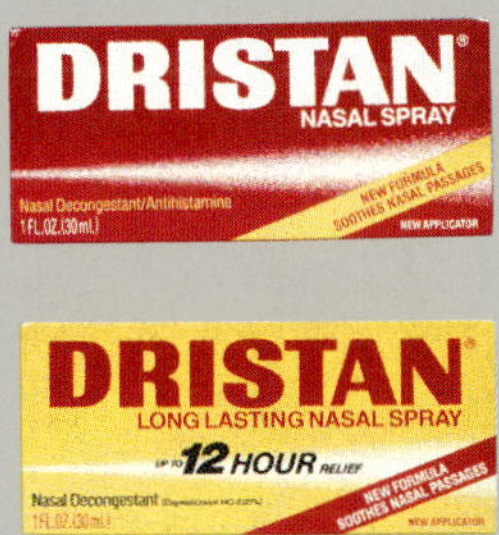

Both Available in Bottles of 15 ml. and 30 ml.

Whitehall

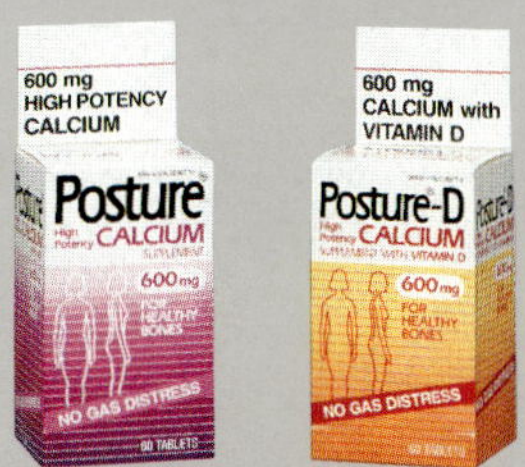

High Potency Calcium Supplement and High Potency Calcium Supplement with Vitamin D

Both available in Bottles of 60

POSTURE® and POSTURE®-D
(elemental calcium/Vitamin D)

Whitehall

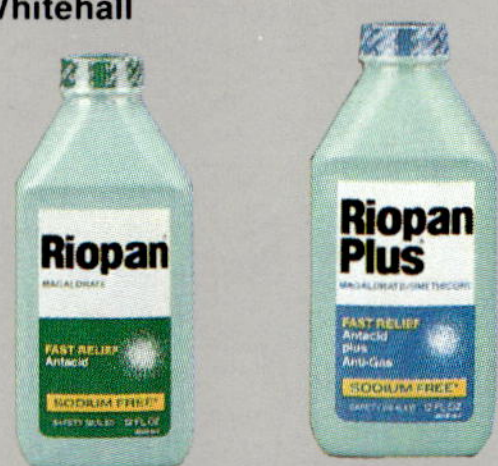

RIOPAN®
Antacid
(magaldrate)

RIOPAN PLUS®
Antacid plus Anti-Gas
(magaldrate and simethicone)

Both products available in 12 fl. oz. Suspension, Chew Tablets, 60's and 100's, and Rollpacks. RIOPAN also available in Swallow Tablets, 60's and 100's.

WINTHROP

Consumer Products

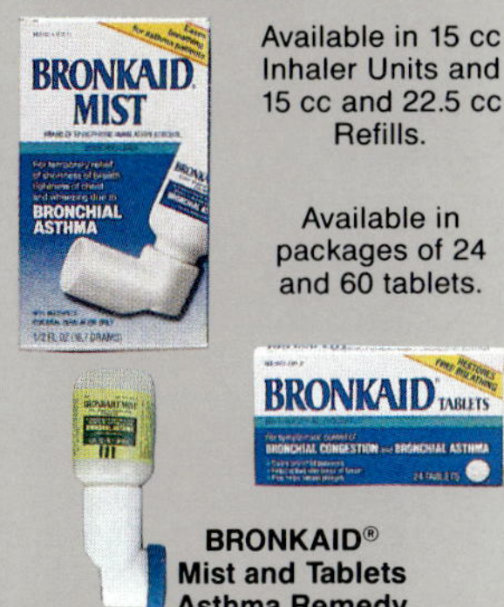

Available in 15 cc Inhaler Units and 15 cc and 22.5 cc Refills.

Available in packages of 24 and 60 tablets.

BRONKAID®
Mist and Tablets
Asthma Remedy

Whitehall

(Shown smaller than actual size)

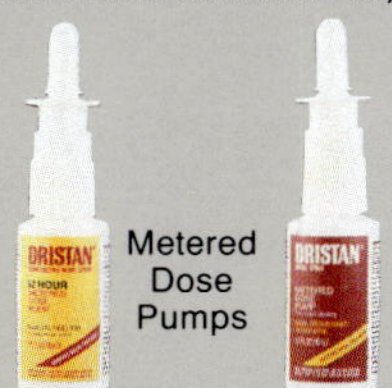

Metered Dose Pumps

12 Hour Regular

Metered Dose Pumps of 15 ml.

DRISTAN®
Nasal Sprays

Whitehall

Ointment
1 oz. and 2 oz. Tubes

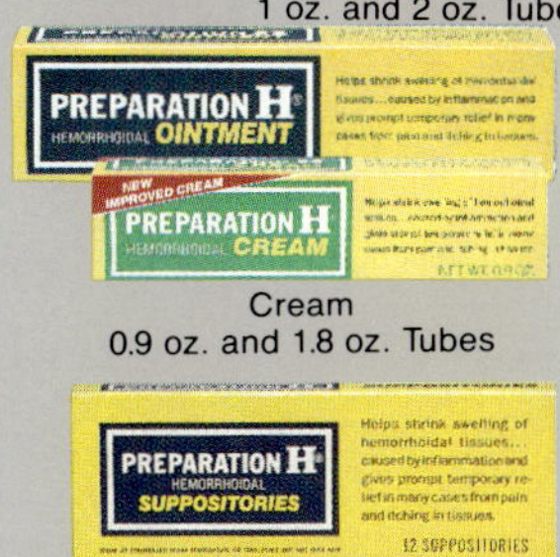

Cream
0.9 oz. and 1.8 oz. Tubes

Suppositories
12s, 24s, 36s and 48s

PREPARATION H®
Hemorrhoidal Ointment, Cream and Suppositories

Whitehall

Available in 12 fl. oz. Suspension and Chew Tablets (60s)

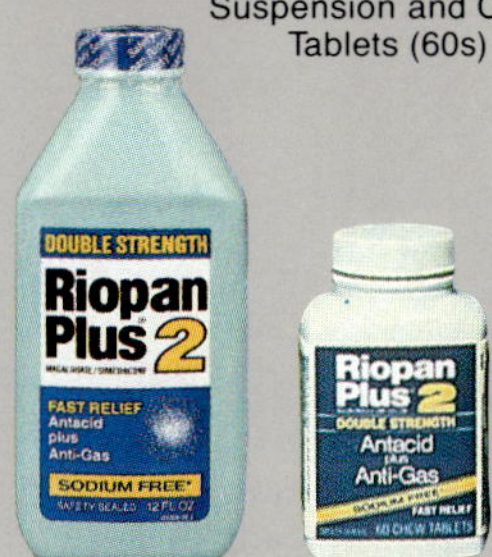

RIOPAN PLUS® 2
High-Potency Antacid plus Anti-Gas
(magaldrate and simethicone)

Winthrop Consumer Products

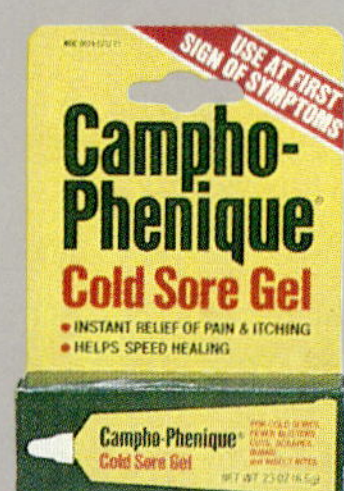

CAMPHO-PHENIQUE®
Cold Sore Gel
.23 oz and .5 oz

Winthrop Consumer Products	Winthrop Consumer Products	WYETH-AYERST	Wyeth-Ayerst

Winthrop Consumer Products

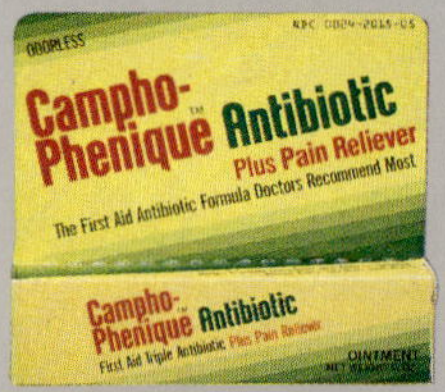

Available in ½ oz and 1 oz tubes and 3.0 oz aerosol spray

CAMPHO-PHENIQUE® First Aid Triple Antibiotic plus Pain Reliever Ointment

Winthrop Consumer Products

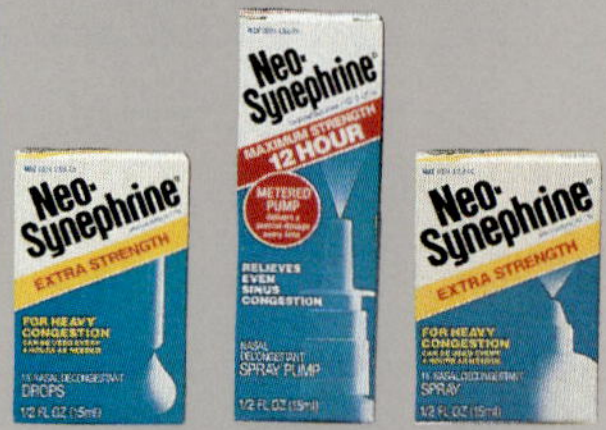

NEO-SYNEPHRINE® Nasal Decongestant

Spray, Spray Pump or Drops

WYETH-AYERST

Tamper-Resistant/Evident Packaging

Statements alerting consumers to the specific type of Tamper-Resistant/Evident Packaging appear on the bottle labels and cartons of all over-the-counter products of Wyeth-Ayerst. This includes plastic cap seals on bottles, individually wrapped tablets or suppositories, and sealed cartons. This packaging has been developed to better protect the consumer.

Wyeth-Ayerst

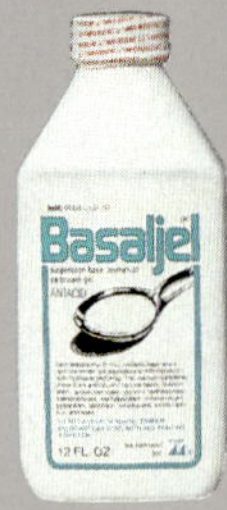

12 Fl. Oz.

BASALJEL® SUSPENSION

Antacid

Winthrop Consumer Products

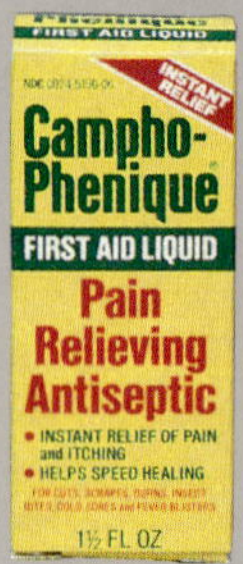

CAMPHO-PHENIQUE® First Aid Liquid
.75 oz, 1.5 oz, 4 oz

Winthrop Consumer Products

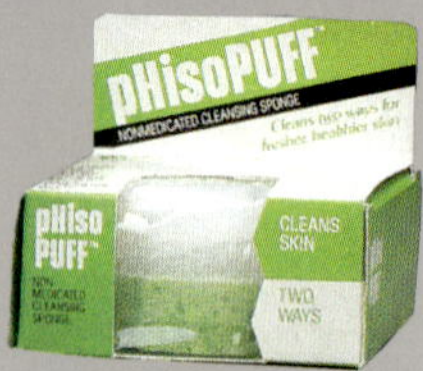

pHisoPUFF® Exfoliating Sponge

Wyeth-Ayerst

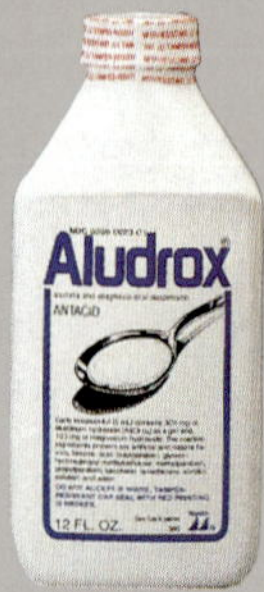

12 Fl. Oz.

ALUDROX® SUSPENSION Antacid

Wyeth-Ayerst

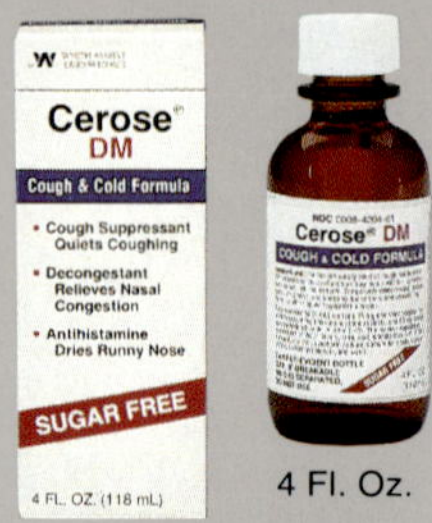

4 Fl. Oz.

CEROSE-DM®

Cough/Cold Formula with Dextromethorphan

Also available in 1-pint bottles

Winthrop Consumer Products

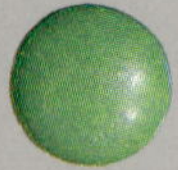

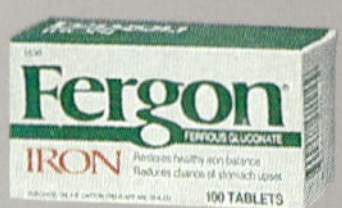

Available in bottles of 100, 500 and 1,000

FERGON® (IRON) Tablets

Winthrop Consumer Products

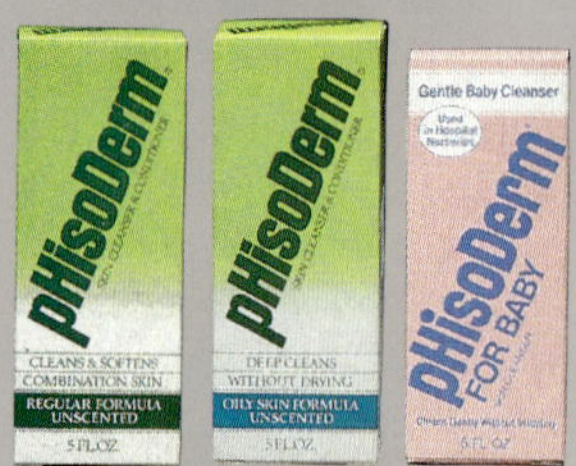

Unscented Regular	Oily Skin Formula	Baby Cleanser 5 oz

Available in 5 oz, 9 oz (regular), 16 oz and Lightly Scented

pHisoDerm®

Wyeth-Ayerst

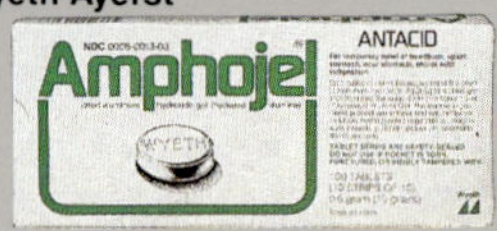

100 tablets

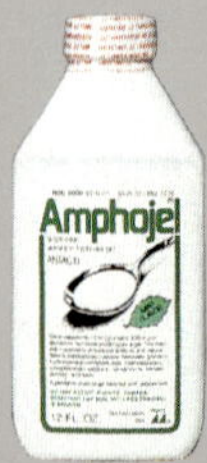

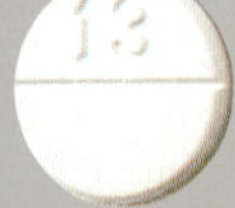

0.6 gram (10 gr.)

AMPHOJEL® TABLETS and SUSPENSION Antacid

12 Fl. Oz.

Also available in 0.3 gram (5 gr.) tablets

Wyeth-Ayerst

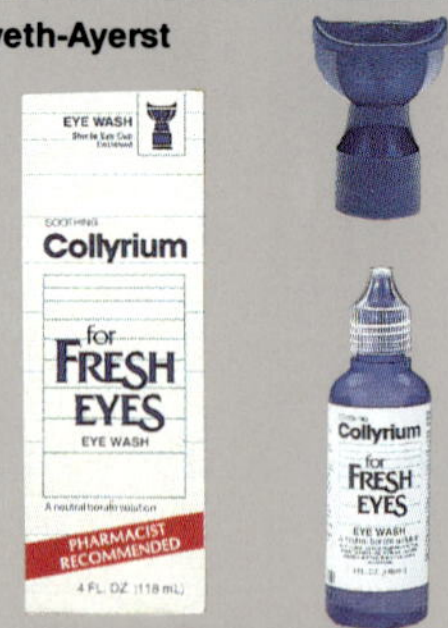

Eye Wash 4 Fl. Oz. (118 ml) with separate eyecup bottle cap.

COLLYRIUM for FRESH EYES Eye Wash

Winthrop Consumer Products

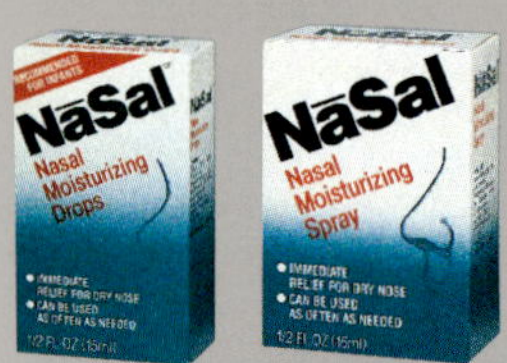

15 ml 15 ml

NāSal™ Nasal Moisturizer Spray and Drops

Winthrop Consumer Products

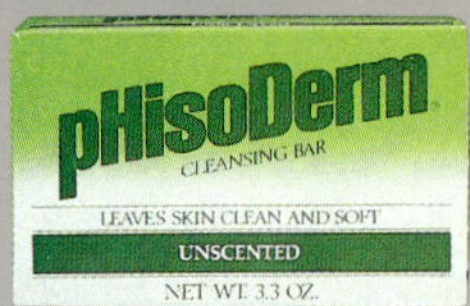

Unscented 3.3 oz

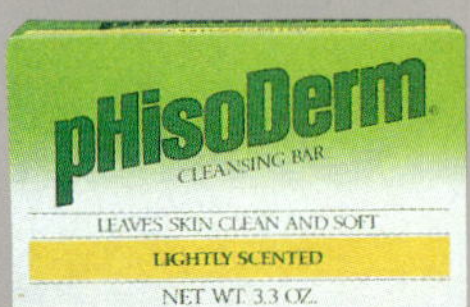

Slightly Scented 3.3 oz

pHisoDerm® CLEANSING BAR

Wyeth-Ayerst

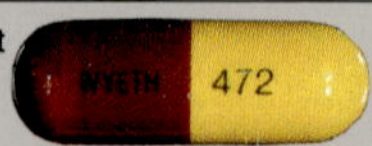

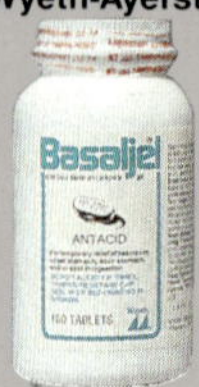

Bottles of 100, 500

Bottles of 100

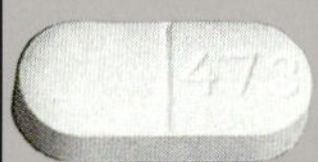

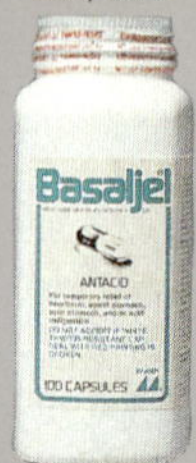

BASALJEL® TABLETS and CAPSULES

Antacid

Wyeth-Ayerst

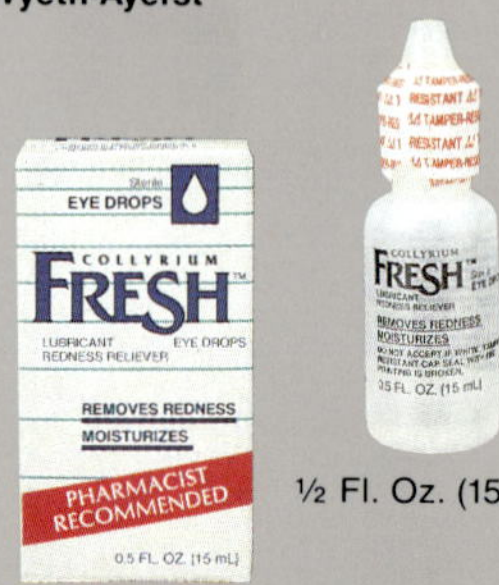

½ Fl. Oz. (15 ml)

COLLYRIUM FRESH™

Eye drops with tetrahydrozoline HCl plus glycerin

Wyeth-Ayerst

Also available in Ready-to-Feed Liquid and Powder

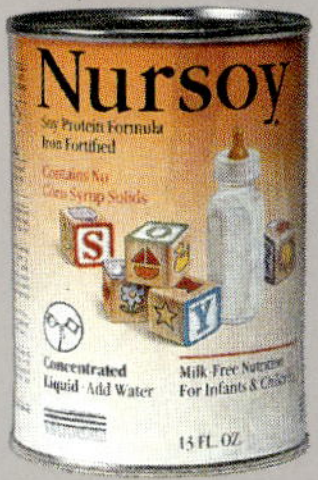

13 Fl. Oz.

Iron Fortified

NURSOY®
SOY PROTEIN ISOLATE FORMULA
Concentrated Liquid

Wyeth-Ayerst

12 Suppositories

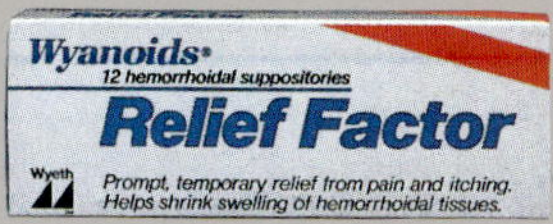

Also available in boxes of 24

WYANOIDS®
RELIEF FACTOR
Hemorrhoidal Suppositories

Wyeth-Ayerst

Also available in Ready-to-Feed Liquid and Powder

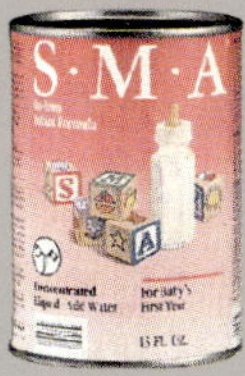

Lo-Iron

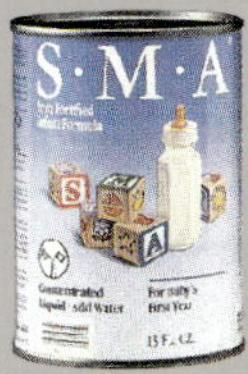

Iron Fortified

13 Fl. Oz.

S • M • A® INFANT FORMULA
Concentrated Liquid

ZILA

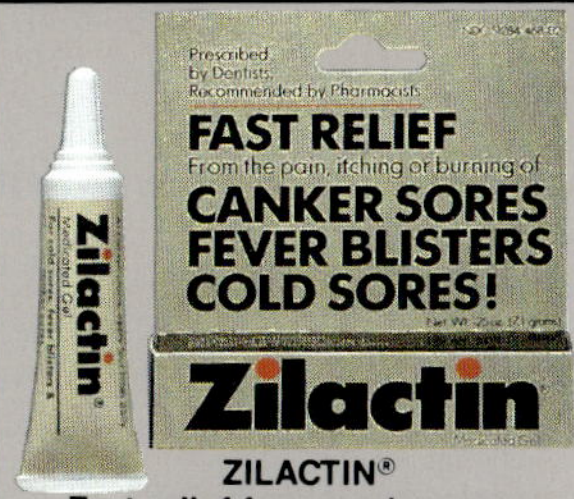

ZILACTIN®
Fast relief from canker sores, fever blisters, and cold sores.

Also available from Zila:
ZilaBrace™ treats brace sores
ZilaDent™ treats denture sores
Zilactol™ treats developing cold sores and fever blisters

MEDICINE CABINET CHECK LIST

Nonprescription drugs

Drug	Reason for purchase	Date purchased	Effect

Conversion Tables

Metric Doses With Approximate Apothecary Equivalents

The approximate dose equivalents represent the quantities usually prescribed by physicians using, respectively, the metric and apothecary system of weights and measures. When prepared dosage forms such as tablets, capsules, etc. are prescribed in the metric system, the pharmacist may dispense the corresponding approximate equivalent in the apothecary system and vice versa. (Note: A milliliter [mL] is the approximate equivalent of a cubic centimeter [cc]). Exact equivalents, which appear in the United States Pharmacopeia and the National Formulary, must be used to calculate quantities in pharmaceutical formulas and prescription compounding:

LIQUID MEASURE		LIQUID MEASURE		LIQUID MEASURE		LIQUID MEASURE	
Metric	Approximate Apothecary Equivalents	Metric	Approximate Apothecary Equivalents	Metric	Approximate Apothecary Equivalents	Metric	Approximate Apothecary Equivalents
1000 mL	1 quart	3 mL	45 minims	30 mL	1 fluid ounce	0.25 mL	4 minims
750 mL	$1\frac{1}{2}$ pints	2 mL	30 minims	15 mL	4 fluid drams	0.2 mL	3 minims
500 mL	1 pint	1 mL	15 minims	10 mL	$2\frac{1}{2}$ fluid drams	0.1 mL	$1\frac{1}{2}$ minims
250 mL	8 fluid ounces	0.75 mL	12 minims	8 mL	2 fluid drams	0.06 mL	1 minim
200 mL	7 fluid ounces	0.6 mL	10 minims	5 mL	$1\frac{1}{4}$ fluid drams	0.05 mL	$\frac{3}{4}$ minim
100 mL	$3\frac{1}{2}$ fluid ounces	0.5 mL	8 minims	4 mL	1 fluid dram	0.03 mL	$\frac{1}{2}$ minim
50 mL	$1\frac{3}{4}$ fluid ounces	0.3 mL	5 minims				

WEIGHT		WEIGHT		WEIGHT		WEIGHT	
Metric	Approximate Apothecary Equivalents	Metric	Approximate Apothecary Equivalents	Metric	Approximate Apothecary Equivalents	Metric	Approximate Apothecary Equivalents
30g	1 ounce	30mg	1/2 grain	500mg	$7\frac{1}{2}$ grains	1.2 mg	1/50 grain
15g	4 drams	25mg	3/8 grain	400mg	6 grains	1 mg	1/60 grain
10g	$2\frac{1}{2}$ drams	20mg	1/3 grain	300mg	5 grains	800 μg	1/80 grain
7.5g	2 drams	15mg	1/4 grain	250mg	4 grains	600 μg	1/100 grain
6g	90 grains	12mg	1/5 grain	200mg	3 grains	500 μg	1/120 grain
5g	75 grains	10mg	1/6 grain	150mg	$2\frac{1}{2}$ grains	400 μg	1/150 grain
4g	60 grains (1 dram)	8mg	1/8 grain	125mg	2 grains	300 μg	1/200 grain
3g	45 grains	6mg	1/10 grain	100mg	$1\frac{1}{2}$ grains	250 μg	1/250 grain
2g	30 grains ($\frac{1}{2}$ dram)	5mg	1/12 grain	75mg	$1\frac{1}{4}$ grains	200 μg	1/300 grain
1.5g	22 grains	4mg	1/15 grain	60mg	1 grain	150 μg	1/400 grain
1g	15 grains	3mg	1/20 grain	50mg	$\frac{3}{4}$ grain	120 μg	1/500 grain
750mg	12 grains	2mg	1/30 grain	40mg	$\frac{2}{3}$ grain	100 μg	1/600 grain
600mg	10 grains	1.5mg	1/40 grain				

Approximate Household Equivalents

For household purposes, an American Standard Teaspoon is defined by the American National Standards Institute as containing 4.93 ± 0.24 mL. The USP states that in view of the almost universal practice of employing teaspoons ordinarily available in the household for administration of medicine, the teaspoon may be regarded as representing 5 mL. Household units of measure often are used to inform patients of the size of a liquid dose. Because of difficulties involved in measuring liquids under normal conditions of use, household spoons are not appropriate when accurate measurement of a liquid dose is required. When accurate measurement of a liquid dose is required, the USP recommends that a calibrated oral syringe or dropper be used.

1 fluid dram = 1 teaspoonful = 5 mL
2 fluid drams = 1 dessertspoonful = 10 mL
4 fluid drams = 1 tablespoonful = 15 mL
2 fluid ounces = 1 wineglassful = 60 mL
4 fluid ounces = 1 teacupful = 120 mL
8 fluid ounces = 1 tumblerful = 240 mL

Pounds—Kilograms (kg) Conversion

1 pound = 0.453592 kg
1 kg = 2.2 pounds

Temperature Conversion Table:

$$9 \times °C = (5 \times °F) - 160$$

Centigrade to Fahrenheit = (°C × 9/5) + 32 = °F
Fahrenheit to Centigrade = (°F − 32) × 5/9 = °C

Milliequivalents per Liter (mEq/L)

$$\text{mEq/L} = \frac{\text{weight of salt (g)} \times \text{valence of ion} \times 1000}{\text{molecular weight of salt}}$$

$$\text{weight of salt (g)} = \frac{\text{mEq/L} \times \text{molecular weight of salt}}{\text{valence of ion} \times 1000}$$

SECTION 6

Product Information Section

This section is made possible through the courtesy of the manufacturers whose products appear on the following pages. The information concerning each product has been prepared, edited and approved by the manufacturer.

Products described in this edition comply with labeling regulations. Copy may include all the essential information necessary for informed usage such as active ingredients, indications, actions, warnings, drug interactions, precautions, symptoms and treatment of oral overdosage, dosage and administration, professional labeling, and how supplied. In some cases additional information has been supplied to complement the foregoing. The Publisher has emphasized to manufacturers the necessity of describing products comprehensively so that all information essential for intelligent and informed use is available. In organizing and presenting the material in this edition the Publisher is providing all the information made available by manufacturers.

In presenting the following material to the medical profession, the Publisher is not necessarily advocating the use of any product.

Abbott Laboratories
Pharmaceutical Products Division
NORTH CHICAGO, IL 60064

DAYALETS® Filmtab®
[*dāy 'a-lets*]
Multivitamin Supplement for adults and children 4 or more years of age

DAYALETS® PLUS IRON Filmtab®
Multivitamin Supplement with Iron for adults and children 4 or more years of age

Description: Dayalets provide 100% of the recommended daily allowances of essential vitamins. Dayalets Plus Iron provides 100% of the recommended daily allowances of essential vitamins plus the mineral iron.
Daily dosage (one Dayalets tablet) provides:

VITAMINS			% U.S. RDA
Vitamin A.. (1.5 mg)..	5000	IU	100%
Vitamin D.. (10 mcg).	400	IU	100%
Vitamin E	30	IU	100%
Vitamin C	60	mg	100%
Folic Acid	0.4	mg	100%
Thiamine (Vitamin B_1)	1.5	mg	100%
Riboflavin (Vitamin B_2)	1.7	mg	100%
Niacin	20	mg	100%
Vitamin B_6	2	mg	100%
Vitamin B_{12}	6	mcg	100%

Ingredients: Ascorbic acid, cellulose, dl-alpha tocopheryl acetate, niacinamide, povidone, pyridoxine hydrochloride, riboflavin, thiamine hydrochloride, vitamin A acetate, vitamin A palmitate, folic acid, FD&C Yellow No. 6, cholecalciferol, and cyanocobalamin in a film-coated tablet with vanillin flavoring and artificial coloring added.
Each Dayalets Plus Iron Filmtab® represents all the vitamins in the Dayalets formula in the same concentrations, plus the mineral iron 18 mg (100% U.S. R.D.A.), as ferrous sulfate. Dayalets Plus Iron contain the same ingredients as Dayalets.
These products contain no sugar and essentially no calories.

Indications: Dietary supplement and supplement with iron for adults and children 4 or more years of age.

Administration and Dosage: One Filmtab tablet daily.

How Supplied: Dayalets® Filmtab® in bottles of 100 tablets (NDC 0074-3925-01).

Dayalets® Plus Iron Filmtab in bottles of 100 tablets (NDC 0074-6667-01).
® Filmtab—Film-sealed tablets, Abbott.

Abbott Laboratories
North Chicago, IL 60064
Ref. 02-6903-8/R9, Ref. 07-8057-7/R8

OPTILETS®-500
[*op 'te-lets*]
High potency multivitamin for use in treatment of multivitamin deficiency.

OPTILETS-M-500®
High potency multivitamin for use in treatment of multivitamin deficiency. Mineral supplementation added.

Description: A therapeutic formula of ten important vitamins, with and without minerals, in a small tablet with the Abbott Filmtab® coating. Each Optilets-500 tablet provides:

Vitamin C (as sodium ascorbate)	500 mg
Niacinamide	100 mg
Calcium Pantothenate	20 mg
Vitamin B_1 (thiamine mononitrate)	15 mg
Vitamin B_2 (riboflavin)	10 mg
Vitamin B_6 (pyridoxine hydrochloride)	5 mg
Vitamin A (as palmitate 1.5 mg, as acetate 1.5 mg—total 3 mg)	10,000 IU
Vitamin B_{12} (cyanocobalamin)	12 mcg
Vitamin D (cholecalciferol)	(10 mcg) 400 IU
Vitamin E (as dl-alpha tocopheryl acetate)	30 IU

Inactive Ingredients: Cellulosic polymers, corn starch, D&C Yellow No. 10, FD&C Yellow No. 6, iron oxide, polyethylene glycol, povidone, stearic acid, talc, titanium dioxide and vanillin.
Each Optilets-M-500 Filmtab contains all the vitamins (vitamin C—ascorbic acid) in the same quantities provided in Optilets-500, plus the following minerals and inactive ingredients:

Magnesium (as oxide)	80 mg
Iron (as dried ferrous sulfate)	20 mg
Copper (as sulfate)	2 mg
Zinc (as sulfate)	1.5 mg
Manganese (as sulfate)	1 mg
Iodine (as calcium iodate)	0.15 mg

Inactive Ingredients: Cellulosic polymers, colloidal silicon dioxide, corn starch, D&C Red No. 7, FD&C Blue No. 1, iron oxide, magnesium stearate, microcrystalline cellulose, polyethylene glycol, povidone, propylene glycol, sorbic acid and titanium dioxide.

Dosage and Administration: Usual adult dosage is one Filmtab tablet daily, or as directed by physician.

How Supplied: Optilets-500 tablets are supplied in bottles of 120 (**NDC** 0074-4287-22). Optilets-M-500 tablets are supplied in bottles of 120 (**NDC** 0074-4286-22).
®Filmtab—Film-sealed Tablets, Abbott.
Abbott Laboratories
North Chicago, IL 60064
Ref. 02-7063-7/R1, Ref. 02-7133-8/R2

SURBEX®
[*sir 'bex*]
Vitamin B-complex

SURBEX® with C
Vitamin B-complex with vitamin C

Description: Each Surbex Filmtab tablet provides:

Niacinamide	30 mg
Calcium Pantothenate	10 mg
Vitamin B_1 (thiamine mononitrate)	6 mg
Vitamin B_2 (riboflavin)	6 mg
Vitamin B_6 (pyridoxine hydrochloride)	2.5 mg
Vitamin B_{12} (cyanocobalamin)	5 mcg

Each Surbex with C Filmtab tablet provides the same ingredients as Surbex, plus 250 mg Vitamin C (as sodium ascorbate).

Inactive Ingredients
Surbex tablets: Cellulosic polymers, corn starch, D&C Yellow No. 10, dibasic calcium phosphate, FD&C Yellow No. 6, magnesium stearate, polyethylene glycol, povidone, propylene glycol, stearic acid, titanium dioxide, and vanillin.
Surbex with C Tablets: Cellulosic polymers, corn starch, D&C Yellow No. 10, FD&C Yellow No. 6, lactose, magnesium stearate, microcrystalline cellulose, polyethylene glycol, povidone, propylene glycol, titanium dioxide, and vanillin.

Indications: Surbex is indicated for treatment of Vitamin B-Complex deficiency.
Surbex with C is indicated for use in treatment of Vitamin B-Complex with Vitamin C deficiency.

Dosage and Administration: Usual adult dosage is one tablet twice daily or as directed by physician.

How Supplied: Surbex is supplied as bright orange-colored tablets in bottles of 100 (NDC 0074-4876-13).
Surbex with C is supplied as yellow-colored tablets in bottles of 100 (NDC 0074-4877-13).
Abbott Laboratories
North Chicago, IL 60064
Ref. 03-1763-5/R12, 03-1616-5/R12

SURBEX-T®
High-potency vitamin B-complex with 500 mg of vitamin C

Description: Each Filmtab® tablet provides:

Vitamin C (ascorbic acid)	500 mg
Niacinamide	100 mg
Calcium Pantothenate	20 mg
Vitamin B_1 (thiamine mononitrate)	15 mg
Vitamin B_2 (riboflavin)	10 mg
Vitamin B_6 (pyridoxine hydrochloride)	5 mg
Vitamin B_{12} (cyanocobalamin)	10 mcg

Inactive Ingredients: Cellulosic polymers, colloidal silicon dioxide, corn starch, D&C Yellow No. 10, FD&C Yellow No. 6, magnesium stearate, microcrystalline cellulose, polyethylene glycol, povidone, propylene glycol, titanium dioxide, and vanillin.

Indications: For use in treatment of Vitamin B-Complex with Vitamin C deficiency.

Dosage and Administration: Usual adult dosage is one Filmtab tablet daily, or as directed by physician.

How Supplied: Orange-colored tablets in bottles of 100 (**NDC** 0074-4878-13). Also supplied in Abbo-Pac® unit dose packages of 100 tablets in strips of 10 tablets per strip (**NDC** 0074-4878-11).
®Filmtab—Film-sealed Tablets, Abbott.
Abbott Laboratories
North Chicago, IL 60064
Ref. 03-1765-7/R13

SURBEX®-750 with IRON
High-potency B-complex with iron, vitamin E and 750 mg vitamin C

Description: Each Filmtab® tablet provides:

VITAMINS

Vitamin C (as sodium ascorbate)	750 mg
Niacinamide	100 mg
Vitamin B_6 (pyridoxine hydrochloride)	25 mg
Calcium Pantothenate	20 mg
Vitamin B_1 (thiamine mononitrate)	15 mg
Vitamin B_2 (riboflavin)	15 mg
Vitamin B_{12} (cyanocobalamin)	12 mcg
Folic Acid	400 mcg
Vitamin E (as dl-alpha tocopheryl acetate)	30 IU
MINERAL	
Elemental Iron (as dried ferrous sulfate)	27 mg

equivalent to 135 mg ferrous sulfate

Inactive Ingredients: Cellulosic polymers, colloidal silicon dioxide, FD&C Red No. 3, corn starch, iron oxide, magnesium stearate, microcrystalline cellulose, polyethylene glycol, povidone, and vanillin.

Indications: For the treatment of vitamin C and B-complex deficiencies and to supplement the daily intake of iron and vitamin E.

Dosage and Administration: Usual adult dosage is one tablet daily or as directed by physician.

How Supplied: Bottles of 50 tablets (**NDC** 0074-8029-50).
Abbott Laboratories
North Chicago, IL 60064
Ref. 03-1800-4/R9

SURBEX®-750 with ZINC
High-potency B-complex with zinc, vitamin E and 750 mg of vitamin C. For persons 12 years of age or older

Description: Daily dose (one Filmtab® tablet) provides:

VITAMINS		**% U.S. R.D.A.***
Vitamin E	30 IU	100%
Vitamin C	750 mg	1250%
Folic Acid	0.4 mg	100%
Thiamine (B_1)	15 mg	1000%
Riboflavin (B_2)	15 mg	882%
Niacin	100 mg	500%
Vitamin B_6	20 mg	1000%
Vitamin B_{12}	12 mcg	200%
Pantothenic Acid	20 mg	200%
MINERAL		
Zinc**	22.5 mg	150%

* % U.S. Recommended Daily Allowance for Adults.
** Equivalent to 100 mg of zinc sulfate.

Ingredients: Ascorbic acid, niacinamide, cellulose, dl-alpha tocopheryl acetate, zinc sulfate, povidone, pyridoxine hydrochloride, calcium pantothenate, riboflavin, thiamine mononitrate, cyanocobalamin, magnesium stearate, colloidal silicon dioxide, folic acid, in a film-coated tablet with vanillin flavoring and artificial coloring added.
Usual Adult Dose: One tablet daily.

How Supplied: Bottles of 50 tablets (**NDC** 0074-8152-50).
Abbott Laboratories
North Chicago, IL 60064
Ref. 03-1767-4/R10

If desired, additional information on any Abbott Product will be provided upon request to Abbott Laboratories.

Adria Laboratories
Division of Erbamont Inc.
7001 POST ROAD
DUBLIN, OH 43017

Professional Labeling

EMETROL®
(Phosphorated Carbohydrate Solution)
For the relief of nausea associated with upset stomach

Description: EMETROL is an oral solution containing balanced amounts of dextrose (glucose) and levulose (fructose) and phosphoric acid with controlled hydrogen ion concentration. Available in original lemon-mint or cherry flavor.

Ingredients: Each 5 mL teaspoonful contains dextrose (glucose), 1.87 g; levulose (fructose), 1.87 g; phosphoric acid, 21.5 mg; and the following inactive ingredients: glycerin, methylparaben, purified water; D&C yellow No. 10 and natural lemon-mint flavor in lemon-mint Emetrol; FD&C red No. 40 and artificial cherry flavor in cherry Emetrol.

Action: EMETROL quickly relieves nausea by local action on the wall of the hyperactive G.I. tract. It reduces smooth-muscle contraction in proportion to the amount used. Unlike systemic antinauseants, EMETROL works almost immediately to control nausea.

Indications: For the relief of nausea associated with upset stomach. For other conditions, take only as directed by your physician.

Advantages:
1. **Fast Action**—works almost immediately by local action on contact with the hyperactive G.I. tract.
2. **Effectiveness**—reduces smooth-muscle contractions in proportion to the amount used—stops nausea.
3. **Safety**—non-toxic—won't mask symptoms of organic pathology.
4. **Convenience**—no ℞ required.
5. **Patient Acceptance**—a low cost that patients appreciate—pleasant lemon-mint or cherry flavor

Usual Adult Dose: One or two tablespoonfuls. Repeat every 15 minutes until distress subsides.

Usual Children's Dose: One or two teaspoonfuls. Repeat dose every 15 minutes until distress subsides.

Important: Never dilute EMETROL or drink fluids of any kind immediately before or after taking a dose.

Caution: Not to be taken for more than one hour (5 doses) without consulting a physician. If upset stomach continues or recurs frequently, consult a physician promptly as it may be a sign of a serious condition.

WARNING: KEEP THIS AND ALL MEDICATIONS OUT OF THE REACH OF CHILDREN. As with any drug, if you are pregnant or nursing a baby, seek the advice of a health professional before using this product.
This product contains fructose and should not be taken by persons with hereditary fructose intolerance (HFI).

This product contains sugar and should not be taken by diabetics except under the advice and supervision of a physician.

In case of accidental overdose, contact a poison control center, emergency medical facility, or physician immediately for advice.

How Supplied: Each 5 mL teaspoonful of EMETROL contains dextrose (glucose), 1.87 g; levulose (fructose), 1.87 g; and phosphoric acid, 21.5 mg in a yellow, lemon-mint or red, cherry-flavored syrup.

Yellow, Lemon-Mint
NDC 0013-2113-45—Bottle of 4 fluid ounces (118 mL)
NDC 0013-2113-65—Bottle of 8 fluid ounces (236 mL)
NDC 0013-2113-51—Bottle of 1 pint (473 mL)

Red, Cherry
NDC 0013-2114-45—Bottle of 4 fluid ounces (118 mL)
NDC 0013-2114-65—Bottle of 8 fluid ounces (236 mL)
NDC 0013-2114-51—Bottle of 1 pint (473 mL)
Store at room temperature.

NOTICE: Each bottle is protected by a printed band around the cap. Do not use if band is damaged or missing.

Shown in Product Identification Section, page 403

Continued on next page

Adria—Cont.

Professional Labeling

MODANE

[*mō 'dāne*]

(phenolphthalein)

Description: MODANE TABLETS (rust red)—Each tablet contains white phenolphthalein 130 mg. Inactive ingredients include acacia, calcium carbonate, calcium sulfate, cornstarch, dibasic calcium phosphate, FD&C Red No. 40 aluminum lake, lactose, magnesium stearate, povidone, shellac, sodium benzoate, starch, sucrose, talc, titanium dioxide, water and carnauba wax.
Phenolphthalein is classified as a stimulant laxative. Chemically phenolphthalein is 3,3-bis(*p*-hydroxyphenyl)phthalide.

Clinical Pharmacology: Phenolphthalein, a stimulant laxative, acts primarily on the large intestine to produce a semifluid stool usually in 4–8 hours. It is dissolved by bile salts and alkaline intestinal secretions and may impart a red color to alkaline feces and urine.

Indications: For temporary relief of constipation.

Contraindications: Sensitivity to phenolphthalein.

Warnings: Do not use any laxative preparations when abdominal pain, nausea, or vomiting are present. Frequent and continued use may cause dependence upon laxatives.
KEEP THIS PRODUCT OUT OF REACH OF CHILDREN.
As with any drug, if the patient is pregnant or nursing a baby, she should consult a health professional before using.

Precautions: Phenolphthalein may color alkaline feces and urine red. If skin rash appears, do not use this product or any other preparation containing phenolphthalein.

Adverse Reactions: Excessive bowel activity, usually diarrhea or abdominal discomfort, nausea, vomiting, cramps, weakness, dizziness, palpitations, sweating and fainting may follow the administration of a laxative. Diarrhea may lead to fluid and electrolyte deficits. Allergic reactions, skin rashes attributed to phenolphthalein, have been reported.

Overdosage: Phenolphthalein is relatively nontoxic. Overdosage may be expected to result in excessive bowel activity. Treatment is symptomatic if the duration of effects is prolonged. Fluid and electrolyte deficits might result from prolonged catharsis.

Dosage and Administration:
MODANE Tablet (rust red)—Adults: One tablet daily, or as directed by a doctor. This strength is not recommended for children.

How Supplied: Each MODANE tablet contains white phenolphthalein 130 mg in a rust red, round, sugar-coated tablet printed with A on one side and 513 on the other. Store at room temperature.
Package of 10 tablets
NDC 0013-5131-07
Package of 30 tablets
NDC 0013-5131-13
Bottle of 100 tablets
NDC 0013-5131-17

Shown in Product Identification Section, page 403

Professional Labeling

MODANE PLUS

[*mō 'dāne plŭs*]

(phenolphthalein and docusate sodium)

Description: Each tablet contains white phenolphthalein 65mg and docusate sodium 100mg. Inactive ingredients include acacia, calcium carbonate, calcium sulfate, croscarmellose sodium, FD&C yellow No. 6 aluminum lake, magnesium stearate, microcrystalline cellulose, povidone, shellac, silica gel, sodium benzoate, sucrose, talc, titanium dioxide, water and carnauba wax.
Phenolphthalein is classified as a stimulant laxative. Chemically phenolphthalein is 3,3-bis(*p*-hydroxyphenyl)phthalide. Docusate sodium is classified as a stool softener. Chemically, docusate sodium is butanedioic acid, sulfo-1,4-bis(2-ethylhexyl) ester, sodium salt. It is an anionic surfactant.

Clinical Pharmacology: Phenolphthalein, a stimulant laxative, acts primarily on the large intestine to produce a semifluid stool usually in 4–8 hours. It is dissolved by bile salts and alkaline intestinal secretions and may impart a red color to alkaline feces and urine.
Docusate sodium, an anionic surfactant, allows increased hydration of the stool for easier passage usually in 24 to 72 hours. Docusate sodium is absorbed to some extent in the duodenum and proximal jejunum.

Indications: For temporary relief of constipation in adults.

Contraindications: Sensitivity to phenolphthalein. Mineral oil administration.

Warnings: Do not use any laxative preparations when abdominal pain, nausea, or vomiting are present. Frequent and continued use may cause dependence upon laxatives.
KEEP THIS PRODUCT OUT OF REACH OF CHILDREN.
As with any drug, if the patient is pregnant or nursing a baby, she should consult a health professional before using.

Precautions: Phenolphthalein may color alkaline feces and urine red. If skin rash appears, do not use this product or any other preparation containing phenolphthalein.
Docusate sodium may increase the intestinal absorption of mineral oil and/or hepatic uptake of other drugs administered concurrently.

Adverse Reactions: Excessive bowel activity, usually diarrhea or abdominal discomfort, nausea, vomiting, cramps, weakness, dizziness, palpitations, sweating and fainting may follow the administration of a laxative. Diarrhea may lead to fluid and electrolyte deficits. Allergic reactions, skin rashes attributed to phenolphthalein, have been reported.

Overdosage: Phenolphthalein is relatively nontoxic. Overdosage may be expected to result in excessive bowel activity. Treatment is symptomatic if the duration of effects is prolonged. Fluid and electrolyte deficits might result from prolonged catharsis.

Dosage and Administration:
Adults: One tablet daily, or as directed by a doctor. This strength is not recommended for children.

How Supplied: Each MODANE PLUS tablet contains white phenolphthalein 65 mg and docusate sodium 100 mg in an orange, round, sugar-coated tablet printed with A on one side and 515 on the other.
Package of 30 tablets
NDC 0013-5151-13
Bottle of 100 tablets
NDC 0013-5151-17
Store at room temperature.

Shown in Product Identification Section, page 403

Allergan Pharmaceuticals

A Division of Allergan, Inc.
2525 DUPONT DRIVE
P.O. BOX 19534
IRVINE, CA 92713-9534

CELLUVISC®

(carboxymethylcellulose sodium) 1%
Lubricant Ophthalmic Solution

Celluvisc® Ophthalmic Solution is a preservative-free ophthalmic lubricant formulated specifically for the patient who needs frequent relief from dryness of the eye:

- Special lubricating formula helps maintain the natural electrolyte balance of your tears.
- Preservative-free for no preservative-induced irritation.
- Single, unit-dose containers for greater convenience.

Contains: Active: Carboxymethylcellulose sodium 1%. Inactives: calcium chloride, potassium chloride, purified water, sodium chloride, and sodium lactate.

FDA APPROVED USES

Indications: FOR USE AS A LUBRICANT TO PREVENT FURTHER IRRITATION OR TO RELIEVE DRYNESS OF THE EYE.

Warnings: To avoid contamination, do not touch tip of container to any surface. Do not reuse. Once opened, discard. If you experience eye pain, changes in vision, continued redness or irritation of the eye, or if the condition worsens or persists for more than 72 hours, discontinue use and consult a doctor. If solution changes color or becomes cloudy, do not use. Keep this and all drugs out of the reach of children. In case of accidental ingestion, seek professional assistance or contact a poison control center immediately.

Directions: Instill 1 or 2 drops in the affected eye(s) as needed.

NOTE: Do not touch unit-dose tip to eye. Celluvisc may cause temporary blurring due to its viscosity.

How Supplied: Celluvisc® (carboxymethylcellulose sodium) 1% Lubricant Ophthalmic Solution is supplied in sterile, preservative-free, disposable, single-use containers of 0.01 fluid ounce each, in the following size:

30 SINGLE-USE CONTAINERS—
NDC 0023-4554-30

Shown in Product Identification Section, page 403

LACRI-LUBE® S.O.P.®
(white petrolatum 56.8%, mineral oil 42.5%)
Lubricant Ophthalmic Ointment

Contains: Actives: white petrolatum 56.8%, mineral oil 42.5%. Inactives: chlorobutanol (chloral deriv.) 0.5% and lanolin alcohols.

FDA APPROVED USES

Indications: FOR USE AS A LUBRICANT TO PREVENT FURTHER IRRITATION OR TO RELIEVE DRYNESS OF THE EYE.

Warnings: To avoid contamination, do not touch tip of container to any surface. Replace cap after using either the 3.5g or 7.0g tube. If you are using the unit-dose product, do not reuse it after it has been opened. Once the product is opened, it should be discarded. If you experience eye pain, changes in vision, continued redness or irritation of the eye, or if the condition worsens or persists for more than 72 hours, discontinue use and consult a doctor. Keep this and all drugs out of the reach of children. In case of accidental ingestion, seek professional assistance or contact a poison control center immediately.

Directions: Pull down the lower lid of the affected eye and apply a small amount (one-fourth inch) of ointment to the inside of the eyelid.

How Supplied: Lacri-Lube® S.O.P.® (white petrolatum 56.8%, mineral oil 42.5%) Lubricant Ophthalmic Ointment is supplied in sterile, disposable unit-dose containers of 0.7 g each and sterile, ophthalmic ointment tubes as follows:

24 UNIT-DOSE CONTAINERS—
NDC 0023-0312-01
3.5 g TUBE—NDC 0023-0312-04
7.0 g TUBE—NDC 0023-0312-07

Shown in Product Identification Section, page 403

LACRI-LUBE® NP
(white petrolatum 57.3%, mineral oil 42.5%)
Lubricant Ophthalmic Ointment

Contains:
Actives:
white petrolatum 57.3%
mineral oil 42.5%
Inactive: lanolin alcohols.

FDA APPROVED USES

> Indications: For use as a lubricant to prevent further irritation or to relieve dryness of the eye.

Warnings: To avoid contamination, do not touch tip of container to any surface. Do not reuse. Once the product is opened, discard. If you experience eye pain, changes in vision, continued redness or irritation of the eye, or if the condition worsens or persists for more than 72 hours, discontinue use and consult a doctor. Keep this and all drugs out of the reach of children. In case of accidental ingestion, seek professional assistance or contact a poison control center immediately.

Directions: Pull down the lower lid of the affected eye and apply a small amount (one-fourth inch) of ointment to the inside of the eyelid.

Note: Do not touch unit-dose tip to eye.

How Supplied: Lacri-Lube® NP (white petrolatum 57.3%, mineral oil 42.5%) Lubricant Ophthalmic Ointment is supplied in sterile, preservative-free, disposable, single-use containers of 0.025 oz (0.7 g) each, in the following size:

SINGLE-USE CONTAINERS—
NDC 0023-0240-01

LACRIL®
(hydroxypropyl methylcellulose 0.5%, gelatin A 0.01%)
Lubricant Ophthalmic Solution

Contains: Actives: Hydroxypropyl methylcellulose 0.5% and gelatin A 0.01%. Inactives: calcium chloride, chlorobutanol (chloral deriv.) 0.5%, dextrose, magnesium chloride, polysorbate 80, potassium chloride, purified water, sodium acetate, sodium borate, sodium chloride, and sodium citrate. May also contain acetic acid to adjust pH.

FDA APPROVED USES

Indications: FOR USE AS A LUBRICANT TO PREVENT FURTHER IRRITATION OR TO RELIEVE DRYNESS OF THE EYE.

Warnings: To avoid contamination, do not touch tip of container to any surface. Replace cap after using. If you experience eye pain, changes in vision, continued redness or irritation of the eye, or if the condition worsens or persists for more than 72 hours, discontinue use and consult a doctor. If solution changes color or becomes cloudy, do not use. Keep this and all drugs out of the reach of children. In case of accidental ingestion, seek professional assistance or contact a poison control center immediately.

Directions: Instill 1 or 2 drops in the affected eye(s) as needed.

Note: Not for use while wearing soft contact lenses.

How Supplied: Lacril® (hydroxypropyl methylcellulose 0.5%, gelatin A 0.01%) Lubricant Ophthalmic Solution is supplied in sterile plastic dropper bottles in the following size:

½ fl oz—NDC 11980-045-15

LIQUIFILM FORTE®
(polyvinyl alcohol) 3.0%
Lubricant Ophthalmic Solution

Contains: Active: Polyvinyl alcohol 3.0%. Inactives: edetate disodium, mono- and dibasic sodium phosphates, purified water, sodium chloride, and thimerosal 0.002%. May also contain hydrochloric acid or sodium hydroxide to adjust pH.

FDA APPROVED USES

Indications: FOR USE AS A LUBRICANT TO PREVENT FURTHER IRRITATION OR TO RELIEVE DRYNESS OF THE EYE.

Warnings: To avoid contamination, do not touch tip of container to any surface. Replace cap after using. If you experience eye pain, changes in vision, continued redness or irritation of the eye, or if the condition worsens or persists for more than 72 hours, discontinue use and consult a doctor. If solution changes color or becomes cloudy, do not use. This product contains thimerosal 0.002% as a preservative. Do not use this product if you are sensitive to mercury. Keep this and all drugs out of the reach of children. In case of accidental ingestion, seek professional assistance or contact a poison control center immediately.

Directions: Instill 1 or 2 drops in the affected eye(s) as needed.

How Supplied: Liquifilm Forte® (polyvinyl alcohol) 3.0% Lubricant Ophthalmic Solution is supplied in sterile plastic dropper bottles in the following sizes:

½ fl oz—NDC 11980-187-15
1 fl oz—NDC 11980-187-30

LIQUIFILM TEARS®
(polyvinyl alcohol) 1.4%
Lubricant Ophthalmic Solution

Contains: Active: Polyvinyl alcohol 1.4%. Inactives: chlorobutanol (chloral deriv.) 0.5%, purified water, and sodium chloride. May also contain hydrochloric acid or sodium hydroxide to adjust pH.

FDA APPROVED USES

Indications: FOR USE AS A LUBRICANT TO PREVENT FURTHER IRRITATION OR TO RELIEVE DRYNESS OF THE EYE.

Warnings: To avoid contamination, do not touch tip of container to any surface. Replace cap after using. If you experience eye pain, changes in vision, continued redness or irritation of the eye, or if the condition worsens or persists for more than 72 hours, discontinue use and consult a doctor. If solution changes color or becomes cloudy, do not use. Keep this and all drugs out of the reach of children.

Continued on next page

Allergan—Cont.

In case of accidental ingestion, seek professional assistance or contact a poison control center immediately.

Directions: Instill 1 or 2 drops in the affected eye(s) as needed.

NOTE: Not for use while wearing soft contact lenses.

How Supplied: Liquifilm Tears® (polyvinyl alcohol) 1.4% Lubricant Ophthalmic Solution is supplied in sterile plastic dropper bottles in the following sizes:

½ fl oz—NDC 11980-025-15
1 fl oz—NDC 11980-025-30

Shown in Product Identification Section, page 403

PREFRIN™ Liquifilm®
(phenylephrine HCl 0.12%, polyvinyl alcohol 1.4%)
Vasoconstrictor (Redness Reliever) and Lubricant Eye Drops

Contains: Actives: Phenylephrine HCl 0.12%, Liquifilm® (polyvinyl alcohol) 1.4%. Inactives: benzalkonium chloride, edetate disodium, mono- and dibasic sodium phosphates, purified water, sodium acetate and sodium thiosulfate. pH may be adjusted with hydrochloric acid or sodium hydroxide.

FDA APPROVED USES

Indications: RELIEVES REDNESS OF THE EYE DUE TO MINOR EYE IRRITATION. FOR USE AS A LUBRICANT TO PREVENT FURTHER IRRITATION OR TO RELIEVE DRYNESS OF THE EYE.

Warnings: If you have glaucoma, do not use this product except under the advice and supervision of a doctor. If you experience eye pain, changes in vision, continued redness or irritation of the eye, or if the condition worsens or persists for more than 72 hours, discontinue use and consult a doctor. Overuse of this product may produce increased redness of the eye. To avoid contamination, do not touch tip of container to any surface. Replace cap after using. If the solution changes color or becomes cloudy, do not use. Pupils may dilate in some individuals. Keep this and all drugs out of the reach of children. In case of accidental ingestion, seek professional assistance or contact a poison control center immediately.

Note: Not for use while wearing soft contact lenses. Bottle filled to ⅔ capacity for proper drop control.

Directions: Instill 1 to 2 drops in the affected eye(s) up to four times daily.

How Supplied: Prefrin™ Liquifilm® (phenylephrine HCl 0.12%, polyvinyl alcohol 1.4%) Vasoconstrictor (Redness Reliever) and Lubricant Eye Drops is supplied in sterile plastic dropper bottles in the following size:

0.7 fl oz—NDC 11980-036-07

Shown in Product Identification Section, page 403

REFRESH®
(polyvinyl alcohol 1.4%, povidone 0.6%)
Lubricant Ophthalmic Solution

Contains: Actives: Polyvinyl alcohol 1.4% and povidone 0.6%. Inactives: purified water and sodium chloride. May also contain hydrochloric acid or sodium hydroxide to adjust pH.

FDA APPROVED USES

Indications: FOR USE AS A LUBRICANT TO PREVENT FURTHER IRRITATION OR TO RELIEVE DRYNESS OF THE EYE.

Warnings: To avoid contamination, do not touch tip of container to any surface. Do not reuse. Once opened, discard. If you experience eye pain, changes in vision, continued redness or irritation of the eye, or if the condition worsens or persists for more than 72 hours, discontinue use and consult a doctor. If solution changes color or becomes cloudy, do not use. Keep this and all drugs out of the reach of children. In case of accidental ingestion, seek professional assistance or contact a poison control center immediately.

Directions: Instill 1 or 2 drops in the affected eye(s) as needed.

Note: Do not touch unit-dose tip to eye.

How Supplied: Refresh® (polyvinyl alcohol 1.4%, povidone 0.6%) Lubricant Ophthalmic Solution is supplied in sterile, preservative-free, disposable, single-use containers of 0.01 fluid ounce each, in the following sizes:

30 SINGLE-USE CONTAINERS—
NDC 0023-0506-01
50 SINGLE-USE CONTAINERS—
NDC 0023-0506-50

Shown in Product Identification Section, page 403

REFRESH® P.M.
(white petrolatum 56.8%, mineral oil 41.5%)
Lubricant Ophthalmic Ointment

Contains: Actives: white petrolatum 56.8%, mineral oil 41.5%. Inactives: lanolin alcohols, purified water and sodium chloride.

FDA APPROVED USES

Indications: FOR USE AS A LUBRICANT TO PREVENT FURTHER IRRITATION OR TO RELIEVE DRYNESS OF THE EYE.

Warnings: To avoid contamination, do not touch tip of container to any surface. Replace cap after using. If you experience eye pain, changes in vision, continued redness or irritation of the eye, or if the condition worsens or persists for more than 72 hours, discontinue use and consult a doctor. Keep this and all drugs out of the reach of children. In case of accidental ingestion, seek professional assistance or contact a poison control center immediately.

Directions: Pull down the lower lid of the affected eye and apply a small amount (one-fourth inch) of ointment to the inside of the eyelid.

Note: Store away from heat. Protect from freezing.

How Supplied: Refresh® P.M. (white petrolatum 56.8%, mineral oil 41.5%) Lubricant Ophthalmic Ointment is supplied in sterile, preservative-free, ophthalmic ointment tubes in the following size:

3.5 g—NDC 0023-0667-04

Shown in Product Identification Section, page 403

RELIEF®
(phenylephrine HCl 0.12%, polyvinyl alcohol 1.4%)
Vasoconstrictor (Redness Reliever) and Lubricant Eye Drops

Contains: Actives: Phenylephrine HCl 0.12%, Liquifilm (polyvinyl alcohol) 1.4%. Inactives: edetate disodium, mono- and dibasic sodium phosphates, purified water, sodium acetate, and sodium thiosulfate. pH adjusted with hydrochloric acid or sodium hydroxide.

FDA APPROVED USES

Indications: RELIEVES REDNESS OF THE EYE DUE TO MINOR EYE IRRITATIONS. FOR USE AS A LUBRICANT TO PREVENT FURTHER IRRITATION OR TO RELIEVE DRYNESS OF THE EYE.

Warnings: To avoid contamination, do not touch tip of container to any surface. Do not reuse. Once opened, discard. If you have glaucoma, do not use this product except under the advice and supervision of a doctor. Pupils may dilate in some individuals. If you experience eye pain, changes in vision, continued redness or irritation of the eye, or if the condition worsens or persists for more than 72 hours, discontinue use and consult a doctor. Overuse of this product may produce increased redness of the eye. If the solution changes color or becomes cloudy, do not use. Keep this and all drugs out of the reach of children. In case of accidental ingestion, seek professional assistance or contact a poison control center immediately.

Note: Do not touch unit-dose tip to eye. Not for use while wearing soft contact lenses.

Directions: Instill 1 to 2 drops in the affected eyes(s) up to four times daily.

How Supplied: Relief® (phenylephrine HCl 0.12%, polyvinyl alcohol 1.4%) Vasoconstrictor (Redness Reliever) and Lubricant Eye Drops is supplied in sterile, preservative-free, disposable, single-use containers of 0.01 fluid ounce each, in the following sizes:

30 SINGLE-USE CONTAINERS—
NDC 0023-0507-01

Shown in Product Identification Section, page 403

TEARS PLUS®
(polyvinyl alcohol 1.4%, povidone 0.6%)
Lubricant Ophthalmic Solution

Contains: Actives: Polyvinyl alcohol 1.4% and povidone 0.6%. Inactives: chlorobutanol (chloral deriv.) 0.5%, purified water and sodium chloride. May also contain hydrochloric acid or sodium hydroxide to adjust pH.

FDA APPROVED USES

Indications: FOR USE AS A LUBRICANT TO PREVENT FURTHER IRRITATION OR TO RELIEVE DRYNESS OF THE EYE.

Warnings: To avoid contamination, do not touch tip of container to any surface. Replace cap after using. If you experience eye pain, changes in vision, continued redness or irritation of the eye, or if the condition worsens or persists for more than 72 hours, discontinue use and consult a doctor. If solution changes color or becomes cloudy, do not use. Keep this and all drugs out of the reach of children. In case of accidental ingestion, seek professional assistance or contact a poison control center immediately.

Directions: Instill 1 or 2 drops in the affected eye(s) as needed.

Note: Not for use while wearing soft contact lenses.

How Supplied: Tears Plus® (polyvinyl alcohol 1.4%, povidone 0.6%) Lubricant Ophthalmic Solution is supplied in sterile, plastic dropper bottles in the following sizes:

½ fl oz—NDC 11980-165-15
1 fl oz—NDC 11980-165-30

Shown in Product Identification Section, page 403

Apothecon

A Bristol-Myers Squibb Company
P.O. BOX 4000
PRINCETON, NJ 08540-4000

Naldecon DX®, EX®, and CX® are distributed by Apothecon. For the Naldecon listing, please see the Bristol Laboratories section.
Theragran Liquid, Theragran Stress Formula, Theragran Tablets and Theragran-M Tablets are distributed by Apothecon. For the Theragran listing, please see E.R. Squibb & Sons, Inc.

Products are indexed by generic and chemical names in the **YELLOW SECTION**

B.F. Ascher & Company, Inc.

15501 WEST 109th STREET
LENEXA, KS 66219
Mailing address:
P.O. BOX 717
SHAWNEE MISSION, KS 66201-0717

AYR® Saline Nasal Mist and Drops
[*ār*]

AYR Mist or Drops restores vital moisture to provide prompt relief for dry, crusted and inflamed nasal membranes due to chronic sinusitis, colds, low humidity, overuse of nasal decongestant drops and sprays, allergies, minor nose bleeds and other minor nasal irritations. AYR provides a soothing way to thin thick secretions and aid their removal from the nose and sinuses. AYR can be used as often as needed without the side effects associated with overuse of decongestant nose drops and sprays.

SAFE AND GENTLE ENOUGH FOR CHILDREN AND INFANTS

AYR Drops are particularly convenient for easy application with infants and children. AYR is formulated to prevent stinging, burning and irritation of delicate nasal tissue, even that of babies.

Directions For Use: SPRAY—Squeeze twice in each nostril as often as needed. Hold bottle upright. To spray, give the bottle short, firm squeezes. Take care not to aspirate nasal contents back into bottle. DROPS—Two to four drops in each nostril every two hours as needed, or as directed by your physician.
AYR is a specially formulated, buffered, isotonic saline solution containing sodium chloride 0.65% adjusted to the proper tonicity and pH with monobasic potassium phosphate/sodium hydroxide buffer to prevent nasal irritation. AYR also contains the non-irritating antibacterial and antifungal preservatives thimerosal and benzalkonium chloride and is formulated with deionized water.

How Supplied: AYR Mist in 50 ml spray bottles, AYR Drops in 50 ml dropper bottles.

Shown in Product Identification Section, page 403

ITCH–X GEL®

Active Ingredients: Benzyl alcohol 10% and pramoxine HCl 1%.
Also contains: Aloe vera gel, carbomer 934, diazolidinyl urea, FD&C blue #1, methylparaben, propylene glycol, propylparaben, SD alcohol 40, styrene/acrylate copolymer, triethanolamine, and water.

Indications: For the temporary relief of pain and itching associated with minor skin irritations, allergic itches, rashes, hives, minor burns, insect bites, sunburns, poison ivy, poison oak, and poison sumac.

Warnings: For external use only. Avoid contact with the eyes. If condition worsens, or if symptoms persist for more than 7 days or clear up and occur again within a few days, discontinue use of this product and consult a physician. KEEP THIS AND ALL DRUGS OUT OF THE REACH OF CHILDREN. In case of accidental ingestion, seek professional assistance or contact a Poison Control Center immediately.

Directions: Adults and children 2 years of age and older: Apply to affected area not more than 3 to 4 times daily. Children under 2 years of age: consult a physician.

How Supplied: 1.25 oz tube

Shown in Product Identification Section, page 403

MOBIGESIC® Analgesic Tablets
[*mō 'bĭ-jē 'zĭk*]

Active Ingredients: Each tablet contains 325 mg of magnesium salicylate with 30 mg of phenyltoloxamine citrate.

Also Contains: Microcrystalline cellulose, magnesium stearate and colloidal silicon dioxide which aid in the formulation of the tablet and its dissolution in the gastrointestinal tract.

Indications: **MOBIGESIC** acts fast to provide relief from the pain and discomfort of simple headaches and colds; for temporary relief of the pain and tension accompanying muscle soreness and fatigue, neuralgia, minor menstrual cramps, T.M.J. and pain of tooth extraction. The unique formula provides relief of pain due to sinusitis and in the fever and inflammation of colds.

Caution: When used for the temporary symptomatic relief of colds, if relief does not occur within 7 days (3 days for fever), discontinue use and consult physician. This preparation may cause drowsiness. Do not drive or operate machinery while taking this medication. Do not administer to children under 6 years of age or exceed recommended dosage unless directed by physician.

Warnings: Keep this and all drugs out of the reach of children. In case of accidental overdose, call your doctor or poison control center immediately. As with any drug, if you are pregnant or nursing a baby, seek the advice of a health professional before using this product.

Usual Dosage: Adults—1 or 2 tablets every four hours, up to 10 tablets daily. Children (6 to 12 years)—1 tablet every 4 hours, up to 5 tablets daily. Do not use more than 10 days unless directed by physician.
Store at room temperature (59°–86°F).

How Supplied: Packages of 18's, 50's and 100's.

Shown in Product Identification Section, page 403

MOBISYL® Analgesic Creme
[*mō 'bĭ-sĭl*]

Active Ingredient: Trolamine salicylate 10%. Also Contains: Glycerin, meth-

Continued on next page

Ascher—Cont.

ylparaben, mineral oil, polysorbate 60, propylparaben, sorbitan stearate, sorbitol, stearic acid, and water.

Description: MOBISYL is a greaseless, odorless, penetrating, non-burning, non-irritating analgesic creme.

Indications: For adults and children, 12 years of age and older, MOBISYL is indicated for the temporary relief of minor aches and pains of muscles and joints, such as simple backache, lumbago, arthritis, neuralgia, strains, bruises and sprains.

Actions: MOBISYL penetrates fast into sore, tender joints and muscles where pain originates. It works to reduce inflammation. Helps soothe stiff joints and muscles and gets you going again.

Warnings: For external use only. Avoid contact with the eyes. Discontinue use if condition worsens or if symptoms persist for more than 7 days, and consult a physician. Do not use on children under 12 years of age except under the advice and supervision of a physician. In case of accidental ingestion, seek professional assistance or contact a Poison Control Center immediately. Close cap tightly. Keep this and all drugs out of the reach of children. Store at room temperature.

Dosage and Administration: Place a liberal amount of MOBISYL Creme in your palm and massage into the area of pain and soreness three or four times a day, especially before retiring. MOBISYL may be worn under clothing or bandages.

How Supplied: MOBISYL is available in 1.25 oz tubes, 3.5 oz tubes, 8 oz jars.

Shown in Product Identification Section, page 403

PEN•KERA® Creme with Keratin Binding Factor
A Therapeutic Creme for Chronic Dry Skin

Ingredients: Water, octyl palmitate, glycerin, mineral oil, polysorbate 60, sorbitan stearate, carbomer 940, triethanolamine, wheat germ glycerides, diazolidinyl urea, polyamino sugar condensate (and) urea, and dehydroacetic acid.

Indications: PEN•KERA Therapeutic Creme for Chronic Dry Skin contains Keratin Binding Factor, a polyamino sugar condensate and urea, which is synthesized to match the same biological components as those found in skin. The Keratin Binding Factor in PEN•KERA Creme replaces the missing elements of dehydrated skin which absorb and retain moisture. The Keratin Binding Factor actually simulates the natural moisturizing mechanism of the skin, relieving itching, flaking, sensitive, dry skin symptoms.
PEN•KERA is fragrance-free, dye-free, paraben-free, lanolin-free and non-greasy for smooth, fast absorption.

Dosage and Administration: Apply in a thin layer. Because it penetrates quickly and is non-greasy, PEN•KERA may be used under make-up or sun screens. Regular use will reduce the frequency of application and quantity required to achieve moisturized skin.

Precautions: FOR EXTERNAL USE ONLY

How Supplied: PEN•KERA Therapeutic Creme is available in 8 oz. bottles (0225-0440-35).

Shown in Product Identification Section, page 403

UNILAX® Softgel Capsules

Active Ingredients: Docusate sodium, USP 230 mg and yellow phenolphthalein, USP 130 mg.

Inactive Ingredients: D&C Yellow No. 10, FD&C Blue No. 1, FD&C Yellow No. 6, gelatin, glycerin, polyethylene glycol 400, sorbitol and titanium dioxide.

Indications: Constipation (irregularity).

Actions: UNILAX® is a dual-acting stool softener and stimulant laxative.

Warnings: Do not use laxative products when abdominal pain, nausea, or vomiting are present. As with all laxatives, frequent or prolonged use may result in dependence. If skin rash appears, do not use this or any other preparation containing phenolphthalein. As with any drug, if you are pregnant or nursing a baby, seek the advice of a health professional before using this product. Keep this and all drugs out of the reach of children. In case of accidental overdose, seek professional assistance or contact a poison control center immediately.

Dosage and Administration: Adults and children 12 years of age and over: Oral dosage is 1 softgel capsule daily (preferably at bedtime) or as directed by a physician. Do not use in children under 12 years of age.

How Supplied: Bottles of 15 and 60 softgel capsules.

Shown in Product Identification Section, page 403

Astra Pharmaceutical Products, Inc.
50 OTIS ST.
WESTBORO, MA 01581-4500

XYLOCAINE® (lidocaine) 2.5%
[*zī'lo-caine*]
OINTMENT

For temporary relief of pain and itching due to minor burns, sunburn, minor cuts, abrasions, insect bites and minor skin irritations.

Composition: Diethylaminoacet-2,6-xylidide 2.5% in a water miscible ointment vehicle consisting of polyethylene glycols and propylene glycol.

Action and Uses: A topical anesthetic ointment for fast, temporary relief of pain and itching due to minor burns, sunburn, minor cuts, abrasions, insect bites and minor skin irritations. The ointment can be easily removed with water. It is ineffective when applied to intact skin.

Administration and Dosage: Apply topically in liberal amounts for adequate control of symptoms. When the anesthetic effect wears off additional ointment may be applied as needed.

Important Warning: *In persistent, severe or extensive skin disorders, advise patient to use only as directed. In case of accidental ingestion advise patient to seek professional assistance or to contact a poison control center immediately. Keep out of the reach of children.*

Caution: *Do not use in the eyes. Not for prolonged use. If the condition for which this preparation is used persists or if a rash or irritation develops, advise patient to discontinue use and consult a physician.*

How Supplied: Available in tube of 35 grams (approximately 1.25 ounces).

Shown in Product Identification Section, page 404

Au Pharmaceuticals, Inc.
P. O. BOX 476
GRAND SALINE, TX 75140

AURUM–The Gold Lotion
Topical Analgesic and Anti-inflammatory
GOLD PLUS–The Gold Lotion
Topical Analgesic and Anti-inflammatory
THERAGOLD–The Gold Lotion
Topical Analgesic and Anti-inflammatory
THERAPEUTIC GOLD–The Gold Lotion
Topical Analgesic and Anti-inflammatory

Active Ingredients: The active ingredients are methyl salicylate 10%; menthol 3%; camphor 2.5%. These are combined in a rich, nonpetroleum base for easy and effective topical application.

Other Selected Ingredients: Special inactive ingredients include 24 KARAT GOLD, Eucalyptus Oil, Jojoba Oil, Ginseng Extract, Urea and Aloe Vera.

Indications: These lotions give fast, deep-penetrating, effective relief from stiff, sore, aching muscles and joints associated with arthritis, bursitis, tendinitis and muscle disorders. These lotions are also effective in reducing inflammation in acute and chronic inflammatory problems within the joints and soft tissues.

Actions: Methyl salicylate, menthol and camphor are classified as counterirritants which combine to provide both heat and cold stimulation to the pain receptors over and around the affected area. The lotions replace the perception of pain with the feeling of heat and/or cold to provide temporary relief of minor aches and pains.

Directions: Apply a liberal amount of lotion to painful area and allow to remain on skin for 30 seconds before rubbing remainder into skin. Apply product 3 or 4 times a day or as needed until pain is relieved, then reduce the frequency to as needed.

Warnings: Use only as directed. For external use only. Avoid contact with eyes, mucous membranes, broken or irritated skin. If condition worsens or persists for more than 7 days without relief, discontinue use of this product and consult a physician. Do not use on children under 2 years of age without consulting a physician.

How Supplied: These products are available in 8 ounce and 2 ounce bottles. National Drug Code Registration #057646

FEMININE GOLD—The Lotion Topical Analgesic

Active Ingredients: The active ingredients are menthol 3%, camphor 2.5%. These are combined in a rich, nonpetroleum base for easy and effective topical application.

Other Selected Ingredients: Special inactive ingredients include 24 KARAT GOLD, Eucalyptus Oil, Jojoba Oil, Ginseng Extract, Urea and Aloe Vera.

Indications: This lotion gives fast, deep-penetrating, effective relief from pain and discomfort of cramps and backache suffered during the menstrual cycle.

Actions: Menthol and camphor are classified as counterirritants which combine to provide both heat and cold stimulation to the pain receptors over and around the affected area. The lotion replaces the perception of pain with the feeling of heat and/or cold to provide temporary relief of minor aches and pains.

Directions: Apply a liberal amount of lotion to painful area and allow to remain on skin for 30 seconds before rubbing remainder into skin. Apply product 3 or 4 times a day or as needed until pain is relieved, then reduce the frequency to as needed.

Warnings: Use only as directed. For external use only. Avoid contact with eyes, mucous membranes, broken or irritated skin. If condition worsens or persists for more than 3 days without relief, discontinue use of this product and consult a physician.

How Supplied: These products are available in 2 ounce bottles. National Drug Code Registration #057646

Ayerst Laboratories
Division of American Home Products Corporation
685 THIRD AVE.
NEW YORK, NY 10017-4071

For information for Ayerst's consumer products, see product listings under Whitehall Laboratories.
Please turn to Whitehall Laboratories, page 749.

Baker Cummins Dermatologicals, Inc.
8800 NORTHWEST 36TH STREET
MIAMI, FL 33178

AQUA-A® Cream

Description: Contains the vitamin A derivative, retinyl palmitate. Moisture-enriched smoothing concentrate. Clinically proven for all skin types.

Ingredients: Water, Caprylic/Capric Triglyceride, Methyl Gluceth-10, Glyceryl Stearate, Squalane, Mineral Oil, PPG-20 Methyl Glucose Ether Distearate, Dimethicone, Stearic Acid, PEG-50 Stearate, Retinyl Palmitate, Sodium Hyaluronate, Lecithin, Sodium Polyglutamate, Ascorbyl Palmitate, Carbomer 934, Dichlorobenzyl Alcohol, Cetyl Alcohol, BHT, Diazolidinyl Urea, Xanthan Gum, Menthol, Sodium Hydroxide, Tetrasodium EDTA.

Directions for Use: Use morning or night or both.

How Supplied: 2 oz. jars

AQUADERM® Combination Treatment/Moisturizer

Description: Aquaderm® Combination Treatment/Moisturizer developed by leading dermatologists to deliver maximum moisturization. Regular daily use of Aquaderm's dual action moisturizer and sunscreen protects and preserves your youthful appearance. This specially developed formula contains sunscreens (SPF 15) that shield your skin from UVA and UVB rays, to protect it from wrinkles and reduce skin damage and possible skin cancer. Aquaderm® Combination Treatment/Moisturizer is safe and effective, hypo-allergenic, non-comedogenic, Paraben-free, and will not leave an artificial-feeling film. Aquaderm® Combination Treatment/Moisturizer is especially suited for patients undergoing Retin-A® therapy, who require maximum moisturization and sun protection. Retin-A® is a registered trademark of Johnson & Johnson.

Ingredients: Octyl Methoxycinnamate, 7.5%, Oybenzone, 6%, Titanium Dioxide, 2%, in a moisturizing cream base.

Indications: Protects against harmful skin-aging rays of the sun.

Warnings: FOR EXTERNAL USE ONLY. Avoid contact with eyes. If irritation develops, discontinue use. Keep this and all drugs out of the reach of children. In case of accidental ingestion, seek professional assistance or contact a Poison Control Center immediately.

Directions for Use: Apply to face and neck as needed. Effective and compatible for daily use under make-up.

How Supplied: 3.5 oz. tube

AQUADERM® Cream

Description: Ultrarich moisturizing cream concentrate. Softens, smooths, protects, absorbs quickly.

Ingredients: Water, Caprylic/Capric Triglyceride, Methyl Gluceth-10, Glyceryl Stearate, Mineral Oil, Squalane, PPG-20 Methyl Glucose Ether Distearate, Dimethicone, Stearic Acid, PEG-50 Stearate, Sodium Hyaluronate, Lecithin, Sodium Polyglutamate, Magnesium Aluminum Silicate, Carbomer 934, Dichlorobenzyl Alcohol, Cetyl Alcohol, BHT, Diazolidinyl Urea, Xanthan Gum, Menthol, Sodium Hydroxide, Tetrasodium EDTA.

Directions for Use: Apply to face or other dry areas morning or night or both.

How Supplied: 4 oz. jar

AQUADERM® Lotion

Description: Ultrarich moisturizing lotion concentrate. Smooths, softens, protects, absorbs quickly. Clinically proven for all skin types.

Ingredients: Water, Caprylic/Capric Triglyceride, Methyl Gluceth-10, Glyceryl Stearate, Dimethicone, Petrolatum, Mineral Oil, PPG-20 Methyl Glucose Ether Distearate, Squalane, PEG-50 Stearate, Stearic Acid, Sodium Hyaluronate, Lecithin, Sodium Polyglutamate, Magnesium Aluminum Silicate, Carbomer 934, Dichlorobenzyl Alcohol, Cetyl Alcohol, BHT, Diazolidinyl Urea, Xanthan Gum, Menthol, Tetrasodium EDTA, Sodium Hydroxide.

Directions for Use: Apply to hands and body morning or night or both.

How Supplied: 7.5 fl. oz. bottle

P&S® Liquid

Ingredients: Mineral Oil, Water, Fragrance, Glycerin, Phenol, Sodium Chloride, D&C Yellow #11, D&C Red #17, D&C Green #6.

Indications: P&S® Liquid, used regularly, helps loosen and remove crusts and scales on the scalp.

Warnings: FOR EXTERNAL USE ONLY. Do not apply to large portions of body surfaces. Discontinue use if excessive skin irritation develops. Avoid contact with eyes or mucous membranes. Keep out of the reach of children. In case of accidental ingestion, seek professional assistance or contact a Poison Control Center immediately.

Continued on next page

Baker Derm.—Cont.

Directions for Use: Apply liberally to scalp lesions each night before retiring. Massage gently to loosen scales and crusts. Leave on overnight and shampoo the next morning. Use daily as needed.

How Supplied: 8 fl. oz. bottle (58174-401-08); 4 fl. oz. bottle (58174-401-04)

P&S® PLUS Tar Gel

Active Ingredients: 8% Coal Tar Solution (equivalent to 1.6% Crude Coal Tar), 2% Salicylic Acid.

Indications: For psoriasis and other scaling conditions. P&S® PLUS relieves the itching, irritation and skin flaking associated with seborrheic dermatitis, psoriasis and dandruff.

Warnings: FOR EXTERNAL USE ONLY. Avoid contact with the eyes; flush with water if product gets into eyes. If irritation develops, discontinue use. If condition worsens or does not improve after regular use of this product as directed, consult a physician. Do not use on children under 2 years of age except as directed by a physician. Use caution in exposing skin to sunlight after applying this product; it may increase your tendency to sunburn for up to 24 hours after application. Do not use product in or around the rectum or in the genital area or groin except on the advice of a physician. Keep this and all drugs out of reach of children. In case of accidental ingestion, seek professional assistance or contact a Poison Control Center immediately.

Directions for Use: Apply to affected areas of skin and scalp daily or as directed by physician.

How Supplied: 3.5 oz. tube (NDC 58174-409-35)

P&S® Shampoo

Active Ingredient: 2% Salicylic Acid.

Indications: P&S® Shampoo relieves the itching, irritation and skin flaking associated with seborrheic dermatitis of the scalp. It also relieves the itching, redness, and scaling associated with psoriasis of the scalp. P&S® Shampoo may be used alone as well as following treatment with P&S® Liquid. Its rich conditioning formula improves hair's manageability and helps prevent tangles.

Warnings: FOR EXTERNAL USE ONLY. Avoid contact with eyes or mucous membranes. If this occurs, rinse thoroughly with water. If condition worsens or does not improve after regular use of this product as directed, consult a physician. Do not use on children under 2 years of age except as directed by a physician. Keep this and all drugs out of reach of children. In case of accidental ingestion, seek professional assistance or contact a Poison Control Center immediately.

Directions for Use: For best results use twice weekly or as directed by a physician. Wet hair, apply to scalp and massage vigorously. Rinse and repeat.

How Supplied: 4 fl. oz. bottle (NDC 58174-407-04)

ULTRA MIDE 25™ Extra Strength Moisturizer

Ingredients: Water, Urea, Mineral Oil, Glycerin, Propylene Glycol, PEG-50 Stearate, Butyrolactone, Hydrogenated Lanolin, Sorbitan Laurate, Glyceryl Stearate, Magnesium Aluminum Silicate, Propylene Glycol Stearate SE, Cetyl Alcohol, Fragrance, Diazolidinyl Urea, Tetrasodium EDTA.

Indications: Extra strength moisturizer. Helps relieve discomfort of extra dry skin. Contains ingredients to soften and moisturize areas of very dry, rough, cracked or calloused skin. The unique formula contains a stabilized form of urea (25%) to help prevent the stinging and irritation often associated with moisturizers containing urea. ULTRA MIDE 25 Lotion contains no parabens.

Warnings: FOR EXTERNAL USE ONLY. Keep out of reach of children. Discontinue use if irritation occurs. Caution should be taken when used near the eyes. In case of accidental ingestion, seek professional assistance or contact a poison control center immediately.

Directions for Use: Apply four times daily, or as directed by a physician. Each application should be rubbed in completely.

How Supplied: 8 fl. oz. bottle (58174-420-08)

X-SEB® Shampoo

Active Ingredient: 4% Salicylic Acid.

Indications: X-SEB® Shampoo relieves the itching and scalp flaking associated with dandruff. Its conditioning formula leaves hair more manageable, with more body.

Warnings: FOR EXTERNAL USE ONLY. Avoid contact with eyes or mucous membranes. If this occurs, rinse thoroughly with water. If condition worsens or does not improve after regular use of this product as directed, consult a physician. Do not use on children under 2 years of age except as directed by a physician. Keep this and all drugs out of the reach of children. In case of accidental ingestion, seek professional assistance or contact a Poison Control Center immediately.

Directions for Use: For best results use twice weekly or as directed by a physician. Wet hair, apply to scalp and massage vigorously. Rinse and repeat.

How Supplied: 4 fl. oz. bottle (NDC 58174-106-04)

X-SEB® PLUS Conditioning Shampoo

Active Ingredients: 1% Pyrithione Zinc, 2% Salicylic Acid.

Indications: For dandruff and seborrheic dermatitis. X-SEB® PLUS Shampoo relieves the itching, irritation and skin flaking associated with dandruff and seborrheic dermatitis. X-SEB® PLUS contains the plus of conditioners to leave hair soft and manageable. Pleasant fragrance.

Warnings: FOR EXTERNAL USE ONLY. Avoid contact with the eyes; if this happens, rinse thoroughly with water. Keep this and all drugs out of the reach of children. In case of accidental ingestion, seek professional assistance or contact a Poison Control Center immediately.

Directions for Use: Wet hair, apply to scalp and massage vigorously. Rinse and repeat. If irritation develops, discontinue use. Use at least twice a week for best results or as directed by a physician.

How Supplied: 4 fl. oz. bottle (NDC 58174-116-04)

X-SEB® T Shampoo

Active Ingredients: 10% Coal Tar Solution (equivalent to 2% Crude Coal Tar), 4% Salicylic Acid.

Indications: X-SEB® T Shampoo relieves the itching, irritation and skin flaking associated with seborrheic dermatitis, psoriasis and dandruff.

Warnings: FOR EXTERNAL USE ONLY. Avoid contact with the eyes; flush with water if product gets in eyes. If irritation develops, discontinue use. If condition worsens or does not improve after regular use of this product as directed, consult a physician. Do not use on children under 2 years of age except as directed by a physician. Use caution in exposing skin to sunlight after applying this product; it may increase your tendency to sunburn for up to 24 hours after application. Keep out of reach of children. In case of accidental ingestion, seek professional assistance or contact a Poison Control Center immediately.

Directions for Use: Wet hair, apply to scalp and massage vigorously. Rinse and repeat or as directed by a physician.

How Supplied: 4 fl. oz. bottle (NDC 58174-105-04)

X-SEB® T PLUS Conditioning Shampoo

Active Ingredients: 10% Coal Tar Solution (equivalent to 2% Crude Coal Tar), 3% Salicylic Acid, 1% Menthol.

Indications: For psoriasis, seborrheic dermatitis and dandruff. X-SEB® T PLUS Shampoo relieves the itching, irritation and skin flaking associated with psoriasis, seborrheic dermatitis, and dandruff. X-SEB® T PLUS contains the plus of conditioners to leave hair soft and manageable. Pleasant color and fragrance.

Warnings: FOR EXTERNAL USE ONLY. Avoid contact with the eyes; if this happens, rinse thoroughly with water. Keep this and all drugs out of the reach of children. In case of accidental ingestion, seek professional assistance or contact a Poison Control Center immediately.

Directions for Use: Wet hair, apply to scalp and massage vigorously. Rinse and repeat. If irritation develops, discontinue use. Use daily until control is achieved. To maintain control, use at least twice a week or as directed by a physician.

How Supplied: 4 fl. oz. bottle (NDC 58174-115-04)

Bausch & Lomb Personal Products Division

1400 N GOODMAN ST.
ROCHESTER, NY 14692-0450

ALLERGY DROPS
Lubricant/Redness Reliever Eye Drops

Description: BAUSCH & LOMB Allergy Drops is a sterile lubricating eye drop that relieves minor irritation caused by allergens—pollen, dust, animal hair, air pollutants, and other common eye irritants. It relieves redness and keeps on working to protect eyes against further irritation.
Unlike other eye drops, BAUSCH & LOMB Allergy Drops contains a special ingredient that provides longer lasting relief from itching, burning, dry, irritated eyes.

Ingredients: Polyethylene glycol 300 (0.2%), naphazoline hydrochloride (0.012%). Also contains: boric acid, disodium edetate, sodium borate, sodium chloride; preserved with benzalkonium chloride (0.01%).

Indications: Relieves redness of the eye due to minor eye irritations. For the temporary relief of burning and irritation due to dryness of the eye and for use as a protectant against further irritation, or to relieve dryness of the eye.

Warnings: To avoid contamination, do not touch tip of container to any surface. Replace cap after using. If solution changes color or becomes cloudy, do not use. If you experience eye pain, changes in vision, continued redness or irritation of the eye, or if the condition worsens or persists for more than 72 hours, discontinue use and consult a doctor. If you have glaucoma, do not use this product except under the advice and supervision of a doctor. Overuse of this product may produce increased redness of the eye.
Keep this and all medication out of the reach of children.
REMOVE CONTACT LENSES BEFORE USING.

Directions: Instill 1 or 2 drops in the affected eye(s) up to four times daily.
Store at room temperature.

How Supplied: In plastic bottles of 0.5 fl oz.

Shown in Product Identification Section, page 404

DRY EYE THERAPY™
Lubricating Eye Drops
Preservative Free

Ingredients: Glycerin 0.3%, with: calcium chloride, magnesium chloride, purified water, potassium chloride, sodium chloride, sodium citrate, sodium phosphate, and zinc chloride.

Indications: For the temporary relief of burning and irritation due to dryness of the eye and for use as a lubricant to prevent further irritation. For the temporary relief of discomfort due to minor irritations of the eye or to exposure to wind or sun.

Description: Bausch & Lomb Dry Eye Therapy, like natural tears, contains a lubricant and four essential nutrients: calcium, zinc, potassium, and magnesium. It provides soothing relief for dry eyes.

Warnings: To avoid contamination, do not touch tip of container to any surface. Do not re-use. Once opened, discard. If you experience eye pain, changes in vision, continued redness or irritation of the eye, or if the condition worsens or persists for more than 72 hours, discontinue use and consult a doctor. If solution changes color or becomes cloudy, do not use.
Use only if single-use container is intact.
Keep this and all drugs out of the reach of children.
Store at room temperature.

Directions:
- Make sure single-use container is intact before use.
- Separate one container from the strip of four.
- Open the single-use container by completely twisting off the top tab.
- Place thumb and forefinger on the marks on the center of the bubble.
- Gently squeeze 1 to 2 drops in the affected eye(s).
- After placing the drops in eye(s), throw away the container. Do not re-use.

Dry Eye Therapy may be used as often as needed.

How Supplied: 32 sterile, single-use containers, each 0.01 fl oz.

Shown in Product Identification Section, page 404

DUOLUBE
Sterile Lubricant Eye Ointment

Description: White petrolatum 80% and mineral oil 20%. Contains no preservatives.

Indications: For use as a lubricant to prevent further irritation or to relieve dryness of the eye.

Directions: Pull down the lower lid of the affected eye and apply a small amount (one-fourth inch) of Duolube ointment to the inside of the eyelid.

Warnings: To avoid contamination, do not touch tip of container to any surface. Replace cap after using. If you experience eye pain, changes in vision, continued redness, irritation of the eye, or if the condition worsens or persists for more than 72 hours, discontinue use and consult a doctor. KEEP OUT OF REACH OF CHILDREN. NOT FOR USE WITH CONTACT LENSES.
DO NOT USE IF BOTTOM RIDGE OF CAP IS EXPOSED PRIOR TO INITIAL USE.
Store at room temperature.

How Supplied: In ⅛-oz (NDC 10119-020-13) tube.

Shown in Product Identification Section, page 404

EYE WASH
Sterile Isotonic Buffered Solution

Description: A sterile, isotonic solution that contains boric acid, purified water, sodium borate and sodium chloride; preserved with disodium edetate 0.025% and sorbic acid 0.1%. CONTAINS NO THIMEROSAL (MERCURY).

Indications: For cleansing the eye to help relieve irritation, burning, stinging and itching by removing loose, foreign material, air pollutants (smog or pollen) or chlorinated water.

Warnings: To avoid contamination, do not touch tip of container to any surface. Replace cap after using. If you experience eye pain, changes in vision, continued redness or irritation of the eye, or if the condition worsens or persists, consult a doctor. Obtain immediate medical treatment for all open wounds in or near the eyes. If solution changes color or becomes cloudy, do not use.
Use only as directed. If you experience any chemical burns, consult a doctor immediately. KEEP OUT OF REACH OF CHILDREN.

Directions: With Eye Cup—Rinse cup with BAUSCH & LOMB® Eye Wash immediately before and after each use. Avoid contamination of rim and inside surfaces of cup. Fill cup one-half full with BAUSCH & LOMB Eye Wash. Apply cup tightly to the affected eye to prevent spillage and tilt head backward. Open eyelids wide and rotate eyeball to thoroughly wash the eye.
NOTE: Enclosed eye cup is sterile if packaging intact.

Directions: Without Eye Cup—Flush the affected eye as needed, controlling the rate of flow of solution by pressure on the bottle.

How Supplied: In plastic dropper bottles of 4 fl oz, packaged with sterile eye cup.

Shown in Product Identification Section, page 404

Continued on next page

Bausch & Lomb—Cont.

MOISTURE DROPS®
Artificial Tears

Description: BAUSCH & LOMB MOISTURE DROPS Artificial Tears quickly provides soothing relief to dry, itchy, burning, irritated eyes. Its unique triple-action formula keeps on working, so your eyes stay moist, healthy, protected against further irritation. And unlike some eye drops, MOISTURE DROPS can be used as often as needed.

Ingredients: Hydroxypropyl methylcellulose (0.5%), dextran 70 (0.1%) and glycerin (0.2%). Also contains: boric acid, disodium edetate, potassium chloride, sodium borate, sodium chloride; preserved with benzalkonium chloride (0.01%).

Indications: For the temporary relief of burning and irritation due to dryness of the eye and for use as a protectant against further irritation, or to relieve dryness of the eye.

Warnings: To avoid contamination, do not touch tip of container to any surface. Replace cap after using. If you experience eye pain, changes in vision, continued redness or irritation of the eye, or if the condition worsens or persists for more than 72 hours, discontinue use and consult a doctor. If solution changes color or becomes cloudy, do not use.
Keep this and all medication out of the reach of children.
REMOVE CONTACT LENSES BEFORE USING.

Directions: Instill 1 or 2 drops in the affected eye(s) as needed.
Store at room temperature.

How Supplied: In plastic bottles of 0.5 and 1.0 fl oz.

Shown in Product Identification Section, page 404

Beach Pharmaceuticals
Division of Beach Products, Inc.
5220 SOUTH MANHATTAN AVE.
TAMPA, FL 33611

BEELITH Tablets
MAGNESIUM SUPPLEMENT
With PYRIDOXINE HCl
Each tablet supplies 362 mg of magnesium (31.83 mEq).

Directions: As a dietary supplement, take one tablet daily or as directed by a physician. Each tablet yields 362 mg of magnesium and supplies 90% of the Adult U.S. Recommended Daily Allowance (RDA) for magnesium and 1000% of the Adult RDA for vitamin B_6.
Each tablet contains magnesium oxide 600 mg and pyridoxine hydrochloride (Vitamin B_6) 25 mg equivalent to B_6 20 mg. *Also, castor oil, hydroxypropyl methylcellulose, magnesium stearate, microcrystalline cellulose, pharmaceutical glaze, povidone, sodium starch glycolate, D&C Yellow #10, FD&C Yellow #6 (Sunset Yellow), and titanium dioxide.*

Drug Interaction Precautions: Do not take this product if you are presently taking a prescription antibiotic drug containing any form of tetracycline.

Warnings: If you have kidney disease, take only under the supervision of a physician. Excessive dosage may cause laxation. **KEEP OUT OF THE REACH OF CHILDREN.** Do not use if protective printed band around cap is broken or missing.

How Supplied: Golden yellow, film coated tablet with the name **BEACH** and the number **1132** printed on each tablet. Packaged in bottles of 100 (NDC 0486-1132-01) tablets.

Storage: Keep tightly closed. Store at 15°–30°C (59°–86°F). Protect from light.
R4/90

Shown on page 404 in the 1991 PHYSICIANS' DESK REFERENCE

Becton Dickinson Consumer Products
ONE BECTON DRIVE
FRANKLIN LAKES, NJ 07417-1883

B-D Glucose Tablets

Indications and Usage: For fast relief from hypoglycemia. B-D Glucose Tablets contain D-Glucose (Dextrose), the most readily absorbed sugar, and are recommended for treatment of hypoglycemia. The tablets are chewable and dissolve quickly in the mouth to facilitate ingestion. Each tablet is 19 calories. When all symptoms have been alleviated, a light meal consisting of a longer acting carbohydrate and protein should be consumed.

Adverse Reactions: No adverse reactions have been reported with appropriate use of glucose. Occasional reports of nausea may be due to the hypoglycemia itself.

Dosage and Administration: The recommended dosage is two (2) to three (3) tablets (10.0 to 15.0 grams of dextrose) at the first sign of hypoglycemia. Repeat dosage as needed to counter additional hypoglycemic episodes that may be caused by longer acting insulins. Dosage may be regulated by taking fewer or more tablets, depending on severity of the reaction, age and body weight. Notify your physician of hypoglycemic episodes. Do not administer to anyone who is unconscious.

How Supplied: Box containing six chewable tablets. Tablets are packaged in durable three tablet blister packs.

Ingredients: Each tablet contains 5.0 grams dextrose. Other ingredients are flavors and tabletting aids: croscarmellose sodium, Type A and magnesium stearate. Contains no preservatives.

EDUCATIONAL MATERIAL

A complete, comprehensive diabetes education teaching system is available to health care professionals. These teaching aids are designed to help the patient and family members understand and manage diabetes. Materials include a series of brochures, patient take-home kits and audio visual aids.

Beiersdorf Inc.
P.O. BOX 5529
NORWALK, CT 06856-5529

AQUAPHOR®
Healing Ointment
NDC Numbers-10356-020-01
10356-020-02
10356-020-06
10356-020-07

Composition: Petrolatum, mineral oil, mineral wax and wool wax alcohol.

Actions and Uses: Aquaphor is a stable, neutral, odorless, anhydrous ointment base. Miscible with water or aqueous solutions, Aquaphor will absorb several times its own weight, forming smooth, creamy water-in-oil emulsions. In its pure form, Aquaphor is recommended for use as a topical preparation to help heal severely dry skin, cracked, chafed skin and minor burns.

Administration and Dosage: Use Aquaphor alone or in compounding virtually any ointment using aqueous solutions or oil-based substances. When used alone, apply Aquaphor liberally to affected area.

Precautions: For external use only. Avoid contact with eyes. Not to be applied over third-degree burns, deep or puncture wounds, infections or lacerations. If condition worsens or does not improve within 7 days, patient should consult a doctor.

How Supplied:
1.75 oz. tube—List No. 45583
3.25 oz. jar—List No. 45584
16 oz. jar—List No. 45585
5 lb. jar—List No. 45586

Shown in Product Identification Section, page 404

BASIS® Facial Cleanser
Normal to Dry Skin

Composition: Contains Triple Purified Water, Glycerin, Lauroamphocarboxyglycinate, Oleic Acid, Coconut Acid, Triethanolamine, Sodium Hydroxide, PEG-7 Glyceryl Cocoate, PEG-4 Rape Seed Amide, Citric Acid, EDTA, Glyceryl Lanolate, Cyclopentadecanolide, BHT.

Actions and Uses: Basis Facial Cleanser is specially formulated to be pure and mild so it pampers your patients' skin while gently cleansing it. It easily removes dirt, impurities, and makeup. Its rich emollients also help maintain the natural moisture level of the skin. Since Basis Facial Cleanser is oil-free, it rinses off completely, leaving behind no soapy residue... just radiantly clean, soft skin.

Administration and Dosage: To be used twice daily by patients with normal to dry skin, as a facial cleanser. Basis Facial Cleanser is gentle enough to be used every day for your patients' morning and evening cleansing needs.

How Supplied: 8 oz. pump bottles.
Shown in Product Identification Section, page 404

BASIS® Soap
Combination Skin

Composition: Contains Sodium Tallowate, Sodium Cocoate, Glycerin, Kaolin, Petrolatum, Titanium Dioxide, Sodium Chloride, Sodium Thiosulfate, Triple Purified Water, Pentasodium Pentetate, Tetrasodium Etidronate, Cyclopentadecanolide, Woolwax Alcohol, Beeswax.

Action and Uses: This non-comedogenic Basis formula is designed to cleanse skin that has both oily and dry patches gently, yet effectively. It's strong enough to cleanse oily patches thoroughly, yet mild enough for even the most sensitive, blemish-prone skin.

Administration and Dosage: To be used twice or three times daily by patients with combination skin, as a facial cleanser. Since it is equally effective on dry and oily areas of the skin, it may also be used in the bath or shower as a gentle allover cleanser.

How Supplied: 1-, 3- and 5-oz. bars.
Shown in Product Identification Section, page 404

BASIS® Soap
Extra Dry Skin

Composition: Contains Sodium Tallowate, Sodium Cocoate, Glycerin, Petrolatum, Sweet Almond Oil, Titanium Dioxide, Sodium Chloride, Sodium Thiosulfate, Triple Purified Water, Pentasodium Pentetate, Tetrasodium Etidronate, Cyclopentadecanolide, Woolwax Alcohol, Beeswax.

Action and Uses: A mild, non-comedogenic soap product formulated specifically to cleanse extra dry skin gently and effectively. Contains extra quantities of pure emollient oils that actually help maintain the skin's natural moisture level while protecting against moisture loss. It rinses away completely—leaving no soapy residue. Basis Extra Dry is an ideal soap for those who must wash often, such as doctors or nurses. It is also a very good choice for elderly patients' dry skin.

Administration and Dosage: To be used twice daily by elderly patients or patients with dry skin, as a moisturizing cleanser—for the face or hands—or to be used all over in the bath or shower.

How Supplied: 1-, 3- and 5-oz. bars.
Shown in Product Identification Section, page 404

BASIS® Soap
Normal to Dry Skin

Composition: Contains Sodium Tallowate, Sodium Cocoate, Glycerin, Petrolatum, Titanium Dioxide, Sodium Chloride, Sodium Thiosulfate, Triple Purified Water, Pentasodium Pentetate, Tetrasodium Etidronate, Cyclopentadecanolide, Woolwax Alcohol, Beeswax.

Action and Uses: A mild, non-comedogenic, non-drying cleanser—gentle enough to use on facial skin, yet effective enough to use all over. Basis leaves no potentially irritating detergent residues and is formulated with pure emollients to help maintain the natural moisture level of your patients' skin.

Administration and Dosage: To be used twice or three times daily by patients with normal or slightly dry skin, as a facial cleanser. For additional benefits, Basis may also be used in the bath or shower for allover cleansing and moisturizing.

How Supplied: 1-, 3- and 5 oz. bars.
Shown in Product Identification Section, page 404

BASIS® Soap
Sensitive Skin

Composition: Contains Sodium Tallowate, Sodium Cocoate, Glycerin, Petrolatum, Titanium Dioxide, Sodium Chloride, Sodium Thiosulfate, Triple Purified Water, Pentasodium Pentetate, Tetrasodium Etidronate, Cyclopentadecanolide, Woolwax Alcohol, Bisabolol, Beeswax.

Action and Uses: Specially formulated to clean, smooth and soothe the skin of patients which tends to sting, itch or blotch after using regular soaps or toiletries—contains bisabolol, a gentle anti-inflammatory agent which reduces the risk of irritation. Also ideal for children's skin.

Administration and Dosage: To be used twice daily by patients with sensitive skin, or children, as a facial cleanser. For additional benefits, patients may also use it in the bath or shower for allover cleansing and moisturizing.

How Supplied: 1-, 3- and 5-oz. bars.
Shown in Product Identification Section, page 404

EUCERIN® Cleansing Bar
[*ū 'sir-in*]
Dry Skin Care

Contains: Disodium Lauryl Sulfosuccinate (and) Sodium Cocoyl Isethionate (and) Cetearyl Alcohol (and) Corn Starch (and) Glyceryl Stearate (and) Paraffin (and) Titanium Dioxide, Water, Disodium Lauryl Sulfosuccinate, Octyldodecanol, Cyclopentadecanolide, Lanolin Alcohol, Bisabolol.

Actions and Uses: Eucerin® Cleansing Bar has been specially formulated for use on sensitive skin, even atopic dermatitis and psoriasis. This formulation contains Eucerite®, a special blend of ingredients that closely resemble the natural oils of the skin, thus providing excellent moisturizing properties. This formulation is fragrance-free and noncomedogenic. Additionally, the pH value of Eucerin Cleansing Bar is neutral so as not to affect the skin's normal acid mantle.

Directions: Use during shower, bath, or regular cleansing, or as directed by physician.

How Supplied:
3 ounce bar
List number 3852
Shown in Product Identification Section, page 404

EUCERIN® Cleansing Lotion
Dry Skin Care

Composition: Water, Sodium Laureth Sulfate, Cocoamphocarboxyglcinate, Cocamidopropyl Betaine, Sodium Laureth Sulfate (and) Glycol Distearate, (and) Cocamide MEA, PEG-7 Glyceryl Cocoate, PEG-5 Lanolate, Citric Acid, PEG-120 Methyl Glucose Dioleate, Lanolin Alcohol, Imidazolidinyl Urea.

Active Ingredient: Eucerite®

Actions and Uses: Eucerin Cleansing Lotion is formulated for the care of dry, sensitive or irritated skin. Its soap-free formula combines gentle cleansing with unique moisturizing ingredients to both clean skin and protect it against dryness. It contains no fragrances, is non-comedogenic, and leaves no soapy residue. It is ideal for atopic dermatitis and psoriasis.

Administration and Dosage: Wash with water; rinse thoroughly.

Precautions: For external use only.

How Supplied: 8 Fluid oz.—List No. 3962
1 Fluid oz.—List No. 3960
Shown in Product Identification Section, page 404

EUCERIN® Creme
[*ū 'sir-in*]
Dry Skin Care
NDC Numbers-10356-090-01
10356-090-05
10356-090-04

Composition: Water, petrolatum, mineral oil, mineral wax, wool wax alcohol, methylchloroisothiazolinone-methylisothiazolinone.

Actions and Uses: A gentle, noncomedogenic, fragrance-free water-in-oil emulsion. Eucerin can be used as treatment for dry skin associated with eczema, psoriasis, chapped or chafed skin, sunburn, windburn, and itching associated with dryness.

Administration and Dosages: Apply freely to affected areas of the skin as of-

Continued on next page

Beiersdorf—Cont.

ten as necessary or as directed by physician.

Precautions: For external use only.

How Supplied:
16 oz. jar—List Number 0090
8 oz. jar—List Number 3774
4 oz. jar—List Number 3797
2 oz. tube—List Number 3868
Shown in Product Identification Section, page 404

EUCERIN® Lotion
[*ū 'sir-in*]
Dry Skin Care
NDC Numbers-10356-793-01
10356-793-04
10356-793-06

Composition: Water, Mineral Oil, Isopropyl Myristate, PEG-40 Sorbitan Peroleate, Lanolin Acid Glycerin Ester, Sorbitol, Propylene Glycol, Cetyl Palmitate, Magnesium Sulfate, Aluminum Stearate, Lanolin Alcohol, BHT, Methylchloroisothiazolinone-Methylisothiazolinone.

Actions and Uses: Eucerin Lotion is a non-comedogenic, fragrance-free, unique water-in-oil formulation that will help to alleviate and soothe excessively dry skin, and provide long-lasting moisturization.

Administration and Dosage: Use daily as preventative care for skin exposed to sun, water, wind, cold or other drying elements.

Precautions: For external use only.

How Supplied:
4 fluid oz. plastic bottle—List Number 3771
8 fluid oz. plastic bottle—List Number 3793
16 fluid oz. plastic bottle—List number 3794
Shown in Product Identification Section, page 404

NIVEA® BATH SILK
Moisturizing Bath Oil

Composition: Soybean Oil, Mineral Oil, Isohexadecane, Octyldodecanol, Fragrance, Cocamide DEA, Castor Oil, Woolwax Alcohol, Aloe Extract, Benzophenone-3, Water, BHT, Propyl Gallate, D&C Green No. 6, D&C Violet No. 2.

Action and Uses: Whereas other bath oils contain only one emollient—mineral oil—Nivea Bath Silk contains *four different types* of emollient oils, thereby replacing four of the major classes of lipids found in human sebum. With repeated application, Nivea Bath Silk has been shown to increase the skin's moisture level over 24 hours. It can be recommended as a convenient whole-body moisturizer in patients with xerosis, before or after radiation therapy, or in infants with skin disorders related to dryness (i.e., cradle cap, etc.).

Administration and Dosage: To be added to the bath according to package instructions, as often as desired, to moisturize skin dried by the effects of bathing. May also be applied directly to the skin when showering. Especially effective when followed by an application of the appropriate Nivea Moisturizer.

How Supplied: 8-oz. bottle.
Shown in Product Identification Section, page 404

NIVEA® BATH SILK
Moisturizing Foam Bath & Shower Gel Extra-Dry Skin

Composition: Soy Protein, Mineral Oil, Isohexadecane, Octyldodecanol, Fragrance, Cocamide DEA, Castor Oil, Woolwax Alcohol, Aloe Extract, Benzophenone-3, Water, BHT, Propyl Gallate, D&C Green No. 6, D&C Violet No. 2.

Action and Uses: Designed to clean gently while helping to retain the skin's natural moisturization level during bathing or showering for extra-dry skin.

Administration and Dosage: To be added to the bath according to package instructions, as often as desired, to help moisturize extra-dry skin. In the shower, Nivea Bath Silk Gel should be applied directly to the skin as a cleanser, then rinsed. Moisturizing is especially effective when followed with an application of the appropriate Nivea moisturizer.

How Supplied: 8-oz. bottle.
Shown in Product Identification Section, page 404

NIVEA® BATH SILK
Moisturizing Foam Bath & Shower Gel Normal-to-Dry Skin

Composition: Sodium Laureth Sulfate, Water, Disodum Laurethsulfosuccinate, Cocamide DEA, Cocamidopropyl Betaine, PEG-7 Glyceryl Cocoate, Glycol Distearate, Cocamide MEA, Fragrance, Soy Protein, Aloe Extract, Imidazolidinyl Urea, Woolwax Alcohol.

Action and Uses: Designed to clean gently while helping retain the skin's natural moisturization level during bathing or showering for normal or slightly dry skin.

Administration and Dosage: To be added to the bath according to package instructions, as often as desired, to help keep the natural moisture level of normal or slightly dry skin. In the shower, Nivea Bath Silk Gel should be applied as a cleanser directly to the skin and then rinsed off. Moisturizing is especially effective when followed with an application of the appropriate Nivea moisturizer.

How Supplied: 8-oz. bottle.
Shown in Product Identification Section, page 404

NIVEA® Moisturizing Creme

Composition: Water, Mineral Oil, Petrolatum, Glycerin, Isohexadecane, Ozokerite, (and) Microcrystalline Wax, Lanolin Alcohol, Paraffin, Panthenol, Magnesium Sulfate, Decyl Oleate, Octyldodecanol, Aluminum Stearate, Sodium Benzoate, Fragrance, Citric Acid, Magnesium Stearate.

Action and Uses: For deep conditioning of dry skin—especially useful on hard to moisturize places such as knees, feet, elbows and hands. Regular use of Nivea Creme has been shown to significantly improve the barrier function of the skin, as shown by reduced stinging reactions to lactic acid; markedly reduced transepidermal water loss; and a significant lowering of the amount of water-extractable amino acids from the skin during washing. Furthermore, Nivea Creme has been demonstrated to increase significantly the moisture level of the skin. Non-comedogenic, so it is ideal for facial use. Especially effective as a winter moisturizer, for moderate dry skin conditions and for aging skin.

Administration and Dosage: To be used twice a day, or as often as needed, on dry skin on the hands, body or face. Particularly effective when used after bathing.

How Supplied: 4- and 6-oz. jars, and 2-oz. tube.
Shown in Product Identification Section, page 404

NIVEA® Extra Enriched Lotion

Composition: Water, Mineral Oil, Isohexadecane, PEG-40 Sorbitan Peroleate, Glycerin, Polyglyceryl-3 Diisostearate, Petrolatum, Isopropyl Palmitate, Cetyl Palmitate, Glyceryl Lanolate, Magnesium Sulfate, Fragrance, Aluminum Stearate, Lanolin Alcohol, Methyldibromoglutaronitrile, Phenoxyethanol.

Action and Uses: For effective and long-lasting moisturizing of very dry skin on the hands and body. Because it is rapidly absorbed and non-comedogenic, Nivea Extra Enriched Lotion is also a good choice for facial use. Efficacy is due to the unique water-in-oil emulsion rather than to any active ingredients which could cause sensitization or unwanted reactions. Moisturization effects last at least 12 hours per application with continued use—longer than with standard oil-in-water formulations. Especially effective as a winter moisturizer, for moderate dry skin conditions and for aging skin.

Administration and Dosage: To be used twice a day, or as often as needed, on the hands, body or face. Particularly effective when used after bathing.

How Supplied: 4-, 8- and 12-oz. bottles.
Shown in Product Identification Section, page 404

NIVEA® Original Formula Lotion

Composition: Water, Mineral Oil, Isopropyl Palmitate, Ceteareth-20, PEG-5 Glyceryl Stearate, Cetearyl Alcohol, Phenoxyethanol, Carbomer, Triethanolamine, Simethicone, Methylparaben, Lanolin Alcohol, Fragrance, Propylparaben.

Action and Uses: Formulated to maintain the moisture content of healthy or slightly dry skin on the hands and body. Suitable for facial use, since it is non-comedogenic. Excellent as a summer moisturizer, when a lighter lotion may be preferred.

Administration and Dosage: To be used twice a day, or as needed to maintain the moisture content of healthy normal skin—or to moisturize slightly dry skin—on the hands, body or face. Particularly effective when used after bathing.

How Supplied: 4-, 8- and 12-oz. bottles.
Shown in Product Identification Section, page 404

NIVEA® Moisturizing Oil

Composition: Water, Mineral Oil, Isopropyl Myristate, PEG-40 Sorbitan Peroleate, Glyceryl Lanolate, Sorbitol, Propylene Glycol, Cetyl Palmitate, Magnesium Sulfate, Aluminum Stearate, Fragrance, Lanolin Alcohol, BHT, Methylchloroisothiazolinone, Methylisothiazolinone.

Action and Uses: Developed as an ultra-effective water-in-oil moisturizing emulsion to replace moisture in severely dry skin. Also useful as a cosmetic for patients who desire a glossy look after moisturizing. An ideal preparation to use for massage, especially for bedridden patients.

Administration and Dosage: For maximum efficacy, Nivea Moisturizing Oil should be applied after the shower or bath to areas of dry skin, while the skin is still damp. Also recommended as an effective overnight treatment. May be used twice daily as an allover moisturizer, or applied as desired to add a cosmetic gloss to the skin.

How Supplied: 4-, 8- and 12-oz. bottles.
Shown in Product Identification Section, page 404

NIVEA® Skin Oil

Composition: Mineral Oil, Water, Lanolin, Petrolatum, Glyceryl Lanolate, Lanolin Alcohol, Fragrance, Sodium Borate, Methylchloroisothiazolinone, Methylisothiazolinone.

Action and Uses: A highly effective moisturizer to soothe and soften even severely dry, chapped, or chafed skin. Its unique formula combines rich creams and emollient oils which form a protective barrier against moisture loss. An excellent recommendation for patients who suffer from dry skin conditions since it effectively seals in moisture.

Administration and Dosage: Nivea® Skin Oil should be applied as often as needed, whenever dry skin is a problem. Recommended after bathing and for year-round use before and after exposure to the sun, wind, or any harsh, drying conditions.

How Supplied: 8-oz. bottles.
Shown in Product Identification Section, page 404

NIVEA® After Tan Moisturizing Lotion

Composition: Water, SD Alcohol 40B, Mineral Oil, Cetearyl Alcohol, PEG-40 Castor Oil, Sodium Cetearyl Sulfate, Isopropyl Palmitate, Cetearyl Octanoate, Glyceryl Stearate, Phenoxyethanol, Methylparaben, Ethylparaben, Propylparaben, Butylparaben, Aloe Extract, Cetearyl Alcohol, Fragrance, Lanolin Alcohol, Imidazolidinyl Urea, Isopropyl Myristate, Triethanolamine, Chamomile Extract, Carbomer, Simethicone, BHT, Citric Acid.

Action and Uses: Aloe and chamomile have a cooling effect on sunburned or parched skin. Moisturizes and soothes skin that has been over-exposed to the sun. Nivea® After Tan Lotion is particularly effective when used after bathing or showering.

Administration and Dosage: Recommended for use after coming in from the sun on sun-exposed or sunburned skin. May be used as often as desired. May be used on the face.

How Supplied: 4-oz. bottle.
Shown in Product Identification Section, page 404

NIVEA® Sun SPF 15

Composition: Active Ingredients: Octyl Methoxycinnamate, Octyl Salicylate, Benzophenone-3, 2-Phenylbenzimidazole-5-Sulfonic Acid.

Action and Uses: Nivea Sun adds effective sunblocking agents to a rich, moisturizing Nivea base. It provides UVA/UVB protection with an SPF of 15, and is waterproof and paba-free. Nivea Sun contains emollients and moisturizers, and is non-comedogenic and lightly scented. Liberal and regular use of this product is an excellent recommendation to help reduce premature aging and wrinkling of the skin, and skin cancer, due to long-term overexposure to the sun.

Administration and Dosage: To be applied liberally before and during exposure to the sun. Should be reapplied after swimming. May also be recommended for year-round use on all sun-exposed areas of the skin.

How Supplied: 4-oz. bottles.
Shown in Product Identification Section, page 404

NIVEA® Visage Facial Nourishing Creme

Composition: Active Ingredients: Octyl Methoxycinnamate, Benzophenone-3 (SPF 5).
Other Ingredients: Water, Trilaurin, Glycerin, Isopropyl Palmitate, Sorbitan Stearate, Cetyl Alcohol, Myristyl Myristate, Cetearyl Octanoate, PEG-20 Stearate, Tocopheryl Acetate (Vitamin E USP), Fragrance, Aloe Extract, Acrylamide/Sodium Acrylate Copolymer, Lanolin Alcohol, BHT, Methylchloroisothiazolinone, Methylisothiazolinone.

Action and Uses: Nivea Visage Creme was specially developed to replenish moisture lost from dried and aging facial skin. The creme form is particularly appropriate for winter moisturizing or for the more dry and sensitive areas of the face. A good choice for patients who have experienced adult-onset acne from using other, heavier products. Also recommended for younger patients who want a rich facial moisturizer that provides UVA/UVB protection.

Administration and Dosage: To be used on aging or extra-dry skin twice daily after washing, morning and evening, as a nourishing, protective moisturizer.

How Supplied: 2-oz. jars.
Shown in Product Identification Section, page 404

NIVEA® Visage Facial Nourishing Lotion

Composition: Active Ingredients: Octyl Methoxycinnamate, Benzophenone-3 (SPF 5).
Other Ingredients: Water, Mineral Oil, Isopropyl Palmitate, Propylene Glycol, DEA-Dihydroxypalmitylphosphate (and) Isopropyl Hydroxypalmityl Ether, Glyceryl Stearate, Caprylic/Capric Triglycerides, Cetearyl Alcohol, Stearic Acid, Tocopheryl Acetate (Vitamin E USP), Phenoxyethanol (and) Methylparaben (and) Ethylparaben (and) Propylparaben (and) Butylparaben, Fragrance, Aloe Extract, Isopropyl Myristate, Triethanolamine, Carbomer, Lanolin Alcohol, Simethicone, Methylparaben.

Actions and Uses: A light, rapidly absorbed moisturizing lotion for the face. Contains Beiersdorf's unique emollient, Eucerite®, other emollients, aloe and Vitamin E for extra moisturization and protection. Also contains an SPF 5 sunscreen to guard against damage and aging caused by UVA and UVB rays. Contains no other active ingredients which could cause sensitization or unwanted reactions. Non-comedogenic, so it will not cause adult-onset acne. Lightly scented. Nivea Visage Lotion was specially developed to replenish moisture lost from dry or aging facial skin. The lotion form is particularly appropriate for light summer moisturizing or for normal or slightly dry areas of the face. Also recommended for younger patients who need UVA/UVB protection.

Administration and Dosage: To be used on facial skin twice daily, morning and evening after washing, as a nourishing, protective moisturizer.

Continued on next page

Beiersdorf—Cont.

How Supplied: 4-oz. bottles.
Shown in Product Identification Section, page 404

Benson Pharmacal Co.

Div. of American Victor Co., Inc.
431 HEMPSTEAD AVENUE
WEST HEMPSTEAD, NY 11552

ALTOCAPS-400 CAPSULES
Vitamin E

Active Ingredient: Each capsule contains 400 mg vitamin E (*dl*-alpha-tocopheryl acetate) equivalent to 400 IU.

Inactive Ingredients: Excipient—soybean oil. Shell Ingredients—gelatin, glycerin, water.

Indication: As a vitamin E supplement.

Action: A main characteristic of vitamin E is its action as an antioxidant, preserving the wall membrane of body cells against adverse oxidation reactions.

Precaution: Keep out of the reach of children.

Dosage: Adults—one capsule daily or as directed by a physician.

How Supplied: Bottles of 25 soft-gel capsules.

ROYGEL 100 MG CAPSULES
Royal Jelly Plus Vitamin B Complex

Description: Royal jelly "Queen Bee Food" is a natural source rich in vitamin B complex, proteins, amino acids, fatty acids, major and trace elements; hence it has a high nutritional value.

Active Ingredients: Each capsule contains royal jelly 100 mg, vitamin B_1 10 mg, vitamin B_2 5 mg, vitamin B_6 1 mg, vitamin C 50 mg, vitamin B_{12} 3 μg, niacinamide 30 mg, pantothenic acid 2 mg.

Inactive Ingredients: Excipients—refined soybean oil, hydrogenated vegetable oil, lecithin, beeswax. Shell Ingredients—gelatin, glycerin, purified water, titanium dioxide, methylparaben, propylparaben, FD&C Yellow No. 10, FD&C Red No. 40.

Indication: As a dietary supplement.

Precaution: Keep out of the reach of children.

Dosage: Adults—one capsule daily in the morning hours or as directed by a physician.

How Supplied: Bottles of 30 soft-gel capsules.

ROYGEL ULTIMA CAPSULES
Royal Jelly, Ginseng, Wheat Germ Oil

Active Ingredients: Each capsule contains royal jelly 100 mg, Korean ginseng powder 250 mg, wheat germ oil 100 mg.

Inactive Ingredients: Excipients—refined soybean oil, hydrogenated vegetable oil, beeswax, lecithin. Shell Ingredients—gelatin, glycerin, purified water, titanium dioxide, FD&C Red No. 40, methylparaben, propylparaben.

Indication: As a dietary supplement.

Precaution: Keep out of the reach of children.

Dosage: Adults—one capsule daily or as directed by a physician.

How Supplied: Bottles of 30 soft-gel capsules.

Blaine Company, Inc.

2700 DIXIE HIGHWAY
FT. MITCHELL, KY 41017

MAG-OX 400

Description: Each tablet contains Magnesium Oxide 400 mg. U.S.P. (Heavy), or 241.3 mg. Elemental Magnesium (19.86 mEq.)

Indications and Usage: Hypomagnesemia, magnesium deficiencies and/or magnesium depletion resulting from malnutrition, restricted diet, alcoholism or magnesium depleting drugs. An antacid. For increasing urinary magnesium excretion.

Warnings: Do not use this product except under the advice and supervision of a physician if you have a kidney disease. May have laxative effect.

Dosage: Adult dose 1 or 2 tablets daily or as directed by a physician.

Professional Labeling: Mag-Ox 400 Tablets for recurring calcium oxalate urinary calculi.
MAGNESIUM OXIDE U.S.P. is indicated in the reduction of crystalluria and calcium oxalate excretion in patients with recurring calcium oxalate lithiasis and to reduce the incidence of calculus formation in idiopathic, recurrent stone formers.

How Supplied: Bottles of 100 and 1000.

URO-MAG

Description: Each capsule contains Magnesium Oxide 140 mg. U.S.P. (Heavy), or 84.5 mg. Elemental Magnesium (6.93 mEq.)

Indications and Usage: Hypomagnesemia, magnesium deficiencies and/or magnesium depletion resulting from malnutrition, restricted diet, alcoholism or magnesium depleting drugs. An antacid. For increasing urinary magnesium excretion.

Warnings: Do not use this product except under the advice and supervision of a physician if you have a kidney disease. May have laxative effect.

Dosage: Adult dose 3-4 capsules daily or as directed by a physician.

Professional Labeling: URO-MAG Capsules for recurring calcium oxalate urinary calculi.
MAGNESIUM OXIDE U.S.P. is indicated in the reduction of crystalluria and calcium oxalate excretion in patients with recurring calcium oxalate lithiasis and to reduce the incidence of calculus formation in idiopathic, recurrent stone formers.

How Supplied: Bottles of 100 and 1000.

EDUCATIONAL MATERIAL

Samples and literature available to physicians upon request.

Block Drug Company, Inc.

257 CORNELISON AVENUE
JERSEY CITY, NJ 07302

ARTHRITIS STRENGTH BC® POWDER

Active Ingredients: Aspirin 742 mg in combination with 222 mg Salicylamide and 36 mg Caffeine per powder.

Indications: Arthritis Strength BC Powder is specially formulated with more of the pain relieving ingredients to provide fast temporary relief of minor arthritis pain and inflammation, neuralgia, neuritis and sciatica; relief of muscular aches, discomfort and fever of colds; and pain of tooth extraction.

Warning: Children and teenagers should not use this medicine for chicken pox or flu symptoms before a doctor is consulted about Reye Syndrome, a rare but serious illness reported to be associated with aspirin. Do not exceed recommended dosage or administer to children, including teenagers, with chicken pox or flu, unless directed by a physician. Do not take this product if you are allergic to aspirin, have asthma, gastric ulcer, or are taking a medication that affects the clotting of blood, except under the advice and supervision of a physician. If pain persists for more than 10 days or redness is present, discontinue use of this product and consult a physician immediately. Keep this and all medication out of children's reach. As with any drug, if you are pregnant or nursing a baby, consult your physician before using this product. IT IS ESPECIALLY IMPORTANT NOT TO USE ASPIRIN DURING THE LAST 3 MONTHS OF PREGNANCY UNLESS SPECIFICALLY DIRECTED TO DO SO BY A DOCTOR BECAUSE IT MAY CAUSE PROBLEMS IN THE UNBORN CHILD OR COMPLICATIONS DURING DELIVERY. Discontinue use if ringing in the ears occurs.
In case of accidental overdosage, contact a physician or poison control center immediately.

Dosage and Administration: Place one powder on tongue and follow with liquid. If you prefer, stir powder into glass of water or other liquid. May be used every three to four hours, up to 4 powders each 24 hours. For children under 12, consult a physician.

How Supplied: Available in tamper resistant cellophane wrapped envelopes of 6 powders, and tamper resistant cellophane wrapped boxes of 24 and 50 powders.

BC COLD POWDER
BC Cold Powder Multi-Symptom Formula
BC Cold Powder Multi-Symptom Non-Drowsy Formula

Active Ingredients: *Multi-Symptom Formula*—Aspirin 650 mg, Phenylpropanolamine Hydrochloride 25 mg, and Chlorpheniramine Maleate 4 mg per powder. *Non-Drowsy Formula*—Aspirin 650 mg and Phenylpropanolamine Hydrochloride 25 mg per powder.

Indications: *BC Cold Powder Multi-Symptom Formula* is for relief of cold symptoms such as body aches, fever, nasal congestion, sneezing, running nose, and watery itchy eyes. *BC Cold Powder Multi-Symptom Non-Drowsy Formula* is for relief of such symptoms as body aches, fever, and nasal congestions.

Warnings: CHILDREN AND TEENAGERS SHOULD NOT USE THIS MEDICINE FOR CHICKEN POX OR FLU SYMPTOMS BEFORE A DOCTOR IS CONSULTED ABOUT REYE SYNDROME, A RARE BUT SERIOUS ILLNESS REPORTED TO BE ASSOCIATED WITH ASPIRIN. KEEP THIS AND ALL MEDICINES OUT OF CHILDREN'S REACH. IN CASE OF ACCIDENTAL OVERDOSE, CONTACT A PHYSICIAN IMMEDIATELY. As with any drug, if you are pregnant or nursing a baby, seek the advice of a health professional before using this product. IT IS ESPECIALLY IMPORTANT NOT TO USE ASPIRIN DURING THE LAST 3 MONTHS OF PREGNANCY UNLESS SPECIFICALLY DIRECTED TO DO SO BY A DOCTOR BECAUSE IT MAY CAUSE PROBLEMS IN THE UNBORN CHILD OR COMPLICATIONS DURING DELIVERY. Do not exceed recommended dosage. If symptoms do not improve within 7 days, or are accompanied by high fever, consult a physician before continuing use. Do not take this product if you have high blood pressure, heart disease, diabetes, or thyroid disease except under the advice and supervision of a physician. Do not take this product if you are presently taking a prescription antihypertensive or antidepressant drug containing a monoamine oxidase inhibitor except under the advice and supervision of a physician. This product contains aspirin and should not be taken by individuals who are sensitive to aspirin. BC Cold Powder Multi-Symptom with antihistamine may cause drowsiness. Avoid alcoholic beverages while taking this product. Use caution when driving a motor vehicle or operating machinery.

Dosage and Administration: *Adults*—one powder into a glass of water or other liquid, or place powder on tongue and follow with liquid. May be used every 4 hours up to 4 times a day. *For children under 12*—consult a physician.

How Supplied: Available in tamper-resistant cellophane-wrapped envelopes of 6 powders, as well as tamper-resistant boxes of 24 powders.

BC® POWDER
[*bee-see*]

Active Ingredients: Aspirin 650 mg per powder, Salicylamide 195 mg per powder and Caffeine 32 mg per powder.

Indications: BC Powder is for relief of simple headache; for temporary relief of minor arthritic pain, neuralgia, neuritis and sciatica; for relief of muscular aches, discomfort and fever of colds; and for relief of normal menstrual pain and pain of tooth extraction.

Warning: Children and teenagers should not use this medicine for chicken pox or flu symptoms before a doctor is consulted about Reye Syndrome, a rare but serious illness reported to be associated with aspirin. Do not exceed recommended dosage or administer to children, including teenagers, with chicken pox or flu, unless directed by a physician. Do not take this product if you are allergic to aspirin, have asthma, gastric ulcer, or are taking a medication that affects the clotting of blood, except under the advice and supervision of a physician. If pain persists for more than 10 days or redness is present, discontinue use of this product and consult a physician immediately. Keep this and all medication out of children's reach. As with any drug, if you are pregnant or nursing a baby, consult your physician before using this product. IT IS ESPECIALLY IMPORTANT NOT TO USE ASPIRIN DURING THE LAST 3 MONTHS OF PREGNANCY UNLESS SPECIFICALLY DIRECTED TO DO SO BY A DOCTOR BECAUSE IT MAY CAUSE PROBLEMS IN THE UNBORN CHILD OR COMPLICATIONS DURING DELIVERY. Discontinue use if ringing in the ears occurs.
In case of accidental overdosage, contact a physician or poison control center immediately.

Dosage and Administration: Stir one powder into a glass of water or other liquid, or, place powder on tongue and follow with liquid. May be used every 3 or 4 hours up to 4 times a day. For children under 12 consult a physician.

How Supplied: Available in tamper resistant cellophane wrapped envelopes of 2 or 6 powders, as well as tamper resistant boxes of 24 and 50 powders.

NYTOL® TABLETS

Active Ingredient: Diphenhydramine Hydrochloride, 25 mg per tablet (NYTOL with DPH) and 50 mg per tablet (Maximum Strength NYTOL).

Indications: Diphenhydramine Hydrochloride is an antihistamine with anticholinergic and sedative effects which induces drowsiness and helps in falling asleep.

Warnings: Do not give children under 12 years of age. If sleeplessness persists continuously for more than 2 weeks, consult your physician. Insomnia may be a symptom of serious underlying medical illness. If pregnant or nursing, consult your physician before taking this or any medicine. Do not take this product if you have asthma, glaucoma, emphysema, chronic pulmonary disorders, shortness of breath, difficulty in breathing or difficulty in urination due to enlargement of the prostate gland unless directed by a physician. Do not take this product if you are taking tranquilizers or sedatives, without first consulting a physician. Avoid alcoholic beverages while taking this product. Keep this and all drugs out of the reach of children. In case of accidental overdose, contact a physician immediately.

Drug Interaction: Alcohol and other drugs which cause CNS depression will heighten the depressant effect of this product. Monoamine oxidase (MAO) inhibitors will prolong and intensify the anticholinergic effects of antihistamines.

Symptoms and Treatment of Oral Overdosage: In adults overdose may cause CNS depression resulting in hypnosis and coma. In children CNS hyperexcitability may follow sedation; the stimulant phase may bring tremor, delirium and convulsions. Gastrointestinal reactions may include dry mouth, appetite loss, nausea and vomiting. Respiratory distress and cardiovascular complications (hypotension) may be evident. Treatment includes inducing emesis, and controlling symptoms.

Dosage and Administration: Take 2 NYTOL with DPH or 1 Maximum Strength NYTOL tablet 20 minutes before bed or as directed by a physician.

How Supplied: Available in tamper resistant packages of 16, 32, and 72 tablets NYTOL with DPH; of 8 and 16 tablets Maximum Strength NYTOL.

PROMISE® SENSITIVE TEETH TOOTHPASTE
Desensitizing Dentifrice

Active Ingredients: 5% Potassium Nitrate in a pleasantly mint-flavored dentifrice.

Promise contains Potassium Nitrate for relief of dentinal hypersensitivity resulting from the exposure of tooth dentin due to periodontal surgery, cervical (gumline) erosion, abrasion or recession which causes pain on contact with hot, cold, or tactile stimuli. The Council on Dental Therapeutics of the ADA has given Promise the ADA Seal of Acceptance as

Continued on next page

Block—Cont.

an effective desensitizing dentifrice for otherwise normal teeth sensitive to hot, cold, or pressure (tactile).

Actions: Promise significantly reduces tooth hypersensitivity, with response to therapy evident after two weeks of use. Controlled double-blind clinical studies provide substantial evidence of the safety and effectiveness of Promise. The current theory on mechanism of action is that the potassium nitrate in Promise has an effect on neural transmission, interrupting the signal which would result in the sensation of pain.

Warning: When you start with Promise, it is important to remember that you have to brush for at least two weeks before relief begins to occur. Greater improvement should occur as regular use continues. If you see no improvement after a month of regular use, consult your dentist.

Dosage and Administration: Use twice a day in place of regular toothpaste or as directed by a dental professional.

How Supplied: Promise Toothpaste is supplied in 1.6 oz. and 3.0 oz. tubes.

ORIGINAL SENSODYNE® TOOTHPASTE
Desensitizing Dentifrice

Description: Each tube contains strontium chloride hexahydrate (10%) in a pleasantly flavored cleansing/polishing dentifrice.

Actions/Indications: Tooth hypersensitivity is a condition in which individuals experience pain from exposure to hot, cold stimuli, from chewing fibrous foods, or from tactile stimuli (e.g. toothbrushing.) Hypersensitivity usually occurs when the protective enamel covering on teeth wears away (which happens most often at the gum line) or if gum tissue recedes and exposes the dentin underneath.
Running through the dentin are microscopic small "tubules" which, according to many authorities, carry the pain impulses to the nerve of the tooth.
Sensodyne provides a unique ingredient—strontium chloride which is believed to be deposited in the tubules where it blocks the pain. The longer Sensodyne is used, the more of a barrier it helps build against pain.
The effect of Sensodyne may not be manifested immediately and may require a few weeks or longer of use for relief to be obtained. A number of clinical studies in the U.S. and other countries have provided substantial evidence of Sensodyne's performance attributes. Complete relief of hypersensitivity has been reported in approximately 65% of users and measurable relief or reduction in hypersensitivity in approximately 90%.
Sensodyne has been commercially available for over 25 years. The ADA Council on Dental Therapeutics has given Sensodyne the Seal of Acceptance as an effective desensitizing dentifrice in otherwise normal teeth sensitive to hot, cold, or pressure (tactile).

Contraindications: Subjects with severe dental erosion should brush properly and lightly with any dentifrice to avoid further removal of tooth structure.

Dosage: Use regularly in place of ordinary toothpaste or as recommended by dental professional.
NOTE: Individuals should be instructed to use SENSODYNE frequently since relief from pain tends to be cumulative. If relief does not occur after 3 months, a dentist should be consulted.

How Supplied: SENSODYNE Toothpaste is supplied in 2.1 oz. and 4.0 oz. tubes and in 4.0 oz. pumps.
(U.S. Patent No. 3,122,483)

MINT SENSODYNE® MINT GEL SENSODYNE® TOOTHPASTES
Desensitizing Dentifrice

Active Ingredients: 5% Potassium Nitrate in a pleasantly mint-flavored dentifrice.
Mint Sensodyne and Mint Gel Sensodyne contain Potassium Nitrate for relief of dentinal hypersensitivity resulting from the exposure of tooth dentin due to periodontal surgery, cervical (gum line) erosion, abrasion or recession which causes pain on contact with hot, cold, or tactile stimuli. Mint Sensodyne has been given the Seal of Acceptance by the ADA Council on Dental Therapeutics as an effective desensitizing dentifrice for otherwise normal teeth sensitive to hot, cold, or pressure (tactile).

Actions: Mint Sensodyne and Mint Gel Sensodyne significantly reduce tooth hypersensitivity, with response to therapy evident after two weeks of use. Controlled double-blind clinical studies provide substantial evidence of the safety and effectiveness of Mint Sensodyne and Mint Gel Sensodyne. The current theory on mechanism of action is that the potassium nitrate has an effect on neural transmission, interrupting the signal which would result in the sensation of pain.

Warning: When used as directed, it is important to remember that you have to brush for at least two weeks before relief begins to occur. If no improvement is seen after one month of use, consult your dentist.

Dosage and Administration: Use twice a day in place of regular toothpaste or as directed by a dental professional.

How Supplied: Mint Sensodyne and Mint Gel Sensodyne Toothpastes are supplied in 2.1 and 4.0 oz. tubes and in 4 oz. pumps.
(U.S. Patent No. 3,863,006)

TEGRIN® MEDICATED SHAMPOO
[tĕg 'rĭn]

Highly effective shampoo for moderate-to-severe dandruff and the relief of flaking, itching, and scaling associated with eczema, seborrhea, and psoriasis. Two commercial product versions are available: a lotion shampoo, in three formulas; herbal, original, and extra conditioning, and a gel concentrate, available in herbal scent.

Description: Each tube of gel shampoo or bottle of lotion shampoo contains 5% coal tar solution in a pleasantly scented, high-foaming, cleansing shampoo base with emollients, conditioners and other formula components.

Actions/Indications: Coal Tar is obtained in the destructive distillation of bituminous coal and is a highly effective agent for the local therapy of a number of dermatological disorders. The action of coal tar is believed to be keratolytic, antiseptic, antipruritic and astringent. The coal tar solution used in the Tegrin products is prepared in such a way as to reduce the pitch and other irritant components found in crude coal tar without reduction in therapeutic potency.
Coal tar solution has been used clinically for many years as a remedy for dandruff and for scaling associated with scalp disorders such as eczema, seborrhea, and psoriasis. Its mechanism of action has not been fully established, but it is believed to retard the rate of turnover of epidermal cells with regular use. A number of clinical studies have demonstrated the performance attributes of Tegrin Shampoo against dandruff and seborrheic dermatitis. In addition to relieving the above symptoms, Tegrin shampoo, used regularly, maintains scalp and hair cleanliness and leaves the hair lustrous and manageable.

Contraindications: For External Use Only—Should irritation develop, discontinue use. Avoid contact with eyes. Keep out of reach of children.

Dosage: Use regularly as a shampoo. Wet hair thoroughly. Rub Tegrin liberally into hair and scalp. Rinse thoroughly. Briskly massage a second application of the shampoo into a rich lather. Rinse thoroughly.

How Supplied: Tegrin Concentrated Gel Shampoo is supplied in 2.5 oz. collapsible tubes.
Tegrin Lotion Shampoo is supplied in 3.75 and 6.6 oz. plastic bottles.

TEGRIN® for Psoriasis Lotion, Cream and Soap
[tĕg 'rĭn]

Description: Each tube of cream or bottle of lotion contains special coal tar solution (5%) and allantoin (1.7%) in a greaseless, stainless vehicle. Tegrin Medicated Soap contains 2.0% coal tar solution.

Actions/Indications: Coal tar is obtained in the destructive distillation of bituminous coal and is a highly effective agent for the local therapy of a number of dermatological disorders. The action of coal tar is believed to be keratolytic, antiseptic, antipruritic and astringent. The coal tar solution used in the Tegrin products is prepared in such a way as to reduce the pitch and other irritant components found in crude coal tar. Allantoin (5-Ureidohydantoin) is a debriding and dispersing agent for psoriatic scales and is believed to accelerate proliferation of normal skin cells. The combination of coal tar and allantoin used in Tegrin has been demonstrated in a number of controlled clinical studies to have a high level of efficacy in controlling the itching and scaling of psoriasis.

Contraindications: Discontinue medication should irritation or allergic reactions occur. Avoid contact with eyes and mucous membranes. Keep out of reach of children.

Dosage and Administration: Apply lotion or cream 2 to 4 times daily as needed, massaging thoroughly into affected areas. Lather with Tegrin Soap in a hot bath before application to help soften heavy scales. Once condition is under control, maintenance therapy should be individually adjusted. Occlusive dressings are not required.

How Supplied: Tegrin Lotion 6 fl. oz., Tegrin Cream 2 oz. and 4.4 oz. tubes, Tegrin Soap 4.5 oz. bars.

Boehringer Ingelheim Pharmaceuticals, Inc.

90 EAST RIDGE
POST OFFICE BOX 368
RIDGEFIELD, CT 06877

DULCOLAX®

[*dul 'co-lax*]
brand of bisacodyl USP
Tablets of 5 mg.................BI-CODE 12
Suppositories of 10 mg..BI-CODE 52
Laxative

Description: Dulcolax is a contact laxative acting directly on the colonic mucosa to produce normal peristalsis throughout the large intestine. Its unique mode of action permits either oral or rectal administration, according to the requirements of the patient. Because of its gentleness and reliability of action, Dulcolax may be used whenever constipation is a problem. In preparation for surgery, proctoscopy, or radiologic examination, Dulcolax provides satisfactory cleansing of the bowel, obviating the need for an enema.
The active ingredient in Dulcolax, bisacodyl, is a colorless, tasteless compound that is practically insoluble in water and alkaline solution. It is designated chemically bis(p-acetoxyphenyl)-2-pyridylmethane.
Each tablet contains bisacodyl USP 5 mg. Also contains acacia, acetylated monoglyceride, carnauba wax, cellulose acetate phthalate, corn starch, D&C Red No. 30 aluminum lake, D&C Yellow No. 10 aluminum lake, dibutyl phthalate, docusate sodium, gelatin, glycerin, iron oxides, kaolin, lactose, magnesium stearate, methylparaben, pharmaceutical glaze, polyethylene glycol, povidone, propylparaben, sodium benzoate, sorbitan monooleate, sucrose, talc, titanium dioxide, white wax.
Each suppository contains bisacodyl USP 10 mg. Also contains hydrogenated vegetable oil.
Dulcolax tablets and suppositories contain less than 0.2 mg per dosage unit which is considered sodium free.

Actions: Dulcolax differs markedly from other laxatives in its mode of action: it is virtually nontoxic, and its laxative effect occurs on contact with the colonic mucosa, where it stimulates sensory nerve endings to produce parasympathetic reflexes resulting in increased peristaltic contractions of the colon. Administered orally, Dulcolax is absorbed to a variable degree from the small bowel but such absorption is not related to the mode of action of the compound. Dulcolax administered rectally in the form of suppositories is negligibly absorbed. The contact action of the drug is restricted to the colon, and motility of the small intestine is not appreciably influenced. Local axon reflexes, as well as segmental reflexes, are initiated in the region of contact and contribute to the widespread peristaltic activity producing evacuation. For this reason, Dulcolax may often be employed satisfactorily in patients with ganglionic blockage or spinal cord damage (paraplegia, poliomyelitis, etc.).

Indications: *Acute Constipation:* Taken at bedtime, Dulcolax tablets are almost invariably effective the following morning. When taken before breakfast, they usually produce an effect within six hours. For a prompter response and to replace enemas, the suppositories, which are usually effective in 15 minutes to one hour, can be used.
Chronic Constipation and Bowel Retraining: Dulcolax is extremely effective in the management of chronic constipation, particularly in older patients. By gradually lengthening the interval between doses as colonic tone improves, the drug has been found to be effective in redeveloping proper bowel hygiene. There is no tendency to "rebound".
Preparation for Radiography: Dulcolax tablets are excellent in eliminating fecal and gas shadows from x-rays taken of the abdominal area. For barium enemas, no food should be given following the administration of the tablets, to prevent reaccumulation of material in the cecum, and a suppository should be given one to two hours prior to examination.
Preoperative Preparation: Dulcolax tablets have been shown to be an ideal laxative in emptying the G.I. tract prior to abdominal surgery or to other surgery under general anesthesia. They may be supplemented by suppositories to replace the usual enema preparation. Dulcolax will not replace the colonic irrigations usually given patients before intracolonic surgery, but is useful in the preliminary emptying of the colon prior to these procedures.
Postoperative Care: Suppositories can be used to replace enemas, or tablets given as an oral laxative, to restore normal bowel hygiene after surgery.
Antepartum Care: Either tablets or suppositories can be used for constipation in pregnancy without danger of stimulating the uterus.
Preparation for Delivery: Suppositories can be used to replace enemas in the first stage of labor provided that they are given at least two hours before the onset of the second stage.
Postpartum Care: The same indications apply as in postoperative care, with no contraindication in nursing mothers.
Preparation for Sigmoidoscopy or Proctoscopy: For unscheduled office examinations, adequate preparation is usually obtained with a single suppository. For sigmoidoscopy scheduled in advance, however, administration of tablets the night before in addition will result in adequate preparation almost invariably.
Colostomies: Tablets the night before or a suppository inserted into the colostomy opening in the morning will frequently make irrigations unnecessary, and in other cases will expedite the procedure.

Contraindication: There is no contraindication to the use of Dulcolax, other than an acute surgical abdomen.

Caution for Patients: Do not use laxative products when abdominal pain, nausea or vomiting are present unless directed by a doctor. As with all medicines, keep these tablets/suppositories out of reach of children. Frequent or continued use of this preparation may result in dependence on laxatives.

Adverse Reactions: As with any laxative, abdominal cramps are occasionally noted, particularly in severely constipated individuals.

Dosage:
Tablets
Tablets must be swallowed whole, not chewed or crushed, and should not be taken within one hour of antacids or milk.
Adults: Two or three (usually two) tablets suffice when an ordinary laxative effect is desired. This usually results in one or two soft, formed stools. Tablets when taken before breakfast usually produce an effect within 6 hours, when taken at bedtime usually in 8–12 hours.
Up to six tablets may be safely given in preparation for special procedures when greater assurance of complete evacuation of the colon is desired. In producing such thorough emptying, these higher doses may result in several loose, unformed stools.
Children: One or two tablets, depending on age and severity of constipation, administered as above. Tablets should not be given to a child too young to swallow them whole.
Suppositories
Adults: One suppository at the time a bowel movement is required. Usually effective in 15 minutes to one hour.
Children: Half a suppository is generally effective for infants and children under

Continued on next page

Boehringer Ingelheim—Cont.

two years of age. Above this age, a whole suppository is usually advisable.
Combined
In preparation for surgery, radiography and sigmoidoscopy, a combination of tablets the night before and a suppository in the morning is recommended (see Indications).

How Supplied: Dulcolax, brand of bisacodyl: Yellow, enteric-coated tablets of 5 mg in boxes of 10, 25, 50 and 100; suppositories of 10 mg in boxes of 4, 8, 16 and 50.

Note: Store Dulcolax suppositories and tablets at temperatures below 77°F (25°C). Avoid excessive humidity.

Also Available: Dulcolax® Bowel Prep Kit. Each kit contains:
1 Dulcolax suppository of 10 mg bisacodyl;
4 Dulcolax tablets of 5 mg bisacodyl;
Complete patient instructions.

Clinical Applications: Dulcolax can be used in virtually any patient in whom a laxative or enema is indicated. It has no effect on the blood picture, erythrocyte sedimentation rate, urinary findings, or hepatic or renal function. It may be safely given to infants and the aged, pregnant or nursing women, debilitated patients, and may be prescribed in the presence of such conditions as cardiovascular, renal, or hepatic diseases.

NŌSTRIL® Nasal Decongestant
[nō 'stril]
phenylephrine HCl, USP

Active Ingredient: phenylephrine HCl 0.25% (¼% Mild strength) or phenylephrine HCl 0.5% (½% Regular strength). Also contains benzalkonium chloride 0.004% as a preservative, boric acid, sodium borate, water.

Indications: For temporary relief of nasal congestion due to the common cold, hay fever, other upper respiratory allergies, or associated with sinusitis.

Actions: NŌSTRIL metered pump spray for nasal decongestion delivers measured, uniform doses. The medication constricts the smaller arterioles of the nasal passages, producing a gentle, predictable, decongestant effect. Nōstril penetrates and shrinks swollen membranes, restoring freer breathing and unclogs sinus passages, bringing the effective medication in contact with inflamed, swollen tissues. It will not hurt tender membranes since it is formulated to match the pH of normal nasal secretions. The one-way pump helps prevent draw-back contamination of the medication.

Warnings: Do not exceed recommended dosage because burning, stinging, sneezing, or increased nasal discharge may occur. Do not use for more than 3 days. If symptoms persist, consult a physician. Use of the dispenser by more than one person may spread infection. Do not use this product if you have heart disease, high blood pressure, thyroid disease, diabetes or difficulty in urination due to enlargement of the prostate gland. Keep this and all drugs out of reach of children.

Symptoms and Treatment of Oral Overdosage: In case of accidental ingestion, seek professional assistance or consult a poison control center immediately.

Dosage and Administration:
¼% Mild—Adults and children 6 to under 12 years of age (with adult supervision): 2 or 3 sprays in each nostril not more often than every 4 hours. Children under 6 years of age: consult a doctor.
½% Regular—Adults: 2 or 3 sprays in each nostril not more often than every 4 hours. Do not give to children under 12 years of age unless directed by a doctor.
Remove protective cap. Hold bottle with thumb at base and nozzle between first and second fingers. With head upright, insert nozzle into nostril. Depress pump 2 or 3 times, all the way down, and sniff deeply. Repeat in other nostril. Before using the first time, prime pump by depressing it firmly several times.

How Supplied: Metered nasal pump spray in white plastic bottles of ½ fl. oz. (15 ml) packaged in tamper-resistant outer cartons.
0.25% (¼% Mild strength) for children 6 years and over and adults who prefer a milder decongestant (NDC 0597-0083-85).
0.5% (½% Regular strength) for adults and children 12 years or older (NDC 0597-0084-85).

NŌSTRILLA® Long Acting
[nō-stril 'a]
Nasal Decongestant
oxymetazoline HCl, USP

Active Ingredient: oxymetazoline HCl 0.05%. Also contains benzalkonium chloride 0.02% as a preservative, glycine, sorbitol solution, water. (Mercury preservatives are not used in this product.)

Indications: For up to 12 hour relief of nasal congestion due to the common cold, hay fever, other upper respiratory allergies, or associated with sinusitis.

Actions: NŌSTRILLA metered pump spray for nasal decongestion delivers measured, uniform doses. The medication constricts the smaller arterioles of the nasal passages, producing a prolonged (up to 12 hours), gentle, predictable, decongestant effect. Nōstrilla penetrates and shrinks swollen membranes, restoring freer breathing and unclogs sinus passages, bringing the effective medication in contact with inflamed, swollen tissues. It will not hurt tender membranes since it is formulated to match the pH of normal nasal secretions. Use at bedtime restores freer nasal breathing through the night. The one-way pump helps prevent draw-back contamination of the medication.

Warnings: Do not exceed recommended dosage because burning, stinging, sneezing or increased nasal discharge may occur. Do not use for more than 3 days. If symptoms persist, consult a physician. Use of the dispenser by more than one person may spread infection. Do not use this product if you have heart disease, high blood pressure, thyroid disease, diabetes or difficulty in urination due to enlargement of the prostate gland unless directed by a doctor. Keep this and all drugs out of reach of children.

Symptoms and Treatment of Oral Overdosage: In case of accidental ingestion, seek professional assistance or contact a poison control center immediately.

Dosage and Administration: Adults and children 6 to under 12 years of age (with adult supervision): 2 or 3 sprays in each nostril not more often than every 10 to 12 hours. Do not exceed 2 applications in any 24-hour period. Children under 6 years of age: consult a doctor.
Remove protective cap. Hold bottle with thumb at base and nozzle between first and second fingers. With head upright, insert nozzle into nostril. Depress pump 2 or 3 times, all the way down, and sniff deeply. Repeat in other nostril. Before using the first time, prime pump by depressing it firmly several times.

How Supplied: Metered nasal pump spray in white plastic bottles of ½ fl. oz. (15 ml) packaged in tamper-resistant outer cartons (NDC 0597-0085-85).

EDUCATIONAL MATERIAL

Bowel Evacuation: An Illustrated Teaching Manual
A nurse's guide to bowel care and retraining.

Boiron
1208 AMOSLAND ROAD
NORWOOD, PA 19074

OSCILLOCOCCINUM®
[ah-sill 'o-cox-see 'num ']

Active Ingredient: Anas Barbariae Hepatis et Cordis Extractum HPUS 200CK

Indications: For the relief of flu-like symptoms such as fever, chills, body aches and pains.

Actions: Like most Homeopathic remedies, Oscillococcinum® acts gently by stimulating the patient's natural defense mechanisms.

Warnings: If symptoms persist for more than three days or worsen, consult your physician. Keep all medication out of reach of children. As with any drug if you are pregnant or nursing a baby, seek professional advice before using this product.

Dosage and Administration: (Adults and Children over 2 years)
At the onset of symptoms, place the entire contents of one tube in your mouth and allow to dissolve under your tongue. Repeat every 6 hours as necessary. For maximum results, Oscillococcinum® should be taken early, at the onset of symptoms, and at least 15 minutes before or 1 hour after meals.

How Supplied: boxes of 3 unit-doses of 0.04 oz. (1 Gram) each (NDC 51979-9756-43) Tamper resistant package.
Manufactured by Boiron, France.
Distributor: Boiron

Shown in Product Identification Section, page 404

EDUCATIONAL MATERIAL

Boiron Product Catalogue
General description of the most popular Boiron remedies and lines.
***Oscillococcinum* ® Brochure**
Brochure on Oscillococcinum® describing clinical research on the product and its general use.
"What's Homeopathy?"
Booklet free to physicians and pharmacists.
"An Introduction to Homeopathy for the Practicing Pharmacist"
A free continuing education booklet for pharmacists.

Bristol Laboratories

A Bristol-Myers Squibb Company
2400 W. LLOYD EXPRESSWAY
EVANSVILLE, IN 47721

Naldecon X-line is now being distributed by Apothecon.

NALDECON CX® ADULT LIQUID Ⓒ

[nal 'dĕ-côn CX]
Nasal Decongestant/
Expectorant/Cough Suppressant

Ⓤ

Description: Each teaspoonful (5 mL) of Naldecon CX Adult Liquid contains:
Phenylpropanolamine hydrochloride .... 12.5 mg
Guaifenesin (glyceryl guaiacolate) .... 200 mg
Codeine phosphate .... 10 mg
(Warning: May be Habit-Forming)
This combination product is antihistamine-free, alcohol-free, and sugar-free.

Inactive Ingredients: Citric acid, FD&C Blue No. 1, FD&C Red No. 40, hydrogenated glucose syrup, natural and artificial flavor, polyethylene glycol, saccharin sodium, sodium benzoate, sodium citrate, and purified water.

Indications: For the temporary relief of nasal congestion due to the common cold (cold), hay fever or other respiratory allergies (allergic rhinitis), or associated with sinusitis. Helps loosen phlegm (sputum) and thin bronchial secretions to rid the bronchial passageways of bothersome mucus. Temporarily quiets cough due to minor throat and bronchial irritation as may occur with a cold or inhaled irritants.

Contraindications: Do not take if hypersensitive to guaifenesin, codeine, or sympathomimetic amines.

Warnings: As with any drug, if you are pregnant or nursing a baby, seek the advice of a health professional before using this product. Do not give this product to children under 12 years of age unless directed by a physician. Do not exceed recommended dosage because at higher doses nervousness, dizziness, or sleeplessness may occur. Do not take this product for more than 7 days. If symptoms do not improve or are accompanied by fever, consult a physician. Do not take this product if you have heart disease, high blood pressure, thyroid disease, diabetes, or difficulty in urination due to enlargement of the prostate gland unless directed by a physician.

Drug Interaction Precaution: Do not take this product if you are presently taking a prescription drug for high blood pressure or depression, without first consulting your physician. A persistent cough may be a sign of a serious condition. If cough persists for more than 1 week, tends to recur, or is accompanied by fever, rash, or persistent headache, consult a physician. Do not take this product for persistent or chronic cough such as occurs with smoking, asthma, chronic bronchitis, or emphysema, or if cough is accompanied by excessive phlegm (sputum) unless directed by a physician. Do not take this product if you have a chronic pulmonary disease or shortness of breath unless directed by a physician. May cause or aggravate constipation. Keep this and all drugs out of the reach of children. In case of accidental overdose, seek professional assistance or contact a Poison Control Center immediately.

Directions: Adults and children 12 years of age and over: Oral dosage is 2 teaspoonfuls every 4 hours, not to exceed 6 doses in 24 hours, or as directed by a physician.

How Supplied: NALDECON CX Adult Liquid—4 ounce and pint bottles.
Store at room temperature. Avoid excessive heat.

NALDECON DX® ADULT LIQUID

[nal 'dĕ-côn DX]
Nasal Decongestant/
Expectorant/Cough Suppressant

Ⓤ

Description: Each teaspoonful (5 mL) of Naldecon DX Adult Liquid contains:
Phenylpropanolamine hydrochloride .... 12.5 mg
Guaifenesin (glyceryl guaiacolate) .... 200 mg
Dextromethorphan hydrobromide .... 10 mg
This combination product is antihistamine-free and sugar-free.

Inactive Ingredients: Alcohol (0.06% V/V), citric acid, FD&C Yellow No. 6, natural and artificial flavor, polyethylene glycol, saccharin sodium, sodium benzoate, sodium citrate, sorbitol solution, and purified water.

Indications: For the temporary relief of nasal congestion due to the common cold (cold), hay fever, or other respiratory allergies (allergic rhinitis), or associated with sinusitis. Helps loosen phlegm (sputum) and thin bronchial secretions to rid the bronchial passageways of bothersome mucus. Temporarily quiets cough due to minor throat and bronchial irritation as may occur with a cold or inhaled irritants.

Contraindications: Do not take if hypersensitive to guaifenesin, dextromethorphan, or sympathomimetic amines.

Warnings: As with any drug, if you are pregnant or nursing a baby, seek the advice of a health professional before using this product. Do not give this product to children under 12 years of age unless directed by a physician. Do not exceed recommended dosage because at higher doses nervousness, dizziness or sleeplessness may occur. Do not take this product for more than 7 days. If symptoms do not improve or are accompanied by fever, consult a physician. Do not take this product if you have heart disease, high blood pressure, thyroid disease, diabetes, or difficulty in urination due to enlargement of the prostate gland unless directed by a physician.

Drug Interaction Precaution: Do not take this product if you are presently taking a prescription drug for high blood pressure or depression, without first consulting your physician. A persistent cough may be a sign of a serious condition. If cough persists for more than 1 week, tends to recur, or is accompanied by fever, rash, or persistent headache, consult a physician. Do not take this product for persistent or chronic cough such as occurs with smoking, asthma, chronic bronchitis, or emphysema, or if cough is accompanied by excessive phlegm (sputum) unless directed by a physician. Keep this and all drugs out of the reach of children. In case of accidental overdose, seek professional assistance or contact a poison control center immediately.

Directions: Adults and children 12 years of age and over: Oral dosage is 2 teaspoonfuls every 4 hours, not to exceed 6 doses in 24 hours, or as directed by a physician.

How Supplied: NALDECON DX Adult Liquid—4 ounce and pint bottles.
Store at room temperature. Avoid excessive heat.

Continued on next page

Bristol—Cont.

NALDECON DX®
[*nal 'dĕ-côn DX*]
CHILDREN'S SYRUP
Nasal Decongestant/ Expectorant/Cough Suppressant

Ⓤ

Description: Each teaspoonful (5 mL) of Naldecon DX Children's Syrup contains:
Phenylpropanolamine hydrochloride ....6.25 mg
Guaifenesin (glyceryl guaiacolate) ....100 mg
Dextromethorphan hydrobromide ....5 mg
This combination product is antihistamine-free.

Inactive Ingredients: Alcohol (5% V/V), FD&C Yellow No. 6, fructose, glycerin, natural and artificial flavors, sodium benzoate, sucrose, tartaric acid, and purified water.

Indications: For the temporary relief of nasal congestion due to the common cold (cold), hay fever, or other respiratory allergies (allergic rhinitis), or associated with sinusitis. Helps loosen phlegm (sputum) and thin bronchial secretions to rid the bronchial passageways of bothersome mucus. Temporarily quiets cough due to minor throat and bronchial irritation as may occur with a cold or inhaled irritants.

Contraindications: Do not take if hypersensitive to guaifenesin, dextromethorphan, or sympathomimetic amines.

Warnings: Do not exceed recommended dosage because at higher doses nervousness, dizziness, or sleeplessness may occur. Do not give this product to children for more than 7 days. If symptoms do not improve or are accompanied by fever, consult a physician. Do not give this product to children who have heart disease, high blood pressure, thyroid disease, or diabetes, unless directed by a physician.

Drug Interaction Precaution: Do not give this product to a child who is taking a prescription drug for high blood pressure or depression, without first consulting the child's physician. A persistent cough may be a sign of a serious condition. If cough persists for more than 1 week, tends to recur, or is accompanied by fever, rash, or persistent headache, consult a physician. Do not give this product for persistent or chronic cough such as occurs with smoking, asthma, chronic bronchitis, or emphysema, or if cough is accompanied by excessive phlegm (sputum) unless directed by a physician. Keep this and all drugs out of the reach of children. In case of accidental overdose, seek professional assistance or contact a poison control center immediately.

Directions: Children 6 to under 12 years of age: Oral dosage is 2 teaspoonfuls every 4 hours, not to exceed 6 doses in 24 hours, or as directed by a physician. Children 2 to under 6 years of age: Oral dosage is 1 teaspoonful every 4 hours, not to exceed 6 doses in 24 hours, or as directed by a physician. Children under 2 years of age: consult a physician.

How Supplied: NALDECON DX Children's Syrup—4 ounce and pint bottles. Store at room temprature. Protect from excessive heat and freezing.

NALDECON DX® PEDIATRIC DROPS
[*nal 'dĕ-côn DX*]
Nasal Decongestant/ Expectorant/Cough Suppressant

Ⓤ

Description: Each 1 mL of Naldecon DX Pediatric Drops contains:
Phenylpropanolamine hydrochloride .... 6.25 mg
Guaifenesin (glyceryl guaiacolate) .... 50 mg
Dextromethorphan hydrobromide .... 5 mg
This combination product is antihistamine-free and sugar-free.

Inactive Ingredients: Citric acid, FD&C Yellow No. 6, natural and artificial flavors, polyethylene glycol 1450, propylene glycol, sodium benzoate, saccharin sodium, sorbitol solution, and purified water.

Indications: For the temporary relief of nasal congestion due to the common cold (cold), hay fever or other respiratory allergies (allergic rhinitis), or associated with sinusitis. Helps loosen phlegm (sputum) and thin bronchial secretions to rid the bronchial passageways of bothersome mucus. Temporarily quiets cough due to minor throat and bronchial irritation as may occur with a cold or inhaled irritants.

Contraindications: Do not take if hypersensitive to guaifenesin, dextromethorphan, or sympathomimetic amines.

Warnings: Take by mouth only. Do not exceed recommended dosage because at higher doses nervousness, dizziness, or sleeplessness may occur. Do not give this product to children for more than 7 days. If symptoms do not improve or are accompanied by fever, consult a physician. Do not give this product to children who have heart disease, high blood pressure, thyroid disease, or diabetes, unless directed by a physician.

Drug Interaction Precaution: Do not give this product to a child who is taking a prescription drug for high blood pressure or depression, without first consulting the child's physician. A persistent cough may be a sign of a serious condition. If cough persists for more than 1 week, tends to recur, or is accompanied by fever, rash, or persistent headache, consult a physician. Do not give this product for persistent or chronic cough such as occurs with smoking, asthma, chronic bronchitis, or emphysema, or if cough is accompanied by excessive phlegm (sputum) unless directed by a physician. Keep this and all drugs out of the reach of children. In case of accidental overdose, seek professional assistance or contact a poison control center immediately.

Directions: Children 2 to under 6 years of age: Oral dosage is 1 mL every 4 hours, not to exceed 6 doses in 24 hours, or as directed by a physician. Children under 2 years of age: consult a physician.

Professional Labeling—Children under 2 years of age: Dosage should be adjusted to age or weight and be administered every 4 hours as shown in the dosage table, not to exceed 6 doses in 24 hours.

Age	Weight	Dosage
1–3 months	8–12 lb	¼ mL
4–6 months	13–17 lb	½ mL
7–9 months	18–20 lb	¾ mL
10–24 months	21+ lb	1.0 mL

Bottle label reads as follows: Children under 2 years of age: Use only as directed by a physician.

How Supplied: NALDECON DX Pediatric Drops—30 mL bottle with calibrated dropper.
Store at room temperature. Protect from freezing.

NALDECON EX® CHILDREN'S SYRUP
[*nal 'dĕ-côn EX*]
Nasal Decongestant/Expectorant

Ⓤ

Description: Each teaspoonful (5 mL) of Naldecon EX Children's Syrup contains:
Phenylpropanolamine hydrochloride ....6.25 mg
Guaifenesin (glyceryl guaiacolate) ....100 mg
This combination product is antihistamine-free and sugar-free.

Inactive Ingredients: Alcohol (5% V/V), D&C Yellow No. 10, glycerin, natural and artificial flavors, propylene glycol, saccharin sodium, sodium benzoate, sorbitol solution, tartaric acid, and purified water.

Indications: For the temporary relief of nasal congestion due to the common cold (cold), hay fever, or other respiratory allergies (allergic rhinitis), or associated with sinusitis. Helps loosen phlegm (sputum) and thin bronchial secretions to rid the bronchial passageways of bothersome mucus.

Contraindications: Do not take if hypersensitive to guaifenesin or sympathomimetic amines.

Warnings: Do not exceed recommended dosage because at higher doses nervousness, dizziness, or sleeplessness may occur. Do not give this product to children for more than 7 days. If symptoms do not improve or are accompanied by fever, consult a physician. Do not give this product to children who have heart disease, high blood pressure, thyroid disease, or diabetes, unless directed by a physician.

Drug Interaction Precaution: Do not give this product to a child who is taking a prescription drug for high blood pressure or depression, without first consulting the child's physician. A persistent cough may be a sign of a serious condition. If cough persists for more than 1 week, tends to recur, or is accompanied by fever, rash, or persistent headache, consult a physician. Do not give this product for persistent or chronic cough such as occurs with smoking, asthma, chronic bronchitis, or emphysema, or if cough is accompanied by excessive phlegm (sputum) unless directed by a physician. Keep this and all drugs out of the reach of children. In case of accidental overdose, seek professional assistance or contact a poison control center immediately. Your physician or pharmacist is the best source of information on this medication.

Directions: Children 6 to under 12 years of age: Oral dosage is 2 teaspoonfuls every 4 hours, not to exceed 6 doses in 24 hours, or as directed by a physician. Children 2 to under 6 years of age: Oral dosage is 1 teaspoonful every 4 hours, not to exceed 6 doses in 24 hours, or as directed by a physician. Children under 2 years of age: consult a physician.

How Supplied: NALDECON EX Children's Syrup—4 ounce and pint bottles. Store at room temperature. Protect from excessive heat and freezing.

NALDECON EX® PEDIATRIC DROPS

[*nal 'dĕ-côn EX*]

Nasal Decongestant/Expectorant

Ⓤ

Description: Each 1 mL of Naldecon EX Pediatric Drops contains:

Phenylpropanolamine hydrochloride ....6.25 mg
Guaifenesin (glyceryl guaiacolate) ....50 mg

This combination product is antihistamine-free.

Inactive Ingredients: Citric acid, D&C Yellow No. 10, natural and artificial flavors, polyethylene glycol 1450, propylene glycol, saccharin sodium, sodium benzoate, sorbitol solution, and purified water.

Indications: For the temporary relief of nasal congestion due to the common cold (cold), hay fever or other respiratory allergies (allergic rhinitis), or associated with sinusitis. Helps loosen phlegm (sputum) and thin bronchial secretions to rid the bronchial passageways of bothersome mucus.

Contraindications: Do not take if hypersensitive to guaifenesin or sympathomimetic amines.

Warnings: Take by mouth only. Do not exceed recommended dosage because at higher doses nervousness, dizziness, or sleeplessness may occur. Do not give this product to children for more than 7 days. If symptoms do not improve or are accompanied by fever, consult a physician. Do not give this product to children who have heart disease, high blood pressure, thyroid disease, or diabetes, unless directed by a physician.

Drug Interaction Precaution: Do not give this product to a child who is taking a prescription drug for high blood pressure or depression, without first consulting the child's physician. A persistent cough may be a sign of a serious condition. If cough persists for more than 1 week, tends to recur, or is accompanied by fever, rash, or persistent headache, consult a physician. Do not give this product for persistent or chronic cough such as occurs with smoking, asthma, chronic bronchitis, or emphysema, or if cough is accompanied by excessive phlegm (sputum) unless directed by a physician. Keep this and all drugs out of the reach of children. In case of accidental overdose, seek professional assistance or contact a poison control center immediately. Your physician or pharmacist is the best source of information on this medication.

Directions: Children 2 to under 6 years of age: Oral dosage is 1 mL every 4 hours, not to exceed 6 doses in 24 hours, or as directed by a physician. Children under 2 years of age: consult a physician.

Professional Labeling—Children under 2 years of age: Dosage should be adjusted to age or weight and be administered every 4 hours as shown in the dosage table, not to exceed 6 doses in 24 hours.

Age	Weight	Dosage
1–3 months	8–12 lb	¼ mL
4–6 months	13–17 lb	½ mL
7–9 months	18–20 lb	¾ mL
10–24 months	21+ lb	1.0 mL

Bottle label reads as follows: Children under 2 years of age: Use only as directed by a physician.

How Supplied: NALDECON EX Pediatric Drops—30 mL bottle with calibrated dropper.
Store at room temperature. Protect from excessive heat and freezing.

NALDECON SENIOR DX®

Expectorant/Cough Suppressant
Cough/Cold Liquid
for Adults 50 and Over

Ⓤ

Description: Each teaspoonful (5 mL) of Naldecon Senior DX Cough/Cold Liquid contains:

Guaifenesin ....200 mg
Dextromethorphan hydrobromide ....15 mg

Inactive Ingredients: Citric acid, FD&C Blue No. 1, FD&C Red No. 40, natural and artificial flavor, polyethylene glycol, saccharin sodium, sodium benzoate, sodium citrate, sorbitol solution, and purified water.

Indications: Non-narcotic cough suppressant for the temporary relief of coughing. Helps loosen phlegm (sputum) and bronchial secretions and rid the bronchial passageways of bothersome mucus.

Contraindications: Do not take if hypersensitive to guaifenesin or dextromethorphan.

Warnings: A persistent cough may be a sign of a serious condition. If cough persists for more than 1 week, tends to recur, or is accompanied by fever, rash, or persistent headache, consult a physician. Do not take this product for persistent or chronic cough such as occurs with smoking, asthma, emphysema, or if cough is accompanied by excessive phlegm (mucus) unless directed by a physician. Do not exceed recommended dose or give this product to children under 12 years of age unless directed by a physician. As with any drug, if you are pregnant or nursing a baby, seek the advice of a health professional before using this product. Keep this and all drugs out of the reach of children. In case of accidental overdose, seek professional assistance or contact a Poison Control Center immediately.

Directions: Adults and children 12 years of age and over: Oral dosage is 2 teaspoonfuls every 4 hours, not to exceed 6 doses in 24 hours, or as directed by a physician. Children under 12 years of age: consult a physician.

How Supplied: Naldecon Senior DX Cough/Cold Liquid—4 ounce and pint bottles.
Store at room temperature.

NALDECON SENIOR EX®

(guaifenesin)
Expectorant
Cough/Cold Liquid
for Adults 50 and Over

Ⓤ

Description: Each teaspoonful (5 mL) of Naldecon Senior EX Cough/Cold Liquid contains:

Guaifenesin ....200 mg

Contains no sugar or alcohol.

Inactive Ingredients: Citric acid, FD&C Blue No. 1, FD&C Red No. 40, natural and artificial flavor, polyethylene glycol, saccharin sodium, sodium benzoate, sodium citrate, sorbitol solution, and purified water.

Indications: Helps loosen phlegm (sputum) and bronchial secretions and rid the bronchial passageways of bothersome mucus.

Contraindications: Do not take if hypersensitive to guaifenesin.

Warnings: A persistent cough may be a sign of a serious condition. If cough persists for more than 1 week, tends to recur, or is accompanied by fever, rash, or persistent headache, consult a physician. Do not take this product for persistent or chronic cough such as occurs with smoking, asthma, emphysema, or if cough is accompanied by excessive phlegm (mucus) unless directed by a physician. Do not exceed recommended dose or give

Continued on next page

Bristol—Cont.

this product to children under 12 years of age unless directed by a physician. As with any drug, if you are pregnant or nursing a baby, seek the advice of a health professional before using this product. Keep this and all drugs out of the reach of children. In case of accidental overdose, seek professional assistance or contact a Poison Control Center immediately.

Directions: Adults and children 12 years and over: Oral dosage is 2 teaspoonfuls every 4 hours, not to exceed 6 doses in 24 hours, or as directed by a physician. Children under 12 years of age: consult a physician.

How Supplied: Naldecon Senior EX Cough/Cold Liquid—4 ounce and pint bottles.
Store at room temperature.

Bristol-Myers Products

(A Bristol-Myers Squibb Company)
345 PARK AVENUE
NEW YORK, NY 10154

ALPHA KERI®
Moisture Rich Body Oil

Composition: Contains mineral oil, Hydroloc™ brand of Westwood's PEG-4 dilaurate, lanolin oil, fragrance, benzophenone-3, D&C green 6.

Indications: ALPHA KERI is a water-dispersible oil for the care of dry skin. ALPHA KERI effectively deposits a thin, uniform, emulsified film of oil over the skin. This film lubricates and softens the skin. ALPHA KERI Moisture Rich Body Oil is an all-over skin moisturizer. Only Alpha Keri contains Hydroloc™—the unique emulsifier that provides a more uniform distribution of the therapeutic oils to moisturize dry skin. ALPHA KERI is valuable as an aid for dry skin and mild skin irritations.

Directions for Use: ALPHA KERI *should always be used with water, either added to water or rubbed on to wet skin.* Because of its inherent cleansing properties it is not necessary to use soap when ALPHA KERI is being used.
For external use only.
Label directions should be followed for use in shower, bath and cleansing.

Precaution: The patient should be warned to guard against slipping in tub or shower.

How Supplied: 4 fl. oz., 8 fl. oz., 12 fl. oz., and 16 fl. oz., plastic bottles. Also available in non-aerosol pump spray, 3.5 oz.

Shown in Product Identification Section, page 405

ALPHA KERI®
Moisture Rich Cleansing Bar
Non-detergent Soap

Composition: Sodium tallowate, sodium cocoate, water, mineral oil, fragrance, PEG-75, glycerin, titanium dioxide, lanolin oil, sodium chloride. May contain: BHT, and/or Trisodium HEDTA, D&C Green 5, D&C Yellow 10.

Indications: ALPHA KERI Moisture Rich Cleansing Bar, rich in emollient oils, thoroughly cleanses as it soothes and softens the skin.

Indications: Adjunctive use in dry skin care.

Directions for Use: To be used as any other soap.

How Supplied: 4 oz. bar.

BUFFERIN®
[*bŭf'fĕr-ĭn*]
Analgesic

Composition:
Active Ingredient: Each coated tablet or caplet contains Aspirin 325 mg in a formulation buffered with Calcium Carbonate, Magnesium Oxide and Magnesium Carbonate.
Other Ingredients: Benzoic Acid, Citric Acid, Corn Starch, FD&C Blue No. 1, Hydroxypropyl Methylcellulose, Magnesium Stearate, Mineral Oil, Polysorbate 20, Povidone, Propylene Glycol, Simethicone Emulsion, Sodium Phosphate, Sorbitan Monolaurate, Titanium Dioxide. May also contain: Carnauba Wax, Zinc Stearate.

Indications: For temporary relief of headaches, pain and fever of colds, muscle aches, minor arthritis pain and inflammation, menstrual pain and toothaches.

Directions: Adults: 2 tablets or caplets with water every 4 hours while symptoms persist, not to exceed 12 tablets or caplets in 24 hours, or as directed by a doctor. Children 6 to under 12 years of age: One tablet or caplet with water every 4 hours, not to exceed 5 tablets or caplets in 24 hours or as directed by a doctor. Children under 6: Consult a doctor.

Warnings: Children and teenagers should not use this medicine for chicken pox or flu symptoms before a doctor is consulted about Reye syndrome, a rare but serious illness reported to be associated with aspirin. KEEP THIS AND ALL OTHER MEDICATIONS OUT OF THE REACH OF CHILDREN. IN CASE OF ACCIDENTAL OVERDOSE, SEEK PROFESSIONAL ASSISTANCE OR CONTACT A POISON CONTROL CENTER IMMEDIATELY. As with any drug, if you are pregnant or nursing a baby, seek the advice of a health professional before using this product. IT IS ESPECIALLY IMPORTANT NOT TO USE ASPIRIN DURING THE LAST 3 MONTHS OF PREGNANCY UNLESS SPECIFICALLY DIRECTED TO DO SO BY A DOCTOR BECAUSE IT MAY CAUSE PROBLEMS IN THE UNBORN CHILD OR COMPLICATIONS DURING DELIVERY. Do not take this product for pain for more than 10 days (for adults) or 5 days (for children) or for fever for more than 3 days unless directed by a doctor. If pain or fever persists or gets worse, if new symptoms occur, or if redness or swelling is present, consult a doctor because these could be signs of a serious condition. Consult a dentist promptly for toothache. Do not give this product to children for the pain of arthritis unless directed by a doctor. Do not take this product if you are allergic to aspirin, have asthma, have stomach problems (such as heartburn, upset stomach or stomach pain) that persist or recur, or if you have ulcers or bleeding problems, unless directed by a doctor. If ringing in the ears or loss of hearing occurs, consult a doctor before taking or giving any more of this product.

Drug Interaction Precaution: This product should not be taken by any adult or child who is taking a prescription drug for anticoagulation (thinning of blood), diabetes, gout or arthritis unless directed by a doctor.

How Supplied: BUFFERIN is supplied as:
Coated circular white tablet with letter "B" debossed on one surface.
NDC 19810-0073-2 Bottle of 12's
NDC 19810-0093-3 Bottle of 30's
NDC 19810-0073-3 Bottle of 36's
NDC 19810-0093-4 Bottle of 50's
NDC 19810-0073-4 Bottle of 60's
NDC 19810-0073-5 Bottle of 100's
NDC 19810-0073-6 Bottle of 200's
NDC 19810-0093-2 Bottle of 275's
NDC 19810-0073-7 Bottle of 1000's for hospital and clinical use.
NDC 19810-0073-9 Boxed 150 × 2 tablet foil pack for hospital and clinical use.
NDC 19810-0073-0 Vials of 10
Coated scored white caplet with letter "B" debossed on each side of scoring.
NDC 19810-0072-7 Bottle of 30's
NDC 19810-0072-1 Bottle of 36's
NDC 19810-0072-8 Bottle of 50's
NDC 19810-0072-2 Bottle of 60's
NDC 19810-0072-3 Bottle of 100's
All consumer sizes have child resistant closures except 100's for tablets and 60's for caplets which are sizes recommended for households without young children.
Store at room temperature.
Also described in *PDR* for prescription drugs.

Professional Labeling

1. BUFFERIN® FOR RECURRENT TRANSIENT ISCHEMIC ATTACKS

Indication: For reducing the risk of recurrent transient ischemic attacks (TIA's) or stroke in men who have had transient ischemia of the brain due to fibrin platelet emboli. There is inadequate evidence that aspirin or buffered aspirin is effective in reducing TIA's in women at the recommended dosage. There is no evidence that aspirin or buffered aspirin is of benefit in the treatment of completed strokes in men or women.

Clinical Trials: The indication is supported by the results of a Canadian study (1) in which 585 patients with threatened stroke were followed in a randomized clinical trial for an average of 26 months to determine whether aspirin or sulfinpyrazone, singly or in combination, was superior to placebo in preventing transient ischemic attacks, stroke, or death. The study showed that, although sulfinpyrazone had no statistically significant effect, aspirin reduced the risk of continuing transient ischemic attacks, stroke, or death by 19 percent and reduced the risk of stroke or death by 31 percent. Another aspirin study carried out in the United States with 178 patients, showed a statistically significant number of "favorable outcomes," including reduced transient ischemic attacks, stroke, and death (2).

Precautions: Patients presenting with signs and symptoms of TIA's should have a complete medical and neurologic evaluation. Consideration should be given to other disorders that resemble TIA's. Attention should be given to risk factors: it is important to evaluate and treat, if appropriate, other diseases associated with TIA's and stroke, such as hypertension and diabetes.

Concurrent administration of absorbable antacids at therapeutic doses may increase the clearance of salicylates in some individuals. The concurrent administration of nonabsorbable antacids may alter the rate of absorption of aspirin, thereby resulting in a decreased acetylsalicylic acid/salicylate ratio in plasma. The clinical significance of these decreases in available aspirin is unknown.

Aspirin at dosages of 1,000 milligrams per day has been associated with small increases in blood pressure, blood urea nitrogen, and serum uric acid levels. It is recommended that patients placed on long-term aspirin treatment be seen at regular intervals to assess changes in these measurements.

Adverse Reactions: At dosages of 1,000 milligrams or higher of aspirin per day, gastrointestinal side effects include stomach pain, heartburn, nausea and/or vomiting, as well as increased rates of gross gastrointestinal bleeding.

Dosage and Administration: Adult oral dosage for men is 1,300 milligrams a day, in divided doses of 650 milligrams twice a day or 325 milligrams four times a day.

References:

(1) The Canadian Cooperative Study Group. "A Randomized Trial of Aspirin and Sulfinpyrazone in Threatened Stroke," *New England Journal of Medicine,* 299:53–59, 1978.

(2) Fields, W.S., et al., "Controlled Trial of Aspirin in Cerebral Ischemia," *Stroke* 8:301–316, 1977.

2. BUFFERIN® FOR MYOCARDIAL INFARCTION

Indication: Aspirin is indicated to reduce the risk of death and/or nonfatal myocardial infarction in patients with a previous infarction or unstable angina pectoris.

Clinical Trials: The indication is supported by the results of six, large, randomized multicenter, placebo-controlled studies[1–7] involving 10,816, predominantly male, post-myocardial infarction (MI) patients and one randomized placebo-controlled study of 1,266 men with unstable angina. Therapy with aspirin was begun at intervals after the onset of acute MI varying from less than 3 days to more than 5 years and continued for periods of from less than one year to four years. In the unstable angina study, treatment was started within 1 month after the onset of unstable angina and continued for 12 weeks and complicating conditions such as congestive heart failure were not included in the study.

Aspirin therapy in MI patients was associated with about a 20 percent reduction in the risk of subsequent death and/or nonfatal reinfarction, a median absolute decrease of 3 percent from the 12 to 22 percent event rates in the placebo groups. In the aspirin-treated unstable angina patients the reduction in risk was about 50 percent, a reduction in the event rate of 5% from the 10% rate in the placebo group over the 12 weeks of the study.

Daily dosage of aspirin in the post-myocardial infarction studies was 300 mg. in one study and 900 and 1500 mg. in five studies. A dose of 325 mg. was used in the study of unstable angina.

Adverse Reactions: Gastrointestinal Reactions: Doses of 1000 mg. per day of aspirin caused gastrointestinal symptoms and bleeding that in some cases were clinically significant. In the largest post-infarction study (The Aspirin Myocardial Infaraction Study (AMIS) with 4,500 people), the percentage incidences of gastrointestinal symptoms for the aspirin (1000 mg. of a standard, solid-tablet formulation) and placebo-treated subjects, respectively, were: stomach pain (14.5%; 4.4%); heartburn (11.9%; 4.8%); nausea and/or vomiting (7.6%; 2.1%); hospitalization for gastrointestinal disorder (4.8%; 3.5%). In the AMIS and other trials, aspirin treated patients had increased rates of gross gastrointestinal bleeding. Symptoms and signs of gastrointestinal irritation were not significantly increased in subjects treated for unstable angina with buffered aspirin in solution.

Cardiovascular and Biochemical: In the AMIS trial, the dosage of 1000 mg. per day of aspirin was associated with small increases in systolic blood pressure (BP) (average 1.5 to 2.1 mm) and diastolic BP (0.5 to 0.6 mm), depending upon whether maximal or last available readings were used. Blood urea nitrogen and uric acid levels were also increased, but by less than 1.0 mg%.

Subjects with marked hypertension or renal insufficiency had been excluded from the trial so that the clinical importance of these observations for such subjects or for any subjects treated over more prolonged periods is not known. It is recommended that patients placed on long-term aspirin treatment, even at doses of 300 mg. per day, be seen at regular intervals to assess changes in these measurements.

Administration and Dosage: Although most of the studies used dosages exceeding 300 mg., two trials used only 300 mg. and pharmacologic data indicate that this dose inhibits platelet function fully. Therefore, 300 mg. or a conventional 325 mg. aspirin dose is a reasonable, routine dose that would minimize gastrointestinal adverse reactions.

References: 1. Elwood P.C., et al., "A Randomized Controlled Trial of Acetylsalicylic Acid in the Secondary Prevention of Mortality from Myocardial Infarction," *British Medical Journal,* 1:436–440, 1974. 2. The Coronary Drug Project Research Group, "Aspirin in Coronary Heart Disease," *Journal of Chronic Disease,* 29:625–642, 1976. 3. Breddin K, et al., "Secondary Prevention of Myocardial Infarction; Comparison of Acetylsalicylic Acid Phenprocoumon and Placebo," *Thromb. Haemost.,* 41:225–236, 1979. 4. Aspirin Myocardial Infarction Study Research Group, "A Randomized, Controlled Trial of Aspirin in Persons Recovered from Myocardial Infarction," *Journal American Medical Association,* 243:661–669, 1980. 5. Elwood P.C., and Sweetnam, P.M., "Aspirin and Secondary Mortality after Myocardial Infarction," *Lancet,* pp. 1313–1315, December 22–29, 1979. 6. The Persantine-Aspirin Reinfarction Study Research Group. "Persantine and Aspirin in Coronary Heart Disease," *Circulation* 62;449–460, 1980. 7. Lewis H.D., et al., "Protective Effects of Aspirin Against Acute Myocardial Infarction and Death in Men with Unstable Angina, Results of a Veterans Administration Cooperative Study," *New England Journal of Medicine,* 309;396–403, 1983.

Shown in Product Identification Section, page 404

Arthritis Strength BUFFERIN®

[*bŭf'fĕr-ĭn*]

Analgesic

Composition:

Active Ingredient: Aspirin (500 mg) in a formulation buffered with Calcium Carbonate, Magnesium Oxide and Magnesium Carbonate.

Other Ingredients: Benzoic Acid, Citric Acid, Corn Starch, FD&C Blue No. 1, Hydroxypropyl Methylcellulose, Magnesium Stearate, Mineral Oil, Polysorbate 20, Povidone, Propylene Glycol, Simethicone Emulsion, Sodium Phosphate, Sorbitan Monolaurate, Titanium Dioxide. May also contain: Carnauba Wax, Zinc Stearate.

Indications: For temporary relief of the minor aches and pains, stiffness, swelling and inflammation of arthritis.

Directions: Adults: 2 caplets with water every 6 hours while symptoms persist,

Continued on next page

Bristol-Myers—Cont.

not to exceed 8 caplets in 24 hours, or as directed by a doctor. Children under 12 years of age: Consult a doctor.

Warnings: Children and teenagers should not use this medicine for chicken pox or flu symptoms before a doctor is consulted about Reye syndrome, a rare but serious illness reported to be associated with aspirin. KEEP THIS AND ALL OTHER MEDICATIONS OUT OF THE REACH OF CHILDREN. IN CASE OF ACCIDENTAL OVERDOSE, SEEK PROFESSIONAL ASSISTANCE OR CONTACT A POISON CONTROL CENTER IMMEDIATELY. As with any drug, if you are pregnant or nursing a baby, seek the advice of a health professional before using this product.
IT IS ESPECIALLY IMPORTANT NOT TO USE ASPIRIN DURING THE LAST 3 MONTHS OF PREGNANCY UNLESS SPECIFICALLY DIRECTED TO DO SO BY A DOCTOR BECAUSE IT MAY CAUSE PROBLEMS IN THE UNBORN CHILD OR COMPLICATIONS DURING DELIVERY. Do not take this product for pain for more than 10 days or for fever for more than 3 days unless directed by a doctor. If pain or fever persists or gets worse, if new symptoms occur, or if redness or swelling is present, consult a doctor because these could be signs of a serious condition. Do not take this product if you are allergic to aspirin, have asthma, have stomach problems (such as heartburn, upset stomach or stomach pain) that persist or recur, or if you have ulcers or bleeding problems, unless directed by a doctor. If ringing in the ears or loss of hearing occurs, consult a doctor before taking any more of this product.

Drug Interaction Precaution: Do not take this product if you are taking a prescription drug for anticoagulation (thinning of blood), diabetes, gout or arthritis unless directed by a doctor.

How Supplied: Arthritis Strength BUFFERIN® is supplied as:
Plain white coated caplet "ASB" debossed on one side.
NDC 19810-0051-1 Bottle of 40's
NDC 19810-0051-2 Bottle of 100's
The 40 caplet size does not have a child resistant closure and is recommended for households without young children.
Store at room temperature.

Shown in Product Identification Section, page 404

Extra Strength BUFFERIN®

[*bŭf'fĕr-ĭn*]

Analgesic

Composition:
Active Ingredient: Aspirin (500 mg) in a formulation buffered with Calcium Carbonate, Magnesium Oxide and Magnesium Carbonate.
Other Ingredients: Benzoic Acid, Citric Acid, Corn Starch, FD&C Blue No. 1, Hydroxypropyl Methylcellulose, Magnesium Stearate, Mineral Oil, Polysorbate 20, Povidone, Propylene Glycol, Simethicone Emulsion, Sodium Phosphate, Sorbitan Monolaurate, Titanium Dioxide. May also contain: Carnauba Wax, Zinc Stearate.

Indications: For temporary relief of headaches, pain and fever of colds, muscle aches, arthritis pain and inflammation, menstrual pain and toothaches.

Directions: Adults: 2 tablets with water every 6 hours while symptoms persist, not to exceed 8 tablets in 24 hours, or as directed by a doctor. Children under 12 years of age: Consult a doctor.

Warnings: Children and teenagers should not use this medicine for chicken pox or flu symptoms before a doctor is consulted about Reye syndrome, a rare but serious illness reported to be associated with aspirin. KEEP THIS AND ALL OTHER MEDICATIONS OUT OF THE REACH OF CHILDREN. IN CASE OF ACCIDENTAL OVERDOSE, SEEK PROFESSIONAL ASSISTANCE OR CONTACT A POISON CONTROL CENTER IMMEDIATELY. As with any drug, if your are pregnant or nursing a baby, seek the advice of a health professional before using this product. IT IS ESPECIALLY IMPORTANT NOT TO USE ASPIRIN DURING THE LAST 3 MONTHS OF PREGNANCY UNLESS SPECIFICALLY DIRECTED TO DO SO BY A DOCTOR BECAUSE IT MAY CAUSE PROBLEMS IN THE UNBORN CHILD OR COMPLICATIONS DURING DELIVERY. Do not take this product for more than 10 days or for fever for more than 3 days unless directed by a doctor. If pain or fever persists or gets worse, if new symptoms occur, or if redness or swelling is present, consult a doctor because these could be signs of a serious condition. Consult a dentist promptly for toothache. Do not take this product if you are allergic to aspirin, have asthma, have stomach problems (such as heartburn, upset stomach or stomach pain) that persist or recur, or if you have ulcers or bleeding problems, unless directed by a doctor. If ringing in the ears or loss of hearing occurs, consult a doctor before taking any more of this product.

Drug Interaction Precaution: Do not take this product if you are taking a prescription drug for anticoagulation (thinning of blood), diabetes, gout or arthritis unless directed by a doctor.

How Supplied: Extra Strength BUFFERIN® is supplied as:
White elongated coated tablet with "ESB" debossed on one side.
NDC 19810-0074-1 Bottle of 30's
NDC 19810-0074-4 Bottle of 50's
NDC 19810-0074-2 Bottle of 60's
NDC 19810-0074-3 Bottle of 100's
All sizes have child resistant closures except 60's which is recommended for households without young children.
Store at room temperature.

Shown in Product Identification Section, page 405

COMTREX®

[*cŏm 'trĕx*]

Multi-Symptom Cold Reliever

Composition: Each tablet, caplet, liquigel and fluidounce (30 ml.) contains:
[See table on next page.]

Indications: COMTREX® provides temporary relief of these major cold symptoms: nasal and sinus congestion, runny nose, sneezing, coughing, fever, minor sore throat pain.

Directions:
Tablets or Caplets: Adults: 2 tablets or caplets every 4 hours while symptoms persist, not to exceed 8 tablets or caplets in 24 hours, or as directed by a doctor. Children 6 to under 12 years of age: One tablet or caplet every 4 hours while symptoms persist, not to exceed 4 tablets or caplets in 24 hours, or as directed by a doctor. Children under 6: Consult a doctor.
Liqui-Gel: Adults: 2 liqui-gels every 4 hours while symptoms persist, not to exceed 12 liqui-gels in 24 hours, or as directed by a doctor. Children 6 to under 12 years of age: 1 liqui-gel every 4 hours while symptoms persist, not to exceed 5 liqui-gels in 24 hours, or as directed by a doctor. Children under 6: Consult a doctor.
Liquid: Adults: One fluidounce (30 ml) in medicine cup provided or 2 tablespoons every 4 hours while symptoms persist, not to exceed 4 doses in 24 hours, or as directed by a doctor. Children 6 to under 12 years of age: ½ fluidounce (15 ml) or one tablespoon every 4 hours while symptoms persist, not to exceed 4 doses in 24 hours, or as directed by a doctor. Children under 6: Consult a doctor.

Warnings: KEEP THIS AND ALL OTHER MEDICATIONS OUT OF THE REACH OF CHILDREN. IN CASE OF ACCIDENTAL OVERDOSE, SEEK PROFESSIONAL ASSISTANCE OR CONTACT A POISON CONTROL CENTER IMMEDIATELY. PROMPT MEDICAL ATTENTION IS CRITICAL FOR ADULTS AS WELL AS FOR CHILDREN EVEN IF YOU DO NOT NOTICE ANY SYMPTOMS. As with any drug, if you are pregnant or nursing a baby, seek the advice of a health professional before using this product. Do not take this product for more than 7 days (for adults) or 5 days (for children), unless directed by a doctor. If symptoms do not improve or are accompanied by a fever that lasts for more than 3 days, or if new symptoms occur, consult a doctor. Do not exceed recommended dosage because at higher doses nervousness, dizziness or sleeplessness may occur. May cause excitability especially in children. A persistent cough may be a sign of a serious condition. If cough persists for more than 7 days, tends to recur, or is accompanied by rash, persistent headache, fever that lasts for more than 3 days, or if new symptoms occur, consult a doctor. Do not take this product for persistent or chronic cough such as occurs with smoking, asthma or emphysema, or if cough is accompanied by excessive phlegm (mu-

	COMTREX Per Tablet or Caplet	COMTREX Liquid-Gel per Liqui-Gel	COMTREX Liquid Per Fl. Ounce
Acetaminophen:	325 mg.	325 mg.	650 mg.
Pseudoephedrine HCl:	30 mg.	—	60 mg.
Phenylpropanolamine HCl:	—	12.5 mg.	—
Chlorpheniramine Maleate:	2 mg.	2 mg.	4 mg.
Dextromethorphan HBr:	10 mg.	10 mg.	20 mg.

Other Ingredients:

Tablet	Caplet		Liqui-Gels	Liquid
Corn Starch	Benzoic Acid	Mineral Oil	D&C Yellow No. 10	Alcohol (20% by volume)
D&C Yellow No. 10 Lake	Carnauba Wax	Polysorbate 20	FD&C Red No. 40	Citric Acid
FD&C Red No. 40 Lake	Corn Starch	Povidone	Gelatin	D&C Yellow No. 10
Magnesium Stearate	D&C Yellow No. 10 Lake	Propylene Glycol	Glycerin	FD&C Blue No. 1
Methylparaben	FD&C Red No. 40 Lake	Propylparaben	Polyethylene Glycol	FD&C Red No. 40
Propylparaben	Hydroxypropyl Methylcellulose	Simethicone Emulsion	Povidone	Flavors
Stearic Acid		Sorbitan Monolaurate	Propylene Glycol	Polyethylene Glycol
May also contain:	Magnesium Stearate	Stearic Acid	Silicon Dioxide	Povidone
Povidone	Methylparaben	Titanium Dioxide	Sorbitol	Sodium Citrate
			Titanium Dioxide	Sucrose
			Water	Water

cus/sputum) unless directed by a doctor. If sore throat is severe, persists for more than 2 days, is accompanied or followed by a fever, headache, rash, nausea or vomiting, consult a doctor promptly. This product should not be taken by persons who have asthma, glaucoma, emphysema, chronic pulmonary disease, high blood pressure, heart disease, thyroid disease, diabetes, shortness of breath, difficulty in breathing or difficulty in urination due to enlargement of the prostate gland unless directed by a doctor. May cause marked drowsiness; alcohol may increase the drowsiness effect. Avoid alcoholic beverages, and do not take this product if you are taking sedatives or tranquilizers without first consulting your doctor. Use caution when driving a motor vehicle or operating machinery.

Drug Interaction Precaution: This product should not be taken by any adult or child who is taking a prescription medication for high blood pressure or depression without first consulting a doctor.

Overdose:

MUCOMYST (acetylcysteine) As An Antidote For Acetaminophen Overdose)

Acetaminophen is rapidly absorbed from the upper gastrointestinal tract with peak plasma levels occurring between 30 and 60 minutes after therapeutic doses and usually within 4 hours following an overdose. The parent compound, which is nontoxic, is extensively metabolized in the liver to form principally the sulfate and glucuronide conjugates which are also nontoxic and are rapidly excreted in the urine. A small fraction of an ingested dose is metabolized in the liver by the cytochrome P-450 mixed function oxidase enzyme system to form a reactive, potentially toxic, intermediate metabolite which preferentially conjugates with hepatic glutathione to form the nontoxic cysteine and mercapturic acid derivatives which are then excreted by the kidney. Therapeutic doses of acetaminophen do not saturate the glucuronide and sulfate conjugation pathways and do not result in the formation of sufficient reactive metabolite to deplete glutathione stores. However, following ingestion of a large overdose (150 mg/kg or greater) the glucuronide and sulfate conjugation pathways are saturated resulting in a larger fraction of the drug being metabolized via the P-450 pathway. The increased formation of reactive metabolite may deplete the hepatic stores of glutathione with subsequent binding of the metabolite to protein molecules within the hepatocyte resulting in cellular necrosis. Acetylcysteine has been shown to reduce the extent of liver injury following acetaminophen overdose. Early symptoms following a potentially hepatotoxic overdose may include: nausea, vomiting, diaphoresis and general malaise. Clinical and laboratory evidence of hepatic toxicity may not be apparent until 48 to 72 hours postingestion. In adults and adolescents, regardless of the quantity of acetaminophen reported to have been ingested, administer MUCOMYST® acetylcysteine immediately. MUCOMYST acetylcysteine therapy should be initiated and continued for a full course of therapy. Its effectiveness depends on early administration, with benefit seen principally in patients treated within 16 hours of the overdose. If acetaminophen plasma assay capability is not available, and the estimated acetaminophen ingestion exceeds 150 mg/kg, MUCOMYST acetylcysteine therapy should be initiated and continued for a full course of therapy.

For full prescribing information, refer to the MUCOMYST package insert. Do not await the results of assays for acetaminophen level before initiating treatment with MUCOMYST acetylcysteine. The following additional procedures are recommended: The stomach should be emptied promptly by lavage or by induction of emesis with syrup of ipecac. A serum acetaminophen assay should be obtained as early as possible, but no sooner than four hours following ingestion. Liver function studies should be obtained initially and repeated at 24-hour intervals.

For additional emergency information call your regional poison center or toll-free (1-800-525-6115) to the Rocky Mountain Poison Center for assistance in diagnosis and for directions in the use of MUCOMYST acetylcysteine as an antidote.

How Supplied:

COMTREX® is supplied as:

Yellow tablet with letter "C" debossed on one surface.

NDC 19810-0790-1 Blister packages of 24's
NDC 19810-0790-2 Bottles of 50's
NDC 19810-0790-3 Vials of 10's

Coated yellow caplet with "Comtrex" printed in red on one side.

NDC 19810-0792-3 Blister packages of 24's
NDC 19810-0792-4 Bottles of 50's

Yellow Liqui-Gel with "Comtrex" printed in red on one side.

NDC 19810-0561-1 Blister packages of 24's
NDC 19810-0561-2 Blister packages of 50's

Clear orange liquid:

NDC 19810-0791-1 6 oz. plastic bottles
NDC 19810-0791-2 10 oz. plastic bottles

Clear Red Cherry Flavored liquid:

NDC 19810-0791-1 6 oz. plastic bottles.

All sizes packaged in child resistant closures except for 24's for tablets, caplets and liqui-gels and 6 oz. orange liquid which are sizes recommended for households without young children. Store caplets, tablets and liquid at room temperature.

Store liqui-gels below 86° F. (30° C.). Keep from freezing.

Shown in Product Identification Section, page 405

ALLERGY-SINUS COMTREX

[cŏm 'trĕx]

Multi-Symptom Allergy/Sinus Formula

Composition:

Active Ingredients: Each coated tablet or caplet contains 500 mg acetaminophen, 30 mg pseudoephedrine HCl, 2 mg chlorpheniramine maleate.

Other Ingredients: Benzoic acid, carnauba wax, corn starch, D&C yellow No. 10 lake, FD&C blue No. 1 lake, FD&C Red No. 40 lake, hydroxypropyl methylcellulose, mineral oil, polysorbate 20, povidone, propylene glycol, simethicone emulsion, sodium citrate, sorbitan monolaurate, stearic acid, titanium dioxide. May also contain: crospovidone, D&C yellow No. 10, erythorbic acid, FD&C blue No. 1, magnesium stearate, methylparaben, microcrystalline cellulose, polysorbate 80, propylparaben, silicon dioxide, wood cellulose.

Continued on next page

Bristol-Myers—Cont.

Indications:
ALLERGY-SINUS COMTREX provides temporary relief of these upper respiratory allergy, hay fever, and sinusitis symptoms: sneezing, itchy, watery eyes, runny nose, headache, nasal and sinus pressure and congestion.

Directions: Adults: 2 tablets or caplets every 6 hours while symptoms persist, not to exceed 8 tablets or caplets in 24 hours, or as directed by a doctor. Children under 12 years of age: Consult a doctor.

Warnings: KEEP THIS AND ALL OTHER MEDICATIONS OUT OF THE REACH OF CHILDREN. IN CASE OF ACCIDENTAL OVERDOSE, SEEK PROFESSIONAL ASSISTANCE OR CONTACT A POISON CONTROL CENTER IMMEDIATELY. PROMPT MEDICAL ATTENTION IS CRITICAL FOR ADULTS AS WELL AS FOR CHILDREN EVEN IF YOU DO NOT NOTICE ANY SIGNS OR SYMPTOMS. As with any drug, if you are pregnant or nursing a baby, seek the advice of a health professional before using this product. Do not take this product for more than 7 days unless directed by a doctor. If symptoms do not improve or are accompanied by a fever that lasts for more than 3 days, or if new symptoms occur, consult a doctor. Do not exceed recommended dosage because at higher doses nervousness, dizziness or sleeplessness may occur. May cause excitability especially in children. This product should not be taken by persons who have asthma, glaucoma, emphysema, chronic pulmonary disease, high blood pressure, heart disease, thyroid disease, diabetes, shortness of breath, difficulty in breathing or difficulty in urination due to enlargement of the prostate gland unless directed by a doctor. May cause drowsiness; alcohol may increase the drowsiness effect. Avoid alcoholic beverages, and do not take this product if you are taking sedatives or tranquilizers without first consulting your doctor. Use caution when driving a motor vehicle or operating machinery.

Drug Interaction Precaution: Do not take this product if you are presently taking a prescription drug for high blood pressure or depression, without first consulting your doctor.

Overdose:
MUCOMYST (acetylcysteine) As An Antidote For Acetaminophen Overdose)
Acetaminophen is rapidly absorbed from the upper gastrointestinal tract with peak plasma levels occurring between 30 and 60 minutes after therapeutic doses and usually within 4 hours following an overdose. The parent compound, which is nontoxic, is extensively metabolized in the liver to form principally the sulfate and glucuronide conjugates which are also nontoxic and are rapidly excreted in the urine. A small fraction of an ingested dose is metabolized in the liver by the cytochrome P-450 mixed function oxidase enzyme system to form a reactive, potentially toxic, intermediate metabolite which preferentially conjugates with hepatic glutathione to form the nontoxic cysteine and mercapturic acid derivatives which are then excreted by the kidney. Therapeutic doses of acetaminophen do not saturate the glucuronide and sulfate conjugation pathways and do not result in the formation of sufficient reactive metabolite to deplete glutathione stores. However, following ingestion of a large overdose (150 mg/kg or greater) the glucuronide and sulfate conjugation pathways are saturated resulting in a larger fraction of the drug being metabolized via the P-450 pathway. The increased formation of reactive metabolite may deplete the hepatic stores of glutathione with subsequent binding of the metabolite to protein molecules within the hepatocyte resulting in cellular necrosis. Acetylcysteine has been shown to reduce the extent of liver injury following acetaminophen overdose. Early symptoms following a potentially hepatotoxic overdose may include: nausea, vomiting, diaphoresis and general malaise. Clinical and laboratory evidence of hepatic toxicity may not be apparent until 48 to 72 hours postingestion. In adults and adolescents, regardless of the quantity of acetaminophen reported to have been ingested, administer MUCOMYST® acetylcysteine immediately. MUCOMYST acetylcysteine therapy should be initiated and continued for a full course of therapy. Its effectiveness depends on early administration, with benefit seen principally in patients treated within 16 hours of the overdose. If acetaminophen plasma assay capability is not available, and the estimated acetaminophen ingestion exceeds 150 mg/kg, MUCOMYST acetylcysteine therapy should be initiated and continued for a full course of therapy.
For full prescribing information, refer to the MUCOMYST package insert. Do not await the results of assays for acetaminophen level before initiating treatment with MUCOMYST acetylcysteine. The following additional procedures are recommended: The stomach should be emptied promptly by lavage or by induction of emesis with syrup of ipecac. A serum acetaminophen assay should be obtained as early as possible, but no sooner than four hours following ingestion. Liver function studies should be obtained initially and repeated at 24-hour intervals.
For additional emergency information call your regional poison center or toll-free (1-800-525-6115) to the Rocky Mountain Poison Center for assistance in diagnosis and for directions in the use of MUCOMYST acetylcysteine as an antidote.

How Supplied: Allergy-Sinus COMTREX® is supplied as:
Coated green tablets with "Comtrex A/S" printed in black on one side.
NDC 19810-0774-1 Blister packages of 24's
NDC 19810-0774-2 Bottles of 50's
Coated green caplets with "A/S" debossed on one surface.
NDC 19810-0081-4 Blister packages of 24's
NDC 19810-0081-5 Bottles of 50's
All sizes packaged in child resistant closures except 24's for tablets and caplets which are sizes recommended for households without young children.
Store at room temperature.

Shown in Product Identification Section, page 405

Cough Formula COMTREX® (NEW FORMULA)
[*cŏm 'trĕx*]
Multi-Symptom Cough Formula

Composition:
Active Ingredients: Each 4 teaspoonfuls (⅔ fl. oz.) contains:
—EXPECTORANT—200 mg Guaifenesin
—COUGH SUPPRESSANT—30 mg Dextromethorphan HBr
—ANALGESIC—500 mg Acetaminophen
—DECONGESTANT—60 mg Pseudoephedrine HCl

Other Ingredients: Alcohol (20% by volume), Citric Acid, FD&C Red No. 40, Flavor, Menthol, Povidone, Saccharin Sodium, Sodium Citrate, Sucrose, Water.

Indications: For temporary relief of cough, nasal and upper chest congestion, minor sore throat pain, and fever and pain due to a chest cold.

BENEFITS OF COUGH FORMULA COMTREX
—Relieves upper chest congestion by loosening phlegm and mucus.
—Relieves your cough for up to 8 hours.
—Relieves muscle pain due to excessive coughing.
—Soothes irritated sore throat.
—Helps clear nasal passages to relieve congestion.

Directions: Adults: ⅔ fluidounce (20 ml) in medicine cup provided or four teaspoons every 4 hours while symptoms persist, not to exceed 4 doses in 24 hours, or as directed by a doctor. Children 6 to under 12 years of age: ⅓ fluidounce (10 ml) in medicine cup provided or 2 teaspoons every 4 hours while symptoms persist, not to exceed 4 doses in 24 hours, or as directed by a doctor. Children under 6: Consult a doctor.

Warnings: KEEP THIS AND ALL OTHER MEDICATIONS OUT OF THE REACH OF CHILDREN. IN CASE OF ACCIDENTAL OVERDOSE, SEEK PROFESSIONAL ASSISTANCE OR CONTACT A POISON CONTROL CENTER IMMEDIATELY. PROMPT MEDICAL ATTENTION IS CRITICAL FOR ADULTS AS WELL AS FOR CHILDREN EVEN IF YOU DO NOT NOTICE ANY SIGNS OR SYMPTOMS. As with any drug, if you are pregnant or nursing a baby, seek the advice of a health professional before using this product. Do not take this product for more than 7 days (for adults) or 5 days (for children) unless directed by a doctor. If symptoms do not improve or are accompanied by a fever that lasts for more than 3 days, or if new symptoms occur, consult a doctor. Do not exceed recommended dosage because at higher doses nervousness, dizziness or sleeplessness may occur. A persistent cough may be a sign of a serious condition. If cough persists for more than 7 days, tends to recur or is accompanied by rash, persistent headache, fever that lasts for more than 3 days, or if new symptoms occur, consult a doctor. Do not take this product for persistent or chronic cough such as occurs with smoking, asthma, chronic bronchitis or emphysema or if cough is accompanied by excessive phlegm (mucus/sputum) unless directed by a doctor. If sore throat is severe, persists for more than two days, is accompanied or followed by a fever, headache, rash, nausea or vomiting, consult a doctor promptly. This product should not be taken by persons who have heart disease, high blood pressure, thyroid disease, diabetes or difficulty in urination due to enlargement of the prostate gland unless directed by a doctor.

Overdose:
MUCOMYST (acetylcysteine) As An Antidote For Acetaminophen Overdose)
Acetaminophen is rapidly absorbed from the upper gastrointestinal tract with peak plasma levels occurring between 30 and 60 minutes after therapeutic doses and usually within 4 hours following an overdose. The parent compound, which is nontoxic, is extensively metabolized in the liver to form principally the sulfate and glucuronide conjugates which are also nontoxic and are rapidly excreted in the urine. A small fraction of an ingested dose is metabolized in the liver by the cytochrome P-450 mixed function oxidase enzyme system to form a reactive, potentially toxic, intermediate metabolite which preferentially conjugates with hepatic glutathione to form the nontoxic cysteine and mercapturic acid derivatives which are then excreted by the kidney. Therapeutic doses of acetaminophen do not saturate the glucuronide and sulfate conjugation pathways and do not result in the formation of sufficient reactive metabolite to deplete glutathione stores. However, following ingestion of a large overdose (150 mg/kg or greater) the glucuronide and sulfate conjugation pathways are saturated resulting in a larger fraction of the drug being metabolized via the P-450 pathway. The increased formation of reactive metabolite may deplete the hepatic stores of glutathione with subsequent binding of the metabolite to protein molecules within the hepatocyte resulting in cellular necrosis. Acetylcysteine has been shown to reduce the extent of liver injury following acetaminophen overdose. Early symptoms following a potentially hepatotoxic overdose may include nausea, vomiting, diaphoresis and general malaise. Clinical and laboratory evidence of hepatic toxicity may not be apparent until 48 to 72 hours postingestion. In adults and adolescents, regardless of the quantity of acetaminophen reported to have been ingested, administer MUCOMYST® acetylcysteine immediately. MUCOMYST acetylcysteine therapy should be initiated and continued for a full course of therapy. Its effectiveness depends on early administration, with benefit seen principally in patients treated within 16 hours of the overdose.
If acetaminophen plasma assay capability is not available, and the estimated acetaminophen ingestion exceeds 150 mg/kg, MUCOMYST acetylcysteine therapy should be initiated and continued for a full course of therapy.
For full prescribing information, refer to the MUCOMYST package insert. Do not await the results of assays for acetaminophen level before initiating treatment with MUCOMYST acetylcysteine. The following additional procedures are recommended: The stomach should be emptied promptly by lavage or by induction of emesis with syrup of ipecac. A serum acetaminophen assay should be obtained as early as possible, but no sooner than four hours following ingestion. Liver function studies should be obtained initially and repeated at 24-hour intervals.
For additional emergency information call your regional poison center or toll-free (1-800-525-6115) to the Rocky Mountain Poison Center for assistance in diagnosis and for directions in the use of MUCOMYST acetylcysteine as an antidote.

How Supplied: Cough Formula COMTREX® is supplied as a clear red raspberry flavored liquid:
NDC 19810-0781-1 4 oz. plastic bottle
NDC 19810-0781-3 8 oz. plastic bottle
The 4 oz. size is not child resistant and is recommended for households without young children.
Store at room temperature.

Shown in Product Identification Section, page 405

CONGESPIRIN® for Children Aspirin Free Chewable Cold Tablets

[*cŏn "gĕs 'pir-in*]

Composition: Each tablet contains acetaminophen 81 mg. (1¼ grains), phenylephrine hydrochloride 1¼ mg. Also Contains: Calcium Stearate, D&C Red No. 30 Aluminum Lake, D&C Yellow No. 10 Aluminum Lake, Ethyl Cellulose, Flavor, Mannitol, Microcrystalline Cellulose, Polyethylene, Saccharin, Calcium, Sucrose.

Indications: A non-aspirin analgesic/nasal decongestant that temporarily reduces fever and relieves aches, pains and nasal congestion associated with colds and "flu."

Warnings: KEEP THIS AND ALL MEDICINES OUT OF CHILDREN'S REACH. IN CASE OF ACCIDENTAL OVERDOSE, CONTACT A PHYSICIAN IMMEDIATELY.

Caution: If child is under medical care, do not administer without consulting physician. Do not exceed recommended dosage. Consult your physician if symptoms persist or if high blood pressure, heart disease, diabetes or thyroid disease is present. Do not administer for more than 10 days unless directed by physician.

Directions:
Under 2, consult your physician.

Age	Dose
2–3 years	2 tablets
4–5 years	3 tablets
6–8 years	4 tablets
9–10 years	5 tablets
11–12 years	6 tablets
over 12 years	8 tablets

Repeat dose in four hours if necessary. Do not give more than four doses per day unless prescribed by your physician.

Overdose:
MUCOMYST (acetylcysteine) As An Antidote For Acetaminophen Overdose)
Acetaminophen is rapidly absorbed from the upper gastrointestinal tract with peak plasma levels occurring between 30 and 60 minutes after therapeutic doses and usually within 4 hours following an overdose. The parent compound, which is nontoxic, is extensively metabolized in the liver to form principally the sulfate and glucuronide conjugates which are also nontoxic and are rapidly excreted in the urine. A small fraction of an ingested dose is metabolized in the liver by the cytochrome P-450 mixed function oxidase enzyme system to form a reactive, potentially toxic, intermediate metabolite which preferentially conjugates with hepatic glutathione to form the nontoxic cysteine and mercapturic acid derivatives which are then excreted by the kidney. Therapeutic doses of acetaminophen do not saturate the glucuronide and sulfate conjugation pathways and do not result in the formation of sufficient reactive metabolite to deplete glutathione stores. However, following ingestion of a large overdose (150 mg/kg or greater) the glucuronide and sulfte conjugation pathways are saturated resulting in a larger fraction of the drug being metabolized via the P-450 pathway. The increased formation of reactive metabolite may deplete the hepatic stores of glutathione with subsequent binding of the metabolite to protein molecules within the hepatocyte resulting in cellular necrosis. Acetylcysteine has been shown to reduce the extent of liver injury following acetaminophen overdose. Early symptoms following a potentially hepatotoxic overdose may include nausea, vomiting, diaphoresis and general malaise. Clinical and laboratory evidence of hepatic toxicity may not be apparent until 48 to 72 hours postingestion. In adults and adolescents, regardless of the quantity of acetaminophen reported to have been ingested, administer MUCOMYST® acetylcysteine immediately. MUCOMYST acetylcysteine therapy should be initiated and continued for a full course of therapy. Its effectiveness depends on early administration, with benefit seen principally in patients treated within 16 hours of the overdose.
If acetaminophen plasma assay capability is not available, and the estimated acetaminophen ingestion exceeds 150

Continued on next page

Bristol-Myers—Cont.

mg/kg, MUCOMYST acetylcysteine therapy should be initiated and continued for a full course of therapy.
For full prescribing information, refer to the MUCOMYST package insert. Do not await the result of assays for acetaminophen level before initiating treatment with MUCOMYST acetylcysteine. The following additional procedures are recommended: The stomach should be emptied promptly by lavage or by induction of emesis with syrup of ipecac. A serum acetaminophen assay should be obtained as early as possible, but no sooner than four hours following ingestion. Liver function studies should be obtained initially and repeated at 24-hour intervals.
For additional emergency information call your regional poison center or toll-free (1-800-525-6115) to the Rocky Mountain Poison Center for assistance in diagnosis and for directions in the use of MUCOMYST acetylcysteine as an antidote.

How Supplied: CONGESPIRIN Aspirin Free Chewable Cold Tablets are supplied as scored orange tablets with "C" on one side.
NDC 19810-0748-1 Bottles of 24's.
Bottles are child resistant.
Store at room temperature.

Shown in Product Identification Section, page 405

Extra-Strength DATRIL®
[*dā'trĭl*]
Analgesic

Composition: Each tablet contains Acetaminophen 500 mg. Other ingredients: Corn Starch, Povidone, Stearic Acid. May also contain: Croscarmellose Sodium, Crospovidone, Erythorbic Acid, Methylparaben, Propylparaben, Wood Cellulose.

Indications: For temporary relief of the pain of headaches, sinusitis, colds or flu, muscular aches, menstrual discomfort, toothaches, and minor arthritis pain and to reduce fever.

Directions: Adults: 2 tablets every 6 hours while symptoms persist, not to exceed 8 tablets in 24 hours, or as directed by a doctor. Children under 12: Consult a doctor.

Warnings: KEEP THIS AND ALL OTHER MEDICATIONS OUT OF THE REACH OF CHILDREN. IN CASE OF ACCIDENTAL OVERDOSE, SEEK PROFESSIONAL ASSISTANCE OR CONTACT A POISON CONTROL CENTER IMMEDIATELY. PROMPT MEDICAL ATTENTION IS CRITICAL FOR ADULTS AS WELL AS FOR CHILDREN EVEN IF YOU DO NOT NOTICE ANY SIGNS OR SYMPTOMS. As with any drug, if you are pregnant or nursing a baby, seek the advice of a health professional before using this product. Do not take this product for pain for more than 10 days or for fever for more than 3 days unless directed by a doctor. If pain or fever persists or gets worse, if new sympoms occur, or if redness or swelling is present, consult a doctor because these could be signs of a serious condition. Consult a dentist promptly for toothache.

Overdose:
MUCOMYST (acetylcysteine) As An Antidote For Acetaminophen Overdose)
Acetaminophen is rapidly absorbed from the upper gastrointestinal tract with peak plasma levels occurring between 30 and 60 minutes after therapeutic doses and usually within 4 hours following an overdose. The parent compound, which is nontoxic, is extensively metabolized in the liver to form principally the sulfate and glucuronide conjugates which are also nontoxic and are rapidly excreted in the urine. A small fraction of an ingested dose is metabolized in the liver by the cytochrome P-450 mixed function oxidase enzyme system to form a reactive, potentially toxic, intermediate metabolite which preferentially conjugates with hepatic glutathione to form the nontoxic cysteine and mercapturic acid derivatives which are then excreted by the kidney. Therapeutic doses of acetaminophen do not saturate the glucuronide and sulfate conjugation pathways and do not result in the formation of sufficient reactive metabolite to deplete glutathione stores. However, following ingestion of a large overdose (150 mg/kg or greater) the glucuronide and sulfate conjugation pathways are saturated resulting in a larger fraction of the drug being metabolized via the P-450 pathway. The increased formation of reactive metabolite may deplete the hepatic stores of glutathione with subsequent binding of the metabolite to protein molecules within the hepatocyte resulting in cellular necrosis. Acetylcysteine has been shown to reduce the extent of liver injury following acetaminophen overdose.
Early symptoms following a potentially hepatotoxic overdose may include: nausea, vomiting, diaphoresis and general malaise. Clinical and laboratory evidence of hepatic toxicity may not be apparent until 48 to 72 hours postingestion. In adults and adolescents, regardless of the quantity of acetaminophen reported to have been ingested, administer MUCOMYST® acetylcysteine immediately. MUCOMYST acetylcysteine therapy should be initiated and continued for a full course of therapy. Its effectiveness depends on early administration, with benefit seen principally in patients treated within 16 hours of the overdose.
If acetaminophen plasma assay capability is not available, and the estimated acetaminophen ingestion exceeds 150 mg/kg, MUCOMYST acetylcysteine therapy should be initiated and continued for a full course of therapy.
For full prescribing information, refer to the MUCOMYST package insert. Do not await the results of assays for acetaminophen level before initiating treatment with MUCOMYST acetylcysteine. The following additional procedures are recommended: The stomach should be emptied promptly by lavage or by induction of emesis with syrup of ipecac. A serum acetaminophen assay should be obtained as early as possible, but no sooner than four hours following ingestion. Liver function studies should be obtained initially and repeated at 24-hour intervals.
For additional emergency information call your regional poison center or toll-free (1-800-525-6115) to the Rocky Mountain Poison Center for assistance in diagnosis and for directions in the use of MUCOMYST acetylcysteine as an antidote.

How Supplied: Extra Strength DATRIL® is supplied as:
White circular tablets with "DATRIL" debossed on one surface.
NDC 19810-0705-1 Bottles of 30's
NDC 19810-0705-2 Bottles of 60's
NDC 19810-0705-3 Bottles of 100's
NDC 19810-0705-6 Vials of 10's
Coated white caplet with "Datril" debossed on one side.
NDC 19810-0799-1 Bottles of 24's
NDC 19810-0799-2 Bottles of 50's
All sizes packaged in child resistant closures except 50's for caplets and 60's for tablets which are sizes recommended for households without young children.
Store at room temperature.

Shown in Product Identification Section, page 405

Aspirin Free EXCEDRIN®

Composition: Each caplet contains Acetaminophen 500 mg. and Caffeine 65 mg. Other Ingredients: Benzoic Acid, Carnauba Wax, Corn Starch, Croscarmellose Sodium, D&C Red No. 27 Lake, D&C Yellow No. 10 Lake, FD&C Blue No. 1 Lake, Hydroxypropyl Methylcellulose, Magnesium Stearate, Methylparaben, Microcrystalline Cellulose, Polyethylene Glycol, Polysorbate 80, Povidone, Propylparaben, Saccharin Sodium, Simethicone Emulsion, Stearic Acid, Titanium Dioxide.

Indications: For temporary relief of the pain of headache, sinusitis, colds, muscular aches, menstrual discomfort, toothaches and minor arthritis pain.

Directions: Adults: 2 caplets every 6 hours while symptoms persist, not to exceed 8 caplets in 24 hours, or as directed by a doctor. Children under 12 years of age: Consult a doctor.

Warnings: KEEP THIS AND ALL OTHER MEDICATIONS OUT OF THE REACH OF CHILDREN. IN CASE OF ACCIDENTAL OVERDOSE, SEEK PROFESSIONAL ASSISTANCE OR CONTACT A POISON CONTROL CENTER IMMEDIATELY. PROMPT MEDICAL ATTENTION IS CRITICAL FOR ADULTS AS WELL AS FOR CHILDREN EVEN IF YOU DO NOT NOTICE ANY SIGNS OR SYMPTOMS. As with any drug, if you are pregnant or nursing a baby, seek the advice of a health professional before using this product. Do not take this product for pain for more than 10 days or for fever for more than 3 days unless directed by a doctor. If pain or fever persists or gets worse, if new symptoms occur, or if redness or swelling is present, consult a doctor because these could be signs of a serious condition. Consult a dentist promptly for toothache.

Overdose:
MUCOMYST (acetylcysteine) As An Antidote For Acetaminophen Overdose)
Acetaminophen is rapidly absorbed from the upper gastrointestinal tract with peak plasma levels occurring between 30 and 60 minutes after therapeutic doses and usually within 4 hours following an overdose. The parent compound, which is nontoxic, is extensively metabolized in the liver to form principally the sulfate and glucuronide conjugates which are also nontoxic and are rapidly excreted in the urine. A small fraction of an ingested dose is metabolized in the liver by the cytochrome P-450 mixed function oxidase enzyme system to form a reactive, potentially toxic, intermediate metabolite which preferentially conjugates with hepatic glutathione to form the nontoxic cysteine and mercapturic acid derivatives which are then excreted by the kidney. Therapeutic doses of acetaminophen do not saturate the glucuronide and sulfate conjugation pathways and do not result in the formation of sufficient reactive metabolite to deplete glutathione stores. However, following ingestion of a large overdose (150 mg/kg or greater) the glucuronide and sulfate conjugation pathways are saturated resulting in a larger fraction of the drug being metabolized via the P-450 pathway. The increased formation of reactive metabolite may deplete the hepatic stores of glutathione with subsequent binding of the metabolite to protein molecules within the hepatocyte resulting in cellular necrosis. Acetylcysteine has been shown to reduce the extent of liver injury following acetaminophen overdose. Early symptoms following a potentially hepatotoxic overdose may include: nausea, vomiting, diaphoresis and general malaise. Clinical and laboratory evidence of hepatic toxicity may not be apparent until 48 to 72 hours postingestion. In adults and adolescents, regardless of the quantity of acetaminophen reported to have been ingested, administer MUCOMYST® acetylcysteine immediately. MUCOMYST acetylcysteine therapy should be initiated and continued for a full course of therapy. Its effectiveness depends on early administration, with benefit seen principally in patients treated within 16 hours of the overdose.
If acetaminophen plasma assay capability is not available, and the estimated acetaminophen ingestion exceeds 150 mg/kg, MUCOMYST acetylcysteine therapy should be initiated and continued for a full course of therapy.
For full prescribing information, refer to the MUCOMYST package insert. Do not await the results of assays for acetaminophen level before initiating treatment with MUCOMYST acetylcysteine. The following additional procedures are recommended: The stomach should be emptied promptly by lavage or by induction of emesis with syrup of ipecac. A serum acetaminophen assay should be obtained as early as possible, but no sooner than four hours following ingestion. Liver function studies should be obtained initially and repeated at 24-hour intervals.
For additional emergency information call your regional poison center or toll-free (1-800-525-6115) to the Rocky Mountain Poison Center for assistance in diagnosis and for directions in the use of MUCOMYST acetylcysteine as an antidote.

How Supplied: Aspirin Free EXCEDRIN® is supplied as: Coated red caplets with "AF Excedrin" printed in white on one side.
NDC 19810-0089-1 Bottles of 24's
NDC 19810-0089-2 Bottles of 50's
NDC 19810-0089-3 Bottles of 100's
All sizes packaged in child resistant closures except 100's which is recommended for households without young children.
Store at room temperature.

Shown in Product Identification Section, page 405

EXCEDRIN® Extra-Strength Analgesic
[ĕx ″cĕd ′rĭn]

Composition:
Each tablet or caplet contains Acetaminophen 250 mg.: Aspirin 250 mg.; and Caffeine 65 mg.
Other ingredients: (Tablets) Hydroxypropylcellulose, Microcrystalline Cellulose, Stearic Acid. (Caplets) Benzoic Acid, FD&C Blue No. 1, Hydroxypropylcellulose, Hydroxypropyl Methylcellulose, Microcrystalline Cellulose, Mineral Oil, Polysorbate 20, Povidone, Propylene Glycol, Simethicone Emulsion, Sorbitan Monolaurate, Stearic Acid, Titanium Dioxide. Caplets may also contain: Carnauba wax.

Indications: For temporary relief of the pain of headache, sinusitis, colds, muscular aches, menstrual discomfort, toothaches and minor arthritis pain.

Directions: Adults: 2 tablets or caplets with water every 6 hours while symptoms persist, not to exceed 8 tablets or caplets in 24 hours, or as directed by a doctor. Children under 12 years of age: Consult a doctor.

Warnings: Children and teenagers should not use this medicine for chickenpox or flu symptoms before a doctor is consulted about Reye syndrome, a rare but serious illness reported to be associated with aspirin. KEEP THIS AND ALL OTHER MEDICATIONS OUT OF THE REACH OF CHILDREN. IN CASE OF ACCIDENTAL OVERDOSE, SEEK PROFESSIONAL ASSISTANCE OR CONTACT A POISON CONTROL CENTER IMMEDIATELY. PROMPT MEDICAL ATTENTION IS CRITICAL FOR ADULTS AS WELL AS FOR CHILDREN EVEN IF YOU DO NOT NOTICE ANY SIGNS OR SYMPTOMS. As with any drug, if you are pregnant or nursing a baby, seek the advice of a health professional before using this product. IT IS ESPECIALLY IMPORTANT NOT TO USE ASPIRIN DURING THE LAST 3 MONTHS OF PREGNANCY UNLESS SPECIFICALLY DIRECTED TO DO SO BY A DOCTOR BECAUSE IT MAY CAUSE PROBLEMS IN THE UNBORN CHILD OR COMPLICATIONS DURING DELIVERY. Do not take this product for pain for more than 10 days or for fever for more than 3 days unless directed by a doctor. If pain or fever persists or gets worse, if new symptoms occur, or if redness or swelling is present, consult a doctor because these could be signs of a serious condition. Consult a dentist promptly for toothache. Do not take this product if you are allergic to aspirin, have asthma, have stomach problems (such as heartburn, upset stomach or stomach pain) that persist or recur, or if you have ulcers or bleeding problems, unless directed by a doctor. If ringing in the ears or loss of hearing occurs, consult a doctor before taking any more of this product.

Drug Interaction Precaution: Do not take this product if you are taking a prescription drug for anticoagulation (thinning of blood), diabetes, gout or arthritis unless directed by a doctor.

Overdose:
MUCOMYST (acetylcysteine As An Antidote For Acetaminophen Overdose)
Acetaminophen is rapidly absorbed from the upper gastrointestinal tract with peak plasma levels occurring between 30 and 60 minutes after therapeutic doses and usually within 4 hours following an overdose. The parent compound, which is nontoxic, is extensively metabolized in the liver to form principally the sulfate and glucuronide conjugates which are also nontoxic and are rapidly excreted in the urine. A small fraction of an ingested dose is metabolized in the liver by the cytochrome P-450 mixed function oxidase enzyme system to form a reactive, potentially toxic, intermediate metabolite which preferentially conjugates with hepatic glutathione to form the nontoxic cysteine and mercapturic acid derivatives which are then excreted by the kidney. Therapeutic doses of acetaminophen do not saturate the glucuronide and sulfate conjugation pathways and do not result in the formation of sufficient reactive metabolite to deplete glutathione stores. However, following ingestion of a larger overdose (150 mg/kg or greater) the glucuronide and sulfate conjugation pathways are saturated resulting in larger fraction of the drug being metabolized via the P-450 pathway. The increased formation of reactive metabolite may deplete the hepatic stores of glutathione with subsequent binding of the metabolite to protein molecules within the hepatocyte resulting in cellular necrosis. Acetylcysteine has been shown to reduce the extent of liver injury following acetaminophen overdose. Early symptoms following a potentially hepatotoxic overdose may include nausea,

Continued on next page

Bristol-Myers—Cont.

vomiting, diaphoresis and general malaise. Clinical and laboratory evidence of hepatic toxicity may not be apparent until 48 to 72 hours postingestion. In adults and adolescents, regardless of the quantity of acetaminophen reported to have been ingested, administer MUCOMYST® acetylcysteine immediately. MUCOMYST acetylcysteine therapy should be initiated and continued for a full course of therapy. Its effectiveness depends on early administration, with benefit seen principally in patients treated within 16 hours of the overdose. If acetaminophen plasma assay capability is not available, and the estimated acetaminophen ingestion exceeds 150 mg/kg, MUCOMYST acetylcysteine therapy should be initiated and continued for a full course of therapy.
For full prescribing information, refer to the MUCOMYST package insert. Do not await the results of assays for acetaminophen level before initiating treatment with MUCOMYST acetylcysteine. The following additional procedures are recommended. The stomach should be emptied promptly by lavage or by induction of emesis with syrup of ipecac. A serum acetaminophen assay should be obtained as early as possible, but no sooner than four hours following ingestion. Liver function studies should be obtained initially and repeated at 24-hour intervals.
For additional emergency information call your regional poison center or toll-free (1-800-525-6115) to the Rocky Mountain Poison Center for assistance in diagnosis and for directions in the use of MUCOMYST acetylcysteine as an antidote.

How Supplied: Extra Strength EXCEDRIN® is supplied as:
White circular tablet with letter "E" debossed on one side.
NDC 19810-0700-2 Bottles of 12's
NDC 19810-0772-9 Bottles of 30's
NDC 19810-0700-4 Bottles of 60's
NDC 19810-0700-5 Bottles of 100's
NDC 19810-0700-6 Bottles of 165's
NDC 19810-0700-7 Bottles of 225's
NDC 19810-0782-2 Bottles of 275's
NDC 19810-0700-1 A metal tin of 12's
NDC 19810-0772-1 Vials of 10's
Coated while caplets with "Excedrin" printed in red on one side.
NDC 19810-0002-1 Bottles of 24's
NDC 19810-0002-2 Bottles of 50's
NDC 19810-0002-8 Bottles of 100's
All sizes packaged in child resistant closures except 100's for tablets, 50's for caplets which are sizes recommended for households without young children.
Store at room temperature.

Shown in Product Identification Section, page 405

EXCEDRIN P.M.®

[*ĕx ″cĕd ′rĭn*]

Analgesic Sleeping Aid

Composition: Each tablet, caplet and fluidounce (30 ml.) contains:
[See table below.]

Indications: For temporary relief of occasional headaches and minor aches and pains with accompanying sleeplessness.

Directions:
Tablets or Caplets:
Adults, 2 tablets or caplets at bedtime if needed or as directed by a doctor.
Liquid:
Adults, 1 fluidounce (2 tablespoons) at bedtime if needed, or as directed by a doctor, using the dosage cup provided.

Warnings: KEEP THIS AND ALL OTHER MEDICATIONS OUT OF THE REACH OF CHILDREN. IN CASE OF ACCIDENTAL OVERDOSE, SEEK PROFESSIONAL ASSISTANCE OR CONTACT A POISON CONTROL CENTER IMMEDIATELY. PROMPT MEDICAL ATTENTION IS CRITICAL FOR ADULTS AS WELL AS FOR CHILDREN EVEN IF YOU DO NOT NOTICE ANY SIGNS OR SYMPTOMS. As with any drug, if you are pregnant or nursing a baby, seek the advice of a health professional before using this product. Do not give this product to children under 12 years of age or use for more than 10 days unless directed by a doctor. Consult a doctor if symptoms persist or get worse or if new ones occur, or if sleeplessness persists continuously for more than 2 weeks because these may be symptoms of serious underlying medical illnesses. Do not take this product if you have asthma, glaucoma, emphysema, chronic pulmonary disease, shortness of breath, difficulty in breathing, or difficulty in urination due to enlargement of the prostate gland unless directed by a doctor. Avoid alcoholic beverages while taking this product. Do not take this product if you are taking sedatives or tranquilizers, without first consulting your doctor.

Overdose:

MUCOMYST (acetylcysteine) As An Antidote For Acetaminophen Overdose)

Acetaminophen is rapidly absorbed from the upper gastrointestinal tract with peak plasma levels occurring between 30 and 60 minutes after therapeutic doses and usually within 4 hours following an overdose. The parent compound, which is nontoxic, is extensively metabolized in the liver to form principally the sulfate and glucuronide conjugates which are also nontoxic and are rapidly excreted in the urine. A small fraction of an ingested dose is metabolized in the liver by the cytochrome P-450 mixed function oxidase enzyme system to form a reactive, potentially toxic, intermediate metabolite which preferentially conjugates with hepatic glutathione to form the nontoxic cysteine and mercapturic acid derivatives which are then excreted by the kidney. Therapeutic doses of acetaminophen do not saturate the glucuronide and sulfate conjugation pathways and do not result in the formation of sufficient reactive metabolite to deplete glutathione stores. However, following ingestion of a large overdose (150 mg/kg or greater) the glucuronide and sulfate conjugation pathways are saturated resulting in a larger fraction of the drug being metabolized via the P-450 pathway. The in-

	EXCEDRIN® PM Per Tablet or Caplet	EXCEDRIN® PM Per Fl. Ounce (30 ml.)
Acetaminophen	500 mg.	1000 mg.
Diphenhydramine Citrate:	38 mg.	—
Diphenhydramine HCl:	—	50 mg

Other Ingredients:

Tablet	Caplet	Liquid
Corn Starch	Benzoic Acid	Alcohol (10% by volume)
D&C Yellow No. 10	Carnauba Wax	Benzoic Acid
D&C Yellow No. 10 Aluminum Lake	Corn Starch	FD&C Blue No. 1
FD&C Blue No. 1	D&C Yellow No. 10	Flavor
FD&C Blue No. 1 Aluminum Lake	D&C Yellow No. 10 Aluminum Lake	Polyethylene Glycol
Magnesium Stearate	FD&C Blue No. 1	Povidone
Methylparaben	FD&C Blue No. 1 Aluminum Lake	Sodium Citrate
Propylparaben	Hydroxypropyl Methylcellulose	Sucrose
Stearic Acid	Methylparaben	Water
	Magnesium Stearate	
	Propylene Glycol	
	Propylparaben	
	Simethicone Emulsion	
	Stearic Acid	
	Titanium Dioxide	

May Also Contain:
Microcrystalline Cellulose
Povidone

creased formation of reactive metabolite may deplete the hepatic stores of glutathione with subsequent binding of the metabolite to protein molecules within the hepatocyte resulting in cellular necrosis. Acetylcysteine has been shown to reduce the extent of liver injury following acetaminophen overdose. Early symptoms following a potentially hepatotoxic overdose may include: nausea, vomiting, diaphoresis and general malaise. Clinical and laboratory evidence of hepatic toxicity may not be apparent until 48 to 72 hours postingestion. In adults and adolescents, regardless of the quantity of acetaminophen reported to have been ingested, administer MUCOMYST® acetylcysteine immediately. MUCOMYST acetylcysteine therapy should be initiated and continued for a full course of therapy. Its effectiveness depends on early administration, with benefit seen principally in patients treated within 16 hours of the overdose.

If acetaminophen plasma assay capability is not available, and the estimated acetaminophen ingestion exceeds 150 mg/kg, MUCOMYST acetylcysteine therapy should be initiated and continued for a full course of therapy.

For full prescribing information, refer to the MUCOMYST package insert. Do not await the results of assays for acetaminophen level before initiating treatment with MUCOMYST acetylcysteine. The following additional procedures are recommended: The stomach should be emptied promptly by lavage or by induction of emesis with syrup of ipecac. A serum acetaminophen assay should be obtained as early as possible, but no sooner than four hours following ingestion. Liver function studies should be obtained initially and repeated at 24-hour intervals.

For additional emergency information call your regional poison center or toll-free (1-800-525-6115) to the Rocky Mountain Poison Center for assistance in diagnosis and for directions in the use of MUCOMYST acetylcysteine as an antidote.

How Supplied: EXCREDRIN P.M.® is supplied as:

Light blue circular tablets with "PM" debossed on one side.

NDC 19810-0763-6 Bottles of 10's
NDC 19810-0763-3 Bottles of 30's
NDC 19810-0763-4 Bottles of 50's
NDC 19810-0763-5 Bottles of 80's
NDC 19810-0763-9 Vials of 10's

Light blue coated caplet with "Excedrin P.M." imprinted on one side.

NDC 19810-0032-2 Bottles of 30's
NDC 19810-0032-3 Bottles of 50's

Light blue wild berry flavored liquid.

NDC 19810-0060-1 6 oz. (177 ml) Plastic Bottle

All sizes packaged in child resistant closures except 50's tablets and caplets which are recommended for households without young children.

Store at room temperature

Shown in Product Identification Section, page 405

Sinus EXCEDRIN®
[ex "cĕd 'rĭn]
Analgesic, Decongestant

Composition: Each coated tablet or caplet contains 500 mg Acetaminophen and 30 mg Pseudoephedrine HCl.

Other Ingredients: Corn Starch, D&C Yellow No. 10 Lake, FD&C Red No. 40 Lake, Hydroxypropyl Methylcellulose, Mineral Oil, Polysorbate 20, Povidone, Propylene Glycol, Simethicone Emulsion, Sorbitan Monolaurate, Stearic Acid, Titanium Dioxide. May also contain: Benzoic Acid, Carnauba Wax.

Indications: For temporary relief of headache, sinus pain and sinus pressure and congestion due to sinusitis or the common cold.

Directions: Adults: 2 tablets or caplets every 6 hours while symptoms persist, not to exceed 8 tablets or caplets in 24 hours, or as directed by a doctor. Children under 12 years of age: Consult a doctor.

Warnings: KEEP THIS AND ALL MEDICATIONS OUT OF THE REACH OF CHILDREN. IN CASE OF ACCIDENTAL OVERDOSE, SEEK PROFESSIONAL ASSISTANCE OR CONTACT A POISON CONTROL CENTER IMMEDIATELY. PROMPT MEDICAL ATTENTION IS CRITICAL FOR ADULTS AS WELL AS FOR CHILDREN EVEN IF YOU DO NOT NOTICE ANY SIGNS OR SYMPTOMS. As with any drug, if you are pregnant or nursing a baby, seek the advice of a health professional before using this product. Do not take this product for more than 10 days unless directed by a doctor. If symptoms do not improve or are accompanied by a fever that lasts for more than 3 days, or if new symptoms occur, consult a doctor. Do not exceed recommended dosage because at higher doses nervousness, dizziness or sleeplessness may occur. Do not take this product if you have heart disease, high blood pressure, thyroid disease, diabetes, or difficulty in urination due to enlargement of the prostate gland unless directed by a doctor.

Drug Interaction Precaution: Do not take this product if you are taking a prescription medication for high blood pressure or depression without first consulting a doctor.

Overdose:
MUCOMYST (acetylcysteine) As An Antidote for Acetaminophen Overdose)

Acetaminophen is rapidly absorbed from the upper gastrointestinal tract with peak plasma levels occurring between 30 and 60 minutes after therapeutic doses and usually within 4 hours following an overdose. The parent compound, which is nontoxic, is extensively metabolized in the liver to form principally the sulfate and glucuronide conjugates which are also nontoxic and are rapidly excreted in the urine. A small fraction of an ingested dose is metabolized in the liver by the cytochrome P-450 mixed function oxidase enzyme system to form a reactive, potentially toxic, intermediate metabolite which preferentially conjugates with hepatic glutathione to form the nontoxic cysteine and mercapturic acid derivatives which are then excreted by the kidney. Therapeutic doses of acetaminophen do not saturate the glucuronide and sulfate conjugation pathways and do not result in the formation of sufficient reactive metabolite to deplete glutathione stores. However, following ingestion of a large overdose (150 mg/kg or greater) the glucuronide and sulfate conjugation pathways are saturated resulting in a larger fraction of the drug being metabolized via the P-450 pathway. The increased formation of reactive metabolite may deplete the hepatic stores of glutathione with subsequent binding of the metabolite to protein molecules within the hepatocyte resulting in cellular necrosis. Acetylcysteine has been shown to reduce the extent of liver injury following acetaminophen overdose. Early symptoms following a potentially hepatotoxic overdose may include: nausea, vomiting, diaphoresis and general malaise. Clinical and laboratory evidence of hepatic toxicity may not be apparent until 48 to 72 hours postingestion. In adults and adolescents, regardless of the quantity of acetaminophen reported to have been ingested, administer MUCOMYST® acetylcysteine immediately. MUCOMYST acetylcysteine therapy should be initiated and continued for a full course of therapy. Its effectiveness depends on early administration, with benefit seen principally in patients treated within 16 hours of the overdose.

If acetaminophen plasma assay capability is not available, and the estimated acetaminophen ingestion exceeds 150 mg/kg, MUCOMYST acetylcysteine therapy should be initiated and continued for a full course of therapy.

For full prescribing information, refer to the MUCOMYST package insert. Do not await the results of assays for acetaminophen level before initiating treatment with MUCOMYST acetylcysteine. The following additional procedures are recommended: The stomach should be emptied promptly by lavage or by induction of emesis with syrup of ipecac. A serum acetaminophen assay should be obtained as early as possible, but no sooner than four hours following ingestion. Liver function studies should be obtained initially and repeated at 24-hour intervals.

For additional emergency information call your regional poison center or toll-free (1-800-525-6115) to the Rocky Mountain Poison Center for assistance in diagnosis and for directions in the use of MUCOMYST acetylcysteine as an antidote.

How Supplied: Sinus EXCEDRIN® is supplied as:

Coated circular orange tablets with "Sinus Excedrin" imprinted in green on one side.

NDC 19810-0080-1 Blister packages of 24's

Continued on next page

Bristol-Myers—Cont.

NDC 19810-0080-2 Bottles of 50's
Coated orange caplets with "Sinus Excedrin" imprinted in green on one side.
NDC 19810-0077-1 Blister packages of 24's
NDC 19810-0077-2 Bottles of 50's
All sizes have child resistant closures except 24's for tablets and caplets which are recommended for households without young children.
Store at room temperature.

Shown in Product Identification Section, page 405

4-WAY® Cold Tablets

Composition: Each tablet contains acetaminophen 325 mg., phenylpropanolamine HCl 12.5 mg., and chlorpheniramine maleate 2 mg. Other Ingredients: Corn Starch, Corn Starch Pregelatinized, Microcrystalline Cellulose, Sodium Starch Glycolate, Stearic Acid, Sucrose.

Indications: For temporary relief of nasal and sinus congestion, runny nose, sneezing, fever, minor sore throat pain, body aches and pain.

Directions:
Adults: 2 tablets every 4 hours while symptoms persist, not to exceed 12 tablets in 24 hours, or as directed by a doctor. Children 6 to under 12 years of age: One tablet every 4 hours while symptoms persist, not to exceed 5 tablets in 24 hours, or as directed by a doctor. Children under 6: Consult a doctor.

Warnings: KEEP THIS AND ALL OTHER MEDICATIONS OUT OF THE REACH OF CHILDREN. IN CASE OF ACCIDENTAL OVERDOSE, SEEK PROFESSIONAL ASSISTANCE OR CONTACT A POISON CONTROL CENTER IMMEDIATELY. PROMPT MEDICAL ATTENTION IS CRITICAL FOR ADULTS AS WELL AS FOR CHILDREN EVEN IF YOU DO NOT NOTICE ANY SIGNS OR SYMPTOMS. As with any drug, if you are pregnant or nursing a baby, seek the advice of a health professional before using this product. Do not take this product for more than 10 days (for adults) or 5 days (for children) unless directed by a doctor. If symptoms do not improve or are accompanied by a fever that lasts for more than 3 days, or if new symptoms occur, consult a doctor. Do not exceed recommended dosage because at higher doses nervousness, dizziness or sleeplessness may occur. May cause excitability especially in children. If sore throat is severe, persists for more than 2 days, is accompanied or followed by a fever, headache, rash, nausea or vomiting, consult a doctor promptly. This product should not be taken by persons who have asthma, glaucoma, emphysema, chronic pulmonary disease, high blood pressure, heart disease, thyroid disease, diabetes, shortness of breath, difficulty in breathing or difficulty in urination due to enlargement of the prostate gland unless directed by a doctor. May cause drowsiness; alcohol may increase the drowsiness effect. Avoid alcoholic beverages, and do not take this product if you are taking sedatives or tranquilizers without first consulting your doctor. Use caution when driving a motor vehicle or operating machinery.

Drug Interaction Precaution: This product should not be taken by any adult or child who is taking a prescription medication for high blood pressure or depression without first consulting a doctor.

Overdose:
MUCOMYST (acetylcysteine) As An Antidote For Acetaminophen Overdose)
Acetaminophen is rapidly absorbed from the upper gastrointestinal tract with peak plasma levels occurring between 30 and 60 minutes after therapeutic doses and usually within 4 hours following an overdose. The parent compound, which is nontoxic, is extensively metabolized in the liver to form principally the sulfate and glucuronide conjugates which are also nontoxic and are rapidly excreted in the urine. A small fraction of an ingested dose is metabolized in the liver by the cytochrome P-450 mixed function oxidase enzyme system to form a reactive, potentially toxic, intermediate metabolite which preferentially conjugates with hepatic glutathione to form the nontoxic cysteine and mercapturic acid derivatives which are then excreted by the kidney. Therapeutic doses of acetaminophen do not saturate the glucuronide and sulfate conjugation pathways and do not result in the formation of sufficient reactive metabolite to deplete glutathione stores. However, following ingestion of a large overdose (150 mg/kg or greater) the glucuronide and sulfate conjugation pathways are saturated resulting in a larger fraction of the drug being metabolized via the P-450 pathway. The increased formation of reactive metabolite may deplete the hepatic stores of glutathione with subsequent binding of the metabolite to protein molecules within the hepatocyte resulting in cellular necrosis. Acetylcysteine has been shown to reduce the extent of liver injury following acetaminophen overdose. Early symptoms following a potentially hepatotoxic overdose may include: nausea, vomiting, diaphoresis and general malaise. Clinical and laboratory evidence of hepatic toxicity may not be apparent until 48 to 72 hours postingestion. In adults and adolescents, regardless of the quantity of acetaminophen reported to have been ingested, administer MUCOMYST® acetylcysteine immediately. MUCOMYST acetylcysteine therapy should be initiated and continued for a full course of therapy. Its effectiveness depends on early administration, with benefit seen principally in patients treated within 16 hours of the overdose. If acetaminophen plasma assay capability is not available, and the estimated acetaminophen ingestion exceeds 150 mg/kg., MUCOMYST acetylcysteine therapy should be initiated and continued for a full course of therapy. For full prescribing information, refer to the MUCOMYST package insert. Do not await the results of assays for acetaminophen level before initiating treatment with MUCOMYST acetylcysteine. The following additional procedures are recommended: The stomach should be emptied promptly by lavage or by induction of emesis with syrup of ipecac. A serum acetaminophen assay should be obtained as early as possible, but no sooner than four hours following ingestion. Liver function studies should be obtained initially and repeated at 24-hour intervals.
For additional emergency information call your regional poison center or toll-free (1-800-525-6115) to the Rocky Mountain Poison Center for assistance in diagnosis and for directions in the use of MUCOMYST acetylcysteine as an antidote.

How Supplied: 4-WAY Cold Tablets are supplied as a white tablet with the number "4" debossed on one surface.
NDC 19810-0040-1 Bottle of 36's
NDC 19810-0040-2 Bottle of 60's
All sizes packaged in child resistant bottle closures.
Store at room temperature.

Shown in Product Identification Section, page 405

4-WAY® Fast Acting Nasal Spray

Composition:
Original Formula: Phenylephrine hydrochloride 0.5%, naphazoline hydrochloride 0.05%, pyrilamine maleate 0.2%, in a buffered isotonic aqueous solution with thimerosal 0.005% added as a preservative. Also Contains: Benzalkonium Chloride, Poloxamer 188, Potassium Phosphate, Sodium Chloride, Sodium Phosphate, Water. Also available in a mentholated formula containing Phenylephrine hydrochloride 0.5%, naphazoline hydrochloride 0.05%, pyrilamine maleate 0.2%, in a buffered isotonic aqueous solution with thimerosal 0.005% added as a preservative. Also Contains: Benzalkonium Chloride, Camphor, Eucalyptol, Menthol, Poloxamer 188, Polysorbate 80, Potassium Phosphate, Sodium Chloride, Sodium Phosphate, Water.

New Formula: Phenylephrine Hydrochloride 0.5% in a buffered isotonic solution. Also contains: Benzalkonium Chloride, Disodium EDTA, Potassium Phosphate, Sodium Chloride, Sodium Phosphate, Water. Also available in a mentholated formula containing Phenylephrine Hydrochloride 0.5% in a buffered isotonic solution. Also contains: Benzalkonium Chloride, Camphor, Disodium EDTA, Eucalyptol, Menthol, Poloxamer 188, Polysorbate 80, Potassium Phosphate, Sodium Chloride, Sodium Phosphate, Water.

Indications: For prompt, temporary relief of nasal congestion due to the common cold, sinusitis, hay fever or other upper respiratory allergies.

Directions and Use Instructions:
Directions: Adults: Spray twice into each nostril not more often than every 4 hours. Do not give to children under 12 years of age unless directed by a doctor.
Use Instructions: For Metered Pump—Remove protective cap. Hold bottle with thumb at base and nozzle between first and second fingers. With head upright, insert metered pump spray nozzle into nostril. Depress pump all the way down, with a firm even stroke and sniff deeply. Repeat in other nostril. Do not tilt head backward while spraying. Wipe tip clean after each use. Note: This bottle is filled to correct level for proper pump action. Before using the first time, remove the protective cap from the tip and prime the metered pump by depressing pump firmly several times.
Use Instructions: For Atomizer—
With head in a normal upright position, put atomizer tip into nostril. Squeeze bottle with firm, quick pressure while inhaling.

Warnings: **KEEP THIS AND ALL OTHER MEDICATIONS OUT OF THE REACH OF CHILDREN. IN CASE OF ACCIDENTAL OVERDOSE OR INGESTION, SEEK PROFESSIONAL ASSISTANCE OR CONTACT A POISON CONTROL CENTER IMMEDIATELY.** Do not exceed recommended dosage because burning, stinging, sneezing, or increase of nasal discharge may occur. The use of this container by more than one person may spread infection. Do not use this product for more than 3 days. If symptoms persist, consult a doctor. Adults and children who have heart disease, high blood pressure, thyroid disease, diabetes, or difficulty in urination due to an enlargement of the prostate gland should not use this product unless directed by a doctor.

How Supplied:
4-WAY® Fast Acting Nasal Spray is supplied as:
Original Regular formula:
NDC 19810-0001-1 Atomizer of ½ fluid ounce.
NDC 19810-0001-2 Atomizer of 1 fluid ounce.
NDC 19810-0001-3 Metered pump of ½ fluid ounce.
Original Mentholated formula:
NDC 19810-0003-1 Atomizer of ½ fluid ounce.
NDC 19810-0003-2 Atomizer of 1 fluid ounce.
New Regular formula:
NDC 19810-0047-1 Atomizer of ½ fluid ounce.
NDC 19810-0047-2 Atomizer of 1 fluid ounce.
NDC 19810-0047-3 Metered pump of ½ fluid ounce.
New Mentholated formula:
NDC 19810-0049-1 Atomizer of ½ fluid ounce.
Store at room temperature.

Shown in Product Identification Section, page 405

4-WAY® Long Lasting Nasal Spray

Composition: Oxymetazoline Hydrochloride 0.05% in a buffered isotonic aqueous solution. **Also Contains:** Benzalkonium Chloride, Glycine, Sorbitol, Water. May also contain: Disodium EDTA, Phenylmercuric Acetate, Sodium Hydroxide.

Indications: For prompt, temporary relief of nasal congestion due to the common cold, sinusitis, hay fever or other upper respiratory allergies.

Directions and Use Instructions:
Directions: Adults and children 6 to under 12 years of age (with adult supervision): 2 or 3 sprays in each nostril not more often than every 10 to 12 hours. Do not exceed 2 applications in any 24-hour period. Children under 6 years of age: Consult a doctor.
Use Instructions: For Metered Pump—Remove protective cap. Hold bottle with thumb at base and nozzle between first and second fingers. With head upright, insert metered pump spray nozzle into nostril. Depress pump all the way down, with a firm even stroke and sniff deeply. Repeat in other nostril. Do not tilt head backward while spraying. Wipe tip clean after each use. Note: This bottle is filled to correct level for proper pump action. Before using the first time, remove the protective cap from the tip and prime the metered pump by depressing pump firmly several times.
Use Instructions: For Atomizer—
With head in a normal, upright position, put atomizer tip into nostril. Squeeze bottle with firm, quick pressure while inhaling.

Warnings: KEEP THIS AND ALL OTHER MEDICATIONS OUT OF THE REACH OF CHILDREN. IN CASE OF ACCIDENTAL OVERDOSE OR INGESTION, SEEK PROFESSIONAL ASSISTANCE OR CONTACT A POISON CONTROL CENTER IMMEDIATELY. Do not exceed recommended dosage because burning, stinging, sneezing, or increase of nasal discharge may occur. The use of this container by more than one person may spread infection. Do not use this product for more than 3 days. If symptoms persist, consult a doctor. Adults and children who have heart disease, high blood pressure, thyroid disease, diabetes, or difficulty in urination due to enlargement of the prostate gland should not use this product unless directed by a doctor.

How Supplied: 4-WAY Long Lasting Nasal Spray is supplied as:
Atomizers and a metered pump:
NDC 19810-0728-1 Atomizers of ½ fluid ounce.
NDC 19810-0728-3 Metered pump of ½ fluid ounce.
NDC 19810-0048-1 Atomizer of ½ fluid ounce.
Store at room temperature.

Shown in Product Identification Section, page 405

KERI LOTION
Skin Lubricant—Moisturizer

Available in two formulations:
KERI Original and KERI Fresh Herbal Scent—recommended for dry skin.

Composition: Mineral oil in water, propylene glycol, glyceryl stearate/PEG-100 stearate, PEG-40 stearate, PEG-4 dilaurate, laureth-4, lanolin oil, methylparaben, propylparaben, fragrance, carbomer-934, triethanolamine, dioctyl sodium sulfosuccinate, quaternium-15. Fresh Herbal scent: FD&C blue 1, D&C yellow 10.

KERI-Silky Smooth—recommended for daily use on dry skin.

Composition: Water, petrolatum, glycerin, dimethicone, steareth-2, cetyl alcohol, benzyl alcohol, laureth-23, carbomer-934, MgAl silicate, fragrance, quaternium-15, sodium hydroxide.

Indications: KERI Lotion lubricates and helps hydrate the skin, making it soft and smooth. It relieves itching, helps maintain a normal moisture balance and supplements the protective action of skin lipids. Indicated for generalized dryness; detergent hands; chapped or chafed skin; "winter-itch," diaper rash; heat rash.

Directions for Use: Apply as often as needed. Use particularly after bathing and exposure to sun, water, soaps and detergents. For external use only.

How Supplied: KERI Lotion Original 6½ oz., 13 oz. and 20 oz. plastic bottles. KERI Lotion Fresh Herbal Scent 6½ oz., 13 oz. and 20 oz. plastic bottles. KERI Silky Smooth 6½ oz., 13 oz. and 20 oz. plastic bottles.

Shown in Product Identification Section, page 406

NO DOZ® Tablets
[*nō 'dōz*]

Composition: Each tablet contains 100 mg. Caffeine. Other Ingredients: Cornstarch, Flavors, Mannitol, Microcrystalline Cellulose, Stearic Acid, Sucrose.

Indications: Helps restore mental alertness or wakefulness when experiencing fatigue or drowsiness.

Directions: Adults 1 or 2 tablets not more often than every 3 to 4 hours.

Warnings: KEEP THIS AND ALL OTHER MEDICATIONS OUT OF THE REACH OF CHILDREN. IN CASE OF ACCIDENTAL OVERDOSE, SEEK PROFESSIONAL ASSISTANCE OR CONTACT A POISON CONTROL CENTER IMMEDIATELY. As with any drug, if you are pregnant or nursing a baby, seek the advice of a health professional before using this product. Do not give to children under 12 years of age. For occasional use only. Not intended for use as a substitute for sleep. If fatigue or drowsiness persists or continues to occur, consult a doctor. The recommended dose of this product contains about as much caf-

Continued on next page

Bristol-Myers—Cont.

feine as a cup of coffee. Limit the use of caffeine-containing medications, foods, or beverages while taking this product because too much caffeine may cause nervousness, irritability, sleeplessness and, occasionally, rapid heart beat.

How Supplied: NO DOZ® is supplied as:
A circular white tablet with "NoDoz" debossed on one side.
NDC 19810-0063-2 Blister pack of 16's
NDC 19810-0063-3 Blister pack of 36's
NDC 19810-0062-5 Bottle of 60's
NDC 19810-0063-1 Vials of 15's
Store at room temperature.

Shown in Product Identification Section, page 406

NO DOZ® Maximum Strength Caplets

Composition: Each caplet contains 200 mg. Caffeine. Other ingredients: Benzoic Acid, Corn Starch, FD&C Blue No. 1, Flavors, Hydroxypropyl Methylcellulose, Microcrystalline Cellulose, Propylene Glycol, Simethicone Emulsion, Stearic Acid, Sucrose, Titanium Dioxide. May also contain: Carnauba Wax, Mineral Oil, Polysorbate 20, Povidone, Sorbitan Monolaurate.

Indications: Helps restore mental alertness or wakefulness when experiencing fatigue or drowsiness.

Directions: Adults: one-half to one caplet not more often than every 3 to 4 hours.

Warnings: KEEP THIS AND ALL OTHER MEDICATIONS OUT OF THE REACH OF CHILDREN. IN CASE OF ACCIDENTAL OVERDOSE, SEEK PROFESSIONAL ASSISTANCE OR CONTACT A POISON CONTROL CENTER IMMEDIATELY. As with any drug, if you are pregnant or nursing a baby, seek the advice of a health professional before using this product. Do not give to children under 12 years of age. For occasional use only. Not intended for use as a substitute for sleep. If fatigue or drowsiness persists or continues to occur, consult a doctor. The recommended dose of this product contains about as much caffeine as a cup of coffee. Limit the use of caffeine-containing medications, foods, or beverages while taking this product because too much caffeine may cause nervousness, irritability, sleeplessness and, occasionally, rapid heart beat.

How Supplied: NO DOZ® Maximum Strength is supplied as: White coated caplets with "NO DOZ" debossed on one side. The opposite side is scored.
NDC 19810-0064-1 Blister Packs of 12's
Store at room temperature.

NUPRIN®
(ibuprofen)
Analgesic

Warning: ASPIRIN SENSITIVE PATIENTS. Do not take this product if you have had a severe allergic reaction to aspirin, e.g.—asthma, swelling, shock or hives, because even though this product contains no aspirin or salicylates, cross-reactions may occur in patients allergic to aspirin. (See ADDITIONAL WARNINGS BELOW)

Composition: Each tablet or caplet contains ibuprofen USP, 200 mg. **Other Ingredients:** Carnauba wax, cornstarch, D&C Yellow No. 10, FD&C Yellow No. 6, hydroxypropyl methylcellulose, propylene glycol, silicon dioxide, stearic acid, titanium dioxide.

Indications: For the temporary relief of minor aches and pains associated with the common cold, headache, toothache, muscular aches, backache, for the minor pain of arthritis, for the pain of menstrual cramps and for reduction of fever.

Additional Warnings: The following warnings are stated on the Nuprin label: Do not take for pain for more than 10 days or for fever for more than 3 days unless directed by a doctor. If pain or fever persists or gets worse, if new symptoms occur, or if the painful area is red or swollen, consult a doctor. These could be signs of serious illness. If you are under a doctor's care for any serious condition, consult a doctor before taking this product. As with aspirin and acetaminophen, if you have any condition which requires you to take prescription drugs or if you have had any problems or serious side effects from taking any non-prescription pain reliever, do not take NUPRIN without first discussing it with your doctor. If you experience any symptoms which are unusual or seem unrelated to the condition for which you took ibuprofen, consult a doctor before taking any more of it. Although ibuprofen is indicated for the same conditions as aspirin and acetaminophen, it should not be taken with them except under a doctor's direction. Do not combine this product with any other ibuprofen-containing product. As with any drug, if you are pregnant or nursing a baby, seek the advice of a health professional before using this product. IT IS ESPECIALLY IMPORTANT NOT TO USE IBUPROFEN DURING THE LAST 3 MONTHS OF PREGNANCY UNLESS SPECIFICALLY DIRECTED TO DO SO BY A DOCTOR BECAUSE IT MAY CAUSE PROBLEMS IN THE UNBORN CHILD OR COMPLICATIONS DURING DELIVERY. Keep this and all drugs out of the reach of children. In case of accidental overdose, seek professional assistance or contact a poison control center immediately.

Caution: Store at room temperature. Avoid excessive heat 40°C (104°F).

Directions: Adults: Take 1 tablet or caplet every 4 to 6 hours while symptoms persist. If pain or fever does not respond to 1 tablet or caplet, 2 tablets or caplets may be used but do not exceed 6 tablets or caplets in 24 hours, unless directed by a doctor. The smallest effective dose should be used. Take with food or milk if occasional and mild heartburn, upset stomach, or stomach pain occurs with use. Consult a doctor if these symptoms are more than mild or if they persist. Children: Do not give this product to children under 12 except under the advice and supervision of a doctor.

How Supplied:
NUPRIN® is supplied as:
Golden yellow round tablets with "NUPRIN" printed in black on one side.
NDC 19810-0767-2 Bottles of 24's
NDC 19810-0767-3 Bottles of 50's
NDC 19810-0767-4 Bottles of 100's
NDC 19810-0767-7 Bottles of 150's
NDC 19810-0767-8 Bottles of 225's
NDC 19810-0767-9 Vials of 10's
Golden yellow caplets with "NUPRIN" printed in black on one side.
NDC 19810-0796-1 Bottles of 24's
NDC 19810-0796-2 Bottles of 50's
NDC 19810-0796-3 Bottles of 100's
All sizes packaged in child resistant closures except 24's for tablets and 24's for caplets, which are sizes recommended for households without young children.
Store at room temperature. Avoid excessive heat 40°C. (104°F.).
Distributed by Bristol-Myers Company

Shown in Product Identification Section, page 406

PAZO® Hemorrhoid Ointment/Suppositories

Composition:
Ointment: Triolyte®, [Bristol-Myers brand of the combination of benzocaine (0.8%) and ephedrine sulphate (0.2%)]; zinc oxide (4.0%); camphor (2.18%). Also Contains: Lanolin, Petrolatum.
Suppositories (per suppository): Triolyte® [Bristol-Myers brand of the combination of benzocaine (15.44 mg) and ephedrine sulfate (3.86 mg)]; zinc oxide (77.2 mg); camphor (42.07 mg). Also Contains: Hydrogenated Vegetable Oil.

Indications: Pazo helps shrink swelling of inflamed hemorrhoid tissue. Provides prompt, temporary relief of burning itch and pain in many cases.

Directions:
Ointment—Apply Pazo well up in rectum night and morning, and after each bowel movement. Repeat as often during the day as may be necessary to maintain comfort. Continue for one week after symptoms subside. When applicator is used, lubricate applicator first with Pazo. Insert slowly, then simply press tube.
Suppositories—Remove foil and insert one Pazo suppository night and morning, and after each bowel movement. Repeat as often during the day as may be necessary to maintain comfort. Continue for one week after symptoms subside.

Warning: If the underlying condition persists or recurs frequently, despite treatment, or if any bleeding or hard irreducible swelling is present, consult your physician.
Keep out of children's reach. Keep in a cool place.

How Supplied: PAZO® ointment is supplied with a plastic applicator as:

NDC 19810-0768-1 One ounce tubes
NDC 19810-0768-2 Two ounce tubes
PAZO® suppositories are silver foil wrapped and supplied as:
NDC 19810-0703-1 Box of 12's
NDC 19810-0703-2 Box of 24's
Keep in a cool place.

Shown in Product Identification Section, page 406

PRESUN® FOR KIDS
Children's Sunscreen

Active Ingredients: Octyl methoxycinnamate, oxybenzone, octyl salicylate. Also contains: Carbomer-940, cetyl alcohol, diazolidinyl urea, dimethicone, methylchloroisothiazolinone and methylisothiazolinone, stearic acid, triethanolamine, water and other ingredients.

Indications: 29 TIMES NATURAL PROTECTION: Used as directed, PRESUN For Kids provides 29 times your child's natural sunburn protection and may help reduce the chance of premature aging and wrinkling of the skin.
NONSTINGING: A non-PABA, fragrance-free formula that is designed not to sting sensitive skin. (Avoid contact with eyes since all sunscreens can cause irritation and stinging of the eye.)
HYPOALLERGENIC: PRESUN For Kids is hypoallergenic and, because the known sensitizers common to most sunscreens have been removed, is suitable for your child's sensitive skin.
WATERPROOF 29: PRESUN For Kids maintains its degree of protection (SPF 29) even after 80 minutes in the water.

Warnings: For external use only. Protect from freezing. *As with all sunscreens:* Apply to a small area; check after 24 hours. Discontinue use if irritation or rash appears. Avoid contact with eyes. In case of contact, flush eyes with water. Keep out of the reach of children. Use on children under six months of age only with the advice of a physician.

Directions for Use: For maximum protection, smooth evenly and liberally onto dry skin before sun exposure. Massage in gently. Reapplication to dry skin after prolonged swimming, excessive perspiration or towel drying is recommended for all-day protection.

How Supplied: 4 oz. plastic bottle.

PRESUN® 8, 15 and 39 CREAMY SUNSCREENS

Active Ingredients: Octyl dimethyl PABA, oxybenzone. Also contains: Carbomer-940, cetyl alcohol, diazolidinyl urea, dimethicone, fragrance, methylchloroisothiazolinone and methylisothiazolinone, stearic acid, triethanolamine, water, and other ingredients.

Indications: 8, 15 or 39 TIMES NATURAL PROTECTION: Used as directed. PRESUN Creamy Sunscreens provide 8, 15 or 39 times your natural sunburn protection and may help reduce the chance of premature aging and wrinkling of the skin as well as skin cancer caused by overexposure to the sun.
WATERPROOF PRESUN Creamy Sunscreen maintains its degree of protection even after 80 minutes in the water.

Warnings: For external use only. Protect from freezing. Do not use if sensitive to *p*-aminobenzoic acid (PABA) or related compounds. *As with all sunscreens:* Apply to a small area; check after 24 hours. Discontinue use if irritation or rash appears. Avoid contact with eyes. In case of contact, flush eyes with water. Keep out of the reach of children. Use on children under six months of age only with the advice of a physician.

Directions for Use: Smooth evenly onto dry skin before sun exposure. Massage in gently. Reapply to dry skin after prolonged swimming, excessive perspiration or towel drying. Repeated applications during prolonged sun exposure are recommended.

How Supplied: 8 Creamy: 4 oz. plastic bottle. 15 Creamy: 4 oz. plastic bottle. 39 Creamy: 4 oz. plastic bottle.

PRESUN® 15 FACIAL SUNSCREEN

Active Ingredients: Octyl dimethyl PABA, oxybenzone. Also contains: Benzyl alcohol, carbomer 934, cetyl alcohol, dimethicone, glyceryl stearate, laureth-23, magnesium aluminum silicate, petrolatum, propylene glycol dioctanoate, quaternium-15, sodium hydroxide, steareth-2 and water.

Indications: 15 TIMES NATURAL PROTECTION: Used as directed, PRESUN 15 Facial Sunscreen provides 15 times your natural *sunburn* protection and may help reduce the chance of premature aging and wrinkling of the skin as well as skin cancer caused by overexposure to the sun.
MOISTURIZES: PRESUN 15 Facial Sunscreen was developed especially for use on the face. The special moisturizers soften and smooth your skin while protecting it from the drying effects of the sun.
SUITABLE UNDER MAKE-UP: A non-greasy cream made especially for daily use under facial make-up and designed not to clog pores or cause acne or blemishes.

Directions for Use: Gently smooth evenly onto dry skin before sun exposure. Reapply to dry skin after swimming, excessive perspiration or towel drying. Repeated applications during prolonged sun exposure are recommended.

Warnings: For external use only. Do not use if sensitive to *p*-aminobenzoic acid (PABA) or related compounds. *As with all sunscreens:* Apply to a small area; check after 24 hours. Discontinue use if irritation or rash appears. Avoid contact with eyes. In case of contact, flush eyes with water. Keep out of reach of children. Use on children under six months of age only with the advice of a physician.

How Supplied: 2 oz. plastic tube.

PRESUN® 23 and PRESUN® FOR KIDS
Spray Mist Sunscreens

Active Ingredients: Octyl dimethyl PABA, octyl methoxycinnamate, oxybenzone, octyl salicylate. Also contains: C_{12-15} alcohols benzoate, cyclomethicone, PG dioctanoate, PVP hexadecene, copolymer, and 19% (w/w) SD alcohol 40.

Indications: 23 TIMES NATURAL PROTECTION: Used as directed, PRESUN 23 and PRESUN For Kids Spray Mist Sunscreens provide 23 times your natural sunburn protection and may help reduce the chance of premature aging and wrinkling of the skin.
WATERPROOF 23: PRESUN 23 and PRESUN For Kids Spray Mist Sunscreens maintain their degree of protection (SPF 23) even after 80 minutes in the water.
Convenience Spray: This revolutionary new spray bottle design is non-aerosol.

Directions for Use: For best results, hold bottle about ten inches away from body while spraying. Massage in gently. Reapplication to dry skin after prolonged swimming, excessive perspiration or towel drying is recommended for all-day protection.

Warnings: For external use only. Do not use if sensitive to *p*-aminobenzoic acid (PABA) or related compounds. Avoid flame. Do not expose to heat or store above 86°F. As with all sunscreens: Apply to a small area; check after 24 hours. Discontinue use if irritation or rash appears. Avoid spraying in the eyes. In case of contact, flush eyes with water. Keep out of reach of children. Use on children under six months of age only with the advice of a physician.

How Supplied: 23 Spray Mist Sunscreen: 3.5 oz. plastic bottle with non-aerosol spray. For Kids Spray Mist Sunscreen: 3.5 oz. plastic bottle with non-aerosol spray.

PRESUN® 15 and 29 SENSITIVE SKIN SUNSCREENS
PABA-FREE Sunscreen Protection

Active Ingredients: Octyl methoxycinnamate, oxybenzone, octyl salicylate. Also contains: Carbomer-940, cetyl alcohol, diazolidinyl urea, dimethicone, methylchloroisothiazolinone and methylisothiazolinone, stearic acid, triethanolamine, water, and other ingredients.

Indications:
15 or 29 TIMES NATURAL PROTECTION: Used as directed, PRESUN 15 or 29 Sensitive Skin Sunscreen provides 15 or 29 times your natural *sunburn* protection and may help reduce the chance of premature aging and wrinkling of the skin as well as skin cancer caused by overexposure to the sun.
PABA-FREE FORMULAS: PABA- and fragrance-free formulas that provide a very high degree of sunburn protection and, because the known sensitizers com-

Continued on next page

Bristol-Myers—Cont.

mon to most sunscreens have been removed, is suitable for sensitive skin.
WATERPROOF: PRESUN Sensitive Skin Sunscreen maintains its degree of protection even after 80 minutes in the water.

Directions for Use: For maximum protection, smooth evenly and liberally onto dry skin before sun exposure. Massage in gently. Reapplication to dry skin after prolonged swimming, excessive perspiration or towel drying is recommended for all-day protection.

Warnings: For external use only. Protect from freezing. *As with all sunscreens:* Apply to a small area; check after 24 hours. Discontinue use if irritation or rash appears. Avoid contact with eyes. In case of contact, flush eyes with water. Keep out of the reach of children. Use on children under six months of age only with the advice of a physician.

How Supplied: 29 Sensitive Skin: 4 oz. (NSN 6505-01-267-1483) plastic bottle.
15 Sensitive Skin: 4 oz. plastic bottle.

Shown in Product Identification Section, page 406

THERAPEUTIC MINERAL ICE

Composition:
Active Ingredient: Menthol 2%
Other Ingredients: Ammonium Hydroxide, Carbomer 934, Cupric Sulfate, FD&C Blue No. 1, Isopropyl Alcohol, Magnesium Sulfate, Sodium Hydroxide, Thymol, Water.

Indications: For the temporary relief of minor aches and pains of muscles and joints associated with arthritis, simple backache, strains, bruises, sprains and sports injuries. **USE ONLY AS DIRECTED. Read all warnings before use.**

Warnings: KEEP OUT OF THE REACH OF CHILDREN. For external use only. Not for internal use. Avoid contact with eyes and mucous membranes. Do not use with other ointments, creams, sprays, or liniments. **Do not use with Heating Pads or Heating Devices.** If condition worsens, or if symptoms persist for more than 7 days, or clear up and occur again within a few days, discontinue use of this product and consult your doctor. Do not apply to wounds or damaged skin. Do not bandage tightly. If you have sensitive skin, consult doctor before use. If skin irritation develops, discontinue use and consult your doctor. As with any drug, if you are pregnant or nursing a baby, seek the advice of a health professional before using this product. Do not use, pour, spill or store near heat or open flame. **Note:** you can always use Mineral Ice as directed, but its use is never intended to replace your doctor's advice.

Directions: Adults and children 2 years of age and older: Clean skin of all other ointments, creams, sprays, or liniments. Apply to affected areas not more than 3 to 4 times daily. May be used with wet or dry bandages or with ice packs. Not greasy. No protective cover needed.
Children: Do not use on children under 2 years of age, except under the advice and supervision of a doctor.

How Supplied: Available in 3.5 oz., 8 oz., and 16 oz. containers.

Shown in Product Identification Section, page 406

THERAPEUTIC MINERAL ICE
Exercise Formula, Pain Relieving Gel

Composition:
Active Ingredient: Menthol 4%.
Other Ingredients: Ammonium Hydroxide, Carbomer 934P or Carbomer 934, Cupric Sulfate, FD&C Blue No. 1, Fragrance Isopropyl Alcohol, Magnesium Sulfate, Sodium Hydroxide, Thymol, Water.

Indications: For the temporary relief of minor aches and pains of muscles and joints associated with strains, sprains, bruises, sports injuries and simple backache. USE ONLY AS DIRECTED. Read all warnings before use.

Warnings: KEEP OUT OF REACH OF CHILDREN. For external use only. Not for internal use. Avoid contact with eyes and mucous membranes. Do not use with other ointments, creams, sprays, or liniments. DO NOT USE WITH HEATING PAD OR HEATING DEVICES. If condition worsens, or if symptoms persist for more than 7 days, or clear up and occur again within a few days, discontinue use of this product and consult your doctor. Do not apply to wounds or damaged skin. Do not bandage tightly. If you have sensitive skin, consult doctor BEFORE use. If skin irritation develops, discontinue use and consult your doctor. As with any drug, if you are pregnant or nursing a baby, seek the advice of a health professional before using this product. Do not use, pour, spill, or store near heat or open flame.
NOTE: You can always use MINERAL ICE® EXERCISE FORMULA as directed, but its use is never intended to replace your doctor's advice.

Directions: Adults and children 2 years of age and older: Clean skin of all other ointments, creams, sprays, or liniments. Apply to affected areas not more than 3 to 4 times daily. May be used with wet or dry bandages or with ice packs. Not greasy. No protective cover needed.
Children: Do not use on children under 2 years of age, except under the advice and supervision of a doctor.

How Supplied: Available in 3 oz. tubes.
STORE AT ROOM TEMPERATURE.
KEEP CAP TIGHTLY CLOSED.

Shown in Product Identification Section, page 406

Products are indexed by generic and chemical names in the **YELLOW SECTION**

Burroughs Wellcome Co.
3030 CORNWALLIS ROAD
RESEARCH TRIANGLE PARK, NC 27709

ACTIDIL® Syrup
ACTIDIL® Tablets
[*ăk 'tuh-dĭl*]

Indications: For the temporary relief of running nose, sneezing, itching of the nose or throat and itchy and watery eyes as may occur in allergic rhinitis (such as hay fever).

Directions: Syrup: Adults and children 12 years of age and over, 2 teaspoonfuls every 4 to 6 hours. Children 6 to under 12 years of age, 1 teaspoonful every 4 to 6 hours. Children under 6 years of age, consult a physician. Do not exceed 4 doses in 24 hours.
Tablets: Adults and children 12 years of age and over, 1 tablet every 4 to 6 hours. Children 6 to under 12 years of age, ½ tablet every 4 to 6 hours. Children under 6 years of age, consult a physician. Do not exceed 4 doses in 24 hours.

Warnings: May cause excitability especially in children. May cause drowsiness. Do not take this product if you have asthma, glaucoma or difficulty in urination due to enlargement of the prostate gland except under the advice and supervision of a physician. Do not give this product to children under 6 years except under the advice and supervision of a physician. As with any drug, if you are pregnant or nursing a baby, seek the advice of a health professional before using this product.

Caution: Avoid driving a motor vehicle or operating heavy machinery. Avoid alcoholic beverages while taking this product.

KEEP THIS AND ALL DRUGS OUT OF THE REACH OF CHILDREN. In case of accidental overdose, seek professional assistance or contact a Poison Control Center immediately.

Syrup

Active Ingredients: Each 5 mL (1 teaspoonful) contains triprolidine hydrochloride 1.25 mg.

Inactive Ingredients: alcohol 4%; methylparaben 0.1% and sodium benzoate 0.1% (added as preservatives), FD&C Yellow No. 6, flavor, glycerin, purified water, and sorbitol.

Store at 15° to 25°C (59° to 77°F) and protect from light.

Tablets

Active Ingredients: Each scored tablet contains triprolidine hydrochloride 2.5 mg.

Inactive Ingredients: Corn and potato starch, lactose, magnesium stearate.

Store at 15° to 25°C (59° to 77°F) in a dry place and protect from light.

How Supplied: Syrup, 1 pint; Tablets, bottle of 100.

Tablets Shown in Product Identification Section, page 406

ACTIFED® Capsules
[*ăk 'tuh-fĕd*]

Product Benefits: Each ACTIFED Capsule contains two important ingredients for relief from symptoms of the common cold, seasonal allergies (hay fever) and sinus congestion.

The **ANTIHISTAMINE** (triprolidine) temporarily dries runny nose and relieves sneezing associated with the common cold, hay fever or other upper respiratory allergies. Also relieves itching of the nose or throat, and itchy, watery eyes due to hay fever.

The **DECONGESTANT** (pseudoephedrine) temporarily relieves nasal congestion due to the common cold, hay fever or other upper respiratory allergies, or associated with sinusitis. Temporarily relieves nasal stuffiness. Reduces the swelling of nasal passages; shrinks swollen membranes; and temporarily restores freer breathing through the nose. Also, helps to decongest sinus openings and passages; relieves sinus pressure.

Each Actifed Capsule Contains: pseudoephedrine hydrochloride 60 mg and triprolidine hydrochloride 2.5 mg. Also contains: corn starch and magnesium stearate. The capsule shell consists of gelatin, D&C Yellow No. 10, FD&C Yellow No. 6, and titanium dioxide. May contain one or more parabens. Printed with edible black ink.

Directions: Adults and children 12 years of age and over, 1 capsule every 4 to 6 hours. Do not exceed 4 capsules in a 24 hour period. Children under 12 years of age, consult a physician.

Warnings: May cause excitability especially in children. Do not give this product to children under 12 years except under the advice and supervision of a physician. May cause drowsiness. Do not exceed recommended dosage because at higher doses nervousness, dizziness, or sleeplessness may occur. If symptoms do not improve within 7 days or are accompanied by high fever, consult a physician before continuing use. Do not take this product if you have high blood pressure, heart disease, diabetes, thyroid disease, asthma, glaucoma or difficulty in urination due to enlargement of the prostate gland except under the advice and supervision of a physician. As with any drug, if you are pregnant or nursing a baby, seek the advice of a health professional before using this product.

Drug Interaction Precaution: Do not take this product if you are presently taking a prescription antihypertensive or antidepressant drug containing a monoamine oxidase inhibitor except under the advice and supervision of a physician.

Caution: Avoid driving a motor vehicle, operating heavy machinery, or drinking alcoholic beverages while taking this product.

KEEP THIS AND ALL DRUGS OUT OF THE REACH OF CHILDREN. In case of accidental overdose, seek professional assistance or contact a Poison Control Center immediately.
Store at 15° to 25°C (59° to 77°F) in a dry place and protect from light.

How Supplied: Boxes of 10, 20.

Shown in Product Identification Section, page 406

ACTIFED® PLUS Caplets
[*ăk 'tuh-fĕd*]

Product Benefits: Each ACTIFED PLUS Caplet contains three important ingredients for maximum strength relief from symptoms of the common cold, seasonal allergies (hay fever) and sinus congestion.
The **ANTIHISTAMINE** (triprolidine) temporarily dries runny nose and relieves sneezing associated with the common cold, hay fever or other upper respiratory allergies. Also relieves itching of the nose or throat, and itchy, watery eyes due to hay fever.
The **DECONGESTANT** (pseudoephedrine) temporarily relieves nasal congestion due to the common cold, hay fever or other upper respiratory allergies, or associated with sinusitis. Temporarily relieves nasal stuffiness. Reduces the swelling of nasal passages; shrinks swollen membranes; and temporarily restores freer breathing through the nose. Also, helps to decongest sinus openings and passages; relieves sinus pressure.
The non-aspirin **ANALGESIC** (acetaminophen) temporarily relieves occasional minor aches, pains and headache, and reduces fever due to the common cold.

Each ACTIFED PLUS Caplet Contains: acetaminophen 500 mg, pseudoephedrine hydrochloride 30 mg and triprolidine hydrochloride 1.25 mg. Also contains: D&C Yellow No. 10 Lake, FD&C Blue No. 1 Lake, hydroxypropyl cellulose, magnesium stearate, microcrystalline cellulose, and povidone.

Directions: Adults and children 12 years and over, 2 caplets every 6 hours, not to exceed 8 caplets in a 24-hour period. Not recommended for children under 12 years of age.

Warnings: May cause excitability especially in children. May cause drowsiness. Do not exceed recommended dosage because at higher doses nervousness, dizziness, or sleeplessness may occur. If symptoms do not improve within 7 days or are accompanied by high fever, consult a physician before continuing use. Do not take this product for more than 10 days. Do not take this product if you have high blood pressure, heart disease, diabetes, thyroid disease, asthma, glaucoma, or difficulty in urination due to enlargement of the prostate gland except under the advice and supervision of a physician. As with any drug, if you are pregnant or nursing a baby, seek the advice of a health professional before using this product.

Drug Interaction Precaution: Do not take this product if you are presently taking a prescription antihypertensive or antidepressant drug containing a monoamine oxidase inhibitor except under the advice and supervision of a physician.

Caution: Avoid driving a motor vehicle, operating heavy machinery, or drinking alcoholic beverages while taking this product.
KEEP THIS AND ALL DRUGS OUT OF THE REACH OF CHILDREN. In case of accidental overdose, seek professional assistance or contact a Poison Control Center immediately.

Store at 15° to 25°C (59° to 77°F) in a dry place and protect from light.

How Supplied: Boxes of 20, 40.

Shown in Product Identification Section, page 406

ACTIFED® 12-Hour Capsules
[*ăk 'tuh-fĕd*]

Indications: For temporary relief of nasal congestion due to the common cold, hay fever or other upper respiratory allergies. Helps decongest sinus openings, sinus passages. For temporary relief of running nose, sneezing, itching of the nose or throat and itchy and watery eyes as may occur in allergic rhinitis (such as hay fever).

Directions: Adults and children 12 years of age and over—One capsule every 12 hours. Do not exceed two capsules in a 24 hour period. Children under 12 years of age, consult a physician.

Warnings: May cause excitability especially in children. Do not give this product to children under 12 years except under the advice and supervision of a physician. May cause drowsiness. Do not exceed recommended dosage because at higher doses nervousness, dizziness or sleeplessness may occur. If symptoms do not improve within 7 days or are accompanied by high fever, consult a physician before continuing use. Do not take this product if you have high blood pressure, heart disease, diabetes, thyroid disease, asthma, glaucoma or difficulty in urination due to enlargement of the prostate gland except under the advice and supervision of a physician. As with any drug, if you are pregnant or nursing a baby, seek the advice of a health professional before using this product.

Drug Interaction Precaution: Do not take this product if you are presently taking a prescription antihypertensive or antidepressant drug containing a monoamine oxidase inhibitor except under the advice and supervision of a physician.

Caution: Avoid driving a motor vehicle or operating heavy machinery. Avoid alcoholic beverages while taking this product.

KEEP THIS AND ALL DRUGS OUT OF THE REACH OF CHILDREN. In

Continued on next page

Burroughs Wellcome—Cont.

case of accidental overdose, seek professional assistance or contact a Poison Control Center immediately.

Active Ingredients: Each capsule contains pseudoephedrine hydrochloride 120 mg and triprolidine hydrochloride 5 mg.

Inactive Ingredients: Corn starch, D&C Yellow No. 10, sucrose, and other ingredients. The capsule shell consists of gelatin, D&C Yellow No. 10, FD&C Yellow No. 6, and titanium dioxide. May contain one or more parabens. Printed with edible black ink.

Store at 15°–25°C (59°–77°F) in a dry place and protect from light.

How Supplied: Boxes of 10, 20.

Shown in Product Identification Section, page 406

ACTIFED® Syrup
[*ăk 'tuh-fĕd*]

Product Benefits: ACTIFED Syrup contains two important ingredients for relief from symptoms of the common cold, seasonal allergies (hay fever) and sinus congestion.
The **ANTIHISTAMINE** (triprolidine) temporarily dries runny nose and relieves sneezing associated with the common cold, hay fever, or other upper respiratory allergies. Also relieves itching of the nose or throat, and itchy, watery eyes due to hay fever.
The **DECONGESTANT** (pseudoephedrine) temporarily relieves nasal congestion due to the common cold, hay fever or other upper respiratory allergies, or associated with sinusitis. Temporarily relieves nasal stuffiness. Reduces the swelling of nasal passages; shrinks swollen membranes; and temporarily restores freer breathing through the nose. Also, helps to decongest sinus openings and passages; relieves sinus pressure.

Each 5 mL (1 teaspoonful) Actifed Syrup Contains: pseudoephedrine hydrochloride 30 mg and triprolidine hydrochloride 1.25 mg. Also contains: methylparaben 0.1% and sodium benzoate 0.1% (added as preservatives), D&C Yellow No. 10, glycerin, purified water, and sorbitol.

Directions: Adults and children 12 years of age and over, 2 teaspoonfuls every 4 to 6 hours. Children 6 to under 12 years of age, 1 teaspoonful every 4 to 6 hours. Children under 6 years of age, consult a physician. Do not exceed 4 doses in 24 hours.

Warnings: May cause excitability especially in children. Do not give this product to children under 6 years except under the advice and supervision of a physician. May cause drowsiness. Do not exceed recommended dosage because at higher doses nervousness, dizziness or sleeplessness may occur. If symptoms do not improve within 7 days or are accompanied by high fever, consult a physician before continuing use. Do not take this product if you have high blood pressure, heart disease, diabetes, thyroid disease, asthma, glaucoma or difficulty in urination due to enlargement of the prostate gland except under the advice and supervision of a physician. As with any drug, if you are pregnant or nursing a baby, seek the advice of a health professional before using this product.

Drug Interaction Precaution: Do not take this product if you are presently taking a prescription antihypertensive or antidepressant drug containing a monoamine oxidase inhibitor except under the advice and supervision of a physician.

Caution: Avoid driving a motor vehicle, operating heavy machinery, or drinking alcoholic beverages while taking this product.

KEEP THIS AND ALL DRUGS OUT OF THE REACH OF CHILDREN. In case of accidental overdose, seek professional assistance or contact a Poison Control Center immediately.
Store at 15° to 25°C (59° to 77°F) and protect from light.

How Supplied: Bottles of 4 fl oz and 1 pint.

Shown in Product Identification Section, page 406

ACTIFED® Tablets
[*ăk 'tuh-fĕd*]

Product Benefits: Each ACTIFED Tablet contains two important ingredients for relief from symptoms of the common cold, seasonal allergies (hay fever) and sinus congestion.
The **ANTIHISTAMINE** (triprolidine) temporarily dries runny nose and relieves sneezing associated with the common cold, hay fever or other upper respiratory allergies. Also relieves itching of the nose or throat, and itchy, watery eyes due to hay fever.
The **DECONGESTANT** (pseudoephedrine) temporarily relieves nasal congestion due to the common cold, hay fever or other upper respiratory allergies, or associated with sinusitis. Temporarily relieves nasal stuffiness. Reduces the swelling of nasal passages; shrinks swollen membranes; and temporarily restores freer breathing through the nose. Also, helps to decongest sinus openings and passages; relieves sinus pressure.

Each Actifed Tablet Contains: pseudoephedrine hydrochloride 60 mg and triprolidine hydrochloride 2.5 mg. Also contains: flavor, hydroxypropyl methylcellulose, lactose, magnesium stearate, polyethylene glycol, potato starch, povidone, sucrose, and titanium dioxide.

Directions: Adults and children 12 years of age and over, 1 tablet every 4 to 6 hours. Children 6 to under 12 years of age, ½ tablet every 4 to 6 hours. Children under 6 years of age, consult a physician. Do not exceed 4 doses in 24 hours.

Warnings: May cause excitability especially in children. Do not give this product to children under 6 years except under the advice and supervision of a physician. May cause drowsiness. Do not exceed recommended dosage because at higher doses nervousness, dizziness or sleeplessness may occur. If symptoms do not improve within 7 days or are accompanied by high fever, consult a physician before continuing use. Do not take this product if you have high blood pressure, heart disease, diabetes, thyroid disease, asthma, glaucoma or difficulty in urination due to enlargement of the prostate gland except under the advice and supervision of a physician. As with any drug, if you are pregnant or nursing a baby, seek the advice of a health professional before using this product.

Drug Interaction Precaution: Do not take this product if you are presently taking a prescription antihypertensive or antidepressant drug containing a monoamine oxidase inhibitor except under the advice and supervision of a physician.

Caution: Avoid driving a motor vehicle, operating heavy machinery, or drinking alcoholic beverages while taking this product.

KEEP THIS AND ALL DRUGS OUT OF THE REACH OF CHILDREN. In case of accidental overdose, seek professional assistance or contact a Poison Control Center immediately.
Store at 15° to 25°C (59° to 77°F) in a dry place and protect from light.

How Supplied: Boxes of 12, 24, 48 and bottles of 100 and 1000; unit dose pack box of 100.

Shown in Product Identification Section, page 406

ACTIFED® PLUS Tablets
[*ăk 'tuh-fĕd*]

Product Benefits: Each ACTIFED PLUS Tablet contains three important ingredients for maximum strength relief from symptoms of the common cold, seasonal allergies (hay fever) and sinus congestion.
The **ANTIHISTAMINE** (triprolidine) temporarily dries runny nose and relieves sneezing associated with the common cold, hay fever or other upper respiratory allergies. Also relieves itching of the nose or throat, and itchy, watery eyes due to hay fever.
The **DECONGESTANT** (pseudoephedrine) temporarily relieves nasal congestion due to the common cold, hay fever or other upper respiratory allergies, or associated with sinusitis. Temporarily relieves nasal stuffiness. Reduces the swelling of nasal passages; shrinks swollen membranes; and temporarily restores freer breathing through the nose. Also, helps to decongest sinus openings and passages; relieves sinus pressure.
The non-aspirin **ANALGESIC** (acetaminophen) temporarily relieves occasional minor aches, pains and headache, and reduces fever due to the common cold.

Each ACTIFED PLUS Tablet Contains: acetaminophen 500 mg, pseudoephedrine hydrochloride 30 mg and triprolidine hydrochloride 1.25 mg. Also contains: D&C Yellow No. 10 Lake, FD&C Blue No. 1 Lake, hydroxypropyl cellulose, magnesium stearate, microcrystalline cellulose and povidone.

Directions: Adults and children 12 years and over, 2 tablets every 6 hours, not to exceed 8 tablets in a 24-hour period. Not recommended for children under 12 years of age.

Warnings: May cause excitability, especially in children. May cause drowsiness. Do not exceed recommended dosage because at higher doses nervousness, dizziness, or sleeplessness may occur. If symptoms do not improve within 7 days or are accompanied by high fever, consult a physician before continuing use. Do not take this product for more than 10 days. Do not take this product if you have high blood pressure, heart disease, diabetes, thyroid disease, asthma, glaucoma, or difficulty in urination due to enlargement of the prostate gland except under the advice and supervision of a physician. As with any drug, if you are pregnant or nursing a baby, seek the advice of a health professional before using this product.

Drug Interaction Precaution: Do not take this product if you are presently taking a prescription antihypertensive or antidepressant drug containing a monoamine oxidase inhibitor except under the advice and supervision of a physician.

Caution: Avoid driving a motor vehicle, operating heavy machinery, or drinking alcoholic beverages while taking this product.

KEEP THIS AND ALL DRUGS OUT OF THE REACH OF CHILDREN. In case of accidental overdose, seek professional assistance or contact a Poison Control Center immediately.

Store at 15° to 25°C (59° to 77°F) in a dry place and protect from light.

How Supplied: Boxes of 20, 40.

Shown in Product Identification Section, page 406

BOROFAX® Ointment

[*bôr 'uh-făks*]

Description: Contains boric acid 5% and lanolin.

Inactive Ingredients: fragrances, glycerin, mineral oil, purified water and sodium borate.

Indications: A soothing application for burns, abrasions, chafing, and for infants' tender skin.

Directions: Apply topically as required.

Keep this and all medicines out of children's reach.

Store at 15° to 25°C (59° to 77°F).

How Supplied: Tube, 1¾ oz.

EMPIRIN® ASPIRIN

[*ĕm 'puh-rŭn*]

For relief of headache, minor muscular aches and pains, toothache, discomfort and fever of colds and flu, pain of the premenstrual and menstrual periods, and temporary relief of minor arthritis pain (see CAUTION below).

Directions: Adults: 1 or 2 tablets with a full glass of water. Repeat every 4 hours as needed, up to 12 tablets a day.
Children: Consult a physician (see WARNINGS).

Caution: In arthritic conditions, if pain persists for more than 10 days or redness is present, consult a physician immediately.

Warnings: Children and teenagers should not use this medicine for chicken pox or flu symptoms before a doctor is consulted about Reye syndrome, a rare but serious illness reported to be associated with aspirin. Keep this and all medicines out of children's reach. In case of accidental overdose, contact a physician immediately.

High or continued fever, severe or persistent sore throat especially when accompanied by high fever, headache, nausea or vomiting, may be serious. Consult your physician. Do not exceed dose unless directed by a physician. Do not take this product if you are allergic to aspirin, have asthma, a gastric ulcer or its symptoms, or are taking a medication that affects the clotting of blood, except under the advice of a physician. As with any drug, if you are pregnant or nursing a baby, seek the advice of a health professional before using this product.

IT IS ESPECIALLY IMPORTANT NOT TO USE ASPIRIN DURING THE LAST 3 MONTHS OF PREGNANCY UNLESS SPECIFICALLY DIRECTED TO DO SO BY A DOCTOR BECAUSE IT MAY CAUSE PROBLEMS IN THE UNBORN CHILD OR COMPLICATIONS DURING DELIVERY.

Active Ingredients: Each tablet contains aspirin 325 mg (5 gr).

Inactive Ingredients: microcrystalline cellulose and potato starch.

Store at 15° to 25°C (59° to 77°F) in a dry place.

How Supplied: Bottles of 50, 100, 250.

Shown in Product Identification Section, page 406

FILTERAY®
Broad Spectrum Sunscreen Lotion

Indications: FILTERAY Broad Spectrum Sunscreen Lotion provides protection from acute and long-term risks associated with UVA and UVB light exposure. FILTERAY screens out the sun's burning rays to prevent sunburn. Overexposure to the sun may lead to premature aging of the skin and skin cancer. The liberal and regular use over the years of this product may help reduce the chance of these harmful effects.

Directions: Shake well before using. Prior to sun exposure, apply liberally and evenly over areas to be protected. To maintain maximal protection, reapply after 40 minutes in the water or after excessive perspiration. There is no recommended dosage for children under six months of age except under the advice and supervision of a physician.

Warnings: Do not use if sensitive to benzocaine, sulfonamides, aniline dyes, aminobenzoic acid (PABA) or related compounds or any other ingredient in this product. Use on children under six months of age only with the advice of a physician.

For external use only. Avoid contact with eyes, eyelids and mouth. If contact with eyes occurs, rinse thoroughly with water. Should skin irritation or rash develop, discontinue use. If irritation or rash persists, consult a physician. Keep out of the reach of children. In case of accidental ingestion, seek professional assistance or contact a Poison Control Center immediately.

Caution: FILTERAY Sunscreen Lotion may stain some fabrics.

Contains: Avobenzone 3.0%, Padimate O (octyl dimethyl p-aminobenzoic acid) 7.0% with: benzyl alcohol; carbomer 934P; cetyl esters wax; edetate disodium; glycerin; imidurea; mineral oil (light); oleth-3 phosphate; purified water; stearyl alcohol (and) ceteareth-20 and white petrolatum. May contain sodium hydroxide or hydrochloric acid to adjust pH.

NOTE: Store at room temperature. Protect from freezing.

How Supplied: 4 oz bottle.

Shown in Product Identification Section, page 406

MAREZINE® Tablets

[*mâr 'uh-zēn*]

FDA APPROVED USES

Indications: For the prevention and treatment of the nausea, vomiting or dizziness associated with motion sickness.

Directions: Adults and children 12 years of age and older: 1 tablet every 4 to 6 hours, not to exceed 4 tablets in 24 hours or as directed by a doctor. Children 6 to under 12 years of age: ½ tablet every 6 to 8 hours, not to exceed 1½ tablets in 24 hours or as directed by a doctor. For prevention, take the first dose one-half hour before departure.

Warnings: Do not take this product if you have asthma, glaucoma, emphysema, chronic pulmonary disease, shortness of breath, difficulty in breathing or difficulty in urination due to enlargement of the prostate gland unless directed by a doctor. Do not give to children under 6 years of age unless directed by a doctor. May cause drowsiness; alcohol, sedatives and tranquilizers may increase

Continued on next page

Burroughs Wellcome—Cont.

the drowsiness effect. Avoid alcoholic beverages while taking this product. Do not take this product if you are taking sedatives or tranquilizers without first consulting your doctor. Use caution when driving a motor vehicle or operating machinery. As with any drug, if you are pregnant or nursing a baby, seek the advice of a health professional before using this product. Keep this and all drugs out of the reach of children. In case of accidental overdose, seek professional assistance or contact a Poison Control Center immediately.

Active Ingredients: Each scored tablet contains cyclizine hydrochloride 50 mg.

Inactive Ingredients: Corn and potato starch, dextrin, lactose, and magnesium stearate.

Store at 15°–25°C (59°–77°F) in a dry place and protect from light.

How Supplied: Box of 12, bottle of 100.

Shown in Product Identification Section, page 406

Maximum Strength NEOSPORIN® Ointment

[*nē 'uh-spō 'rŭn*]

Indications: First aid to help prevent infection in minor cuts, scrapes and burns.

Directions: Clean the affected area. Apply a small amount of this product (an amount equal to the surface area of the tip of a finger) on the area 1 to 3 times daily. May be covered with sterile bandage.

Warnings: For external use only. Do not use in the eyes or apply over large areas of the body. In case of deep or puncture wounds, animal bites, or serious burns, consult a physician. Stop use and consult a physician if the condition persists or gets worse. Do not use longer than 1 week unless directed by a physician. Keep this and all drugs out of the reach of children. In case of accidental ingestion, seek professional assistance or contact a Poison Control Center immediately.

Each Gram Contains: polymyxin B sulfate 10,000 units, bacitracin zinc 500 units and neomycin 3.5 mg in a special white petrolatum base.

Store at 15° to 25°C (59° to 77°F).

How Supplied: ½ oz tube (with applicator tip).

Professional Labeling: Consult *1991 Physicians' Desk Reference®.*

Shown in Product Identification Section, page 407

NEOSPORIN® Cream

[*nē 'uh-spō 'rŭn*]

Indications: First aid to help prevent infection in minor cuts, scrapes, and burns.

Directions: Clean the affected area. Apply a small amount of this product (an amount equal to the surface area of the tip of a finger) on the area 1 to 3 times daily. May be covered with sterile bandage.

Warnings: For external use only. Do not use in the eyes or apply over large areas of the body. In case of deep or puncture wounds, animal bites, or serious burns, consult a physician. Stop use and consult a physician if the condition persists or gets worse. Do not use longer than 1 week unless directed by a physician. Keep this and all drugs out of the reach of children. In case of accidental ingestion, seek professional assistance or contact a Poison Control Center immediately.

Each Gram Contains: polymyxin B sulfate 10,000 units and neomycin 3.5 mg. Also contains: methylparaben 0.25% (added as a preservative), emulsifying wax, mineral oil, polyoxyethylene polyoxypropylene compound, propylene glycol, purified water and white petrolatum.

Store at 15° to 25°C (59° to 77°F).

How Supplied: ½ oz tube (with applicator tip); 1/32 oz (approx.) foil packets packed 144 per carton.

Professional Labeling: Consult *1991 Physicians' Desk Reference®.*

Shown in Product Identification Section, page 407

NEOSPORIN® Ointment

[*nē 'uh-spō 'rŭn*]

Indications: First aid to help prevent infection in minor cuts, scrapes and burns.

Directions: Clean the affected area. Apply a small amount of this product (an amount equal to the surface area of the tip of a finger) on the area 1 to 3 times daily. May be covered with sterile bandage.

Warnings: For external use only. Do not use in the eyes or apply over large areas of the body. In case of deep or puncture wounds, animal bites, or serious burns, consult a physician. Stop use and consult a physician if the condition persists or gets worse. Do not use longer than 1 week unless directed by a physician. Keep this and all drugs out of the reach of children. In case of accidental ingestion, seek professional assistance or contact a Poison Control Center immediately.

Each Gram Contains: polymyxin B sulfate 5,000 units, bacitracin zinc 400 units and neomycin 3.5 mg in a special white petrolatum base.

Store at 15° to 25°C (59° to 77°F).

How Supplied: Tubes, ½ oz (with applicator tip), 1 oz; 1/32 oz (approx.) foil packets packed 144 per carton.

Professional Labeling: Consult *1991 Physicians' Desk Reference®.*

Shown in Product Identification Section, page 407

NIX™
Permethrin
Lice Treatment

Product Benefits: Nix Creme Rinse kills lice and their unhatched eggs with only one application. Nix protects against head lice reinfestation for a full 14 days. The unique creme rinse formula leaves hair manageable and easy to comb.

Indications: For the treatment of head lice.

Directions for Use: Nix Creme Rinse should be used after hair has been washed with your regular shampoo, rinsed with water and towel dried. A sufficient amount should be applied to saturate hair and scalp (especially behind the ears and on the nape of the neck). Leave on hair for 10 minutes but no longer. Rinse with water. A single application is sufficient. Retreatment is required in less than 1% of patients. If live lice are observed seven days or more after the first application of this product, a second treatment should be given. For proper head lice management, remove nits with the nit comb provided.

Head lice live on the scalp and lay small white eggs (nits) on the hair shaft close to the scalp. The nits are most easily found on the nape of the neck or behind the ears. All personal headgear, scarfs, coats, and bed linen should be disinfected by machine washing in hot water and drying, using the hot cycle of a dryer for at least 20 minutes. Personal articles of clothing or bedding that cannot be washed may be dry-cleaned, sealed in a plastic bag for a period of about 2 weeks, or sprayed with a product specifically designed for this purpose. Personal combs and brushes may be disinfected by soaking in hot water (above 130°F) for 5 to 10 minutes. Thorough vacuuming of rooms inhabited by infected patients is recommended.

Warnings: For external use only. Itching, redness, or swelling of the scalp may occur. If skin irritation persists or infection is present or develops, discontinue use and consult a doctor. Do not use near the eyes or permit contact with mucous membranes. If product gets into the eyes, immediately flush with water. Consult a doctor if infestation of eyebrows or eyelashes occurs. This product may cause breathing difficulty or an asthmatic episode in susceptible persons. This product should not be used on children less than 2 months of age. As with any drug, if you are pregnant or nursing a baby, seek the advice of a health professional before using this product. Keep this and all drugs out of the reach of children. In case of accidental ingestion, seek professional assistance or contact a Poison Control Center immediately.

Each Fluid Ounce Contains: permethrin 280 mg (1%). Inactive ingredients are: balsam canada, cetyl alcohol, citric acid. FD&C Yellow No. 6, fragrance, hydrolyzed animal protein, hydroxyethylcellulose, polyoxyethylene 10

cetyl ether, propylene glycol, and stearalkonium chloride. Also contains: isopropyl alcohol 5.6 g (20%) and added as preservatives, imidazolidinyl urea 56 mg (0.2%), methylparaben 56 mg (0.2%), and propylparaben 22 mg (0.08%).
Store at 15° to 25°C (59° to 77°F.)

How Supplied: Bottles of 2 fl oz and Family Pack of 2 bottles, 2 fl oz each.

Shown in Product Identification Section, page 407

POLYSPORIN® Ointment

[*pŏl 'ē-spō 'rŭn*]

Indications: First aid to help prevent infection in minor cuts, scrapes and burns.

Directions: Clean the affected area. Apply a small amount of this product (an amount equal to the surface area of the tip of a finger) on the area 1 to 3 times daily. May be covered with a sterile bandage.

Warnings: For external use only. Do not use in the eyes or apply over large areas of the body. In case of deep or puncture wounds, animal bites, or serious burns, consult a physician. Stop use and consult a physician if the condition persists or gets worse. Do not use longer than 1 week unless directed by a physician. Keep this and all drugs out of the reach of children. In case of accidental ingestion, seek professional assistance or contact a Poison Control Center immediately.

Each Gram Contains: Aerosporin® (Polymyxin B Sulfate) 10,000 units and bacitracin zinc 500 units in a special white petrolatum base.

Store at 15° to 25°C (59° to 77°F).

How Supplied: Tubes, ½ oz with applicator tip, 1 oz; 1/32 oz (approx.) foil packets packed in cartons of 144.

Shown in Product Identification Section, page 407

POLYSPORIN® Powder

[*pŏl 'ē-spō 'rŭn*]

Indications: First aid to help prevent infection in minor cuts, scrapes and burns.

Directions: Clean the affected area. Apply a light dusting of the powder on the area 1 to 3 times daily. May be covered with a sterile bandage.

Warnings: For external use only. Do not use in the eyes or apply over large areas of the body. In case of deep or puncture wounds, animal bites, or serious burns, consult a physician. Stop use and consult a physician if the condition persists or gets worse.
Do not use longer than 1 week unless directed by a physician. Keep this and all drugs out of the reach of children. In case of accidental ingestion, seek professional assistance or contact a Poison Control Center immediately.

Each Gram Contains: polymyxin B sulfate 10,000 units and bacitracin zinc 500 units in a lactose base.
Store at 15° to 25°C (59° to 77°F). Do not store under refrigeration.

How Supplied: 0.35 oz (10 g) shaker-vial.

Shown in Product Identification Section, page 407

POLYSPORIN® Spray

[*pŏl 'ē-spō 'rŭn*]

Indications: First aid to help prevent infection in minor cuts, scrapes and burns.

Directions: Clean the affected area. SHAKE WELL before each spraying. Remove cap and press button to spray affected area. Hold container upright when spraying. Use two to three second intermittent sprays from a distance of about eight inches. Spray a small amount of this product on the area 1 to 3 times daily. May be covered with a sterile bandage.

Warnings: Avoid spraying in eyes. Contents under pressure. Do not puncture or incinerate. Do not store at temperatures above 120°F. **FLAMMABLE. Do not use near fire, flame, or while smoking.** Use only as directed. Intentional misuse by deliberately concentrating and inhaling the contents can be harmful or fatal. For external use only. Do not use in the eyes or apply over large areas of the body. In case of deep or puncture wounds, animal bites, or serious burns, consult a physician. Stop use and consult a physician if the condition persists or gets worse. Do not use longer than 1 week unless directed by a physician. Keep this and all drugs out of the reach of children. In case of accidental ingestion, seek professional assistance or contact a Poison Control Center immediately.

Each 90 gram can contains: polymyxin B sulfate 200,000 units and bacitracin zinc 10,000 units. Also contains: isopropyl myristate. Propellant—isobutane. Each 1 second spray delivers approximately 690 units polymyxin B sulfate and 34 units bacitracin zinc.

Store at 15° to 25°C (59° to 77°F).

How Supplied: 3.17 oz (90 g) spray can.

Shown in Product Identification Section, page 407

Children's SUDAFED® Liquid

[*sū 'duh-fĕd*]

Each 5 mL (1 teaspoonful) contains pseudoephedrine hydrochloride 30 mg. Also contains: methylparaben 0.1% and sodium benzoate 0.1% (added as preservatives), citric acid, FD&C Red No. 40, flavor, glycerin, purified water, sorbitol and sucrose.

Indications: For temporary relief of nasal congestion due to the common cold, hay fever or other upper respiratory allergies, and nasal congestion associated with sinusitis; promotes nasal and/or sinus drainage.

Directions: To be given every 4 to 6 hours. Do not exceed 4 doses in 24 hours. Children 6 to under 12 years of age, 1 teaspoonful. Children 2 to under 6 years of age, ½ teaspoonful. For children under 2 years of age, consult a physician.

Warnings: Do not exceed recommended dosage because at higher doses nervousness, dizziness or sleeplessness may occur. Do not give this product to children for more than 7 days. If symptoms do not improve or are accompanied by high fever, consult a physician. Do not give this product to children who have heart disease, high blood pressure, thyroid disease or diabetes unless directed by a physician.

Drug Interaction Precaution: Do not give this product to a child who is taking a prescription drug for high blood pressure or depression, without first consulting the child's physician.

KEEP THIS AND ALL MEDICINES OUT OF CHILDREN'S REACH. In case of accidental overdose, seek professional assistance or contact a Poison Control Center immediately.

Store at 15° to 25°C (59° to 77°F) and protect from light.

How Supplied: Bottles of 4 fl oz.

Shown in Product Identification Section, page 407

SUDAFED® Cough Syrup

[*sū 'duh-fĕd*]

Each 5 mL (1 teaspoonful) contains pseudoephedrine hydrochloride 15 mg, dextromethorphan hydrobromide 5 mg and guaifenesin 100 mg. Also contains: alcohol 2.4%, methylparaben 0.1% and sodium benzoate 0.1% (added as preservatives), citric acid, D&C Yellow No. 10, FD&C Blue No. 1, flavor, glycerin, purified water, saccharin sodium, sodium chloride and sucrose.

Indications: For temporary relief of cough due to minor throat and bronchial irritation as may occur with the common cold or inhaled irritants. For temporary relief of nasal congestion due to the common cold. Helps loosen phlegm (sputum) and thin bronchial secretions to rid the bronchial passageways of bothersome mucus.

Directions: To be given every 4 hours. Do not exceed 4 doses in 24 hours. Adults and children 12 years of age and over, 4 teaspoonfuls. Children 6 to under 12 years of age, 2 teaspoonfuls. Children 2 to under 6 years of age, 1 teaspoonful. For children under 2 years of age, consult a physician.

Warnings: Do not give this product to children under 2 years of age unless directed by a physician. Do not exceed recommended dosage because at higher doses nervousness, dizziness or sleeplessness may occur. Do not take this product

Continued on next page

Burroughs Wellcome—Cont.

for persistent or chronic cough such as occurs with smoking, asthma, chronic bronchitis, or emphysema, or where cough is accompanied by excessive phlegm (sputum) unless directed by a physician. A persistent cough may be a sign of a serious condition. If cough persists for more than 1 week, tends to recur, or is accompanied by fever, rash, or persistent headache, consult a physician. Do not take this preparation if you have high blood pressure, heart disease, diabetes, thyroid disease, or difficulty in urination due to enlargement of the prostate gland, except under the advice and supervision of a physician. As with any drug, if you are pregnant or nursing a baby, seek the advice of a health professional before using this product.

Drug Interaction Precaution: Do not take this product if you are presently taking a prescription antihypertensive or antidepressant drug containing a monoamine oxidase inhibitor except under the advice and supervision of a physician.

KEEP THIS AND ALL DRUGS OUT OF THE REACH OF CHILDREN. In case of accidental overdose, seek professional assistance or contact a Poison Control Center immediately.

Store at 15° to 25°C (59° to 77°F).
DO NOT REFRIGERATE.

How Supplied: Bottles of 4 fl oz and 8 fl oz.

Shown in Product Identification Section, page 407

SUDAFED® Tablets 30 mg

[*sū 'duh-fĕd*]

Each tablet contains pseudoephedrine hydrochloride 30 mg. Also contains: acacia, carnauba wax, dibasic calcium phosphate, FD&C Red No. 40 Lake and Yellow No. 6 Lake, magnesium stearate, polysorbate 60, potato starch, povidone, sodium benzoate, stearic acid, sucrose and titanium dioxide.

Indications: For temporary relief of nasal congestion due to the common cold, hay fever or other upper respiratory allergies, and nasal congestion associated with sinusitis; promotes nasal and/or sinus drainage.

Directions: To be given every 4 to 6 hours. Do not exceed 4 doses in 24 hours. Adults and children 12 years of age and over, 2 tablets. Children 6 to under 12 years of age, 1 tablet. Children 2 to under 6 years of age, use Children's Sudafed Liquid. For children under 2 years of age, consult a physician.

Warnings: Do not exceed recommended dosage because at higher doses nervousness, dizziness or sleeplessness may occur. If symptoms do not improve within 7 days, or are accompanied by a high fever, consult a physician before continuing use. Do not take this preparation if you have high blood pressure, heart disease, diabetes, thyroid disease, or difficulty in urination due to enlargement of the prostate gland, except under the advice and supervision of a physician. As with any drug, if you are pregnant or nursing a baby, seek the advice of a health professional before using this product.

Drug Interaction Precaution: Do not take this product if you are presently taking a prescription antihypertensive or antidepressant drug containing a monoamine oxidase inhibitor except under the advice and supervision of a physician.

KEEP THIS AND ALL MEDICINES OUT OF CHILDREN'S REACH. In case of accidental overdose, seek professional assistance or contact a Poison Control Center immediately.

Store at 15° to 25°C (59° to 77°F) in a dry place and protect from light.

How Supplied: Boxes of 24, 48. Bottles of 100. Institutional Pack, Carton of 500 x 2.

Shown in Product Identification Section, page 407

SUDAFED® Tablets 60 mg (Adult Strength)

[*sū 'duh-fĕd*]

Each tablet contains pseudoephedrine hydrochloride 60 mg. Also contains: acacia, carnauba wax, corn starch, dibasic calcium phosphate, hydroxypropyl methylcellulose, magnesium stearate, polysorbate 60, sodium starch glycolate, stearic acid, sucrose, titanium dioxide, and white shellac. Printed with edible red ink.

Indications: For temporary relief of nasal congestion due to the common cold, hay fever or other upper respiratory allergies, and nasal congestion associated with sinusitis; promotes nasal and/or sinus drainage.

Directions: To be given every 4 to 6 hours. Do not exceed 4 doses in 24 hours. Adults and children 12 years of age and over, 1 tablet. Children 6 to under 12 years of age, use Sudafed 30 mg Tablets. Children 2 to under 6 years of age, use Children's Sudafed Liquid. For children under 2 years of age, consult a physician.

Warnings: Do not exceed recommended dosage because at higher doses nervousness, dizziness or sleeplessness may occur. If symptoms do not improve within 7 days, or are accompanied by a high fever, consult a physician before continuing use. Do not take this preparation if you have high blood pressure, heart disease, diabetes, thyroid disease, or difficulty in urination due to enlargement of the prostate gland, except under the advice and supervision of a physician. As with any drug, if you are pregnant or nursing a baby, seek the advice of a health professional before using this product.

Drug Interaction Precaution: Do not take this product if you are presently taking a prescription antihypertensive or antidepressant drug containing a monoamine oxidase inhibitor, except under the advice and supervision of a physician.

KEEP THIS AND ALL MEDICINES OUT OF CHILDREN'S REACH. In case of accidental overdose, seek professional assistance or contact a Poison Control Center immediately.

Store at 15° to 25°C (59° to 77°F) in a dry place and protect from light.

How Supplied: Bottles of 100.

Shown in Product Identification Section, page 407

SUDAFED PLUS® Liquid

[*sū 'duh-fĕd*]

Each 5 mL (1 teaspoonful) contains pseudoephedrine hydrochloride 30 mg and chlorpheniramine maleate 2 mg. Also contains: methylparaben 0.1% and sodium benzoate 0.1% (added as preservatives), citric acid, D&C Yellow No. 10, FD&C Yellow No. 6, flavor, glycerin, purified water and sucrose.

Indications: For the temporary relief of nasal/sinus congestion associated with the common cold; also sneezing; watery, itchy eyes; runny nose and other hay fever/upper respiratory allergy symptoms.

Directions: To be given every 4 to 6 hours. Do not exceed 4 doses in 24 hours. Adults and children 12 years of age and over, 2 teaspoonfuls. Children 6 to under 12 years of age, 1 teaspoonful. Children under 6 years of age, consult a physician.

Warnings: May cause excitability, especially in children. Do not give to children under 6 years except as directed by a physician. May cause drowsiness. Do not exceed recommended dosage because at higher doses nervousness, dizziness or sleeplessness may occur. If symptoms do not improve within 7 days, or are accompanied by a high fever, consult a physician before continuing use. Do not take this product if you have high blood pressure, heart disease, diabetes, thyroid disease, asthma, glaucoma or difficulty in urination due to enlargement of the prostate gland except under the advice and supervision of a physician. As with any drug, if you are pregnant or nursing a baby, seek the advice of a health professional before using this product.

Drug Interaction Precaution: Do not take this product if you are presently taking a prescription antihypertensive or antidepressant drug containing a monoamine oxidase inhibitor except under the advice and supervision of a physician.

Caution: Avoid driving a motor vehicle or operating heavy machinery. Avoid alcoholic beverages while taking this product.

KEEP THIS AND ALL MEDICINES OUT OF CHILDREN'S REACH. In case of accidental overdose, seek professional assistance or contact a Poison Control Center immediately.

Store at 15° to 25°C (59° to 77°F) and protect from light.

How Supplied: Bottles of 4 fl oz.
Shown in Product Identification Section, page 407

SUDAFED PLUS® Tablets
[*sū 'duh-fĕd*]

Each scored tablet contains pseudoephedrine hydrochloride 60 mg and chlorpheniramine maleate 4 mg. Also contains: lactose, magnesium stearate, potato starch and povidone.

Indications: For the temporary relief of nasal/sinus congestion associated with the common cold; also sneezing; watery, itchy eyes; runny nose and other hay fever/upper respiratory allergy symptoms.

Directions: To be given every 4 to 6 hours. Do not exceed 4 doses in 24 hours. Adults and children 12 years of age and over, 1 tablet. Children 6 to under 12 years of age, ½ tablet. Children under 6 years of age, consult a physician.

Warnings: May cause excitability, especially in children. Do not give to children under 6 years except as directed by a physician. May cause drowsiness. Do not exceed recommended dosage because at higher doses nervousness, dizziness or sleeplessness may occur. If symptoms do not improve within 7 days, or are accompanied by a high fever, consult a physician before continuing use. Do not take this product if you have high blood pressure, heart disease, diabetes, thyroid disease, asthma, glaucoma or difficulty in urination due to enlargement of the prostate gland except under the advice and supervision of a physician. As with any drug, if you are pregnant or nursing a baby, seek the advice of a health professional before using this product.

Drug Interaction Precaution: Do not take this product if you are presently taking a prescription antihypertensive or antidepressant drug containing a monoamine oxidase inhibitor except under the advice and supervision of a physician.

Caution: Avoid driving a motor vehicle or operating heavy machinery. Avoid alcoholic beverages while taking this product.

KEEP THIS AND ALL MEDICINES OUT OF CHILDREN'S REACH. In case of accidental overdose, seek professional assistance or contact a Poison Control Center immediately.

Store at 15° to 25°C (59° to 77°F) in a dry place and protect from light.

How Supplied: Boxes of 24, 48.
Shown in Product Identification Section, page 407

SUDAFED® SINUS Caplets
[*sū 'dah-fĕd " 'sī-nəs*]

Product Benefits:

- Maximum allowable levels of non-aspirin pain reliever and nasal decongestant provide temporary relief of sinus headache pain, pressure and nasal congestion due to colds or hay fever and other allergies.
- Contains no ingredients which may cause drowsiness.

Directions: Adults and children 12 years and over, 2 caplets every 6 hours, not to exceed 8 caplets in a 24-hour period. Not recommended for children under 12 years of age.

Each Caplet Contains: acetaminophen 500 mg and pseudoephedrine hydrochloride 30 mg. Also contains FD&C Yellow No. 6 Lake, magnesium stearate, microcrystalline cellulose, povidone and sodium starch glycolate.

Warnings: Do not exceed recommended dosage because at higher doses nervousness, dizziness, or sleeplessness may occur. If symptoms do not improve within 7 days or are accompanied by high fever, consult a physician before continuing use. Do not take this product for more than 10 days. Do not take this product if you have high blood pressure, heart disease, diabetes, thyroid disease, or difficulty in urination due to enlargement of the prostate gland except under the advice and supervision of a physician. As with any drug, if you are pregnant or nursing a baby, seek the advice of a health professional before using this product.

Drug Interaction Precaution: Do not take this product if you are presently taking a prescription antihypertensive or antidepressant drug containing a monoamine oxidase inhibitor except under the advice and supervision of a physician.

KEEP THIS AND ALL DRUGS OUT OF THE REACH OF CHILDREN. In case of accidental overdose, seek professional assistance or contact a Poison Control Center immediately.

Store at 15°–25°C (59°–77°F) in a dry place and protect from light.

How Supplied: Boxes of 24 and 48.
Shown in Product Identification Section, page 407

SUDAFED® SINUS Tablets
[*sū 'dah-fĕd " 'sī-nəs*]

Product Benefits:

- Maximum allowable levels of non-aspirin pain reliever and nasal decongestant provide temporary relief of sinus headache pain, pressure and nasal congestion due to colds or hay fever and other allergies.
- Contains no ingredients which may cause drowsiness.

Directions: Adults and children 12 years and over, 2 tablets every 6 hours, not to exceed 8 tablets in a 24-hour period. Not recommended for children under 12 years of age.

Each Tablet Contains: Acetaminophen 500 mg and pseudoephedrine hydrochloride 30 mg. Also contains FD&C Yellow No. 6 Lake, magnesium stearate, microcrystalline cellulose, povidone and sodium starch glycolate.

Warnings: Do not exceed recommended dosage because at higher doses nervousness, dizziness, or sleeplessness may occur. If symptoms do not improve within 7 days or are accompanied by high fever, consult a physician before continuing use. Do not take this product for more than 10 days. Do not take this product if you have high blood pressure, heart disease, diabetes, thyroid disease, or difficulty in urination due to enlargement of the prostate gland except under the advice and supervision of a physician. As with any drug, if you are pregnant or nursing a baby, seek the advice of a health professional before using this product.

Drug Interaction Precaution: Do not take this product if you are presently taking a prescription antihypertensive or antidepressant drug containing a monoamine oxidase inhibitor except under the advice and supervision of a physician.

KEEP THIS AND ALL DRUGS OUT OF THE REACH OF CHILDREN. In case of accidental overdose, seek professional assistance or contact a Poison Control Center immediately.

Store at 15°–25°C (59°–77°F) in a dry place and protect from light.

How Supplied: Boxes of 24 and 48.
Shown in Product Identification Section, page 407

SUDAFED® 12 Hour Capsules
[*sū 'duh-fĕd*]

Each capsule contains pseudoephedrine hydrochloride 120 mg. Also contains: corn starch, sucrose and other ingredients. The capsule shell consists of gelatin, FD&C Blues No. 1 and 2, and Red No. 3. May contain one or more parabens. Printed with edible black ink.

Indications: For temporary relief of nasal congestion due to the common cold, hay fever, or other upper respiratory allergies, and nasal congestion associated with sinusitis; promotes nasal and/or sinus drainage.

Directions: Adults and children 12 years and over—One capsule every 12 hours, not to exceed two capsules in 24 hours. Sudafed 12 Hour is not recommended for children under 12 years of age.

Warnings: Do not exceed recommended dosage because at higher doses nervousness, dizziness, or sleeplessness may occur. If symptoms do not improve within 7 days, or are accompanied by a high fever, consult a physician before continuing use. Do not take this preparation if you have high blood pressure, heart disease, diabetes, thyroid disease, or difficulty in urination due to enlargement of the prostate gland, except under the advice and supervision of a physician. As with any drug, if you are pregnant or nursing a baby, seek the advice of a health professional before using this product.

Drug Interaction Precaution: Do not take this product if you are presently taking a prescription antihypertensive

Continued on next page

Burroughs Wellcome—Cont.

or antidepressant drug containing a monoamine oxidase inhibitor, except under the advice and supervision of a physician.

KEEP THIS AND ALL DRUGS OUT OF THE REACH OF CHILDREN. In case of accidental overdose, seek professional assistance or contact a Poison Control Center immediately.

Store at 15°–25°C (59°–77°F) in a dry place and protect from light.

How Supplied: Boxes of 10, 20, 40.

Shown in Product Identification Section, page 407

WELLCOME® LANOLINE

[*lăn 'ō-lŭn*]

Description: Lanolin with solid and liquid petrolatum, fragrances, and glycerin.

Indications: A soothing and softening application for dry, rough skin and a protective application against the effects of harsh weather.

Directions: Apply topically to the hands and face as required.

Keep this and all medicines out of children's reach.

Store at 15°–25°C (59°–77°F).

How Supplied: Tubes, $1\frac{3}{4}$ oz.

Campbell Laboratories Inc.

300 EAST 51st STREET
P.O. BOX 812, F.D.R. STATION
NEW YORK, NY 10150

HERPECIN-L® Cold Sore Lip Balm

[*her "puh-sin-el "*]

PRODUCT OVERVIEW

Key Facts: HERPECIN-L Lip Balm is a convenient, easy-to-use treatment for perioral herpes simplex infections.

Major Uses: HERPECIN-L not only treats cold sores, sun and fever blisters, but with prophylactic use, its sunscreens also protect to help prevent them. Users report early use at the prodromal stages of an attack will often abort the lesions and prevent scabbing. Prescribe: Apply "early and often."

Safety Information: For topical use only. A rare sensitivity may occur.

PRESCRIBING INFORMATION

HERPECIN-L® Cold Sore Lip Balm

Composition: A soothing, emollient, lip balm incorporating allantoin, the sunscreen, octyl-dimethyl-PABA (Padimate O), in a balanced, slightly acidic lipid base that includes petrolatum and titanium dioxide at a cosmetically acceptable level. (No caines, antibiotics, phenol or camphor.) (NDC 38083-777-31)

Actions and Uses: HERPECIN-L® relieves dryness and chapping by providing a lipid barrier to help restore normal moisture balance to the lips. Skin protectants help to soften the crusts and scabs of "cold sores." The sunscreen is effective in 2900-3200 AU range while titanium dioxide, though at low levels, helps to block, scatter and reflect the sun's rays. (With moderate to generous applications, SPF will range from 7 to 15.)

Administration: (1) *Recurrent "cold sores, sun and fever blisters":* Simply put, use **soon** and **often.** Frequent sufferers report that with *prophylactic* use (BID/PRN), attacks are fewer and less severe. Most recurrent herpes labialis patients are aware of the prodromal symptoms: tingling, itching, burning. At this stage, or if the lesion has already developed, HERPECIN-L should be applied liberally as often as convenient —at least *every hour.* (2) *Outdoor protection:* Apply before and during sun exposure, after swimming and again at bedtime (h.s.). (3) *Dry, chapped lips:* Apply as needed.

Adverse Reactions: If sensitive to any of the ingredients, discontinue use.

Contraindications: None.

How Supplied: 2.8 gm. swivel tubes.

Samples Available: Yes. (Request on professional letterhead or Rx pad.)

Chattem Consumer Products

Division of Chattem, Inc.
1715 WEST 38TH STREET
CHATTANOOGA, TN 37409

FLEX-ALL 454® PAIN RELIEVING GEL

Active Ingredient: Menthol 7%.

Inactive Ingredients: Alcohol, Allantoin, Aloe Vera Gel, Boric Acid Carbomer 940, Diazolidinyl Urea, Eucalyptus Oil, Glycerin, Iodine, Methylparaben, Methyl Salicylate, Peppermint Oil, Polysorbate 60, Potassium Iodide, Propylene Glycol, Propylparaben, Thyme Oil, Triethanolamine, Water, 97-116.

Indications: To relieve the pain of minor arthritis, simple backache, strains, sprains, bruises, and cramps.

Actions: Flex-all is classified as a counterirritant which provides relief of deep-seated pain through cutaneous stimulation rather than through a direct analgesic effect.

Warnings: For external use only. Keep out of reach of children. If swallowed, call a physician or contact a poison control center. Keep away from eyes and mucous membranes, broken or irritated skin. Do not bandage tightly or use heating pad. If skin redness or irritation develops, or pain lasts more than 10 days, discontinue use and call a physician.

Dosage and Administration: Apply generously to painful muscles and joints and gently massage until Flex-all 454 disappears. Use before and after exercise. Repeat as needed for temporary relief of minor arthritis pain, simple backache, strains, sprains, bruises, and cramps.

How Supplied: Available in 2 oz., 4 oz. and 8 oz. bottles.

NORWICH® EXTRA-STRENGTH ASPIRIN

Aspirin (acetylsalicylic acid) tablets

Active Ingredient: Each tablet contains 500 mg (7.7 grains) of pure aspirin.

Inactive Ingredients: Starch, Hydroxypropyl Methylcellulose, Polyethylene Glycol.

Actions: Analgesic and antipyretic.

Indications: For fast, effective relief of headache, minor aches and pains, and for reduction of fever, as well as temporary relief of minor aches and pains of arthritis, muscular aches, colds and flu, and menstrual discomfort.

Warnings: Children and teenagers should not use this medicine for chicken pox or flu symptoms before a doctor is consulted about Reye syndrome, a rare but serious illness reported to be associated with aspirin. As with any drug, if you are pregnant or nursing a baby, seek the advice of a health professional before using this product. IT IS ESPECIALLY IMPORTANT NOT TO USE ASPIRIN DURING THE LAST 3 MONTHS OF PREGNANCY UNLESS SPECIFICALLY DIRECTED TO DO SO BY A DOCTOR BECAUSE IT MAY CAUSE PROBLEMS IN THE UNBORN CHILD OR COMPLICATIONS DURING DELIVERY. Keep this and all medicines out of reach of children. In case of accidental overdose, seek professional assistance or contact a poison control center immediately.

Caution: If pain persists for more than 10 days or if redness is present, or in conditions affecting children under 12, consult physician immediately. If asthmatic or taking medicines for anticoagulation (thinning the blood), diabetes, gout, or arthritis, consult physician before use. Discontinue if ringing in the ears occurs.

Treatment of Oral Overdosage: IN CASE OF ACCIDENTAL OVERDOSE, SEEK PROFESSIONAL ASSISTANCE OR CONTACT A POISON CONTROL CENTER IMMEDIATELY.

Dosage and Administration: Adults: Initial dose 2 tablets followed by 1 tablet every 3 hours or 2 tablets every 6 hours, not to exceed 8 tablets in any 24-hour period, or as directed by a physician. NOT RECOMMENDED FOR CHILDREN UNDER 12.

Professional Labeling: Same as outlined under Indications.

How Supplied: In child-resistant bottles of 150 tablets.

NORWICH® REGULAR STRENGTH ASPIRIN
Aspirin (acetylsalicylic acid) tablets

Active Ingredient: Each tablet contains 325 mg (5 grains) of pure aspirin.

Inactive Ingredients: Starch, Hydroxypropyl Methylcellulose, Polyethylene Glycol.

Actions: Analgesic and antipyretic.

Indications: For fast, effective relief of headache, minor aches and pains, and for reduction of fever, as well as temporary relief of minor aches and pains of arthritis, muscular aches, colds and flu, and menstrual discomfort.

Warnings: Children and teenagers should not use this medicine for chicken pox or flu symptoms before a doctor is consulted about Reye syndrome, a rare but serious illness reported to be associated with aspirin. As with any drug, if you are pregnant or nursing a baby, seek the advice of a health professional before using this product. IT IS ESPECIALLY IMPORTANT NOT TO USE ASPIRIN DURING THE LAST 3 MONTHS OF PREGNANCY UNLESS SPECIFICALLY DIRECTED TO DO SO BY A DOCTOR BECAUSE IT MAY CAUSE PROBLEMS IN THE UNBORN CHILD OR COMPLICATIONS DURING DELIVERY. Keep this and all medicines out of reach of children. In case of accidental overdose, seek professional assistance or contact a poison control center immediately.

Caution: If pain persists for more than 10 days or if redness is present, or in conditions affecting children under 12, consult physician immediately. Do not take if you have ulcers, ulcer symptoms or bleeding problems. If asthmatic or taking medicines for anticoagulation (thinning the blood), diabetes, gout, or arthritis, consult physician before use. Discontinue if ringing in the ears occurs.

Treatment of Oral Overdosage: IN CASE OF ACCIDENTAL OVERDOSE, SEEK PROFESSIONAL ASSISTANCE OR CONTACT A POISON CONTROL CENTER IMMEDIATELY.

Dosage and Administration: Adults: 1 or 2 tablets every 3–4 hours up to 6 times a day. Children: under 3 years, consult physician; 3–6 years, ½–1 tablet; over 6 years, 1 tablet. May be taken every 3–4 hours up to 3 times a day.

Professional Labeling: Same as outlined under Indications.

How Supplied: In child-resistant bottles of 500 tablets, 250 tablets and 100 tablets.

NULLO® Deodorant Tablets

Active Ingredient: Each tablet contains 33.3 mg. Chlorophyllin Copper Complex.

Indications: Control of body odors including odor due to problems of bowel control, colostomy and ileostomy.

Warnings: Keep this and all drugs out of reach of children. Contains iron. In case of accidental overdose, seek professional assistance or contact a poison control center immediately. If cramps or diarrhea occur, reduce the dosage. If symptoms persist, consult your doctor. IF PRINTED CAP SEAL IS BROKEN OR MISSING, DO NOT USE.

Drug Interaction: None has ever been reported.

Toxicity: None has ever been reported.

Directions for Use: Dosage requirements will vary depending on cause of odor, dietary habits, etc. For odor control due to problems of fecal incontinence, colostomy and ileostomy, swallow one or two tablets three times a day before meals until odor is eliminated (from 2 to 7 days). If odor is not controlled, take 3 tablets three times a day before meals as required. Once odor is controlled, take one tablet three times a day or as needed. The smallest effective dose should be used. Do not exceed 9 tablets daily. Children under 12 years of age, consult a doctor. In addition, for colostomy and ileostomy odors, place one or two tablets in empty pouch each time it is reused or changed.

Side Effects: Few side effects have been reported following the administration of chlorophyllin copper complex in oral doses of up to 800 mg. (in divided doses) daily for varying durations, each exceeding one week. Temporary mild diarrhea has occurred with a few humans along with the expected green coloration of the stool. One case of abdominal cramps and one case of excessive gas were reported.

How Supplied: Tamper-resistant bottles containing 30, 60, and 135 tablets.

PRĒMSYN PMS®
[preem 'sin pms]
Premenstrual Syndrome Capsules/Caplets

Active Ingredients: Each capsule and caplet contain Acetaminophen 500 mg., Pamabrom 25 mg., and Pyrilamine Maleate 15 mg.

Indications: PRĒMSYN PMS® has been clinically proven to safely and effectively relieve premenstrual tension, irritability, nervousness, edema, backaches, legaches, and headaches that often accompany premenstrual syndrome.

Warning: KEEP THIS AND ALL DRUGS OUT OF THE REACH OF CHILDREN. In case of accidental overdose, seek professional assistance or contact a poison control center immediately.

Precautions: If drowsiness occurs, do not drive or operate machinery. As with any drug, if pregnant or nursing a baby, seek the advice of a health professional before using this product.

Dosage and Administration: Two capsules or caplets at first sign of premenstrual discomfort and repeat every three or four hours as needed, not to exceed 8 capsules/caplets in a 24-hour period.

How Supplied: Tamper-resistant bottles of 20 and 40 capsules and caplets.

Product Identification Marks: White caplet with PRĒMSYN PMS debossed on one surface. Grey and red capsules, film sealed with PRĒMSYN PMS printed on capsule.

EDUCATIONAL MATERIAL

NULLO®
Odor Control Following Ostomy Surgery
An information leaflet for patients with a colostomy, ileostomy, or urostomy. It contains basic information on odor, odor control, diet, and deodorants. Free to physicians, pharmacists, and patients.
Incontinence, Prevalence • Types • Causes • Treatment Options • Daily Management
An information leaflet for persons experiencing temporary or long-term bladder control problems. It contains facts about incontinence, types of urinary incontinence, treatment options, and support groups for incontinent people. Free to physicians, pharmacists, health professionals, and patients.
Nullo® Internal Deodorant Tablets
The 12-page booklet provides the results of clinical studies in odor control for fecal incontinence, urinary incontinence, colostomy, and ileostomy. Free to physicians, pharmacists, and health professionals.

PRĒMSYN PMS®
Pamabrom and Pyrilamine Maleate, Two of the Active Ingredients in PREMSYN PMS®
The 22-page booklet presents information about the ingredients in PRĒMSYN PMS®. The booklet includes results of basic pharmacology and clinical studies. Free to physicians and pharmacists.
PMS: Premenstrual Syndrome, A Review for Health Professionals
This 16-page booklet is directed to the health professional. It is a review of premenstrual syndrome, the mechanism, the varying symptoms, and modes of treatment, including dietary tips and a daily symptom diary. Free to physicians and pharmacists.
***PMS: Premenstrual Syndrome* (3-Month Symptom Diary)**
Two-page symptom diary to determine if the patient does have PMS. The diary covers three months using various symbols for symptoms and instructions for use. Free to physicians, pharmacists, clinics, and patients.
***PMS: Premenstrual Syndrome* (Slide Lecture Kit)**
***PMS, You're Not Alone* (30-Minute Videotape)**
Both are used by health professionals as instructional tools for educating either individual patients or groups of patients,

Continued on next page

Chattem—Cont.

other health professionals, and community groups. These can be obtained by writing Chattem, Inc.

PMS—Practical Advice for the Period Before Your Period
This booklet is written to the woman who suffers from PMS. It describes PMS, the various symptoms associated with the syndrome, a three-month symptom dairy and treatments including dietary tips, stress reduction and exercise. Free to physicians, pharmacists and other health professionals for distribution to patients.

Church & Dwight Co., Inc.
469 N. HARRISON STREET
PRINCETON, NJ 08540

ARM & HAMMER®
Pure Baking Soda

Active Ingredient: Sodium Bicarbonate U.S.P.

Indications: For alleviation of acid indigestion, also known as heartburn or sour stomach. Not a remedy for other types of stomach complaints such as nausea, stomachache, abdominal cramps, gas pains, or stomach distention caused by overeating and/or overdrinking. In the latter case, one should not ingest solids, liquids or antacid but rather refrain from all physical activity and—if uncomfortable—call a physician.

Actions: ARM & HAMMER® Pure Baking Soda provides fast-acting, effective neutralization of stomach acids. Each level ½ teaspoon dose will neutralize 20.9 mEq of acid.

Warnings: Except under the advice and supervision of a physician: (1) do not take more than eight level ½ teaspoons per person up to 60 years old or four level ½ teaspoons per person 60 years or older in a 24-hour period, (2) do not use this product if you are on a sodium restricted diet, (3) do not use the maximum dose for more than two weeks, (4) do not ingest food, liquid or any antacid when stomach is overly full to avoid possible injury to the stomach.

Dosage and Administration: Level ½ teaspoon in ½ glass (4 fl. oz.) of water every two hours up to maximum dosage or as directed by a physician. Accurately measure level ½ teaspoon. Each level ½ teaspoon contains 20.9 mEq (.476 gm) sodium.

How Supplied: Available in 8 oz., 16 oz., 32 oz., and 64 oz. boxes.

OTIX™ DROPS
EAR WAX REMOVAL AID

Description: OTIX™ DROPS with Cotton Ear Plugs is an external ear wax removal aid that contains the active ingredient carbamide peroxide, 6.5%. OTIX™ DROPS Complete Ear Wax Removal Kit includes cotton ear plugs and a soft rubber bulb ear irrigator. Application of carbamide peroxide drops followed by warm water irrigation is an effective, medically recommended way to loosen excessive ear wax. OTIX™ DROPS is the only ear wax removal brand that supplies cotton ear plugs, which are recommended for use as a means to keep each product application in the ear for several minutes.

Indication: For occasional use as an aid to gently soften, loosen and remove excessive ear wax.

Ingredients: Carbamide Peroxide 6.5% in a base of Anhydrous Glycerin and Glyceryl Succinate.

Actions: OTIX™ DROPS patent pending formulation provides the foaming action of hydrogen peroxide with the solvent action of glycerin. In the bottle the carbamide peroxide is stabilized with the unique stabilizer glyceryl succinate. When contact is made with natural enzymes in the ear, oxygen is released. This oxygen release results in a foaming action which together with the solvent action of glycerin helps loosen and remove impacted ear wax. It is usually necessary to remove the loosened wax by gently flushing the ear with warm water using a soft rubber bulb ear irrigator.

Directions: FOR USE IN THE EAR ONLY. Adults and children over 12 years of age: Tilt head sideways and place 5 to 10 drops into ear. Tip of applicator should not enter ear canal. Keep drops in ear for several minutes by keeping head tilted or placing cotton in the ear. Use twice daily for up to 4 days if needed, or as directed by a physician. Any wax remaining after treatment may be removed by gently flushing the ear with warm water, using a soft rubber bulb ear irrigator. Children under 12 years of age: Consult a physician.

Warnings: Do not use if you have ear drainage or discharge, ear pain, irritation, or rash in the ear or are dizzy; consult a physician. Do not use if you have an injury or perforation (hole) of the eardrum or after ear surgery, unless directed by a physician.
Do not use for more than 4 days; if excessive ear wax remains after use of this product, consult a physician. Avoid contact with the eyes. Keep this and all drugs out of the reach of children. In case of accidental ingestion, consult a physician.

Caution: Avoid exposing bottle to excessive heat and direct sunlight.

How Supplied:
For Patients
OTIX™ DROPS with Cotton Ear Plugs and OTIX™ DROPS Complete Ear Wax Removal Kit with Cotton Ear Plugs and Rubber Bulb Irrigator each contain a ½ fl. oz. bottle which will provide 30 to 60 applications. Both are available in the eye/ear sections of leading food and drug stores.

For Physicians
OTIX™ DROPS is also available in a 0.03 fl. oz. unit dose application for professional use only.

CIBA Consumer Pharmaceuticals
Division of CIBA-GEIGY Corporation
RARITAN PLAZA III
EDISON, NJ 08837

ACUTRIM® 16 HOUR* STEADY CONTROL APPETITE SUPPRESSANT TABLETS
Caffeine Free

ACUTRIM® II—MAXIMUM STRENGTH APPETITE SUPPRESSANT TABLETS
Caffeine Free

ACUTRIM LATE DAY® STRENGTH APPETITE SUPPRESSANT TABLETS
Caffeine Free

Description:
ACUTRIM® tablets deliver their maximum strength dosage of appetite suppressant at a precisely controlled, even rate.
This steady release is scientifically targeted to effectively distribute the appetite suppressant all day.
ACUTRIM makes it easier to follow the kind of reduced calorie diet needed for best weight control results.
A diet plan developed by an expert dietitian is included in the package for your personal use as a further aid.

Formula: Each ACUTRIM® tablet contains: Active Ingredient—phenylpropanolamine HCl 75 mg (appetite suppressant).
Inactive Ingredients—ACUTRIM® 16 HOUR* Steady Control: Cellulose Acetate, Hydroxypropyl Methylcellulose, Stearic Acid—ACUTRIM® II MAXIMUM STRENGTH: Cellulose Acetate, D&C Yellow #10, FD&C Blue #1, FD&C Yellow #6, Hydroxypropyl Methylcellulose, Povidone, Propylene Glycol, Stearic Acid, Titanium Dioxide—ACUTRIM LATE DAY® Strength: Cellulose Acetate, FD&C Yellow #6, Hydroxypropyl Methylcellulose, Isopropyl Alcohol, Propylene Glycol, Riboflavin, Stearic Acid, Titanium Dioxide.

*Extent of duration relates solely to blood levels.

Dosage: For best results, take one tablet daily directly after breakfast. Do not take more than one tablet every 24 hours. Recommended dosage may be used up to three months.

Caution: Do not give this product to children under 12. Do not exceed recommended dosage. If nervousness, dizziness, or sleeplessness occurs, stop taking this medication and consult your physician. If you are being treated for high blood pressure or depression, or have heart disease, diabetes, or thyroid disease, do not take this product, except under the supervision of a physician. If you are taking a cough/cold allergy medication containing any form of phenylpropanolamine, do not take this product.

Warning: As with any drug, if you are pregnant or nursing a baby, seek the advice of a health professional before using this product.

KEEP THIS AND ALL MEDICATION OUT OF THE REACH OF CHILDREN. In case of accidental overdose, seek professional assistance or contact a poison control center immediately.

Drug Interaction Precaution: If you are taking any prescription drugs, or any type of nasal decongestant, antihypertensive or antidepressant drug, do not take this product, except under the supervision of a physician.

How Supplied: Tamper-evident blister packages of 20 and 40 tablets. Do not use if individual seals are broken.

DO NOT STORE ABOVE 86°F
PROTECT FROM MOISTURE

12/86

Shown in Product Identification Section, page 407

EXTRA STRENGTH DOAN'S®
Analgesic Caplets

Indications: For temporary relief of minor backache.

Directions: Adults—Two caplets 3 or 4 times daily, not to exceed 8 caplets during a 24-hour period or as directed by a physician. Not intended for use by children or teenagers except under the advice of a physician. If pain persists for more than 10 days, discontinue use and consult your physician.

Warning: Children and teenagers should not use this medicine for symptoms of chicken pox, flu or other viral illnesses before a doctor is consulted about Reye's syndrome, a rare but serious illness. As with any drug, if you are pregnant or nursing a baby, seek the advice of a health professional before using this product. Do not use this product if you are under medical care or are allergic to aspirin or salicylates, except under the advice and supervision of your physician. **Keep this and all medicines out of the reach of children.** In case of accidental overdose, seek professional assistance or consult a Poison Control Center immediately.

Active Ingredient: Each caplet contains Magnesium Salicylate 500 mg. **Also Contains:** Hydroxypropyl methylcellulose, magnesium stearate, microcrystalline cellulose, polyethylene glycol, polysorbate 80, propylene glycol, stearic acid and titanium dioxide.

How Supplied: Tamper-evident blister packages of 24 and 48 caplets. Do not use if individual seals are broken.
Store at 15°–30°C (59°–86°F). Protect from moisture.

Shown in Product Identification Section, page 407

REGULAR STRENGTH DOAN'S®
Analgesic Caplets

Indications: For temporary relief of minor backache.

Directions: Adults—Two caplets every 4 hours as needed, not to exceed 12 caplets during a 24-hour period or as directed by a physician. Not intended for use by children or teenagers except under the advice of a physician. If pain persists for more than 10 days, discontinue use and consult your physician.

Warning: Children and teenagers should not use this medicine for symptoms of chicken pox, flu or other viral illnesses before a doctor is consulted about Reye's syndrome, a rare but serious illness. As with any drug, if you are pregnant or nursing a baby, seek the advice of a health professional before using this product. Do not use this product if you are under medical care or are allergic to aspirin or salicylates, except under the advice and supervision of your physician. **Keep this and all medicines out of the reach of children.** In case of accidental overdose, seek professional assistance or consult a Poison Control Center immediately.

Active Ingredient: Each caplet contains Magnesium Salicylate 325 mg. **Also Contains:** Magnesium Stearate, Microcrystalline Cellulose, Opadry Olive Green, Polyethylene Glycol, Purified Water, Stearic Acid.

How Supplied: Tamper-evident blister packages of 24 and 48 caplets. Do not use if individual seals are broken.
Store at 15°–30°C (59°–86°F). Protect from moisture.

Shown in Product Identification Section, page 407

EUCALYPTAMINT®
100% All Natural Ointment
External Analgesic

Description: An all-natural, deep-penetrating topical analgesic that provides hours of soothing relief.

Active Ingredient: Natural Menthol (15%)

Inactive Ingredients: Lanolin and Eucalyptus Oil

Indications: For the temporary relief of minor aches and pains of muscles and joints associated with arthritis, backache, strains, bruises, and sprains.

Directions: Adults and children 2 years of age and older: Gently massage a conservative amount into affected area not more than 3 to 4 times daily. Children under 2 years of age: Consult a physician. For best results, gently massage ointment into affected area and loosely cover with a warm moist towel.

Warning: FOR EXTERNAL USE ONLY. Avoid contact with eyes. Do not apply to wounds or damaged skin. Do not bandage tightly. If condition worsens, or if symptoms persist for more than 7 days, discontinue use of this product and consult a physician. Keep this and all drugs out of the reach of children. In case of accidental ingestion, seek professional assistance or contact a Poison Control Center immediately.

How Supplied: Eucalyptamint is supplied in 2 oz. and 4 oz. bottles.

Shown in Product Identification Section, page 407

FIBERALL® Chewable Tablets
[fi 'ber-all]
Lemon Creme Flavor

Description: Fiberall Chewable Tablets are a bulk-forming, nonirritant laxative which contains less than 1.5 grams of sugar per tablet. The active ingredient is polycarbophil, a bulk-forming man-made fiber. The smooth gelatinous bulk formed by Fiberall Chewable Tablets encourages peristaltic activity and a more normal elimination of the bowel contents.
The recommended dose of one tablet contains the equivalent to 1 gram of polycarbophil.
Inactive Ingredients: Crospovidone, dextrose, flavors, magnesium stearate and yellow No. 10 aluminum lake. Each dose contains less than 1 mg of sodium, 225 mg of calcium and less than 6 calories.

Indications: Fiberall Chewable Tablets are indicated for the management of chronic constipation, temporary constipation caused by illness or pregnancy, irritable bowel syndrome, and for constipation related to duodenal ulcer or diverticulosis. Fiberall Chewable Tablets are also indicated for stool softening in patients with hemorrhoids or after anorectal surgery.

Actions: After the tablet is chewed it readily disperses and acts without irritants or stimulants. Polycarbophil absorbs water in the gastrointestinal tract to form a gelatinous bulk which encourages a more normal bowel movement.

Dosage and Administration: *Adults and children 12 years and older:* chew and swallow 1 tablet, 1–4 times a day. *Children 6 to under 12 years:* one-half the usual adult dose or as recommended by a physician. *Children under 6:* consult a physician. **Drink a full glass (8 fl oz) of liquid with each dose.** Drinking additional liquid helps Fiberall work even more effectively. Continued use for 2 to 3 days may be desired for maximum laxative benefit.

Contraindications: Fecal impaction or intestinal obstruction. Any disease state in which consumption of extra calcium is contraindicated.

Continued on next page

The full prescribing information for each CIBA Consumer Pharmaceuticals product is contained herein and is that in effect as of December 1, 1990.

Drug Interactions: This product contains calcium, which may interact with some forms of TETRACYCLINE if taken concomitantly. The tetracycline product should be taken 1 hour before or 2–3 hours after taking a Fiberall Chewable Tablet.

How Supplied: Boxes containing 18 tablets.

FIBERALL® Fiber Wafers
[fi 'ber-all]
Fruit & Nut

Description: Fiberall Fiber Wafers are a bulk-forming, nonirritant laxative. The active ingredient is psyllium hydrophilic mucilloid, a dietary fiber extracted from the seed husk of blond psyllium seed *(Plantago ovata).* The smooth gelatinous bulk formed by Fiberall Wafers encourages peristaltic activity and a more normal elimination of the bowel contents.
One (1) Fiberall Fiber Wafer contains 3.4 g of psyllium hydrophilic mucilloid in a good-tasting wafer form, of which approximately 2.2 g is soluble fiber. One wafer is equivalent to one teaspoonful of Fiberall Powder.
Inactive Ingredients: Baking powder, brown sugar, butter flavor, cinnamon, corn syrup, crisp rice, dried ground apricots, flour, glycerin, granulated sugar, granulated walnuts, lecithin, margarine, molasses, oats, salt, vegetable oil shortening (soybean and cottonseed oil), water and wheat bran. Fiberall Fiber Wafers contain approximately 79 calories and 110 mg of sodium per wafer.

Indications: Fiberall Fiber Wafers are indicated for the management of chronic constipation, temporary constipation caused by illness or pregnancy, irritable bowel syndrome, and for constipation related to duodenal ulcer or diverticulosis. Fiberall Wafers are also indicated for stool softening in patients with hemorrhoids or after anorectal surgery.

Actions: The homogenous high-fiber formula of Fiberall Fiber Wafers, eaten with 8 oz of a beverage of the patient's choice, acts without irritants or stimulants in the gastrointestinal tract.

Dosage and Administration: The recommended dosage for adults is one to two Fiberall Fiber Wafers 1 to 3 times daily, with a full 8 oz glass of water or other liquid with each wafer. The recommended daily dose for children 6 to 12 years old is one-half the usual adult dose (with liquid), or as recommended by a physician. For children under 6, consult a physician. Drinking additional liquid is recommended and helps Fiberall work even more effectively. Two to three days' usage may be required for optimal laxative benefits.

Contraindications: Fecal impaction or intestinal obstruction.

Precaution: As with any grain product, inhaled or ingested psyllium powder may cause an allergic reaction in individuals sensitive to it.

How Supplied: Boxes containing 14 wafers.

Shown in Product Identification Section, page 407

FIBERALL® Fiber Wafers
[fi 'ber-all]
Oatmeal Raisin

Description: Fiberall Fiber Wafers are a bulk-forming, nonirritant laxative. The active ingredient is psyllium hydrophilic mucilloid, a dietary fiber extracted from the seed husk of blond psyllium seed *(Plantago ovata).* The smooth gelatinous bulk formed by Fiberall Fiber Wafers encourages peristaltic activity and a more normal elimination of the bowel contents.
One (1) Fiberall Fiber Wafer contains 3.4 g of psyllium hydrophilic mucilloid in a good-tasting wafer form, of which approximately 2.2 g is soluble fiber. One wafer is equivalent to one teaspoonful of Fiberall powder.
Inactive Ingredients: baking powder, cinnamon, cinnamon flavor, cloves, corn syrup, flour, glycerin, granulated sugar, lecithin, molasses, oats, raisins, vegetable oil shortening (soybean and cottonseed oil), water and wheat bran. Oatmeal Raisin Fiberall Fiber Wafers contain approximately 78 calories and 30 mg of sodium per wafer.

Indications: Fiberall Fiber Wafers are indicated for the management of chronic constipation, temporary constipation caused by illness or pregnancy, irritable bowel syndrome, and for constipation related to duodenal ulcer or diverticulosis. Fiberall Wafers are also indicated for stool softening in patients with hemorrhoids or after anorectal surgery.

Actions: The homogenous high-fiber formula of Fiberall Fiber Wafers, eaten with 8 oz of a beverage of the patient's choice, acts without irritants or stimulants in the gastrointestinal tract.

Dosage and Administration: The recommended dosage for adults is one to two Fiberall Fiber Wafers 1 to 3 times daily, with a full 8 oz glass of water or other liquid with each wafer. The recommended daily dose for children 6 to 12 years old is one-half the usual adult dose (with liquid) or as recommended by a physician. For children under 6, consult a physician. Drinking additional liquid is recommended and helps Fiberall work even more effectively. Two to three days' usage may be required for optimal laxative benefits.

Contraindications: Fecal impaction or intestinal obstruction.

Precaution: As with any grain product, inhaled or ingested psyllium powder may cause an allergic reaction in individuals sensitive to it.

How Supplied: Boxes containing 14 wafers.

Shown in Product Identification Section, page 407

FIBERALL® Powder, Natural Flavor
[fi 'ber-all]

Description: Fiberall is a bulk-forming, nonirritant laxative which contains no sugar. The active ingredient is psyllium hydrophilic mucilloid, a dietary fiber extracted from the seed husk of blond psyllium seed *(Plantago ovata).* The smooth gelatinous bulk formed by Fiberall encourages peristaltic activity and a more normal elimination of the bowel contents.
The recommended dose of one slightly rounded teaspoonful (5 g) contains 3.4 g psyllium hydrophilic mucilloid, of which approximately 2.2 g is soluble fiber.
Inactive Ingredients: Citric acid, flavor, polysorbate 60 and wheat bran. Each dose contains less than 10 mg of sodium, less than 60 mg of potassium, and provides less than 6 calories.

Indications: Fiberall is indicated for the management of chronic constipation, temporary constipation caused by illness or pregnancy, irritable bowel syndrome, and for constipation related to duodenal ulcer or diverticulosis. Fiberall is also indicated for stool softening in patients with hemorrhoids or after anorectal surgery.

Actions: The homogenous, high-fiber formula of Fiberall is readily dispersed in liquids and acts without irritants or stimulants in the gastrointestinal tract.

Dosage and Administration: The recommended dosage for adults is one slightly rounded teaspoonful (5 g) stirred into an 8 oz glass of cool water or other liquid and taken orally one to three times daily according to the individual response. The recommended daily dose for children 6 to 12 years old is one-half the usual adult dose (with liquid) or as recommended by a physician. For children under 6, consult a physician. Drinking additional liquid is recommended and helps Fiberall work even more effectively. Two to three days' usage may be required for maximum laxative benefits.

Contraindications: Fecal impaction or intestinal obstruction.

Precaution: As with any grain product, inhaled or ingested psyllium powder may cause an allergic reaction in individuals sensitive to it.

How Supplied: Powder, in 10 or 15 oz containers.

Shown in Product Identification Section, page 407

FIBERALL® Powder, Orange Flavor
[fi 'ber-all]

Description: Fiberall is a bulk-forming, nonirritant laxative which contains no sugar. The active ingredient is psyllium hydrophilic mucilloid, a dietary fiber extracted from the seed husk of blond psyllium seed *(Plantago ovata)*. The smooth gelatinous bulk formed by Fiberall encourages peristaltic activity and a more normal elimination of the lower bowel contents.

The recommended dose of one rounded teaspoonful (5.9 g) contains 3.4 g psyllium hydrophilic mucilloid, of which approximately 2.2 g is soluble fiber.

Inactive Ingredients: Beta-carotene, citric acid, flavors, polysorbate 60, saccharin, wheat bran and yellow No. 6 lake. Each dose contains less than 10 mg of sodium, less than 60 mg of potassium, and provides less than 10 calories.

Indications: Fiberall is indicated for the management of chronic constipation, temporary constipation caused by illness or pregnancy, irritable bowel syndrome, and for constipation related to duodenal ulcer or diverticulosis. Fiberall is also indicated for stool softening in patients with hemorrhoids or after anorectal surgery.

Actions: The homogenous, high-fiber formula of Fiberall is readily dispersed in liquids and acts without irritants or stimulants in the gastrointestinal tract.

Dosage and Administration: The recommended dosage for adults is one rounded teaspoonful (5.9 g) stirred into an 8 oz glass of cool water or other liquid and taken orally one to three times daily according to the individual response. The recommended daily dose for children 6 to 12 years old is one-half the usual adult dose (with liquid) or as recommended by a physician. For children under 6, consult a physician. Drinking additional liquid is recommended and helps Fiberall work even more effectively. Two to three days' usage may be required for maximum laxative benefits.

Contraindications: Fecal impaction or intestinal obstruction.

Precaution: As with any grain product, inhaled or ingested psyllium powder may cause an allergic reaction in individuals sensitive to it.

How Supplied: Powder, in 10 and 15 oz containers.

Shown in Product Identification Section, page 407

NUPERCAINAL®
Hemorrhoidal and Anesthetic Ointment
Pain-Relief Cream

Caution:
Nupercainal products are not for prolonged or extensive use and should never be applied in or near the eyes. If the symptom being treated does not subside, or rash, irritation, swelling, pain, bleeding or other symptoms develop or increase, discontinue use and consult a physician.
Consult labels before using.
Keep this and all medications out of reach of children.

NUPERCAINAL SHOULD NOT BE SWALLOWED. IN CASE OF ACCIDENTAL INGESTION CONSULT A PHYSICIAN OR POISON CONTROL CENTER IMMEDIATELY.

Indications: Nupercainal Ointment and Cream are fast-acting, long-lasting pain relievers that you can use for a number of painful skin conditions. **Nupercainal Hemorrhoidal and Anesthetic Ointment** is for hemorrhoids as well as for general use. **Nupercainal Pain-Relief Cream** is for general use only. The **Cream** is half as strong as the **Ointment.**

How to use Nupercainal Anesthetic Ointment (for general use). This soothing Ointment helps lubricate dry, inflamed skin and gives fast, temporary relief of pain, itching and burning. It is recommended for sunburn, nonpoisonous insect bites, minor burns, cuts and scratches. **DO NOT USE THIS PRODUCT IN OR NEAR YOUR EYES.**

Apply to affected areas gently. If necessary, cover with a light dressing for protection. Do not use more than 1 ounce of Ointment in a 24-hour period for an adult. Do not use more than one-quarter of an ounce in a 24-hour period for a child. If irritation develops, discontinue use and consult your doctor.

How to use Nupercainal Hemorrhoidal and Anesthetic Ointment for fast, temporary relief of pain and itching due to hemorrhoids (also known as piles).

Remove cap from tube and set it aside. Attach the white plastic applicator to the tube. Squeeze the tube until you see the Ointment begin to come through the little holes in the applicator. Using your finger, lubricate the applicator with the Ointment. Now insert the entire applicator gently into the rectum. Give the tube a good squeeze to get enough Ointment into the rectum for comfort and lubrication. Remove applicator from rectum and wipe it clean. Apply additional Ointment to anal tissues to help relieve pain, burning, and itching. For best results use Ointment morning and night and after each bowel movement. After each use detach applicator, and wash it off with soap and water. Put cap back on tube before storing. In case of rectal bleeding, discontinue use and consult your doctor.

Pain-Relief Cream for general use. This Cream is particularly effective for fast, temporary relief of pain and itching associated with sunburn, cuts, scrapes, scratches, minor burns and nonpoisonous insect bites. **DO NOT USE THIS PRODUCT IN OR NEAR YOUR EYES.**

Apply liberally to affected area and rub in gently. This Cream is water-washable, so be sure to reapply after bathing, swimming or sweating. If irritation develops, discontinue use and consult your doctor.

Nupercainal Hemorrhoidal and Anesthetic Ointment contains 1% dibucaine USP. Also contains acetone sodium bisulfite, lanolin, light mineral oil, purified water, and white petrolatum. Available in tubes of 1 and 2 ounces. Store between 59°–86°F.

Nupercainal Pain-Relief Cream contains 0.5% dibucaine USP. Also contains acetone sodium bisulfite, fragrance, glycerin, potassium hydroxide, purified water, stearic acid, and trolamine. Available in $1\frac{1}{2}$ ounce tubes.

Dibucaine USP is officially classified as a "topical anesthetic" and is one of the strongest and longest lasting of all topical pain relievers. It is not a narcotic.

C86-62 (Rev. 11/86)

Shown in Product Identification Section, page 408

NUPERCAINAL®
Suppositories

Indications: Nupercainal Rectal Suppositories give temporary relief of itching, burning, and discomfort associated with hemorrhoids or other anorectal disorders.

Each suppository contains 2.1 gram cocoa butter and .25 gram zinc oxide. Also contains acetone sodium bisulfite and bismuth subgallate.

Directions: ADULTS—Tear off one suppository and remove foil wrapper before inserting into the rectum. Gently insert the suppository rectally, rounded end first. Use one suppository in the morning, night and after each bowel movement. Do not use more than six in a 24-hour period. CHILDREN UNDER 12 YEARS OF AGE—Consult a physician.

WARNING: IF ACCIDENTALLY SWALLOWED, CONSULT A PHYSICIAN OR POISON CONTROL CENTER IMMEDIATELY.

Nupercainal suppositories are not for prolonged use. If irritation develops at site of application or in case of rectal bleeding, discontinue use and consult a physician. As with any drug, if you are pregnant or nursing a baby, seek the advice of a health professional before using this product.

Keep this and all medications out of reach of children.

Nupercainal Suppositories are available in packages of 12 and 24.

Do not store above 86 °F.

C86-42 (Rev. 9/86)

Shown in Product Identification Section, page 408

OTRIVIN®
xylometazoline hydrochloride USP
Decongestant
Nasal Spray and Nasal Drops 0.1%
Pediatric Nasal Drops 0.05%

One application provides rapid and long-lasting relief of nasal congestion for up to 10 hours.

Quickly clears stuffy noses due to common cold, sinusitis, hay fever.

Continued on next page

The full prescribing information for each CIBA Consumer Pharmaceuticals product is contained herein and is that in effect as of December 1, 1990.

CIBA Consumer—Cont.

Nasal congestion can make life miserable—you can't breathe, smell, taste, or sleep comfortably. That is why Otrivin is so helpful. It clears away that stuffy feeling, usually within 5 to 10 minutes, and your head feels clear for hours.
Otrivin has been prescribed by doctors for many years. Here is how you use it:
Nasal Spray 0.1%—for adults and children 12 years and older. Spray 2 or 3 times into each nostril every 8–10 hours. With head upright, squeeze sharply and firmly while inhaling (sniffing) through the nose.
Nasal Drops 0.1%—for adults and children 12 years and older. Put 2 or 3 drops into each nostril every 8 to 10 hours. Tilt head as far back as possible. Immediately bend head forward toward knees, hold for a few seconds, then return to upright position.
Do not give Nasal Spray 0.1% or Nasal Drops 0.1% to children under 12 years except under the advice and supervision of a physician.
Pediatric Nasal Drops 0.05%—for children 2 to 12 years of age. Put 2 or 3 drops into each nostril every 8 to 10 hours. Tilt head as far back as possible. Immediately bend head forward toward knees, hold a few seconds, then return to upright position.
Do not give this product to children under 2 years except under the advice and supervision of a physician.
Otrivin Nasal Spray/Nasal Drops contain 0.1% xylometazoline hydrochloride, USP. Also contains benzalkonium chloride, potassium chloride, potassium phosphate monobasic, purified water, sodium chloride and sodium phosphate dibasic. They are available in an unbreakable plastic spray package of ½ fl oz (15 ml) and in a plastic dropper bottle of .66 fl oz (20 ml).
Otrivin Pediatric Nasal Drops contain 0.05% xylometazoline hydrochloride, USP. Also contains benzalkonium chloride, potassium chloride, potassium phosphate monobasic, purified water, sodium chloride and sodium phosphate dibasic. It is available in a plastic dropper bottle of .66 fl oz (20 ml).

Warnings: Do not exceed recommended dosage, because symptoms such as burning, stinging, sneezing, or increase of nasal discharge may occur. Do not use this product for more than 3 days. If symptoms persist, consult a physician. The use of this dispenser by more than one person may cause infection.
Keep this and all medicines out of the reach of children. Overdosage in young children may cause marked sedation. In case of accidental ingestion, seek professional assistance or contact a Poison Control Center immediately.
Store between 33°–86°F.

C86-44 (9/86)

Shown in Product Identification Section, page 408

PRIVINE®
naphazoline hydrochloride, USP
0.05% Nasal Solution
0.05% Nasal Spray

Caution: Do not use Privine if you have glaucoma. Privine is an effective nasal decongestant **when you use it in the recommended dosage.** If you use too much, too long, or too often, Privine may be harmful to your nasal mucous membranes and cause burning, stinging, sneezing or an increased runny nose.
Do not use Privine by mouth.
Keep this and all medications out of the reach of children. Do not use Privine with children under 12 years of age, except with the advice and supervision of a doctor.
OVERDOSAGE IN YOUNG CHILDREN MAY CAUSE MARKED SEDATION AND IF SEVERE, EMERGENCY TREATMENT MAY BE NECESSARY.
IF NASAL STUFFINESS PERSISTS AFTER 3 DAYS OF TREATMENT, DISCONTINUE USE AND CONSULT A DOCTOR.
Privine is a nasal decongestant that comes in two forms: Nasal Solution (in a bottle with a dropper) and Nasal Spray (in a plastic squeeze bottle). Both are for prompt, and prolonged relief of nasal congestion due to common colds, sinusitis, hay fever, etc.
How to use Nasal Solution. Squeeze rubber bulb to fill dropper with proper amount of medication. For best results, tilt head as far back as possible and put two drops of solution into your right nostril. Then lean head forward, inhaling and turning your head to the left. Refill dropper by squeezing bulb. Now tilt head as far back as possible and put two drops of solution into your left nostril. Then lean head forward, inhaling, and turning your head to the right.
Use only 2 drops in each nostril. Do not repeat this dosage more than every 3 hours.
The Privine dropper bottle is designed to make administration of the proper dosage easy and to prevent accidental overdosage. Privine will not cause sleeplessness, so you may use it before going to bed.

Important: After use, be sure to rinse the dropper with very hot water. This helps prevent contamination of the bottle with bacteria from nasal secretions. Use of the dispenser by more than one person may spread infection.

Note: Privine Nasal Solution may be used on contact with glass, plastic, stainless steel and specially treated metals used in atomizers. Do not let the solution come in contact with reactive metals, especially aluminum. If solution becomes discolored, it should be discarded.
How to use Nasal Spray. For best results do **not** shake the plastic squeeze bottle.
Remove cap. With head held upright, spray twice into each nostril. Squeeze the bottle sharply and firmly while sniffing through the nose.
For best results use every 4 to 6 hours. Do not use more often than every 3 hours. Avoid overdosage. Follow directions for use carefully.
Privine Nasal Solution contains 0.05% naphazoline hydrochloride USP. It also contains benzalkonium chloride, disodium edetate dihydrate, hydrochloric acid, purified water, sodium chloride, and trolamine. It is available in bottles of .66 fl. oz. (20 ml) with dropper, and bottles of 16 fl. oz. (473 ml).
Privine Nasal Spray contains 0.05% naphazoline hydrochloride USP. It also contains benzalkonium chloride, disodium edetate dihydrate, hydrochloric acid, purified water, sodium chloride, and trolamine. It is available in plastic squeeze bottles of ½ fl. oz. (15 ml).
Store the nasal solution and nasal spray between 59°–86°F.

C86-43 (Rev. 9/86)

Shown in Product Identification Section, page 408

Q-VEL®
Muscle Relaxant Pain Reliever

Active Ingredient: Quinine Sulfate 1 gr. (64.8 mg).

Contains: Vitamin E (400 I.U. *dl*-alpha tocopheryl acetate) in a lecithin base.

Indications: For prevention and temporary relief of night leg cramps.

Warnings: Do not take if pregnant, nursing a baby or of childbearing potential, if sensitive to quinine, or under 12 years of age. Discontinue use and consult your physician if ringing in the ears, deafness, diarrhea, nausea, skin rash, bruising or visual disturbances occur. In case of accidental overdose, seek medical assistance or contact Poison Control Center at once. Keep this and all medicine out of reach of children.

Dosage: To prevent night leg cramps take 2 soft caplets after the evening meal plus 2 at bedtime. For relief in case of sudden attack, take 2 soft caplets at once plus 2 after ½ hour if needed. Do not exceed 4 soft caplets daily.

How Supplied: Bottles of 16, 30 and 50 softgels.
Store at 15°–30°C (59°–86°F) and protect from moisture.

Shown in Product Identification Section, page 408

SLOW FE®
Slow Release Iron Tablets

Description: SLOW FE supplies ferrous sulfate for the treatment of iron deficiency and iron deficiency anemia with a significant reduction in the incidence of the common side effects of oral iron. The wax matrix delivery system of SLOW FE is designed to maximize the release of ferrous sulfate in the duodenum and the jejunum where it is best tolerated and absorbed. SLOW FE has been clinically shown to be associated with a lower incidence of constipation, diarrhea and abdominal discomfort when compared to regular iron tablets and the leading capsule.

Formula: Each tablet contains 160 mg. dried ferrous sulfate USP, equivalent to 50 mg. elemental iron. Also contains cetostearyl alcohol, colloidal silicon dioxide, hydroxypropyl methylcellulose, shellac, lactose, magnesium stearate, polyethylene glycol.

Dosage: ADULTS—one or two tablets daily or as recommended by a physician. A maximum of four tablets daily may be taken. CHILDREN—one tablet daily. Tablets must be swallowed whole.

Warning: The treatment of any anemic condition should be on the advice and under the supervision of a physician. As oral iron products interfere with absorption of oral tetracycline antibiotics, these products should not be taken within two hours of each other. As with any drug, if you are pregnant or nursing a baby, seek the advice of a health professional before using this product.

Keep this and all medicines out of reach of children. In case of accidental overdose, contact your physician or poison control center immediately.

Tamper-Resistant Packaging.

How Supplied: Blister packages of 30, 60 and bottles of 100. Do Not Store Above 86°F. Protect From Moisture.

Shown in Product Identification Section, page 408

SUNKIST CHILDREN'S CHEWABLE MULTIVITAMINS—REGULAR

Vitamin Ingredients: Each tablet contains:
[See table above.]

Indication: Dietary supplementation.

Dosage and Administration: One chewable tablet daily for children two years and older.

Warning: Phenylketonurics: Contains Phenylalanine

How Supplied: SUNKIST Children's Multivitamins-Regular are supplied in bottles of 60 chewable tablets with child resistant caps.

Shown in Product Identification Section, page 408

SUNKIST CHILDREN'S CHEWABLE MULTIVITAMINS—PLUS EXTRA C

Vitamin Ingredients: Each tablet contains the ingredients of the Regular vitamin product plus extra Vitamin C (a total of 250 mg).

Indication: Dietary supplementation.

Dosage and Administration: One chewable tablet daily for adults and children two years and older.

Warning: Phenylketonurics: Contains Phenylalanine.

How Supplied: SUNKIST Children's Multivitamins Plus Extra C are supplied in bottles of 60 chewable tablets with child resistant caps.

VITAMINS	QUANTITY PER TABLET	PERCENT U.S. RDA FOR CHILD. 2 TO 4 YRS OF AGE (1 TABLET)	PERCENT U.S. RDA FOR ADULTS & CHILD. OVER 4 YRS OF AGE (1 TABLET)
Vitamin A (as Palmitate + Beta Carotene)	2500 IU	100	50
Vitamin D-3	400 IU	100	100
Vitamin E	15 IU	150	50
Vitamin C	60 mg	150	100
Folic Acid	0.3 mg	150	75
Niacinamide	13.5 mg	150	68
Vitamin B-6	1.05 mg	150	53
Vitamin B-12	4.5 mcg	150	75
Vitamin B-1	1.05 mg	150	70
Vitamin B-2	1.20 mg	150	71
Vitamin K-1	5 mcg	*	*

*Recognized as essential in human nutrition, but no U.S. RDA established.

Shown in Product Identification Section, page 408

SUNKIST CHILDREN'S CHEWABLE MULTIVITAMINS—PLUS IRON

Vitamin Ingredients: Each tablet contains the vitamins of the Regular product plus 15 mg of Iron.

Indication: Dietary supplementation.

Dosage and Administration: One chewable tablet daily for children two years and older.

Warning: Phenylketonurics: Contains Phenylalanine.

Precaution: Contains iron, which can be harmful in large doses. Close tightly and keep out of reach of children. In case of overdose, contact a physician or poison control center immediately.

How Supplied: SUNKIST Children's Multivitamins Plus Iron are supplied in bottles of 60 chewable tablets with child resistant caps.

Shown in Product Identification Section, page 408

SUNKIST CHILDREN'S CHEWABLE MULTIVITAMINS—COMPLETE

Vitamin Ingredients: Each tablet contains the following ingredients:
[See table on next page.]

Indication: Dietary supplementation.

Dosage and Administration: Children ages 2 to 4 one-half chewable tablet daily; One chewable tablet daily for children four years and older.

Warning: Phenylketonurics: Contains Phenylalanine.

Precautions: Contains iron, which can be harmful in large doses. Close tightly and keep out of reach of children. In case of overdose, contact a physician or poison control center immediately.

How Supplied: SUNKIST Children's Multivitamins Complete are supplied in bottles of 60 chewable tablets with child resistant caps.

Shown in Product Identification Section, page 408

SUNKIST® VITAMIN C
Citrus Complex
Chewable Tablets
Easy to Swallow Caplets

Description: All Sunkist Vitamin C chewable tablets have a delicious orange flavor unlike any other Vitamin C tablet. Each 60 mg chewable tablet contains 100% of the U.S. RDA* of Vitamin C. Each 250 mg chewable tablet contains 417% of the U.S. RDA* of Vitamin C. Each 500 mg chewable tablet contains 833% of the U.S. RDA* of Vitamin C.

Each 500 mg easy to swallow caplet contains 833% of the U.S. RDA* of Vitamin C.

Sunkist Vitamin C chewable tablets and easy to swallow caplets do not contain artificial flavors, colors or preservatives.

*U.S. Recommended Daily Allowance for adults and children over 4 years of age.

Indication: Dietary supplement.

How Supplied: 60 mg Chewable Tablets—Rolls of 11.
250 mg and 500 mg Chewable Tablets—Bottles of 60.
500 mg Easy to Swallow Caplets—Bottles of 60.

Store in a cool dry place.

Sunkist® is a registered trademark of Sunkist Growers, Inc., Sherman Oaks, CA 91423.©

(12/86)

Shown in Product Identification Section, page 408

The full prescribing information for each CIBA Consumer Pharmaceuticals product is contained herein and is that in effect as of December 1, 1990.

Products are indexed alphabetically in the **PINK SECTION**

Colgate-Palmolive Company

A Delaware Corporation
300 PARK AVENUE
NEW YORK, NY 10022

COLGATE® JUNIOR FLUORIDE GEL TOOTHPASTE

Active Ingredient: Sodium Fluoride (NaF) 0.24% in a fruit-flavored toothpaste base.

Other Ingredients: Sorbitol, Glycerin, Hydrated Silica, Water, PEG-12, Sodium Lauryl Sulfate, Sodium Benzoate, Flavor, Cellulose Gum, Sodium Saccharin, Titanium Dioxide, FD&C Blue No. 1, D&C Yellow No. 10.

Indications: This toothpaste, with its anti-cavity ingredient Sodium Fluoride, provides clinically proven fluoride protection. It has been specially formulated to appeal to children 12 and under.

Actions: Clinical tests have shown Colgate® with Sodium Fluoride to be an effective aid in the reduction of the incidence of cavities. It is approved as a decay-preventive agent by the American Dental Association.

Contraindications: Sensitivity to any ingredient in the product.

Directions: Brush regularly as part of a dental health program.

How Supplied: 2.7 oz., 4.5 oz., 6.4 oz., and 8.2 oz. tubes. Also available in 4.5 oz. pump.

Shown in Product Identification Section, page 408

COLGATE Fluoride FLUORIDE GEL

Active Ingredient: Sodium Fluoride (NaF) 0.24% in a spearmint flavored gel toothpaste base.

Other Ingredients: Sorbitol, Glycerin, Hydrated Silica, Water, PEG-12, Sodium Lauryl Sulfate, Flavor, Sodium Benzoate, Cellulose Gum, Sodium Saccharin, Titanium Dioxide, FD&C Blue No. 1.

Indications: The gel toothpaste with the anti-cavity ingredient Sodium Fluoride providing maximum fluoride protection by a toothpaste and a fresh clean taste for the whole family.

Actions: Clinical tests have shown COLGATE® with Sodium Fluoride to be an effective aid in the reduction of the incidence of cavities. It is approved as a decay-preventive dentifrice by the American Dental Association.

Contraindications: Sensitivity to any ingredient in this product.

Directions: Brush regularly as part of a dental health program.

How Supplied: 1.4 oz., 2.6 oz., 4.6 oz., 6.4 oz., 8.2 oz. tubes. Also available in 4.5 and 6.4 oz. pumps.

Shown in Product Identification Section, page 408

COLGATE MFP® FLUORIDE TOOTHPASTE

Active Ingredient: Sodium Monofluorophosphate (MFP®) 0.76% in a doublemint flavored toothpaste base.

Other Ingredients: Dicalcium Phosphate Dihydrate, Water, Glycerin, Sodium Lauryl Sulfate, Cellulose Gum, Flavor, Sodium Benzoate, Tetrasodium Pyrophosphate, Sodium Saccharin.

Indications: The toothpaste with the anti-cavity ingredient MFP® Fluoride providing maximum fluoride protection by a toothpaste.

Actions: Clinical tests have shown COLGATE® with MFP® Fluoride to be an effective aid in the reduction of the incidence of cavities. It is approved as a decay-preventive dentifrice by the American Dental Association.

Contraindications: Sensitivity to any ingredient in this product.

Directions: Brush regularly as part of a dental health program.

How Supplied: 1.50 oz., 3.0 oz., 5.0 oz., 7.0 oz., 9.0 oz. tubes. Also available in 4.9 and 6.4 oz. pumps with Sodium Fluoride (NaF) 0.24%.

Shown in Product Identification Section, page 408

COLGATE® MOUTHWASH TARTAR CONTROL FORMULA

Ingredients: Water, SD Alcohol 38-B (15.3%), Glycerin, Tetrapotassium Pyrophosphate, Poloxamer 336, Poloxamer 407, Tetrasodium Pyrophosphate, Benzoic Acid, PVM/MA Copolymer, Flavor, Sodium Saccharin, Sodium Fluoride, FD&C Blue #1, FD&C Yellow #5.

Indications: Highly effective in the inhibition of supragingival calculus, Colgate Mouthrinse Tartar Control Formula also provides effective breath odor control.

Actions: Clinical studies have shown that Colgate's exclusive combination of pyrophosphate and PVM/MA copolymer reduces calculus build-up by up to 37.7%.

Contraindications: Sensitivity to any ingredient in the product.

Directions: Adults and children 6 years of age and older. Use twice daily after brushing teeth with a toothpaste. Vigorously swish 10 ml. (2 teaspoons; or up to mark on cap) of rinse between teeth for 1 minute and then expectorate. Do not swallow rinse. Do not eat or drink for 30 minutes after rinsing. Children under 6 years of age: Consult a dentist or physician. Children under 12 years of age should be supervised in the use of this product.

How Supplied: 2 oz., 6 oz., 24 oz. and 32 oz. plastic bottles with dose-measure cap.

Shown in Product Identification Section, page 409

COLGATE® TARTAR CONTROL FORMULA

Active Ingredient: Sodium Fluoride 0.24% in a mint flavored toothpaste base.

Other Ingredients: Water, Hydrated Silica, Sorbitol, Glycerine, PEG-12, Tetrapotassium Pyrophosphate, Tetrasodium Pyrophosphate, Sodium Lauryl Sulfate, Flavor, PVM/MA Copolymer, Titanium Dioxide, Carrageenan,

		PERCENT U.S. RDA	
VITAMINS	QUANTITY PER TABLET	FOR CHILD. 2 TO 4 YRS OF AGE (½ TABLET)	FOR ADULTS & CHILD. OVER 4 YRS OF AGE (1 TABLET)
Vitamin A (as Palmitate + Beta Carotene)	5000 IU	100	100
Vitamin D-3	400 IU	50	100
Vitamin E	30 IU	150	100
Vitamin C	60 mg	75	100
Folic Acid	0.4 mg	100	100
Biotin	40 mcg	13	13
Pantothenic Acid	10 mg	100	100
Niacinamide	20 mg	111	100
Vitamin B-6	2 mg	143	100
Vitamin B-12	6 mcg	100	100
Vitamin B-1	1.5 mg	107	100
Vitamin B-2	1.7 mg	106	100
Vitamin K-1	10 mcg	*	*
MINERALS			
Iron	18 mg	90	100
Magnesium	20 mg	5	5
Iodine	150 mcg	107	100
Zinc	10 mg	63	67
Manganese	1 mg	*	*
Calcium	100 mg	6	10
Phosphorus	78 mg	5	8
Copper	2 mg	100	100

*Recognized as essential in human nutrition, but no U.S. RDA established.

Sodium Saccharin. CONTAINS NO SUGAR.

Indications: This toothpaste with the anti-cavity ingredient sodium fluoride provides maximum fluoride protection by a toothpaste and is highly effective in inhibiting the formation of calculus. Repeated clinical studies have demonstrated an average 46% inhibition of calculus buildup.

Actions: Clinical tests have shown Colgate Tartar Control Formula to be effective in the reduction of calculus accumulation. It is also approved as a decay preventive dentifrice by the American Dental Association.

Contraindications: Sensitivity to any ingredient in the product.

Directions: Brush regularly as part of a dental health program.

How Supplied: 1.3 oz., 2.6 oz., 4.6 oz., 6.4 oz., and 8.2 oz. tubes. Also available in 4.5 oz. Pump.

Shown in Product Identification Section, page 409

COLGATE® TARTAR CONTROL GEL

Active Ingredient: Sodium Fluoride 0.24% in a mint flavored gel toothpaste base.

Other Ingredients: Water, Hydrated Silica, Sorbitol, Glycerine, PEG-12, Tetrapotassium Pyrophosphate, Tetrasodium Pyrophosphate, Sodium Lauryl Sulfate, Flavor, PVM/MA Copolymer, Carrageenan, Sodium Saccharin, FD&C Blue No. 1. CONTAINS NO SUGAR.

Indications: This gel toothpaste with the anti-cavity ingredient sodium fluoride provides maximum fluoride protection by a toothpaste and is highly effective in inhibiting the formation of calculus. Repeated clinical studies have demonstrated an average 46% inhibition of calculus buildup.

Actions: Clinical tests have shown Colgate Tartar Control Gel to be effective in the reduction of calculus accumulation. It is also approved as a decay preventive dentifrice by the American Dental Association.

Contraindications: Sensitivity to any ingredient in the product.

Directions: Brush regularly as part of a dental health program.

How Supplied: 1.3 oz., 2.6 oz., 4.6 oz., 6.4 oz., and 8.2 oz. tubes. Also available in 4.5 oz. Pump.

Shown in Product Identification Section, page 408

FLUORIGARD ANTI-CAVITY FLUORIDE RINSE

Fluorigard is accepted by the American Dental Association.

Active Ingredient: Sodium Fluoride (0.05%) in a neutral solution.

Other Ingredients: Water, Glycerin, SD Alcohol 38-B (6%), Poloxamer 338, Poloxamer 407, Sodium Benzoate, Sodium Saccharin, Benzoic Acid, Flavor, FD & C Blue No. 1, FD & C Yellow No. 5.

Indications: Good tasting Fluorigard Anti-Cavity Fluoride Rinse is fluoride in liquid form. It helps get cavity-fighting fluoride to back teeth, as well as front teeth; even floods those dangerous spaces between teeth where brushing might miss. 70% of all cavities happen in back teeth and between teeth.

Actions: Fluorigard Anti-Cavity Fluoride Rinse is a 0.05% Sodium Fluoride solution which has been proven effective in reducing cavities.

Contraindications: Sensitivity to any ingredient in this product.

Warnings: Do not swallow. For rinsing only. Not to be used by children under 6 years of age unless recommended by a dentist. Keep out of reach of young children. If an amount considerably larger than recommended for rinsing is swallowed, give as much milk as possible and contact a physician immediately.

Directions: Use once daily after thoroughly brushing teeth. For persons 6 years of age and over, fill measuring cap to 10 ml. level (2 teaspoons), rinse around and between teeth for one minute, then spit out. For maximum benefit, use every day and do not eat or drink for at least 30 minutes afterward. Rinsing may be most convenient at bedtime. This product may be used in addition to a fluoride toothpaste.

How Supplied: 6 oz., 12 oz., 18 oz. in shatterproof plastic bottles.
1 Gallon Professional Size for use in dentists' offices only.

Shown in Product Identification Section, page 409

Products are indexed by product category in the **BLUE SECTION**

Age	Initial Dose	Maximum Dose per 24 hours
Adults and children over 12 years	4 tsp or 4 Tablets	12 tsp or 12 Tablets
Children 6–12 years	2 tsp or 2 Tablets	6 tsp or 6 Tablets
Children 3–6 years	1 tsp or 1 Tablet	3 tsp or 3 Tablets
Infants and children under 3 years	Only as directed by a physician	

Columbia Laboratories, Inc.

4000 HOLLYWOOD BLVD.
HOLLYWOOD, FL 33021

DIASORB®

[*dī 'ă-zorb*]

Nonfibrous Activated Attapulgite Liquid and Tablets

Description: Diasorb relieves cramps and pain associated with diarrhea. It is available as a pleasant-tasting cola-flavored liquid and as easy-to-swallow tablets. Diasorb is safe for children.

Active Ingredient: Each liquid teaspoonful and tablet contains 750 mg nonfibrous activated attapulgite.

Inactive Ingredients: *Liquid*—Benzoic acid, citric acid, flavor, glycerin, magnesium aluminum silicate, methylparaben, polysorbate, propylene glycol, propylparaben, saccharin, sodium hypochlorite solution, sorbitol, xanthan gum, and water. *Tablet*—D&C Red No. 30 aluminum lake, distilled acetylated monoglycerides, ethylcellulose, gelatin, hydroxypropyl methylcellulose, magnesium stearate, mannitol, titanium dioxide, and water.

Directions for Use: Take the full recommended starting dose at the first sign of diarrhea, and repeat after each subsequent bowel movement. Do not exceed maximum recommended dose per day. Shake liquid well before using. **Swallow tablets with water. Do not chew.**

Warning: Do not use for more than 2 days or in the presence of fever or in infants or children under 3, unless directed by a physician. In case of accidental overdose, seek professional assistance or contact a poison control center immediately. **Store at room temperature.**
KEEP THIS AND ALL MEDICATIONS OUT OF THE REACH OF CHILDREN.

Dosage: See Table for recommended dosage for acute diarrhea.
[See table above.]

How Supplied: *Liquid*—In plastic bottles of 4 fl oz (120 mL).
Tablets—Packaged in blister packs of 24.

Shown in Product Identification Section, page 409

Continued on next page

Columbia—Cont.

LEGATRIN®
[*lega-trin*]

Active Ingredient: Quinine Sulfate, 162.5 mg per tablet.

Other Ingredients: Calcium phosphate dibasic, cellulose, croscarmellose sodium, FD&C blue No. 2 aluminum lake, FD&C red No. 40 aluminum lake, gelatin, hydroxypropyl cellulose, hydroxypropyl methylcellulose, magnesium stearate, polyethylene glycol 400, silica, starch, stearic acid, titanium dioxide.

Indications: For prevention and temporary relief of night leg cramps, muscle spasms, restless legs.

Warnings: Discontinue use and consult a physician immediately if swelling, bruising, skin rash, skin discoloration or bleeding occurs. These symptoms may indicate a serious condition. Discontinue use if ringing in the ears, deafness, diarrhea, nausea or visual disturbances occur. In case of accidental overdose, seek medical assistance or contact Poison Control Center immediately. Do not take if pregnant, nursing a baby, allergic or sensitive to quinine or under 12 years of age. Keep this and all medication out of reach of children.

Dosage: When a leg cramp occurs, take two tablets at once. To help prevent future night leg cramp attacks, take two tablets two hours before bedtime. Do not exceed two tablets daily. Consult a physician if symptoms persist longer than ten days.

How Supplied: Blister packages of 30 and 50 tablets.

Shown in Product Identification Section, page 409

REPLENS® vaginal moisturizer
[*ree 'plenz*]

Description: Replens relieves vaginal dryness, discomfort and painful intercourse for up to 72 hours with a single application. Replens non-hormonal vaginal moisturizer liberates water to continuously hydrate vaginal tissue. Replens is non-staining, fragrance free, unflavored, non-greasy and non-irritating.

Actions: When used as directed, Replens helps relieve vaginal dryness, discomfort and painful intercourse by providing continuous hydration to the vaginal cells.

Ingredients: Purified water, glycerin, mineral oil, polycarbophil, Carbomer 934P, hydrogenated palm oil glyceride, methylparaben, and sorbic acid.

Warnings: Keep out of the reach of children. Replens is not a contraceptive. Does not contain spermicide.

Dosage: Use 3 times a week.

How Supplied: Replens is available in boxes containing 3 and 12 pre-filled disposable applicators. Each applicator contains 2.5 grams.

Shown in Product Identification Section, page 409

Combe, Inc.
**1101 WESTCHESTER AVE.
WHITE PLAINS, NY 10604**

**GYNECORT 5® 0.5%
Hydrocortisone Feminine Itch Relief Creme**

Active Ingredients: 0.5% Hydrocortisone Acetate

Indications: GYNECORT 5® antipruritic creme medication was specifically formulated for the effective relief of external feminine genital itching and itching associated with minor skin irritations. GYNECORT is a highly emollient white vanishing cream which is soothing to delicate vulval tissue. It is hypoallergenic (contains no potentially irritating perfume), greaseless and non-staining.

Action: Hydrocortisone Acetate is an anti-inflammatory corticosteroid whose mechanism of action has been widely investigated. Current thinking points to the following modes of action: (1) controlling the rate of protein synthesis; (2) reducing the amounts of prostaglandin substrate available for the enzyme. Corticosteroids are also known to reduce immune hypersensitivity by reducing the inflammatory response. GYNECORT 5 calms the body's reaction to skin disturbances and so helps natural healing. Also provides external relief of external rectal itching.

Warning: For external use only. Avoid contact with the eyes. If condition worsens or if symptoms persist for more than 7 days, or clear up and recur within a few days, do not use GYNECORT 5 or any other hydrocortisone product, unless a doctor has been consulted. Do not use if you have a vaginal discharge. Consult a physician. Do not use for the treatment of diaper rash. Consult a doctor. Keep this and all drugs out of reach of children. In case of accidental ingestion, seek professional assistance or contact a Poison Control Center immediately.

Dosage and Administration: Adults and children 2 years of age and older. Apply to affected area not more than 3 or 4 times daily. Children under 2 years of age; do not use, consult a physician.

How Supplied: Available in ½ oz. tubes.

References:

1. Goodman and Gilman, *the Pharmacological Basis of Therapeutics.* Page 1487, 5th Ed., MacMillian, 1975.
2. Su-Chen L. Hong, Lawrence Levine, *J. Bio. Chem.*, Vol 251, No 18, pp, 5814–5816, 1976.
3. Ryszard J. Gryglewski, et al. *Prostaglandins,* Vol. 10, No. 2, pp. 343–55, August, 1975.

Shown in Product Identification Section, page 409

LANABIOTIC®

Active Ingredients: Each gram contains Bacitracin 500 units Neomycin Sulfate 5 mg., Polymyxin B Sulfate 10,000 units, Lidocaine 40 mg.

Indications: Applied to minor cuts, scrapes, scratches, burns and other minor wounds LANABIOTIC® Ointment helps prevent infection, aids natural healing with the maximum strength triple antibiotic ingredients available without a prescription. LANABIOTIC also contains Lidocaine to stop pain fast. It aids healing, provides temporary pain relief and protects irritated skin. It is soothing to the minor wound site and will not sting.

Actions: The three ingredients provide broad-spectrum topical antibiotic action against both gram-positive and gram-negative organisms. The Lidocaine pain reliever is quickly absorbed into the skin's damaged nerve endings, and nerve conductance is temporarily blocked, so pain disappears. The gentle occlusive base helps soften dry lesions and provides temporary protection for the wound site. The low melting point of the base provides even, quick spreading without caking.

Warnings: For external use only. Do not use in the eyes or apply over large areas of the body. In case of deep puncture wounds, animal bites, or serious burns, consult a doctor. Stop use and consult a doctor if the condition persists or gets worse. Do not use longer than 1 week unless directed by a doctor. Keep this and all medicines out of reach of children. In case of accidental ingestion, seek professional assistance or contact a Poison Control Center immediately.

Directions: Clean the affected area. Apply a small amount (an amount equal to the surface area of the tip of a finger) directly to the affected areas and cover with sterile gauze if desired. May be applied 1 to 3 times daily as the condition indicates.
Do not use longer than 1 week.

How Supplied: Available in ½ oz. and 1 oz. tubes.

Shown in Product Identification Section, page 409

LANACANE® Creme Medication

Active Ingredients: Benzocaine; Benzethonium Chloride

Indication: LANACANE® Creme Medication is specially formulated to give prompt, temporary relief from dry skin itching, external feminine and rectal itching, heat rash, insect bites, sunburn, chafing, poison ivy, poison oak, poison sumac, chapping sore detergent hands, minor burns and other irritated skin conditions. LANACANE checks bacteria.

Actions: Benzocaine is a well-known anesthetic of low toxicity considered to be one of the safest and most widely used of the over-the-counter topical anesthetics. Temporary anesthesia is elicited by penetrating the cutaneous barriers and blocking sensory receptors for the perception of pain and itching.

Warnings: For external use only. Avoid contact with the eyes. As with all topical medication; if condition worsens, or if symptoms persist for more than 7 days or clear up and occur again within a few days, discontinue use of this product and consult a physician. Keep out of reach of children. In case of accidental ingestion, seek professional assistance or contact a Poison Control Center immediately.

Drug Interaction Precaution: Benzocaine has been known to occasionally cause allergic dermatitis. Cross-reactions have infrequently been reported in other Para-Amino Compounds.

Dosage and Administration: Apply LANACANE Creme Medication liberally to the affected area. Adults and children 2 years of age and older, repeat as needed 3 or 4 times daily. Children under 2 years of age, consult a physician.

How Supplied: Available in 1 and 2 oz. tubes.

Shown in Product Identification Section, page 409

LANACANE® Spray Medication

Active Ingredients (to deliver): Benzocaine 20%, Benzethonium Chloride 0.1%

Indications: LANACANE® Spray Medication offers prompt, cooling, and temporary relief from sunburn along with antimicrobial action to help prevent infection in first aid uses such as cuts, insect bites and minor burns.

Actions: Benzocaine is a well-known anesthetic of low toxicity considered to be one of the safest and most widely used of the over-the-counter topical anesthetics. Temporary anesthesia is elicited by penetrating the cutaneous barriers and blocking sensory receptors for the perception of pain and itching. Benzethonium Chloride is antimicrobial. This non-aqueous aerosol system is an easily applied product and also provides a cooling anti-pruritic action to the skin on application.

Warning: For external use only. Do not spray into eyes, mouth, rectal or vaginal area. Not for deep puncture wounds or serious burns. As with all topical medications; if condition worsens, if a rash or irritation develops, or if symptoms persist for more than 7 days or clear up and occur again within a few days, discontinue use of this product and consult a physician. Do not puncture or incinerate. Do not store at temperatures above 120 F, nor use near fire or throw into fire. Use only as directed. Intentional misuse by deliberately concentrating and inhaling the contents can be harmful or fatal. Keep out of reach of children. In case of accidental ingestion, seek professional assistance or contact a Poison Control Center immediately.

Drug Interaction Precaution: Benzocaine has been known to occasionally cause allergic dermatitis. Cross-reactions have infrequently been reported with Para-Amino Compounds such as paraphenylenediamine, a hair dye, sulfa drugs and sun screens containing paraaminobenzoic acid esters.

Directions: Adults and children 2 years of age and older; apply to affected area not more than 3 to 4 times daily. Children under 2 years of age; consult a physician. Hold can 4 to 6 inches from skin, spray a protective film over the affected area. Rub in gently if desired.

How Supplied: Available in 4 oz. aerosol can.

Shown in Product Identification Section, page 409

LANACORT 5® Anti-Itch Hydrocortisone 0.5% Creme and Ointment

Active Ingredients: 0.5% Hydrocortisone Acetate

Indications: Lanacort 5® blends hydrocortisone acetate with a soothing aloe-containing moisturizing creme (or ointment) to provide temporary relief of itching associated with minor skin irritations, inflammation and rashes due to eczema (symptoms are redness, itching and flaking), psoriasis, seborrheic dermatitis, soaps, detergents, insect bites, cosmetics, jewelry, poison ivy, poison oak, poison sumac and for external feminine and rectal itching.

Actions: Hydrocortisone Acetate is an anti-inflammatory corticosteroid[1,2] whose mechanism of action has been widely investigated. Current thinking points to the following modes of action: (1) controlling the rate of protein synthesis; (2) reducing the amounts of prostaglandin substrate available for the enzyme.[3] Corticosteroids are also known to reduce immune hypersensitivity by reducing the inflammatory response.[1]

Warning: For external use only. Avoid contact with the eyes. If condition worsens or if symptoms persist for more than 7 days, or clear up and occur again within a few days, discontinue use of this product and consult a physician. Do not use for external feminine itching if an unusual or abnormal vaginal discharge is present. Consult a physician. Do not use for the treatment of diaper rash. Consult a physician. Keep out of reach of children. In case of accidental ingestion, seek professional assistance or contact a Poison Control Center immediately.

Dosage and Administration: Adults and children 2 years of age and older: Apply to affected area not more than 3 to 4 times daily. Children under 2 years of age; consult a physician.

How Supplied: Available in ½ and 1 oz. tubes. Ointment in ½ oz. tubes.

References:

1. Goodman and Gilman, *the pharmacological basis of Therapeutics,* page 1487, 5th Ed. MacMillan, 1975.
2. Su-Chen L. Hong Lawrence Levine, *J. Bio. Chem.* Vol. 251, No. 18, pp. 5814–5816, 1976.
3. Ryszard J. Gryglewski, et al., *Prostaglandins,* Vol. 10, No. 2 pp. 343–55, August 1975.

Shown in Product Identification Section, page 409

ODOR-EATERS Antifungal Spray Powder

Active Ingredients: Tolnaftate 1%

Description: An antifungal aerosol spray powder that contains Tolnaftate, a clinically proven ingredient that kills athlete's foot fungi on contact.

Indication: Athlete's foot fungi.

Actions and Uses: With clinically proven Tolnaftate, ODOR-EATERS Antifungal Spray Powder kills athlete's foot fungi on contact and prevents reinfection with daily use. It also soothes and cools burning and itching feet—and helps to control foot odor.

Directions: Thoroughly wash and dry infected areas twice daily. Shake can well. Hold at a convenient angle and apply spray from 4 to 6 inches away. Spray liberally between toes, and feet and into shoes. After symptoms disappear, continue treatment to prevent reinfection.

Warnings: For external use only. Do not use on children under 2 years of age except under advice and supervision of a doctor. Avoid spraying in eyes. If irritation occurs or symptoms do not improve in 4 weeks discontinue use and consult your physician. Contents under pressure. Do not puncture or incinerate. Do not store at temperatures above 120 F. Flammable mixture: do not use near fire or flame. Use only as directed. Intentional misuse by deliberately concentrating and inhaling the contents can be harmful or fatal. Keep out of reach of children. In case of accidental ingestion, seek professional assistance or contact a Poison Control Center immediately.

How Supplied: Available in 3 oz. aerosol can.

Shown in Product Identification Section, page 409

VAGISIL® Creme Medication

Active Ingredients: Benzocaine, Resorcin

Indications: VAGISIL® Creme Medication has been formulated to give prompt effective relief from the discomfort of minor itching, burning, and other irritations of the external feminine genitalia (vulva). VAGISIL forms a cooling, protective film over irritated tissues to reduce the chance of further irritation. Lightly scented, stainless, greaseless.

Continued on next page

Combe—Cont.

Actions: Benzocaine is a well-known anesthetic of low toxicity considered to be one of the safest and most widely used of the over-the-counter topical anesthetics. Temporary anesthesia is elicited by penetrating the cutaneous barriers and blocking sensory receptors for the perception of pain and itching. Resorcin activity is mildly keratolytic and antipruritic.

Warnings: For external use only. Avoid contact with the eyes. If condition worsens or if symptoms persist for more than 7 days, or clear up and occur again within a few days, discontinue use and consult a physician. Do not use if an unusual or abnormal discharge is present, including a discharge suspected of being caused by a yeast infection except under the supervision of a physician. A doctor should be seen by the patient if a yeast infection is suspected, for only a doctor can diagnose and treat a yeast infection. Keep this and all drugs out of reach of children. In case of accidental ingestion, seek professional assistance or contact a Poison Control Center immediately.

Drug Interaction Precaution: Benzocaine has been known to occasionally cause allergic dermatitis. Cross-reactions have infrequently been reported with other Para-Amino Compounds such as para-phenylenediamine a hair dye, sulfa drugs and sun screens containing para-aminobenzoic acid esters.

Dosage and Administration: Adults and children 2 years of age and older; apply to affected area not more than 3 to 4 times daily. Children under 2 years of age; consult a physician.

How Supplied: Available in 1 and 2 oz. tubes.

Shown in Product Identification Section, page 409

VAGISIL® Feminine Powder

Active Ingredients: None

Indications: VAGISIL® Feminine Powder is the first powder designed specifically for the external vaginal (vulval) area. Cornstarch-based, it offers several special advantages over traditional talcum powders in absorbing moisture to control wetness from discharge or perspiration, the major causes of itching and irritations. VAGISIL Feminine Powder also absorbs odor to help promote freshness. VAGISIL Feminine Powder contains microencapsulated mineral oil and, hence, provides a barrier against moisture to help protect against irritation and chafing.

Actions: Microfine cornstarch offers as much as 25 times the moisture absorptive capacity of talc. Mineral oil provides an exclusive moisture barrier to help soothe sensitive skin and protect against irritation. VAGISIL Feminine Powder is 100% talc-free as gynecologists recommend.

Warning: Keep out of reach of children.

Directions: Safe and gentle enough to use as often as you like.

How Supplied: Available in 7 oz. and 11 oz. containers.

Shown in Product Identification Section, page 409

Copley Pharmaceutical Inc.

25 JOHN RD
CANTON, MA 02021

LICE·ENZ FOAM
Shampoo Aerosol
Lice Killing Shampoo Kit

Description: Lice·Enz Foam shampoo is supplied as a metered aerosol delivery system for ease of application to the patient for the treatment of lice infestation.

Active Ingredients: Pyrethrins 0.3%, Piperonyl Butoxide, 3.0%; inert ingredients, 96.7%.

Indications: Lice·Enz is indicated for the treatment of human pediculosis—head lice, body lice, pubic lice and their eggs. Lice·Enz is specially formulated for head lice in children. The mousse application allows complete control of the amount of pesticide the child is exposed to; no messy shampoo to drip onto the child. Lice·Enz is user friendly and easy to apply.

Actions: Lice·Enz is a pediculicide for control of head lice, pubic lice and body lice and their nits.
SHOULD NOT BE USED BY RAGWEED-SENSITIZED PERSONS.
KEEP THIS AND ALL DRUGS OUT OF THE REACH OF CHILDREN.
CAUTIONS: For external use only. Harmful if swallowed. Do not inhale. Keep out of eyes and avoid contact with mucous membranes.

First Aid: In case this product should get in eyes, flush immediately with water. In case of infection or skin irritation, discontinue use and consult a physician. Consult a physician if infestation of eyebrows and eyelashes occur. Avoid contamination of food or foodstuffs. Use only as directed. Intentional misuse by deliberately concentrating and inhaling the contents can be harmful or fatal.

Physical or Chemical Hazard: Contents under pressure. Do not use or store near heat or open flame. Do not puncture or incinerate container. Exposure to temperatures above 120°F may cause bursting.

Storage: Store away from heat, sparks and open flame in original container and in an area inaccessible to children.

Disposal: Do not reuse empty container. Replace cap and discard container in trash. Do not incinerate or puncture.

Directions for Use: It is a violation of Federal Law to use this product in a manner inconsistent with its labeling. 1. Shake well. Apply as much LICE·ENZ FOAM as needed to the hair and scalp or any other infested areas until entirely wet. Do not use on eyelashes or eyebrows. 2. Massage LICE·ENZ FOAM into scalp and allow it to remain for no more than 10 minutes. 3. Wash hair thoroughly with warm water and shampoo or soap. 4. If desired, apply creme rinse to ease the nit removal process. 5. Comb hair with special no-nit comb to remove dead lice and eggs. 6. After combing, rinse hair thoroughly. 7. Repeat treatment in 7–10 days if reinfestation has occurred. 8. Do not exceed two consecutive applications within 24 hours. To help eliminate infestation, it is important to sterilize all clothing and bedding of infested person at time of treatment.
Note: The manufacturer of this product endorses the National Pediculosis Association's "No Nit Policy."

How Supplied: LICE·ENZ FOAM aerosol is supplied in a 2-ounce aerosol container (ozone-friendly propellant).

Literature Available: Additional patient literature available upon request.

Shown in Product Identification Section, page 409

Fisons Consumer Health Division

Fisons Corporation
P.O. BOX 1212
ROCHESTER, NY 14603

AMERICAINE® HEMORRHOIDAL OINTMENT
[*a-mer 'i-kān*]

Active Ingredient: Benzocaine 20%.

Other Ingredients: Benzethonium Chloride; Polyethylene Glycol 300; Polyethylene Glycol 3350.

Indications: For the temporary relief of local pain, itching and soreness associated with hemorrhoids and anorectal inflammation.

Warnings: If condition worsens, or does not improve within 7 days, consult a physician. Do not exceed the recommended daily dosage unless directed by a physician. In case of bleeding, consult a physician promptly. Do not put this product into the rectum by using fingers or any mechanical device or applicator. Certain persons can develop allergic reactions to ingredients in this product. If the symptom being treated does not subside or if redness, irritation, swelling, pain, or other symptoms develop or increase, discontinue use and consult a physician. **Keep this and all drugs out of the reach of children.** In case of accidental ingestion, seek professional assistance or contact a Poison Control Center immediately.

Directions: *Adults:* When practical, cleanse the affected area with mild soap and warm water and rinse thoroughly. Gently dry by patting or blotting with toilet tissue or a soft cloth before application of this product. Apply externally to the affected area up to 6 times daily. *Children under 12 years of age:* Consult a physician.

How Supplied: *Hemorrhoidal Ointment*—1 oz. tube.

Shown in Product Identification Section, page 409

AMERICAINE® TOPICAL ANESTHETIC SPRAY AND FIRST AID OINTMENT

[*a-mer 'i-kān*]

Active Ingredient: Benzocaine 20%.

Other Ingredients: *Spray*—Butane (propellant); Isobutane (propellant); Polyethylene Glycol 200; Propane (propellant). *Ointment*—Benzethonium chloride; Polyethylene Glycol 300; Polyethylene Glycol 3350.

Indications: For the temporary relief of pain and itching associated with minor cuts, scrapes, burns, sunburn, insect bites, or minor skin irritations.

Warnings: For external use only. Avoid contact with the eyes. If condition worsens, or if symptoms persist for more than 7 days or clear up and occur again within a few days, discontinue use of this product and consult a physician. Keep this and all drugs out of the reach of children. In case of accidental ingestion, seek professional assistance or contact a Poison Control Center immediately. *For Spray only*—Contents under pressure. Do not puncture or incinerate. Flammable mixture; do not use near fire or flame. Do not store at temperature above 120°F. Use only as directed. Intentional misuse by deliberately concentrating and inhaling the contents can be harmful or fatal.

Directions: Adults and children 2 years of age and older: Apply liberally to affected area not more than 3 to 4 times daily. Children under 2 years of age: Consult a physician.

How Supplied: *Topical Anesthetic Spray*—2/3 oz., 2 oz. and 4 oz. aerosol containers. *First Aid Ointment*—3/4 oz. tube, which is a clear, fragrance-free gel formula that is nonstaining, easy to apply, and is easily removed with soap and water.

Shown in Product Identification Section, page 409

ALLEREST® MAXIMUM STRENGTH TABLETS, CHILDREN'S CHEWABLE TABLETS, HEADACHE STRENGTH TABLETS, SINUS PAIN FORMULA TABLETS, 12 HOUR CAPLETS AND NO DROWSINESS ALLEREST™ TABLETS

[*al 'e-rest*]

Active Ingredients:
acetaminophen
- Headache Strength, 325 mg
- No Drowsiness, 325 mg
- Sinus Pain Formula, 500 mg

chlorpheniramine maleate
- Maximum Strength, 2 mg
- Children's Chewables, 1 mg
- Sinus Pain Formula, 2 mg
- Headache Strength, 2 mg
- 12 Hour Caplets, 12 mg

phenylpropanolamine HCl
- Children's Chewables, 9.4 mg
- 12 Hour Caplets, 75 mg

pseudoephedrine HCl
- No Drowsiness, 30 mg
- Maximum Strength, 30 mg
- Sinus Pain Formula, 30 mg
- Headache Strength, 30 mg

Other Ingredients:
Allerest Tablets— Blue 1; Dibasic Calcium Phosphate; Magnesium Stearate; Microcrystalline Cellulose; Povidone; Pregelatinized Starch; Sodium Starch Glycolate.
Children's Chewable Tablets—Calcium Stearate; Citric Acid; Flavor; Magnesium Trisilicate Mannitol; Saccharin Sodium; Sorbitol.
Headache Strength and No Drowsiness Tablets—Magnesium Stearate; Microcrystalline Cellulose; Povidone; Pregelatinized Starch.
Sinus Pain Formula Tablets—Magnesium Stearate; Microcrystalline Cellulose; Povidone; Pregelatinized Starch; Sodium Starch Glycolate.
12 Hour Caplets—Carnauba Wax; Colloidal Silicon Dioxide; Lactose; Methylcellulose; Polyethylene Glycol; Povidone; Red 30; Stearic Acid; Titanium Dioxide; Yellow 6.

Indications: Allerest is indicated for symptomatic relief of hay fever, pollen allergies, upper respiratory allergies (allergic rhinitis), sinusitis and nasal passage congestion. Those symptoms include headache pain, sneezing, runny nose, itchy/watery eyes, and itching of the nose and throat.

Actions: Allerest contains the antihistamine chlorpheniramine maleate which acts to suppress the symptoms of allergic rhinitis. In addition, it may contain the decongestant phenylpropanolamine hydrochloride or pseudoephedrine hydrochloride which acts to reduce swelling of the upper respiratory tract mucosa. Headache Strength and Sinus Pain Formula also contain acetaminophen to relieve headache pain.
No Drowsiness Allerest contains the decongestant pseudoephedrine hydrochloride and the analgesic acetaminophen to relieve headache pain and nasal congestion without causing drowsiness.

Contraindications: Known hypersensitivity to the ingredients in this drug.

Warnings: Allerest should be used with caution in patients with high blood pressure, heart disease, diabetes, thyroid disease, asthma, glaucoma, emphysema, chronic pulmonary disease, shortness of breath, difficulty in breathing, or difficulty in urination due to enlargement of the prostate gland. Since antihistamines may cause drowsiness, patients should be instructed not to operate a car or machinery. Products containing analgesics should not be taken for more than 10 days in adults and 5 days in children under 12. **Keep this and all drugs out of the reach of children.** In case of accidental ingestion, seek professional assistance or contact a Poison Control Center immediately.

Drug Interaction Precaution: Not to be taken by patients currently taking a prescription antihypertensive or antidepressant drug containing a monoamine oxidase inhibitor except under the advice and supervision of a physician.
Antihistamines and oral nasal decongestants have additive effects with alcohol and other CNS depressants.

Adverse Reactions: Drowsiness; excitability, especially in children; nervousness; dizziness and sleeplessness.

Overdosage: Acetaminophen in massive overdosage may cause hepatotoxicity.

Dosage and Administration:
Tablets and Headache Strength—**Adults and children 12 years of age and over:** 2 tablets every 4 to 6 hours, not exceed 8 tablets in 24 hours. **Children 6 to under 12 years of age:** 1 tablet every 4 to 6 hours, not to exceed 4 tablets in 24 hours. Dosage for children under 6 should be individualized under the supervision of a physician. *Children's Chewable Tablets*—**Children 6 to under 12 years of age:** 2 tablets every 4 hours, not to exceed 8 tablets in 24 hours. **Children under 6:** consult a physician. *Sinus Pain Formula*—**Adults:** 2 tablets every 6 hours. Not to exceed 8 tablets in 24 hours. Not recommended for children 12 and under. *12 Hour Caplets*-—**Adults and children over 12 years of age:** 1 caplet every 12 hours. Do not exceed 2 caplets in 24 hours. *No Drowsiness:*—**Adults and children 12 years of age and over:** 2 tablets every 4 hours, not to exceed 8 tablets in 24 hours. **Children 6 to under 12 years of age:** 1 tablet every 4 hours, not to exceed 4 tablets in 24 hours.

How Supplied: *Tablets*—packaged on blister cards in 24, 48 and 72 count cartons. *Children's Chewable Tablets*—packaged on blister cards in 24 count cartons. *Headache Strength Tablets*—packaged on blister cards in 24 count cartons. *Sinus Pain Formula Tablets*—packaged on blister cards in 20 count cartons. *12 Hour Caplets*—packaged on blister cards in 10 count cartons.

Continued on next page

Fisons—Cont.

No Drowsiness Tablets—packaged on blister cards in 20 count cartons.

Shown in Product Identification Section, page 409

CaldeCORT® ANTI-ITCH CREAM AND SPRAY; CaldeCORT Light® CREAM

[*kal 'de-kort*]

Active Ingredient: *Cream, Light Cream*—Hydrocortisone Acetate (equivalent to Hydrocortisone 0.5%). *Spray*—Hydrocortisone 0.5%.

Other Ingredients: *Cream*—Glyceryl Monostearate; Lanolin Alcohol; Methylparaben; Mineral Oil; Polyoxyl 40 Stearate; Propylparaben; Sodium Metabisulfite; Sorbitol Solution; Stearyl Alcohol; Water; White Petrolatum; White Wax. *Light Cream*—Aloe Vera Gel; Isopropyl Myristate; Methylparaben; Polysorbate 60; Propylparaben; Sorbitan Monostearate; Sorbitol Solution; Stearic Acid; Water. *Spray*—Isobutane (propellant); Isopropyl Myristate; SD Alcohol 40-B 89.5% by volume.

Indications: For the temporary relief of itching associated with minor skin irritations, inflammation and rashes due to eczema, insect bites, poison ivy, poison oak, poison sumac, soaps, detergents, cosmetics and jewelry; and for external genital itching.

Actions: Antidermatitis cream and spray for the temporary relief from itching and minor skin irritations in a gentle, greaseless, fragrance-free formula.

Warnings: For external use only. Avoid contact with the eyes. If condition worsens, or if symptoms persist for more than 7 days or clear up and occur again within a few days, discontinue use and consult a doctor. Do not use if you have a vaginal discharge. Consult a doctor. Keep this and all drugs out of the reach of children. In case of accidental ingestion, seek professional assistance or contact a Poison Control Center immediately. *For Spray only*—Avoid contact with the eyes or on other mucous membranes. Contents under pressure. Do not puncture or incinerate. Flammable mixture, do not use near fire or flame. Do not store at temperature above 120°F. Use only as directed. Intentional misuse by deliberately concentrating and inhaling the contents can be harmful or fatal.

Directions: Adults and children 2 years of age and older: Apply to affected area not more than 3 to 4 times daily. Children under 2 years of age: Consult a doctor.

How Supplied: *Anti-Itch Cream*—½ and 1 oz. tubes. *Anti-Itch Spray*—1½ oz. can. *Light Cream*—½ oz. tubes.

Shown in Product Identification Section, page 409

CALDESENE® MEDICATED POWDER AND OINTMENT

[*kal 'de-sēn*]

Active Ingredients: *Powder*—Calcium Undecylenate 10%. *Ointment*—Petrolatum 53.9%; Zinc Oxide 15%.

Other Ingredients: *Powder* — Fragrance; Talc. *Ointment*—Cod Liver Oil; Fragrance; Lanolin Oil; Methylparaben; Propylparaben; Talc.

Indications: Caldesene Medicated Powder is indicated to help heal, relieve and prevent diaper rash, prickly heat and chafing. Caldesene Ointment helps treat and prevent diaper rash, protects against urine and other irritants, soothes chafed skin, and promotes healing.

Actions: Only Caldesene Medicated Powder contains calcium undecylenate, an antifungal/antibacterial that inhibits growth of the organisms frequently associated with diaper rash (including *S aureus, S epidermidis, E coli, and P aeruginosa*). Also forms a protective coating to repel moisture, soothe and comfort minor skin irritations, help heal and prevent chafing and prickly heat. Caldesene Ointment forms a protective skin coating to repel moisture and promote healing of diaper rash, while its natural ingredients protect irritated skin against wetness and other irritants. Additionally, the mild astringent action of zinc oxide helps heal local irritation and inflammation. Unlike other ointments containing zinc oxide, Caldesene Ointment has a mild fragrance and is easily removed from the diaper area with soap and water.

Warnings: For external use only. Avoid contact with eyes. If condition worsens or does not improve within 7 days, consult a doctor. Do not apply ointment over deep or puncture wounds, infections and lacerations. Keep this and all drugs out of the reach of children. In case of accidental ingestion, seek professional assistance or contact a Poison Control Center immediately.

Directions: Cleanse and thoroughly dry affected area. Smooth on Caldesene 3–4 times daily, after every bath or diaper change, or as directed by a physician.

How Supplied: *Medicated Powder*—2.0 oz. and 4.0 oz. shaker containers. *Medicated Ointment*—1.25 oz. collapsible tubes.

Shown in Product Identification Section, page 409

CRUEX® ANTIFUNGAL POWDER, SPRAY POWDER AND CREAM

[*kru 'ex*]

Active Ingredients: *Powder*—Calcium Undecylenate 10%. *Spray Powder* — Total Undecylenate 19%, as Undecylenic Acid and Zinc Undecylenate. *Cream*—Total Undecylenate 20%, as Undecylenic Acid and Zinc Undecylenate.

Other Ingredients: *Powder*—Colloidal Silicon Dioxide; Fragrance; Isopropyl Myristate; Talc. *Spray Powder*—Fragrance; Isobutane (propellant); Isopropyl Myristate; Menthol; Talc; Trolamine. *Cream*—Anhydrous Lanolin; Fragrance; Glycol Stearate SE; Methylparaben; PEG-6 Stearate; PEG-8 Laurate; Propylparaben; Sorbitol Solution; Stearic Acid; Trolamine; Water; White Petrolatum.

Indications: For the treatment of Jock Itch (tinea cruris) and relief of itching, chafing, burning rash and irritation in the groin area. Cruex powders also absorb perspiration.

Actions: Antifungal Powder, Spray Powder and Cream are proven clinically effective in the treatment of superficial fungus infections of the skin.

Warnings: Do not use on children under 2 years of age except under the advice and supervision of a doctor. For external use only. If irritation occurs, or if there is no improvement within 2 weeks, discontinue use and consult a doctor or pharmacist. Keep this and all drugs out of the reach of children. In case of accidental ingestion, seek professional assistance or contact a Poison Control Center immediately. *For Spray Powder only*—Avoid spraying in eyes or on other mucous membranes. Contents under pressure. Do not puncture or incinerate. Flammable mixture, do not use near a fire or flame. Do not store at temperature above 120° F. Use only as directed. Intentional misuse by deliberately concentrating and inhaling the contents can be harmful or fatal.

Directions: Cleanse skin with soap and water and dry thoroughly. Apply Cruex to affected area morning and night, before and after athletic activity, or as directed by a doctor. Best results are usually obtained with 2 weeks' use of this product. If satisfactory results have not occurred within this time, consult a doctor or pharmacist. Children under 12 years of age should be supervised in the use of this product. This product is not effective on the scalp or nails.

How Supplied: *Powder*—1.5 oz. plastic squeeze bottle. *Spray Powder*—1.8 oz., 3.5 oz. and 5.5 oz. aerosol containers. *Cream*—½ oz. tube.

Shown in Product Identification Section, page 410

DELSYM®
(dextromethorphan polistirex)
12-Hour Cough Relief

Active Ingredients: Each teaspoonful (5 mL) contains dextromethorphan polistirex equivalent to 30 mg dextromethorphan hydrobromide.

Other Ingredients: Citric acid, ethylcellulose, FD&C Yellow No. 6, flavor, high fructose corn syrup, methylparaben, polyethylene glycol 3350, polysorbate 80, propylene glycol, propylparaben, purified water, sucrose, tragacanth, vegetable oil, xanthan gum.

Indications: Temporarily relieves cough due to minor throat and bronchial irritation as may occur with the common cold or inhaled irritants.

Warnings: Do not take this product for persistent or chronic cough such as occurs with smoking, asthma, emphysema, or if cough is accompanied by excessive phlegm (mucus) unless directed by a physician. A persistent cough may be a sign of a serious condition. If cough persists for more than 1 week, tends to recur, or is accompanied by fever, rash, or persistent headache, consult a physician. As with any drug, if you are pregnant or nursing a baby, seek the advice of a health professional before using this product. Keep this and all drugs out of the reach of children. In case of accidental overdose, seek professional assistance or contact a Poison Control Center immediately.

Directions: Shake Bottle Well Before Using. Dose as follows or as directed by a physician.
Adults and Children 12 years of age and over: 2 teaspoonfuls every 12 hours, not to exceed 4 teaspoonfuls in 24 hours.
Children 6 to under 12 years of age: 1 teaspoonful every 12 hours, not to exceed 2 teaspoonfuls in 24 hours.
Children 2 to under 6 years of age: ½ teaspoonful every 12 hours, not to exceed 1 teaspoonful in 24 hours.
Children under 2 years of age: Consult a physician.

How Supplied: 3 fl. oz. bottles
NDC 0585-0842-61
Fisons Corporation
Rochester, NY 14623 USA

DESENEX® ANTIFUNGAL POWDER, SPRAY POWDER, CREAM, OINTMENT, AND PENETRATING FOAM; SOAP; FOOT & SNEAKER DEODORANT SPRAY

[dess 'i-nex]

Active Ingredients: *Powder, Spray Powder*—Total Undecylenate 19%, as Undecylenic Acid and Zinc Undecylenate. *Cream*—Total Undecylenate 20%, as Undecylenic Acid and Zinc Undecylenate. *Ointment*—Total Undecylenate 22%, as Undecylenic Acid and Zinc Undecylenate. *Penetrating Foam*—Undecylenic Acid 10%. *Foot & Sneaker Deodorant Spray*—Aluminum Chlorohydrex.

Other Ingredients: *Powder* — Fragrance; Talc. *Spray Powder*—Fragrance; Isobutane (propellant); Isopropyl Myristate; Menthol; Talc; Trolamine. *Cream, Ointment*—Anhydrous Lanolin; Fragrance; Glycol Stearate SE; Methylparaben; PEG-6 Stearate; PEG-8 Laurate; Propylparaben; Sorbitol Solution; Stearic Acid; Trolamine; Water; White Petrolatum. *Penetrating Foam*—Emulsifying Wax; Fragrance; Isobutane (propellant); Isopropyl Alcohol 35.2% by volume; Sodium Benzoate; Trolamine; Water. *Foot & Sneaker Deodorant Spray*—Colloidal Silicon Dioxide; Diisopropyl Adipate; Fragrance; Isobutane (propellant); Menthol; SD Alcohol 40-B (23.6% w/w); Talc; Tartaric Acid.

Indications: Desenex Antifungal Products cure athlete's foot (tinea pedis) and body ringworm (tinea corporis) exclusive of the nails and scalp. Relieves itching and burning. Desenex Foot & Sneaker Deodorant Spray helps stop odor and absorbs moisture.

Actions: Desenex Antifungal Powders, Cream, Ointment, and Penetrating Foam are proven effective in the treatment of superficial fungus infections of the skin caused by the three major types of dermatophytic fungi (T. rubrum, T. mentagrophytes, E. floccosum). Penetrating Foam quickly dissolves into a highly concentrated liquid. Foot & Sneaker Deodorant Spray is specially formulated with a unique combination of ingredients including a deodorant, antiperspirant and a moisture-absorbing powder. So it cools, soothes your feet and helps keep them dry and comfortable.

Warnings: Do not use on children under 2 years of age except under the advice and supervision of a doctor. For external use only. Avoid contact with the eyes. If irritation occurs, or if there is no improvement within 4 weeks, discontinue use and consult a doctor. Keep this and all drugs out of the reach of children. In case of accidental ingestion, seek professional assistance or contact a Poison Control Center immediately. *For Spray Powder, Penetrating Foam and Foot & Sneaker Deodorant Spray only*—Avoid spraying in eyes or on other mucous membranes. Contents under pressure. Do not puncture or incinerate. Flammable mixture, do not use near fire or flame. Do not store at temperature above 120° F. Use only as directed. Intentional misuse by deliberately concentrating and inhaling the contents can be harmful or fatal.

Directions: *Powder, Spray Powder, Cream, Ointment, and Penetrating Foam*—Cleanse skin with soap and water and dry thoroughly. Apply over affected area morning and night or as directed by a doctor, paying special attention to the spaces between the toes. It is also helpful to wear well-fitting, ventilated shoes and to change shoes and socks at least once daily. Best results are usually obtained with 4 weeks' use of this product. If satisfactory results have not occurred within this time, consult a doctor. Children under 12 years of age should be supervised in the use of this product. This product is not effective on the scalp or nails. For persistent cases of athlete's foot, use Desenex Ointment or Cream at night and Desenex Powder or Spray Powder during the day. *Soap*—Use in conjunction with Desenex Antifungal Products. *Foot & Sneaker Deodorant Spray*—Spray on soles of feet and between toes daily. For maximum effectiveness, spray in your shoes or sneakers after wearing to keep them fresh and pleasantly scented.

How Supplied: *Powder*—1.5 oz. and 3.0 oz. shaker containers. *Spray Powder*—2.7 oz. and 5.5 oz. aerosol containers. *Cream*—½ oz. tube. *Ointment*—½ oz. and 1 oz. tubes. *Penetrating Foam*—1.5 oz. aerosol container. *Soap*—3.25 oz. bar. *Foot & Sneaker Deodorant Spray*—3.0 oz. aerosol container.

Shown in Product Identification Section, page 410

ISOCLOR® Timesule®

[īs 'ō-klōr]

Capsules

Description: Isoclor® Timesule® Capsules combine a nasal decongestant with an antihistamine in a special sustained release capsule without dyes, artificial coloring or preservatives.
Each Isoclor Timesule Capsule contains 8 mg chlorpheniramine maleate, USP, and 120 mg pseudoephedrine hydrochloride, USP, in a special form providing therapeutic effects up to12 hours.

Indications: For temporary relief of nasal congestion due to the common cold, hay fever, or other upper respiratory allergies, or associated with sinusitis. Helps decongest sinus openings, sinus passages. Reduces swelling of nasal passages, shrinks swollen membranes, and temporarily restores freer breathing through the nose. Alleviates runny nose, sneezing, itching of the nose or throat, and itchy and watery eyes as may occur in allergic rhinitis (such as hay fever).

Directions: Adults and children 12 years and older—one capsule every 12 hours. Do not exceed two capsules in 24 hours.

Drug Interaction Precaution: Do not take this product if you are currently taking a prescription drug for high blood pressure or depression without first consulting your physician.

Warnings: Do not exceed recommended dosage because at higher doses nervousness, dizziness, or sleeplessness may occur. Do not give this product to children under 12 years except under the advice and supervision of a physician. Do not take this product if you have asthma, glaucoma, emphysema, chronic pulmonary disease, shortness of breath, difficulty in breathing, difficulty in urination due to enlargement of the prostate gland, high blood pressure, heart disease, diabetes, or thyroid disease except under the advice and supervision of a physician. If symptoms do not improve within seven days or are accompanied by a high fever, consult a physician before continuing use. May cause drowsiness; alcohol may increase the drowsiness effect. May cause excitability especially in children. As with any drug, if you are pregnant or nursing a baby, seek the advice of a health professional before using this product.
Avoid driving a motor vehicle or operating heavy machinery. Avoid alcoholic beverages while taking this product.
Keep this and all drugs out of the reach of children. In case of accidental overdose, seek professional assistance or contact a Poison Control Center immediately.

Inactive Ingredients: Castor wax, ethylcellulose, gelatin capsule, mineral

Continued on next page

Fisons—Cont.

oil, silicone oil, sugar spheres, white petrolatum.

How Supplied: Packaged on blister cards in cartons of 10's and 20's, and bottles of 100 and 500.
Store at room temperature (15°–30°C, 59°–86°F).
Protect from excessive moisture.
Isoclor® and Timesule® are registered trademarks of Fisons Corporation.
Distributed by:
FISONS
Consumer Health
Rochester, NY 14623 USA

Shown in Product Identification Section, page 410

SINAREST® TABLETS, EXTRA STRENGTH TABLETS AND NO DROWSINESS SINAREST™ TABLETS

[sīn 'a-rest]

Active Ingredients:
acetaminophen:
Tablets, 325 mg
Extra Strength, 500 mg
No Drowsiness, 500 mg
chlorpheniramine maleate
Tablets, 2 mg
Extra Strength, 2 mg
pseudoephedrine HCl
No Drowsiness, 30 mg
Tablets, 30 mg
Extra Strength, 30 mg

Other Ingredients: *All Tablets*—Magnesium Stearate; Microcrystalline Cellulose; Povidone; Pregelatinized Starch. *Extra Strength Tablets and No Drowsiness Tablets only*—Sodium Starch Glycolate. *Sinarest Tablets and Extra Strength Tablets only*—Yellow 10; Yellow 6.

Indications: Sinarest is indicated for symptomatic relief from the headache pain, pressure and nasal congestion associated with sinusitis and allergic rhinitis.

Actions: Sinarest Tablets and Extra Strength Sinarest contain an antihistamine (chlorpheniramine maleate) and a decongestant (pseudoephedrine hydrochloride) for the relief of sinus and nasal passage congestion as well as an analgesic (acetaminophen) to relieve pain and discomfort. No Drowsiness Sinarest contains a decongestant (pseudoephedrine hydrochloride) and an analgesic (acetaminophen) for the relief of headache pain, sinus pressure and nasal congestion without causing drowsiness.

Contraindications: Known hypersensitivity to any of the ingredients in this compound.

Warnings: Sinarest should be used with caution in patients with high blood pressure, heart disease, diabetes, thyroid disease, asthma, glaucoma, emphysema, chronic pulmonary disease, shortness of breath, difficulty in breathing, or difficulty in urination due to enlargement of the prostate gland. Since antihistamines may cause drowsiness, patients should be instructed not to operate a car or machinery. Products containing analgesics should not be taken for more than 10 days in adults and 5 days in children under 12. **Keep this and all drugs out of the reach of children.** In case of accidental ingestion, seek professional assistance or contact a Poison Control Center immediately.

Drug Interaction Precautions: Not to be taken by patients currently taking a prescription drug for high blood pressure or depression except under the advice and supervision of a physician. Antihistamines and oral nasal decongestants have additive effects with alcohol and other CNS depressants.

Adverse Reactions: Drowsiness; excitability, especially in children; nervousness; dizziness; sleeplessness.

Overdosage: Acetaminophen in massive overdosage may cause hepatotoxicity.

Dosage and Administration:
Tablets—Adults and children 12 years of age and older: 2 tablets every 4 hours, not to exceed 8 tablets in 24 hours. Children 6 to under 12 years of age: 1 tablet every 4 hours, not to exceed 4 tablets in 24 hours. Dosage for children under 6 should be individualized under the supervision of a physician. *Extra Strength Tablets*—Adults and children 12 years of age and older: 2 tablets every 6 hours, not to exceed 8 tablets in 24 hours. Not recommended for children under 12. *No Drowsiness Tablets*—Adults and children 12 years of age and older: 2 tablets every 6 hours, not to exceed 8 tablets in 24 hours. Not recommended for children under 12.

How Supplied: *Tablets*—Blister packages of 20, 40 and 80 tablets. *Extra Strength tablets*—package of 24 tablets. *No Drowsiness tablets*—blister package of 20 tablets.

TING® ANTIFUNGAL CREAM, POWDER, SPRAY LIQUID, and SPRAY POWDER

Active Ingredient: Tolnaftate, 1%.

Other Ingredients: *Cream*—BHT, fragrance, polyethylene glycol 400, polyethylene glycol 3350, titanium dioxide. *Powder*—Corn starch, fragrance, talc. *Spray Liquid*—BHT, fragrance, isobutane (propellant), polyethylene glycol 400, SD alcohol 40-B (41% w/w). *Spray Powder*—BHT, fragrance, isobutane (propellant), PPG-12-buteth-16, SD alcohol 40-B (14% w/w), talc.

Indications: Cures athlete's foot and jock itch with a clinically proven ingredient. Relieves itching and burning. Prevents recurrence of athlete's foot with daily use.

Actions: Ting soothes itching, burning, chafing, and irritation. It kills superficial fungi of the skin which cause athlete's foot. And, because Ting contains tolnaftate, daily use prevents reinfection of athlete's foot.

Warnings: Do not use on children under 2 years of age except under the advice and supervision of a doctor. For external use only. If irritation occurs, or if there is no improvement within 4 weeks for athlete's foot, or within 2 weeks for jock itch, discontinue use and consult a doctor or pharmacist. Keep this and all drugs out of the reach of children. In case of accidental ingestion, seek professional assistance or contact a Poison Control Center immediately. *For Spray Liquid and Spray Powder only*—Avoid spraying on eyes or on other mucous membranes. Contents under pressure; do not puncture or incinerate. Flammable mixture, do not use near fire or flame. Do not store at temperature above 120°F. Use only as directed. Intentional misuse by deliberately concentrating and inhaling contents can be harmful or fatal.

Directions: Cleanse skin with soap and water and dry thoroughly. Apply over affected area morning and night or as directed by a doctor. For athlete's foot pay special attention to the spaces between the toes. It is also helpful to wear well-fitting, ventilated shoes and to change shoes and socks at least once daily. Best results in athlete's foot are usually obtained within 4 weeks' use of this product, and in jock itch, with two weeks' use. If unsatisfactory results have not occurred within these times, consult a doctor or pharmacist. Children under 12 years of age should be supervised in the use of this product. This product is not effective on the scalp or nails. To prevent recurrence of athlete's foot, apply Ting to feet once or twice daily following the above directions.

How Supplied: *Cream*—½ oz. tube, *Powder*—1.5 oz. shaker container, *Spray Liquid and Spray Powder*—3.0 oz. aerosol containers.

Shown in Product Identification Section, page 410

EDUCATIONAL MATERIAL

Americaine® Hemorrhoidal Ointment
Comforting Facts On a Painful Subject
Booklet with cents-off coupon describing hemorrhoidal conditions, with instructions on self-treatment, and when to consult a doctor.
Samples
To order FREE booklets and Americaine® Hemorrhoidal patient samples, write to Fisons Consumer Health.

Americaine® Topical Anesthetic
Make It All Better
Booklet with cents-off coupon featuring basic information on child safety/accident prevention, with instructions on self-treatment of minor pain and itching, and when to consult a doctor. To order FREE booklet, write to Fisons Consumer Health.

Caldesene®
Health and Safety Tips
Booklets with cents-off coupon and basic information on prevention of diaper rash, with instructions on home treatment, and when to consult a doctor (English and Spanish).
Samples
To order FREE booklets and Caldesene® Medicated Powder and Caldesene® Ointment patient samples, write to Fisons Consumer Health.

Fleming & Company
1600 FENPARK DR.
FENTON, MO 63026

CHLOR-3
Medicinal Condiment

Active Ingredients: A troika of sodium chloride (50% 24.3 mEq/half tsp. iodized); potassium chloride (30% 11.5 mEq/half tsp.); magnesium chloride (20% 5.6 mEq/half tsp.).

Indications: The first medicinal condiment to restore needed K^+ & Mg^{++} lost during diuresis, at the expense of Na^+. To restore electrolytes lost by overcooking foods, or to add to diets that lack green vegetables, bananas, etc. And to replace conventional salting of foods in culinary and gourmet arts.

Symptoms and Treatment of Oral Overdosage: Hyperkalemia and hypermagnesemia are not end-stage results of usage.

How Supplied: In 8-oz plastic shaker, tamper-evident bottles.

IMPREGON Concentrate

Active Ingredient: Tetrachlorosalicylanilide 2%

Indications: Diaper Rash Relief, 'Staph' control, Mold inhibitor.

Actions: This is a bacteriostatic/fungistatic agent for home usage and hospital usage.

Warnings: Impregon should not be exposed to direct sunlight for long periods after applications.

Precaution: Addition of bleach prior to diaper treatment negates application effects.

Dosage and Administration: One capful (5ml) per gallon of water to impregnate diapers in the diaper pail. Dilutions for many home areas accompany the full package.

Note: For disposable-type diapers, add one teaspoonful to 8 oz of water to a 'Windex-type' sprayer. Spray middle half area of diapers until damp, and allow to dry before using, to prevent rashes.

How Supplied: Four ounce amber plastic bottles.

MAGONATE TABLETS
MAGONATE LIQUID
Magnesium Gluconate (Dihydrate)

Active Ingredients: Each tablet contains magnesium gluconate (dihydrate) 500mg (27mg of Mg^{++}). Each 5cc of Magonate Liquid contains magnesium gluconate (dihydrate) 1000mg (54mg of Mg^{++}).

Indications: Alcoholism; digitalis toxicity; cardiac arrhythmias; extrinsic asthma; dysmenorrhea; eclampsia; hypertension; insomnia; muscle twitching; tremors; anxiety; pancreatitis, and toxicity of chemotherapy.

Precaution: Excessive dosage may cause loose stools.

Dosage and Administration: Magonate is recommended during and for three weeks after a course in chemotherapy, then monitored regularly.
Adults and children over 12 yrs.—one or two tablets or ½ to 1 teaspoon of liquid t.i.d. Under 12 yrs.—one tablet or ½ teaspoon of liquid t.i.d. Dosage may be increased in severe cases.

How Supplied: Magonate Tablets are supplied in bottles of 100 and 1000 tablets. Magonate Liquid is supplied in pints and gallons.

MARBLEN Suspensions and Tablet

Composition: A modified 'Sippy Powder' antacid containing magnesium and calcium carbonates.

Action and Uses: The peach/apricot (pink) or unflavored (green) antacid suspensions are sugar-free and neutralize 18 mEq acid per teaspoonful with a low sodium content of 18mg per fl. oz. Each pink tablet consumes 18.0 mEq acid.

Administration and Dosage: One teaspoonful rather than a tablespoonful or one tablet to reduce patient cost by ⅔.

How Supplied: Plastic pints and bottles of 100 and 1000.

NEPHROX SUSPENSION
(aluminum hydroxide)
Antacid Suspension

Composition: A watermelon flavored aluminum hydroxide (320mg as gel)/mineral oil (10% by volume) antacid per teaspoonful.

Action and Uses: A sugar-free/saccharin-free pink suspension containing no magnesium and low sodium (19mg/oz). Extremely palatable and especially indicated in renal patients. Each teaspoon consumes 9 mEq acid.

Administration and Dosage: Two teaspoonfuls or as directed by a physician.

Caution: To be taken only at bedtime. Do not use at any other time or administer to infants, expectant women, and nursing mothers except upon the advice of a physician as this product contains mineral oil.

How Supplied: Plastic pints and gallons.

NICOTINEX Elixir
nicotinic acid

Composition: Contains niacin 50 mg./tsp. in a sherry wine base (amber color).

Action and Uses: Produces flushing when tablets fail. To increase micro-circulation of inner-ear in Meniere's, tinnitus and labyrinthine syndromes. For 'cold hands & feet', and as a vehicle for additives.

Administration and Dosage: One or two teaspoonsful on fasting stomach.

Side Effects: Patients should be warned of dermal flush. Ulcer and gout patients may be affected by 14% alcoholic content.

Contraindications: Severe hypotension and hemorrhage.

How Supplied: Plastic pints and gallons.

OCEAN MIST
(buffered saline)

Composition: Special isotonic saline, buffered with sodium bicarbonate to proper pH so as not to irritate the nose.

Action and Uses: Rhinitis medicamentosa, rhinitis sicca and atrophic rhinitis. For patients 'hooked on nose drops' and glaucoma patients on diuretics having dry nasal capillaries. OCEAN may be used as a mist or drop.

Administration and Dosage: One or two squeezes in each nostril.

Supplied: Plastic 45cc spray bottles and pints.

PURGE
(flavored castor oil)

Composition: Contains 95% castor oil (USP) in a sweetened lemon flavored base that completely masks the odor and taste of the oil.

Indications: Preparation of the bowel for x-ray, surgery and proctological procedures, IVPs, and constipation.

Dosage: Infants—1–2 teaspoonfuls. Children—adjust between infant and adult dose. Adult—2–4 tablespoonfuls.

Precaution: Not indicated when nausea, vomiting, abdominal pain or symptoms of appendicitis occur. Pregnancy, use only on advice of physician.

Supplied: Plastic 1 oz. & 2 oz. bottles.

Products are indexed by generic and chemical names in the **YELLOW SECTION**

Flex Aid, Inc.

a Division of NDL Products, Inc.
2313 N.W. 30th PLACE
POMPANO BEACH, FL 33069

ELASTIC SPLINT WRIST BRACE

Indications: Supports weak or injured wrists.

Actions: Supports hand/wrist at doctor recommended 30° angle for proper healing. Physician/Therapist can contour removable alloy splint to any desired angle.

How Supplied: Individually boxed; Sized Small–X-Large; Left- and Right-Hand style available.

Shown in Product Identification Section, page 410

ELASTIC SUPPORT HOISERY

Description: Sheerest Support Pantyhose, 14 mm Hg compression

Indications: For relief of discomfort due to tired aching legs, varicose veins, swelling and pregnancy.

Actions: Compression is graduated—strongest (14 mm Hg) at the ankle, gradually reducing upward. Promotes blood circulation.

How Supplied: Individually boxed; Sized Small–X-Large; Colors: Beige and Taupe.

Shown in Product Identification Section, page 410

NEOPRENE KNEE SUPPORT

Description: Neoprene Knee Support, with Open Patella

Indications: Provides support and compression for weak or injured knees.

Actions: Neoprene construction retains body heat promoting blood circulation. Supports knee without restricting movement or applying pressure on patella.

How Supplied: Individually boxed; Sized Small–X-Large.
For Free Full-Color Product Brochure write: FLEX AID, P.O. BOX 1917 POMPANO BEACH, FL 33061.

Shown in Product Identification Section, page 410

G&W Laboratories

111 COOLIDGE STREET
SOUTH PLAINFIELD, NJ 07080

Shown in Product Identification Section, page 410

Products are cross-indexed by generic and chemical names in the **YELLOW SECTION**

Glenbrook Laboratories

Division of Sterling Drug Inc.
90 PARK AVENUE
NEW YORK, NY 10016

Children's BAYER® Chewable Aspirin
Aspirin (Acetylsalicylic Acid)

Active Ingredients: Children's Bayer Chewable Aspirin—Aspirin $1\frac{1}{4}$ grains (81 mg) per orange flavored chewable tablet.

Inactive Ingredients: Dextrose excipient, FD&C Yellow No. 6, flavor, saccharin sodium, starch.

Actions and Uses: Analgesic, antipyretic, anti-inflammatory. For effective, gentle relief of painful discomforts, sore throat; fever of colds; headache; teething pain, toothache; and other minor aches and pains.

Warnings: Children and teenagers should not use this medicine for chicken pox or flu symptoms before a doctor is consulted about Reye syndrome, a rare but serious illness reported to be associated with aspirin. Keep this and all drugs out of the reach of children. In case of accidental overdose, seek professional assistance or contact a poison control center immediately. As with any drug, if you are pregnant or nursing a baby, seek the advice of a health professional before using this product. **IT IS ESPECIALLY IMPORTANT NOT TO USE ASPIRIN DURING THE LAST THREE MONTHS OF PREGNANCY UNLESS SPECIFICALLY DIRECTED TO DO SO BY A DOCTOR BECAUSE IT MAY CAUSE PROBLEMS IN THE UNBORN CHILD OR COMPLICATIONS DURING DELIVERY.**
IMPORTANT NOTICE: Do not take this product if you are allergic to aspirin, have asthma, stomach problems that persist or recur, gastric ulcers or bleeding, or if you are taking a prescription drug for arthritis, anticoagulation (thinning of the blood), diabetes, or gout unless directed by a doctor. If ringing in the ears or loss of hearing occurs, consult a doctor before taking any more of this product.

Administration and Dosage: The following dosages are those provided in the packaging, as appropriate for self-medication.
Children's Dose: To be administered only under adult supervision. For children under 3 consult physician.

Age (Years)	Weight (lb)	Dosage
3 up to 4	32 to 35	2 tablets
4 up to 6	36 to 45	3 tablets
6 up to 9	46 to 65	4 tablets
9 up to 11	66 to 76	5 tablets
11 up to 12	77 to 83	6 tablets
12 and over	84 and over	8 tablets

Indicated dosage may be repeated every four hours up to but not more than five times a day. Larger dosage may be prescribed by a physician.
Ways to Administer: CHEW, then follow with a half glass of water, milk or fruit juice.
SWALLOW WHOLE with a half a glass of water, milk or fruit juice.
DISSOLVE ON TONGUE, follow with a half a glass of water, milk or fruit juice.
DISSOLVE TABLET in a little water, milk or fruit juice and drink the solution.
CRUSHED in a teaspoonful of water—followed with part of a glass of water.

How Supplied: Children's Bayer Chewable Aspirin $1\frac{1}{4}$ grains (81 mg)—
NDC 12843-131-05, bottle of 36 tablets with child-resistant safety closure.

Shown in Product Identification Section, page 410

Genuine BAYER® Aspirin
Aspirin (Acetylsalicylic Acid)
Tablets and Caplets

Active Ingredients: Each Bayer-Aspirin contains aspirin 5 grains (325 mg) in a thin, inert, hydroxypropyl methylcellulose coating for easier swallowing. This is not an enteric coating and does not alter the onset of action of Genuine Bayer Aspirin.

Inactive Ingredients: Starch and Triacetin.

Actions and Uses: Analgesic, antipyretic, anti-inflammatory. For relief of headache; painful discomfort and fever of colds and flu; sore throats; muscular aches and pains; temporary relief of minor pains of arthritis, rheumatism†, bursitis, lumbago, sciatica; toothache, teething pains, and pain following dental procedures; neuralgia and neuritic pain; functional menstrual pain; minor painful discomfort; painful discomfort and fever accompanying immunizations.

†**Caution:** If pain persists for more than 10 days, or redness is present, or in conditions affecting children under 12 years of age, consult a physician immediately.

Warnings: Children and teenagers should not use this medicine for chicken pox or flu symptoms before a doctor is consulted about Reye syndrome, a rare but serious illness reported to be associated with aspirin. Keep this and all drugs out of the reach of children. In case of accidental overdose, seek professional assistance or contact a poison control center immediately. As with any drug, if you are pregnant or nursing a baby, seek the advice of a health professional before using this product. **IT IS ESPECIALLY IMPORTANT NOT TO USE ASPIRIN DURING THE LAST 3 MONTHS OF PREGNANCY UNLESS SPECIFICALLY DIRECTED TO DO SO BY A DOCTOR BECAUSE IT MAY CAUSE PROBLEMS IN THE UNBORN CHILD OR COMPLICATIONS DURING DELIVERY.**

IMPORTANT NOTICE: Do not take this product if you are allergic to aspirin, have asthma, stomach problems that persist or recur, gastric ulcers or bleeding, or if you are taking a prescription drug for arthritis, anticoagulation (thinning of the blood), diabetes, or gout unless directed by a doctor. If ringing in the ears or loss of hearing occurs, consult a doctor before taking any more of this product.

Administration and Dosage: The following dosages are those provided in the packaging, as appropriate for self-medication. Larger or more frequent dosage may be necessary as appropriate to the condition or needs of the patient.

The hydroxypropyl methylcellulose coating makes Genuine Bayer Aspirin particularly appropriate for those who must take frequent doses of aspirin and for those who have difficulty in swallowing uncoated tablets and caplets.

Usual Adult Dose: One or two tablets/caplets with water. May be repeated every four hours as necessary up to 12 tablets/caplets a day.

FOR ANTIPLATELET USE: RECURRENT TIA

There is evidence that aspirin is safe and effective for reducing the risk of recurrent transient ischemic attacks or stroke in men who have had transient ischemia of the brain due to fibrin platelet emboli. There is no evidence that aspirin is effective in reducing TIAs in women, or that it is of benefit in the treatment of completed strokes in men or women. Patients presenting with signs and symptoms of TIAs should have a complete medical and neurologic evaluation. Consideration should be given to other disorders which resemble TIAs.

It is important to evaluate and treat, if appropriate, other diseases associated with TIAs and stroke, such as hypertension and diabetes.

Dosage: The recommended dosage for this new indication is 1,300 mg/day (650 mg twice a day or 325 mg four times a day).

Precautions: A complete medical and neurologic evaluation should be performed on the male patient with recurrent TIA prior to instituting antiplatelet therapy with aspirin. The differential diagnosis should include consideration of disorders that resemble TIAs. An assessment of the presence and need for treatment of other diseases associated with TIAs or stroke, such as diabetes and hypertension, should be made.

IN MI PROPHYLAXIS

Aspirin is indicated to reduce the risk of death and/or nonfatal myocardial infarction in patients with a previous infarction or unstable angina pectoris.

Clinical Trials: The indication is supported by the results of six, large, randomized multicenter, placebo-controlled studies[1–6] by the word-studies involving 10,816, predominantly male, post-myocardial infarction (MI) patients and one randomized placebo-controlled study[7] by the word study of 1,266 men with unstable angina. Therapy with aspirin was begun at intervals after the onset of acute MI varying from less than 3 days to more than 5 years and continued for periods of from less than 1 year to 4 years. In the unstable angina study, treatment was started within 1 month after the onset of unstable angina and continued for 12 weeks and complicating conditions, such as congestive heart failure, were not included in the study.

Aspirin therapy in MI patients was associated with about a 20 percent reduction in the risk of subsequent death and/or nonfatal reinfarction, a median absolute decrease of 3 percent from the 12 to 22 percent event rates in the placebo groups. In aspirin-treated unstable angina patients the reduction in risk was about 50 percent, a reduction in event rate of 5 percent from the 10 percent rate in the placebo group over the 12 weeks of the study.

Daily dosage of aspirin in the post-myocardial infarction studies was 300 mg in one study and 900—1500 mg in five studies. A dose of 325 mg was used in the study of unstable angina.

Adverse Reactions: Gastrointestinal Reactions: Doses of 1000 mg per day of aspirin caused gastrointestinal symptoms and bleeding that in some cases were clinically significant. In the largest post-infarction study (the Aspirin Myocardial Infarction Study [AMIS] trial with 4,500 people), the percentage incidences of gastrointestinal symptoms for the aspirin (1000 mg of a standard, solid-tablet formulation) and placebo-treated subjects, respectively, were: stomach pain (14.5%; 4.4%); heartburn (11.9%; 4.8%); nausea and/or vomiting (7.6%; 2.1%) hospitalization for Gl disorder (4.9%; 3.5%). In the AMIS and other trials, aspirin-treated patients had increased rates of gross gastrointestinal bleeding. Symptoms and signs of gastrointestinal irritation were not significantly increased in subjects treated for unstable angina with buffered aspirin in solution.

Cardiovascular and Biochemical: In the AMIS trial, the dosage of 1000 mg per day of aspirin was associated with small increases in systolic blood pressure (BP) (average 1.5 to 2.1 mm) and diastolic BP (0.5 to 0.6 mm), depending upon whether maximal or last available readings were used. Blood urea nitrogen and uric acid levels were also increased, but by less than 1.0 mg%. Subjects with marked hypertension or renal insufficiency had been excluded from the trial so that the clinical importance of these observations for such subjects or for any subjects treated over more prolonged periods is not known. It is recommended that patients placed on long-term aspirin treatment, even at doses of 300 mg per day, be seen at regular intervals to assess changes in these measurements.

Sodium in Buffered Aspirin for Solution Formulations: One tablet daily of buffered aspirin in solution adds 553 mg of sodium to that in the diet and may not be tolerated by patients with active sodium-retaining states such as congestive heart or renal failure. This amount of sodium adds about 30 percent to the 70 to 90 meq intake suggested as appropriate for dietary treatment of essential hypertension in the 1984 Report of the Joint National Committee on Detection, Evaluation, and Treatment of High Blood Pressure.[8]

Dosage and Administration: Although most of the studies used dosages exceeding 300 mg, two trials used only 300 mg, daily, and pharmacologic data indicate that this dose inhibits platelet function fully. Therefore, 300 mg or a conventional 325 mg aspirin dose daily, is a reasonable routine dose that would minimize gastrointestinal adverse reactions. This use of aspirin applies to both solid, oral dosage forms (buffered and plain aspirin) and buffered aspirin in solution.

REFERENCES

(1) Elwood, P.C., et al., A Randomized Controlled Trial of Acetylsalicylic Acid in the Secondary Prevention of Mortality from Myocardial Infarction, *British Medical Journal,* 1:436–440, 1974.

(2) The Coronary Drug Project Research Group, "Aspirin in Coronary Heart Disease," *Journal of Chronic Disease,* 29:625–642, 1976.

(3) Breddin, K., et al., "Secondary Prevention of Myocardial Infarction: A Comparison of Acetylsalicylic Acid, Phenprocoumon or Placebo," *Homeostasis,* 470:263–268, 1979.

(4) Aspirin Myocardial Infarction Study Research Group, "A Randomized, Controlled Trial of Aspirin in Persons Recovered from Myocardial Infarction," *Journal American Medical Association* 245:661–669, 1980.

(5) Elwood, P.C., and Sweetnam P.M., "Aspirin and Secondary Mortality after Myocardial Infarction," *Lancet,* pp. 1313–1315, December 22–29, 1979.

(6) The Persantine-Aspirin Reinfarction Study Research Group, "Persantine and Aspirin in Coronary Heart Disease," *Circulation,* 62: 449–460, 1980.

(7) Lewis, H.D., et al., "Protective Effects of Aspirin Against Acute Myocardial Infarction and Death in Men with Unstable Angina. Results of a Veterans Administration Cooperative Study," *New England Journal of Medicine* 309:396–403, 1983.

(8) "1984 Report of the Joint National Committee on Detection, Evaluation and Treatment of High Blood Pressure," U.S. Department of Health and Human Services and United States Public Health Service, National Institutes of Health.

How Supplied:

Genuine Bayer Aspirin 5 grains (325 mg)—

NDC 12843-101-10, packs of 12 tablets.
NDC 12843-101-11, bottles of 24 tablets.
NDC 12843-101-17, bottles of 50 tablets.
NDC 12843-101-12, bottles of 100 tablets.
NDC 12843-101-20, bottles of 200 tablets.
NDC 12843-101-13, bottles of 300 tablets.
NDC 12843-102-38, bottles of 50 caplets.
NDC 12843-102-39, bottles of 100 caplets.
NDC 12843-102-20, bottles of 200 caplets.
Child-resistant safety closures on 12's,

Continued on next page

Glenbrook—Cont.

24's, 50's, 200's, 300's tablets and 50's and 200's caplets. Bottles of 100's tablets and caplets available without safety closure for households without small children.

Shown in Product Identification Section, page 410

Maximum BAYER® Aspirin Aspirin (Acetylsalicylic Acid) Tablets and Caplets

Active Ingredients: Maximum Bayer Aspirin—Aspirin 500 mg (7.7 grains) contains a thin, inert, hydroxypropyl methylcellulose coating for easier swallowing. This is not an enteric coating and does not alter the onset of action of Bayer Aspirin.

Inactive Ingredients: Starch and triacetin.

Actions and Uses: Analgesic, antipyretic, anti-inflammatory. For relief of headache; painful discomfort and fever of colds and flu; sore throats; muscular aches and pains; temporary relief of minor pains of arthritis, rheumatism†, bursitis, lumbago, sciatica; toothache, teething pains, and pain following dental procedures; neuralgia and neuritic pain; functional menstrual pain; minor painful discomforts; painful discomfort and fever accompanying immunizations.

†**Caution:** If pain persists for more than 10 days or redness is present, or in conditions affecting children under 12 years of age, consult a physician immediately.

Warnings: Children and teenagers should not use this medicine for chicken pox or flu symptoms before a doctor is consulted about Reye syndrome, a rare but serious illness reported to be associated with aspirin. Keep this and all drugs out of the reach of children. In case of accidental overdose, seek professional assistance or contact a poison control center immediately. As with any drug, if you are pregnant or nursing a baby, seek the advice of a health professional before using this product. **IT IS ESPECIALLY IMPORTANT NOT TO USE ASPIRIN DURING THE LAST 3 MONTHS OF PREGNANCY UNLESS SPECIFICALLY DIRECTED TO DO SO BY A DOCTOR BECAUSE IT MAY CAUSE PROBLEMS IN THE UNBORN CHILD OR COMPLICATIONS DURING DELIVERY.**

IMPORTANT NOTICE: Do not take this product if you are allergic to aspirin, have asthma, stomach problems that persist or recur, gastric ulcers or bleeding, or if you are taking a prescription drug for arthritis, anticoagulation (thinning of the blood), diabetes, or gout unless directed by a doctor. If ringing in the ears or loss of hearing occurs, consult a doctor before taking any more of this product.

Administration and Dosage: The following dosages are those provided on the packaging, as appropriate for self-medication. Larger or more frequent dosage may be necessary as appropriate for the condition or needs of the patient.

The hydroxypropyl methylcellulose coating makes Maximum Bayer Aspirin particularly appropriate for those who must take frequent doses of aspirin and for those who have difficulty in swallowing uncoated tablets/caplets.

Maximum Bayer Aspirin—500 mg (7.7 grains) tablets/caplets.

Usual Adult Dose: One or two tablets/caplets with water. May be repeated every four hours as necessary up to 8 tablets/caplets a day.

How Supplied:

Maximum Bayer Aspirin 500 mg (7.7 grains)

NDC 12843-161-53, bottles of 30 tablets.
NDC 12843-161-56, bottles of 60 tablets.
NDC 12843-161-58, bottles of 100 tablets.
NDC 12843-202-30, bottles of 30 caplets.
NDC 12843-202-56, bottles of 60 caplets.

Child-resistant safety closures on 30's bottles of tablets and caplets, 60's, bottles of caplets, and 100's bottles of tablets. Bottle of 60's tablets available without safety closure for households without young children.

Shown in Product Identification Section, page 410

8-Hour BAYER® Timed-Release Aspirin Aspirin (acetylsalicylic acid)

Active Ingredients: Each oblong white scored caplet contains 10 grains (650 mg) of aspirin in microencapsulated form.

Inactive Ingredients: Guar gum, microcrystalline cellulose, starch and other ingredients.

Indications: 8-Hour Bayer Timed-Release Aspirin is indicated for the temporary relief of low-grade pain amenable to relief with salicylates, such as in rheumatoid arthritis, osteoarthritis, spondylitis, bursitis and other forms of rheumatism, as well as in many common musculoskeletal disorders. It possesses the same advantages for other types of prolonged aches and pains, such as minor injuries, dental pain and dysmenorrhea. Its long-lasting effectiveness should also make it valuable as an analgesic in simple headache, colds, grippe, flu and other similar conditions in which aspirin is indicated for symptomatic relief, either by itself or as an adjunct to specific therapy.

Caution: If pain persists for more than 10 days, or redness is present, or in conditions affecting children under 12 years, consult a physician immediately.

Warnings: Children and teenagers should not use this medicine for chicken pox or flu symptoms before a doctor is consulted about Reye syndrome, a rare but serious illness reported to be associated with aspirin. Keep this and all drugs out of the reach of children. In case of accidental overdose, seek professional assistance or contact a poison control center immediately. As with any drug, if you are pregnant or nursing a baby, seek the advice of a health professional before using this product. **IT IS ESPECIALLY IMPORTANT NOT TO USE ASPIRIN DURING THE LAST 3 MONTHS OF PREGNANCY UNLESS SPECIFICALLY DIRECTED TO DO SO BY A DOCTOR BECAUSE IT MAY CAUSE PROBLEMS IN THE UNBORN CHILD OR COMPLICATIONS DURING DELIVERY.**

Administration and Dosage: Two 8-Hour Bayer Timed-Release Aspirin caplets q. 8 h. provide effective long-lasting pain relief. This two-caplet (20 grain or 1300 mg) dose of timed-release aspirin promptly produces salicylate blood levels greater than those achieved by a 10-grain (650 mg) dose of regular aspirin, and in the second 4-hour period produces a salicylate blood level curve which approximates that of two successive 10-grain (650 mg) doses of regular aspirin at 4-hour intervals. The 10-grain (650 mg) scored 8-Hour Bayer Timed-Release Aspirin caplets permit administration of aspirin in multiples of 5 grains (325 mg) allowing individualization of dosage to meet the specific needs of the patient. For the convenience of patients on a regular aspirin dosage schedule, two 10-grain (650 mg) 8-Hour Bayer Timed-Release Aspirin caplets may be administered with water every 8 hours. Whenever necessary, two caplets (20 grains or 1300 mg) should be given before retiring to provide effective analgesic and anti-inflammatory action—for relief of pain throughout the night and lessening of stiffness upon arising. Do not exceed 6 caplets in 24 hours. 8-Hour Bayer Timed-Release Aspirin has been made in a special caplet to permit easy swallowing. However, for patients who do have difficulty, 8-Hour Bayer Timed-Release Aspirin caplets may be gently crumbled in the mouth and swallowed with water without loss of timed-release effect. There is no bitter "aspirin" taste. For children under 12, consult physician.

Side Effects: Side effects encountered with regular aspirin may be encountered with 8-Hour Bayer Timed-Release Aspirin. Tinnitus and dizziness are the ones most frequently encountered.

Contraindications and Precautions: 8-Hour Bayer Timed-Release Aspirin is contraindicated in patients with marked aspirin hypersensitivity, and should be given with extreme caution to any patient with a history of adverse reaction to salicylates. It may cautiously be tried in patients intolerant to aspirin because of gastric irritation, but the usual precautions for any form of aspirin should be observed in patients with gastric ulcers, bleeding tendencies, asthma, or hypoprothrombinemia.

How Supplied:

NDC 12843-191-72, Caplets in Bottle of 30's.

NDC 12843-191-74, Caplets in Bottle of 72's.

NDC 12843-191-76, Caplets in Bottle of 125's.

All sizes packaged in child-resistant safety closure except 72's, which is a size recommended for households without young children.

Shown in Product Identification Section, page 410

BAYER® PLUS
Buffered Aspirin

Active Ingredients: Each Bayer Plus contains aspirin (325 mg), in a formulation buffered with Calcium Carbonate, Magnesium Carbonate, and Magnesium Oxide.

Inactive Ingredients: Corn Starch, Ethylcellulose, FD&C Blue #2, Hydroxypropyl Methylcellulose, Microcrystalline Cellulose, Pharmaceutical Glaze, Sodium Starch Glycolate, Talc, Zinc Stearate.

Actions and Uses: Analgesic, antipyretic, anti-inflammatory. For relief of headache; painful discomfort and fever of colds and flu; muscular aches and pains; temporary relief of minor pains of arthritis, rheumatism†, bursitis, lumbago, sciatica; toothache, teething pains, and pain following dental procedures; neuralgia and neuritic pain; functional menstrual pain; minor painful discomfort; painful discomfort and fever accompanying immunizations.

†Caution: If pain persists for more than 10 days, or redness is present, or in conditions affecting children under 12 years of age, consult a physician immediately.

Warnings: Children and teenagers should not use this medicine for chicken pox or flu symptoms before a doctor is consulted about Reye syndrome, a rare but serious illness reported to be associated with aspirin. Keep this and all drugs out of the reach of children. In case of accidental overdose, seek professional assistance or contact a poison control center immediately. As with any drug, if you are pregnant or nursing a baby, seek the advice of a health professional before using this product. **IT IS ESPECIALLY IMPORTANT NOT TO USE ASPIRIN DURING THE LAST 3 MONTHS OF PREGNANCY UNLESS SPECIFICALLY DIRECTED TO DO SO BY A DOCTOR BECAUSE IT MAY CAUSE PROBLEMS IN THE UNBORN CHILD OR COMPLICATIONS DURING DELIVERY.**

IMPORTANT NOTICE: Do not take this product if you are allergic to aspirin, have asthma, stomach problems that persist or recur, gastric ulcers or bleeding, or if you are taking a prescription drug for arthritis, anticoagulation (thinning of the blood), diabetes, or gout unless directed by a doctor. If ringing in the ears or loss of hearing occurs, consult a doctor before taking any more of this product.

Administration and Dosage: The following dosages are those provided in the packaging, as appropriate for self-medication. Larger or more frequent dosage may be necessary as appropriate to the condition or needs of the patient.

The hydroxypropyl methylcellulose coating makes Bayer® Plus particularly appropriate for those who must take frequent doses of aspirin and for those who have difficulty in swallowing uncoated tablets and caplets.

Usual Adult Dose: One or two tablets with water. May be repeated every four hours as necessary up to 12 tablets a day.

FOR ANTIPLATELET USE: RECURRENT TIA

There is evidence that aspirin is safe and effective for reducing the risk of recurrent transient ischemic attacks or stroke in men who have had transient ischemia of the brain due to fibrin platelet emboli. There is no evidence that aspirin is effective in reducing TIAs in women, or that it is of benefit in the treatment of completed strokes in men or women. Patients presenting with signs and symptoms of TIAs should have a complete medical and neurologic evaluation. Consideration should be given to other disorders which resemble TIAs.

It is important to evaluate and treat, if appropriate, other diseases associated with TIAs and stroke, such as hypertension and diabetes.

Dosage: The recommended dosage for this new indication is 1,300 mg/day (650 mg twice a day or 325 mg four times a day).

Precautions: A complete medical and neurologic evaluation should be performed on the male patient with recurrent TIA prior to instituting antiplatelet therapy with aspirin. The differential diagnosis should include consideration of disorders that resemble TIAs. An assessment of the presence and need for treatment of other diseases associated with TIAs or stroke, such as diabetes and hypertension, should be made.

IN MI PROPHYLAXIS

Aspirin is indicated to reduce the risk of death and/or nonfatal myocardial infarction in patients with a previous infarction or unstable angina pectoris.

Clinical Trials: The indication is supported by the results of six, large, randomized multicenter, placebo-controlled studies[1–6] by the word-studies involving 10,816, predominantly male, post–myocardial infarction (MI) patients and one randomized placebo-controlled study[7] by the word study of 1,266 men with unstable angina. Therapy with aspirin was begun at intervals after the onset of acute MI varying from less than 3 days to more than 5 years and continued for periods of from less than 1 year to 4 years. In the unstable angina study, treatment was started within 1 month after the onset of unstable angina and continued for 12 weeks and complicating conditions, such as congestive heart failure, were not included in the study.

Aspirin therapy in MI patients was associated with about a 20 percent reduction in the risk of subsequent death and/or nonfatal reinfarction, a median absolute decrease of 3 percent from the 12 to 22 percent event rates in the placebo groups. In aspirin-treated unstable angina patients the reduction in risk was about 50 percent, a reduction in event rate of 5 percent from the 10 percent rate in the placebo group over the 12 weeks of the study.

Daily dosage of aspirin in the post–myocardial infarction studies was 300 mg in one study and 900—1500 mg in five studies. A dose of 325 mg was used in the study of unstable angina.

Adverse Reactions: Gastrointestinal Reactions: Doses of 1000 mg per day of aspirin caused gastrointestinal symptoms and bleeding that in some cases were clinically significant. In the largest post-infarction study (the Aspirin Myocardial Infarction Study [AMIS] trial with 4,500 people), the percentage incidences of gastrointestinal symptoms for the aspirin (1000 mg of a standard, solid-tablet formulation) and placebo-treated subjects, respectively, were: stomach pain (14.5%; 4.4%); heartburn (11.9%; 4.8%); nausea and/or vomiting (7.6%; 2.1%) hospitalization for Gl disorder (4.9%; 3.5%). In the AMIS and other trials, aspirin-treated patients had increased rates of gross gastrointestinal bleeding. Symptoms and signs of gastrointestinal irritation were not significantly increased in subjects treated for unstable angina with buffered aspirin in solution.

Cardiovascular and Biochemical: In the AMIS trial, the dosage of 1000 mg per day of aspirin was associated with small increases in systolic blood pressure (BP) (average 1.5 to 2.1 mm) and diastolic BP (0.5 to 0.6 mm), depending upon whether maximal or last available readings were used. Blood urea nitrogen and uric acid levels were also increased, but by less than 1.0 mg%. Subjects with marked hypertension or renal insufficiency had been excluded from the trial so that the clinical importance of these observations for such subjects or for any subjects treated over more prolonged periods is not known. It is recommended that patients placed on long-term aspirin treatment, even at doses of 300 mg per day, be seen at regular intervals to assess changes in these measurements.

Sodium in Buffered Aspirin for Solution Formulations: One tablet daily of buffered aspirin in solution adds 553 mg of sodium to that in the diet and may not be tolerated by patients with active sodium-retaining states such as congestive heart or renal failure. This amount of sodium adds about 30 percent to the 70 to 90 meq intake suggested as appropriate for dietary treatment of essential hypertension in the 1984 Report of the Joint National Committee on Detection, Evaluation, and Treatment of High Blood Pressure.[8]

Dosage and Administration: Although most of the studies used dosages exceeding 300 mg, two trials used only 300 mg, daily, and pharmacologic data indicate that this dose inhibits platelet function fully. Therefore, 300 mg or a conventional 325 mg aspirin dose daily, is a reasonable routine dose that would minimize gastrointestinal adverse reactions.

Continued on next page

Glenbrook—Cont.

This use of aspirin applies to both solid, oral dosage forms (buffered and plain aspirin) and buffered aspirin in solution.

REFERENCES

(1) Elwood, P.C., et al., A Randomized Controlled Trial of Acetylsalicylic Acid in the Secondary Prevention of Mortality from Myocardial Infarction, *British Medical Journal,* 1:436–440, 1974.

(2) The Coronary Drug Project Research Group, "Aspirin in Coronary Heart Disease," *Journal of Chronic Disease,* 29:625–642, 1976.

(3) Breddin, K., et al., "Secondary Prevention of Myocardial Infarction: A Comparison of Acetylsalicylic Acid, Phenprocoumon or Placebo," *Homeostasis,* 470:263–268, 1979.

(4) Aspirin Myocardial Infarction Study Research Group, "A Randomized, Controlled Trial of Aspirin in Persons Recovered from Myocardial Infarction," *Journal American Medical Association* 245:661–669, 1980.

(5) Elwood, P.C., and Sweetnam P.M., "Aspirin and Secondary Mortality after Myocardial Infarction," *Lancet,* pp. 1313–1315, December 22–29, 1979.

(6) The Persantine-Aspirin Reinfarction Study Research Group, "Persantine and Aspirin in Coronary Heart Disease," *Circulation,* 62: 449–460, 1980.

(7) Lewis, H.D., et al., "Protective Effects of Aspirin Against Acute Myocardial Infarction and Death in Men with Unstable Angina. Results of a Veterans Administration Cooperative Study," *New England Journal of Medicine* 309:396–403, 1983.

(8) "1984 Report of the Joint National Committee on Detection, Evaluation and Treatment of High Blood Pressure," U.S. Department of Health and Human Services and United States Public Health Service, National Institutes of Health.

How Supplied:
Bayer® Plus Aspirin (325 mg)—
NDC 12843-104-01, bottles of 8 tablets
NDC 12843-104-02, bottles of 24 tablets
NDC 12843-104-03, bottles of 50 tablets
NDC 12843-104-04, bottles of 100 tablets
Child resistant closures on 8's, 24's and 50's tablets. Bottles of 100's tablets available without safety closure for households without young children.

Shown in Product Identification Section, page 410

Therapy BAYER® Aspirin Delayed-Release Enteric Aspirin (Acetylsalicylic Acid) Caplets Antiarthritic, Antiplatelet

Composition: Therapy BAYER is 325 mg enteric-coated aspirin available in caplet form. The enteric coating prevents disintegration in the stomach and promotes dissolution in the duodenum, where there is a more neutral-to-alkaline environment. This action aids in protecting the stomach against injuries that may occur as a result of ingesting non-enteric-coated aspirin (see **Safety**).

Inactive Ingredients: D&C Yellow No. 10, FD&C Yellow No. 6, hydroxypropyl methylcellulose, methacrylic acid, copolymer, starch, titanium dioxide, triacetin, polysorbate 80, and sodium lauryl sulfate.

Indications: Therapy BAYER is an anti-inflammatory, analgesic, and antiplatelet agent indicated for the relief of painful discomfort and muscular aches and pains associated with conditions requiring long-term aspirin therapy, e.g., arthritis or rheumatism and for situations where compliance with aspirin is hindered by the gastrointestinal side effects of non-enteric-coated or buffered aspirin.

Dosage: For analgesic or anti-inflammatory indications, the OTC maximum dosage for aspirin is 4,000 mg per day in divided doses, i.e., two 325 mg caplets every 4 hours or three 325 mg caplets every six hours. For antiplatelet effect dosage, see the **Antiplatelet Effect** section.

Caution: If pain persists for more than 10 days or redness is present, or in conditions affecting children under 12 years of age, consult a physician immediately.

Consumer Warning: Children and teenagers should not use this medicine for chicken pox or flu symptoms before a doctor is consulted about Reye syndrome, a rare but serious illness reported to be associated with aspirin. Keep this and all drugs out of the reach of children. In case of accidental overdose, seek professional assistance or contact a poison control center immediately. As with any drug, if you are pregnant or nursing a baby, seek the advice of a health professional before using this product. **IT IS ESPECIALLY IMPORTANT NOT TO USE ASPIRIN DURING THE LAST 3 MONTHS OF PREGNANCY UNLESS SPECIFICALLY DIRECTED TO DO SO BY A DOCTOR BECAUSE IT MAY CAUSE PROBLEMS IN THE UNBORN CHILD OR COMPLICATIONS DURING DELIVERY.**

IMPORTANT NOTICE: Do not take this product if you are allergic to aspirin, have asthma, stomach problems that persist or recur, gastric ulcers or bleeding, or if you are taking a prescription drug for arthritis, anticoagulation (thinning of the blood), diabetes, or gout unless directed by a doctor. If ringing in the ears or loss of hearing occurs, consult a doctor before taking any more of this product.

Professional Warning: Occasional reports have documented individuals with impaired gastric emptying in whom there may be retention of one or more enteric-coated aspirin caplets over time. This phenomenon may occur as a result of outlet obstruction from ulcer disease alone or combined with hypotonic gastric peristalsis. Because of the integrity of the enteric coating in an acidic environment, these caplets may accumulate and form a bezoar in the stomach. Individuals with this condition may present with complaints of early satiety or of vague upper abdominal distress. Diagnosis may be made by endoscopy or by abdominal films, which show opacities suggestive of a mass of small caplets.[1] Management may vary according to the condition of the patient. Options include gastrotomy and alternating slightly basic and neutral lavage.[2] While there have been no clinical reports, it has been suggested that such individuals may also be treated with parenteral cimetidine (to reduce acid secretion) and then given sips of slightly basic liquids to effect gradual dissolution of the enteric coating. Progress may be followed with plasma salicylate levels or via recognition of tinnitus by the patient.

It should be kept in mind that individuals with a history of partial or complete gastrectomy may produce reduced amounts of acid and therefore have less acidic gastric pH. Under these circumstances, the benefits offered by the acid-resistant enteric coating may not exist.

Safety: The safety of enteric-coated aspirin has been demonstrated in a number of endoscopic studies comparing enteric-coated aspirin and plain aspirin, as well as plain buffered and "arthritis-strength" preparations. In these studies, endoscopies were performed in healthy volunteers before and after either two-day or 14-day administration of aspirin doses of 3,900 or 4,000 mg/day. Compared to all the other preparations, the enteric-coated aspirin produced significantly less damage to the gastric mucosa. There was also statistically less duodenal damage when compared with the plain, i.e., non-enteric-coated, aspirin.

Bioavailability: A single-dose bioavailability study[3] has demonstrated that plasma acetylsalicylic acid and salicylic acid concentrations resulting from Therapy BAYER are equivalent to those from plain aspirin, i.e., non-enteric-coated aspirin. As expected, enteric coating on Therapy BAYER results in delayed absorption (peak achieved at approximately five hours postdosing) relative to plain aspirin. Dissolution of the enteric coating occurs at a neutral-to-base pH and is therefore dependent on gastric emptying into the duodenum. With continued dosing, appropriate therapeutic plasma levels are maintained.

Antiplatelet Effect: IN MI PROPHYLAXIS

Indication: Aspirin is indicated to reduce the risk of death and/or nonfatal myocardial infarction in patients with a previous infarction or unstable angina pectoris.

Clinical Trials: The indication is supported by the results of six large randomized, multicenter, placebo-controlled studies[4–10] involving 10,816, predominantly male, post–myocardial infarction (MI) patients and one randomized placebo-controlled study of 1,266 men with unstable angina. Therapy with aspirin was begun at intervals after the onset of acute MI varying from less than three days to more than five years and continuing for periods of from less than 1 year to 4 years. In the unstable angina study,

treatment was started within 1 month after the onset of unstable angina and continued for 12 weeks, and complicating conditions, such as congestive heart failure, were not included in the study. Aspirin therapy in MI patients was associated with about a 20% reduction in the risk of subsequent death and/or nonfatal reinfarction, a median absolute decrease of 3% from the 12% to 22% event rates in the placebo groups. In the aspirin-treated unstable angina patients the reduction in risk was about 50%, a reduction in event rate of 5% from the 10% rate in the placebo group over the 12 weeks of the study.
Daily dosage of aspirin in the post-myocardial infarction studies was 300 mg in one study and 900–1,500 mg in five studies. A dose of 325 mg was used in the study of unstable angina.

Adverse Reactions: Gastrointestinal reactions: Doses of 1,000 mg per day of aspirin caused gastrointestinal symptoms and bleeding that, in some cases were clinically significant. In the largest postinfarction study (the Aspirin Myocardial Infarction Study [AMIS] with 4,500 people), the percentage of incidences of gastrointestinal symptoms for the aspirin (1,000 mg of a standard, solid-tablet formulation) and placebo-treated subjects, respectively, were: stomach pain (14.5%; 4.4%); heartburn (11.9%; 4.8%); nausea and/or vomiting (7.6%; 2.1%), hospitalization for GI disorder (4.9%; 3.5%). In the AMIS and other trials, aspirin-treated patients had increased rates of gross gastrointestinal bleeding. Symptoms and signs of gastrointestinal irritation were not significantly increased in subjects treated for unstable angina with buffered aspirin in solution.

Cardiovascular and Biochemical: In the AMIS trial, the dosage of 1,000 mg per day of aspirin was associated with small increases in systolic blood pressure (BP) (average 1.5 to 2.1 mm) and diastolic BP (0.5 to 0.6 mm), depending upon whether maximal or last available readings were used. Blood urea nitrogen and uric acid levels were also increased but by less than 1.0 mg percent. Subjects with marked hypertension or renal insufficiency had been excluded from the trial so that the clinical importance of these observations for such subjects or for any subjects treated over more prolonged periods is not known. It is recommended that patients placed on long-term aspirin treatment, even at doses of 300 mg per day, be seen at regular intervals to assess changes in these measurements.

Sodium in Buffered Aspirin for Solution Formulations: One tablet daily of buffered aspirin in solution adds 553 mg of sodium to that in the diet and may not be tolerated by patients with active sodium-retaining states, such as congestive heart or renal failure. This amount of sodium adds about 30% to the 70 to 90 meq intake suggested as appropriate for dietary treatment of essential hypertension in the 1984 Report of the Joint National Committee on Detection, Evaluation, and Treatment of High Blood Pressure.[11]

Dosage and Administration: Although most of the studies used dosages exceeding 300 mg, two trials used only 300 mg daily, and pharmacologic data indicate that this dose inhibits platelet function fully. Therefore, 300 mg or a conventional 325 mg aspirin dose daily, is a reasonable routine dose that would minimize gastrointestinal adverse reactions. This use of aspirin applies to both solid oral dosage forms (buffered and plain aspirin) and buffered aspirin in solution.

For Recurrent TIAs in Men: There is evidence that aspirin is safe and effective for reducing the risk of recurrent transient ischemic attacks (TIAs) or stroke in men who have had transient ischemia of the brain due to fibrin platelet emboli. There is no evidence that aspirin is effective in reducing TIAs in women or is of benefit in the treatment of completed strokes in men or women.
Patients presenting with signs and/or symptoms of TIAs should have a complete medical and neurologic evaluation. Consideration should be given to other disorders that may resemble TIAs. It is important to evaluate and treat, if appropriate, other diseases associated with TIAs and stroke, such as hypertension and diabetes.

Dosage: The recommended dosage for this new indication is 1300 mg/day (650 mg b.i.d. or 325 mg q.i.d.). Store at controlled room temperature (59°–86°F).

References: 1. Bogacz, K, Caldron, P: Enteric-coated aspirin bezoar: Elevation of serum salicylate level by barium study. *Am J Med* 1987;83:783–786. 2. Baum, J: Enteric-coated aspirin and the problem of gastric retention. *J Rheumatol* 1984; 11:250–251. 3. Data on file, Glenbrook Laboratories. 4. Elwood, PC, et al: A randomized controlled trial of acetylsalicylic acid in the secondary prevention of mortality from myocardial infarction. *Br Med J* 1974;1:436–440. 5. The Coronary Drug Project Research Group: Aspirin in coronary heart disease. *J Chronic Dis* 1976;29:625–642. 6. Breddin, K, et al: Secondary prevention of myocardial infarction: A comparison of acetylsalicylic acid, phenprocoumon or placebo. *Homeostasis* 1979; 470:263–268. 7. Aspirin Myocardial Infarction Study Research Group: A randomized, controlled trial of aspirin in persons recovered from myocardial infarction. *JAMA* 1980;245:661–669. 8. Elwood, PC, Sweetnam, PM: Aspirin and secondary mortality after myocardial infarction. *Lancet,* December 22–29, 1979, pp 1313–1315. 9. The Persantine-Aspirin Reinfarction Study Research Group: Persantine and aspirin in coronary heart disease. *Circulation* 1980;62:449–460. 10. Lewis, HD, et al: Protective effects of aspirin against acute myocardial infarction and death in men with unstable angina: Results of a Veterans Administration Cooperative Study. *N Eng J Med* 1983;309:396–403. 11. *1984 Report of the Joint National Committee on Detection, Evaluation and Treatment of High Blood Pressure,* U.S. Dept of Health and Human Services and US Public Health Service, National Institutes of Health.

How Supplied: Therapy BAYER 325 mg caplets in bottles of 50, 100.

Shown in Product Identification Section, page 410

HALEY'S M-O®

Active Ingredients: A suspension of magnesium hydroxide in purified water plus mineral oil. Haley's M-O contains 304 mg per teaspoon (5 mL) of magnesium hydroxide and 1.25 mL of mineral oil.

Inactive Ingredients: Purified water. For flavored Haley's M-O only, D&C Red No. 28, flavor, purified water, saccharin sodium.

Indications: For the relief of occasional constipation or irregularity accompanied by hemorrhoids.

Action at Laxative Dosage: Haley's M-O is a mild saline laxative which acts by drawing water into the gut, increasing intraluminal pressure, and increasing intestinal motility. This product generally produces bowel movement in ½ to 6 hours.

Administration and Dosage: As a laxative, especially for hemorrhoid sufferers, adults 1–2 tbsp at bedtime and upon arising. For constipation relief, adults 2 tbsp at bedtime and upon arising; children 6–12, minimum single dose; 1 tsp, maximum daily dose; 1 tbsp. For adults and children, as bowel function improves reduce dose gradually.

Caution: Do not take this product if you are presently taking a stool softener laxative unless directed by a doctor. Do not take with meals.

Warnings: Do not use laxative products when abdominal pain, nausea or vomiting are present unless directed by a doctor. If you have noticed a sudden change in bowel habits that persists over a period of 2 weeks, consult a doctor before using a laxative. Laxative products should not be used for a period longer than 1 week unless directed by a doctor. Rectal bleeding, or failure to have a bowel movement after use of a laxative may indicate a serious condition; discontinue use and consult your doctor. Do not administer to children under 6 years of age, to pregnant women, to bedridden patients, or to persons with difficulty swallowing. As with any drug, if you are nursing a baby, seek the advice of a health professional before using this product. Keep this and all drugs out of the reach of children. In case of accidental overdose, seek professional assistance or contact a poison control center immediately.

How Supplied: Haley's M-O is available in regular and flavored liquids:

Continued on next page

Glenbrook—Cont.

Regular
12 fl oz NDC 12843-350-46; 26 fl oz NDC 12843-350-47.
Flavored
12 fl oz NDC 12843-360-68; 26 fl oz NDC 12843-360-69.

Shown in Product Identification Section, page 410

Regular Strength MIDOL® Multi-Symptom Menstrual Formula

Active Ingredients: Each caplet contains: acetaminophen 325 mg and pyrilamine maleate 12.5 mg.

Inactive Ingredients: Croscarmellose sodium, hydroxypropyl methylcellulose, magnesium stearate, microcrystalline cellulose, pregelatinized starch and triacetin.

Action and Uses: For relief of multiple symptoms suffered during menstrual cycle: cramps, headache, tension, irritability, and backache.
Unlike general pain relievers, which contain only analgesics, Teen Strength Midol Multi-Symptom Menstrual Formula has a combination of ingredients (an analgesic and tension reliever) specially formulated to give:

1. Relief from cramps, headaches, backaches and muscle aches.
2. Relief of irritability, anxiety and tension.

Caution: May cause drowsiness. Use caution when driving or operating machinery. Alcohol, sedatives or tranquilizers may increase drowsiness.

Warnings: Keep this and all drugs out of the reach of children. In case of accidental overdose, seek professional assistance or contact a poison control center immediately. As with any drug, if you are pregnant or nursing a baby, seek the advice of a health professional before using this product.

Dosage: Take 2 caplets with water. Repeat every four hours as needed up to a maximum of 12 caplets per day. Under age 12: Consult your physician.

How Supplied:
White, capsule-shaped caplets.
NDC 12843-156-16, professional dispenser, 250 2-caplet packets for sample use.
NDC 12843-156-17, bottle of 12 caplets.
NDC 12843-156-18, bottle of 30 caplets.
NDC 12843-156-19, bottles of 60 caplets.
Child-resistant safety closures on bottles of 12 and 60 Caplets.

Shown in Product Identification Section, page 411

Maximum Strength MIDOL® PMS Premenstrual Syndrome Formula

Active Ingredients: Each caplet contains acetaminophen 500 mg, pamabrom 25 mg, pyrilamine maleate 15 mg.

Inactive Ingredients: Croscarmellose sodium, hydrogenated vegetable oil, hydroxypropyl methylcellulose, magnesium stearate, microcrystalline cellulose, pregelatinized starch, talc and triacetin.

Action and Uses: Relieves the symptoms of premenstrual syndrome (PMS). Contains maximum strength medication for all these premenstrual symptoms: tension, irritability, anxiety, bloating, water-weight gain, cramps, backache, and headache. Unlike general pain relievers, which contain only analgesics, Midol PMS contains a combination of ingredients (an analgesic, diuretic, and a tension reliever) for the physical and emotional symptoms associated with PMS.

Dosage: Take 2 caplets with water. Repeat every 4 hours as needed, up to a maximum of 8 caplets per day. Under age 12: Take under the advice of your physician.

Caution: May cause drowsiness. Use caution when driving or operating machinery. Alcohol, sedatives or tranquilizers may increase drowsiness.

Warnings: Keep this and *all* drugs out of the reach of children. In case of accidental overdose, seek professional assistance or contact a poison control center immediately. As with any drug, if you are pregnant or nursing a baby, seek the advice of a health professional before using this product.

How Supplied:
White capsule-shaped caplets.
NDC 12843-163-46, bottles of 16 caplets.
NDC 12843-163-47, bottles of 32 caplets.
Child-resistant safety closure on bottles of 32 caplets.

Shown in Product Identification Section, page 411

MIDOL® 200 CRAMP RELIEF FORMULA Ibuprofen Tablets, USP 200 mg Menstrual Pain/Cramp Reliever

Warning: Aspirin-Sensitive Patients —Do not take this product if you have had a severe allergic reaction to aspirin, eg, asthma, swelling, shock or hives, because even though this product contains no aspirin or salicylates, cross-reactions may occur in patients allergic to aspirin.

Indications: For the temporary relief of painful menstrual cramps (dysmenorrhea); also headaches, backaches and muscular aches and pains associated with Premenstrual Syndrome.

Directions:
Adults: Take 1 tablet every 4 to 6 hours at the onset of menstrual symptoms and while pain persists. If pain does not respond to 1 tablet, 2 tablets may be used but do not exceed 6 tablets in 24 hours, unless directed by a doctor. The smallest effective dose should be used. Take with food or milk if occasional and mild heartburn, upset stomach, or stomach pain occurs with use. Consult a doctor if these symptoms are more than mild or if they persist. *Children:* Do not give this product to children under 12 except under the advice and supervision of a doctor.

Warnings: Do not take for pain for more than 10 days unless directed by a doctor. If pain persists or gets worse, or if new symptoms occur, consult a doctor. These could be signs of serious illness. If you are under a doctor's care for any serious condition, consult a doctor before taking this product. As with aspirin and acetaminophen, if you have any condition which requires you to take prescription drugs or if you have had any problems or serious side effects from taking any nonprescription pain reliever, do not take this product without first discussing it with your doctor. If you experience any symptoms which are unusual or seem unrelated to the condition for which you took ibuprofen, consult a doctor before taking any more of it. Although ibuprofen is indicated for the same conditions as aspirin and acetaminophen, it should not be taken with them except under a doctor's direction. Do not combine this product with any other ibuprofen-containing product. As with any drug, if you are pregnant or nursing a baby, seek the advice of a health professional before using this product. **IT IS ESPECIALLY IMPORTANT NOT TO USE IBUPROFEN DURING THE LAST 3 MONTHS OF PREGNANCY UNLESS SPECIFICALLY DIRECTED TO DO SO BY A DOCTOR BECAUSE IT MAY CAUSE PROBLEMS IN THE UNBORN CHILD OR COMPLICATIONS DURING DELIVERY.** Keep this and *all* drugs out of the reach of children. In case of accidental overdose, seek professional assistance or contact a poison control center immediately.
Ibuprofen is used for the relief of painful menstrual cramps and the pain associated with Premenstrual Syndrome. Ibuprofen has been proven more effective in relieving menstrual pain and cramps than aspirin and is gentler on the stomach. Ibuprofen had been widely prescribed for years and is now available in nonprescription strength.

Active Ingredients: Each tablet contains ibuprofen USP 200 mg.

Inactive Ingredients: Calcium phosphate, cellulose, magnesium stearate, silicon dioxide, sodium lauryl sulfate, sodium starch glycolate, stearic acid, titanium dioxide.
Store at room temperature; avoid excessive heat 40°C (104°F).

How Supplied:
White tablets NDC 12843-154-50, bottles of 16 tablets.
NDC 12843-154-51, bottles of 32 tablets.
Child-resistant safety closure on bottles of 32 tablets.

Shown in Product Identification Section, page 411

Maximum Strength
MIDOL®
Multi-Symptom Menstrual Formula

Active Ingredients: Each caplet contains acetaminophen 500 mg and pyrilamine maleate 15 mg.

Inactive Ingredients: Croscarmellose sodium, hydroxypropyl methylcellulose, magnesium stearate, microcrystalline cellulose, pregelatinized starch and triacetin.

Action and Uses: Maximum strength medication for the relief of multiple symptoms suffered during menstrual cycle: cramps, headache, tension, irritability and backache.
Unlike general pain relievers, which contain only analgesics, Midol Maximum Strength Multi-Symptom Menstrual Formula has a combination of ingredients (an analgesic and tension reliever) specially formulated to give:
1. Maximum strength relief from cramps, plus relief of headaches, backaches and muscle aches.
2. Maximum relief of irritability, anxiety and tension.

Caution: May cause drowsiness. Use caution when driving or operating machinery. Alcohol, sedatives or tranquilizers may increase drowsiness.

Warnings: Keep this and all drugs out of the reach of children. In case of accidental overdose, seek professional assistance or contact a poison control center immediately. As with any drug, if you are pregnant or nursing a baby, seek the advice of a health professional before using this product.

Dosage: Take 2 caplets with water. Repeat every 4 hours, as needed, up to a maximum of 8 caplets per day.
Under age 12: Consult your physician.

How Supplied: White capsule-shaped caplets.
NDC 12843-157-16, professional dispenser, 250 2-caplet packets for sample use.
NDC 12843-157-17, bottles of 8 caplets.
NDC 12843-157-18, bottles of 16 caplets.
NDC 12843-157-19, bottles of 32 caplets.
Child-resistant safety closures on bottles of 8 and 32 caplets.

Shown in Product Identification Section, page 411

Children's PANADOL®
Acetaminophen Chewable Tablets, Liquid, Drops.

Description: Each Children's PANADOL Chewable Tablet contains 80 mg acetaminophen in a fruit-flavored sugar-free tablet. Children's PANADOL Acetaminophen Liquid is fruit-flavored, red in color, and is alcohol-free, sugar-free and aspirin-free. Each ½ teaspoonful contains 80 mg of acetaminophen. Infant's PANADOL Drops are fruit-flavored, red in color, and are alcohol-free, sugar-free and aspirin-free. Each 0.8 mL (one calibrated dropperful) contains 80 mg acetaminophen.

Actions and Indications: Acetaminophen, the active ingredient in Children's PANADOL, is the analgesic/antipyretic most widely recommended by pediatricians for fast, effective relief of children's fevers. It also relieves the aches and pains of colds and flu, earaches, headaches, teething, immunizations, tonsillectomy, and childhood illnesses.
Children's PANADOL Tablets, Liquid, and Drops are aspirin-free and contain no alcohol or sugar. The pleasant-tasting formulations are not likely to upset or irritate children's stomachs.

Usual Dosage: Dosing is based on single doses in the range of 10–15 mg/kg body weight. Doses may be repeated every four hours up to 4 or 5 times daily, but not to exceed 5 doses in 24 hours. To be administered to children under 2 years only on advice of a physician.
Children's PANADOL Chewable Tablets: 2–3 yr, 24–35 lb, 2 tablets; 4–5 yr, 36–47 lb, 3 tablets; 6–8 yr, 48–59 lb, 4 tablets; 9–10 yr, 60–71 lb, 5 tablets; 11–12 yr, 72–95 lb, 6 tablets. May be repeated every 4 hours, up to 5 times in a 24-hour period.
Children's PANADOL Liquid: (a special 3 teaspoon cup for accurate measurement is provided). 0–4 mo, 6–11 lb, ¼ teaspoonful; 4–11 mo, 12–17 lb, ½ teaspoonful; 12–23 mo, 18–23 lb, ¾ teaspoonful; 2–3 yr, 24–35 lb, 1 teaspoonful; 4–5 yr, 36–47 lb, 1½ teaspoonfuls; 6–8 yr, 48–59 lb, 2 teaspoonfuls; 9–10 yr, 60–71 lb, 2½ teaspoonfuls; 11–12 yr, 72–95 lb, 3 teaspoonfuls. May be repeated every 4 hours up to 5 times in a 24-hour period. May be administered alone or mixed with formula, milk, juice, cereal, etc.
Infant's PANADOL Drops: 0–4 mo, 6–11 lb, ½ dropperful (0.4 mL); 4–11 mo, 12–17 lb, 1 dropperful (0.8 mL); 12–23 mo, 18–23 lb, 1½ dropperfuls (1.2 mL); 2–3 yr, 24–35 lb, 2 dropperfuls (1.6 mL); 4–5 yr, 36–47 lb, 3 dropperfuls (2.4 mL); 6–8 yr, 48–59 lb, 4 dropperfuls (3.2 mL). May be repeated every 4 hours, up to 5 times in a 24-hour period. May be administered alone or mixed with formula, milk, juice, cereal, etc.

Warnings: Since Children's PANADOL Acetaminophen Chewable Tablets, Liquid, and Drops are available without a prescription as an analgesic/antipyretic, the following appears on the package labels: "WARNINGS: Do not take this product for more than 5 days. If symptoms persist or new ones occur, consult a physician. If fever persists for more than 3 days, or recurs, consult a physician. Keep this and *all* drugs out of the reach of children. In case of accidental overdose, seek professional assistance or contact a poison control center immediately. High fever, severe or persistent sore throat, cough, headache, nausea or vomiting may be serious; consult a physician."
Tamper Resistant: Children's PANADOL Acetaminophen Chewable Tablets packaging provides tamper-resistant features on both the outer carton and bottle. The following copy appears on the end flaps of this carton—"Purchase only if carton end flaps are sealed." "Use only if seal under bottle cap with white G/W print is intact. The outer carton of the liquid and drops contain the following copy: "Purchase only if overwrap printed with red Panda bears is intact."
Children's PANADOL Liquid and Drops provide tamper-resistant features on the carton. The following copy appears on the carton—"Purchase only if Red Tear Tape and Plastic Overwrap are intact," and bottle—"Use only if Carton Overwrap and Red Tear Tape Are Intact."

Composition:
Tablets: Active Ingredient: Acetaminophen. Inactive Ingredients: FD&C Red No. 3, flavor, mannitol, saccharin sodium, starch, stearic acid and other ingredients.
Liquid: Active Ingredient: Acetaminophen. Inactive Ingredients: Benzoic acid, FD&C Red No. 40, flavor, glycerin, polyethylene glycol, potassium sorbate, propylene glycol, purified water, saccharin sodium, sorbitol solution. May also contain sodium chloride or sodium hydroxide.
Drops: Active Ingredient: Acetaminophen. Inactive Ingredients: Citric acid, FD&C Red No. 40, flavors, glycerin, parabens, polyethylene glycol, propylene glycol, purified water, saccharin sodium, sodium chloride, sodium citrate.

How Supplied: Chewable Tablets (colored pink and scored)—bottles of 30. Liquid (colored red)—bottles of 2 fl. oz. and 4 fl. oz. Drops (colored red)—bottles of ½ oz. (15 mL).
All packages listed above have child-resistant safety caps and tamper-resistant features.

Shown in Product Identification Section, page 411

Junior Strength PANADOL®

Description: Each Junior Strength PANADOL® Caplet contains 160 mg of acetaminophen.

Actions and Indications: Acetaminophen, the active ingredient in Junior Strength PANADOL®, is the analgesic/antipyretic most widely recommended by pediatricians for fast, effective relief of children's fevers. It also relieves the aches and pains of colds and flu, earaches, headaches, teething, immunizations, tonsillectomy, menstrual discomfort, and childhood illness.
Junior Strength PANADOL® Caplets are aspirin-free, sugar-free.

Usual Dosage: Dosing is based on single doses in the range of 10–15 mg/kg body weight. Doses may be repeated every 4 hours up to 4 or 5 times daily, but not to exceed 5 doses in 24 hours. To be administered to children under 2 years only on the advice of a physician.
2–3 yr, 24–35 lb, 1 caplet; 4–5 yr, 36–47 lb, 1½ caplets; 6–8 yr, 48–59 lb, 2 caplets; 9–10 yr, 60–71 lb, 2½ caplets; 11–12 yr, 72–95 lb, 3 caplets. Over 12 yr, 96 lb and

Continued on next page

Glenbrook—Cont.

over, 4 caplets. Dosage may be repeated every 4 hours, up to 5 times in a 24-hour period.

Inactive Ingredients: Hydroxypropyl methylcellulose, potassium sorbate, povidone, pregelatinized starch, starch, stearic acid, talc, triacetin.

Warnings: If symptoms persist or new ones occur, consult physician. If fever persists for more than 3 days, or recurs, consult a physician. Do not take this product for more than 5 days. Keep this and all drugs out of the reach of children. In case of accidental overdose, seek professional assistance or contact a poison control center immediately. As with any drug, if you are pregnant, or nursing a baby, seek the advice of a health professional before using this product.

How Supplied: Swallowable caplets (white)—blister-pack of 30. Package has child-resistant and tamper-resistant features.
NDC 12843-216-14

Shown in Product Identification Section, page 411

Maximum Strength PANADOL® Tablets and Caplets

Active Ingredients: Each Maximum Strength PANADOL micro-thin coated tablet and caplet contains acetaminophen 500 mg.

Inactive Ingredients: Hydroxypropyl methylcellulose, potassium sorbate, povidone, pregelatinized starch, starch, stearic acid, talc, triacetin.

Actions: PANADOL acetaminophen has been clinically proven as a fast, effective analgesic (pain reliever) and antipyretic (fever reducer). PANADOL acetaminophen is a nonaspirin product designed to provide relief without stomach upset. Its patented micro-thin coating makes each 500 mg tablet or caplet easy to swallow.

Indications: For the temporary relief from pain of headaches, colds or flu, sinusitis, backaches, muscle aches, and menstrual discomfort. Also to reduce fever and for temporary relief of minor arthritis pain and headache.

Precautions: If a rare sensitivity reaction occurs, the drug should be stopped. PANADOL acetaminophen has rarely been found to produce any side effects. It is usually well tolerated by aspirin-sensitive patients.
Severe recurrent pain or high continued fever may indicate a serious condition. Under these circumstances consult a physician.

Warnings: As with other products available without prescription, the following appears on the label of PANADOL acetaminophen: Do not give to children under 12 or use for more than 10 days unless directed by a physician. Keep this and all drugs out of the reach of children. In case of accidental overdose, seek professional assistance or contact a poison control center immediately. As with any drug, if you are pregnant or nursing a baby, seek the advice of a health professional before using this product.

Usual Dosage: *Adults:* Two tablets or caplets every 4 hours as needed. Do not exceed 8 tablets or caplets in 24 hours unless directed by a physician.

Overdosage: In massive overdosage acetaminophen may cause hepatic toxicity in some patients. Clinical and laboratory evidence of overdosage may be delayed up to 7 days. Under circumstances of suspected overdose, contact your regional poison control center immediately.

How Supplied: Tablets and caplets (white, micro-thin coated, imprinted "PANADOL" and "500"). Tablets packaged in tamper-evident bottles of 30 and 60. Caplets packaged in tamper-evident bottles of 24, 50.

Shown in Product Identification Section, page 411

PHILLIPS'® LAXCAPS®

Active Ingredients: A combination of phenolphthalein (90 mg) and docusate sodium (83 mg) per gelatin capsule.

Inactive Ingredients: FD&C Blue No. 1, Red No. 3, Red No. 40 and Yellow No. 6, gelatin, glycerin, PEG 400 and 3350, propylene glycol and sorbitol.

Indications: For relief of occasional constipation (irregularity).

Action: Phenolphthalein is a stimulant laxative which increases the peristaltic activity of the intestine. Docusate sodium is a stool softener which allows easier passage of the stool. This product generally produces bowel movement in 6 to 12 hours.

Administration and Dosage: Adults and children 12 and over take one (1) or two (2) capsules daily with a full glass (8 oz) of liquid, or as directed by a physician. For children under 12, consult your physician.

Warnings: Do not take any laxative if abdominal pain, nausea, vomiting, change in bowel habits persisting for over 2 weeks, rectal bleeding or kidney disease is present. Laxative products should not be used for a period longer than one week, unless directed by a physician. If there is a failure to have a bowel movement after use, discontinue and consult your doctor. If a skin rash appears do not take this or any other preparation which contains phenolphthalein. Keep this and all drugs out of the reach of children. In case of accidental overdose, seek professional assistance or contact a Poison Control Center immediately. As with any drug, if you are pregnant or nursing a baby, seek the advice of a health professional before using this product.

How Supplied: Blister packs for safety:
8's NDC 12843-384-18
24's NDC 12843-384-19

Shown in Product Identification Section, page 411

PHILLIPS' ® MILK OF MAGNESIA

Active Ingredients: A suspension of magnesium hydroxide in purified water meeting all USP specifications. Phillips' Milk of Magnesia contains 400 mg per teaspoon (5 mL) of magnesium hydroxide.

Inactive Ingredients: Purified water, and for Mint Flavored Phillips' Milk of Magnesia only—flavor, mineral oil and saccharin sodium.

Indications: For relief of occasional constipation (irregularity), relief of acid indigestion, sour stomach and heartburn.

Action at Laxative Dosage: Phillips' Milk of Magnesia is a mild saline laxative which acts by drawing water into the gut, increasing intraluminal pressure, and increasing intestinal motility. This product generally produces bowel movement in ½ to 6 hours.
At Antacid Dosage: Phillips' Milk of Magnesia is an effective acid neutralizer.

Administration and Dosage: As a laxative, adults and children 12 years and older, 2–4 tbsp; children 6–11, 1–2 tbsp; children 2–5, 1–3 tsp followed by a full glass (8 oz) of liquid. Children under 2, consult a physician.
As an antacid, 1–3 tsp with a little water, up to four times a day, or as directed by your physician.

Cautions: Antacids may interact with certain prescription drugs. If you are taking a prescription drug do not take this product without checking with your physician.

Laxative Warnings: Do not take any laxative if abdominal pain, nausea, vomiting, change in bowel habits persisting for over 2 weeks, rectal bleeding, or kidney disease is present. Laxative products should not be used for a period longer than 1 week, unless directed by a doctor. If there is a failure to have a bowel movement after use, discontinue and consult your doctor.

Antacid Warnings: Do not take more than the maximum recommended daily dosage in a 24-hour period (see Directions), or use the maximum dosage of this product for more than two weeks, or use this product if you have kidney disease, except under the advice and supervision of a physician. May have laxative effect.

General Warnings: As with any drug, if you are pregnant or nursing a baby, seek the advice of a health professional before using this product. Keep this and all drugs out of reach of children. In case of accidental overdose, seek professional assistance or contact a poison control center immediately.

How Supplied: Phillips' Milk of Magnesia is available in regular and mint flavor in bottles of:
Regular
4 fl oz NDC 12843-353-01, 12 fl oz NDC 12843-353-02, 26 fl oz NDC 12843-353-03.

Mint
4 fl oz NDC 12843-363-04, 12 fl oz NDC 12843-363-05, 26 fl oz NDC 12843-363-06.
Also available in tablet form and concentrated liquid form.

Shown in Product Identification Section, page 411

CONCENTRATED PHILLIPS'® MILK OF MAGNESIA

Active Ingredients: A suspension of magnesium hydroxide in purified water meeting all USP specifications. Concentrated Phillips' Milk of Magnesia contains 800 mg per teaspoon (5 ml) of magnesium hydroxide.

Inactive Ingredients: Avicel, Citric Acid, FD&C Red #28, Flavor Glycerin, Propylene Glycol, Purified Water, Sorbitol, Sugar, Xanthan Gum.

Indications: For relief of occasional constipation (irregularity), relief of acid indigestion, sour stomach and heartburn.

Action at Laxative Dosage: Concentrated Phillips' Milk of Magnesia is a mild saline laxative which acts by drawing water into the gut, increasing intraluminal pressure, and increasing intestinal motility. This product generally produces bowel movement in ½ hour to 6 hours. *At Antacid Dosage*: Concentrated Phillips' Milk of Magnesia is an effective acid neutralizer.

Laxative Warnings: Do not take any laxative if abdominal pain, nausea, vomiting, change in bowel habits (that persists for over two weeks), rectal bleeding, or kidney disease are present. Laxative products should not be used for a period longer than 1 week, unless directed by a physician. If there is a failure to have a bowel movement after use, discontinue and consult a doctor.

Antacid Warnings: Do not take more than the maximum recommended daily dosage in a 24 hour period (see directions), or use the maximum dosage of this product for more than two weeks, or use this product if you have kidney disease, except under the advice and supervision of a physician. May have laxative effect.

General Warnings: As with any drug, if you are pregnant or nursing a baby, seek the advice of a health professional before using this product. Keep this and all drugs out of reach of children. In case of accidental overdose seek professional assistance or contact a poison control center immediately.

Drug Interaction: Antacids may interact with certain prescription drugs. If you are presently taking a prescription drug, do not take this product without checking with your physician.

Dosage and Administration: As a laxative, adults and children 12 years and older, 1–2 tbsp.; children 6–11, ½–1 tbsp.; children 2–5, ½ to 1½ tsp. followed by a full glass (8 oz.) of liquid. Children under 2, consult a physician.
As an antacid, adults and children 12 years and older, ½ to 1½ tsp. with a little water, up to four times a day or as directed by a physician.

How Supplied: Concentrated Phillips' Milk of Magnesia is available in strawberry creme (NDC 12843-347-10) and orange vanilla creme (NDC 12843-346-08) flavors in bottles of 8 fl. oz.

Shown in Product Identification Section, page 411

PHILLIPS'® MILK OF MAGNESIA TABLETS

Active Ingredients: Each Tablet contains 311 mg of magnesium hydroxide.

Inactive Ingredients: Flavor, starch, sucrose. Product description not USP.

Indications: For relief of acid indigestion, sour stomach, heartburn and occasional constipation (irregularity).

Action at Laxative Dosage: Phillips' Milk of Magnesia Tablets offer the same mild saline laxative ingredient as liquid Phillips' Milk of Magnesia in a convenient, chewable tablet form. It acts by drawing water into the gut, increasing intraluminal pressure, and increasing intestinal motility. This product generally produces bowel movement in ½ to 6 hours.
At Antacid Dosage: Phillips' Milk of Magnesia Tablets are effective acid neutralizers.

Administration and Dosage:
As an Antacid —Adults chew thoroughly 2 to 4 tablets up to 4 times a day. Children 7 to 14 years, 1 tablet up to 4 times a day or as directed by a physician.
As a Laxative —Adults and children 12 years of age and older chew thoroughly 6 to 8 tablets. Children 6 to 11, 3 to 4 tablets; children 2 to 5, 1 to 2 tablets, preferably before bedtime and follow with a full glass (8 oz) of liquid. Children under 2, consult a physician.

Laxative Warnings: Do not take any laxative if abdominal pain, nausea, vomiting, change in bowel habits (that persists for over 2 weeks), rectal bleeding, or kidney disease are present. Laxative products should not be used for a period longer than 1 week, unless directed by a doctor. If there is a failure to have a bowel movement after use, discontinue and consult your doctor.

Antacid Warnings: Do not take more than the maximum recommended daily dosage in a 24-hour period (see Directions), or use the maximum dosage of this product for more than two weeks, or use this product if you have kidney disease, except under the advice and supervision of a physician. May have laxative effect.

General Warnings: As with any drug, if you are pregnant or nursing a baby, seek the advice of a health professional before using this product. Keep this and *all* drugs out of reach of children. In case of accidental overdose, seek professional assistance or contact a poison control center immediately.

How Supplied: Phillips' Milk of Magnesia Tablets are available in a mint flavored chewable tablet in blister packs of: 24. NDC 12843-373-19, Bottle of 100. NDC 12843-373-12, Bottle of 200. NDC 12843-373-09.
Also available in liquid form.

Shown in Product Identification Section, page 411

STRI-DEX® DUAL TEXTURED PADS REGULAR STRENGTH STRI-DEX® DUAL TEXTURED PADS MAXIMUM STRENGTH

Active Ingredients:
Stri-Dex® Regular Strength: Salicylic acid 0.5%, SD alcohol 25% (w/w).
Stri-Dex® Maximum Strength: Salicylic acid 2.0%, SD alcohol 40% (w/w).

Inactive Ingredients:
Stri-Dex® Regular Strength: Citric acid, fragrance, menthol, purified water, simethicone emulsion, sodium carbonate, sodium dodecylbenzenesulfonate, sodium xylenesulfonate.
Stri-Dex® Maximum Strength: Ammonium xylenesulfonate, citric acid, fragrance, menthol, purified water, simethicone emulsion, sodium carbonate, sodium dodecylbenzenesulfonate.

Indications: For the treatment of acne. Reduces the number of acne pimples and blackheads, and allows the skin to heal. Helps prevent new acne pimples from forming.

Directions: Cleanse the skin thoroughly before using Stri-Dex medicated pad.
Use the deep cleaning textured side first to open pores and loosen the oil and dirt that can clog them. Then use the soothing soft side to wipe away oil and dirt and leave behind a tough pimple fighting medicine that will treat your pimples and help prevent new ones from forming.
Use the pad to wipe the entire affected area one to three times daily. Because excessive drying of the skin may occur, start with one application daily, then gradually increase to two or three times daily if needed or as directed by a doctor.

Warnings: FOR EXTERNAL USE ONLY: Using other topical acne medications at the same time or immediately following use of this product may increase dryness or irritation of the skin. If this occurs, only one medication should be used unless directed by a doctor.
Persons with very sensitive skin or known allergy to salicylic acid should not use this medication. If irritation or excessive dryness and/or peeling occurs, reduce frequency of use or dosage. If excessive itching, dryness, redness, or swelling occurs, discontinue use. If these symptoms persist, consult a physician promptly.
Keep away from eyes, lips, and other mucous membranes. Keep this and all drugs out of reach of children. In the case of accidental ingestion, seek professional as-

Continued on next page

Glenbrook—Cont.

sistance or contact a Poison Control Center immediately.

Dosage and Administration: See Labeling instructions for use.

How Supplied:
Stri-Dex Regular Strength is available in
NDC 12843-085-32—32 Pads
NDC 12843-085-50—50 Pads
Stri-Dex Maximum Strength is available in:
NDC 12843-098-32—32 Pads
NDC 12843-098-50—50 Pads

Shown in Product Identification Section, page 411

VANQUISH® Analgesic Caplets

Active Ingredients: Each caplet contains aspirin 227 mg, acetaminophen 194 mg, caffeine 33 mg, dried aluminum hydroxide gel 25 mg, magnesium hydroxide 50 mg.

Inactive Ingredients: Acacia, colloidal silicon dioxide, hydrogenated vegetable oil, microcrystalline cellulose, powdered cellulose, sodium lauryl sulfate, starch, talc.

Action and Uses: A buffered analgesic, antipyretic for relief of headache; muscular aches and pains; neuralgia and neuritic pain; toothache; pain following dental procedures; for painful discomforts and fever of colds and flu; sinusitis; functional menstrual pain, headache and pain due to cramps; temporary relief from minor pains of arthritis†, rheumatism, bursitis, lumbago, sciatica.

†Caution: If pain persists for more than 10 days, or redness is present or in conditions affecting children under 12 years of age, consult a physician immediately.

Warnings: Children and teenagers should not use this medicine for chicken pox or flu symptoms before a doctor is consulted about Reye syndrome, a rare but serious illness reported to be associated with aspirin. Keep this and all drugs out of the reach of children. In case of accidental overdose, seek professional assistance or contact a poison control center immediately. As with any drug, if you are pregnant or nursing a baby, seek the advice of a health professional before using this product. **IT IS ESPECIALLY IMPORTANT NOT TO USE ASPIRIN DURING THE LAST THREE MONTHS OF PREGNANCY UNLESS SPECIFICALLY DIRECTED TO DO SO BY A DOCTOR BECAUSE IT MAY CAUSE PROBLEMS IN THE UNBORN CHILD OR COMPLICATIONS DURING DELIVERY.**
IMPORTANT NOTICE: Do not take this product if you are allergic to aspirin, have asthma, stomach problems that persist or recur, gastric ulcers or bleeding, or if you are taking a prescription drug for arthritis, anticoagulation (thinning of the blood), diabetes, or gout unless directed by a doctor. If ringing in the ears or loss of hearing occurs, consult a doctor before taking any more of this product.

Usual Adult Dosage: Two caplets with water. May be repeated every four hours if necessary up to 12 tablets per day. Larger or more frequent doses may be prescribed by physician if necessary.

Contraindications: Hypersensitivity to salicylates and acetaminophen. (To be used with caution during anticoagulant therapy or in asthmatic patients).

How Supplied:
White, capsule-shaped caplets in bottles of:
30 Caplets—NDC 12843-171-44
60 Caplets—NDC 12843-171-46
100 Caplets—NDC 12843-171-48

Shown in Product Identification Section, page 411

Herald Pharmacal, Inc.
6503 WARWICK ROAD
RICHMOND, VA 23225

AQUA GLYCOLIC LOTION

Description: Aqua Glycolic lotion is a high-potency moisturizer containing 12 per cent partially neutralized Glycolic Acid in an unscented lanolin-free lotion base.

How Supplied: 4 oz. bottles and 8 oz. bottles

AQUA GLYCOLIC SHAMPOO®

Description: Cosmetically elegant shampoo, non-irritating, containing Glycolic Acid, leaves hair soft, manageable, helps eliminate itching, leaves scalp free from scale.

How Supplied: 8 oz. bottles and 16 oz. bottles

AQUA GLYDE CLEANSER®

Description: A cleanser for acne and other oily skin conditions. Contains special denatured alcohol #40, purified water, and Glycolic Acid.

How Supplied: 8 oz. plastic bottles.

AQUARAY® 20 SUNSCREEN

Description: AQUARAY Sunscreen is free of the sensitizing ingredients PABA, Padimate O, fragrance, lanolin, alcohol and parabens. It offers a wide range of protection from both UVA and UVB sun rays.

How Supplied: 4 fl. oz. bottles.

CAM LOTION®

Description: Lipid-free, soap-free skin cleanser for atopic dermatitis and other diseases aggravated by oily, greasy substances of animal and vegetable origin.

How Supplied: 8 and 16 oz. bottles.

Hoechst-Roussel Pharmaceuticals Inc.
SOMERVILLE, NJ 08876-1258

FESTAL® II
Digestive Aid

Composition: Each film-coated tablet contains lipase 6,000 USP units, amylase 30,000 USP units, protease 20,000 USP units and the following inactive ingredients: colloidal silicon dioxide NF, methacrylic acid copolymer NF, microcrystalline cellulose NF, opaque black, pharmaceutical glaze, polyethylene glycol NF, povidone USP, sodium chloride USP, sodium hydroxide NF, talc USP and titanium dioxide USP.

Actions and Uses: Festal® II provides a high degree of protected digestive activity in a formula of standardized enzymes. Enteric coating of the tablet prevents release of ingredients in the stomach so that high enzymatic potency is delivered to the site in the intestinal tract where digestion normally takes place.
Festal® II is indicated in any condition where normal digestion is impaired by insufficiency of natural digestive enzymes, or when additional digestive enzymes may be beneficial. These conditions often manifest complaints of discomfort due to excess intestinal gas, such as bloating, cramps and flatulence. The following are conditions or situations where Festal® II may be helpful: pancreatic insufficiency, chronic pancreatitis, pancreatic necrosis, and removal of gas prior to x-ray examination.
Keep this and all medication out of the reach of children.

Dosage: Usual adult dose is one or two tablets with each meal, or as directed by a physician. Store at controlled room temperature (59°–86°F). Store in a well-closed container in a dry place.

Contraindications: Festal® II should not be given to patients sensitive to protein of porcine origin.

How Supplied: Bottles of 100 white, film-coated enteric-coated tablets for oral use.
Festal REG TM Hoechst AG

ICN Pharmaceuticals, Inc.
ICN PLAZA
3300 HYLAND AVENUE
COSTA MESA, CA 92626

FOTOTAR® CREAM
[fōtō 'tar]
2% Coal Tar USP
(Equivalent to 10% Coal Tar Solution, USP)
Therapeutic Coal Tar Cream
FOR EXTERNAL USE ONLY
AVAILABLE WITHOUT A PRESCRIPTION

Description: Fototar® Cream contains Eldotar® (equivalent to 2% Coal Tar USP), in an emollient moisturizing cream base containing purified water, white petrolatum, mineral oil, microcrystalline cellulose, PEG 8, stearyl alcohol, glyceryl stearate PEG 100 stearate blend, coceth 6, imidazolidinyl urea, methylparaben, and propylparaben.

Clinical Pharmacology: The mechanism of action of coal tar products is largely unknown. Coal tars have antiseptic qualities, because they contain many substituted phenols. Coal tars also act as mild irritants and have a keratoplastic and antipruritic action. Coal tars have a photosensitizing effect and have been used for years with sunlight or ultraviolet (UV) radiation (Goeckerman Therapy) for the treatment of psoriasis. Coal tars have been successfully used in the treatment of seborrhea, eczema, psoriasis, lichen simplex chronicus, and other chronic skin diseases with lichenification. Pharmaceutical compounding of the crude coal tars has not lessened their therapeutic effectiveness and has increased patient acceptability.

Indications: Fototar is indicated in chronic skin disorders that are responsive to coal tars such as psoriasis, infantile and atopic eczema, seborrhea, lichen simplex chronicus, and other chronic skin disorders exhibiting lichenification. Fototar is useful in the Goeckerman program (tars plus UV radiation) in the treatment of psoriasis or other conditions responding to this combined therapy.

Contraindications:
A. Fototar is contraindicated in patients with a history of sensitivity to this product or with a history of sensitivity to coal tar products.
B. Fototar should not be used on patients who have a disease characterized by photosensitivity such as lupus erythematosus or allergy to sunlight.

Warnings:
A. Fototar should not be applied to inflamed or broken skin except on the advice of a physician.
B. Since Fototar is photosensitizing, care must be exercised in exposing the areas of application to excessive UV or sunlight for 24 hours. In the Goeckerman treatment of psoriasis or other skin conditions, care must be taken against overexposure of the areas of application during therapeutic UV radiation or subsequent to such treatment because serious burns may result. Sunscreening or sunblocking agents or protective clothing for at least 24 hours after treatment is recommended to protect the treated areas against additional UV exposure from sunlight.
C. Fototar contains a coal tar derivative. Coal tar preparations should not be used in patients with an exacerbation of psoriasis since this may precipitate total body exfoliation.
D. In psoriatic patients receiving Goeckerman therapy, care should be taken that Fototar application and/or subsequent sunlight exposure be avoided over normal skin since this may cause the appearance of new psoriatic lesions in areas of skin trauma (Koebner Phenomenon).
E. Contact with the eyes should be avoided.
F. Staining of clothing may occur which is normally removed by standard laundry methods. Use on the scalp may cause temporary staining of light colored hair.

Precautions:
A. Patients should be advised of the photosensitizing effect of Fototar.
B. Laboratory tests—none required.
C. Carcinogenesis. Skin cancer following the use of Fototar has not been seen. The use of crude coal tar combined with UV radiation in the production of skin cancer has been studied with conflicting results. Stern, et al, 1980, estimated an increased risk for such cancer in patients with high exposure to tar and ultraviolet radiation compared with those lacking high exposure. They recommended continued surveillance for tumors among psoriatic patients who receive long-term tar and/or UV radiation therapy. However, Pittelkow, et al, 1981, did a 25 year follow-up study on patients receiving combined crude coal tar and UV radiation for psoriasis at the Mayo Clinic and found the incidence of skin cancer not appreciably increased above the expected incidence for the general population, and concluded that this combined regimen (Goeckerman) could be used with minimal risk for skin cancer in the treatment of psoriasis.
D. Pregnancy Category C. Animal reproduction studies have not been conducted with Fototar. It is not known whether Fototar can cause fetal harm when administered to a pregnant woman or can affect reproductive capacity. Fototar should be given to a pregnant woman only if clearly indicated.
E. Nursing Mothers. The absorption of Fototar in nursing mothers has not been studied and caution should be exercised when Fototar is administered to a nursing woman.
F. Pediatric Use. Safety and effectiveness of Fototar in children have not been established.

Adverse Reactions:
A. SEE WARNINGS
B. Chemical folliculitis has been observed in areas of skin which have received long term coal tar applications. This phenomenon has not been observed with the use of Fototar, but its possibility should be borne in mind. This reaction normally clears if coal tar is discontinued or frequency of application reduced.

Overdosage:
A. SEE WARNINGS about use on normal skin.
B. If Fototar is accidentally ingested, call a physician or a poison control center for instructions.

Dosage and Administration: Fototar should be rubbed in the desired area well prior to UV radiation. After several minutes, the excess cream remaining on the skin can be patted with paper tissues to remove the excess.

How Supplied: Fototar is supplied in 3.0 ounce (85 gm) tubes (NDC 0187-0526-03) and in 1-lb. (453.6 gm) jars (NDC 0187-0526-05).
Fototar Cream should be stored at room temperature (15–30°C) (59–86°F).

Shown in Product Identification Section, page 411

INSTA-GLUCOSE
[*n-sta glū-cose*]
Liquid Glucose

Active Ingredient: Liquid Glucose NF, 30 grams. Each 31 g tube contains 24 g carbohydrate.

Indications: For relief from insulin reaction and hypoglycemia, Insta-Glucose is readily absorbed into the bloodstream from the digestive tract. The liquid gel is pleasant tasting and easy to swallow.

Dosage and Administration: The recommended dosage is one entire 31 g unit dose tube of Insta-Glucose (24 g carbohydrate). One tube will usually treat a mild to moderate insulin reaction. Notify your physician or diabetes specialist immediately to report occurrence of hypoglycemia.

How Supplied: Three 31 g unit dose tubes in a Tri-Pak container. 5-year shelf life. NDC #0187-0746-33

Shown in Product Identification Section, page 411

EDUCATIONAL MATERIAL

STAYING IN CONTROL
A guide to insulin reaction and hypoglycemia. This pamphlet describes common causes of hypoglycemia as well as stages, symptoms and treatment as recommended by the American Diabetes Assn.

Inter-Cal Corporation
421 MILLER VALLEY RD.
PRESCOTT, AZ 86301

ESTER-C®
(Calcium Ascorbate)

Description: Each Ester-C tablet contains 500 mg Vitamin C in the form of Calcium Ascorbate 550 mg, vegetable-derived cellulose, stearic acid, and magnesium stearate. Ester-C contains no preservatives, sugars, artificial colorings, or flavorings.
As the calcium salt of L-ascorbic acid, Ester-C has an empirical formula of $CaC_{12}H_{14}O_{12}$ and a formula weight of 390.3.

Continued on next page

Inter-Cal—Cont.

Actions: Vitamin C has been found to be essential for the prevention of scurvy. In humans, an exogenous source of the vitamin is required for collagen formation and tissue repair. Ascorbate ion is reversibly oxidized to dehydroascorbate ion in the body. Both of these are active forms of the vitamin and are considered to play important roles in biochemical oxidation-reduction reactions. The vitamin is involved in tyrosine metabolism, carbohydrate metabolism, iron metabolism, folic acid-folinic acid conversion, synthesis of lipids and proteins, resistance to infections, and cellular respiration.

Indications and Usage: Vitamin C and its salts, such as Calcium Ascorbate, are recommended as nutritional supplements in the prevention of scurvy. In scurvy, collagenous structures are primarily affected, and lesions develop in blood vessels and bones. Symptoms of mild deficiency may include faulty development of teeth and bones, bleeding gums, gingivitis, and loose teeth. An increased need for the vitamin exists in febrile states, chronic illness and infection, e.g., rheumatic fever, pneumonia, tuberculosis, whooping cough, diphtheria, sinusitis, etc. Additional increases in the daily intake of ascorbate are indicated in burns, delayed healing of bone fractures and wounds, and hemovascular disorders. Immature and premature infants require relatively larger amounts of Vitamin C.

Contraindications: Because of its calcium content, Ester-C is contraindicated in hypercalcemic states, e.g., from dosing with parathyroid hormone or overdosage of Vitamin D.
Diabetics, persons prone to recurrent renal calculi, those undergoing stool occult blood tests, and those on anticoagulant therapy should not take excessive doses of Vitamin C over extended periods of time.

Precautions: Because of its calcium content, Ester-C should be used with caution by those undergoing treatment with digitalis or cardiotonic glycosides such as digitoxin and digoxin.
Laboratory Tests—Diabetics taking more than 500 mg of Vitamin C may generate false readings in their urinary glucose tests. To avoid false-negative results, forms of the vitamin should not be taken as supplements for 48 to 72 hours before amine-dependent stool occult blood tests are conducted.
Drug Interactions—There is limited evidence suggesting that Vitamin C may influence the intensity and duration of action of bishydroxycoumarin.
Usage in Pregnancy—Pregnancy Category C—Animal reproduction studies have not been carried out with Ester-C tablets. It is also not known whether Ester-C can cause fetal harm when administered to a pregnant woman or can affect reproductive capacity.
Nursing Mothers—Caution should be exercised when Ester-C tablets are recommended for nursing mothers.

Adverse Reactions: There are no known adverse reactions following ingestion of Ester-C tablets. The gastric disturbances characteristic of large doses of ascorbic acid are absent or greatly diminished when the pH-neutral form of calcium ascorbate present in Ester-C tablets is utilized as the source of Vitamin C supplementation.

Dosage and Administration: The minimum U.S. Recommended Daily Allowance for Vitamin C for the prevention of diseases such as scurvy is 60 mg per day. Optimum daily allowances, e.g., for the maintenance of increased plasma and cellular reserves, are significantly greater. For adults, the recommended average preventative dose of the vitamin is 70 to 150 mg daily. The recommended average optimum dose of Ester-C is 550 to 1650 mg (1 to 3 tablets) daily.
For frank scurvy, doses of 300 mg to one gram of Vitamin C daily have been recommended. Normal adults, however, have received as much as six grams of the vitamin without evidence of toxicity.
For enhancement of wound healing, doses of the vitamin approximating two Ester-C tablets daily for a week or ten days both preoperatively and postoperatively are generally considered adequate, although considerably larger amounts may be recommended. In the treatment of burns, the daily number of Ester-C tablets recommended is governed by the extent of tissue injury. For severe burns, daily doses of 2 to 4 tablets (approximately one to two grams of Vitamin C) are recommended.
In other conditions in which the need for increased Vitamin C is recognized, three to five times the optimum allowance appears to be adequate.

How Supplied: 550 mg tablets of Ester-C in plastic bottles of 100, 250, 90, and 225's. 4 oz. and 8 oz. powders, 275 mg tablet also available.
Store at room temperature.
U.S. Patent granted April 18, 1989; No. 4,822,816.

Literature revised: December, 1989.
Mfd. by Inter-Cal Corp.
Prescott, AZ 86301

Jackson-Mitchell Pharmaceuticals, Inc.
P.O. BOX 5425
SANTA BARBARA, CA 93150

MEYENBERG GOAT MILK
[my 'en-berg]
Concentrated liquid • powder

Composition: A natural, mammalian milk more closely related to the structure of human milk than cow milk. Does not contain alpha S_1 casein. More easily digested.
Standard dilution (adults and babies over 6 months) supplies 20 calories/fl oz).
EVAPORATED supplemented with folic acid and Vitamin D. POWDER, folic acid only.
NOTE: ***Not a complete formula.*** Vitamin supplement recommended if sole source of nutrition.

Action and Uses: For cow milk and/or soy milk sensitive adults and children.

Preparation: Adults—20 calories/fl oz with concentrated liquid—1 part to 1 part water. Refrigerate. Baby Formula—should be refrigerated and used within 48 hours.

MEYENBERG Evaporated GOAT MILK Fortified with Folic Acid and Vitamin D

	Evap. Milk	Water	Calories Fl. Oz.*
First or transitional dilution	1 part	2 parts	14
Standard dilution	1 part	1 part	20

*Increase calorie value as desired by the addition of a carbohydrate.

MEYENBERG Powdered GOAT MILK Fortified with Folic Acid

RECOMMENDED FOR BABIES OVER 1 YEAR BECAUSE OF FLAVOR

	Pwdr. Milk	Water	Calories Fl. Oz.*
Standard dilution	1 Tbsp.	2 Fl. Oz.	20

EDUCATIONAL MATERIAL

Is It Really Milk Allergy?
Brochure.
Meyenberg Story
Brochure.

Johnson & Johnson
Consumer Products, Inc
GRANDVIEW ROAD
SKILLMAN, NJ 08558

JOHNSON'S MEDICATED DIAPER RASH OINTMENT

Description: JOHNSON'S Medicated Diaper Rash Ointment special formula contains skin protectants that *seal out wetness as it heals,* so JOHNSON'S helps keep rash from spreading and protects against further irritation.

Active Ingredient: Zinc oxide—active skin protectant.

Other Ingredients: Petrolatum—emollient base, provides occlusive barrier against wetness.
Trihydroxystearin—vehicle that suspends zinc oxide in petrolatum for better dispersal and added smoothness
Bisabolol—emollient and anti-irritant
Benzethonium chloride—antimicrobial preservative

Indications: Most cases of diaper rash begin with a baby's tender skin being exposed to wetness in a warm, enclosed diaper. Unlike dry skin, wet, warm skin is susceptible to even minor forms of irritation like friction between the diaper and baby's skin or chafing between skin folds. Wet skin is also easily irritated by contact with the bacteria and enzymes in stool.

Actions: Since wetness is the usual starting point for diaper rash, prevention and treatment is generally pretty straightforward. The steps identified below are widely recommended by pediatricians for effectively handling the most common forms of diaper rash. When following these steps, you should see significant healing progress within the first few days.

Recommended Steps for Treating Diaper Rash

1. Check your baby's diaper more frequently and change it at the first sign of wetness.
2. Allow the rash area to get as much exposure to air as possible.
3. When cleaning the diaper area after each change, use only warm water or a mild baby soap. Avoid scrubbing, as this can further irritate tender skin. Rinse well and pat dry.
4. Gently apply a medicated ointment to the rash area after each diaper change. This will help soothe and heal the rash while protecting the skin from further wetness.
5. At nighttime, apply a thick coating of medicated ointment on and around the rash area (since wetness protection is especially important) and change your baby's diaper once during the night until the rash has healed.

Directions for Use: At the first sign of redness, apply ointment evenly over the affected area. Reapply after each diaper change until rash symptoms disappear. For daily diaper rash protection, apply ointment after each diaper change or between infrequent changes (like bedtime).

Warning: For external use only. Avoid contact with eyes. If condition worsens or does not improve within 7 days, consult your doctor. Keep out of reach of children.

How Supplied: JOHNSON'S Medicated Diaper Rash Ointment is available in 2 oz. flip-top tubes.

Shown in Product Identification Section, page 411

Johnson & Johnson ◦ Merck
Consumer Pharmaceuticals Company
CAMP HILL ROAD
FORT WASHINGTON, PA 19034

ALternaGEL™
[*al-tern 'a-jel*]
Liquid
High-Potency Aluminum Hydroxide Antacid

Description: ALternaGEL is available as a white, pleasant-tasting, high-potency aluminum hydroxide liquid antacid.

Ingredients: Each 5 mL teaspoonful contains: Active: 600 mg aluminum hydroxide (equivalent to dried gel, USP) providing 16 milliequivalents (mEq) of acid-neutralizing capacity (ANC), and less than 2.5 mg (0.109 mEq) of sodium and no sugar. Inactive: butylparaben, flavors, propylparaben, purified water, simethicone, and other ingredients.

Indications: ALternaGEL is indicated for the symptomatic relief of hyperacidity associated with peptic ulcer, gastritis, peptic esophagitis, gastric hyperacidity, hiatal hernia, and heartburn.
ALternaGEL will be of special value to those patients for whom magnesium-containing antacids are undesirable, such as patients with renal insufficiency, patients requiring control of attendant G.I. complications resulting from steroid or other drug therapy, and patients experiencing the laxation which may result from magnesium or combination antacid regimens.

Directions: One to two teaspoonfuls, as needed, between meals and at bedtime, or as directed by a physician: May be followed by a sip of water if desired. Concentrated product. Shake well before using. Keep tightly closed.

Warnings: As with all medications, ALternaGEL should be kept out of the reach of children. ALternaGEL may cause constipation.
Except under the advice and supervision of a physician: do not take more than 18 teaspoonfuls in a 24-hour period, or use the maximum dose of ALternaGEL for more than two weeks.

Drug Interaction Precaution: ALternaGEL should not be taken concurrently with an antibiotic containing any form of tetracycline.

How Supplied: ALternaGEL is available in bottles of 12 fluid ounces and 5 fluid ounces, and 1 fluid ounce hospital unit doses. NDC 16837-860

Shown in Product Identification Section, page 412

DIALOSE® Capsules
[*di 'a-lose*]
Stool Softener Laxative

Description: DIALOSE is a sodium-free, nonhabit forming, stool softener containing docusate potassium in capsules of 100 mg.
The docusate in DIALOSE is a highly efficient surfactant which facilitates absorption of water by the stool to form a soft, easily evacuated mass. Unlike stimulant laxatives, DIALOSE does not interfere with normal peristalsis, neither does it cause griping nor sensations of urgency.

Ingredients: Each capsule contains: Active: docusate potassium. Inactive: Blue 1, gelatin, lactose, magnesium stearate, Red 28, Red 40, silicon dioxide, titanium dioxide.

Indications: DIALOSE is an effective aid to soften or prevent formation of hard stools in a wide range of conditions that may lead to constipation. DIALOSE helps to eliminate straining associated with obstetric, geriatric, cardiac, surgical, anorectal, or proctologic conditions. In cases of mild constipation, the fecal softening action of DIALOSE can prevent constipation from progressing and relieve painful defecation.

Directions: *Adults:* Adjust dosage as needed, one capsule one to three times daily. *Children:* 6 years and over—One capsule at bedtime, or as directed by physician. *Children:* under 6 years—As directed by physician. It is helpful to increase the daily intake of fluids by taking a glass of water with each dose.

Warnings: As with any drug, if you are pregnant or nursing a baby, seek the advice of a health professional before using this product. Keep out of the reach of children.

How Supplied: Bottles of 36 and 100 pink capsules, identified "DIALOSE". Also available in 100 capsule unit dose boxes (10 strips of 10 capsules each). NDC 16837-867

Shown in Product Identification Section, page 412

DIALOSE® PLUS Capsules
[*di 'a-lose Plus*]
Stool Softener/Stimulant Laxative

Description: DIALOSE PLUS provides a sodium-free formulation of docusate potassium in capsules of 100 mg and casanthranol, 30 mg.

Continued on next page

J & J ○ Merck—Cont.

Ingredients: Each capsule contains: Active: docusate potassium, casanthranol. Inactive: gelatin, lactose, magnesium stearate, Red 33, silicon dioxide, titanium dioxide, Yellow 10.

Indications: DIALOSE PLUS is indicated for the treatment of constipation characterized by lack of moisture in the intestinal contents, resulting in hardness of stool and decreased intestinal motility. DIALOSE PLUS combines the advantages of the stool softener, docusate potassium, with the peristaltic activating effect of casanthranol.

Directions: *Adults:* Initially, one capsule two times a day. *Children:* As directed by physician. When adequate bowel function is restored, the dose may be adjusted to meet individual needs. It is helpful to increase the daily intake of fluids by taking a glass of water with each dose.

Warnings: As with any drug, if you are pregnant or nursing a baby, seek the advice of a health professional before using this product. And, as with any laxative, DIALOSE PLUS should not be used when abdominal pain, nausea, or vomiting are present. Frequent or prolonged use may result in dependence on laxatives. Keep out of the reach of children.

How Supplied: Bottles of 36, 100, and 500 yellow capsules, identified "DIALOSE PLUS". Also available in 100 capsule unit dose boxes (10 strips of 10 capsules each). NDC 16837-865

Shown in Product Identification Section, page 412

EFFER-SYLLIUM®

[ef'fer-sil'lium]

Natural Fiber Bulking Agent

Description: EFFER-SYLLIUM is a tan, granular powder. Each rounded teaspoonful, or individual packet (7 g) contains psyllium hydrocolloid, 3 g.

Ingredients: Active: psyllium hydrocolloid. Inactive: citric acid, ethyl vanillin, lemon and lime flavors, potassium bicarbonate, potassium citrate, saccharin calcium, starch, sucrose.

EFFER-SYLLIUM contains less than 5 mg sodium per rounded teaspoonful and is considered dietetically sodium free.

Indications: EFFER-SYLLIUM is indicated to restore normal bowel habits in chronic constipation, to promote normal elimination in irritable bowel syndrome, and to ease passage of stools in presence of anorectal disorders. EFFER-SYLLIUM produces a soft, lubricating bulk which promotes natural elimination.

EFFER-SYLLIUM is not a one-dose, fast-acting bowel regulator. Administration for several days may be needed to establish regularity.

Directions:
Adults: One rounded teaspoonful, or one packet, in a glass of water one to three times a day, or as directed by physician. *Children, 6 years and over:* One level teaspoonful, or one-half packet (3.5 g) in one-half glass of water at bedtime, or as directed by physician. *Children, under 6 years:* As directed by physician.

Instructions: Pour EFFER-SYLLIUM into a *dry* glass, add water and stir briskly. Drink immediately. To avoid caking, always use a *dry* spoon to remove EFFER-SYLLIUM from its container. Replace cap tightly. Keep in a dry place.

Caution: People sensitive to psyllium powder should avoid inhalation as it may cause an allergic reaction such as wheezing.

Warning: As with all medications, keep out of the reach of children.

How Supplied: Bottles of 9 oz and 16 oz, and individual convenience packets (7 g each) packaged in boxes of 24. NDC 16837-440.

Shown in Product Identification Section, page 412

FERANCEE®

[fer'an-see]

Chewable Hematinic

Two Tablets Daily Provide:

	US RDA*	
Iron	744%	134 mg
Vitamin C	500%	300 mg

*Percentage of US Recommended Daily Allowances for adults and children 4 or more years of age.

Ingredients: Active: ferrous fumarate, sodium ascorbate, ascorbic acid. Inactive: confectioner's sugar, flavors, magnesium stearate, mannitol, povidone, saccharin calcium, starch, Yellow 5 (tartrazine), Yellow 6.

Indications: A pleasant-tasting hematinic for iron deficiency anemias, well-tolerated FERANCEE is particularly useful when chronic blood loss, onset of menses, or pregnancy create additional demands for iron supplementation. Available information indicates a low incidence of staining of the teeth by ferrous fumarate, alone or in combination with ascorbic acid. The peach-cherry flavored chewable tablets dissolve quickly in the mouth and may be either chewed or swallowed.

Directions:
Adults: Two tablets daily, or as directed by physician.
Chidren over 6 years of age: One tablet daily, or as directed by physician.
Children under 6 years of age: As directed by physician.

Warnings: As with any drug, if you are pregnant or nursing a baby, seek the advice of a health professional before using this product. Keep out of the reach of children. In case of accidental overdose, seek professional assistance or contact a Poison Control Center immediately.

How Supplied: FERANCEE is supplied in bottles of 100 brown and yellow, two-layer tablets. A child-resistant cap is standard on each bottle as a safeguard against accidental ingestion by children. Keep in a dry place. Replace cap tightly. NDC 16837-650.

FERANCEE®-HP Tablets

[fer-an-see hp]

High Potency Hematinic

One Tablet Daily Provides:

	US RDA*	
Iron	611%	110 mg
Vitamin C	1000%	600 mg

*Percentage of US Recommended Daily Allowances for adults and children 4 or more years of age.

Ingredients: Active: ferrous fumarate, sodium ascorbate, ascorbic acid. Inactive: flavor, hydrogenated vegetable oil, microcrystalline cellulose, povidone, Red 40, and other ingredients.

Indications: FERANCEE-HP is a high potency formulation of iron and vitamin C and is intended for use as either:

(1) a maintenance hematinic for those patients needing a daily iron supplement to maintain normal hemoglobin levels, or
(2) intensive therapy for the acute and/or severe iron deficiency anemia where a high intake of elemental iron is required.

The use of well-tolerated ferrous fumarate provides high levels of elemental iron with a low incidence of gastric distress. The inclusion of 600 mg of vitamin C per tablet serves to maintain more of the iron in the absorbable ferrous state.

Precautions: Because FERANCEE-HP contains 110 mg of elemental iron per tablet, it is recommended that its use be limited to adults, ie over 12 years of age.

Directions: One tablet per day after a meal or as directed by a physician. Should be sufficient to maintain normal hemoglobin levels in most patients with a history of recurring iron deficiency anemia. Not recommended for children under 12 years of age.
For acute and/or severe iron deficiency anemia, two or three tablets per day taken one tablet per dose after meals. (Each tablet provides 110 mg elemental iron).

Warnings: As with all medications, keep out of the reach of children. In case of accidental overdose, seek professional assistance or contact a Poison Control Center immediately.

How Supplied: FERANCEE-HP is supplied in bottles of 60 red, film coated, oval shaped tablets.
NDC 16837-863.
Note: A child-resistant safety cap is standard on each bottle of 60 tablets as a safeguard against accidental ingestion by children.

Shown in Product Identification Section, page 412

KASOF® Capsules
[kay 'sof]
High Strength Stool Softener
Laxative

Ingredients: Each capsule contains: Active: docusate potassium, 240 mg. Inactive: Blue 1, gelatin, glycerin, methylparaben, polyethylene glycol, propylparaben, purified water, Red 40, sorbitol, Yellow 10.

Indications: KASOF provides a highly efficient wetting action to restore moisture to the bowel, thus softening the stool to prevent straining. The action of KASOF does not interfere with normal peristalsis and generally does not cause griping or extreme sensation of urgency. KASOF is sodium-free, containing a unique potassium formulation, without the problems associated with sodium intake. KASOF is especially valuable for the severely constipated, as well as patients with anorectal disorders, such as hemorrhoids and anal fissures. KASOF is ideal for patients with any condition that can be complicated by straining at stool, for example, cardiac patients. The simple, one-a-day dosage helps assure patient compliance in maintaining normal bowel function.

Directions: Adults: One KASOF capsule daily for several days, or until bowel movements are normal and gentle. It is helpful to increase the daily intake of fluids by drinking a glass of water with each dose.
Store in a closed container, protect from freezing and avoid excessive heat (104°F).

Warnings: As with any drug, if you are pregnant or nursing a baby, seek the advice of a health professional before using this product. Keep out of the reach of children.

How Supplied: KASOF is available in bottles of 30 and 60 brown, gelatin capsules, identified "KASOF".
NDC 16837-380.

Shown in Product Identification Section, page 412

MYLANTA®
[my-lan 'ta]
Liquid and Tablets
Antacid/Anti-Gas

Ingredients: Each chewable tablet or each 5 mL (one teaspoonful) of liquid contains: Active: Aluminum hydroxide (Dried Gel, USP in tablet and equiv. to Dried Gel, USP in liquid) 200 mg, Magnesium hydroxide 200 mg, Simethicone 20 mg. Inactive: Tablets: dextrates, flavors, magnesium stearate, mannitol, sorbitol, starch, Yellow 10. Liquid: butylparaben, carboxymethylcellulose sodium, flavors, hydroxypropyl methylcellulose, microcrystalline cellulose, propylparaben, purified water, sorbitol solution with no added sugar.
Sodium Content: MYLANTA contains an insignificant amount of sodium per daily dose and is considered dietetically sodium free. Typical values are 0.68 mg (0.03 mEq) sodium per 5 mL teaspoonful of liquid and 0.77 mg (0.03 mEq) per tablet.
Acid Neutralizing Capacity: Two teaspoonfuls of MYLANTA liquid will neutralize 25.4 mEq of acid. Two MYLANTA tablets will neutralize 23.0 mEq.

Indications: MYLANTA, a well-balanced combination of two antacids and simethicone, provides consistently dependable relief of symptoms associated with gastric hyperacidity, and mucus-entrapped air or "gas". These indications include:

Common heartburn (pyrosis)
Hiatal hernia
Peptic esophagitis
Gastritis
Peptic ulcer

The exceptionally pleasant tasting liquid and soft, easy-to-chew tablets encourage patients' acceptance, thereby minimizing the skipping of prescribed doses. MYLANTA is appropriate whenever there is a need for effective relief of temporary gastric hyperacidity and mucus-entrapped gas.

Directions: *Liquid:* Shake well, 2–4 teaspoonfuls between meals and at bedtime or as directed by a physician. *Tablets:* 2–4 tablets, well chewed, between meals and at bedtime or as directed by a physician.

Warnings: Keep this and all drugs out of the reach of children.
Except under the advice and supervision of a physician: Do not take more than 24 teaspoonfuls or 24 tablets in a 24 hour period or use the maximum dose for more than two weeks. Do not use this product if you have kidney disease. Magnesium hydroxide and other magnesium salts, in the presence of renal insufficiency, may cause central nervous system depression and other symptoms of hypermagnesemia.

Drug Interaction Precaution: Do not use this product for any patient receiving a prescription antibiotic containing any form of tetracycline.

How Supplied: MYLANTA is available as a white, pleasant tasting liquid suspension, and as a two-layer yellow and white chewable tablet, identified on yellow layer "MYLANTA". Liquid supplied in 5 oz, 12 oz and 24 oz bottles. Tablets supplied in boxes of individually wrapped 100's, economy size bottles of 180, consumer convenience pocket packs of 48, roll packs of 12 tablets each and 3-roll packs containing 36 tablets. Also available for hospital use in liquid unit doses of 1 oz, and bottles of 5 oz.
NDC 16837-610 (liquid). NDC 16387-620 (tablets).

Shown in Product Identification Section, page 412

MYLANTA® DOUBLE STRENGTH
[my-lan 'ta]
Liquid and Tablets
Double Strength Antacid/Anti-Gas

Ingredients: Each chewable tablet or each 5 mL (one teaspoonful) of liquid contains: Active: Aluminum hydroxide (Dried Gel, USP in tablet and equiv. to Dried Gel, USP in liquid) 400 mg
Magnesium hydroxide 400 mg
Simethicone 40 mg
Tablets: Blue 1, cereal solids, confectioner's sugar, flavors, glycerin, lactose, mannitol, starch, Yellow 10. Liquid: butylparaben, carboxymethylcellulose sodium, flavors, hydroxypropyl methylcellulose, microcrystalline cellulose, potassium citrate, propylparaben, purified water, sorbitol solution with no added sugar.
Sodium Content: MYLANTA-DOUBLE STRENGTH contains an insignificant amount of sodium per daily dose. Typical values are 1.14 mg (0.05 mEq) sodium per 5 mL teaspoonful of liquid and 1.3 mg (0.06 mEq) per tablet.
Acid Neutralizing Capacity: Two teaspoonfuls of MYLANTA-DOUBLE STRENGTH liquid will neutralize 50.8 mEq of acid. Two MYLANTA-DOUBLE STRENGTH tablets will neutralize 46.0 mEq.

Indications: MYLANTA-DOUBLE STRENGTH is a double strength antacid with an anti-gas ingredient for the relief of heartburn, acid indigestion, sour stomach and accompanying gas.The exceptionally pleasant tasting liquid and soft, easy-to-chew tablets encourage patient acceptance, thereby minimizing the skipping of prescribed doses. MYLANTA-DOUBLE STRENGTH provides consistently dependable relief of the symptoms of peptic ulcer and other problems related to acid hypersecretion. The high potency of MYLANTA-DOUBLE STRENGTH is achieved through its concentration of noncalcium antacid ingredients. Thus MYLANTA-DOUBLE STRENGTH can produce both rapid and long lasting neutralization without the acid rebound associated with calcium carbonate. The balanced formula of aluminum and magnesium hydroxides minimizes undesirable bowel effects. Simethicone is effective for the relief of concomitant distress caused by mucus-entrapped gas and swallowed air.

Directions: Liquid: Shake well, 2–4 teaspoonfuls between meals and at bedtime, or as directed by a physician. Tablets: 2–4 tablets, well-chewed, between meals and at bedtime, or as directed by a physician.
Because patients with peptic ulcer vary greatly in both acid output and gastric emptying time, the amount and schedule of dosages should be varied accordingly.

Warnings: Keep this and all drugs out of the reach of children.
Except under the advice and supervision of a physician: Do not take more than 12 teaspoonfuls or 12 tablets in a 24 hour period or use the maximum dose for more than two weeks. Do not use this product if you have kidney disease. Magnesium hydroxide and other magnesium salts, in the presence of renal insufficiency, may cause central nervous system depression and other symptoms of hypermagnesemia.

Continued on next page

Drug Interaction Precaution: Do not use this product for any patient receiving a prescription antibiotic containing any form of tetracycline.

How Supplied: MYLANTA-DOUBLE STRENGTH is available as a white, pleasant tasting liquid suspension, and a two-layer green and white chewable tablet, identified "MYLANTA DS". Liquid supplied in 5 oz, 12 oz and 24 oz bottles. Tablets supplied in boxes of 60 individually wrapped chewable tablets, consumer convenience pocket packs of 24, 8 tablet rollpacks, and 3-roll packs containing 24 tablets. Also available for hospital use in liquid unit dose bottles of 1 oz, and bottles of 5 oz.
NDC 16837-652 (liquid). NDC 16837-651 (tablets).

Shown in Product Identification Section, page 412

MYLICON® Tablets and Drops

[my 'li-con]

Antiflatulent

Ingredients: Each tablet or 0.6 mL of drops contains: Active: simethicone, 40 mg. Inactive: Tablets: calcium silicate, lactose, povidone, saccharin calcium. Drops: carbomer 934P, citric acid, flavors, hydroxypropyl methylcellulose, purified water, Red 3, saccharin calcium, sodium benzoate, sodium citrate.

Indications: For relief of the painful symptoms of excess gas in the digestive tract. Such gas is frequently caused by excessive swallowing of air or by eating foods that disagree. If condition persists consult your physician. MYLICON is a valuable adjunct in the treatment of many conditions in which the retention of gas may be a problem, such as: postoperative gaseous distention, air swallowing, functional dyspepsia, peptic ulcer, spastic or irritable colon, diverticulosis. The defoaming action of MYLICON relieves flatulence by dispersing and preventing the formation of mucus-surrounded gas pockets in the gastrointestinal tract. MYLICON acts in the stomach and intestines to change the surface tension of gas bubbles enabling them to coalesce; thus the gas is freed and is eliminated more easily by belching or passing flatus.
Infants: MYLICON drops are also useful for relief of the painful symptoms of excess gas associated with such conditions as colic, lactose intolerance, or air swallowing.

Directions:
Tablets—One or two tablets four times daily after meals and at bedtime. May also be taken as needed up to 12 tablets daily or as directed by a physician. TABLETS SHOULD BE CHEWED THOROUGHLY.
Drops—Adults and Children 0.6 mL four times daily after meals and at bedtime or as directed by a physician. Shake well before using.
Infants (under 2 years): Initially, 0.3 mL four times daily, after meals and at bedtime, or as directed by a physician. The dosage can also be mixed with 1 oz of cool water, infant formula, or other suitable liquids to ease administration. Dosage should not exceed 12 doses per day.

Warnings: Keep this and all drugs out of the reach of children.

How Supplied: Bottles of 100 and 500 white, scored, chewable tablets, identified MYLICON, and dropper bottles of 30 mL (1 fl oz) pink, pleasant tasting liquid. Also available in 100 tablet unit dose boxes (10 strips of 10 tablets each).
NDC 16837-450 (tablets).
NDC 16837-630 (drops).

Shown in Product Identification Section, page 412

MYLICON®-80 Tablets

[my 'li-con]

High-Capacity Antiflatulent

Ingredients: Each tablet contains: Active: simethicone, 80 mg. Inactive: flavor, cereal solids, lactose, mannitol, povidone, Red 3, talc.

Indications: For relief of the painful symptoms of excess gas in the digestive tract. Such gas is frequently caused by excessive swallowing of air or by eating foods that disagree. If condition persists, consult your physician. MYLICON-80 is a high capacity antiflatulent for adjunctive treatment of many conditions in which the retention of gas may be a problem, such as the following: air swallowing, functional dyspepsia, postoperative gaseous distention, peptic ulcer, spastic or irritable colon, diverticulosis.
MYLICON-80 has a defoaming action that relieves flatulence by dispersing and preventing the formation of mucus-surrounded gas pockets in the gastrointestinal tract. MYLICON-80 acts in the stomach and intestines to change the surface tension of gas bubbles enabling them to coalesce; thus, the gas is freed and is eliminated more easily by belching or passing flatus.

Directions: One tablet four times daily after meals and at bedtime. May also be taken as needed up to 6 tablets daily or as directed by a physician. TABLETS SHOULD BE CHEWED THOROUGHLY.

Warnings: Keep this and all drugs out of the reach of children.

How Supplied: Economical bottles of 100 and convenience packages of individually wrapped 12 and 48 pink, scored, chewable tablets identified MYLICON 80. Also available in 100 tablet unit dose boxes (10 strips of 10 tablets each).
NDC 16837-858.

Shown in Product Identification Section, page 412

MYLICON®-125 Tablets

[my 'li-con]

Maximum Strength Antiflatulent

Ingredients: Each tablet contains: Active: simethicone, 125 mg. Inactive: cereal solids, flavor, lactose, mannitol, povidone, Red 3, talc.

Indications: MYLICON-125 is useful for relief of the painful symptoms of excess gas in the digestive tract. Such gas is frequently caused by excessive swallowing of air or by eating foods that disagree. If condition persists, consult your physician. MYLICON-125 is the strongest possible antiflatulent for adjunctive treatment of many conditions in which the retention of gas may be a problem, such as the following: air swallowing, functional dyspepsia, postoperative gaseous distention, peptic ulcer, spastic or irritable colon, diverticulosis. MYLICON-125 has a defoaming action that relieves flatulence by dispersing and preventing the formation of mucus-surrounded gas pockets in the gastrointestinal tract. MYLICON-125 acts in the stomach and intestines to change the surface tension of gas bubbles enabling them to coalesce; thus, the gas is freed and is eliminated more easily by belching or passing flatus.

Directions: One tablet four times daily after meals and at bedtime or as directed by physician. TABLETS SHOULD BE CHEWED THOROUGHLY.

Warnings: Keep this and all drugs out of the reach of children.

How Supplied: Convenience packages of individually wrapped 12 and 60 dark pink, scored chewable tablets identified MYLICON 125. NDC 16837-455.

Shown in Product Identification Section, page 412

OREXIN® SOFTAB® Tablets

[or 'ex-in]

High Potency Vitamin Supplement

One Tablet Daily Provides:

VITAMINS:	US RDA*	
B_1 (thiamin)	540%	8.1 mg
B_6 (pyridoxine hydrochloride)	205%	4.1 mg
B_{12} (cyanocobalamin)	417%	25 mcg

*Percentage of US Recommended Daily Allowances for adults and children 4 or more years of age.

Ingredients: Active: thiamin mononitrate, pyridoxine hydrochloride, cyanocobalamin. Inactive: flavor, mannitol, saccharin calcium, sodium chloride, starch.

Indications: OREXIN is a high-potency vitamin supplement providing vitamins B_1, B_6, and B_{12}.
OREXIN SOFTAB tablets are specially formulated to dissolve quickly in the mouth. They may be chewed or swallowed. Dissolve tablet in a teaspoonful of water or fruit juice if liquid is preferred.

Directions: One tablet daily or as directed by a physician.

Warnings: Keep this and all drugs out of the reach of children.

How Supplied: Bottles of 100 pale pink SOFTAB tablets, identified OREXIN.
NDC 16837-280.
Shown in Product Identification Section, page 412

PROBEC®–T Tablets
[pro 'bec-t]
Vitamin B Complex Supplement

One Tablet Daily Provides:

VITAMINS:	US RDA*	
C	1000%	600 mg
B_1 (thiamin)	813%	12.2 mg
B_2 (riboflavin)	588%	10 mg
Niacin	500%	100 mg
B_6 (pyridoxine hydrochloride)	205%	4.1 mg
B_{12} (cyanocobalamin)	83%	5 mcg
Pantothenic Acid	184%	18.4 mg

*Percentage of US Recommended Daily Allowances for adults and children 4 or more years of age.

DOSAGE: One tablet a day with a meal or as directed by physician.

Ingredients: Active: sodium ascorbate, niacinamide, calcium pantothenate, ascorbic acid, thiamin mononitrate, riboflavin, pyridoxine hydrochloride, cyanocobalamin. Inactive: calcium sulfate, carnauba wax, magnesium oxide, pharmaceutical glaze, povidone, Red 30, sucrose, titanium dioxide, white wax, Yellow 10.

Indications: PROBEC-T is a high-potency B complex supplement with 600 mg of vitamin C in easy to swallow odorless tablets.

Directions: One tablet a day with a meal or as directed by physician.

Warnings: As with all medications, keep out of the reach of children.

How Supplied: Bottles of 60, peach colored, capsule-shaped tablets.
NDC 16837-840.
Shown in Product Identification Section, page 412

THE STUART FORMULA® Tablets
Multivitamin/Multimineral Supplement

One Tablet Daily Provides:

VITAMINS:	US RDA*	
A	100%	5,000 IU
D	100%	400 IU
E	50%	15 IU
C	100%	60 mg
Folic Acid	100%	0.4 mg
B_1 (thiamin)	80%	1.2 mg
B_2 (riboflavin)	100%	1.7 mg
Niacin	100%	20 mg
B_6 (pyridoxine hydrochloride)	100%	2 mg
B_{12} (cyanocobalamin)	100%	6 mcg
MINERALS:	**US RDA**	
Calcium	16%	160 mg
Phosphorus	12%	125 mg
Iodine	100%	150 mcg
Iron	100%	18 mg
Magnesium	25%	100 mg

*Percentage of US Recommended Daily Allowances for adults and children 4 or more years of age.

Ingredients: Each tablet contains: Active: dibasic calcium phosphate, magnesium oxide, ascorbic acid, ferrous fumarate, dl-alpha tocopheryl acetate, folic acid, niacinamide, vitamin A palmitate, cyanocobalamin, pyridoxine hydrochloride, riboflavin, thiamin mononitrate, ergocalciferol, potassium iodide. Inactive: calcium sulfate, carnauba wax, pharmaceutical glaze, povidone, sodium starch glycolate, starch, sucrose, titanium dioxide, white wax.

Indications: The STUART FORMULA tablet provides a well-balanced multivitamin/multimineral formula intended for use as a daily dietary supplement for adults and children over age four.

Directions: One tablet daily or as directed by physician.

Warnings: Keep this and all drugs out of the reach of children. In case of accidental overdose, seek professional assistance or contact a Poison Control Center immediately.

How Supplied: Bottles of 100 and 250 white round tablets. Child-resistant safety caps are standard on both bottles as a safeguard against accidental ingestion by children.
NDC 16837-866.
Shown in Product Identification Section, page 412

STUARTINIC® Tablets
[stu "are-tin 'ic]
Hematinic

One Tablet Daily Provides:

	US RDA*	
Iron	556%	100 mg
VITAMINS:		
C	833%	500 mg
B_1 (thiamin)	327%	4.9 mg
B_2 (riboflavin)	353%	6 mg
Niacin	100%	20 mg
B_6 (pyridoxine hydrochloride)	40%	0.8 mg
B_{12} (cyanocobalamin)	417%	25 mcg
Pantothenic Acid	92%	9.2 mg

*Percentage of US Recommended Daily Allowances for adults and children 4 or more years of age.

Ingredients: Active: ferrous fumarate, ascorbic acid, sodium ascorbate, niacinamide, calcium pantothenate, thiamin mononitrate, riboflavin, pyridoxine hydrochloride, cyanocobalamin. Inactive: flavor, hydrogenated vegetable oil, microcrystalline cellulose, povidone, Yellow 6, Yellow 10, and other ingredients.

Indications: STUARTINIC is a complete hematinic for patients with history of iron deficiency anemia who also lack proper amounts of vitamin C and B-complex vitamins due to inadequate diet. The use of well-tolerated ferrous fumarate in STUARTINIC provides a high level of elemental iron with a low incidence of gastric distress. The inclusion of 500 mg of Vitamin C per tablet serves to maintain more of the iron in the absorbable ferrous state. The B-complex vitamins improve nutrition where B-complex deficient diets contribute to the anemia.

Warnings: As with any drug, if you are pregnant or nursing a baby, seek the advice of a health professional before using this product. Keep out of the reach of children. In case of accidental overdose, seek professional assistance or contact a Poison Control Center immediately.

Dosage: One tablet daily taken after a meal or as directed by physician. Because of the high amount of iron per tablet, STUARTINIC is not recommended for children under 12 years of age.

How Supplied: STUARTINIC is supplied in bottles of 60 yellow, film coated, oval shaped tablets. NDC 16837-862.

Note: A child-resistant safety cap is standard on each 60 tablet bottle as a safeguard against accidental ingestion by children.
Shown in Product Identification Section, page 412

Kremers Urban Company

See SCHWARZ PHARMA.

Lactaid Inc.
P.O. BOX 111
PLEASANTVILLE, NJ
08232-0111

BEANO™

PRODUCT OVERVIEW

Key Facts: Beano™ alpha galactosidase enyzme hydrolyzes raffinose, verbascose and stachyose into the digestible sugars, sucrose, fructose, glucose and galactose. Beano Drops are added to food immediately prior to eating, for *in vivo* treatment of the food during digestion.

Major Uses: As a gas and bloat preventive. Beano™ enyzme has been shown to be effective in both clinical and anecdotal studies with humans when consuming foods with high alpha-linked sugars content, as well as with direct challenges of alpha-linked sugars themselves. Use results in substantially reduced breath hydrogen emissions and marked reduction or elimination of symptoms, compared with identical challenges without Beano.

Continued on next page

Lactaid—Cont.

Safety Information: Beano™ enyzme should be discontinued in anyone who develops hypersensitivity to the enzyme. No such reports to date.

PRESCRIBING INFORMATION

BEANO™

Description: Each 5 drop dosage contains not less than 175 GALU (galactose units) of alpha-D-galactosidase derived from *Aspergillus niger* fungus. The enzyme is in a liquid carrier of water and glycerol. Approximately 5 drops on the first portion of food consumed will deal with the entire subsequent portion; will hydrolyze the complex sugars, raffinose, stachyose and verbascose into the simple sugars, glucose, galactose and fructose, and the easily digestible disaccharide, sucrose. This happens simultaneously with normal digestion. In some cases, more or less enzyme than 5 drops will be required, and this is a function of the quantity of food eaten, the levels of alpha-linked sugars in the food and the gas-producing propensity of the person.

Action: Hydrolysis converts raffinose, stachyose and verbascose into their sugar components: glucose, galactose, sucrose and fructose. Raffinose yields sucrose + galactose; stachyose yields sucrose + galactose; verbascose yields glucose + fructose + galactose.

Indications: Gassiness and/or bloat as a result of eating a variety of grains, cereals, nuts, seeds, vegetables containing the sugars raffinose, stachyose and/or verbascose. This includes all or most legumes and all or most cruciferous vegetables. Examples of such foods are oats, wheat, beans of all kinds, chick-peas, peas, lentils, peanuts, soy-content foods, pistachios, broccoli, brussels sprouts, cabbage, carrots, corn, leeks, onions, parsnips, squash. Note: Most vegetables also contain fiber, which is gas productive in some people, but usually far less so than the alpha-linked sugars. Beano™ has no effect on fiber.

Usage: 3–8 drops per average serving, higher or lower levels depending on symptoms.

How Supplied: Beano™ is supplied in a stable liquid form, 12- and 75-serving sizes, at 5 drops per dose.

Toxicity: None known

Adverse Reactions: None known; enzyme is derived from *Asperigillus niger,* a mold, and it is conceivable that mold-sensitive persons could react. Penicillin-sensitive persons might be particularly suspect. No such reports to date.

Drug Interactions: None known. Beano™ is classified as a food, not a drug.

Precautions: Diabetics should be aware that the sugars in these vegetables will now be metabolically available and must be taken into account. No reports received of any diabetics' reactions. **Galactosemics should not use without physician's advice,** since one of the breakdown sugars is galactose.

For more information and samples, please write or call toll-free 1-800-257-8650.

Shown in Product Identification Section, page 413

LACTAID®
[*lăkt 'ād*]
Lactaid Drops and Lactaid Caplets (lactase enzyme)

PRODUCT OVERVIEW

Key Facts: Lactaid® lactase enzyme hydrolyzes lactose into digestible sugars: glucose and galactose. Lactaid Drops are added to milk for *in vitro* treatment; Lactaid Caplets are taken orally for *in vivo* hydrolysis.

Major Uses: Lactaid lactase enzyme (liquid and caplets) have proven to be clinically effective for lactose-intolerant people when consuming milk and/or dairy foods, by permitting consumption of lactose-containing foods without gas, cramps, bloating and/or diarrhea.

Safety Information: Lactaid enzyme should be discontinued in anyone who develops hypersensitivity to the enzyme.

PRESCRIBING INFORMATION

LACTAID®
[*lăkt 'ād*]
Lactaid Drops and Lactaid Caplets (lactase enzyme)

Description:
Drops: Each 5 drop dosage contains not less than 1250 NLU (Neutral Lactase Units) of beta-D-galactosidase derived from *Kluyveromyces lactis* yeast. The enzyme is in a liquid carrier of glycerol (50%), water (30%), and inert yeast dry matter (20%). 5 drops hydrolyze approximately 70% of the lactose in 1 quart of milk at refrigerator temperature, at 40°F (4°C) in 24 hours, or will do the same in 2 hours at 85°F (30°C). Additional time and/or enzyme required for 100% lactose conversion. 1 U.S. quart of milk will contain approximately 50 gm lactose prior to lactose hydrolysis and will contain 15 gm or less, after 70% conversion.

Action: Hydrolysis converts the lactose into its simple sugar components: glucose and galactose.

Indications: Lactase insufficiency in the patient, suspected from GI disturbances after consumption of milk or milk-content products: e.g., bloat, distension, flatulence, diarrhea; or identified by a lactose tolerance test.

Usage: Added to milk. 5–15 drops per quart of milk depending on level of lactose conversion desired.

Other Uses: *In vivo* activity has been demonstrated, indicating usage in tube feedings and other lactose-content solid and liquid foods, with addition at time of consumption.

How Supplied: Lactase enzyme in a stable liquid form, in sales units of 12, 30 and 75 one-quart dosages at 5 drops per dose.

Caplets: Each caplet contains not less than 3350 FCC lactase units of beta-D-galactosidase from *Aspergillus oryzae.* One to two caplets taken with a meal will normally handle a lactose challenge equal to 1 glass of milk. In severe cases, 3 caplets may be required.

Toxicity: None

Drug Interactions: None. Both liquid and caplets are classified as food, not drugs.

Warnings: Should hypersensitivity occur, discontinue use.

Precautions: Diabetics should be aware that the milk sugar will now be metabolically available and must be taken into account (17.5 gm glucose and 17.5 gm galactose per quart at 70% hydrolysis). No reports received of any diabetics' reactions. Galactosemics may not have milk in any form, lactase enzyme modified or not.

Adverse Reactions: The most frequently reported adverse reactions to Lactaid lactase caplets are gastrointestinal in nature, sometimes mimicking the symptoms of lactose intolerance and sometimes involving violent vomiting. Such reactions believed to be allergic. Persons sensitive to penicillin and other molds may be particularly susceptible. Discontinue immediately and convert to *in vivo* use of liquid. No reactions of any kind observed from Lactaid liquid drops. Total reactions to caplets estimated at under 0.1% (1/10 of 1%) of users.

How Supplied: In bottles of 100, bottles of 12 and boxes of 25 2-caplet "take along" packets.

Other Lactose Reduced Products: In most areas of the U.S.: Fresh lactose reduced lowfat milk from dairies, ready to drink, sold in food markets. Lactose hydrolysis level: 70%. If desired, further conversion of the dairy-treated milk can be done at home or institution with the Lactaid liquid enzyme. Also in some areas: Lactaid lactose reduced cottage cheese and American process cheese.
Any person or institution unable to locate Lactaid enzyme locally can order direct from Lactaid Inc. retail or wholesale. Samples and full product information to doctors, institutions and nutritionists on request.
Call toll-free 1-800-522-8243.

Shown in Product Identification Section, page 413

EDUCATIONAL MATERIAL

Brochures

Patient brochure—"Why Lactaid? The Problem with Milk and the Answer"

Professional brochure—"Lactaid Specially Digestible Milk and Dairy Products as Part of a Nutritional Program"

Samples

Dispensing samples of Lactaid Caplets and Lactaid Drops.

PATIENT STARTER KITS

Contains patient brochure, 12 Lactaid Caplets and Lactaid Drops for treating 4 quarts of milk.

All literature, samples and patient starter kits are available free to physicians and dietitians.

Lavoptik Company, Inc.

661 WESTERN AVENUE N.
ST. PAUL, MN 55103

LAVOPTIK® Eye Wash

Description: Isotonic LAVOPTIK Eye Wash is a buffered solution designed to help physically remove contaminants from the surface of the eye and lids. Formulated to buffer contaminants toward the safe range and help restore normal salts and water ratios in the tears.

Contents: Each 100 ml

Sodium Chloride	0.49 gram
Sodium Biphosphate	0.40 gram
Sodium Phosphate	0.45 gram
Preservative Agent	
Benzalkonium Chloride	0.005 gram

Precautions: If you experience severe eye pain, headache, rapid change in vision (side or straight ahead); sudden appearance of floating objects, acute redness of the eyes, pain on exposure to light or double vision consult a physician at once. If symptoms persist or worsen after use of this product, consult a physician. If solution changes color or becomes cloudy do not use. Keep this and all medicines out of reach of children. Keep container tightly closed. Do not use if safety seal is broken at time of purchase.

Administration: 6 ounce size with Eye Cup.

Rinse cup with clean water immediately before and after each use, avoid contamination of rim and inside surfaces of cup. Apply cup, half-filled with LAVOPTIK Eye Wash tightly to the eye. Tilt head backward. Open eyelids wide, rotate eyeball and blink several times to insure thorough washing. Discard washings. Repeat other eye. Tightly cap bottle.

32 ounce size.

Break seal as you remove cap and pour directly on contaminated area.

How Supplied: 6 ounce bottle with eyecup, NDC 10651-01040.

32 ounce bottle, NDC 10651-01019.

Products are indexed by generic and chemical names in the **YELLOW SECTION**

Lederle Laboratories

A Division of American Cyanamid Co.
ONE CYANAMID PLAZA
WAYNE, NJ 07470

LEDERMARK®
Product Identification Code

Many Lederle tablets and capsules bear an identification code. A current listing appears in the Product Information Section of the 1991 PDR for prescription drugs.

CALTRATE®, JR.
[*căl-trāte*]
Calcium Supplement For Children Chewable Orange Flavored

- Nature's most concentrated form of calcium®
- Made with pure calcium carbonate
- No lactose, no salt, no starch
- Great orange taste. Nonchalky.
- Plus Vitamin D to help absorb calcium.
- Children 4–10 years old need 1000 mg of calcium (U.S. RDA) every day to help keep teeth and bones strong.

ONE TABLET DAILY CONTAINS:

	Children 4+ % U.S. RDA
750 mg Calcium Carbonate which provides 300 mg elemental calcium	30%
60 I.U. Vitamin D	15%

Inactive Ingredients: Dextrose, *dl*-Alpha Tocopheryl, Gelatin, Magnesium Stearate, Malto Dextrin, Mannitol, Orange Flavor, Silica Gel, Sorbitol, Stearic Acid, Sucrose, Yellow 6, and other ingredients.

Recommended Intake: One or two tablets daily or as directed by a physician.

Warnings: Keep out of the reach of children.

How Supplied: Bottle of 60—
NDC 0005-5516-19
Store at Room Temperature.

22043
D2

Shown in Product Identification Section, page 413

CALTRATE® 600
[*căl-trāte*]
High Potency Calcium Supplement Nature's Most Concentrated Form of Calcium®
No Sugar, No Salt, No Lactose, No Cholesterol, No Preservatives, Film-Coated for Easy Swallowing

Inactive Ingredients: Croscarmellose Sodium, Hydroxypropyl Methylcellulose, Magnesium Stearate, Microcrystalline Cellulose, PVPP, Sodium Lauryl Sulfate, and Titanium Dioxide.

TWO TABLETS DAILY PROVIDE:

	For Adults— Percentage of U.S. Recommended Daily Allowance (U.S. RDA)
3000 mg Calcium Carbonate which provides 1200 mg elemental calcium	120%

Recommended Intake: One or two tablets daily or as directed by the physician.

Warnings: Keep this and all medications out of the reach of children.

How Supplied: Bottle of 60—
NDC 0005-5510-19
Store at Room Temperature.

26276
D14

Shown in Product Identification Section, page 413

CALTRATE® 600+Iron & Vitamin D
[*căl-trāte*]
High Potency Calcium Supplement Nature's Most Concentrated Form of Calcium®
No Sugar, No Salt, No Lactose, No Cholesterol, Film-Coated for Easy Swallowing

ONE TABLET DAILY CONTAINS:

	Adults— % U.S. RDA
1500 mg Calcium Carbonate which provides 600 mg elemental calcium	60%
18 mg elemental Iron in the Optisorb® Time-Release System (as ferrous fumarate)	100%
125 I.U. Vitamin D	31%

Inactive Ingredients: Blue 2, Croscarmellose Sodium, Hydroxypropyl Cellulose, Magnesium Stearate, Microcrystalline Cellulose, Polysorbate 80, Povidone, PVPP, Red 40, Sodium Lauryl Sulfate, Titanium Dioxide, and Triethyl Citrate.

- CALTRATE + Iron contains pure calcium and time-release iron for diets deficient in both minerals.
- Plus Vitamin D to help absorb calcium.

Recommended Intake: One or two tablets daily or as directed by the physician.

Warnings: Keep out of the reach of children.

How Supplied: Bottle of 60—
NDC 0005-5523-19
Store at Room Temperature.

27466
D8

Shown in Product Identification Section, page 413

Continued on next page

Lederle—Cont.

CALTRATE® 600 + Vitamin D
[*căl-trāte*]
High Potency Calcium Supplement
Nature's Most Concentrated Form of Calcium®
No Sugar, No Salt, No Lactose, No Cholesterol, Film-Coated for Easy Swallowing

Inactive Ingredients: Blue 2, Croscarmellose Sodium, FD&C Yellow No. 6, Hydroxypropyl Methylcellulose, Magnesium Stearate, Microcrystalline Cellulose, Povidone, PVPP, Red 40, Sodium Lauryl Sulfate, and Titanium Dioxide.
TWO TABLETS DAILY PROVIDE:

	Adults— % U.S. RDA
3000 mg Calcium Carbonate which provides 1200 mg elemental calcium	120%
Vitamin D 250 I.U.	62%

Recommended Intake: One or two tablets daily or as directed by the physician.

Warnings: Keep out of the reach of children.

How Supplied: Bottle of 60—
NDC-0005-5509-19
Store at Room Temperature.

26277
D11

Shown in Product Identification Section, page 413

CENTRUM®
[*sĕn-trŭm*]
High Potency Multivitamin/Multimineral Formula, Advanced Formula From A to Zinc®

Each tablet contains:

	For Adults Percentage of U.S. Recommended Daily Allowance (U.S. RDA)
Vitamin A (as Acetate and Beta Carotene)	5000 I.U. (100%)
Vitamin E (as *dl*-Alpha Tocopheryl Acetate)	30 I.U. (100%)
Vitamin C (as Ascorbic Acid)	60 mg (100%)
Folic Acid	400 mcg (100%)
Vitamin B_1 (as Thiamine Mononitrate)	1.5 mg (100%)
Vitamin B_2 (as Riboflavin)	1.7 mg (100%)
Niacinamide	20 mg (100%)
Vitamin B_6 (as Pyridoxine Hydrochloride)	2 mg (100%)
Vitamin B_{12} (as Cyanocobalamin)	6 mcg (100%)
Vitamin D	400 I.U. (100%)
Biotin	30 mcg (10%)
Pantothenic Acid (as Calcium Pantothenate)	10 mg (100%)
Calcium (as Dibasic Calcium Phosphate)	162 mg (16%)
Phosphorus (as Dibasic Calcium Phosphate)	125 mg (13%)
Iodine (as Potassium Iodide)	150 mcg (100%)
Iron (as Ferrous Fumarate)	18 mg (100%)
Magnesium (as Magnesium Oxide)	100 mg (25%)
Copper (as Cupric Oxide)	2 mg (100%)
Zinc (as Zinc Oxide)	15 mg (100%)
Manganese (as Manganese Sulfate)	2.5 mg*
Potassium (as Potassium Chloride)	40 mg*
Chloride (as Potassium Chloride)	36.3 mg*
Chromium (as Chromium Chloride)	25 mcg*
Molybdenum (as Sodium Molybdate)	25 mcg*
Selenium (as Sodium Selenate)	25 mcg*
Vitamin K_1 (as Phytonadione)	25 mcg*
Nickel (as Nickelous Sulfate)	5 mcg*
Tin (as Stannous Chloride)	10 mcg*
Silicon (as Metasilicates and Oxides)	2 mg*
Vanadium (as Sodium Metavanadate)	10 mcg*
Boron (as Borates)	150 mcg*

*No U.S. RDA established.

Inactive Ingredients: Acacia Gum, Dextrose, FD&C Yellow No. 6, Hydroxypropyl Methylcellulose, Lactose, Magnesium Stearate, Methylparaben, Microcrystalline Cellulose, Modified Food Starch, Mono- and Di-glycerides, Potassium Sorbate, Propylparaben, PVPP, Silica Gel, Sodium Benzoate, Sorbic Acid, Stearic Acid, and Sucrose.

Recommended Intake: Adults, 1 tablet daily.

How Supplied:
Light peach, engraved CENTRUM C1.
Bottle of 60—NDC 0005-4239-19
Combopack*—NDC 0005-4239-30
*Bottles of 100 plus 30
Store at Room Temperature.

26287
D33

Shown in Product Identification Section, page 413

CENTRUM® Liquid
High Potency
Multivitamin-Multimineral Formula

Each 15 mL (1 tablespoon) contains:

		For Adults—Percentage of U.S. Recommended Daily Allowance (U.S. RDA)
Vitamin A (as Palmitate)	2500 I.U.	(50%)
Vitamin E (as *dl*-Alpha Tocopheryl Acetate)	30 I.U.	(100%)
Vitamin C (as Ascorbic Acid)	60 mg	(100%)
Vitamin B_1 (as Thiamine Hydrochloride)	1.5 mg	(100%)
Vitamin B_2 (as Riboflavin)	1.7 mg	(100%)

CENTRUM, JR.®
Children's Chewable Vitamin/Mineral Formula + Extra C

EACH TABLET CONTAINS:	Quantity per tablet	Percentage of U.S. Recommended Daily Allowance (U.S. RDA) For Children 2 to 4 (½ tablet)	For Children Over 4 (1 tablet)
VITAMINS			
Vitamin A (as Acetate)	5,000 I.U.	(100%)	(100%)
Vitamin D	400 I.U.	(50%)	(100%)
Vitamin E (as Acetate)	30 I.U.	(150%)	(100%)
Vitamin C (as Ascorbic Acid and Sodium Ascorbate)	300 mg	(375%)	(500%)
Folic Acid	400 mcg	(100%)	(100%)
Biotin	45 mcg	(15%)	(15%)
Thiamine (as Thiamine Mononitrate)	1.5 mg	(107%)	(100%)
Pantothenic Acid (as Calcium Pantothenate)	10 mg	(100%)	(100%)
Riboflavin	1.7 mg	(107%)	(100%)
Niacinamide	20 mg	(111%)	(100%)
Vitamin B_6 (as Pyridoxine Hydrochloride)	2 mg	(143%)	(100%)
Vitamin B_{12} (as Cyanocobalamin)	6 mcg	(100%)	(100%)
Vitamin K_1 (as Phytonadione)	10 mcg*		
MINERALS			
Iron (as Ferrous Fumarate)	18 mg	(90%)	(100%)
Magnesium (as Magnesium Oxide)	40 mg	(10%)	(10%)
Iodine (as Potassium Iodide)	150 mcg	(107%)	(100%)
Copper (as Cupric Oxide)	2 mg	(100%)	(100%)
Phosphorous (as Tribasic Calcium Phosphate)	50 mg	(3.12%)	(5.0%)
Calcium (as Tribasic Calcium Phosphate)	108 mg	(6.75%)	(10.8%)
Zinc (as Zinc Oxide)	15 mg	(93%)	(100%)
Manganese (as Manganese Sulfate)	1 mg*		
Molybdenum (as Sodium Molybdate)	20 mcg*		
Chromium (as Chromium Chloride)	20 mcg*		

*Recognized as essential in human nutrition but no U.S. RDA established.

Niacinamide	20 mg	(100%)
Vitamin B_6 (as Pyridoxine Hydrochloride)	2 mg	(100%)
Vitamin B_{12} (as Cyanocobalamin)	6 mcg	(100%)
Vitamin D_2	400 I.U.	(100%)
Biotin	300 mcg	(100%)
Pantothenic Acid (Panthenol)	10 mg	(100%)
Iodine (as Potassium Iodide)	150 mcg	(100%)
Iron (as Ferrous Gluconate)	9 mg	(50%)
Zinc (as Zinc Gluconate)	3 mg	(20%)
Manganese (as Manganese Chloride)	2.5 mg	*
Chromium (as Chromium Chloride)	25 mcg	*
Molybdenum (as Sodium Molybdate)	25 mcg	*

*No U.S. RDA established.

Inactive Ingredients: Alcohol 6.6%, Artificial and Natural Flavors, Citric Acid, Glycerin, Polysorbate 80, Sodium Benzoate, and Sucrose.

Recommended Intake: Adults, 1 tablespoonful (15 mL) daily.

Keep this and all medication out of the reach of children.

How Supplied: 8 oz Bottle—
NDC 0005-4343-61

Store at Controlled Room Temperature 15°–30°C (59°–86°F).
PROTECT FROM FREEZING.

23317
D3

Shown in Product Identification Section, page 413

CENTRUM, JR.®
[*sĕn-trŭm*]

Children's Chewable Vitamin/Mineral Formula+Extra C Tablets

Nutritional Support From Head to Toe®

[See table on preceding page]

Inactive Ingredients: Acacia, Artificial Flavorings, Blue 1, Blue 2, Colloidal Silicon Dioxide, Dextrins, Dextrose, Gelatin, Hydrogenated Vegetable Oil, Hydrolyzed Protein, Lactose, Magnesium Stearate, Methylparaben, Microcrystalline Cellulose, Modified Food Starch, Mono- and Di-glycerides, Potassium Sorbate, Povidone, Propylparaben, Red 40, Sodium Benzoate, Sorbic Acid, Stearic Acid, Sucrose, Yellow 6.

Warnings: CONTAINS IRON, WHICH CAN BE HARMFUL IN LARGE DOSES. CLOSE TIGHTLY AND KEEP OUT OF THE REACH OF CHILDREN. IN CASE OF ACCIDENTAL OVERDOSE, CONTACT A PHYSICIAN OR POISON CONTROL CENTER IMMEDIATELY.

How Supplied: Bottle of 60—
NDC 0005-4249-19
Store at Room Temperature.

27120
D8

Shown in Product Identification Section, page 413

CENTRUM, JR.®
[*sĕn-trŭm*]

Children's Chewable Vitamin/Mineral Formula+Extra Calcium

Nutritional Support From Head to Toe®

[See table below.]

Inactive Ingredients:
Acacia, Artificial Flavorings, Colloidal Silicon Dioxide, Dextrins, Dextrose, Gelatin, Hydrogenated Vegetable Oil, Hydrolyzed Protein, Lactose, Magnesium Stearate, Methylparaben, Microcrystalline Cellulose, Modified Food Starch, Mono- and Di-glycerides, Potassium Sorbate, Propylparaben, Red 40, Sodium Benzoate, Sodium Starch Glycolate, Sorbic Acid, Stearic Acid, Sucrose.

Warnings: CONTAINS IRON, WHICH CAN BE HARMFUL IN LARGE DOSES. CLOSE TIGHTLY AND KEEP OUT OF THE REACH OF CHILDREN. IN CASE OF ACCIDENTAL OVERDOSE, CONTACT A PHYSICIAN OR POISON CONTROL CENTER IMMEDIATELY.

Recommended Intake: 2 to 4 years of age: chew one-half tablet daily. Over 4 years of age: chew one tablet daily.

How Supplied: Bottle of 60—
NDC 0005-4222-19
Store at Room Temperature. Rev. 12/87

21340

Shown in Product Identification Section, page 413

CENTRUM, JR.®
Children's Chewable
Vitamin/Mineral Formula + Extra Calcium

EACH TABLET CONTAINS:	Quantity per tablet	Percentage of U.S. Recommended Daily Allowance (U.S. RDA): For Children 2 to 4 (½ tablet)	For Children Over 4 (1 tablet)
VITAMINS			
Vitamin A (as Acetate)	5,000 I.U.	(100%)	(100%)
Vitamin D	400 I.U.	(50%)	(100%)
Vitamin E (as Acetate)	30 I.U.	(150%)	(100%)
Vitamin C (as Ascorbic Acid)	60 mg	(75%)	(100%)
Folic Acid	400 mcg	(100%)	(100%)
Biotin	45 mcg	(15%)	(15%)
Thiamine (as Thiamine Mononitrate)	1.5 mg	(107%)	(100%)
Pantothenic Acid (as Calcium Pantothenate)	10 mg	(100%)	(100%)
Riboflavin	1.7 mg	(107%)	(100%)
Niacinamide	20 mg	(111%)	(100%)
Vitamin B_6 (as Pyridoxine Hydrochloride)	2 mg	(143%)	(100%)
Vitamin B_{12} (as Cyanocobalamin)	6 mcg	(100%)	(100%)
Vitamin K_1 (as Phytonadione)	10 mcg*		
MINERALS			
Iron (as Ferrous Fumarate)	18 mg	(90%)	(100%)
Magnesium (as Magnesium Oxide)	40 mg	(10%)	(10%)
Iodine (as Potassium Iodide)	150 mcg	(107%)	(100%)
Copper (as Cupric Oxide)	2 mg	(100%)	(100%)
Phosphorus (as Dibasic Calcium Phosphate)	50 mg	(3.12%)	(5.0%)
Calcium (as Dibasic Calcium Phosphate and Calcium Carbonate)	160 mg	(10%)	(16%)
Zinc (as Zinc Oxide)	15 mg	(93%)	(100%)
Manganese (as Manganese Sulfate)	1 mg*		
Molybdenum (as Sodium Molybdate)	20 mcg*		
Chromium (as Chromium Chloride)	20 mcg*		

*Recognized as essential in human nutrition but no U.S. RDA established.

Continued on next page

Lederle—Cont.

CENTRUM, JR.®
[*sĕn-trŭm*]
Children's Chewable Vitamin/Mineral Formula + Iron Tablets
Nutritional Support From Head to Toe®

[See table below.]

Inactive Ingredients: Acacia, Artificial Flavorings, Blue 1, Blue 2, Colloidal Silicon Dioxide, Dextrins, Dextrose, Gelatin, Hydrogenated Vegetable Oil, Hydrolyzed Protein, Lactose, Magnesium Stearate, Methylparaben, Microcrystalline Cellulose, Modified Food Starch, Mono- and Di-glycerides, Potassium Sorbate, Propylparaben, Red 40, Sodium Benzoate, Sodium Starch Glycolate, Sorbic Acid, Stearic Acid, Sucrose, Yellow 6.

Recommended Intake: 2 to 4 years of age: Chew one-half tablet daily. Over 4 years of age: Chew one tablet daily.

Warnings: CONTAINS IRON, WHICH CAN BE HARMFUL IN LARGE DOSES. CLOSE TIGHTLY AND KEEP OUT OF THE REACH OF CHILDREN. IN CASE OF ACCIDENTAL OVERDOSE, CONTACT A PHYSICIAN OR POISON CONTROL CENTER IMMEDIATELY.

How Supplied: Assorted Flavors—Uncoated Tablet—Partially Scored —Engraved Lederle C2 and CENTRUM, JR.
Bottle of 60—NDC 0005-4234-19
Store at room temperature.

27118
D9

Shown in Product Identification Section, page 413

CENTRUM® SILVER™
Specially Formulated Multivitamin-Multimineral for Adults 50+

Each tablet contains:

		For Adults—Percentage of U.S. Recommended Daily Allowance (U.S. RDA)
Vitamin A (as Acetate and Beta Carotene)	6000 I.U.	(120%)
Vitamin B_1	1.5 mg	(100%)
Vitamin B_2	1.7 mg	(100%)
Vitamin B_6	3 mg	(150%)
Vitamin B_{12}	25 mcg	(416%)
Biotin	30 mcg	(10%)
Folic Acid	200 mcg	(50%)
Niacinamide	20 mg	(100%)
Pantothenic Acid	10 mg	(100%)
Vitamin C	60 mg	(100%)
Vitamin D	400 I.U.	(100%)
Vitamin E	45 I.U.	(150%)
Vitamin K_1	10 mcg*	
Calcium	200 mg	(20%)
Copper	2 mg	(100%)
Iodine	150 mcg	(100%)
Iron	9 mg	(50%)
Magnesium	100 mg	(25%)
Phosphorus	48 mg	(5%)
Zinc	15 mg	(100%)
Chloride	72 mg*	
Chromium	100 mcg*	
Manganese	2.5 mg*	
Molybdenum	25 mcg*	
Nickel	5 mcg*	
Potassium	80 mg*	
Selenium	25 mcg*	
Silicon	10 mcg*	
Vanadium	10 mcg*	

*No U.S. RDA established.

Inactive Ingredients: Blue 2, Crospovidone, Gelatin, Hydroxypropyl Methylcellulose, Lactose, Magnesium Stearate, Microcrystalline Cellulose, Polyethylene Glycol, Polysorbate 80, Red 40, Silica Gel, Stearic Acid, Titanium Dioxide, and Yellow 6.

Gel-Tabs™ —Specially coated supplement to assure ease of swallowing.

Recommended Intake:
Adults, 1 tablet daily.

How Supplied: Bottle of 60—NDC 0005-4177-19
Store at Room Temperature.

27453
D1

Shown in Product Identification Section, page 413

Dual Action
FERRO-SEQUELS®
[*fĕrrō-sēēquals*]
High Potency Iron Supplement
Time-Release Iron Plus
Clinically Proven Anticonstipant
Easy-to-Swallow Tablets
Low Sodium, No Sugar

Active Ingredients: Each tablet contains 150 mg of ferrous fumarate equivalent to 50 mg of elemental iron and 100 mg of docusate sodium (DSS).

Inactive Ingredients: Blue 1, Corn Starch, Crospovidone, Hydroxypropyl Methylcellulose, Lactose, Magnesium

CENTRUM, JR.®
Children's Chewable Vitamin/Mineral Formula + Iron

EACH TABLET CONTAINS:	Quantity per tablet	Percentage of U.S. Recommended Daily Allowance (U.S. RDA) For Children 2 to 4 (½ tablet)	For Children Over 4 (1 tablet)
VITAMINS			
Vitamin A (as Acetate)	5,000 I.U.	(100%)	(100%)
Vitamin D	400 I.U.	(50%)	(100%)
Vitamin E (as Acetate)	30 I.U.	(150%)	(100%)
Vitamin C (as Ascorbic Acid)	60 mg	(75%)	(100%)
Folic Acid	400 mcg	(100%)	(100%)
Biotin	45 mcg	(15%)	(15%)
Thiamine (as Thiamine Mononitrate)	1.5 mg	(107%)	(100%)
Pantothenic Acid (as Calcium Pantothenate)	10 mg	(100%)	(100%)
Riboflavin	1.7 mg	(107%)	(100%)
Niacinamide	20 mg	(111%)	(100%)
Vitamin B_6 (as Pyridoxine Hydrochloride)	2 mg	(143%)	(100%)
Vitamin B_{12} (as Cyanocobalamin)	6 mcg	(100%)	(100%)
Vitamin K_1 (as Phytonadione)	10 mcg*		
MINERALS			
Iron (as Ferrous Fumarate)	18 mg	(90%)	(100%)
Magnesium (as Magnesium Oxide)	40 mg	(10%)	(10%)
Iodine (as Potassium Iodide)	150 mcg	(107%)	(100%)
Copper (as Cupric Oxide)	2 mg	(100%)	(100%)
Phosphorus (as Dibasic Calcium Phosphate)	50 mg	(3.12%)	(5.0%)
Calcium (as Dibasic Calcium Phosphate and Calcium Carbonate)	108 mg	(6.75%)	(10.8%)
Zinc (as Zinc Oxide)	15 mg	(93%)	(100%)
Manganese (as Manganese Sulfate)	1 mg*		
Molybdenum (as Sodium Molybdate)	20 mcg*		
Chromium (as Chromium Chloride)	20 mcg*		

*Recognized as essential in human nutrition but no U.S. RDA established.

Stearate, Microcrystalline Cellulose, Modified Food Starch, Povidone, Silica Gel, Sodium Lauryl Sulfate, Titanium Dioxide, and Yellow 10.

Warning: As with any drug, if you are pregnant or nursing a baby, seek the advice of a health professional before using this product. Keep this and all medications out of the reach of children. In case of accidental overdose, seek professional assistance or contact a Poison Control Center immediately.

Recommended Intake: One tablet, once or twice daily or as prescribed by a physician.

How Supplied: Boxes of 30—
NDC 0005-5267-68
Bottle of 30—NDC 0005-5267-13
Bottle of 100—NDC 0005-5267-23
Unit Dose Pack 10×10—
NDC 0005-5267-60
Green, capsule-shaped, film-coated tablets
Engraved LL and F2
Store at Room Temperature.

27533
D3

Shown in Product Identification Section, page 414

FIBERCON®

[fī-bĕr-cŏn]

Calcium Polycarbophil
Bulk-Forming Fiber Laxative

Safe and effective, Less than one calorie per tablet, Sodium- and Preservative-free, Film-coated for easy swallowing, Calcium rich, No chemical stimulants.

Active Ingredient: Each tablet contains 625 mg calcium polycarbophil.

Inactive Ingredients: Calcium Carbonate, Caramel, Crospovidone, Hydroxypropyl Methylcellulose, Magnesium Stearate, Microcrystalline Cellulose, Povidone and Silica Gel.

Indications: Relief of constipation (irregularity).

Actions: Increases bulk volume and water content of the stool.

Warnings: If you have noticed a sudden change in bowel habits that persists over a period of 2 weeks, consult a physician before using a laxative. If the recommended use of this product for 1 week has no effect, discontinue use and consult a physician.
Do not use laxative products when abdominal pain, nausea or vomiting is present except under the direction of a physician. Discontinue use and consult a physician if rectal bleeding occurs after use of any laxative product.
For chronic or continued constipation consult your physician.

Interaction Precaution: Contains calcium. Take this product at least 1 hour before or 2 hours after taking an oral dose of a prescription antibiotic containing any form of tetracycline.
KEEP THIS AND ALL MEDICINES OUT OF THE REACH OF CHILDREN.
STORE AT CONTROLLED ROOM TEMPERATURE 15°–30°C (59°–86°F).
PROTECT CONTENTS FROM MOISTURE.

Recommended Intake: Adults and children 12 years and older: swallow two tablets one to four times a day. Children 6 to 12 years: swallow one tablet one to three times a day. Children under 6 years: consult a physician. See package insert for additional information.
A FULL GLASS (8 fl oz) OF LIQUID SHOULD BE TAKEN WITH EACH DOSE.

How Supplied:
Film coated tablets, scored, engraved *LL* and F66.
Package of 36 tablets, NDC 0005-2500-02
Package of 60 tablets, NDC 0005-2500-86
Package of 90 tablets, NDC 0005-2500-33
Bottle of 500 tablets, NDC 0005-2500-31
Unit Dose Pkg, NDC 0005-2500-28

27982
D7

Shown in Product Identification Section, page 413

FILIBON®

[fĭ-lĭ-bōn]

Multivitamin-Multimineral Supplement for Pregnant or Lactating Women Prenatal Tablets

Each tablet contains:

	For Pregnant or Lactating Women Percentage of U.S. Recommended Daily Allowance (U.S. RDA)
Vitamin A (as Acetate)	5000 I.U. (63%)
Vitamin D_2	400 I.U. (100%)
Vitamin E (as *dl*-Alpha Tocopheryl Acetate)	30 I.U. (100%)
Vitamin C (as Ascorbic Acid)	60 mg (100%)
Folic Acid	0.4 mg (50%)
Vitamin B_1 (as Thiamine Mononitrate)	1.5 mg (88%)
Vitamin B_2 (as Riboflavin)	1.7 mg (85%)
Niacinamide	20 mg (100%)
Vitamin B_6 (as Pyridoxine Hydrochloride)	2 mg (80%)
Vitamin B_{12} (as Cyanocobalamin)	6 mcg (75%)
Calcium (as Calcium Carbonate)	125 mg (10%)
Iodine (as Potassium Iodide)	150 mcg (100%)
Iron (as Ferrous Fumarate)	18 mg (100%)
Magnesium (as Magnesium Oxide)	100 mg (22%)

Inactive Ingredients: Ethylcellulose, Hydroxypropyl Methylcellulose, Lactose, Magnesium Stearate, Microcrystalline Cellulose, Povidone, Pregelatinized Starch, Red 40, Silicon Dioxide, Sodium Lauryl Sulfate, Sodium Starch Glycolate, Titanium Dioxide and Stearic Acid.

Recommended Intake: 1 daily, or as prescribed by the physician.

How Supplied: Capsule-shaped tablets (film-coated, pink) engraved *LL* F4—bottle of 100 NDC-0005-4294-23
Store at Room Temperature.

22892
D11

GEVRABON®

[jĕv-ra băn]

Vitamin-Mineral Supplement

Composition: Each fluid ounce (30 mL) contains:

	For Adults— Percentage of U.S. Recommended Daily Allowance (U.S. RDA)
Vitamin B_1 (as Thiamine Hydrochloride)	5 mg (333%)
Vitamin B_2 (as Riboflavin-5-Phosphate Sodium)	2.5 mg (147%)
Niacinamide	50 mg (250%)
Vitamin B_6 (Pyridoxine Hydrochloride)	1 mg (50%)
Vitamin B_{12} (as Cyanocobalamin)	1 mcg (17%)
Pantothenic Acid (as D-Pantothenyl Alcohol)	10 mg (100%)
Iodine (as Potassium Iodide)	100 mcg (67%)
Iron (as Ferrous Gluconate)	15 mg (83%)
Magnesium (as Magnesium Chloride)	2 mg (0.5%)
Zinc (as Zinc Chloride)	2 mg (13%)
Choline (as Tricholine Citrate)	100 mg.*
Manganese (as Manganese Chloride)	2 mg.*

*Recognized as essential in human nutrition but no U.S. RDA established.

Alcohol 18%

Inactive Ingredients: Alcohol, citric acid, glycerin, sherry wine, sucrose.

Indications: For use as a nutritional supplement. Shake well.

Warning: As with any drug, if you are pregnant or nursing a baby, seek the advice of a health professional before using this product. Keep this preparation out of the reach of children.

Administration and Dosage: Adult: One ounce (30 mL) daily or as prescribed by the physician as a nutritional supplement.

Important Note: In time a slight natural deposit, characteristic of the sherry wine base, may occur. This does not indicate in any way a loss of quality.

How Supplied: Syrup (sherry flavor) decanters of 16 fl oz—NDC 0005-5250-35
Keep Out of Direct Sunlight
Store at Room Temperature, 15°–30°C (59°–86°F).
DO NOT FREEZE.

16520
D4

Continued on next page

Lederle—Cont.

GEVRAL®

[jěv-ral]

Multivitamin and Multimineral Supplement

TABLETS

Composition: Each tablet contains:

	For Adults—Percentage of U.S. Recommended Daily Allowance (U.S. RDA)
Vitamin A (as Acetate)	5000 I.U. (100%)
Vitamin E (as *dl*-Alpha Tocopheryl Acetate)	30 I.U. (100%)
Vitamin C (as Ascorbic Acid)	60 mg (100%)
Folic Acid	0.4 mg (100%)
Vitamin B_1 (as Thiamine Mononitrate)	1.5 mg (100%)
Vitamin B_2 (as Riboflavin)	1.7 mg (100%)
Niacinamide	20 mg (100%)
Vitamin B_6 (as Pyridoxine Hydrochloride)	2 mg (100%)
Vitamin B_{12} (as Cyanocobalamin)	6 mcg (100%)
Calcium (as Dibasic Calcium Phosphate)	162 mg (16%)
Phosphorus (as Dibasic Calcium Phosphate)	125 mg (13%)
Iodine (as Potassium Iodide)	150 mcg (100%)
Iron (as Ferrous Fumarate)	18 mg (100%)
Magnesium (as Magnesium Oxide)	100 mg (25%)

Inactive Ingredients: Blue 2, Ethylcellulose, Gelatin, Hydrolyzed Protein, Hydroxypropyl Methylcellulose, Lactose, Magnesium Stearate, Methylparaben, Microcrystalline Cellulose, Modified Food Starch, Mono- and Di-glycerides, Polacrilin, Potassium Sorbate, Propylparaben, PVPP, Red 30, Silica Gel, Sodium Benzoate, Sorbic Acid, Stearic Acid, Sucrose, Titanium Dioxide, and Yellow 6.

Indications: Supplementation of the diet.

Administration and Dosage: One tablet daily or as prescribed by the physician.
Keep this and all medications out of the reach of children.

How Supplied: Capsule-shaped tablets (film-coated, brown) engraved LL G1—Bottle of 100—NDC 0005-4289-23

Store at Room Temperature.

A SPECTRUM® Product

22788
D15

GEVRAL® T

[jěv-ral t]

High Potency Multivitamin and Multimineral Supplement

TABLETS

Each tablet contains:

	For Adults—Percentage of U.S. Recommended Daily Allowance (U.S. RDA)
Vitamin A (as Acetate)	5000 I.U. (100%)
Vitamin E (as *dl*-Alpha Tocopheryl Acetate)	45 I.U. (150%)
Vitamin C (as Ascorbic Acid)	90 mg (150%)
Folic Acid	0.4 mg (100%)
Vitamin B_1 (as Thiamine Mononitrate)	2.25 mg (150%)
Vitamin B_2 (as Riboflavin)	2.6 mg (153%)
Niacinamide	30 mg (150%)
Vitamin B_6 (as Pyridoxine Hydrochloride)	3 mg (150%)
Vitamin B_{12} (as Cyanocobalamin)	9 mcg (150%)
Vitamin D_2	400 I.U. (100%)
Calcium (as Dibasic Calcium Phosphate)	162 mg (16%)
Phosphorus (as Dibasic Calcium Phosphate)	125 mg (13%)
Iodine (as Potassium Iodide)	225 mcg (150%)
Iron (as Ferrous Fumarate)	27 mg (150%)
Magnesium (as Magnesium Oxide)	100 mg (25%)
Copper (as Cupric Oxide)	1.5 mg (75%)
Zinc (as Zinc Oxide)	22.5 mg (150%)

Inactive Ingredients: BHA, BHT, Blue 2, Gelatin, Hydrolyzed Protein, Hydroxypropyl Methylcellulose, Lactose, Magnesium Stearate, Methylparaben, Microcrystalline Cellulose, Modified Food Starch, Mono- and Di-glycerides, Polacrilin, Polysorbate 60, Potassium Sorbate, Propylparaben, PVPP, Red 40, Silica Gel, Sodium Benzoate, Sodium Lauryl Sulfate, Sorbic Acid, Stearic Acid, Sucrose, Titanium Dioxide, and other ingredients.

Indications: For the treatment of vitamin and mineral deficiencies.

Dosage: 1 tablet daily or as prescribed by physician.
Keep this and all medications out of the reach of children.
Store at Room Temperature.

How Supplied: Tablets (film coated, maroon). Printed LL G2—bottle of 100 NDC 0005-4286-23
A SPECTRUM® Product

Rev. 10/86
14170

INCREMIN®

[ĭn-cre-mĭn]

WITH IRON SYRUP

Vitamins + Iron

DIETARY SUPPLEMENT

(Cherry Flavored)

Composition: Each teaspoonful (5 mL) contains:

Elemental Iron (as Ferric Pyrophosphate)	30 mg
L-Lysine HCl	300 mg
Thiamine HCl (B_1)	10 mg
Pyridoxine HCl (B_6)	5 mg
Vitamin B_{12} (Cyanocobalamin)	25 mcg
Sorbitol	3.50 gm
Alcohol	0.75%

Inactive Ingredients: Alcohol, Flavorings, Red 33, Sodium Benzoate, Sorbic Acid.

Each teaspoonful (5 mL) supplies the following Minimum Daily Requirements:

	Child under 6	Child over 6	Adults
Vitamin B_1	20 MDR	13⅓ MDR	10 MDR
Iron	4 MDR	3 MDR	3 MDR

Indications: For the prevention and treatment of iron deficiency anemia in children and adults.

Warning: As with any drug, if you are pregnant or nursing a baby, seek the advice of a health professional before using this product.
Keep this and all medications out of the reach of children.

Administration and Dosage: or as prescribed by a physician.
Children: One teaspoonful (5 mL) daily for the prevention of iron deficiency anemia.
Adults: One teaspoonful (5 mL) daily for the prevention of iron deficiency anemia.

Notice: To protect from light always dispense in this container or in an amber bottle.
Store at Room Temperature.

How Supplied: Syrup (cherry flavor)—bottles of 4 fl. oz—NDC 0005-5604-58 and 16 fl. oz—NDC 0005-5604-65

Rev. 9/85
16846

NEOLOID®

[nēē-o-loid]

Emulsified Castor Oil

Peppermint Flavored

Composition: Emulsified Castor Oil USP 36.4% (w/w) with 0.1% (w/w) Sodium Benzoate and 0.2% (w/w) Potassium Sorbate added as preservatives, emulsifying and flavoring agents in water. Also contains the following inactive ingredients: Citric Acid, Glyceryl Monostearate, Polysorbate 80, Propylene Glycol, Sodium Alginate, Sodium Saccharin, Stearic Acid, Tenox II. NEOLOID is an emulsion with an exceptionally bland, pleasant taste.

Indications: For the treatment of isolated bouts of constipation.

SHAKE WELL

Administration and Dosage:
Infants—½ to 1½ teaspoonfuls
Children—Adjust between infant and adult dose.
Adult—Average dose, 2 to 4 tablespoonfuls or as prescribed by a physician.

Precautions: Not to be used when abdominal pain, nausea, vomiting, or other symptoms of appendicitis are present. Frequent or continued use of this preparation may result in dependence on laxatives. Do not use during pregnancy except on a physician's advice. Keep this and all drugs out of the reach of children.

Warning: As with any drug, if you are pregnant or nursing a baby, seek the advice of a health professional before using this product. In case of accidental overdose, seek professional assistance or contact a Poison Control Center immediately.

How Supplied: Bottles of 4 fl oz (118 mL) (peppermint flavor)
NDC-0005-5442-58
Store at Room Temperature.
DO NOT FREEZE.

16838
D4

PERITINIC®
[peri-tin-ic]
Hematinic with Vitamins and Fecal Softener
Tablets
Film Coated

Each tablet contains:
Elemental Iron
(as Ferrous Fumarate)..............100 mg
Docusate Sodium USP (DSS)
(to counteract the constipating effect of iron).......100 mg
Vitamin B_1
(as Thiamine Mononitrate).......7.5 mg (7½ MDR)
Vitamin B_2 (Riboflavin)................7.5 mg (6¼ MDR)
Vitamin B_6
(Pyridoxine Hydrochloride).......7.5 mg
Vitamin B_{12}
(Cyanocobalamin) ....50 mcg
Vitamin C (Ascorbic Acid)...........200 mg (6⅔ MDR)
Niacinamide....................................30 mg (3 MDR)
Folic Acid ....0.05 mg
Pantothenic Acid
(as D-Pantothenyl Alcohol)........15 mg
MDR = Adult Minimum Daily Requirement

Inactive Ingredients: Alginic Acid, Amberlite Resin, Blue 2, Ethyl Cellulose, FD&C Yellow No. 6,* Hydroxypropyl Methylcellulose, Lactose, Magnesium Stearate, Modified Food Starch, Povidone, Red 40, Silica Gel, Titanium Dioxide, and other ingredients.
*Contains FD&C Yellow No. 6 (Sunset Yellow) as a color additive.

Warning: As with any drug, if you are pregnant or nursing a baby, seek the advice of a health professional before using this product. In case of accidental overdose, seek professional assistance or contact a Poison Control Center immediately. Keep out of the reach of children.

Action and Uses: In the prevention of nutritional anemias, certain vitamin deficiencies, and iron-deficiency anemias.

Administration and Dosage:
Adults: 1 or 2 tablets daily.

How Supplied: Tablets (maroon, capsule-shaped, film coated) P8—bottle of 60 NDC 0005-5124-19

18649
D15

STRESSTABS® Advanced Formula
[strĕss-tăbs]
High Potency
Stress Formula Vitamins

Each tablet contains:

		For Adults—Percentage of U.S. Recommended Daily Allowance (U.S. RDA)
Vitamin E (as *dl*-Alpha Tocopheryl Acetate)	30 I.U.	(100%)
Vitamin C (as Ascorbic Acid)	500 mg	(833%)
B VITAMINS		
Folic Acid	400 mcg	(100%)
Vitamin B_1 (as Thiamine Mononitrate)	10 mg	(667%)
Vitamin B_2 (as Riboflavin)	10 mg	(588%)
Niacinamide	100 mg	(500%)
Vitamin B_6 (as Pyridoxine Hydrochloride)	5 mg	(250%)
Vitamin B_{12} (as Cyanocobalamin)	12 mcg	(200%)
Biotin	45 mcg	(15%)
Pantothenic Acid (as Calcium Pantothenate USP)	20 mg	(200%)

Inactive Ingredients: Calcium Carbonate, Magnesium Stearate, Microcrystalline Cellulose, Modified Food Starch, Silica Gel, Stearic Acid, and Yellow 6.

Store at Room Temperature.

Recommended Intake: Adults, 1 tablet daily or as directed by the physician.

How Supplied:
Bottle of 30—NDC 0005-4124-13
Bottle of 60—NDC 0005-4124-19
Unit Dose Pack 10 × 10s—NDC 0005-4124-60

27196
D17

Shown in Product Identification Section, page 414

STRESSTABS® + IRON Advanced Formula
[strĕss-tăbs]
High Potency
Stress Formula Vitamins

Each tablet contains:

		For Adults—Percentage of U.S. Recommended Daily Allowance (U.S. RDA)
Vitamin E (as *dl*-Alpha Tocopheryl Acetate)	30 I.U.	(100%)
Vitamin C (as Ascorbic Acid)	500 mg	(833%)
B VITAMINS		
Folic Acid	400 mcg	(100%)
Vitamin B_1 (as Thiamine Mononitrate)	10 mg	(667%)
Vitamin B_2 (as Riboflavin)	10 mg	(588%)
Niacinamide	100 mg	(500%)
Vitamin B_6 (as Pyridoxine Hydrochloride)	5 mg	(250%)
Vitamin B_{12} (as Cyanocobalamin)	12 mcg	(200%)
Biotin	45 mcg	(15%)
Pantothenic Acid (as Calcium Pantothenate USP)	20 mg	(200%)
Iron (as Ferrous Fumarate)	27 mg	(150%)

Inactive Ingredients: Calcium Carbonate, Magnesium Stearate, Microcrystalline Cellulose, Modified Food Starch, Red 40, Silica Gel, Stearic Acid, and Yellow 6.

Recommended Intake: Adults, 1 tablet daily or as directed by physician.

How Supplied: Capsule-shaped tablets (film-coated, orange-red, scored). Engraved LL S2.
Bottle of 30—NDC 0005-4126-13
Bottle of 60—NDC 0005-4126-19
Store at Room Temperature.

27403
D15

Shown in Product Identification Section, page 414

STRESSTABS® + ZINC Advanced Formula
[strĕss-tăbs]
High Potency
Stress Formula Vitamins

Each tablet contains:

		For Adults—Percentage of U.S. Recommended Daily Allowance (U.S. RDA)
Vitamin E (as *dl*-Alpha Tocopheryl Acetate)	30 I.U.	(100%)
Vitamin C (as Ascorbic Acid)	500 mg	(833%)
B VITAMINS		
Folic Acid	400 mcg	(100%)
Vitamin B_1 (as Thiamine Mononitrate)	10 mg	(667%)
Vitamin B_2 (as Riboflavin)	10 mg	(588%)
Niacinamide	100 mg	(500%)
Vitamin B_6 (as Pyridoxine Hydrochloride)	5 mg	(250%)
Vitamin B_{12} (as Cyanocobalamin)	12 mcg	(200%)
Biotin	45 mcg	(15%)
Pantothenic Acid (as Calcium Pantothenate USP)	20 mg	(200%)
Copper (as Cupric Oxide)	3 mg	(150%)
Zinc (as Zinc Sulfate)	23.9 mg	(159%)

Inactive Ingredients: Calcium Carbonate, Magnesium Stearate, Microcrystalline Cellulose, Modified Food Starch, Silica Gel, Stearic Acid, and Yellow 6.

Recommended Intake: Adults, 1 tablet daily or as directed by the physician.

Continued on next page

Lederle—Cont.

How Supplied: Capsule-shaped Tablet (film coated, peach color). Engraved LL S3.
Bottle of 30—NDC 0005-4125-13
Bottle of 60—NDC 0005-4125-19
Store at Room Temperature.

27402
D17

Shown in Product Identification Section, page 414

ZINCON®
[zinc-ŏn]
Dandruff Shampoo

Contains: Pyrithione zinc (1%), water, sodium methyl cocoyl taurate, cocamide MEA, sodium chloride, magnesium aluminum silicate, sodium cocoyl isethionate, fragrance, glutaraldehyde, D&C green #5, citric acid or sodium hydroxide to adjust pH if necessary.

Indications: Relieves the itching and scalp flaking associated with dandruff. Relieves the itching, irritation, and skin flaking associated with seborrheic dermatitis of the scalp.

Directions: For best results use twice a week. Wet hair, apply to scalp and massage vigorously. Rinse and repeat. SHAKE WELL BEFORE USING.

Warnings: Keep this and all drugs out of the reach of children. For external use only. Avoid contact with the eyes—if this happens, rinse thoroughly with water. If condition worsens or does not improve after regular use of this product as directed, consult a doctor. Do not use on children under 2 years of age except as directed by a doctor.

How Supplied:
4 oz Bottle—NDC 0005-5455-58
8 oz Bottle—NDC 0005-5455-61

13918
D4

Shown in Product Identification Section, page 414

EDUCATIONAL MATERIAL

Calcium Supplements: The Differences Are Real
8-page pamphlet describing why today's women need to supplement their diet with calcium.

Healthy Regularity . . . and the Fiber Action Advantage
8-page pamphlet describing the role of fiber in maintaining good digestive health.

Write to: Lederle Promotional Center
2200 Bradley Hill Road
Blauvelt, NY 10913

If desired, additional information on any Lederle product will be provided by contacting Lederle Professional Services Dept.

Luyties Pharmacal Company
P.O. BOX 8080
ST. LOUIS, MO 63156

YELLOLAX
[yel 'o-laks]

Description: YELLOLAX is a combination of time proven Yellow-phenolphthalein, and the Homeopathic ingredients, Bryonia and Hydrastis. Clinically YELLOLAX is an oral laxative. Each tablet contains two grains of yellow phenolphthalein and the Bryonia and Hydrastis approximately one fortieth grain each.

Action: Yellow-phenolphthalein is an effective and safe laxative, which is not contraindicated in pregnancy. Homeopathic Bryonia is used to treat constipation and the pain associated with constipation. Homeopathic Bryonia tends to increase mucous membrane moisture. Homeopathic Hydrastis is also included in the treatment of constipation because the Homeopathic Hydrastis provides some relief of constipation and the associated pain and headaches by relaxing mucous membranes and encouraging their secretion. YELLOLAX has been safely used in pregnancy, children, and as conjunctive treatment with hemorrhoidal complications.

Indications: YELLOLAX is indicated in the management of simple constipation. YELLOLAX is also indicated in those conditions which require a gentle laxative.

Contraindications: YELLOLAX and all laxatives are contraindicated in appendicitis. All laxatives containing phenolphthalein are contraindicated in patients who have hypersensitivity to phenolphthalein.

Warnings: Do not use laxatives in cases of severe colic, nausea and other symptoms of appendicitis. Do not use laxatives habitually nor continually. If condition persists consult physician. Keep this and all medication out of the reach of children. DO NOT exceed the recommended dosage.

Caution: Frequent or prolonged use may result in laxative dependence. If skin rash appears, discontinue use.

Side Effects: The phenolphthalein may impart a red color to the urine, (phenolphthalein is also used as a pH indicator), this is normal.

Dosage: For adults one or two tablets chewed before retiring. For children over six a quarter tablet to half tablet before retiring. Tablets should be well chewed. For younger children consult physician.

Supplied: Compressed tablets packed in glass bottles of 36 (NDC 0618-0832-55) and 100 (NDC 0618-0832-12), and in repackers of 1000 tablets.

Homoeopathic
Luyties also manufactures a complete line of homoeopathic products. If more information is needed contact them direct.

EDUCATIONAL MATERIAL

Packets are available containing descriptive literature on products manufactured by Luyties Pharmacal Company, company history, and pricing information.

Macsil, Inc.
1326 FRANKFORD AVENUE
PHILADELPHIA, PA 19125

BALMEX® BABY POWDER

Composition: Contains: Active Ingredient—zinc oxide; Inactive Ingredients—corn starch, calcium carbonate, BALSAN® (especially purified balsam Peru).

Action and Uses: Absorbent, emollient, soothing—for diaper irritation, intertrigo, and other common dermatological conditions. In acute, simple miliaria, itching ceases in minutes and lesions dry promptly. For routine use after bathing and each diaper change.

How Supplied: 8 oz. shaker-top plastic containers.

BALMEX® EMOLLIENT LOTION
Gentle and effective scientifically compounded infant's skin conditioner.

Composition: Contains a special lanolin oil (non-sensitizing, dewaxed, moisturizing fraction of lanolin), BALSAN® (specially purified balsam Peru) and silicone.

Action and Uses: The special Lanolin Oil aids nature lubricate baby's skin to keep it smooth and supple. Balmex Emollient Lotion is also highly effective as a physiologic conditioner on adult's skin.

How Supplied: Available in 6 oz. dispenser-top plastic bottles.

BALMEX® OINTMENT

Composition: Contains: Active Ingredients—Bismuth Subnitrate, Zinc Oxide; Inactive Ingredients—Balsan (Specially Purified Balsam Peru), Benzoic Acid, Beeswax, Mineral Oil, Silicone, Synthetic White Wax, Purified Water, and other ingredients.

Action and Uses: Emollient, protective, anti-inflammatory, promotes healing—for diaper rash, minor burns, sunburn, and other simple skin conditions; also decubitus ulcers, skin irritations associated with ileostomy and colostomy drainage. Nonstaining, readily washes out of diapers and clothing.

How Supplied: 1, 2, 4 oz. tubes; 1 lb. plastic jars (½ oz. tubes for Hospitals only). Balmex Ointment-All Commercial Sizes-Safety Sealed.

Marion Merrell Dow Inc.

Consumer Products Division
10123 ALLIANCE ROAD
P.O. BOX 429553
CINCINNATI, OHIO 45242-9553

CĒPACOL®/CĒPACOL MINT
[*sē 'pə-cŏl*]
Mouthwash/Gargle

Description: Cēpacol Mouthwash contains: Ceepryn® (cetylpyridinium chloride) 0.05%. Also contains: Alcohol 14%, Edetate Disodium, FD&C Yellow No. 5 (tartrazine) as a color additive, Flavors, Glycerin, Polysorbate 80, Saccharin, Sodium Biphosphate, Sodium Phosphate, and Water.
Cēpacol Mint Mouthwash contains: Ceepryn® (cetylpyridinium chloride) 0.05%. Also contains: Alcohol 14.5%, D&C Yellow No. 10, FD&C Green No. 3, Flavor, Glucono Delta-Lactone, Glycerin, Poloxamer 407, Saccharin Sodium, Sodium Gluconate, and Water.

Actions: Cēpacol/Cēpacol Mint is a soothing, pleasant-tasting mouthwash/gargle. It kills germs that cause bad breath for a fresher, cleaner mouth.
Cēpacol/Cēpacol Mint has a low surface tension, approximately ½ that of water. This property is the basis of the spreading action in the oral cavity as well as its foaming action. Cēpacol/Cēpacol Mint leaves the mouth feeling fresh and clean and helps provide soothing, temporary relief of dryness and minor mouth irritations.

Uses: Recommended as a mouthwash and gargle for daily oral care; as an aromatic mouth freshener to provide a clean feeling in the mouth; as a soothing, foaming rinse to freshen the mouth.
Used routinely before dental procedures, helps give patient confidence of not offending with mouth odor. Often employed as a foaming and refreshing rinse before, during, and after instrumentation and dental prophylaxis. Convenient as a mouth-freshening agent after taking dental impressions. Helpful in reducing the unpleasant taste and odor in the mouth following gingivectomy.
Used in hospitals as a mouthwash and gargle for daily oral care. Also used to refresh and soothe the mouth following emesis, inhalation therapy, and intubations, and for swabbing the mouths of patients incapable of personal care.

Warning: Keep out of the reach of children.

Directions for Use: Rinse vigorously before or after brushing or any time to freshen the mouth. Particularly useful after meals or before social engagements. Cēpacol/Cēpacol Mint leaves the mouth feeling refreshingly clean.
Use full strength every two or three hours as a soothing, foaming gargle, or as directed by a physician or dentist. May also be mixed with warm water.
Product label directions are as follows: Use full strength. Rinse mouth thoroughly before or after brushing or whenever desired or use as directed by a physician or dentist.

How Supplied:
Cēpacol Mouthwash: 12 oz, 18 oz, 24 oz, and 32 oz. 4 oz trial size.
Shown in Product Identification Section, page 414

CĒPACOL®
[*sē 'pə-cŏl*]
Dry Throat Lozenges
Cherry Flavor

Description: Each lozenge contains Menthol 3.6 mg. Also contains: Benzyl Alcohol, Cetylpyridinium Chloride, D&C Red No. 33, FD&C Red No. 40, Flavor, Liquid Glucose, and Sucrose.

Actions: Menthol provides a cooling sensation to aid in symptomatic relief of minor throat irritations.

Indications: Cēpacol Cherry Flavor Lozenges provide temporary relief of occasional dry, scratchy throat.

Warnings: If sore throat is severe, persists for more than 2 days, is accompanied or followed by fever, headache, rash, nausea, or vomiting, consult a physician promptly. If sore mouth symptoms do not improve in 7 days, see your dentist or physician promptly. Do not administer to children under 6 years of age unless directed by physician or dentist. Keep this and all drugs out of the reach of children. In case of accidental overdose, seek professional assistance or contact a Poison Control Center immediately. As with any drug, if you are pregnant or nursing a baby, seek the advice of a health professional before using this product.

Dosage and Administration: Adults and children 6 years of age and older: Allow product to dissolve slowly in the mouth. May be repeated every 2 hours as needed or as directed by a dentist or physician. Do not exceed 10 lozenges per day.

How Supplied:
18 lozenges in 2 pocket packs of 9 each. Store at room temperature, below 86°F (30°C). Protect contents from humidity.
Shown in Product Identification Section, page 414

CĒPACOL®
[*sē-pə-cŏl*]
Dry Throat Lozenges
Honey-Lemon Flavor

Description: Each lozenge contains Menthol 3.6 mg. Also contains: Benzyl Alcohol, Caramel, Cetylpyridinium Chloride, FD&C Yellow No. 6, D&C Yellow No. 10, Flavors, Liquid Glucose, and Sucrose.

Actions: Menthol provides a cooling sensation to aid in symptomatic relief of minor throat irritations.

Indications: Cēpacol Honey-Lemon Flavor Lozenges provide temporary relief of occasional dry, scratchy throat.

Warnings: If sore throat is severe, persists for more than 2 days, is accompanied or followed by fever, headache, rash, nausea, or vomiting, consult a physician promptly. If sore mouth symptoms do not improve in 7 days, see your dentist or physician promptly. Do not administer to children under 6 years of age unless directed by physician or dentist. Keep this and all drugs out of the reach of children. In case of accidental overdose, seek professional assistance or contact a Poison Control Center immediately. As with any drug, if you are pregnant or nursing a baby, seek the advice of a health professional before using this product.

Dosage and Administration: Adults and children 6 years of age and older: Allow product to dissolve slowly in the mouth. May be repeated every 2 hours as needed or as directed by a dentist or physician.

How Supplied:
18 lozenges in 2 pocket packs of 9 each. Store at room temperature, below 86°F (30°C). Protect contents from humidity.
Shown in Product Identification Section, page 414

CĒPACOL®
[*sē-pə-cŏl*]
Dry Throat Lozenges
Menthol-Eucalyptus Flavor

Description: Each lozenge contains Menthol 5.0 mg. Also contains: Benzyl Alcohol, Cetylpyridinium Chloride, Eucalyptol, Liquid Glucose, and Sucrose.

Actions: Menthol provides a cooling sensation to aid in symptomatic relief of minor throat irritations.

Indications: Cēpacol Menthol-Eucalyptus Flavor Lozenges provide temporary relief of occasional dry, scratchy throat.

Warnings: If sore throat is severe, persists for more than 2 days, is accompanied or followed by fever, headache, rash, nausea, or vomiting, consult a physician promptly. If sore mouth symptoms do not improve in 7 days, see your dentist or physician promptly. Do not administer to children under 6 years of age unless directed by physician or dentist. Keep this and all drugs out of the reach of children. In case of accidental overdose, seek professional assistance or contact a Poison Control Center immediately. As with any drug, if you are pregnant or nursing a baby, seek the advice of a health professional before using this product.

Dosage and Administration: Adults and children 6 years of age and older: Allow product to dissolve slowly in the mouth. May be repeated every 2 hours as needed or as directed by a dentist or physician.

How Supplied:
18 lozenges in 2 pocket packs of 9 each. Store at room temperature, below 86°F (30°C). Protect contents from humidity.
Shown in Product Identification Section, page 414

Continued on next page

Marion Merrell Dow—Cont.

CĒPACOL®
[sē 'pə-cŏl]
Dry Throat Lozenges
Original Flavor

Description: Each lozenge contains Ceepryn® (cetylpyridinium chloride) 0.07%, Benzyl Alcohol 0.3%. Also contains: FD&C Yellow No. 5 (tartrazine) as a color additive, Flavor, Glucose, and Sucrose.

Actions: Cetylpyridinium chloride (Ceepryn) is a cationic quaternary ammonium compound, which is a surface-active agent. Aqueous solutions of cetylpyridinium chloride have a surface tension lower than that of water.
Cetylpyridinium chloride in the concentration used in Cēpacol is nonirritating to tissues.

Indications: For soothing, temporary relief of dryness of the mouth and throat.

Warnings: Severe sore throat or sore throat accompanied by high fever, headache, nausea, or vomiting, or any sore throat or mouth irritations persisting more than 2 days may be serious. Consult a physician promptly. Persons with a high fever or persistent cough should not use this preparation unless directed by a physician. Do not administer to children under 6 years of age unless directed by a physician or dentist. If sensitive to any of the ingredients, do not use. Keep this and all drugs out of the reach of children. In case of accidental overdose, seek professional assistance or contact a Poison Control Center immediately. As with any drug, if you are pregnant or nursing a baby, seek the advice of a health professional before using this product.

Dosage and Administration: Adults and children 6 years and older, dissolve 1 lozenge in the mouth every 2 hours, if needed. For children under 6 years, consult a physician or dentist.

How Supplied:
Trade Package: 18 lozenges in 2 pocket packs of 9 each.
Professional Package: 648 lozenges in 72 blisters of 9 each.
Store at room temperature, 59°–86°F (15°–30°C). Protect contents from humidity.

Shown in Product Identification Section, page 414

CĒPACOL®
[sē 'pə-cŏl]
Anesthetic Lozenges (Troches)

Description: Each lozenge contains Benzocaine 10 mg, Ceepryn® (cetylpyridinium chloride) 0.07%. Also contains: FD&C Blue No. 1, FD&C Yellow No. 5 (tartrazine) as a color additive, Flavors, Glucose, and Sucrose.

Actions: Cetylpyridinium chloride (Ceepryn) is a cationic quaternary ammonium compound, which is a surface-active agent. Aqueous solutions of cetylpyridinium chloride have a surface tension lower than that of water.
Cetylpyridinium chloride in the concentration used in Cēpacol is nonirritating to tissues.
Cēpacol Anesthetic Lozenges stimulate salivation to relieve dryness of the mouth and provide a mild anesthetic effect for pain relief.

Indications: For fast, temporary relief of minor sore throat pain. For temporary relief of minor pain and discomfort associated with tonsillitis and pharyngitis.

Warnings: If sore throat is severe, persists for more than 2 days, is accompanied or followed by fever, headache, rash, nausea, or vomiting, consult a physician promptly. Keep this and all drugs out of the reach of children. In case of accidental overdose, seek professional assistance or contact a Poison Control Center immediately. As with any drug, if you are pregnant or nursing a baby, seek the advice of a health professional before using this product.

Dosage and Administration: Adults and children 6 years and older, dissolve 1 lozenge in the mouth every 2 hours, if needed. For children under 6 years, consult a physician or dentist.

How Supplied:
Trade Package: 18 troches in 2 pocket packs of 9 each.
Professional Package: 324 troches in 36 blisters of 9 each.
Store at room temperature, below 86°F (30°C). Protect contents from humidity.

Shown in Product Identification Section, page 414

CĒPASTAT®
[sē 'pə-stăt]
Sore Throat Lozenges
Cherry Flavor and Extra Strength

Description: Each Cherry Flavor lozenge contains: Phenol 14.5 mg. Also contains: Antifoam Emulsion, D&C Red No. 33, FD&C Yellow No. 6, Flavor, Gum Crystal, Mannitol, Menthol, Saccharin Sodium, and Sorbitol.
Each Extra Strength lozenge contains: Phenol 29 mg. Also contains: Antifoam Emulsion, Caramel, Eucalyptus Oil, Gum Crystal, Mannitol, Menthol, Saccharin Sodium, and Sorbitol.

Actions: Phenol is a recognized topical anesthetic. The sugar-free formula should not promote tooth decay as sugar-based lozenges can.

Indications: For fast, temporary relief of minor sore throat pain.

Warnings*: If sore throat is severe, persists for more than 2 days, is accompanied or followed by fever, headache, rash, nausea, or vomiting, consult a physician promptly. If sore mouth symptoms do not improve in 7 days, see your dentist or physician promptly. Keep this and all drugs out of the reach of children. In case of accidental overdose, seek professional assistance or contact a Poison Control Center immediately. As with any drug, if you are pregnant or nursing a baby, seek the advice of a health professional before using this product.

Note to Diabetics*: Each lozenge contributes approximately 8 calories from 2 grams of sorbitol.

Dosage and Administration:
Lozenges–Cherry Flavor
Adults and children 12 years of age and older: Allow the lozenge to dissolve slowly in the mouth. May be repeated every 2 hours, not to exceed 18 lozenges per day, or as directed by a dentist or physician. Children 6 to under 12 years of age: Allow lozenge to dissolve slowly in the mouth. May be repeated every 2 hours, not to exceed 10 lozenges per day, or as directed by a dentist or physician. Children under 6 years of age: Consult a dentist or physician.
Lozenges–Extra Strength
Adults and children 12 years of age and older: Allow the lozenge to dissolve slowly in the mouth. May be repeated every 2 hours, not to exceed 18 lozenges per day, or as directed by a dentist or physician. Children 6 to under 12 years of age: Allow lozenge to dissolve slowly in the mouth. May be repeated every 2 hours, not to exceed 10 lozenges per day, or as directed by a dentist or physician. Children under 6 years of age: Consult a dentist or physician.

How Supplied:
Lozenges–Cherry Flavor
Trade package: Boxes of 18 lozenges as 2 pocket packs of 9 lozenges each. Professional package: 648 lozenges in 72 blisters of 9 lozenges each.
Lozenges–Extra Strength
Trade package: Boxes of 18 lozenges as 2 pocket packs of 9 lozenges each. Professional package: 648 lozenges in 72 blisters of 9 lozenges each.
Store at room temperature, below 86°F (30°C). Protect contents from humidity.

*This section appears on the label for the consumer.

Shown in Product Identification Section, page 414

Orange Flavor
CITRUCEL®
[sĭt 'rə-sĕl]
(Methylcellulose)
Bulk-forming Fiber Laxative

Description: Each 19 g adult dose (approximately one heaping measuring tablespoonful) contains Methylcellulose 2 g. Each 9.5 g child's dose (approximately 1 level measuring tablespoonful) contains Methylcellulose 1 g. Also contains: Citric Acid, FD&C Yellow No. 6, Orange Flavors (Natural and Artificial), Potassium Citrate, Riboflavin, Sucrose, and Other Ingredients. Each adult dose contains approximately 3 mg of sodium, 105 mg of potassium, and contributes 60 calories from 15 g of Sucrose.

Actions: Promotes elimination by providing additional fiber (bulk) to the diet. This product generally produces bowel movement in 12 to 72 hours.

Indications: For relief of constipation (irregularity). May also be used for relief of constipation associated with other bowel disorders such as irritable bowel syndrome, diverticular disease, and hemorrhoids as well as for bowel management during postpartum, postsurgical, and convalescent periods.

Contraindications: Intestinal obstruction, fecal impaction, known hypersensitivity to formula ingredients.

Precautions: Patients should be instructed to consult their physician before using any laxative if they have noticed a sudden change in bowel habits which persists for two weeks. Unless directed by a physician, patients should be advised not to use laxative products when abdominal pain, nausea, or vomiting is present. Patients should also be advised to discontinue use and consult a physician if rectal bleeding or failure to have a bowel movement occurs after use of any laxative product.

Dosage and Administration: Adults and children 12 years and older: *one heaping measuring* tablespoonful stirred briskly into 8 ounces of cold water or fruit juice, one to three times a day and administered promptly. Children 6 to under 12 years: *one level measuring* tablespoonful stirred briskly into 4 ounces of cold water, one to three times a day and administered promptly. Children under 6 years: use only as directed by a physician.
Continued use for two or three days may be necessary for full benefit.
Administering additional water is helpful.

How Supplied:
16 oz, 24 oz, and 30 oz containers.
Boxes of 20 single-dose packets.
Store below 86°F (30°C). Protect contents from humidity; keep tightly closed.

Shown in Product Identification Section, page 414

Regular Flavor CITRUCEL®
[*sĭt 'rə-sĕl*]
(Methylcellulose)
Bulk-forming Fiber Laxative

Description: Each 5.50 g adult dose (approximately one level measuring tablespoonful) contains Methylcellulose 2 g. Each 2.75 g child's dose (approximately one rounded measuring teaspoonful) contains Methylcellulose 1 g. Also contains: Malic Acid, Maltodextrin, Natural Citrus Flavor, Potassium Citrate, Riboflavin, Sucrose, and Other Ingredients. Each 5.50 g dose contains approximately 3 mg of sodium, 80 mg of potassium, and contributes 12 calories (from Maltodextrin and Sucrose).

Actions: Promotes elimination by providing additional fiber (bulk) to the diet. This product generally produces bowel movement in 12 to 72 hours.

Indications: For relief of constipation (irregularity). May also be used for relief of constipation associated with other bowel disorders such as irritable bowel syndrome, diverticular disease, and hemorrhoids as well as for bowel management during postpartum, postsurgical, and convalescent periods.

Contraindications: Intestinal obstruction, fecal impaction, known hypersensitivity to formula ingredients.

Precautions: Patients should be instructed to consult their physician before using any laxative if they have noticed a sudden change in bowel habits which persists for two weeks. Unless directed by a physician, patients should be advised not to use laxative products when abdominal pain, nausea or vomiting is present. Patients should also be advised to discontinue use and consult a physician if rectal bleeding or failure to have a bowel movement occurs after use of any laxative product.

Dosage and Administration: Adults and children 12 years and older: *one level measuring* tablespoonful *stirred immediately and briskly* into 8 ounces of cold water or fruit juice, one to three times a day and administered promptly. Children 6 to under 12 years: *one rounded measuring* teaspoonful *stirred immediately and briskly* into 4 ounces of cold water or fruit juice, one to three times a day and administered promptly. Children under 6 years: use only as directed by a physician.
Continued use for two or three days may be necessary for full benefit.
Administering additional water is helpful.

How Supplied:
7 oz and 10 oz containers.
Store below 86°F (30°C). Protect contents from humidity; keep tightly closed.

Shown in Product Identification Section, page 414

DEBROX® Drops
[*dē 'brŏx*]

Description: Carbamide peroxide 6.5%. Also contains citric acid, glycerin, propylene glycol, sodium stannate, water, and other ingredients.

Actions: DEBROX®, used as directed, cleanses the ear with sustained microfoam. DEBROX Drops foam on contact with earwax due to the release of oxygen.

Indications: DEBROX Drops provide a safe, nonirritating method of softening and removing earwax.

Directions: FOR USE IN THE EAR ONLY. Adults and children over 12 years of age: tilt head sideways and place 5 to 10 drops into ear. Tip of applicator should not enter ear canal. Keep drops in ear for several minutes by keeping head tilted or placing cotton in the ear. Use twice daily for up to four days if needed, or as directed by a doctor. Any wax remaining after treatment may be removed by gently flushing the ear with warm water, using a soft rubber bulb ear syringe. Children under 12 years of age: consult a doctor.

Warnings: Do not use if you have ear drainage or discharge, ear pain, irritation or rash in the ear, or are dizzy, unless directed by a physician. Do not use if you have an injury or perforation (hole) of the eardrum or after ear surgery unless directed by a physician. Do not use for more than four consecutive days. If excessive earwax remains after use of this product, consult a physician. Consult a physician prior to use in children under 12.

Cautions: Avoid exposing bottle to excessive heat and direct sunlight. Keep color tip on bottle when not in use. Avoid contact with eyes. Keep this and all drugs out of the reach of children. In case of accidental ingestion, seek professional assistance or contact a poison control center immediately.

How Supplied: DEBROX Drops are available in ½- or 1-fl-oz plastic squeeze bottles with applicator spouts.

Issued 1/89

Shown in Product Identification Section, page 414

GAVISCON® Antacid Tablets
[*găv 'ĭs-kŏn*]

Composition: Each chewable tablet contains the following active ingredients:
Aluminum hydroxide dried gel... 80 mg
Magnesium trisilicate .... 20 mg
and the following inactive ingredients: alginic acid, calcium stearate, flavor, sodium bicarbonate, starch (may contain cornstarch), and sucrose.

Actions: Unique formulation produces soothing foam which floats on stomach contents. Foam containing antacid precedes stomach contents into the esophagus when reflux occurs to help protect the sensitive mucosa from further irritation. GAVISCON® acts locally without neutralizing entire stomach contents to help maintain integrity of the digestive process. Endoscopic studies indicate that GAVISCON Antacid Tablets are equally as effective in the erect or supine patient.

Indications: GAVISCON is specifically formulated for the temporary relief of heartburn (acid indigestion) due to acid reflux. GAVISCON is not indicated for the treatment of peptic ulcers.

Directions: Chew two to four tablets four times a day or as directed by a physician. Tablets should be taken after meals and at bedtime or as needed. For best results follow by a half glass of water or other liquid. DO NOT SWALLOW WHOLE.

Warnings: Do not take more than 16 tablets in a 24-hour period or 16 tablets daily for more than 2 weeks, except under the advice and supervision of a physician. Do not use this product except under the advice and supervision of a physician if you are on a sodium-restricted diet. Each GAVISCON Tablet contains approximately 0.8 mEq sodium.

Continued on next page

Marion Merrell Dow—Cont.

Drug Interaction Precautions: Do not take this product if you are presently taking a prescription antibiotic drug containing any form of tetracycline.
Store at a controlled room temperature in a dry place.
Keep this and all drugs out of the reach of children. In case of accidental overdose, seek professional assistance or contact a poison control center immediately.

How Supplied: Available in bottles of 100 tablets and in foil-wrapped 2s in boxes of 30 tablets.

Issued 2/87

Shown in Product Identification Section, page 414

GAVISCON® EXTRA STRENGTH RELIEF FORMULA Antacid Tablets

[*găv 'ĭs-kŏn*]

Composition: Each chewable tablet contains the following active ingredients:
Aluminum hydroxide .... 160 mg
Magnesium carbonate .... 105 mg
and the following inactive ingredients: alginic acid, calcium stearate, flavor, mannitol, sodium bicarbonate, stearic acid, and sucrose.

Directions: Chew 2 to 4 tablets four times a day or as directed by a physician. Tablets should be taken after meals and at bedtime or as needed. For best results follow by a half glass of water or other liquid. DO NOT SWALLOW WHOLE.

> **FDA Approved Uses:** For the relief of heartburn, sour stomach, and/or acid indigestion, and upset stomach associated with heartburn, sour stomach, and/or acid indigestion.

Warnings: Do not take more than 16 tablets in a 24-hour period or 16 tablets daily for more than 2 weeks, except under the advice and supervision of a physician. Do not use this product except under the advice and supervision of a physician if you are on a sodium-restricted diet. Each tablet contains approximately 1.3 mEq sodium.

Drug Interaction Precautions: Do not take this product if you are presently taking a prescription antibiotic drug containing any form of tetracycline.
Store at a controlled room temperature in a dry place.
Keep this and all drugs out of the reach of children.
In case of accidental overdose, seek professional assistance or contact a poison control center immediately.

How Supplied: Available in bottles of 100 tablets.

Issued 4/87

Shown in Product Identification Section, page 414

GAVISCON® EXTRA STRENGTH RELIEF FORMULA Liquid Antacid

[*găv 'ĭs-kŏn*]

Composition: Each 2 teaspoonfuls (10 mL) contains the following active ingredients:
Aluminum hydroxide.....................508 mg
Magnesium carbonate...................475 mg
And the following inactive ingredients: butylparaben, edetate disodium, flavor, glycerin, propylparaben, saccharin sodium, simethicone emulsion, sodium alginate, sorbitol solution, water, and xanthan gum.

> **FDA Approved Uses:** For the relief of heartburn, sour stomach and/or acid indigestion, and upset stomach associated with heartburn, sour stomach and/or acid indigestion.

Directions: SHAKE WELL BEFORE USING. Take 2 to 4 teaspoonfuls four times a day or as directed by a physician. GAVISCON Extra Strength Relief Formula Liquid should be taken after meals and at bedtime, followed by half a glass of water. Dispense product only by spoon or other measuring device.

Warnings: Except under the advice and supervision of a physician, do not take more than 16 teaspoonfuls in a 24-hour period or 16 teaspoonfuls daily for more than 2 weeks. May have laxative effect. Do not use this product if you have a kidney disease; do not use this product if you are on a sodium-restricted diet. Each teaspoonful contains approximately 0.9 mEq sodium.

Drug Interaction Precautions: Do not take this product if you are presently taking a prescription antibiotic drug containing any form of tetracycline.
Keep tightly closed. Avoid freezing. Store at a controlled room temperature.
Keep this and all drugs out of the reach of children.
In case of accidental overdose, seek professional assistance or contact a poison control center immediately.

How Supplied: Available in 12 fl oz (355 mL) bottles.

Issued 2/89

Shown in Product Identification Section, page 414

GAVISCON® Liquid Antacid

[*găv 'ĭs-kŏn*]

Composition: Each tablespoonful (15 ml) contains the following active ingredients:
Aluminum hydroxide .... 95 mg
Magnesium carbonate .... 412 mg
And the following inactive ingredients: D&C Yellow #10, edetate disodium, FD&C Blue #1, flavor, glycerin, paraben preservatives, saccharin sodium, sodium alginate, sorbitol solution, water, and xanthan gum.

> **FDA Approved Uses:** For the relief of heartburn, sour stomach and/or acid indigestion, and upset stomach associated with heartburn, sour stomach and/or acid indigestion.

Directions: SHAKE WELL BEFORE USING. Take 1 or 2 tablespoonfuls four times a day or as directed by a physician. GAVISCON Liquid should be taken after meals and at bedtime, followed by half a glass of water. Dispense product only by spoon or other measuring device.

Warnings: Except under the advice and supervision of a physician, do not take more than 8 tablespoonfuls in a 24-hour period or 8 tablespoonfuls daily for more than 2 weeks. May have laxative effect. Do not use this product if you have a kidney disease; do not use this product if you are on a sodium-restricted diet. Each tablespoonful of GAVISCON Liquid contains approximately 1.7 mEq sodium.

Drug Interaction Precautions: Do not take this product if you are presently taking a prescription antibiotic drug containing any form of tetracycline.
Keep tightly closed. Avoid freezing. Store at a controlled room temperature.
Keep this and all drugs out of the reach of children.
In case of accidental overdose, seek professional assistance or contact a poison control center immediately.

How Supplied: Bottles of 12 fluid ounce (355 ml) and 6 fluid ounce (177 ml).

Issued 2/87

Shown in Product Identification Section, page 414

GAVISCON®-2 Antacid Tablets

[*găv 'ĭs-kŏn*]

Composition: Each chewable tablet contains the following active ingredients:
Aluminum hydroxide dried gel...160 mg
Magnesium trisilicate .... 40 mg
and the following inactive ingredients: alginic acid, calcium stearate, flavor, sodium bicarbonate, starch (may contain cornstarch), and sucrose.

Indications: GAVISCON® is specifically formulated for the temporary relief of heartburn (acid indigestion) due to acid reflux. GAVISCON is not indicated for the treatment of peptic ulcers.

Directions: Chew one to two tablets four times a day or as directed by a physician. Tablets should be taken after meals and at bedtime or as needed. For best results follow by a half glass of water or other liquid. DO NOT SWALLOW WHOLE.

Warnings: Do not take more than eight tablets in a 24-hour period or eight tablets daily for more than 2 weeks, except under the advice and supervision of a physician. Do not use this product except under the advice and supervision of a physician if you are on a sodium-restricted diet. Each GAVISCON-2 Tablet contains approximately 1.6 mEq sodium.

Drug Interaction Precautions: Do not take this product if you are presently taking a prescription antibiotic drug containing any form of tetracycline.
Store at a controlled room temperature in a dry place.
Keep this and all drugs out of the reach of children. In case of accidental overdose, seek professional assistance or contact a poison control center immediately.

How Supplied: Boxes of 48 foil-wrapped tablets.

Issued 2/87

Shown in Product Identification Section, page 415

GLY-OXIDE® Liquid
[*glī-ok 'sīd*]

Description: GLY-OXIDE® Liquid contains carbamide peroxide 10%. Also contains citric acid, flavor, glycerin, propylene glycol, sodium stannate, water, and other ingredients.

Actions: GLY-OXIDE® Liquid has an oxygen-rich formula that works to relieve the pain of canker sores by cleaning and debriding damaged tissue so natural healing can occur.

Administration: Do not dilute. Apply directly from bottle. Replace color tip on bottle when not in use.

Indications: For local treatment and hygienic prevention of minor oral inflammation such as canker sores, denture irritation, and postdental procedure irritation. Place several drops on affected area four times daily, after meals and at bedtime, or as directed by a dentist or physician; expectorate after two or three minutes. Or place 10 drops onto tongue, mix with saliva, swish for several minutes, and expectorate.
As an adjunct to oral hygiene (orthodontics, dental appliances) after regular brushing, swish 10 or more drops vigorously. Continue for two to three minutes; expectorate.
When normal oral hygiene is inadequate or impossible (total care geriatrics, etc), swish 10 or more drops vigorously after meals and expectorate.

Precautions: Severe or persistent oral inflammation, denture irritation, or gingivitis may be serious. If these conditions or unexpected side effects occur, consult a dentist or physician immediately.
Avoid contact with eyes. Protect from heat and direct light. Keep this and all drugs out of the reach of children. In case of accidental overdose, seek professional assistance or contact a poison control center immediately.

How Supplied: GLY-OXIDE® Liquid is available in ½-fl-oz and 2-fl-oz nonspill, plastic squeeze bottles with applicator spouts.

Issued 2/89

Shown in Product Identification Section, page 415

NOVAHISTINE® DMX
[*nō "vă-hĭs 'tēn*]
Cough/Cold Formula & Decongestant

Description: Each 5 mL teaspoonful of NOVAHISTINE DMX contains: Dextromethorphan Hydrobromide 10 mg, Guaifenesin 100 mg, Pseudoephedrine Hydrochloride 30 mg. Also contains: Alcohol 10%, FD&C Red No. 40, FD&C Yellow No. 6, Flavors, Glycerin, Hydrochloric Acid, Invert Sugar, Saccharin Sodium, Sodium Chloride, Sorbitol, and Water.
Dextromethorphan hydrobromide, a synthetic nonnarcotic antitussive, is the dextrorotatory isomer of 3-methoxy-*N*-methylmorphinan. Guaifenesin is the glyceryl ether of guaiacol. Pseudoephedrine hydrochloride is the salt of a pharmacologically active stereoisomer of ephedrine (1-phenyl-2-methylamino-1-propanol).

Actions: Dextromethorphan hydrobromide suppresses the cough reflex by a direct effect on the cough center in the medulla of the brain. Although it is chemically related to morphine, it produces no analgesia or addiction. Its antitussive activity is about equal to that of codeine.
Pseudoephedrine hydrochloride is an orally effective nasal decongestant. It is a sympathomimetic amine with peripheral effects similar to epinephrine and central effects similar to, but less intense than, amphetamines. Therefore, it has the potential for excitatory side effects. Pseudoephedrine hydrochloride at the recommended oral dosage has little or no pressor effect in normotensive adults. Patients taking pseudoephedrine orally have not been reported to experience the rebound congestion sometimes experienced with frequent, repeated use of topical decongestants. Pseudoephedrine is not known to produce drowsiness.
Guaifenesin acts as an expectorant by increasing respiratory tract fluid which reduces the viscosity of tenacious secretions, thus making expectoration easier.

Indications: NOVAHISTINE DMX is indicated for temporary relief of cough and nasal congestion. It is useful when exhausting, nonproductive cough accompanies respiratory tract congestion and in the symptomatic relief of upper respiratory congestion associated with the common cold, influenza, bronchitis, and sinusitis.

Contraindications: NOVAHISTINE DMX is contraindicated in patients with severe hypertension, severe coronary artery disease, and in patients on MAO inhibitor therapy. Patient idiosyncrasy to adrenergic agents may be manifested by insomnia, dizziness, weakness, tremor, or arrhythmias.
Nursing mothers: Pseudoephedrine is contraindicated in nursing mothers because of the higher than usual risk for infants from sympathomimetic amines.
Hypersensitivity: NOVAHISTINE DMX is contraindicated in patients with hypersensitivity or idiosyncrasy to sympathomimetic amines, dextromethorphan, or to other formula ingredients.

Warnings: At dosages higher than the recommended dose, nervousness, dizziness, sleeplessness, nausea, or headache may occur. Do not take for more than 7 days. A persistent cough may be a sign of a serious condition. If symptoms do not improve, recur, or are accompanied by fever, rash, or persistent headache, patients should be advised to consult their physician before continuing use. Do not use for persistent or chronic cough such as occurs with smoking, asthma, chronic bronchitis or emphysema, or where cough is accompanied by excessive phlegm (sputum) unless directed by a physician. Sympathomimetic amines should be used judiciously and sparingly in patients with hypertension, diabetes mellitus, ischemic heart disease, increased intraocular pressure, hyperthyroidism, or prostatic hypertrophy. Sympathomimetics may produce central nervous system stimulation with convulsions or cardiovascular collapse with accompanying hypotension. See Contraindications.
Use in elderly: The elderly (60 years and older) are more likely to have adverse reactions to sympathomimetics. Overdosage of sympathomimetics in this age group may cause hallucinations, convulsions, CNS depression, and death.
Use in children: NOVAHISTINE DMX should not be used in children under 2 years except under the advice and supervision of a physician.
Use in pregnancy: Safety for use during pregnancy has not been established. As with any drug, if you are pregnant or nursing a baby, seek the advice of a health professional before using this product.
If sensitive to any of the ingredients, do not use.
Keep this and all drugs out of the reach of children. In case of accidental overdose, seek professional assistance or contact a Poison Control Center immediately.

Precautions: Drugs containing pseudoephedrine should be used with caution in patients with diabetes, hypertension, cardiovascular disease, and hyperreactivity to ephedrine. See Contraindications.

Adverse Reactions: Adverse reactions occur infrequently with usual oral doses of NOVAHISTINE DMX. When they occur, adverse reactions may include gastrointestinal upset and nausea.
Because of the pseudoephedrine in NOVAHISTINE DMX, hyperreactive individuals may display ephedrine-like reactions such as tachycardia, palpitations, headache, dizziness or nausea. Sympathomimetic drugs have been associated with certain untoward reactions including fear, anxiety, tenseness, restlessness, tremor, weakness, pallor, respiratory difficulty, dysuria, insomnia, hallucinations, convulsions, CNS depres-

Continued on next page

Marion Merrell Dow—Cont.

sion, arrhythmias, and cardiovascular collapse with hypotension.

Note: Guaifenesin interferes with the colorimetric determination of 5-hydroxyindoleacetic acid (5-HIAA) and vanillylmandelic acid (VMA).

Drug Interactions: NOVAHISTINE DMX should not be used in patients taking a prescription drug for hypertension or depression without the advice of a physician. MAO inhibitors and beta-adrenergic blockers increase the effects of pseudoephedrine (sympathomimetics). Sympathomimetics may reduce the antihypertensive effects of methyldopa, mecamylamine, reserpine, and veratrum alkaloids.

Dosage and Administration: Adults and children 12 years and over, 2 teaspoonfuls every 4 hours. Children 6 to under 12 years, 1 teaspoonful every 4 hours. Children 2 to under 6 years, ½ teaspoonful every 4 hours. Not more than 4 doses every 24 hours. For children under 2 years of age, give only as directed by a physician.

How Supplied: As a red syrup in 4 fluid ounce bottles.
Keep tightly closed. Protect from excessive heat and light. Avoid freezing.

Shown in Product Identification Section, page 415

NOVAHISTINE® Elixir

[*nō″vă-hĭs′tēn*]

Cold & Hay Fever Formula

Description: Each 5 ml teaspoonful of NOVAHISTINE Elixir contains: Chlorpheniramine Maleate 2 mg, Phenylephrine Hydrochloride 5 mg. Also contains: Alcohol 5%, D&C Yellow No. 10, FD&C Blue No. 1, Flavors, Glycerin, Sodium Chloride, Sorbitol, and Water. Although considered sugar-free, each 5 ml contributes approximately 7 calories from sorbitol.

Actions: Phenylephrine is a nasal decongestant. Its effects are similar to epinephrine, but it is less potent on a weight basis, and has a longer duration of action. Phenylephrine produces peripheral effects similar to epinephrine, but has little or no central nervous system stimulation. After oral administration, nasal decongestion may occur within 15 or 20 minutes and persist for 2 to 4 hours.
Chlorpheniramine maleate, an antihistaminic effective for the symptomatic relief of allergic rhinitis, possesses anticholinergic and sedative effects. Chlorpheniramine antagonizes many of the pharmacologic actions of histamine. It prevents released histamine from dilating capillaries and causing edema of the respiratory mucosa.

Indications: For the temporary relief of nasal congestion and eustachian tube congestion associated with the common cold, sinusitis, and hay fever (allergic rhinitis). Also provides temporary relief of runny nose, sneezing, itching of nose or throat, and itchy, watery eyes due to the common cold, hay fever (allergic rhinitis) or other upper respiratory allergies. May be given concomitantly, when indicated, with analgesics and antibiotics.

Contraindications: NOVAHISTINE Elixir is contraindicated in patients with severe hypertension, severe coronary artery disease, and in patients on MAO inhibitor therapy. Patient idiosyncrasy to adrenergic agents may be manifested by insomnia, dizziness, weakness, tremor, or arrhythmias.
NOVAHISTINE Elixir is also contraindicated in patients with narrow-angle glaucoma, urinary retention, peptic ulcer, asthma, emphysema, chronic pulmonary disease, shortness of breath, or difficulty in breathing.
Nursing mothers: Phenylephrine is contraindicated in nursing mothers.
Hypersensitivity: NOVAHISTINE Elixir is also contraindicated in patients with hypersensitivity or idiosyncrasy to sympathomimetic amines, antihistamines or to other formula ingredients.

Warnings: At dosages higher than the recommended dose, nervousness, dizziness, sleeplessness, nausea, or headache may occur. If symptoms do not improve within 7 days or are accompanied by high fever, patients should be advised to consult their physician before continuing use. Sympathomimetic amines should be used judiciously and sparingly in patients with hypertension, diabetes mellitus, ischemic heart disease, increased intraocular pressure, hyperthyroidism, or prostatic hypertrophy. Sympathomimetics may produce central nervous system stimulation with convulsions or cardiovascular collapse with accompanying hypotension. See Contraindications.
Use in elderly: The elderly (60 years and older) are more likely to have adverse reactions to sympathomimetics. Overdosage of sympathomimetics in this age group may cause hallucinations, convulsions, CNS depression, and death.
Use in children: May cause excitability. NOVAHISTINE Elixir should not be used in children under 6 years except under the advice and supervision of a physician.
Use in pregnancy: Safety for use during pregnancy has not been established. As with any drug, if you are pregnant or nursing a baby, seek the advice of a health professional before using this product.
If sensitive to any of the ingredients, do not use.
Keep this and all drugs out of the reach of children. In case of accidental overdose, seek professional assistance or contact a Poison Control Center immediately.

Precautions: Caution should be exercised if used in patients with high blood pressure, heart disease, diabetes or thyroid disease. The antihistamine may cause drowsiness, and ambulatory patients who operate machinery or motor vehicles should be cautioned accordingly.

Adverse Reactions: Drugs containing sympathomimetic amines have been associated with certain untoward reactions, including fear, anxiety, tenseness, restlessness, tremor, weakness, pallor, respiratory difficulty, dysuria, insomnia, hallucinations, convulsions, CNS depression, arrhythmias, and cardiovascular collapse with hypotension. Individuals hyperreactive to phenylephrine may display ephedrine-like reactions such as tachycardia, palpitation, headache, dizziness, or nausea.
Phenylephrine is considered safe and relatively free of unpleasant side effects when taken at recommended dosage.
Patients sensitive to antihistamine drugs may experience mild sedation. Other side effects from antihistamines may include dry mouth, dizziness, weakness, anorexia, nausea, vomiting, headache, nervousness, polyuria, heartburn, diplopia, dysuria, and, very rarely, dermatitis.

Drug Interactions: NOVAHISTINE Elixir should not be used in patients taking a prescription drug for hypertension or depression without the advice of a physician. MAO inhibitors and beta-adrenergic blockers increase the effects of sympathomimetics. Sympathomimetics may reduce the antihypertensive effects of methyldopa, mecamylamine, reserpine, and veratrum alkaloids. Antihistamines have been shown to enhance one or more of the effects of tricyclic antidepressants, barbiturates, alcohol, and other central nervous system depressants.

Dosage and Administration: Adults and children 12 years and older, 2 teaspoonfuls every 4 hours; children 6 to under 12 years, 1 teaspoonful every 4 hours; children 2 to under 6 years, ½ teaspoonful every 4 hours.
For children under 2 years, at the discretion of the physician.
Product label dosage is as follows: Adults and children 12 years and older, 2 teaspoonfuls every 4 hours. Children 6 to under 12 years, 1 teaspoonful every 4 hours. Not more than 6 doses every 24 hours. For children under 6 years, give only as directed by a physician.

How Supplied: NOVAHISTINE Elixir, as a green liquid in 4 fluid ounce bottles.
Keep tightly closed. Protect from excessive heat and light. Avoid freezing.

Shown in Product Identification Section, page 415

OS-CAL® 500 Chewable Tablets

[*ăhs′kăl*]

(calcium supplement)

Each Tablet Contains: 1,250 mg of calcium carbonate.
Elemental calcium....................... 500 mg

Ingredients: calcium carbonate, dextrose monohydrate, maltodextrin, microcrystalline cellulose, magnesium stearate, Bavarian cream flavor, sodium chloride, and coconut cream flavor.

Directions: One tablet two to three times a day with meals, or as recommended by your physician.

Two Tablets Provide: 1,000 mg calcium, 100% of U.S. RDA for adults and children 12 or more years of age.

Three Tablets Provide: 1,500 mg calcium, 115% of U.S. RDA for pregnant and lactating women.

Store at room temperature. Keep out of reach of children.

How Supplied: OS-CAL® 500 Chewable Tablets is available in bottles of 60 tablets.

Issued 10/87

Shown in Product Identification Section, page 415

OS-CAL® 500 Tablets
[*ăhs 'kăl*]
(calcium supplement)

Each Tablet Contains: 1,250 mg of calcium carbonate from oyster shell, an organic calcium source.
Elemental calcium .... 500 mg

Ingredients: oyster shell powder, corn syrup solids, talc, hydroxypropyl methylcellulose, cornstarch, sodium starch glycolate, calcium stearate, polysorbate 80, pharmaceutical glaze, titanium dioxide, methyl propyl paraben, polyethylene glycol, polyvinylpyrrolidone, carnauba wax, D&C Yellow #10, acetylated monoglyceride, edetate disodium, FD&C Blue #1, and simethicone emulsion.

Directions: One tablet two or three times a day with meals, or as recommended by your physician.

Two Tablets Provide: 1,000 mg calcium, 100% of U.S. RDA for adults and children 12 or more years of age.

Three Tablets Provide: 1,500 mg calcium, 115% of U.S. RDA for pregnant and lactating women.

Store at room temperature. Keep out of reach of children.

How Supplied: OS-CAL® 500 is available in bottles of 60 and 120 tablets.

Issued 10/87

Shown in Product Identification Section, page 415

OS-CAL® 250+D Tablets
[*ăhs 'kăl*]
(calcium supplement with vitamin D)

Each Tablet Contains: 625 mg of calcium carbonate from oyster shell, an organic calcium source.
Elemental calcium .... 250 mg
Vitamin D .... 125 USP Units

Ingredients: oyster shell powder, corn syrup solids, talc, cornstarch, hydroxypropyl methylcellulose, calcium stearate, polysorbate 80, titanium dioxide, methyl propyl paraben, polyethylene glycol, pharmaceutical glaze, vitamin D, polyvinylpyrrolidone, carnauba wax, D&C Yellow #10, acetylated monoglyceride, edetate disodium, FD&C Blue #1, simethicone emulsion, and edible gray ink.

Directions: One tablet three times a day with meals, or as recommended by your physician.

Three Tablets Provide:

		% U.S. RDA for Adults
Calcium	750 mg	75%
Vitamin D	375 Units	94%

Store at room temperature. Keep out of reach of children.

How Supplied: OS-CAL® 250+D is available in bottles of 100, 240, 500, and 1,000 tablets.

Issued 10/87

Shown in Product Identification Section, page 415

OS-CAL® 500+D Tablets
[*ăhs 'kăl*]
(calcium supplement with vitamin D)

Each Tablet Contains: 1,250 mg of calcium carbonate from oyster shell, an organic calcium source.
Elemental calcium .... 500 mg
Vitamin D .... 125 USP Units

Ingredients: oyster shell powder, corn syrup solids, talc, hydroxypropyl methylcellulose, cornstarch, sodium starch glycolate, calcium stearate, polysorbate 80, pharmaceutical glaze, titanium dioxide, methyl propyl paraben, polyethylene glycol, polyvinylpyrrolidone, vitamin D, carnauba wax, D&C Yellow #10, acetylated monoglyceride, edetate disodium, FD&C Blue #1, and simethicone emulsion.

Directions: One tablet two or three times a day with meals, or as recommended by your physician.

Two Tablets Provide: 1,000 mg calcium, 100% of U.S. RDA for adults and children 12 or more years of age and 64% of vitamin D.

Three Tablets Provide: 1,500 mg calcium, 115% of U.S. RDA for pregnant and lactating women and 94% of vitamin D.
Store at room temperature. Keep out of reach of children.

How Supplied: OS-CAL® 500+D is available in bottles of 60 and 120.

Issued 10/87

Shown in Product Identification Section, page 415

OS–CAL® FORTIFIED Tablets
[*ăhs 'kăl*]
(multivitamin and minerals supplement with added calcium)

Each Tablet Contains:
Vitamin A (palmitate) 1668 USP Units
Vitamin D .... 125 USP Units
Thiamine mononitrate (vitamin B_1) .... 1.7 mg
Riboflavin (vitamin B_2) .... 1.7 mg
Pyridoxine hydrochloride (vitamin B_6) .... 2.0 mg
Ascorbic acid (vitamin C) .... 50.0 mg
dl-alpha-tocopherol acetate (vitamin E) .... 0.8 IU
Niacinamide .... 15.0 mg
Calcium (from oyster shell) .... 250.0 mg
Iron (as ferrous fumarate) .... 5.0 mg
Magnesium (as oxide) .... 1.6 mg
Manganese (as sulfate) .... 0.3 mg
Zinc (as sulfate) .... 0.5 mg

Ingredients: oyster shell powder, ascorbic acid, corn syrup solids, niacinamide, D&C Yellow #10 Aluminum Lake, ferrous fumarate, calcium stearate, FD&C Blue #1 Aluminum Lake, cornstarch, vitamin A palmitate, polysorbate 80, magnesium oxide, pyridoxine, thiamine, riboflavin, vitamin E, pharmaceutical glaze, methyl paraben, zinc sulfate, manganese sulfate, propylparaben, povidone, vitamin D, hydroxypropyl methylcellulose, carnauba wax, titanium dioxide, ethylcellulose, and acetylated monoglyceride.

Indication: Multivitamin and mineral supplement with added calcium.

Dosage: One tablet three times daily with meals or as directed by physician. In case of accidental overdose, seek professional assistance or contact a poison control center immediately.

Keep out of reach of children.
Store at room temperature.

How Supplied: Bottles of 100 tablets.

Issued 6/89

Shown in Product Identification Section, page 415

OS-CAL® PLUS Tablets
[*ăhs 'kăl*]
(multivitamin and multimineral supplement)

Each Tablet Contains:
Elemental calcium (from oyster shell) .... 250 mg
Vitamin D .... 125 USP Units
Vitamin A (palmitate) 1666 USP Units
Vitamin C (ascorbic acid) .... 33.0 mg
Vitamin B_2 (riboflavin) .... 0.66 mg
Vitamin B_1 (thiamine mononitrate) .... 0.5 mg
Vitamin B_6 (pyridoxine HCl) 0.5 mg
Niacinamide .... 3.33 mg
Iron (as ferrous fumarate) ..... 16.6 mg
Zinc (as the sulfate) .... 0.75 mg
Manganese (as the sulfate) .... 0.75 mg

Ingredients: oyster shell powder, corn syrup solids, ferrous fumarate, ascorbic acid, calcium stearate, cornstarch, hydroxypropyl methylcellulose, polysorbate 80, titanium dioxide, vitamin A palmitate, niacinamide, ethylcellulose, manganese sulfate, methyl propyl paraben, zinc sulfate, pharmaceutical glaze, acetylated monoglyceride, riboflavin, thiamine mononitrate, pyridoxine hydrochloride, povidone, vitamin D, carnauba wax, and D&C Red #33.

Indications: As a multivitamin and multimineral supplement.

Dosage: One (1) tablet three times a day before meals or as directed by a physician. For children under 4 years of age, consult a physician.

Continued on next page

Marion Merrell Dow—Cont.

Store at room temperature.
Keep out of reach of children. In case of accidental overdose, seek professional assistance or contact a poison control center immediately.

How Supplied: Bottles of 100 tablets.

Issued 10/87

Shown in Product Identification Section, page 415

SINGLET® For Adults

[*sĭng-lət*]

Decongestant/Antihistamine/ Analgesic (pain reliever)/Antipyretic (fever reducer)

Description: Each pink Singlet tablet contains Pseudoephedrine Hydrochloride 60 mg, Chlorpheniramine Maleate 4 mg, and Acetaminophen 650 mg. Also contains: D&C Red No. 27, D&C Yellow No. 10, FD&C Blue No. 1, Hydroxypropyl Cellulose, Hydroxypropyl Methylcellulose 2910, Magnesium Stearate, Microcrystalline Cellulose, Polyethylene Glycol 8000, Pregelatinized Corn Starch, Sodium Starch Glycolate, Sucrose, and Titanium Dioxide.

Indications: For the temporary relief of nasal congestion, runny nose, occasional sinus headache, fever, sneezing, watery eyes or itching of the nose, throat, and eyes due to colds, hay fever, or other upper respiratory allergies.

Warnings: Do not take this product for more than 7 days. Unless directed by a physician, do not take this product if you have asthma, glaucoma, emphysema, chronic pulmonary disease, heart disease, high blood pressure, thyroid disease, diabetes, shortness of breath, difficulty in breathing, difficulty in urination due to enlargement of the prostate gland, or if you are presently taking a prescription drug for high blood pressure or depression. Do not exceed recommended dosage because severe liver damage, nervousness, dizziness, or sleeplessness may occur. May cause excitability. Consult your physician if symptoms persist, if new symptoms occur, or if redness or swelling is present, because these could be signs of a serious condition. Consult your physician if fever persists for more than 3 days (72 hours) or recurs. May cause drowsiness; alcohol, sedatives, and tranquilizers may increase the drowsiness effect. Avoid alcoholic beverages while taking this product. Do not take this product if you are taking sedatives or tranquilizers without first consulting your physician. Use caution when driving a motor vehicle or operating machinery. If sensitive to any of the ingredients, do not use.
As with any drug, if you are pregnant or nursing a baby, seek the advice of a health professional before using this product. KEEP THIS AND ALL DRUGS OUT OF THE REACH OF CHILDREN. In case of accidental overdose, seek professional assistance or contact a Poison Control Center immediately. Prompt medical attention is critical for adults as well as for children even if you do not notice any signs or symptoms.

Dosage and Administration: Adults and children 12 years and older: one tablet 3 to 4 times a day, taken with water, while symptoms persist. Do not take more than 1 tablet within a 4-hour period. Do not exceed 4 tablets in 24 hours. Children under 12 years of age: consult a physician.

Storage: Protect from excessive heat and moisture.

How Supplied: Bottles of 100.

THROAT DISCS® Throat Lozenges

[*thrōt dĭsks*]

Description: Each lozenge contains sucrose, starch (may contain cornstarch), acacia, glycyrrhiza extract (licorice), gum tragacanth, anethole, linseed, cubeb oleoresin, anise oil, peppermint oil, capsicum, and mineral oil.

Indications: Effective for soothing, temporary relief of minor throat irritations from hoarseness and coughs due to colds.

Precautions: For severe or persistent cough or sore throat, or sore throat accompanied by high fever, headache, nausea, and vomiting, consult physician promptly. Not recommended for children under 3 years of age.

Directions: Allow lozenge to dissolve slowly in mouth. One or two should give the desired relief.

How Supplied: Boxes of 60 lozenges.

Issued 9/88

Shown in Product Identification Section, page 415

Marlyn Health Care

6324 FERRIS SQUARE
SAN DIEGO, CA 92121

MARLYN FORMULA 50®

PRODUCT OVERVIEW

Key Facts: MARLYN FORMULA 50 is a combination of amino acids and B6 in a gelatin capsule which provides protein "building blocks" important to growth and development of all protein containing tissue including nails, hair and skin.

Major Uses: Dermatologists recommend Formula 50 not only for splitting, peeling nails but also prescribe it in conjunction with their favorite topical cream for control of nail fungus. OB-Gyns recommend it for help in controlling excessive hair fall-out after child birth.
The recommended daily dose is six capsules daily.

Safety Information: There are no known contraindications or adverse reactions.

PRESCRIBING INFORMATION

MARLYN FORMULA 50®

Composition: Each capsule contains:

Amino Acids	0.3 Gm*
Vitamin B6 (pyridoxine HCl)	1.0 mg.

*Approximate analysis of the amino acids: indispensable amino acids (lysine, tryptophan, phenylalanine, methionine, threonine, leucine, isoleucine, valine), 35.30%; semi-dispensable amino acids (arginine, histidine, tyrosine, cystine, glycine), 19.18%; dispensable amino acids (glutamic acid, alanine, aspartic acid, serine, proline), 45.56%.
Amino acids: Protein "building blocks" important to growth and development of all protein containing tissue including nails, hair, and skin.

Dosage and Administration: The recommended daily dose is 6 capsules daily.

Supply: Bottles of 100, 250 and 1000 capsules.

MARLYN FORMULA 50 MEGA FORTE

PRODUCT OVERVIEW

Key Facts: MARLYN FORMULA 50 MEGA FORTE is a combination of amino acids and B6 in a gelatin capsule which provides protein "building blocks" important to growth and development of all protein containing tissues including nails, hair, and skin. In addition FORMULA 50 MEGA FORTE has the added advantages of Silicon, L-Cysteine and natural Mucopolysaccharides (from bovine cartilage.)

Major Uses: Dermatologists recommend FORMULA 50 MEGA FORTE not only for splitting, peeling nails but also prescribe it in conjunction with their favorite topical cream for control of nail fungus. OB-Gyns recommend it for help in controlling excessive hair fall-out after child birth.
The recommended daily dose is six capsules daily.

Safety Information: There are no known contraindications or adverse reactions.

PRESCRIBING INFORMATION

MARLYN FORMULA 50 MEGA FORTE

Each 6 capsules contain:

Amino Acids	1980 mg
Vitamin B_6	6 mg
Silicon (from Amino Acid Chelate)	90 mg
L-Cysteine HCl	120 mg
(Natural Extract) Mucopolysaccharides	60 mg
(from Bovine cartilage extract)	

Approximate analysis of amino acids: indispensable amino acids: (lysine, tryptophan, phenylalanine, methionine, threonine, leucine, isoleucine, valine) 35.30%; semi-dispensable amino acids; (arginine, histidine, tyrosine, cystine, glycine, 19.18%; dispensable amino acids (glutamic acids, alanine, aspartic acid, serine, proline), 45.56%.
Amino Acids; Protein "building blocks" important to growth and development of

all protein containing tissue including nails, hair, and skin.

Dosage and Administration: The recommended daily dose is 6 capsules daily.

Supply: Bottles of 100, 240, 500 and 1000.

McNeil Consumer Products Company

Division of McNeil-PPC, Inc.
FORT WASHINGTON, PA 19034

IMODIUM® A-D
(loperamide hydrochloride)

Description: Each 5 ml (teaspoon) of Imodium A-D liquid contains loperamide hydrochloride 1 mg. Imodium A-D liquid is stable, cherry flavored, and clear in color.
Each caplet of Imodium AD contains 2 mg of loperamide and is scored and colored green.

Actions: Imodium A-D contains a clinically proven antidiarrheal medication. Loperamide HCl acts by slowing intestinal motility and by affecting water and electrolyte movement through the bowel.

Indication: Imodium A-D is indicated for the control and symptomatic relief of acute nonspecific diarrhea.

Usual Dosage: Adults: Take four teaspoonfuls or two caplets after first loose bowel movement. If needed, take two teaspoonfuls or one caplet after each subsequent loose bowel movement. Do not exceed eight teaspoonfuls or four caplets in any 24 hour period, unless directed by a physician.
9–11 years old (60–95 lbs.): Two teaspoonfuls or one caplet after first loose bowel movement, followed by one teaspoonful or one-half caplet after each subsequent loose bowel movement. Do not exceed six teaspoonfuls or three caplets a day.
6–8 years old (48–59 lbs.): Two teaspoonfuls or one caplet after first loose bowel movement, followed by one teaspoonful or one-half caplet after each subsequent loose bowel movement. Do not exceed four teaspoonfuls or two caplets a day.
Professional Dosage Schedule for children two–five years old (24–47 lbs): one teaspoon after first loose bowel movement, followed by one after each subsequent loose bowel movement. Do not exceed three teaspoonfuls a day.

Warnings: DO NOT USE FOR MORE THAN TWO DAYS UNLESS DIRECTED BY A PHYSICIAN. Do not use if diarrhea is accompanied by high fever (greater than 101°F), or if blood is present in the stool, or if you have had a rash or other allergic reaction to loperamide HCl. If you are taking antibiotics or have a history of liver disease, consult a physician before using this product. As with any drug, if you are pregnant or nursing a baby, seek the advice of a physician before using this product. Keep this and all drugs out of the reach of children. In case of accidental overdose, seek professional assistance or contact a poison control center immediately. Store at room temperature.

Overdosage: Overdosage of loperamide HCl in man may result in constipation, CNS depression and nausea. A slurry of activated charcoal administered promptly after ingestion of loperamide hydrochloride can reduce the amount of drug which is absorbed. If vomiting occurs spontaneously upon ingestion, a slurry of 100 grams of activated charcoal should be administered orally as soon as fluids can be retained. If vomiting has not occurred, and CNS depression is evident, gastric lavage should be performed followed by administration of 100 gms of the activated charcoal slurry through the gastric tube. In the event of overdosage, patients should be monitored for signs of CNS depression for at least 24 hours. Children may be more sensitive to central nervous system effects than adults. If CNS depression is observed, naloxone may be administered. If responsive to naloxone, vital signs must be monitored carefully for recurrence of symptoms of drug overdose for at least 24 hours after the last dose of naloxone.

Inactive Ingredients:
Liquid: Alcohol (5.25%), citric acid, flavors, glycerin, methylparaben, propylparaben and purified water.
Caplets: Corn starch, lactose, magnesium stearate, microcrystalline cellulose, FD&C Blue #1 and D&C yellow #10.

How Supplied:
Cherry flavored liquid (clear) 2 fl. oz., 3 fl. oz., and 4 fl. oz. tamper resistant bottles with child resistant safety caps and special dosage cups.
Green Scored caplets in 6's and 12's blister packaging which is tamper resistant and child resistant.

Shown in Product Identification Section, page 417

MEDIPREN®
Ibuprofen Caplets and Tablets
Pain Reliever/Fever Reducer

WARNING
ASPIRIN SENSITIVE PATIENTS: Do not take this product if you have had a severe allergic reaction to aspirin (e.g., asthma, swelling, shock or hives) because even though this product contains no aspirin or salicylates, cross-reactions may occur in patients allergic to aspirin.

Description: Each MEDIPREN Caplet or Tablet contains ibuprofen 200 mg.

Indications: For the temporary relief of minor aches and pains associated with the common cold, headache, toothaches, muscular aches, backache, for the minor pain of arthritis, for the pain of menstrual cramps, and for reduction of fever.

Usual Dosage: Adults: One Caplet or Tablet every 4 to 6 hours while symptoms persist. If pain or fever does not respond to 1 Caplet or Tablet, 2 Caplets or Tablets may be used but do not exceed 6 Caplets or Tablets in 24 hours, unless directed by a doctor. The smallest effective dose should be used. Take with food or milk if occasional and mild heartburn, upset stomach, or stomach pain occurs with use. Consult a doctor if these symptoms are more than mild or if they persist.
Children: Do not give this product to children under 12 except under the advice and supervision of a doctor.

Warnings: Do not take for pain for more than 10 days or for fever for more than 3 days unless directed by a doctor. If pain or fever persists or gets worse, if new symptoms occur, or if the painful area is red or swollen, consult a doctor. These could be signs of serious illness. If you are under a doctor's care for any serious condition, consult a doctor before taking this product. As with aspirin and acetaminophen, if you have any condition which requires you to take prescription drugs or if you have had any problems or serious side effects from taking any non-prescription pain reliever, do not take this product without first discussing it with your doctor. If you experience any symptoms which are unusual or seem unrelated to the condition for which you took ibuprofen, consult a doctor before taking any more of it. Although ibuprofen is indicated for the same conditions as aspirin and acetaminophen, it should not be taken with them except under a doctor's direction. Do not combine this product with any other ibuprofen containing product. As with any drug, if you are pregnant or nursing a baby, seek the advice of a health professional before using this product. IT IS ESPECIALLY IMPORTANT NOT TO USE IBUPROFEN DURING THE LAST 3 MONTHS OF PREGNANCY UNLESS SPECIFICALLY DIRECTED TO DO SO BY A DOCTOR BECAUSE IT MAY CAUSE PROBLEMS IN THE UNBORN CHILD OR COMPLICATIONS DURING DELIVERY. Keep this and all drugs out of the reach of children.

Overdosage: In case of accidental overdose, contact a physician or poison control center.

Storage: Store at room temperature; avoid excessive heat 40°C (104°F).

Inactive Ingredients: Colloidal silicon dioxide, glyceryl triacetate, hydroxypropyl methylcellulose, microcrystalline cellulose, pregelatinized starch, sodium lauryl sulfate, sodium starch glycolate, titanium dioxide, Red #40.

How Supplied: Coated Caplets (colored white, imprinted "MEDIPREN")—bottles of 24's, 50's, and 125's. Coated Tablets (colored white, imprinted "MEDIPREN")—bottles of 24's and 50's.

Shown in Product Identification Section, page 415

Continued on next page

McNeil Consumer—Cont.

PEDIACARE® Allergy Formula
PEDIACARE® Cough-Cold Formula Liquid and Chewable Tablets
PEDIACARE® NightRest Cough-Cold Formula Liquid
PEDIACARE® Infants' Oral Decongestant Drops

Description: Each 5 ml of PEDIACARE Allergy Formula contains chlorpheniramine maleate 1 mg. Each 5 ml of PEDIACARE Cough-Cold Formula Liquid contains pseudoephedrine hydrochloride 15 mg, chlorpheniramine maleate 1 mg and dextromethorphan hydrobromide 5 mg. Each PEDIACARE Cough-Cold Formula Chewable Tablet contains pseudoephedrine hydrochloride 7.5 mg, chlorpheniramine maleate 0.5 mg and dextromethorphan hydrobromide 2.5 mg. Each 0.8 ml oral dropper of PEDIACARE Infants' Oral Decongestant Drops contains pseudoephedrine hydrochloride 7.5 mg. PEDIACARE NightRest contains pseudoephedrine hydrochloride 15 mg, chlorpheniramine maleate 1 mg and dextromethorphan hydrobromide 7.5 mg per 5 ml. PEDIACARE Cough-Cold Formula Liquid and Infants' Drops are stable, cherry flavored and red in color. PEDIACARE Allergy Formula Liquid is grape flavored and purple in color. PEDIACARE Cough-Cold Formula Chewable Tablets are fruit flavored and pink in color.

Actions: PEDIACARE Products are available in four different formulas, allowing you to select the ideal product to temporarily relieve the patient's symptoms. PEDIACARE Allergy Formula contains an antihistamine to relieve children's allergy symptoms. PEDIACARE Cough-Cold Formula Liquid and Chewable Tablets contain both of the above ingredients plus a cough suppressant, dextromethorphan hydrobromide, to provide temporary relief of nasal congestion, runny nose, sneezing and coughing due to the common cold, hay fever or other upper respiratory allergies. PEDIACARE NightRest Cough-Cold Formula Liquid contains a decongestant, pseudoephedrine hydrochloride, an antihistamine, chlorpheniramine maleate, and a cough suppressant, dextromethorphan hydrobromide, to provide temporary relief of coughs, nasal congestion, runny nose and sneezing due to the common cold. PEDIACARE NightRest may be used day or night to relieve cough and cold symptoms. PEDIACARE Infants' Oral Decongestant Drops contain a decongestant, pseudoephedrine hydrochloride, to provide temporary relief of nasal congestion due to the common cold, hay fever or other upper respiratory allergies.

Professional Dosage: A calibrated dosage cup is provided for accurate dosing of the PEDIACARE Liquid formulas. A calibrated oral dropper is provided for accurate dosing of PEDIACARE Infants' Drops. All doses of PEDIACARE Allergy Formula Liquid, PEDIACARE Cough-Cold Formula Liquid and Chewable Tablets and PEDIACARE Infants' Drops may be repeated every 4–6 hours, not to exceed 4 doses in 24 hours. PEDIACARE NightRest Liquid may be repeated every 6–8 hrs, not to exceed 4 doses in 24 hours. [See table below.]

" **Warnings:** Do not use if carton is opened, or if printed plastic bottle wrap or foil inner seal is broken. Keep this and all medication out of the reach of children. In case of accidental overdosage, contact a physician or poison control center immediately."

The following information appears on the appropriate package labels:

PEDIACARE Allergy Formula Liquid: May cause drowsiness. May cause excitability, especially in children. Do not give this product to children who have asthma or glaucoma unless directed by a doctor.

PEDIACARE Cough-Cold Formula Liquid, NightRest Cough-Cold Formula Liquid and Chewable Tablets: Do not exceed the recommended dosage because nervousness, dizziness or sleeplessness may occur. Do not give this product to children for more than 7 days. If symptoms do not improve, or are accompanied by fever, consult a doctor. A persistent cough may be a sign of a serious condition. If cough persists for more than one week, tends to recur or is accompanied by fever, rash, or persistent headache, consult a doctor. Do not give this product for persistent or chronic cough such as occurs with asthma or if cough is accompanied by excessive phlegm (mucus) unless directed by a doctor. This preparation may cause drowsiness or, in some cases, excitability. Do not give this product to children who have heart disease, high blood pressure, thyroid disease, glaucoma or asthma unless directed by a doctor.

Drug Interaction Precaution: Do not give this product to a child who is taking a prescription drug for high blood pressure or depression, without first consulting the child's doctor.

PEDIACARE Infants' Oral Decongestant Drops: "Do not exceed the recommended dosage because at higher doses nervousness, dizziness or sleeplessness may occur. Do not give this product to children who have heart disease, high blood pressure, thyroid disease or diabetes unless directed by a physician. Do not give this product to children for more than seven days. If symptoms do not improve or are accompanied by fever, consult a physician. Do not give this product to children who are taking a prescription drug for high blood pressure or depression without first consulting a physician. Take by mouth only. Not for nasal use."

PEDIACARE Cough-Cold Formula Liquid: Inactive Ingredients: Benzoic acid, citric acid, flavors, glycerin, polyethylene glycol, propylene glycol, sodium benzoate, sorbitol, sucrose, purified water, Red #33, Blue #1 and Red #40.

PEDIACARE NightRest Cough-Cold Formula Liquid: Inactive ingredients Benzoic acid, citric acid, flavors, glycerin, polyethylene glycol, propylene glycol, sodium benzoate, sorbitol, sucrose, purified water. Red #33, Blue #1 and Red #40.

PEDIACARE Cough-Cold Formula Chewable Tablets also contain the warning, "Phenylketonurics: contains phenylalanine 3 mg per tablet,"and the inactive ingredient listing, "Inactive Ingredients: Aspartame, cellulose, citric acid, dextrose, flavors, magnesium stearate, magnesium trisilicate, mannitol, starch, sucrose and Red #7."

PEDIACARE Infants' Oral Decongestant Drops: "Inactive Ingredients: Benzoic acid, citric acid, flavors, glycerin, polyethylene glycol, propylene glycol, purified water, sodium benzoate, sorbitol, sucrose and Red #40."

Overdosage: Acute dextromethorphan overdose usually does not result in serious signs and symptoms unless massive amounts have been ingested. Signs and symptoms of a substantial overdose may include nausea and vomiting, visual disturbances, CNS disturbances, and urinary retention. Symptoms from pseudo-

Age Group	0–3 mos	4–11 mos	12–23 mos	2–3 yrs	4–5 yrs	6–8 yrs	9–10 yrs	11 yrs	Dosage
Weight (lbs)	6–11 lb	12–17 lb	18–23 lb	24–35 lb	36–47 lb	48–59 lb	60–71 lb	72–95 lb	
PEDIACARE Infants' Drops*	½ dropper (0.4 ml)	1 dropper (0.8 ml)	1½ droppers (1.2 ml)	2 droppers (1.6 ml)					q4–6h
PEDIACARE Allergy Formula Liquid**				1 tsp	1½ tsp	2 tsp	2½ tsp	3 tsp	q4–6h
PEDIACARE Cough-Cold Formula Liquid**				1 tsp	1½ tsp	2 tsp	2½ tsp	3 tsp	q4–6h
Chewable Tablets**				2 tabs	3 tabs	4 tabs	5 tabs	6 tabs	q4–6h
PEDIACARE NightRest Liquid**						2 tsp	2 tsp	2 tsp	q6–8h

*Administer to children under 2 years only on the advice of a physician.
**Administer to children under 6 years only on the advice of a physician.

ephedrine overdose consist most often of mild anxiety, tachycardia and/or mild hypertension. Symptoms usually appear within 4 to 8 hours of ingestion and are transient, usually requiring no treatment. Chlorpheniramine toxicity should be treated as you would an antihistamine/anticholinergic overdose and is likely to be present within a few hours after acute ingestion.

How Supplied: PEDIACARE Cough-Cold Liquid and NightRest Cough-Cold Formula Liquid (colored red)—bottles of 4 fl. oz. with child-resistant safety cap and calibrated dosage cup. PEDIACARE Allergy Liquid (colored purple)—bottles of 4 fl. oz. with child resistant safety cap and calibrated dosage cup. PEDIACARE Cough-Cold Formula Chewable Tablets (pink, scored)—bottles of 24 with child-resistant safety cap. PEDIACARE Infants' Drops (colored red)—bottles of ½ fl. oz. with calibrated dropper.

Shown in Product Identification Section, page 416

MAXIMUM STRENGTH SINE-AID®
Sinus Headache Caplets and Tablets

Description: Each MAXIMUM STRENGTH SINE-AID® Caplet or tablet contains acetaminophen 500 mg and pseudoephedrine hydrochloride 30 mg.

Actions: MAXIMUM STRENGTH SINE-AID® Caplets and tablets contain a clinically proven analgesic-antipyretic and a decongestant. Maximum allowable non-prescription levels of acetaminophen and pseudoephedrine provide temporary relief of sinus congestion and pain. Acetaminophen is equal to aspirin in analgesic and antipyretic effectiveness and it is unlikely to produce many of the side effects associated with aspirin and aspirin-containing products. Acetaminophen produces analgesia by elevation of the pain threshold and antipyresis through action on the hypothalamic heat-regulating center. Pseudoephedrine hydrochloride is a sympathomimetic amine that promotes sinus cavity drainage by reducing nasopharyngeal mucosal congestion.

Indications: MAXIMUM STRENGTH SINE-AID® Caplets and Tablets provide effective symptomatic relief from sinus headache pain and congestion. SINE-AID® is particularly well-suited in patients with aspirin allergy, hemostatic disturbances (including anticoagulant therapy), and bleeding diatheses (e.g., hemophilia) and upper gastrointestinal disease (e.g., ulcer, gastritis, hiatus hernia).

Precautions: If a rare sensitivity occurs, the drug should be discontinued. Although pseudoephedrine is virtually without pressor effect in normotensive patients, it should be used with caution in hypertensives.

Usual Dosage: Adult dosage: Two caplets or tablets every four to six hours. Do not exceed eight caplets or tablets in any 24 hour period.

"**WARNING:** Do not exceed the recommended dosage because at higher doses nervousness, dizziness or sleeplessness may occur. Do not administer to children under 12. Do not take this product if you have heart disease, high blood pressure, thyroid disease, diabetes or difficulty in urination due to enlargement of the prostate gland unless directed by a doctor. Do not take this product for more than 7 days. If symptoms do not improve or are accompanied by high fever, consult a physician. **Do not use if carton is opened, or if printed red neck wrap or printed foil inner seal is broken. Keep this and all medication out of the reach of children. As with any drug, if you are pregnant or nursing a baby, seek the advice of a health professional before using this product. In case of accidental overdosage, contact a physician or poison control center immediately.**"

Drug Interaction Precaution: Do not take this product if you are presently taking a prescription drug for high blood pressure or depression without first consulting your doctor.

Overdosage: Acetaminophen in massive overdosage may cause hepatic toxicity in some patients. In adults and adolescents, hepatic toxicity has rarely been reported following ingestion of acute overdoses of less than 10 grams. Fatalities are infrequent (less than 3–4% of untreated cases) and have rarely been reported with overdoses of less than 15 grams. In children, an acute overdosage of less than 150 mg/kg has not been associated with hepatic toxicity.
Early symptoms following a potentially hepatotoxic overdose may include: nausea, vomiting, diaphoresis and general malaise. Clinical and laboratory evidence of hepatic toxicity may not be apparent until 48 to 72 hours postingestion.
In adults and adolescents, regardless of the quantity of acetaminophen reported to have been ingested, administer MUCOMYST® acetylcysteine immediately if 24 hours or less have elapsed from the reported time of ingestion. For full prescribing information, refer to the MUCOMYST package insert. Do not await results of assays for acetaminophen level before initiating treatment with MUCOMYST acetylcysteine. The following additional procedures are recommended: The stomach should be emptied promptly by lavage or by induction of emesis with syrup of ipecac. A serum acetaminophen assay should be obtained as early as possible, but no sooner than four hours following ingestion. Liver function studies should be obtained initially and repeated at 24-hour intervals.
Serious toxicity or fatalities are extremely infrequent in children, possibly due to differences in the way they metabolize acetaminophen. In children, the maximum potential amount ingested can be more easily estimated. If more than 150 mg/kg or an unknown amount was ingested, obtain an acetaminophen plasma level. The acetaminophen plasma level should be obtained as soon as possible, but no sooner than 4 hours following the ingestion. Induce emesis using syrup of ipecac. If the plasma level is obtained and falls above the broken line on the acetaminophen overdose nomogram, the MUCOMYST acetylcysteine therapy should be initiated and continued for a full course of therapy. If acetaminophen plasma assay capability is not available, and the estimated acetaminophen ingestion exceeds 150 mg/kg, MUCOMYST acetylcysteine therapy should be initiated and continued for a full course of therapy.
For additional emergency information, call your regional poison center or call the Rocky Mountain Poison Center toll-free (1-800-525-6115).
Symptoms from pseudoephedrine overdose consist most often of mild anxiety, tachycardia and/or mild hypertension. Symptoms usually appear within 4 to 8 hours of ingestion and are transient, usually requiring no treatment.

Inactive Ingredients: Tablets: Cellulose, magnesium stearate, sodium starch glycolate, starch.
Caplets: Cellulose, hydroxypropyl methylcellulose, magnesium stearate, polyethylene glycol, sodium starch glycolate, starch, titanium dioxide, Blue #1, and Red #40.

How Supplied: Caplets (colored white imprinted "Maximum SINE-AID")—tamper-resistant bottles of blister pack of 24 and 50.
Tablets (colored white embossed "Sine-Aid")—blister package of 24 and tamper-resistant bottles of 50 and 100.

Shown in Product Identification Section, page 416

CHILDREN'S TYLENOL®
acetaminophen
Chewable Tablets, Elixir, Drops

Description: Infants' TYLENOL acetaminophen Drops are stable, alcohol-free, fruit-flavored and orange in color. Each 0.8 ml (one calibrated dropperful) contains 80 mg acetaminophen. Children's TYLENOL Elixir is stable and alcohol-free, cherry-flavored, and red in color or grape-flavored, and purple in color. Each 5 ml contains 160 mg acetaminophen. Each Children's TYLENOL Chewable Tablet contains 80 mg acetaminophen in a grape- or fruit-flavored tablet.

Actions: Acetaminophen is a clinically proven analgesic/antipyretic. Acetaminophen produces analgesia by elevation of the pain threshold and antipyresis through action on the hypothalamic heat-regulating center. Acetaminophen is equal to aspirin in analgesic and antipyretic effectiveness and it is unlikely to produce many of the side effects associated with aspirin and aspirin-containing products.

Indications: Children's TYLENOL Chewable Tablets, Elixir and Drops are designed for treatment of infants and chil-

Continued on next page

McNeil Consumer—Cont.

dren with conditions requiring temporary relief of fever and discomfort due to colds and "flu," and of simple pain and discomfort due to teething, immunizations and tonsillectomy.

Precautions: If a rare sensitivity reaction occurs, the drug should be stopped.

Usual Dosage: All dosages may be repeated every 4 hours, but not more than 5 times daily. Administer to children under 2 years only on the advice of a physician. Children's TYLENOL Chewable Tablets: 2–3 years: two tablets; 4–5 years: three tablets; 6–8 years: four tablets; 9–10 years: five tablets; 11–12 years: six tablets.
Children's TYLENOL Elixir: (special cup for measuring dosage is provided) 4–11 months: one-half teaspoon; 12–23 months: three-quarters teaspoon; 2–3 years: one teaspoon; 4–5 years: one and one-half teaspoons; 6–8 years: 2 teaspoons; 9–10 years: two and one-half teaspoons; 11–12 years: three teaspoons.
Infants' TYLENOL Drops: 0–3 months: 0.4 ml.; 4–11 months: 0.8 ml.; 12–23 months: 1.2 ml.; 2–3 years: 1.6 ml.; 4–5 years: 2.4 ml.
Warning: Keep this and all medication out of reach of children. In case of accidental overdose, contact a physician or poison control center immediately. Consult your physician if fever persists for more than 3 days or if pain continues for more than 5 days. Store at room temperature.
NOTE: In addition to the above:
Children's TYLENOL® Drops—Do not use if printed carton overwrap or printed plastic bottle wrap is broken or missing or if carton is opened.
Children's TYLENOL Elixir—Do not use if printed carton overwrap is broken or missing or if carton is opened. Do not use if printed plastic bottle wrap or printed foil inner seal is broken. Not a USP elixir.
Children's TYLENOL Chewables—Do not use if carton is opened or if printed plastic bottle wrap or printed foil inner seal is broken. Phenylketonurics: contains phenylalanine 3 mg per tablet.

Overdosage: Acetaminophen in massive overdosage may cause hepatic toxicity in some patients. In adults and adolescents, hepatic toxicity has rarely been reported following ingestion of acute overdoses of less than 10 grams. Fatalities are infrequent (less than 3–4% of untreated cases) and have rarely been reported with overdoses of less than 15 grams. In children, an acute overdosage of less than 150 mg./kg. has not been associated with hepatic toxicity.
Early symptoms following a potentially hepatotoxic overdose may include: nausea, vomiting, diaphoresis and general malaise. Clinical and laboratory evidence of hepatic toxicity may not be apparent until 48 to 72 hours postingestion. In adults and adolescents, regardless of the quantity of acetaminophen reported to have been ingested, administer MUCOMYST® acetylcysteine immediately if 24 hours or less have elapsed from the reported time of ingestion. For full prescribing information, refer to the MUCOMYST package insert. Do not await results of assays for acetaminophen level before initiating treatment with MUCOMYST acetylcysteine. The following additional procedures are recommended: The stomach should be emptied promptly by lavage or by induction of emesis with syrup of ipecac. A serum acetaminophen assay should be obtained as early as possible, but no sooner than four hours following ingestion. Liver function studies should be obtained initially and repeated at 24-hour intervals.
Serious toxicity or fatalities are extremely infrequent in children, possibly due to differences in the way they metabolize acetaminophen. In children, the maximum potential amount ingested can be more easily estimated. If more than 150 mg./kg. or an unknown amount was ingested, obtain an acetaminophen plasma level. The acetaminophen plasma level should be obtained as soon as possible, but no sooner than 4 hours following the ingestion. Induce emesis using syrup of ipecac. If the plasma level is obtained and falls above the broken line on the acetaminophen overdose nomogram, the MUCOMYST acetylcysteine therapy should be initiated and continued for a full course of therapy. If acetaminophen plasma assay capability is not available, and the estimated acetaminophen ingestion exceeds 150 mg./kg., MUCOMYST acetylcysteine therapy should be initiated and continued for a full course of therapy.
For additional emergency information, call your regional poison center or call the Rocky Mountain Poison Center toll free (1-800-525-6115).

Inactive Ingredients: Children's TYLENOL Chewable Tablets—Aspartame, Cellulose, Citric Acid, Ethylcellulose, Flavors, Hydroxypropyl Methylcellulose, Mannitol, Starch, Magnesium Stearate, Red #7 and Blue #1 (Grape only).
Children's TYLENOL Elixir—Benzoic Acid, Citric Acid, Flavors, Glycerin, Polyethylene Glycol, Propylene Glycol, Sodium Benzoate, Sorbitol, Sucrose, Purified Water, Red #40. In addition to the above ingredients cherry-flavored elixir contains Red #33 and grape-flavored elixir contains malic acid and Blue #1.
Infant's TYLENOL Drops—Flavors, Propylene Glycol, Saccharin, Purified Water, Yellow #6.

How Supplied: Chewable Tablets (pink colored fruit, purple colored grape, scored, imprinted "TYLENOL")—Bottles of 30 and child-resistant blister packs of 48 (fruit only). Elixir (cherry colored red and grape colored purple)—bottles of 2 and 4 fl. oz. Drops (colored orange)—bottles of ½ oz. (15 ml.) with calibrated plastic dropper.
All packages listed above have child-resistant safety caps.

Shown in Product Identification Section, pages 415 and 416

Junior Strength TYLENOL® acetaminophen Coated Caplets

Description: Each Junior Strength Caplet or chewable tablet contains 160 mg acetaminophen in a small, coated, capsule-shaped tablet or a chewable tablet.

Actions: Acetaminophen is a clinically proven analgesic/antipyretic. Acetaminophen produces analgesia by elevation of the pain threshold and antipyresis through action on the hypothalamic heat-regulating center. Acetaminophen is equal to aspirin in analgesic and antipyretic effectiveness and it is unlikely to produce many of the side effects associated with aspirin and aspirin-containing products.

Indications: Junior Strength TYLENOL Caplets are designed for easy swallowability in older children and young adults. Both Junior Strength TYLENOL Caplets and Junior Strength Chewable Tablets provide fast, effective temporary relief of fever and discomfort due to colds and "flu," and pain and discomfort due to simple headaches, minor muscle aches, sprains and overexertion.

Precautions: If a rare sensitivity reaction occurs, the drug should be stopped.

Usual Dosage: Caplets should be taken with liquid. Chewable tablets should be well chewed. All dosages may be repeated every 4 hours, but not more than 5 times daily. For ages: 6–8 years: two Caplets or tablets; 9–10 years: two and one-half Caplets or tablets; 11 years: three Caplets or tablets; 12–14 years: four Caplets or tablets.
Warning: Do not use if carton is opened or if a blister unit is broken. Keep this and all medications out of the reach of children. In case of accidental overdosage, contact a physician or poison control center immediately. Consult your physician if fever persists for more than three days or if pain continues for more than five days. As with any drug, if you are pregnant or nursing a baby, seek the advice of a health professional before using this product. In addition the caplet package states: Not for children who have difficulty swallowing tablets. In addition the chewable tablet package states: Phenylketonurics: contains phenylalanine 5 mg per tablet.

Overdosage: Acetaminophen in massive overdosage may cause hepatic toxicity in some patients. In adults and adolescents, hepatic toxicity has rarely been reported following ingestion of acute overdosage of less than 10 grams. Fatalities are infrequent (less than 3–4% of untreated cases) and have rarely been reported with overdoses of less than 15 grams. In children, an acute overdosage of less than 150 mg/kg has not been associated with hepatic toxicity.
Early symptoms following a potentially hepatotoxic overdose may include: nausea, vomiting, diaphoresis and general malaise. Clinical and laboratory evidence of hepatic toxicity may not be ap-

parent until 48 to 72 hours postingestion. In adults and adolescents, regardless of the quantity of acetaminophen reported to have been ingested, administer MUCOMYST® acetylcysteine immediately if 24 hours or less have elapsed from the reported time of ingestion. For full prescribing information, refer to the MUCOMYST package insert. Do not await the results of assays for acetaminophen level before initiating treatment with MUCOMYST acetylcysteine. The following additional procedures are recommended: The stomach should be emptied promptly by lavage or by induction of emesis with syrup of ipecac. A serum acetaminophen assay should be obtained as early as possible, but no sooner than four hours following ingestion. Liver function studies should be obtained initially and repeated at 24-hour intervals.

Serious toxicity or fatalities are extremely infrequent in children, possibly due to differences in the way they metabolize acetaminophen. In children, the maximum potential amount ingested can be more easily estimated. If more than 150 mg/kg or an unknown amount was ingested, obtain an acetaminophen plasma level. The acetaminophen plasma level should be obtained as soon as possible, but no sooner than 4 hours following the ingestion. Induce emesis using syrup of ipecac. If the plasma level is obtained and falls above the broken line on the acetaminophen overdose nomogram, the MUCOMYST acetylcysteine therapy should be initiated and continued for a full course of therapy. If acetaminophen plasma assay capability is not available, and the estimated acetaminophen ingestion exceeds 150 mg/kg, MUCOMYST acetylcysteine therapy should be initiated and continued for a full course of therapy.

For additional emergency information, call your regional poison center or call the Rocky Mountain Poison Center toll-free (1-800-525-6115).

Inactive Ingredients: Caplets: Cellulose, Ethylcellulose, Magnesium Stearate, Sodium Lauryl Sulfate, Sodium Starch Glycolate, Starch.

Tablets: Aspartame, Cellulose, Citric Acid, Ethylcellulose, Flavors, Magnesium Stearate, Mannitol, Starch, Blue #1 and Red #7.

How Supplied: Coated Caplets (colored white, coated, scored, imprinted "TYLENOL 160"). Package of 30.

Chewable tablets (colored purple, imprinted "TYLENOL 160"). Package of 24. All packages are safety sealed and use child-resistant blister packaging.

Shown in Product Identification Section, page 416

Regular Strength TYLENOL® acetaminophen Tablets and Caplets

Description: Each Regular Strength TYLENOL Tablet or Caplet contains acetaminophen 325 mg.

Actions: Acetaminophen is a clinically proven analgesic and antipyretic. Acetaminophen produces analgesia by elevation of the pain threshold and antipyresis through action on the hypothalamic heat-regulating center. Acetaminophen is equal to aspirin in analgesic and antipyretic effectiveness and it is unlikely to produce many of the side effects associated with aspirin and aspirin-containing products.

Indications: Acetaminophen acts safely and quickly to provide temporary relief from: simple headache; minor muscular aches; the minor aches and pains associated with bursitis, neuralgia, sprains, overexertion, menstrual cramps; and from the discomfort of fever due to colds and "flu." Also for temporary relief of minor aches and pains of arthritis and rheumatism. Acetaminophen is particularly well suited as an analgesic-antipyretic in the presence of aspirin allergy, hemostatic disturbances (including anticoagulant therapy), and bleeding diatheses (e.g., hemophilia) and upper gastrointestinal disease (e.g., ulcer, gastritis, hiatus hernia).

Precautions: If a rare sensitivity reaction occurs, the drug should be discontinued.

Usual Dosage: Adults: One to two tablets or caplets three or four times daily. Children (6 to 12): One-half to one tablet 3 or 4 times daily. (Junior Strength TYLENOL acetaminophen Swallowable Tablets, Chewable Tablets, Elixir and Drops are available for greater convenience in younger patients.)

Warning: Do not take for pain for more than 10 days (for adult) or 5 days (for children) and do not take for fever for more than 3 days unless directed by a doctor. **Do not use if printed red neck wrap or printed foil inner seal is broken. Keep this and all medications out of the reach of children. As with any drug, if you are pregnant or nursing a baby, seek the advice of a health professional before using this product. In case of accidental overdosage, contact a doctor or poison control center immediately.**

Overdosage: Acetaminophen in massive overdosage may cause hepatic toxicity in some patients. In adults and adolescents, hepatic toxicity has rarely been reported following ingestion of acute overdoses of less than 10 grams. Fatalities are infrequent (less than 3–4% of untreated cases) and have rarely been reported with overdoses of less than 15 grams. In children, an acute overdosage of less than 150 mg/kg has not been associated with hepatic toxicity.

Early symptoms following a potentially hepatotoxic overdose may include: nausea, vomiting, diaphoresis and general malaise. Clinical and laboratory evidence of hepatic toxicity may not be apparent until 48 to 72 hours postingestion. In adults and adolescents, regardless of the quantity of acetaminophen reported to have been ingested, administer MUCOMYST® acetylcysteine immediately if 24 hours or less have elapsed from the reported time of ingestion. For full prescribing information, refer to the MUCOMYST package insert. Do not await results of assays for acetaminophen level before initiating treatment with MUCOMYST acetylcysteine. The following additional procedures are recommended: The stomach should be emptied promptly by lavage or by induction of emesis with syrup of ipecac. A serum acetaminophen assay should be obtained as early as possible, but no sooner than four hours following ingestion. Liver function studies should be obtained initially and repeated at 24-hour intervals.

Serious toxicity or fatalities are extremely infrequent in children, possibly due to differences in the way they metabolize acetaminophen. In children, the maximum potential amount ingested can be more easily estimated. If more than 150 mg/kg or an unknown amount was ingested, obtain an acetaminophen plasma level. The acetaminophen plasma level should be obtained as soon as possible, but no sooner than 4 hours following the ingestion. Induce emesis using syrup of ipecac. If the plasma level is obtained and falls above the broken line on the acetaminophen overdose nomogram, the MUCOMYST acetylcysteine therapy should be initiated and continued for a full course of therapy. If acetaminophen plasma assay capability is not available, and the estimated acetaminophen ingestion exceeds 150 mg/kg, MUCOMYST acetylcysteine therapy should be initiated and continued for a full course of therapy.

For additional emergency information, call your regional poison center or call the Rocky Mountain Poison Center toll-free (1-800-525-6115).

Inactive Ingredients: Tablets—Calcium Stearate or Magnesium Stearate, Cellulose, Docusate Sodium and Sodium Benzoate or Sodium Lauryl Sulfate, and Starch. Caplets—Cellulose, Hydroxpropyl Methylcellulose, Magnesium Stearate, Polyethylene Glycol, Sodium Starch Glycolate and Starch.

How Supplied: Tablets (colored white, scored, imprinted "TYLENOL")—tins and vials of 12, and tamper-resistant bottles of 24, 50, 100 and 200. Caplets (colored white, "TYLENOL")—tamper-resistant bottles of 24, 50, 100. For additional pain relief, Extra-Strength TYLENOL® Tablets and Caplets, 500 mg, and Extra-Strength TYLENOL® Adult Liquid Pain Reliever are available (colored green; 1 fl. oz. = 1000 mg.)

Shown in Product Identification Section, page 415

Extra-Strength TYLENOL® acetaminophen Caplets, Gelcaps, Tablets

Description: Each Extra-Strength TYLENOL Caplet, Gelcap or Tablet contains acetaminophen 500 mg.

Continued on next page

McNeil Consumer—Cont.

Actions: Acetaminophen is a clinically proven analgesic and antipyretic. Acetaminophen produces analgesia by elevation of the pain threshold and antipyresis through action on the hypothalamic heat-regulating center. Acetaminophen is equal to aspirin in analgesic and antipyretic effectiveness and it is unlikely to produce many of the side effects associated with aspirin and aspirin-containing products.

Indications: For the temporary relief of minor aches, pains, headaches and fever.

Precautions: If a rare sensitivity reaction occurs, the drug should be discontinued.

Usual Dosage: Adults: Two Caplets, Gelcaps or Tablets 3 or 4 times daily. No more than a total of eight Caplets, Gelcaps or Tablets in any 24-hour period.
Warning: Do not take for more than 10 days or for fever for more than 3 days unless directed by a doctor. Severe or recurrent pain or high or continued fever may be indicative of serious illness. Under these conditions, consult a doctor. **Do not use if printed red neck wrap or printed foil inner seal is broken. Keep this and all medication out of the reach of children. As with any drug, if you are pregnant or nursing a baby, seek the advice of a health professional before using this product. In case of accidental overdosage, contact a doctor or poison control center immediately.**

Overdosage: Acetaminophen in massive overdosage may cause hepatic toxicity in some patients. In adults and adolescents, hepatic toxicity has rarely been reported following ingestion of acute overdosage of less than 10 grams. Fatalities are infrequent (less than 3–4% of untreated cases) and have rarely been reported with overdoses of less than 15 grams. In children, an acute overdosage of less than 150 mg/kg has not been associated with hepatic toxicity.
Early symptoms following a potentially hepatotoxic overdose may include: nausea, vomiting, diaphoresis and general malaise. Clinical and laboratory evidence of hepatic toxicity may not be apparent until 48 to 72 hours postingestion.
In adults and adolescents, regardless of the quantity of acetaminophen reported to have been ingested, administer MUCOMYST® acetylcysteine immediately if 24 hours or less have elapsed from the reported time of ingestion. For full prescribing information, refer to the MUCOMYST package insert. Do not await the results of assays for acetaminophen level before initiating treatment with MUCOMYST acetylcysteine. The following additional procedures are recommended: The stomach should be emptied promptly by lavage or by induction of emesis with syrup of ipecac. A serum acetaminophen assay should be obtained as early as possible, but no sooner than four hours following ingestion. Liver function studies should be obtained initially and repeated at 24-hour intervals.
Serious toxicity or fatalities are extremely infrequent in children, possibly due to differences in the way they metabolize acetaminophen. In children, the maximum potential amount ingested can be more easily estimated. If more than 150 mg/kg or an unknown amount was ingested, obtain an acetaminophen plasma level. The acetaminophen plasma level should be obtained as soon as possible, but no sooner than 4 hours following the ingestion. Induce emesis using syrup of ipecac. If the plasma level is obtained and falls above the broken line on the acetaminophen overdose nomogram, the MUCOMYST acetylcysteine therapy should be initiated and continued for a full course of therapy. If acetaminophen plasma assay capability is not available, and the estimated acetaminophen ingestion exceeds 150 mg/kg, MUCOMYST acetylcysteine therapy should be initiated and continued for a full course of therapy.
For additional emergency information, call your regional poison center or call the Rocky Mountain Poison Center toll-free (1-800-525-6115).

Inactive Ingredients: Tablets—Calcium Stearate or Magnesium Stearate, Cellulose, Docusate Sodium and Sodium Benzoate or Sodium Lauryl Sulfate and Starch.
Caplets — Cellulose, Hydroxypropyl Methylcellulose, Magnesium Stearate, Polyethylene Glycol, Sodium Starch Glycolate, Starch and Red #40.
Gelcaps—Benzyl Alcohol, Butylparaben, Castor Oil, Cellulose, Edetate Calcium Disodium, Gelatin, Hydroxypropyl Methylcellulose, Magnesium Stearate, Methylparaben, Propylparaben, Sodium Lauryl Sulfate, Sodium Propionate, Sodium Starch Glycolate, Starch, Titanium Dioxide, Blue #1 and #2, Red #40 and Yellow #10.

How Supplied: Tablets (colored white, imprinted "TYLENOL" and "500")—vials of 10 and tamper-resistant bottles of 30, 60, 100, and 200.
Caplets (colored white, imprinted "TYLENOL 500 mg")—vials of 10 and tamper-resistant bottles of 24, 50, 100, 175, and 250's.
Gelcaps (colored yellow and red, imprinted "Tylenol 500") tamper-resistant bottles of 24, 50 and 100. For adults who prefer liquids or can't swallow solid medication, Extra-Strength TYLENOL® Adult Liquid Pain Reliever, mint flavored, is also available (colored green; 1 fl. oz. = 1000 mg).

Shown in Product Identification Section, page 415

Extra-Strength TYLENOL® acetaminophen Adult Liquid Pain Reliever

Description: Each 15 ml. (½ fl. oz. or one tablespoonful) contains 500 mg acetaminophen (alcohol 7%).

Actions: TYLENOL acetaminophen is a clinically proven analgesic and antipyretic. Acetaminophen produces analgesia by elevation of the pain threshold and antipyresis through action on the hypothalamic heat-regulating center. Acetaminophen is equal to aspirin in analgesic and antipyretic effectiveness and it is unlikely to produce many of the side effects associated with aspirin and aspirin-containing products.

Indications: Acetaminophen provides temporary relief of minor aches, pains, headaches and fevers.

Precautions: If a rare sensitivity reaction occurs, the drug should be discontinued.

Usual Dosage: Extra-Strength TYLENOL Adult Liquid Pain Reliever is an adult preparation for those adults who prefer liquids or can't swallow solid medication. Not for use in children under 12. Measuring cup is marked for accurate dosage. Extra-Strength Dose—1 fl. oz. (30 ml or 2 tablespoonsful, 1000 mg), which is equivalent to two 500 mg Extra-Strength TYLENOL Tablets or Caplets. Take every 4–6 hours, no more than 4 doses in any 24-hour period.
"**Warning:** Do not exceed recommended dosage. Consult a physician for use longer than 10 days. Severe or recurrent pain or high or continued fever may be indicative of serious illness. Under these conditions, consult a physician. **Do not use if printed plastic overwrap or printed foil inner seal is broken. Keep this and all medication out of the reach of children. As with any drug, if you are pregnant or nursing a baby, seek the advice of a health professional before using this product. In case of accidental overdosage, contact a doctor or poison control center immediately.**"

Overdosage: Acetaminophen in massive overdosage may cause hepatic toxicity in some patients. In adults and adolescents, hepatic toxicity has rarely been reported following ingestion of acute overdosage of less than 10 grams. Fatalities are infrequent (less than 3–4% of untreated cases) and have rarely been reported with overdoses of less than 15 grams. In children, an acute overdosage of less than 150 mg/kg has not been associated with hepatic toxicity.
Early symptoms following a potentially hepatotoxic overdose may include: nausea, vomiting, diaphoresis and general malaise. Clinical and laboratory evidence of hepatic toxicity may not be apparent until 48 to 72 hours postingestion.
In adults and adolescents, regardless of the quantity of acetaminophen reported to have been ingested, administer MUCOMYST® acetylcysteine immediately if 24 hours or less have elapsed from the reported time of ingestion. For full prescribing information, refer to the MUCOMYST package insert. Do not await the results of assays for acetaminophen level before initiating treatment with MUCOMYST acetylcysteine. The following additional procedures are

recommended: The stomach should be emptied promptly by lavage or by induction of emesis with syrup of ipecac. A serum acetaminophen assay should be obtained as early as possible, but no sooner than four hours following ingestion. Liver function studies should be obtained initially and repeated at 24-hour intervals.
Serious toxicity or fatalities are extremely infrequent in children, possibly due to differences in the way they metabolize acetaminophen. In children, the maximum potential amount ingested can be more easily estimated. If more than 150 mg/kg or an unknown amount was ingested, obtain an acetaminophen plasma level. The acetaminophen plasma level should be obtained as soon as possible, but no sooner than 4 hours following the ingestion. Induce emesis using syrup of ipecac. If the plasma level is obtained and falls above the broken line on the acetaminophen overdose nomogram, the MUCOMYST acetylcysteine therapy should be initiated and continued for a full course of therapy. If acetaminophen plasma assay capability is not available, and the estimated acetaminophen ingestion exceeds 150 mg/kg, MUCOMYST acetylcysteine therapy should be initiated and continued for a full course of therapy.
For additional emergency information, call your regional poison center or call the Rocky Mountain Poison Center toll-free (1-800-525-6115).

Inactive Ingredients: Alcohol, Citric Acid, Flavors, Glycerin, Polyethylene Glycol, Purified Water, Sodium Benzoate, Sorbitol, Sucrose, Yellow #6 (Sunset Yellow), Yellow #10 and Blue #1.

How Supplied: Mint-flavored liquid (colored green), 8 fl. oz. tamper-resistant bottle with child-resistant safety cap and special dosage cup.

CHILDREN'S TYLENOL COLD®
Chewable Cold Tablets and Liquid Cold Formula

Description: Each Children's Tylenol Cold Chewable Grape-Flavored Tablet contains acetaminophen 80 mg, chlorpheniramine maleate 0.5 mg and pseudoephedrine hydrochloride 7.5 mg. Children's Tylenol Cold Liquid Formula is grape flavored, and contains no alcohol. Each teaspoon (5 ml) contains acetaminophen 160 mg, chlorpheniramine maleate 1 mg, and pseudoephedrine hydrochloride 15 mg.

Actions: Children's Tylenol Cold Chewable Tablets and Liquid combine the analgesic-antipyretic acetaminophen with the decongestant pseudoephedrine hydrochloride and the antihistamine chlorpheniramine maleate to help relieve nasal congestion, dry runny noses and prevent sneezing as well as to relieve the fever, aches, pains and general discomfort associated with colds and upper respiratory infections.
Acetaminophen is equal to aspirin in analgesic and antipyretic effectiveness and it is unlikely to produce the side effects often associated with aspirin or aspirin-containing products.

Indications: Provides fast, effective temporary relief of nasal congestion, runny nose, sneezing, minor aches and pains, headaches and fever due to the common cold, hay fever or other upper respiratory allergies.

Usual Dosage: Administer to children under 6 years only on the advice of a physician. Children's Tylenol Cold Chewable Tablets: 2–5 years—2 tablets, 6–11 years—4 tablets.
Children's Tylenol Cold Liquid Formula: 2–5 years—1 teaspoonful; 6–11 years—2 teaspoonsful. Measuring cup is provided and marked for accurate dosing.
Doses may be repeated every 4-6 hours as needed, not to exceed 4 doses in 24 hours.
The Warnings are identical for the two dosage forms except the Liquid Cold Formula does not contain the phenylketonurics statement since the product does not contain aspartame.

Warning: Do not use if carton is opened, or if printed plastic bottle wrap or printed foil inner seal is broken.
Keep this and all medication out of the reach of children. In case of accidental overdosage, contact a physician or poison control center immediately. Phenylketonurics: contains phenylalanine, 4 mg per tablet. Do not exceed the recommended dosage because nervousness, dizziness or sleeplessness may occur. If fever persists for more than three days, or if symptoms do not improve or new ones occur within five days or are accompanied by high fever, consult a physician before continuing use. This preparation may cause drowsiness, or in some cases, excitability. Do not give this product to children who have heart disease, high blood pressure, thyroid disease, diabetes, glaucoma or asthma or are taking a prescription drug for high blood pressure or depression, except under the advice and supervision of a physician.

Overdosage: Acetaminophen in massive overdosage may cause hepatic toxicity in some patients. In adults and adolescents, hepatic toxicity has rarely been reported following ingestion of acute overdosage of less than 10 grams. Fatalities are infrequent (less than 3–4% of untreated cases) and have rarely been reported with overdoses of less than 15 grams. In children, an acute overdosage of less than 150 mg/kg has not been associated with hepatic toxicity.
Early symptoms following a potentially hepatotoxic overdose may include: nausea, vomiting, diaphoresis and general malaise. Clinical and laboratory evidence of hepatic toxicity may not be apparent until 48 to 72 hours postingestion.
In adults and adolescents, regardless of the quantity of acetaminophen reported to have been ingested, administer MUCOMYST® acetylcysteine immediately if 24 hours or less have elapsed from the reported time of ingestion. For full prescribing information, refer to the MUCOMYST package insert. Do not await the results of assays for acetaminophen level before initiating treatment with MUCOMYST acetylcysteine. The following additional procedures are recommended: The stomach should be emptied promptly by lavage or by induction of emesis with syrup of ipecac. A serum acetaminophen assay should be obtained as early as possible, but no sooner than four hours following ingestion. Liver function studies should be obtained initially and repeated at 24-hour intervals.
Serious toxicity or fatalities are extremely infrequent in children, possibly due to differences in the way they metabolize acetaminophen. In children, the maximum potential amount ingested can be more easily estimated. If more than 150 mg/kg or an unknown amount was ingested, obtain an acetaminophen plasma level. The acetaminophen plasma level should be obtained as soon as possible, but no sooner than 4 hours following the ingestion. Induce emesis using syrup of ipecac. If the plasma level is obtained and falls above the broken line on the acetaminophen overdose nomogram, the MUCOMYST acetylcysteine therapy should be initiated and continued for a full course of therapy. If acetaminophen plasma assay capability is not available, and the estimated acetaminophen ingestion exceeds 150 mg/kg, MUCOMYST acetylcysteine therapy should be initiated and continued for a full course of therapy.
For additional emergency information, call your regional poison center or call the Rocky Mountain Poison Center toll-free (1-800-525-6115).
Chlorpheniramine toxicity should be treated as you would an antihistamine/anticholinergic overdose and is likely to be present within a few hours after acute ingestion.
Symptoms from pseudoephedrine overdose consist most often of mild anxiety, tachycardia and/or mild hypertension. Symptoms usually appear within 4 to 8 hours of ingestion and are transient, usually requiring no treatment.

Inactive Ingredients: Chewable Tablets—Aspartame, citric acid, ethylcellulose, flavors, magnesium stearate, mannitol, microcrystalline cellulose, pregelatinized starch, sucrose, Blue #1 and Red #7.
Liquid—Benzoic acid, citric acid, flavors, glycerin, malic acid, polyethylene glycol, propylene glycol, sodium benzoate, sorbitol, sucrose, purified water, Blue #1 and Red #40.

How Supplied: Chewable Tablets (colored purple, scored, imprinted "Tylenol Cold" on one side and "TC" on opposite side)—bottles of 24. Cold Formula—bottles (colored purple) of 4 fl. oz.

Shown in Product Identification Section, page 417

Continued on next page

McNeil Consumer—Cont.

Fast Acting Effervescent TYLENOL® Cold Medication Tablets

Description: Each Effervescent TYLENOL Cold Tablet contains acetaminophen 325 mg., chlorpheniramine maleate 2 mg., and phenylpropanolamine hydrochloride 12.5 mg.

Actions: TYLENOL Cold Medication Tablets contain a clinically proven analgesic-antipyretic, decongestant and antihistamine. Acetaminophen produces analgesia by elevation of the pain threshold and antipyresis through action on the hypothalamic heat-regulating center. Acetaminophen is equal to aspirin in analgesic and antipyretic effectiveness and it is unlikely to produce many of the side effects associated with aspirin and aspirin-containing products. Phenylpropanolamine is a sympathomimetic amine which provides temporary relief of nasal congestion. Chlorpheniramine is an antihistamine which helps provide temporary relief of runny nose, sneezing and watery and itchy eyes.

Indications: TYLENOL Cold Medication provides effective temporary relief of runny nose, sneezing, watery and itchy eyes, nasal congestion, and aches, pains, sore throat and fever due to a cold or "flu."

Precautions: If a rare sensitivity reaction occurs, the drug should be stopped. Although phenylpropanolamine is virtually without pressor effect in normotensive patients, it should be used with caution in hypertensives.

Usual Dosage:
Effervescent TYLENOL® Cold must be dissolved in water before taking.
ADULTS (12 years and over): 2 tablets every 4 hours, not to exceed 12 tablets in 24 hours.
CHILDREN (6–11): 1 tablet every 4 hours, not to exceed 6 tablets in 24 hours.
"**WARNINGS:** Do not administer to children under 6. Do not take this product for more than 7 days (Adults) or 5 days (Children) or for fever for more than 3 days unless directed by a doctor. Do not exceed recommended dosage because at higher doses nervousness, dizziness or sleeplessness may occur. May cause excitability, especially in children. May cause drowsiness; alcohol may increase the drowsiness effect. Avoid alcoholic beverages while taking this product. Use caution when driving a motor vehicle or operating machinery. Do not take this product if you have asthma, glaucoma, emphysema, chronic pulmonary disease, shortness of breath, difficulty in breathing, heart disease, high blood pressure, thyroid disease, diabetes or difficulty in urination due to enlargement of the prostate gland unless directed by a doctor. DO NOT USE IF GLUED CARTON FLAP IS OPENED OR IF FOIL PACK IS TORN OR BROKEN. **KEEP THIS AND ALL MEDICATION OUT OF THE REACH OF CHILDREN. AS WITH ANY DRUG, IF YOU ARE PREGNANT OR NURSING A BABY, SEEK THE ADVICE OF A HEALTH PROFESSIONAL BEFORE USING THIS PRODUCT. IN CASE OF ACCIDENTAL OVERDOSAGE, CONTACT A PHYSICIAN OR POISON CONTROL CENTER IMMEDIATELY. DO NOT TAKE THIS PRODUCT IF YOU ARE ON A SODIUM RESTRICTED DIET, EXCEPT UNDER THE ADVICE AND SUPERVISION OF A DOCTOR. EACH TABLET CONTAINS 525 MG. OF SODIUM.**
DRUG INTERACTION PRECAUTION: Do not take this product if you are presently taking a prescription drug for high blood pressure or depression without first consulting your doctor."

Overdosage: Acetaminophen in massive overdosage may cause hepatic toxicity in some patients. In adults and adolescents, hepatic toxicity has rarely been reported following ingestion of acute overdosage of less than 10 grams. Fatalities are infrequent (less than 3–4% of untreated cases) and have rarely been reported with overdoses of less than 15 grams. In children, an acute overdosage of less than 150 mg/kg has not been associated with hepatic toxicity.
Early symptoms following a potentially hepatotoxic overdose may include: nausea, vomiting, diaphoresis and general malaise. Clinical and laboratory evidence of hepatic toxicity may not be apparent until 48 to 72 hours postingestion.
In adults and adolescents, regardless of the quantity of acetaminophen reported to have been ingested, administer MUCOMYST® acetylcysteine immediately if 24 hours or less have elapsed from the reported time of ingestion. For full prescribing information, refer to the MUCOMYST package insert. Do not await results of assays for acetaminophen level before initiating treatment with MUCOMYST acetylcysteine. The following additional procedures are recommended: The stomach should be emptied promptly by lavage or by induction of emesis with syrup of ipecac. A serum acetaminophen assay should be obtained as early as possible, but no sooner than four hours following ingestion. Liver function studies should be obtained initially and repeated at 24-hour intervals.
Serious toxicity or fatalities are extremely infrequent in children, possibly due to differences in the way they metabolize acetaminophen. In children, the maximum potential amount ingested can be more easily estimated. If more than 150 mg/kg or an unknown amount was ingested, obtain an acetaminophen plasma level. The acetaminophen plasma level should be obtained as soon as possible, but no sooner than 4 hours following the ingestion. Induce emesis using syrup of ipecac. If the plasma level is obtained and falls above the broken line on the acetaminophen overdose nomogram, the MUCOMYST acetylcysteine therapy should be initiated and continued for a full course of therapy. If acetaminophen plasma assay capability is not available, and the estimated acetaminophen ingestion exceeds 150 mg/kg, MUCOMYST acetylcysteine therapy should be initiated and continued for a full course of therapy.
For additional emergency information, call your regional poison center or call the Rocky Mountain Poison Center toll-free, (1-800-525-6115).
Symptoms from phenylpropanolamine overdose consist most often of mild anxiety, tachycardia and/or mild hypertension. Symptoms usually appear within 4 to 8 hours of ingestion and are transient, usually requiring no treatment.
Inactive Ingredients: Citric Acid, Flavor, Potassium Benzoate, Povidone, Saccharin, Sodium Bicarbonate, Sodium Carbonate, Sodium Docusate, Sorbitol.

How Supplied: Tablets: carton of 20 tablets in 10 foil twin packs; carton of 36 tablets in 18 foil twin packs.

Shown in Product Identification Section, page 416

Hot Medication TYLENOL® Cold & Flu Medication Packets

Description: Each packet of TYLENOL Cold & Flu contains acetaminophen 650 mg., chlorpheniramine maleate 4 mg., pseudoephedrine hydrochloride 60 mg. and dextromethorphan hydrobromide 30 mg.

Actions: TYLENOL Cold and Flu Medication contains a clinically proven analgesic-antipyretic, decongestant, cough suppressant and antihistamine. Acetaminophen produces analgesia by elevation of the pain threshold and antipyresis through action on the hypothalamic heat-regulating center. Acetaminophen is equal to aspirin in analgesic and antipyretic effectiveness and it is unlikely to produce many of the side effects associated with aspirin and aspirin-containing products. Pseudoephedrine hydrochloride is a sympathomimetic amine which provides temporary relief of nasal congestion. Dextromethorphan is a cough suppressant which provides temporary relief of coughs due to minor throat irritations that may occur with the common cold. Chlorpheniramine is an antihistamine which helps provide temporary relief of runny nose, sneezing and watery and itchy eyes.

Indications: TYLENOL Cold and Flu Medication provides effective temporary relief of runny nose, sneezing, watery and itchy eyes, nasal congestion, coughing, and aches, pains, sore throat and fever due to a cold or "flu."

Precautions: If a rare sensitivity reaction occurs, the drug should be stopped. Although pseudoephedrine is virtually without pressor effect in normotensive patients, it should be used with caution in hypertensives.

Usual Dosage: Adults (12 years and over): Dissolve one packet in 6 oz. cup of hot water. Sip while hot. Sweeten to taste, if desired. May repeat every 6 hours, not to exceed 4 doses in 24 hours.

"**WARNINGS:** Not recommended for children under 12. Do not take this product for more than 7 days or for fever for more than 3 days unless directed by a doctor. If symptoms do not improve or are accompanied by fever, consult a doctor. A persistent cough may be a sign of a serious condition. If cough persists for more than 1 week, tends to recur or is accompanied by fever, rash or persistent headache, consult a doctor. Do not take this product for persistent or chronic cough such as occurs with smoking, asthma, emphysema, or if cough is accompanied by excessive phlegm (mucus) unless directed by a doctor. Do not exceed recommended dosage because at higher doses nervousness, dizziness, or sleeplessness may occur. May cause excitability, expecially in children. Do not take this product if you have asthma, glaucoma, heart disease, high blood pressure, emphysema, chronic pulmonary disease, shortness of breath, difficulty in breathing, diabetes, thyroid disease or difficulty in urination due to enlargement of the prostate gland unless directed by a doctor. May cause drowsiness, alcohol may increase the drowsiness effect. Avoid alcoholic beverages while taking this product. Use caution when driving a motor vehicle or operating machinery.

DO NOT USE IF GLUED CARTON FLAP IS OPENED OR IF FOIL PACKET IS TORN OR BROKEN. KEEP THIS AND ALL MEDICATION OUT OF THE REACH OF CHILDREN. AS WITH ANY DRUG, IF YOU ARE PREGNANT OR NURSING A BABY, SEEK THE ADVICE OF A HEALTH PROFESSIONAL BEFORE USING THIS PRODUCT. IN CASE OF ACCIDENTAL OVERDOSAGE, CONTACT A PHYSICIAN OR POISON CONTROL CENTER IMMEDIATELY. PHENYLKETONURICS: CONTAINS PHENYLALANINE 11 MG PER PACKET.

DRUG INTERACTION PRECAUTION: Do not take this product if you are presently taking a prescription drug for high blood pressure or depression without first consulting your doctor."

Overdoasge: Acetaminophen in massive overdosage may cause hepatic toxicity in some patients. In adults and adolescents, hepatic toxicity has rarely been reported following ingestion of acute overdosage of less than 10 grams. Fatalities are infrequent (less than 3–4% of untreated cases) and have rarely been reported with overdoses of less than 15 grams. In children, an acute overdosage of less than 150 mg/kg has not been associated with hepatic toxicity.

Early symptoms following a potentially hepatotoxic overdose may include: nausea, vomiting, diaphoresis and general malaise. Clinical and laboratory evidence of hepatic toxicity may not be apparent until 48 to 72 hours postingestion. In adults and adolescents, regardless of the quantity of acetaminophen reported to have been ingested, administer MUCOMYST® acetylcysteine immediately if 24 hours or less have elapsed from the reported time of ingestion. For full prescribing information, refer to the MUCOMYST package insert. Do not await results of assays for acetaminophen level before initiating treatment with MUCOMYST acetylcysteine. The following additional procedures are recommended: The stomach should be emptied promptly by lavage or by induction of emesis with syrup of ipecac. A serum acetaminophen assay should be obtained as early as possible, but no sooner than four hours following ingestion. Liver function studies should be obtained initially and repeated at 24-hour intervals.

Serious toxicity or fatalities are extremely infrequent in children, possibly due to differences in the way they metabolize acetaminophen. In children, the maximum potential amount ingested can be more easily estimated. If more than 150 mg/kg or an unknown amount was ingested, obtain an acetaminophen plasma level. The acetaminophen plasma level should be obtained as soon as possible, but no sooner than 4 hours following the ingestion. Induce emesis using syrup of ipecac. If the plasma level is obtained and falls above the broken line on the acetaminophen overdose nomogram, the MUCOMYST acetylcysteine therapy should be initiated and continued for a full course of therapy. If acetaminophen plasma assay capability is not available, and the estimated acetaminophen ingestion exceeds 150 mg/kg, MUCOMYST acetylcysteine therapy should be initiated and continued for a full course of therapy.

For additional emergency information, call your regional poison center or call the Rocky Mountain Poison Center toll-free, (1-800-525-6115).

Symptoms from pseudoephedrine overdose consist most often of mild anxiety, tachycardia and/or mild hypertension. Symptoms usually appear within 4 to 8 hours of ingestion and are transient, usually requiring no treatment.

Acute dextromethorphan overdose usually does not result in serious signs and symptoms unless massive amounts have been ingested. Signs and symptoms of a substantial overdose may include nausea and vomiting, visual disturbances, CNS disturbances, and urinary retention.

Chlorpheniramine toxicity should be treated as you would an antihistamine/anticholinergic overdose and is likely to be present within a few hours after acute ingestion.

Inactive Ingredients: Aspartame, Citric Acid, Flavors, Sodium Citrate, Starch, Sucrose, Tribasic Calcium Phosphate, Red #40 and Yellow #10.

How Supplied: Packets of powder (yellow colored) cartons of 6 foil packets and cartons of 12 tamper-resistant foil cartons.

Shown in Product Identification Section, page 416

Multisymptom TYLENOL® Cold Medication Tablets and Caplets

Description: Each TYLENOL Cold Tablet or Caplet contains acetaminophen 325 mg., chlorpheniramine maleate 2 mg., pseudoephedrine hydrochloride 30 mg. and dextromethorphan hydrobromide 15 mg.

Actions: TYLENOL Cold Medication Tablets and Caplets contain a clinically proven analgesic-antipyretic, decongestant, cough suppressant and antihistamine. Acetaminophen produces analgesia by elevation of the pain threshold and antipyresis through action on the hypothalamic heat-regulating center. Acetaminophen is equal to aspirin in analgesic and antipyretic effectiveness and it is unlikely to produce many of the side effects associated with aspirin and aspirin-containing products. Pseudoephedrine hydrochloride is a sympathomimetic amine which provides temporary relief of nasal congestion. Dextromethorphan is a cough suppressant which provides temporary relief of coughs due to minor throat irritations that may occur with the common cold. Chlorpheniramine is an antihistamine which helps provide temporary relief of runny nose, sneezing and watery and itchy eyes.

Indications: TYLENOL Cold Medication provides effective temporary relief of runny nose, sneezing, watery and itchy eyes, nasal congestion, coughing, and aches, pains and fever due to a cold or "flu."

Precautions: If a rare sensitivity reaction occurs, the drug should be stopped. Although pseudoephedrine is virtually without pressor effect in normotensive patients, it should be used with caution in hypertensives.

Usual Dosage: Adults: Two tablets or caplets every 6 hours, not to exceed 8 tablets or caplets in 24 hours. Children (6–12 years): One caplet or tablet every 6 hours, not to exceed 4 tablets or caplets in 24 hours for 5 days.

WARNING: Do not administer to children under 6 or exceed the recommended dosage because nervousness, dizziness or sleeplessness may occur. May cause excitability especially in children. Do not take this product for more than 7 days. If fever persists for more than three days, or if symptoms do not improve or are accompanied by high fever, consult a physician. A persistent cough may be a sign of a serious condition. If cough persists for more than 1 week, tends to recur or is accompanied by fever, rash or persistent headache, consult a physician. Do not take this product for persistent or chronic cough such as occurs with smoking, asthma, emphysema or if cough is accompanied by excessive phlegm (mucus) unless directed by a physician. This preparation may cause drowsiness; alcohol may increase the drowsiness effect. Avoid alcoholic beverages when taking this product. Use caution when driving a

Continued on next page

McNeil Consumer—Cont.

motor vehicle or operating machinery. Do not take this product if you have heart disease, high blood pressure, thyroid disease, diabetes, asthma, glaucoma, emphysema, chronic pulmonary disease, shortness of breath, difficulty in breathing, or difficulty in urination due to enlargement of the prostate gland or are taking a prescription drug for high blood pressure or depression, unless directed by a doctor. **Do not use if carton is opened, or if printed green neck wrap or printed foil inner seal is broken. Keep this and all medication out of the reach of children. As with any drug, if you are pregnant or nursing a baby, seek the advice of a health professional before using this product. In case of accidental overdosage, contact a physician or poison control center immediately.**

Drug Interaction Precaution: Do not take this product if you are presently taking a prescription drug for high blood pressure or depression without first consulting your physician.

Overdosage: Acetaminophen in massive overdosage may cause hepatic toxicity in some patients. In adults and adolescents, hepatic toxicity has rarely been reported following ingestion of acute overdosage of less than 10 grams. Fatalities are infrequent (less than 3–4% of untreated cases) and have rarely been reported with overdoses of less than 15 grams. In children, an acute overdosage of less than 150 mg/kg has not been associated with hepatic toxicity.

Early symptoms following a potentially hepatotoxic overdose may include: nausea, vomiting, diaphoresis and general malaise. Clinical and laboratory evidence of hepatic toxicity may not be apparent until 48 to 72 hours postingestion.

In adults and adolescents, regardless of the quantity of acetaminophen reported to have been ingested, administer MUCOMYST® acetylcysteine immediately if 24 hours or less have elapsed from the reported time of ingestion. For full prescribing information, refer to the MUCOMYST package insert. Do not await results of assays for acetaminophen level before initiating treatment with MUCOMYST acetylcysteine. The following additional procedures are recommended: The stomach should be emptied promptly by lavage or by induction of emesis with syrup of ipecac. A serum acetaminophen assay should be obtained as early as possible, but no sooner than four hours following ingestion. Liver function studies should be obtained initially and repeated at 24-hour intervals.

Serious toxicity or fatalities are extremely infrequent in children, possibly due to differences in the way they metabolize acetaminophen. In children, the maximum potential amount ingested can be more easily estimated. If more than 150 mg/kg or an unknown amount was ingested, obtain an acetaminophen plasma level. The acetaminophen plasma level should be obtained as soon as possible, but no sooner than 4 hours following the ingestion. Induce emesis using syrup of ipecac. If the plasma level is obtained and falls above the broken line on the acetaminophen overdose nomogram, the MUCOMYST acetylcysteine therapy should be initiated and continued for a full course of therapy. If acetaminophen plasma assay capability is not available, and the estimated acetaminophen ingestion exceeds 150 mg/kg, MUCOMYST acetylcysteine therapy should be initiated and continued for a full course of therapy.

For additional emergency information, call your regional poison center or call the Rocky Mountain Poison Center toll-free (1-800-525-6115).

Chlorpheniramine toxicity should be treated as you would an antihistamine/anticholinergic overdose and is likely to be present within a few hours after acute ingestion.

Symptoms from pseudoephedrine overdose consist most often of mild anxiety, tachycardia and/or mild hypertension. Symptoms usually appear within 4 to 8 hours of ingestion and are transient, usually requiring no treatment.

Acute dextromethorphan overdose usually does not result in serious signs and symptoms unless massive amounts have been ingested. Signs and symptoms of a substantial overdose may include nausea and vomiting, visual disturbances, CNS disturbances, and urinary retention.

Inactive Ingredients: Tablets: Cellulose, Starch, Magnesium Stearate, Yellow #6 and Yellow #10. Caplets: Cellulose, Glyceryl Triacetate, Hydroxypropyl Methylcellulose, Magnesium Stearate, Sodium Starch Glycolate, Starch, Titanium Dioxide, Blue #1 and Yellow #6 and #10.

How Supplied: Tablets (colored yellow, imprinted "TYLENOL Cold")—blister packs of 24 and tamper-resistant bottles of 50. Caplets (light yellow, imprinted "TYLENOL Cold")—blister packs of 24 and tamper-resistant bottles of 50.

Shown in Product Identification Section, page 416

TYLENOL® Cold Medication No Drowsiness Formula Caplets

Description: Each TYLENOL Cold Medication No Drowsiness Formula Caplet contains acetaminophen 325 mg., pseudoephedrine hydrochloride 30 mg. and dextromethorphan hydrobromide 15 mg.

Actions: TYLENOL Cold Medication No Drowsiness Formula Caplets contain a clinically proven analgesic-antipyretic, decongestant and cough suppressant. Acetaminophen produces analgesia by elevation of the pain threshold and antipyresis through action on the hypothalamic heat-regulating center. Acetaminophen is equal to aspirin in analgesic and antipyretic effectiveness and it is unlikely to produce many of the side effects associated with aspirin and aspirin-containing products. Pseudoephedrine hydrochloride is a sympathomimetic amine which provides temporary relief of nasal congestion. Dextromethorphan is a cough suppressant which provides temporary relief of coughs due to minor throat irritations that may occur with the common cold.

Indications: TYLENOL Cold Medication No Drowsiness Formula provides effective temporary relief of the nasal congestion, coughing, and aches, pains and fever due to a cold or "flu."

Precautions: If a rare sensitivity reaction occurs, the drug should be stopped. Although pseudoephedrine is virtually without pressor effect in normotensive patients, it should be used with caution in hypertensives.

Usual Dosage:

Adults: Two caplets every 6 hours, not to exceed 8 caplets in 24 hours. Children (6–12 years): One caplet every 6 hours, not to exceed 4 tablets or caplets in 24 hours for 5 days.

WARNING: Do not administer to children under 6 or exceed the recommended dosage because nervousness, dizziness or sleeplessness may occur. Do not take this product for more than 7 days. If fever persists for more than three days, or if symptoms do not improve or are accompanied by high fever, consult a physician. A persistent cough may be a sign of a serious condition. If cough persists for more than 1 week, tends to recur or is accompanied by fever, rash or persistent headache, consult a physician. Do not take this product for persistent or chronic cough such as occurs with smoking, asthma, emphysema or if cough is accompanied by excessive phlegm (mucus) unless directed by a physician. Do not take this product if you have heart disease, high blood pressure, thyroid disease, diabetes, or difficulty in urination due to enlargement of the prostate gland unless directed by a physician.

DO NOT USE IF CARTON IS OPENED OR IF A BLISTER UNIT IS BROKEN. KEEP THIS AND ALL MEDICATION OUT OF THE REACH OF CHILDREN. AS WITH ANY DRUG, IF YOU ARE PREGNANT OR NURSING A BABY, SEEK THE ADVICE OF HEALTH PROFESSIONAL BEFORE USING THIS PRODUCT. IN THE CASE OF ACCIDENTAL OVERDOSAGE CONTACT A PHYSICIAN OR POISON CONTROL CENTER IMMEDIATELY.

DRUG INTERACTION PRECAUTION: Do not take this product if you are presently taking a prescription drug for high blood pressure or depression without first consulting your physician.

Overdosage: Acetaminophen in massive overdosage may cause hepatic toxicity in some patients. In adults and adolescents, hepatic toxicity has rarely been reported following ingestion of acute overdosage of less than 10 grams. Fatalities are infrequent (less than 3–4% of untreated cases) and have rarely been reported with overdosage of less than 15 grams. In children, an acute overdosage

of less than 150 mg/kg has not been associated with hepatic toxicity.
Early symptoms following a potentially hepatotoxic overdose may include: nausea, vomiting, diaphoresis and general malaise. Clinical and laboratory evidence of hepatic toxicity may not be apparent until 48 to 72 hours postingestion.
In adults and adolescents, regardless of the quantity of acetaminophen reported to have been ingested, administer MUCOMYST® acetylcysteine immediately if 24 hours or less have elapsed from the reported time of ingestion. For full prescribing information, refer to the MUCOMYST package insert. Do not await results of assays for acetaminophen level before initiating treatment with MUCOMYST acetylcysteine. The following additional procedures are recommended: The stomach should be emptied promptly by lavage or by induction of emesis with syrup of ipecac. A serum acetaminophen assay should be obtained as early as possible, but no sooner than four hours following ingestion. Liver function studies should be obtained initially and repeated at 24–hour intervals.
Serious toxicity or fatalities are extremely infrequent in children, possibly due to differences in the way they metabolize acetaminophen. In children, the maximum potential amount ingested can be more easily estimated. If more than 150 mg/kg or an unknown amount was ingested, obtain an acetaminophen plasma level. The acetaminophen plasma level should be obtained as soon as possible, but no sooner than 4 hours following the ingestion. Induce emesis using syrup of ipecac. If the plasma level is obtained and falls above the broken line on the acetaminophen overdose nomogram, the MUCOMYST acetylcysteine therapy should be initiated and continued for a full course of therapy. If acetaminophen plasma assay capability is not available, and the estimated acetaminophen ingestion exceeds 150 mg/kg, MUCOMYST acetylcysteine therapy should be initiated and continued for a full course of therapy.
For additional emergency information, call your regional poison center or call the Rocky Mountain Poison Center toll-free (1-800-525-6115).
Symptoms from pseudoephedrine overdose consist most often of mild anxiety, tachycardia and/or mild hypertension. Symptoms usually appear within 4 to 8 hours of ingestion and are transient, usually requiring no treatment.
Acute dextromethorphan overdose usually does not result in serious signs and symptoms unless massive amounts have been ingested. Signs and symptoms of a substantial overdose may include nausea and vomiting, visual disturbances, CNS disturbances, and urinary retention.

Inactive Ingredients: Cellulose, Glyceryl Triacetate, Hydroxypropyl Methylcellulose, Magnesium Stearate, Sodium Starch Glycolate, Starch, Titanium Dioxide, Blue #1 and Yellow #10.

How Supplied: Caplets (colored white, imprinted TYLENOL "cold")—blister packs of 24 and tamper-resistant bottles of 50.

Shown in Product Identification Section, page 416

TYLENOL® Cold Night Time Medication Liquid

Description: Each 30 ml (1 fl. oz.) contains acetaminophen 650 mg., diphenhydramine hydrochloride 50 mg., pseudoephedrine hydrochloride 60 mg., and dextromethorphan hydrobromide 30 mg. (alcohol 10%).

Actions: TYLENOL Cold Night Time Medication Liquid contains a clinically proven analgesic-antipyretic, decongestant, cough suppressant and antihistamine. Acetaminophen produces analgesia by elevation of the pain threshold and antipyresis through action on the hypothalamic heat-regulating center. Acetaminophen is equal to aspirin in analgesic and antipyretic effectiveness and it is unlikely to produce many of the side effects associated with aspirin and aspirin-containing products. Pseudoephedrine hydrochloride is a sympathomimetic amine which provides temporary relief of nasal congestion. Dextromethorphan is a cough suppressant which provides temporary relief of coughs due to minor throat irritations that may occur with the common cold. Diphenhydramine is an antihistamine which helps provide temporary relief of runny nose, sneezing and watery and itchy eyes.

Indications: TYLENOL Cold Night Time Medication Liquid provides effective temporary relief of runny nose, sneezing, watery and itchy eyes, nasal congestion, coughing, and aches, pains, sore throat and fevers due to a cold or "flu."

Precautions: If a rare sensitivity reaction occurs, the drug should be stopped. Although pseudoephedrine is virtually without pressor effect in normotensive patients, it should be used with caution in hypertensives.

Usual Dosage: Measuring cup is provided and marked for accurate dosing. Adults (12 years and over): 1 fluid ounce (2 tbsp.) in measuring cup provided every 6 hours, not to exceed 4 doses in 24 hours. Not recommended for children.

WARNINGS: Do not take this product for more than 7 days or for fever for more than 3 days unless directed by a doctor. If symptoms do not improve or are accompanied by fever, consult a doctor. A persistent cough may be a sign of a serious condition. If cough persists for more than 1 week, tends to recur or is accompanied by fever, rash or persistent headache, consult a doctor. Do not take this product for persistent or chronic cough such as occurs with smoking, asthma, emphysema, or if cough is accompanied by excessive phlegm (mucus) unless directed by a doctor. Do not exceed recommended dosage because at higher doses nervousness, dizziness or sleeplessness may occur. May cause excitability, especially in children. Do not take this product if you have asthma, glaucoma, heart disease, high blood pressure, emphysema, chronic pulmonary disease, shortness of breath, difficulty in breathing, diabetes, thyroid disease or difficulty in urination due to enlargement of the prostate gland, or if you are taking sedatives or tranquilizers, unless directed by a doctor. May cause marked drowsiness; alcohol, sedatives and tranquilizers may increase the drowsiness effect. Avoid alcoholic beverages while taking this product. Use caution when driving a motor vehicle or operating machinery.
DO NOT USE IF CARTON IS OPENED OR IF PRINTED PLASTIC WRAP OR PRINTED FOIL INNER SEAL IS BROKEN. KEEP THIS AND ALL MEDICATION OUT OF THE REACH OF CHILDREN. AS WITH ANY DRUG, IF YOU ARE PREGNANT OR NURSING A BABY, SEEK THE ADVICE OF A HEALTH PROFESSIONAL BEFORE USING THIS PRODUCT. IN CASE OF ACCIDENTAL OVERDOSAGE, CONTACT A PHYSICIAN OR POISON CONTROL CENTER IMMEDIATELY.
DRUG INTERACTION PRECAUTION: Do not take this product if you are presently taking a prescription drug for high blood pressure or depression without first consulting your doctor.

Overdosage: Acetaminophen in massive overdosage may cause hepatic toxicity in some patients. In adults and adolescents, hepatic toxicity has rarely been reported following ingestion of acute overdosage of less than 10 grams. Fatalities are infrequent (less than 3–4% of untreated cases) and have rarely been reported with overdoses of less than 15 grams. In children, an acute overdosage of less than 150 mg/kg has not been associated with hepatic toxicity.
Early symptoms following a potentially hepatotoxic overdose may include: nausea, vomiting, diaphoresis and general malaise. Clinical and laboratory evidence of hepatic toxicity may not be apparent until 48 to 72 hours postingestion.
In adults and adolescents, regardless of the quantity of acetaminophen reported to have been ingested, administer MUCOMYST® acetylcysteine immediately if 24 hours or less have elapsed from the reported time of ingestion. For full prescribing information, refer to the MUCOMYST package insert. Do not await results of assays for acetaminophen level before initiating treatment with MUCOMYST acetylcysteine. The following additional procedures are recommended: The stomach should be emptied promptly by lavage or by induction of emesis with syrup of ipecac. A serum acetaminophen assay should be obtained as early as possible, but no sooner than four hours following ingestion. Liver function studies should be obtained initially and repeated at 24-hour intervals.

Continued on next page

McNeil Consumer—Cont.

Serious toxicity or fatalities are extremely infrequent in children, possibly due to differences in the way they metabolize acetaminophen. In children, the maximum potential amount ingested can be more easily estimated. If more than 150 mg/kg or an unknown amount was ingested, obtain an acetaminophen plasma level. The acetaminophen plasma level should be obtained as soon as possible, but no sooner than 4 hours following the ingestion. Induce emesis using syrup of ipecac. If the plasma level is obtained and falls above the broken line on the acetaminophen overdose nomogram, the MUCOMYST acetylcysteine therapy should be initiated and continued for a full course of therapy. If acetaminophen plasma assay capability is not available, and the estimated acetaminophen ingestion exceeds 150 mg/kg, MUCOMYST acetylcysteine therapy should be initiated and continued for a full course of therapy.

For additional emergency information, call your regional poison center or call the Rocky Mountain Poison Center toll-free, (1-800-525-6115).

Diphenhydramine toxicity should be treated as you would an antihistamine/anticholinergic overdose and is likely to be present within a few hours after acute ingestion.

Symptoms from pseudoephedrine overdose consist most often of mild anxiety, tachycardia and/or mild hypertension. Symptoms usually appear within 4 to 8 hours of ingestion and are transient, usually requiring no treatment.

Acute dextromethorphan overdose usually does not result in serious signs and symptoms unless massive amounts have been ingested. Signs and symptoms of a substantial overdose may include nausea and vomiting, visual disturbances, CNS disturbances, and urinary retention.

Inactive Ingredients: Alcohol (10%), Citric Acid, Flavors, Glycerin, Polyethylene Glycol, Purified Water, Sodium Benzoate, Sucrose, Red #40, Red #33 and Blue #1.

How Supplied: Cherry flavored (colored red) in 5 oz. bottles with child-resistant safety cap, special dosage cup graded in ounces and tablespoons, and tamper-resistant packaging.

Shown in Product Identification Section, page 416

Maximum-Strength TYLENOL® Allergy Sinus Medication Caplets and Gelcaps

Description: Each TYLENOL® Allergy Sinus Caplet and Gelcap contains acetaminophen 500 mg, chlorpheniramine maleate 2 mg, and pseudoephedrine hydrochloride 30 mg.

Actions: TYLENOL® Allergy Sinus Caplets and Gelcaps contain a clinically proven analgesic-antipyretic, decongestant, and antihistamine. Acetaminophen produces analgesia by elevation of the pain threshold and antipyresis through action on the hypothalamic heat-regulating center. Acetaminophen is equal to aspirin in analgesic and antipyretic effectiveness, and it is unlikely to produce many of the side effects associated with aspirin and aspirin-containing products. Pseudoephedrine hydrochloride is a sympathomimetic amine which provides temporary relief of nasal congestion. Chlorpheniramine is an antihistamine which helps provide temporary relief of runny nose, sneezing and watery and itchy eyes.

Indications: TYLENOL® Allergy Sinus provides effective temporary relief of these upper respiratory allergy, hay fever and sinusitis symptoms: sneezing, itchy, watery eyes, runny nose, itching of the nose or throat, nasal and sinus congestion and sinus pain and headaches.

Precautions: If a rare sensitivity reaction occurs, the drug should be stopped. Although pseudoephedrine is virtually without pressor effect in normotensive patients, it should be used with caution in hypertensives.

Usual Dosage: Adults: Two caplets or gelcaps every 6 hours, not to exceed 8 caplets or gelcaps in 24 hours.

"**WARNING:** Do not administer to children under 12 or exceed the recommended dosage because nervousness, dizziness, or sleeplessness may occur. May cause excitability, especially in children. This preparation may cause drowsiness; alcohol may increase the drowsiness effect. Avoid alcoholic beverages when taking this product. Use caution when driving a motor vehicle or operating machinery. Do not take this product if you have heart disease, high blood pressure, thyroid disease, diabetes, asthma, glaucoma, emphysema, chronic pulmonary disease, shortness of breath, difficulty in breathing or difficulty in urination due to enlargement of prostate gland unless directed by a doctor. Do not take this product for more than 7 days. If symptoms do not improve or are accompanied by a high fever, consult a physician." **DO NOT USE IF CARTON IS OPEN OR IF A BLISTER UNIT IS BROKEN. KEEP THIS AND ALL MEDICATION OUT OF THE REACH OF CHILDREN. AS WITH ANY DRUG, IF YOU ARE PREGNANT OR NURSING A BABY, SEEK THE ADVICE OF A HEALTH PROFESSIONAL BEFORE USING THIS PRODUCT. IN THE CASE OF ACCIDENTAL OVERDOSE, CONTACT A PHYSICIAN OR POISON CONTROL CENTER IMMEDIATELY. DRUG INTERACTION PRECAUTION:** Do not take this product if you are presently taking a prescription drug for high blood pressure or depression without first consulting your doctor.

Overdosage: Acetaminophen in massive overdosage may cause hepatic toxicity in some patients. In adults and adolescents, hepatic toxicity has rarely been reported following ingestion of acute overdosage of less than 10 grams. Fatalities are infrequent (less than 3–4% of untreated cases) and have rarely been reported with overdoses of less than 15 grams. In children, an acute overdosage of less than 150 mg/kg has not been associated with hepatic toxicity.

Early symptoms following a potentially hepatotoxic overdose may include: nausea, vomiting, diaphoresis and general malaise. Clinical and laboratory evidence of hepatic toxicity may not be apparent until 48 to 72 hours postingestion. In adults and adolescents, regardless of the quantity of acetaminophen reported to have been ingested, administer MUCOMYST® acetylcysteine immediately if 24 hours or less have elapsed from the reported time of ingestion. For full prescribing information, refer to the MUCOMYST package insert. Do not await results of assays for acetaminophen level before initiating treatment with MUCOMYST acetylcysteine. The following additional procedures are recommended: The stomach should be emptied promptly by lavage or by induction of emesis with syrup of ipecac. A serum acetaminophen assay should be obtained as early as possible, but no sooner than four hours following ingestion. Liver function studies should be obtained initially and repeated at 24-hour intervals.

Serious toxicity or fatalities are extremely infrequent in children, possibly due to differences in the way they metabolize acetaminophen. In children, the maximum potential amount ingested can be easily estimated. If more than 150 mg/kg or an unknown amount was ingested, obtain an acetaminophen plasma level. The acetaminophen plasma level should be obtained as soon as possible, but no sooner than 4 hours following ingestion. Induce emesis using syrup of ipecac. If the plasma level is obtained and falls above the broken line on the acetaminophen overdose nomogram, the MUCOMYST acetylcysteine therapy should be initiated and continued for a full course of therapy. If acetaminophen plasma assay capability is not available, and the estimated acetaminophen ingestion exceeds 150 mg/kg, MUCOMYST acetylcysteine therapy should be initiated and continued for a full course of therapy.

For additional emergency information, call your regional poison center or call the Rocky Mountain Poison Control Center toll-free (1-800-525-6115).

Chlorpheniramine toxicity should be treated as you would an antihistamine/anticholinergic overdose and is likely to be present within a few hours after acute ingestion.

Symptoms from pseudophedrine overdose consist most often of mild anxiety, tachycardia and/or hypertension. Symptoms usually appear within 4 to 8 hours of ingestion and are transient, usually requiring no treatment.

Inactive Ingredients: Caplets: cellulose, hydroxypropyl cellulose, hydroxypropyl methylcellulose, magnesium stearate, polyethylene glycol, sodium starch glycolate, starch, titanium dioxide, blue #1, yellow #6, yellow #10.

Gelcaps: benzyl alcohol, butyl paraben, castor oil, cellulose, edetate calcium disodium, gelatin, hydroxypropyl methylcellulose, magnesium stearate, methylparaben, propylparaben, sodium lauryl sulfate, sodium propionate, sodium starch glycolate, starch, titanium dioxide, blue #1 and #2 and yellow #10.

How Supplied: Caplets: (dark yellow, imprinted "TYLENOL Allergy Sinus")—Blister packs of 24 and tamper-resistant bottles of 50.
Gelcaps: (green and yellow, imprinted "TYLENOL A/S" on green and yellow halves)—Blister packs of 20 and tamper-resistant bottles of 40.

Shown in Product Identification Section, page 416

Maximum-Strength TYLENOL® Sinus Medication Tablets, Caplets and Gelcaps

Description: Each Maximum-Strength TYLENOL® Sinus Medication tablet, caplet or gelcap contains acetaminophen 500 mg and pseudoephedrine hydrochloride 30 mg.

Actions: TYLENOL Sinus Medication contains a clinically proven analgesic-antipyretic and a decongestant. Maximum allowable non-prescription levels of acetaminophen and pseudoephedrine provide temporary relief of sinus headache and congestion. Acetaminophen is equal to aspirin in analgesic and antipyretic effectiveness and it is unlikely to produce many of the side effects associated with aspirin and aspirin-containing products.
Acetaminophen produces analgesia by elevation of the pain threshold and antipyresis through action on the hypothalamic heat-regulating center. Pseudoephedrine hydrochloride is a sympathomimetic amine which promotes sinus cavity drainage by reducing nasopharyngeal mucosal congestion.

Indications: Maximum-Strength TYLENOL Sinus Medication provides effective symptomatic relief from sinus headache pain and congestion. Maximum-Strength TYLENOL Sinus Medication is particularly well-suited in patients with aspirin allergy, hemostatic disturbances (including anticoagulant therapy), and bleeding diatheses (e.g., hemophilia) and upper gastrointestinal disease (e.g., ulcer, gastritis, hiatus hernia).

Precautions: If a rare sensitivity occurs, the drug should be discontinued. Although pseudoephedrine is virtually without pressor effect in normotensive patients, it should be used with caution in hypertensives.

Usual Dosage: Adult dosage: Two tablets or caplets every four to six hours. Do not exceed eight tablets or caplets in any 24-hour period.
WARNING: Do not administer to children under 12 or exceed the recommended dosage because at higher doses nervousness, dizziness, or sleeplessness may occur. Do not take this product for more than 7 days. If symptoms do not improve or are accompanied by fever, consult a physician. Do not take this product if you have heart disease, high blood pressure, thyroid disease, diabetes, or difficulty in urination due to enlargement of the prostate gland unless directed by a doctor.
DRUG INTERACTION PRECAUTION: Do not take this product if you are presently taking a prescription drug for high blood pressure or depression without first consulting your doctor.
Do not use if carton is opened or if blister unit is broken or if printed green neck wrap or printed foil inner seal is broken. Keep this and all medication out of the reach of children. As with any drug, if you are pregnant or nursing a baby, seek the advice of a health professional before using this product. In case of accidental overdosage, contact a physician or poison control center immediately.

Overdosage: Acetaminophen in massive overdosage may cause hepatic toxicity in some patients. In adults and adolescents, hepatic toxicity has rarely been reported following ingestion of acute overdosage of less than 10 grams. Fatalities are infrequent (less than 3–4% of untreated cases) and have rarely been reported with overdoses of less than 15 grams. In children, an acute overdosage of less than 150 mg/kg has not been associated with hepatic toxicity.
Early symptoms following a potentially hepatotoxic overdose may include: nausea, vomiting, diaphoresis and general malaise. Clinical and laboratory evidence of hepatic toxicity may not be apparent until 48 to 72 hours postingestion. In adults and adolescents, regardless of the quantity of acetaminophen reported to have been ingested, administer MUCOMYST® acetylcysteine immediately if 24 hours or less have elapsed from the reported time of ingestion. For full prescribing information, refer to the MUCOMYST package insert. Do not await the results of assays for acetaminophen level before initiating treatment with MUCOMYST acetylcysteine. The following additional procedures are recommended: The stomach should be emptied promptly by lavage or by induction of emesis with syrup of ipecac. A serum acetaminophen assay should be obtained as early as possible, but no sooner than four hours following ingestion. Liver function studies should be obtained initially and repeated at 24-hour intervals.
Serious toxicity or fatalities are extremely infrequent in children, possibly due to differences in the way they metabolize acetaminophen. In children, the maximum potential amount ingested can be more easily estimated. If more than 150 mg/kg or an unknown amount was ingested, obtain an acetaminophen plasma level. The acetaminophen plasma level should be obtained as soon as possible, but no sooner than 4 hours following the ingestion. Induce emesis using syrup of ipecac. If the plasma level is obtained and falls above the broken line on the acetaminophen overdose nomogram, the MUCOMYST acetylcysteine therapy should be initiated and continued for a full course of therapy. If acetaminophen plasma assay capability is not available, and the estimated acetaminophen ingestion exceeds 150 mg/kg, MUCOMYST acetylcysteine therapy should be initiated and continued for a full course of therapy.
For additional emergency information, call your regional poison center or call the Rocky Mountain Poison Center toll-free (1-800-525-6115).
Symptoms from pseudoephedrine overdose consist most often of mild anxiety, tachycardia and/or mild hypertension. Symptoms usually appear within 4 to 8 hours of ingestion and are transient, usually requiring no treatment.

Inactive Ingredients: Caplets—Cellulose, Hydroxypropyl Methylcellulose, Magnesium Stearate, Polysorbate 80, Sodium Starch Glycolate, Starch, Titanium Dioxide, Blue #1, Red #40 and Yellow #10.
Tablets—Cellulose, Magnesium Stearate, Sodium Lauryl Sulfate, Starch, Yellow #6, Yellow #10, and Blue #1.
Gelcaps—Benzyl alcohol, butylparaben, castor oil, cellulose, edetate calcium disodium, gelatin, hydroxypropyl methylcellulose, iron oxide black, magnesium stearate, methylparaben, propylparaben, sodium lauryl sulfate, sodium propionate, sodium starch glycolate, starch, titanium dioxide, Blue #1 and Yellow #10.

How Supplied: Tablets (colored light green, imprinted "Maximum-Strength TYLENOL Sinus")—tamper-resistant bottles of 24 and 50.
Caplets (light green coating, printed "TYLENOL Sinus" in dark green) tamper-resistant bottles of 24 and 50.
Gelcaps (colored green and white), imprinted "TYLENOL Sinus" in tamper-resistant packages of 20 and 40.

Shown in Product Identification Section, page 416

Mead Johnson Nutritionals

A Bristol-Myers Squibb Company
2400 W. LLOYD EXPRESSWAY
EVANSVILLE, IN 47721

Casec® Calcium Caseinate Powder
Ce-Vi-Sol® Vitamin C Supplement Drops for Infants
Criticare HN® Ready-To-Use High Nitrogen Elemental Diet
Enfamil® Infant Formula[1]
Enfamil® With Iron Infant Formula[1]
Enfamil Infant Formula Nursette®
Fer-In-Sol® Iron Supplement Drops, Syrup, Capsules
Isocal® Nutritionally Complete Liquid Tube-Feeding Formula
Isocal® HCN High Calorie and Nitrogen Nutritionally Complete Liquid Tube-Feeding Formula

Continued on next page

Mead Johnson Nutr.—Cont.

Isocal® HN High Nitrogen, Nutritionally Complete Liquid Tube-Feeding Formula
Lonalac® Powder, Low-Sodium, High-Protein Beverage Mix
MCT Oil, Medium Chain Triglycerides
Moducal® Dietary Carbohydrate
Nutramigen® Hypoallergenic Protein Hydrolysate Formula[1]
Portagen® Iron-Fortified Nutritionally Complete Powder with Medium Chain Triglycerides
ProSobee® Soy Isolate Formula[1]
ProSobee® Soy Isolate Formula Nursette®[1]

[1]Concentrated liquid, powder, and ready to use

Special Metabolic Diets:
Lofenalac® Iron Fortified Low Phenylalanine Diet Powder
Low Methionine Diet Powder (Product 3200K)
Low PHE-TYR Diet Powder (Product 3200AB)
Mono- and Disaccharide-Free Diet Powder (Product 3232A)
MSUD Diet Powder
Phenyl-Free® Phenylalanine-Free Diet Powder
Pregestimil® Iron Fortified Protein Hydrolysate Formula with Medium Chain Triglycerides

Special Metabolic Modules:
HIST 1
HIST 2
HOM 1
HOM 2
LYS 1
LYS 2
MSUD 1
MSUD 2
OS 1
OS 2
PKU 1
PKU 2
PKU 3
Protein-Free Diet Powder (Product 80056)
TYR 1
TYR 2
UCD 1
UCD 2
Sustacal® Nutritionally Complete Liquid, Powder, Pudding
Sustacal® with Fiber Nutritionally Complete Liquid Food with Soy Fiber
Sustacal® HC High-Calorie, Nutritionally Complete Food
Sustagen® High-Calorie, High-Protein Nutritional Supplement
TraumaCal® High-Nitrogen, Nutritionally Complete Formula for Metabolically Stressed Patients
Trind® Liquid, Antihistamine, Nasal Decongestant, Sugar-Free
Trind-DM® Liquid, Cough Suppressant, Antihistamine, Nasal Decongestant, Sugar-Free
Ultracal® High-Nitrogen, Nutritionally Complete Liquid Tube-Feeding Formula with Dietary Fiber

Detailed information may be obtained by contacting Mead Johnson Nutritionals Medical Affairs Department at (812) 429-6437.

POLY-VI-SOL®
[*pahl-ē-vī-sahl"*]
Vitamin drops • chewable tablets

Composition: Usual daily doses supply:
[See table below.]

Action and Uses: Daily vitamin supplementation for infants and children. Chewable tablets useful also for adults.

Administration and Dosage: Usual doses or as indicated.

How Supplied: Poly-Vi-Sol® vitamin drops: (with 'Safti-Dropper' marked to deliver 1.0 mL)
0087-0402-02 Bottles of 1 fl oz (30 mL)
0087-0402-03 Bottles of 1⅔ fl oz (50 mL)
6505-00-104-8433 (50 mL) (Defense)

POLY-VI-SOL® Vitamin drops, chewable tablets	Drops 1.0 mL	% U.S. RDA for Infants	Chewable Tablets 1 tablet	% U.S. RDA Children Age 2–3 Years	% U.S. RDA Adults and Children Age 4 Years or More
Vitamin A, IU	1500	100	2500	100	50
Vitamin D, IU	400	100	400	100	100
Vitamin E, IU	5	100	15	150	50
Vitamin C, mg	35	100	60	150	100
Folic acid, mg	—	—	0.3	150	75
Thiamine, mg	0.5	100	1.05	150	70
Riboflavin, mg	0.6	100	1.2	150	70
Niacin, mg	8	100	13.5	150	68
Vitamin B_6, mg	0.4	100	1.05	150	53
Vitamin B_{12}, μg	2	100	4.5	150	75

Poly-Vi-Sol® chewable vitamins tablets:
0087-0412-03 Bottles of 100
Poly-Vi-Sol® chewable vitamins tablets in Circus Shapes:
0087-0414-02 Bottles of 100
0087-0414-06 Bottles of 60

Shown in Product Identification Section, page 417

POLY-VI-SOL® with Iron Chewable Tablets	Chewable Tablets 1 tablet	% U.S. RDA Children Age 2–3 Years	% U.S. RDA Adults and Children Age 4 Years or More
Vitamin A, IU	2500	100	50
Vitamin D, IU	400	100	100
Vitamin E, IU	15	150	50
Vitamin C, mg	60	150	100
Folic acid, mg	0.3	150	75
Thiamine, mg	1.05	150	70
Riboflavin, mg	1.2	150	70
Niacin, mg	13.5	150	68
Vitamin B_6, mg	1.05	150	53
Vitamin B_{12}, μg	4.5	150	75
Iron, mg	12	120	67
Copper, mg	0.8	80	40
Zinc, mg	8	100	53

POLY-VI-SOL® with Iron
[*pahl-ē-vī-sahl"*]
Chewable vitamins and minerals

Composition: Each tablet supplies same vitamins as Poly-Vi-Sol tablets plus 12 mg iron, 8 mg zinc, and 0.8 mg copper.

Action and Uses: Daily vitamin and mineral supplement for adults and children.

Administration and Dosage: 1 tablet daily.

How Supplied: Poly-Vi-Sol® chewable vitamins with Iron tablets.
0087-0455-02 Bottles of 100
Poly-Vi-Sol® chewable vitamins with Iron tablets in Circus Shapes.
0087-0456-02 Bottles of 100
0087-0456-06 Bottles of 60
[See table above.]

Shown in Product Identification Section, page 417

POLY-VI-SOL® with Iron
[*pahl-ē-vī'sahl"*]
Vitamin and Iron drops

Composition: Each 1.0 mL supplies:

		% U.S. RDA Infants
Vitamin A, IU	1500	100
Vitamin D, IU	400	100
Vitamin E, IU	5	100
Vitamin C, mg	35	100
Thiamine, mg	0.5	100
Riboflavin, mg	0.6	100
Niacin, mg	8	100
Vitamin B_6, mg	0.4	100
Iron, mg	10	67

Action and Uses: Daily vitamin and iron supplement for infants.

Administration and Dosage: Drop into mouth with 'Safti-Dropper.' Dose: 1.0 mL daily, or as indicated.

When an infant or child is taking iron, stools may appear darker in color. This is to be expected and should be no cause for concern. When drops containing iron are given to infants or young children, some darkening of the plaque on the teeth may occur. This is not serious or permanent as it does not affect the enamel. The stains can be removed or prevented by rubbing the teeth with a little baking soda or powder on a toothbrush or small cloth once or twice a week.

How Supplied: Poly-Vi-Sol® vitamin and iron drops (with dropper marked to deliver 1 mL)

0087-0405-01 Bottles of 1⅔ fl oz (50 mL)

Shown in Product Identification Section, page 417

RICELYTE™

[*rīs ′līt*]

Rice-based oral electrolyte maintenance solution

Ricelyte rapidly replenishes fluid and electrolytes lost in diarrhea. It is designed for oral administration and provides electrolytes and rice carbohydrate in a balanced formulation.

Composition: Water, rice syrup solids, natural fruit flavors, sodium chloride, potassium citrate, sodium citrate, citric acid.

Concentrations of Electrolytes:

	Per liter
Sodium (mEq)	50
Potassium (mEq)	25
Chloride (mEq)	45
Citrate (mEq)	34
Rice Syrup Solids (g)	30
Calories	126

Indications: Oral feedings of Ricelyte may be used to supply water and electrolytes for maintenance during diarrhea; and to replace mild to moderate fluid losses.

Intake and Administration: Feed by nursing bottle, cup, straw, or spoon. Ricelyte should be initiated as soon as diarrhea is recognized and continued until after the last soft, watery stool. Intake should approximate the normal fluid intake plus 4 to 8 fluid ounces for each watery stool. Recommended approximate intakes by weight of the infant or child are shown in the accompanying table.

For older children and adults two or more quarts per day may be necessary. Intake should be adjusted on the basis of clinical findings, amount of fluid loss, patient's usual fluid intake, and other relevant factors such as thirst.

Contraindications: Ricelyte should not be used:

—in the presence of severe, continuing diarrhea or other critical fluid losses requiring parenteral fluid therapy

—in intractable vomiting, adynamic ileus, intestinal obstruction, or perforated bowel

—when renal function is depressed (anuria, oliguria) or homeostatic mechanisms are impaired

Precautions: Urgent needs in severe fluid imbalances must be met parenterally. Ricelyte should be used on a doctor's orders and should be discontinued when the diarrhea has ceased. Ricelyte does not meet the caloric requirements of infants and children. Additional food or formula should be given as instructed by the doctor.

Opened bottles of Ricelyte should be resealed, refrigerated, and used within 48 hours.

Features: Ricelyte is ready to use—no mixing or dilution is necessary.

—Ricelyte is balanced to provide the necessary electrolytes and fluid

—Natural fruit flavor

—No artificial colors or flavors

—No fruit juice

How Supplied: Ricelyte is available in one-liter plastic bottles. It is also available in the Hospital Feeding System in 8 fl oz Nursette® Disposable Bottles.

Ricelyte™ ADMINISTRATION GUIDE
For Maintenance Therapy*

1.5–2.3 fl oz/lb Per Day		or 100–150 mL/kg Per Day	
Weight lb	Ricelyte fl oz	Weight kg	Ricelyte mL
7	11–16	3.2	320– 480
13	20–30	5.9	590– 885
17	26–39	7.7	770–1155
20	30–46	9.1	910–1365
23	35–53	10.5	1050–1575
25	38–58	11.4	1140–1710
28	42–64	12.7	1270–1905
32	48–74	14.5	1450–2175
38	57–87	17.3	1730–2595

* *Ongoing Loss Replacement:* For every diarrheal stool, the caregiver should give an additional 4 to 8 fl oz (120 to 240 mL).

- For breast-fed infants, allow breast milk *ad lib.* For formula-fed infants, alternate Ricelyte with equal amounts of lactose-free formula, like ProSobee®, or half-strength lactose-containing formula, like Enfamil®
- Avoid products such as carbonated or fruit-flavored drinks which have a high carbohydrate content.

Reference: Adapted from Santosham M., et al, *Ped Rev.* 1987; 8:273 as presented in The Harriet Lane Handbook, ed 12, 1990:274.

Shown in Product Identification Section, page 417

TEMPRA®

[*tem ′prah*]

Acetaminophen

Drops • syrup • chewable tablets

For infants and children

Description: Tempra is acetaminophen, a safe and effective analgesic-antipyretic. It is not a salicylate. It contains no phenacetin or caffeine. It has no effect on prothrombin time. Tempra offers prompt, non-irritating therapy. Because it provides significant freedom from side effects, it is particularly valuable for patients who do not tolerate aspirin well.

Tempra drops contain no alcohol.

Tempra syrup contains no alcohol.

Tempra chewable tablets are sugar-free.

Indications and Usage: Tempra drops, syrup and chewable tablets are useful for reducing fever and for the temporary relief of minor aches, pains and discomfort associated with the common cold or "flu," inoculations or vaccination. Tempra syrup is valuable in reducing pain following tonsillectomy and adenoidectomy. When Tempra is used by pregnant or nursing women, there are no known adverse effects upon fetal development or nursing infants.

Note: A prescription is not required for Tempra drops, syrup or tablets as an analgesic. To prevent its misuse by the layman, the following information appears on the package label:

Warnings: If fever persists for more than 3 days (72 hours) or if pain continues for more than 5 days, consult your physician.

Phenylketonurics: Each 80 mg tablet contains 3.3 mg phenylalanine. Each 160 mg tablet contains 6.6 mg phenylalanine.

Precaution: Acetaminophen has been reported to potentiate the effect of orally administered anticoagulants and may enhance the elimination of chloramphenicol. Therapeutic drug monitoring should be considered whenever these drugs are used concurrently.

Adverse Reactions: Infrequent, nonspecific side effects have been reported with the therapeutic use of acetaminophen.

Overdosage: Acetaminophen in massive overdosage may cause hepatic toxicity in some patients. In adults and adolescents, hepatic toxicity has rarely been reported following ingestion of acute overdoses of less than 10 grams. Fatalities are infrequent (less than 3–4% of untreated cases) and have rarely been reported with overdoses of less than 15 grams. In children, an acute overdosage of less than 150 mg/kg has not been associated with hepatic toxicity.

Early symptoms following a potentially hepatotoxic overdose may include: nausea, vomiting, diaphoresis and general malaise. Clinical and laboratory evidence of hepatic toxicity may not be apparent until 48 to 72 hours postingestion.

In adults and adolescents, regardless of the quantity of acetaminophen reported to have been ingested, administer MUCOMYST® acetylcysteine immediately if 24 hours or less have elapsed from the reported time of ingestion. For full prescribing information, refer to the MUCOMYST package insert. Do not await results of assays for acetaminophen level before initiating treatment with MUCOMYST acetylcysteine. The following additional procedures are recommended: The stomach should be emptied promptly by lavage or by induc-

Continued on next page

tion of emesis with syrup of ipecac. A serum acetaminophen assay should be obtained as early as possible, but no sooner than four hours following ingestion. Liver function studies should be obtained initially and repeated at 24-hour intervals.

Serious toxicity or fatalities are extremely infrequent in children, possibly due to differences in the way they metabolize acetaminophen. In children, the maximum potential amount ingested can be more easily estimated. If more than 150 mg/kg or an unknown amount was ingested, obtain an acetaminophen plasma level. The acetaminophen plasma level should be obtained as soon as possible, but no sooner than 4 hours following the ingestion. Induce emesis using syrup of ipecac. If the plasma level is obtained and falls above the broken line on the nomogram, the MUCOMYST acetylcysteine therapy should be initiated and continued for a full course of therapy. If acetaminophen plasma assay capability is not available, and the estimated acetaminophen ingestion exceeds 150 mg/kg, MUCOMYST acetylcysteine therapy should be initiated and continued for a full course of therapy.

For additional emergency information, call your regional poison center or toll-free (1-800-525-6115) to the Rocky Mountain Poison Center for assistance in diagnosis and for directions on the use of MUCOMYST acetylcysteine as an antidote.

Dosage and Administration:
Every 4 hours as needed but not more than 5 times daily.
(See table below.)
Drops are given with calibrated 'Safti-Dropper' or mixed with water or fruit juices. Syrup is given by teaspoon.

How Supplied: Tempra® (acetaminophen) drops: (with calibrated 'Safti-Dropper') grape-flavored
NDC 0087-0730-01 Bottles of 15 mL
Tempra® (acetaminophen) syrup: grape-flavored
NDC 0087-0733-04 Bottles of 4 fl oz
NDC 0087-0733-03 Bottles of 16 fl oz
Tempra chewables: grape-flavored, no sucrose
NDC 0087-0738-01 Bottles of 30 (80 mg) tablets
NDC 0087-0749-01 Bottles of 30 (160 mg) tablets
No Rx required.
Dosage may be given every 4 hours as needed but not more than 5 times daily.
DROPS: Each 0.8 mL dropper contains 80 mg acetaminophen.
SYRUP: Each 5 mL teaspoon contains 160 mg acetaminophen.
CHEWABLES: Each regular tablet contains 80 mg acetaminophen. Each Double Strength tablet contains 160 mg acetaminophen.
* If child is significantly under- or overweight, dosage may need to be adjusted accordingly.
† Ask your doctor before administering to children under the age of 2 years.

Shown in Product Identification Section, page 417

TEMPRA®

Age	Approximate Weight Range*	Drops	Syrup	Chewables 80 mg	Chewables 160 mg
		Drops			
†Under 4 mo	Under 12 lb	½ dropper	¼ tsp	—	—
†4 to 11 mo	12–17 lb	1 dropper	½ tsp	—	—
†12 to 23 mo	18–23 lb	1½ droppers	¾ tsp	—	—
2 to 3 yr	24–35 lb	2 droppers	1 tsp	2 tablets	—
4 to 5 yr	36–47 lb	3 droppers	1½ tsp	3 tablets	—
6 to 8 yr	48–59 lb	—	2 tsp	4 tablets	2 tablets
9 to 10 yr	60–71 lb	—	2½ tsp	5 tablets	2½ tablets
11 yr	72–95 lb	—	3 tsp	6 tablets	3 tablets
12 yr & older	96 lb & over	—	4 tsp	8 tablets	4 tablets

TRI-VI-SOL®
[*trī-vī-sahl"*]
Vitamins A, D and C drops

	Drops 1.0 mL	% U.S. RDA for Infants
Vitamin A, IU	1500	100
Vitamin D, IU	400	100
Vitamin C, mg	35	100

Action and Uses: Tri-Vi-Sol drops provide vitamins A, D and C.

How Supplied: Tri-Vi-Sol® drops: (with 'Safti-Dropper' marked to deliver 1 mL)
0087-0403-02 Bottles of 1 fl oz (30 mL)
0087-0403-03 Bottles of 1⅔ fl oz (50 mL)

Shown in Product Identification Section, page 417

TRI-VI-SOL® with Iron
[*trī-vī-sahl"*]
Vitamins A, D, C and Iron drops

Composition: Each 1.0 mL supplies same vitamins as in Tri-Vi-Sol® vitamin drops (see above) plus 10 mg iron.

Action and Uses: Tri-Vi-Sol with Iron vitamins A, D, C and Iron for infants and children.

Administration and Dosage: Drop into mouth with 'Safti-Dropper.' Dose: 1.0 mL daily, or as indicated.

How Supplied: Tri-Vi-Sol® vitamin drops with Iron (with dropper marked to deliver 1 mL)
0087-0453-03 Bottles of 1⅔ fl oz (50 mL)

Shown in Product Identification Section, page 417

Mead Johnson Pharmaceuticals
A Bristol-Myers Squibb Company
2400 W. LLOYD EXPRESSWAY
EVANSVILLE, IN 47721-0001

COLACE®
[*kōlās*]
docusate sodium, Mead Johnson
capsules • syrup • liquid (drops)

Description: Colace (docusate sodium) is a stool softener.
Colace Capsules, 50 mg, contain the following inactive ingredients: citric acid, D&C Red No. 33, FD&C Red No. 40, non-porcine gelatin, edible ink, polyethylene glycol, propylene glycol, and purified water.
Colace Capsules, 100 mg, contain the following inactive ingredients: citric acid, D&C Red No. 33, FD&C Red No. 40, FD&C Yellow No. 6, non-porcine gelatin, edible ink, polyethylene glycol, propylene glycol, titanium dioxide, and purified water.
Colace Liquid, 1%, contains the following inactive ingredients: citric acid, D&C Red No. 33, methylparaben, poloxamer, polyethylene glycol, propylene glycol, propylparaben, sodium citrate, vanillin, and purified water.
Colace Syrup, 20 mg/5 mL, contains the following inactive ingredients: alcohol, citric acid, D&C Red No. 33, FD&C Red No. 40, flavor (natural), menthol, methylparaben, peppermint oil, poloxamer, polyethylene glycol, propylparaben, sodium citrate, sucrose, and purified water.

Actions and Uses: Colace, a surface-active agent, helps to keep stools soft for easy, natural passage and is not a laxative, thus, not habit forming. Useful in constipation due to hard stools, in painful anorectal conditions, in cardiac and other conditions in which maximum ease of passage is desirable to avoid difficult or painful defecation, and when peristaltic stimulants are contraindicated.
Note: When peristaltic stimulation is needed due to inadequate bowel motility, see Peri-Colace® (laxative and stool softener).

Contraindications: There are no known contraindications to Colace.

Side Effects: The incidence of side effects—none of a serious nature—is exceedingly small. Bitter taste, throat irritation, and nausea (primarily associated with the use of the syrup and liquid) are the main side effects reported. Rash has occurred.

Administration and Dosage: *Orally*—Suggested daily Dosage: *Adults and older children:* 50 to 200 mg *Children 6 to 12:* 40 to 120 mg *Children 3 to 6:* 20 to 60 mg. *Infants and children under 3:* 10 to 40 mg. The higher doses are recommended for initial therapy. Dosage should be adjusted to individual response. The effect on stools is usually apparent 1 to 3 days after the first dose. Give Colace liquid in half a glass of milk or fruit juice or in infant formula, to mask bitter taste. *In enemas* —Add 50 to 100 mg Colace (5 to 10 mL Colace liquid) to a retention or flushing enema.

Warning: As with any drug, if you are pregnant or nursing a baby, seek the advice of a health professional before using this product.

How Supplied: Colace capsules, 50 mg
NDC 0087-0713-01 Bottles of 30
NDC 0087-0713-02 Bottles of 60
NDC 0087-0713-03 Bottles of 250
NDC 0087-0713-05 Bottles of 1000
NDC 0087-0713-07 Cartons of 100 single unit packs
Colace capsules, 100 mg
NDC 0087-0714-01 Bottles of 30
NDC 0087-0714-02 Bottles of 60
NDC 0087-0714-03 Bottles of 250
NDC 0087-0714-05 Bottles of 1000
NDC 0087-0714-07 Cartons of 100 single unit packs
Note: Colace capsules should be stored at controlled room temperature (59°–86°F or 15°–30°C)
Colace liquid, 1% solution; 10 mg/mL (with calibrated dropper)
NDC 0087-0717-04 Bottles of 16 fl oz
NDC 0087-0717-02 Bottles of 30 mL
NSN 6505-00-045-7786 Bottles of 30 mL (M)
Colace syrup, 20 mg/5-mL teaspoon; contains not more than 1% alcohol
NDC 0087-0720-01 Bottles of 8 fl oz
NDC 0087-0720-02 Bottles of 16 fl oz

Shown in Product Identification Section, page 417

PERI-COLACE® capsules • syrup (casanthranol and docusate sodium)

Description: Peri-Colace is a combination of the mild stimulant laxative casanthranol, and the stool-softener Colace® (docusate sodium). Each capsule contains 30 mg of casanthranol and 100 mg of Colace; the syrup contains 30 mg of casanthranol and 60 mg of Colace per 15-mL tablespoon (10 mg of casanthranol and 20 mg of Colace per 5-mL teaspoon) and 10% alcohol.
Peri-Colace Capsules contain the following inactive ingredients: D&C Red No. 33, FD&C Red No. 40, non-porcine gelatin, edible ink, polyethylene glycol, propylene glycol, titanium dioxide, and purified water.
Peri-Colace Syrup contains the following inactive ingredients: alcohol, citric acid, flavors, methyl salicylate, methylparaben, poloxamer, polyethylene glycol, propylparaben, sodium citrate, sorbitol solution, sucrose, and purified water.

Action and Uses: Peri-Colace provides gentle peristaltic stimulation and helps to keep stools soft for easier passage. Bowel movement is induced gently—usually overnight or in 8 to 12 hours. Nausea, griping, abnormally loose stools, and constipation rebound are minimized. Useful in management of chronic or temporary constipation.
Note: To prevent hard stools when laxative stimulation is not needed or undesirable, see Colace (stool softener).

Side Effects: The incidence of side effects—none of a serious nature—is exceedingly small. Nausea, abdominal cramping or discomfort, diarrhea, and rash are the main side effects reported.

Administration and Dosage:
Adults —1 or 2 capsules, or 1 or 2 tablespoons syrup at bedtime, or as indicated. In severe cases, dosage may be increased to 2 capsules or 2 tablespoons twice daily, or 3 capsules at bedtime. *Children* —1 to 3 teaspoons of syrup at bedtime, or as indicated.

Warnings: Do not use when abdominal pain, nausea, or vomiting are present. Frequent or prolonged use of this preparation may result in dependence on laxatives. As with any drug, if you are pregnant or nursing a baby, seek the advice of a health professional before using this product.

Overdosage: In addition to symptomatic treatment, gastric lavage, if timely, is recommended in cases of large overdosage.

How Supplied: Peri-Colace® Capsules
NDC 0087-0715-01 Bottles of 30
NDC 0087-0715-02 Bottles of 60
NDC 0087-0715-03 Bottles of 250
NDC 0087-0715-05 Bottles of 1000
NDC 0087-0715-07 Cartons of 100 single unit packs
Note: Peri-Colace capsules should be stored at controlled room temperatures (59°–86°F or 15°–30°C).
Peri-Colace® Syrup
NDC 0087-0721-01 Bottles of 8 fl oz
NDC 0087-0721-02 Bottles of 16 fl oz

Shown in Product Identification Section, page 417

Menley & James Laboratories

A Division of WKW, Inc.
COMMONWEALTH CORPORATE CENTER
100 TOURNAMENT DRIVE, SUITE 110
HORSHAM, PA 19044

A.R.M.® Allergy Relief Medicine Maximum Strength Caplets

Product Information: A.R.M. combines two important medicines in one safe, fast-acting caplet:

- The highest level of antihistamine available without prescription—for better relief of sneezing, runny nose and itchy, weepy eyes.
- A clinically proven sinus decongestant to help ease breathing and drain sinus congestion for hours.

Formula: Active Ingredients: Each caplet contains Chlorpheniramine Maleate, 4 mg., Phenylpropanolamine Hydrochloride, 25 mg. **Inactive Ingredients (listed for individuals with specific allergies):** Carnauba Wax, D&C Yellow 10, FD&C Yellow 6 (Sunset Yellow) as a color additive, Gelatin, Hydroxypropyl Methylcellulose, Lactose, Magnesium Stearate, Polyethylene Glycol, Sodium Starch Glycolate, Starch.

Directions: One caplet every 4 hours, not to exceed 6 caplets daily.
Children (6–12 years): one-half the adult dose. Children under 6 years use only as directed by physician.

TAMPER-RESISTANT PACKAGE FEATURES FOR YOUR PROTECTION:

- The carton has been sealed at the factory with a clear overwrap printed with "safety sealed."
- Each caplet is encased in a clear plastic cell with a foil back.
- The name A.R.M. appears on each caplet (see product illustration on front of carton).
- **DO NOT USE THIS PRODUCT IF ANY OF THESE TAMPER-RESISTANT FEATURES ARE MISSING OR BROKEN. IF YOU HAVE ANY QUESTIONS, PLEASE CALL 1-800-321-1834 TOLL FREE.**

Warning: Do not exceed recommended dosage. If symptoms do not improve within 7 days, or are accompanied by high fever, consult a physician before continuing use. Stop use if dizziness, sleeplessness or nervousness occurs. If you have or are being treated for depression, high blood pressure, glaucoma, diabetes, asthma, difficulty in urination due to enlarged prostate, heart disease or thyroid disease, use only as directed by physician. Do not take this product if you are taking another medication containing phenylpropanolamine.
Avoid alcoholic beverages while taking this product. Do not drive or operate heavy machinery. May cause drowsiness. May cause excitability, especially in children. Keep this and all drugs out of reach of children. In case of accidental overdose, seek professional assistance or contact a poison control center immediately. As with any drug, if you are pregnant or nursing a baby, seek the advice of a health professional before using this product. Store at controlled room temperature (59°–86°F.).

How Supplied: Consumer packages of 20 and 40 caplets.

Shown in Product Identification Section, page 417

ACNOMEL® CREAM acne therapy

Description: Cream—sulfur, 8%; resorcinol, 2%; alcohol, 11% (w/w); nongreasy, dries oily skin, easy to apply.

Inactive Ingredients: Bentonite, Fragrance, Iron Oxides, Potassium Hydroxide, Propylene Glycol, Titanium Dioxide, Purified Water.

Indications: Acnomel Cream is effective in the treatment of pimples and blemishes due to acne.

Continued on next page

Menley & James—Cont.

Directions: Wash and dry affected areas thoroughly. Apply a thin coating of Acnomel Cream once or twice daily, making sure it does not get into the eyes or on eyelids. Do not rub in. If a marked chapping effect occurs, discontinue use temporarily.

Warning: Acnomel should not be applied to acutely inflamed area. If undue skin irritation develops or increases, discontinue use and consult physician. Keep this and all drugs out of reach of children. In case of accidental ingestion, seek professional assistance or contact a poison control center immediately. Keep tube tightly closed to prevent drying. Store at controlled room temperature (59°–86°F.).

How Supplied: Cream—in specially lined 1 oz. tubes.

Shown in Product Identification Section, page 417

AQUA CARE® CREAM
With 10% Urea
Effective Medication for Dry Skin Relief

Product Information: AQUA CARE, with 10% urea, is a topical cream formulated to restore nature's moisture balance to rough, dry skin. The special urea ingredient penetrates the surface of the skin to both restore lost moisture and soften dry, rough skin.

Formula: Purified water, urea 10%, cetyl esters wax, DEA-oleth-3 phosphate, petrolatum, trolamine, glycerin, carbomer 934, mineral oil and lanolin alcohol, lanolin oil, benzyl alcohol, and fragrance.

Directions: Apply two or three times daily to affected area or as your physician directs.

Warning: Discontinue use if irritation occurs.
Store at controlled room temperature (59°–86°F.).
FOR EXTERNAL USE ONLY

How Supplied: Available in 2.5 oz. tubes.

Shown in Product Identification Section, page 417

AQUA CARE® LOTION
With 10% Urea
Effective Medication for Dry Skin Relief

Product Information: AQUA CARE, with 10% urea, is a topical lotion formulated to restore nature's moisture balance to rough, dry skin. The special urea ingredient penetrates the surface of the skin to both restore lost moisture and soften dry, rough skin.

Formula: 10% urea with purified water, mineral oil, petrolatum, propylene glycol stearate, sorbitan stearate, cetyl alcohol, lactic acid, magnesium aluminum silicate, sodium lauryl sulfate, methylparaben and propylparaben.

Directions: Apply two or three times daily to affected area or as your physician directs.

Warning: Discontinue use if irritation occurs.
Store at controlled room temperature (59°–86°F.).
FOR EXTERNAL USE ONLY

How Supplied: Available in 8 oz. bottles.

Shown in Product Identification Section, page 417

ASTHMAHALER® Mist
epinephrine bitartrate bronchodilator
Alcohol Free Formula

Active Ingredients: Contains epinephrine bitartrate 7 mg per ml in inert propellant.

Inactive Ingredients: Cetylpyridinium Chloride, Propellants 11, 12, & 114, Sorbitan Trioleate.

Indications: For temporary relief of shortness of breath, tightness of chest, and wheezing due to bronchial asthma.

Warnings: Do not use this product unless a diagnosis of asthma has been made by a doctor. Do not use this product if you have heart disease, high blood pressure, thyroid disease, diabetes, or difficulty in urination due to enlargement of the prostate gland unless directed by a doctor. Do not use this product if you have ever been hospitalized for asthma or if you are taking any prescription drug for asthma unless directed by a doctor.
As with any drug, if you are pregnant or nursing a baby, seek the advice of a health professional before using this product.
Keep this and all medication out of the reach of children. In case of accidental overdose, consult a physician immediately.
DO NOT USE THIS PRODUCT MORE FREQUENTLY OR AT HIGHER DOSES THAN RECOMMENDED UNLESS DIRECTED BY A DOCTOR. Excessive use may cause nervousness and rapid heart beat, and possibly, adverse effects on the heart.
DO NOT CONTINUE TO USE THIS PRODUCT, BUT SEEK MEDICAL ASSISTANCE IMMEDIATELY IF SYMPTOMS ARE NOT RELIEVED WITHIN 20 MINUTES OR BECOME WORSE.

Drug Interaction Precaution: Do not use this product if you are presently taking a prescription drug for high blood pressure or depression, without first consulting your doctor.
Contents under pressure. Do not puncture or incinerate container. Do not expose to heat or store at temperature above 120°F.

Dosage and Administration: For oral inhalation only. Each inhalation contains the equivalent of 0.16 milligram of epinephrine base.
Dosage: Inhalation dosage for adults and children 4 years of age and older: Start with one inhalation, then wait at least 1 minute. If not relieved, use once more. Do not use again for at least 3 hours. Use of this product by children should be supervised by an adult. Children under 4 years of age: consult a doctor.

Directions: Shake well before each use.

1. Remove plastic dust cap, take mouthpiece off metal vial and fit other end of mouthpiece onto top of vial, turn vial upside down. Shake well.
2. Breathe out fully and place mouthpiece well into mouth, aimed at the back of the throat.
3. As you begin to breathe in deeply, press the vial firmly down into the adapter with the index finger. This releases one dose.
4. Release pressure on vial and remove unit from mouth. Hold the breath as long as possible, then breathe out slowly.

The plastic mouthpiece should be cleaned daily. Remove metal vial and wash adapter with soap and hot water and rinse thoroughly. Dry and replace with vial.

How Supplied: ½ fl. oz. (15 ml). Available as combination package metal vial plus plastic mouthpiece, or as refill metal vial only.

ASTHMANEFRIN®
Solution "A" Bronchodilator

Active Ingredients: Racepinephrine hydrochloride equivalent to 1% epinephrine base.

Inactive Ingredients: Benzoic Acid, Chlorobutanol, Glycerin, Hydrochloric Acid, Sodium Bisulfite, Sodium Chloride, Water.

Indications: For temporary relief of shortness of breath, tightness of chest, and wheezing due to bronchial asthma.

Warnings: Do not use this product unless a diagnosis of asthma has been made by a doctor. Do not use this product if you have heart disease, high blood pressure, thyroid disease, diabetes, or difficulty in urination due to enlargement of the prostate gland unless directed by a doctor. Do not use this product if you have ever been hospitalized for asthma or if you are taking any prescription drug for asthma unless directed by a doctor.
As with any drug, if you are pregnant or nursing a baby, seek the advice of a physician before using this product.
Keep this and all medication out of the reach of children.
Store at room temperature; avoid excessive heat.
DO NOT USE THIS PRODUCT MORE FREQUENTLY OR AT HIGHER DOSES THAN RECOMMENDED UNLESS DIRECTED BY A DOCTOR. Excessive use may cause nervousness and rapid heart beat, and possibly, adverse effects on the heart. **DO NOT CONTINUE TO USE THIS PRODUCT, BUT**

SEEK MEDICAL ASSISTANCE IMMEDIATELY IF SYMPTOMS ARE NOT RELIEVED WITHIN 20 MINUTES OR BECOME WORSE.
Do not use this product if it is brown in color or cloudy.

Drug Interaction Precaution: Do not use this product if you are presently taking a prescription drug for high blood pressure or depression, without first consulting your doctor.

Dosage and Administration: Inhalation dosage for adults and children 4 years of age and older: 1 to 3 inhalations not more often than every 3 hours. The use of this product by children should be supervised by an adult. Children under 4 years of age: consult a doctor.

Directions: For use in hand-held rubber bulb nebulizer. Pour at least 8 drops of solution into AsthmaNefrin Nebulizer.
Care of Solution: Refrigerate once bottle has been opened.

How Supplied: ½ fl. oz. (15 ml) and 1 fl. oz. (30 ml) Solutions. FOR USE WITH ASTHMANEFRIN® NEBULIZER.

BENZEDREX® INHALER
Nasal Decongestant

Description: Each inhaler packed with propylhexedrine, 250 mg. Inactive ingredients: Lavender Oil, Menthol.

Indications: For temporary relief of nasal congestion in colds and hay fever; also for ear block and pressure pain during air travel.

Directions: Insert in nostril. Close other nostril. Inhale twice. Treat other nostril the same way. Avoid excessive use.
Inhaler loses potency after 2 or 3 months' use but some aroma may linger.

Warning: Ill effects may result if taken internally. In the case of accidental overdose or ingestion of contents, seek professional assistance or contact a poison control center immediately. Keep this and all drugs out of reach of children.
As with any drug, if you are pregnant or nursing a baby, seek the advice of a health professional before using.
TAMPER-RESISTANT PACKAGE FEATURES FOR YOUR PROTECTION:
- The carton has been sealed at the factory with a clear overwrap printed with "safety sealed."
- Inhaler sealed with imprinted cellophane.
- **DO NOT USE THIS PRODUCT IF ANY OF THESE TAMPER-RESISTANT FEATURES ARE MISSING OR BROKEN. IF YOU HAVE ANY QUESTIONS, PLEASE CALL 1-800-321-1834 TOLL FREE.**

How Supplied: In single plastic tubes.
Shown in Product Identification Section, page 417

CONGESTAC®
Congestion Relief Medicine
Decongestant/Expectorant
Caplets

Product Information: Helps you breathe easier by temporarily relieving nasal congestion associated with the common cold, sinusitis, hay fever and allergies. Also helps relieve chest congestion by loosening phlegm and clearing bronchial passages of excess mucus. Contains no antihistamines which may overdry or make you drowsy.

Formula: Active Ingredients: Each caplet contains Pseudoephedrine Hydrochloride 60 mg., Guaifenesin 400 mg. **Inactive Ingredients (listed for individuals with specific allergies):** Cellulose, Croscarmellose Sodium, Hydroxypropyl Methylcellulose, Magnesium Stearate, Polyethylene Glycol, Povidone, Silica Gel, Starch.

Directions: One caplet every 4 hours not to exceed 4 caplets in 24 hours. Children (6 to 12 years): one-half the adult dose (break caplet in half). Children under 6 years use only as directed by physician.
TAMPER-RESISTANT PACKAGE FEATURES FOR YOUR PROTECTION:
- The carton has been sealed at the factory with a clear overwrap printed with "safety sealed."
- Each caplet is encased in a clear plastic cell with a foil back.
- The letter "C" appears on each caplet (see product illustration on front of carton).
- **DO NOT USE THIS PRODUCT IF ANY OF THESE TAMPER-RESISTANT FEATURES ARE MISSING OR BROKEN. IF YOU HAVE ANY QUESTIONS, PLEASE CALL 1-800-321-1834 TOLL FREE.**

Warning: Do not exceed recommended dosage. If symptoms do not improve within 7 days or are accompanied by high fever, rash, shortness of breath or persistent headache, consult a physician before continuing use. Do not use if you have high blood pressure, heart disease, diabetes, thyroid disease or a persistent or chronic cough, except under the advice and supervision of a physician. Keep this and all drugs out of reach of children. In case of accidental overdose, seek professional assistance or contact a poison control center immediately. As with any drug, if you are pregnant or nursing a baby, seek the advice of a health professional before using this product.

Drug Interaction Precaution: Do not take this product if you are presently taking a prescription antihypertensive or antidepressant drug containing a monoamine oxidase inhibitor except under the advice and supervision of a physician.

Store at controlled room temperature (59°–86°F.).
The Congestac horizontal color bar is a trademark.

How Supplied: In consumer packages of 12 and 24 caplets.
Shown in Product Identification Section, page 417

FEMIRON® Multi-Vitamins and Iron
[fem 'i 'ern]

Active Ingredients: Iron (from ferrous fumarate) 20 mg; Vitamin A 5,000 I.U.; Vitamin D 400 I.U.; Thiamine (Vitamin B_1) 1.5 mg; Riboflavin (Vitamin B_2) 1.7 mg; Niacinamide 20 mg; Ascorbic Acid (Vitamin C) 60 mg; Pyridoxine (Vitamin B_6) 2 mg; Cyanocobalamin (Vitamin B_{12}) 6 mcg; Pantothenic Acid 10 mg; Folic Acid .4 mg; and Tocopherol Acetate (Vitamin E) 15 I.U.

Inactive Ingredients: Alginic acid, blue 2, carnauba wax, dibasic calcium phosphate, flavor, hydroxypropyl methylcellulose, magnesium stearate, polyethylene glycol, red 40, silicon dioxide, sodium lauryl sulfate, starch, titanium dioxide, white wax.

Indications: For use as an iron and vitamin supplement.

Actions: Helps ensure adequate intake of iron and vitamins.

Warning: Keep out of reach of children.

Precaution: Alcoholics and individuals with chronic liver or pancreatic disease may have enhanced iron absorption with the potential for iron overload. NOTE: Unabsorbed iron may cause some darkening of the stool.

Symptoms and Treatment of Oral Overdosage: Toxicity and symptoms are primarily due to iron overdose. Abdominal pain, nausea, vomiting and diarrhea may occur, with possible subsequent acidosis and cardiovascular collapse with severe poisoning. **Treatment:** Induce vomiting immediately. Administer milk, eggs to reduce gastric irritation. Contact a physician immediately.

Dosage and Administration: Women: One tablet daily.
TAMPER-RESISTANT PACKAGE FEATURE:
- Bottle has imprinted seal under cap.
- **DO NOT USE IF SEAL IS BROKEN OR MISSING. IF YOU HAVE ANY QUESTIONS, PLEASE CALL 1-800-321-1834 TOLL FREE.**

How Supplied: Bottles of 35, 60, and 90 tablets. Femiron Iron Supplement (no added vitamins) is also available.
Shown in Product Identification Section, page 417

HOLD®
4 Hour Cough Suppressant Lozenge

Active Ingredient: 5.0 mg. dextromethorphan HBr per lozenge. **Inactive Ingredients:** Corn syrup, flavors, magnesium trisilicate, sucrose, vegetable oil, Yellow 10.

Continued on next page

Menley & James—Cont.

Indications: Suppresses coughs for up to 4 hours.

Actions: Dextromethorphan is the most widely used, non-narcotic/non-habit forming antitussive. A 10-20 mg. dose has been recognized as being effective in relieving the discomfort of coughs up to 4 hours by reducing cough intensity and frequency.

Warnings: Do not take this product for persistent or chronic cough such as occurs with smoking, asthma, chronic bronchitis, or emphysema, or where cough is accompanied by excessive phlegm (sputum), unless directed by a doctor. A persistent cough may be a sign of a serious condition. If cough persists for more than 1 week, tends to recur, or is accompanied by fever, rash or persistent headache, consult a doctor. Do not give this product to children under 6 years of age unless directed by a doctor. As with any drug, if you are pregnant or nursing a baby, seek the advice of a health professional before using this product. Keep this and all drugs out of the reach of children. In case of accidental overdose, seek professional assistance or contact a poison control center immediately.

Dosage and Administration: Adults (12 years and older): Take 2 lozenges one after the other, every 4 hours as needed. Children (6-12 years): One lozenge every 4 hours as needed. Let dissolve fully.

How Supplied: 10 individually wrapped lozenges come packaged in a plastic tube container.

Shown in Product Identification Section, page 418

LIQUIPRIN®
Infants' Drops and Children's Elixir (acetaminophen)

Description: Liquiprin is a nonsalicylate analgesic and antipyretic particularly suitable for infants and children. Liquiprin Drops is a raspberry-flavored, reddish pink solution. Liquiprin Elixir is a cherry-flavored, reddish solution. Neither contains alcohol.

Active Ingredient:
Liquiprin Drops: Acetaminophen 80 mg per 1.66 ml (top mark on dropper).
Liquiprin Elixir: Acetaminophen 80 mg per ½ teaspoon.

Inactive Ingredients: Artificial Cherry and other artificial and natural flavors, Citric Acid, D&C Red #33, FD&C Red #40, Dextrose, Fructose, Glycerin, Methylparaben, Polyethylene Glycol, Propylparaben, Sodium Citrate, Sodium Gluconate, Sucrose, Water.

Actions: Liquiprin Children's Elixir and Infants' Drops safely and effectively reduces fever and pain in infants and children without the hazards of salicylate therapy (e.g., gastric mucosal irritation).

Warnings: Do not give this product for pain for more than 5 days or for fever for more than 3 days unless directed by a doctor. If pain or fever persists or gets worse, if new symptoms occur, or if redness or swelling is present, consult a doctor because these could be signs of a serious condition.

Indications: Liquiprin is indicated for use in the treatment of infants and children with conditions requiring reduction of fever and/or relief of pain such as mild upper respiratory infections (tonsillitis, common cold, flu), teething, headache, myalgia, postimmunization reactions, posttonsillectomy discomfort and gastroenteritis. As adjunctive therapy with antibiotics or sulfonamides, Liquiprin may be useful as an analgesic and antipyretic in bacterial or viral infections, such as bronchitis, pharyngitis, tracheobronchitis, sinusitis, pneumonia, otitis media and cervical adenitis.

Precautions and Adverse Reactions: If a sensitivity reaction occurs, the drug should be discontinued. Liquiprin has rarely been found to produce side effects. It is usually well tolerated by patients who are sensitive to products containing aspirin.

Usual Dosage:
Liquiprin Drops and Elixir may be given alone or mixed with milk, juices, applesauce or other beverages and foods. All dosages may be repeated every 4 hours, if pain and fever persist, but not to exceed 5 times daily or as directed by physician.
Liquiprin Drops should be administered in the following dosages:
0–3 months: 40 mg—½ dropperful
4–11 months: 80 mg—1 dropperful
12–23 months: 120 mg—1½ dropperfuls
2–3 years, 24–35 lbs.: 160 mg—2 dropperfuls
4–5 years, 36–47 lbs.: 240 mg—3 dropperfuls
Liquiprin Elixir should be administered in the following dosages:
Under 2 years, use Liquiprin Drops.
2–3 years, 24–35 lbs.: 1 teaspoonful
4–5 years, 36–47 lbs.: 1½ teaspoonfuls
6–8 years, 48–59 lbs.: 2 teaspoonfuls
9–10 years, 60–71 lbs.: 2½ teaspoonfuls
11–12 years, 72–95 lbs.: 3 teaspoonfuls

How Supplied: Liquiprin Drops is available in a 1.16 fl. oz. (35 ml) plastic bottle with a calibrated dropper and child-resistant cap, and safety-sealed package.
Liquiprin Elixir is available in a 4 fl. oz. plastic bottle with a pre-marked measuring cup and child-resistant cap, and safety-sealed package.

Shown in Product Identification Section, page 418

ORNEX®
decongestant/analgesic Caplets

Product Information: For temporary relief of nasal congestion, headache, aches, pains and fever due to colds, sinusitis and flu.

NO ANTIHISTAMINE DROWSINESS

Formula: Active Ingredients: Each caplet contains Pseudoephedrine Hydrochloride 30 mg., Acetaminophen 325 mg.
Inactive Ingredients (listed for individuals with specific allergies): Cellulose, Crospovidone, FD&C Blue 1, Hydroxypropyl Methylcellulose, Magnesium Stearate, Polyethylene Glycol, Polysorbate 80, Povidone, Starch, Titanium Dioxide, and trace amounts of other inactive ingredients.

Directions: Adults—TWO CAPLETS every 4 hours, not to exceed 8 caplets in any 24-hour period. Children (6 to 12 years)—ONE CAPLET every 4 hours, not to exceed 4 caplets in 24 hours.

TAMPER-RESISTANT PACKAGE FEATURES FOR YOUR PROTECTION:
- The carton has been sealed at the factory with a clear overwrap printed with "safety sealed."
- Each caplet is encased in a clear plastic cell with a foil back.
- The name ORNEX appears on each caplet (see product illustration on front of carton).
- **DO NOT USE THIS PRODUCT IF ANY OF THESE TAMPER-RESISTANT FEATURES ARE MISSING OR BROKEN. IF YOU HAVE ANY QUESTIONS, PLEASE CALL 1-800-321-1834 TOLL FREE.**

Warnings: Do not exceed recommended dosage. Do not give to children under 6 or use for more than 10 days, unless directed by physician. If you have or are being treated for depression, high blood pressure, diabetes, heart disease or thyroid disease, use only as directed by physician. Stop use if dizziness, sleeplessness or nervousness occurs. This package is for households without young children. Keep this and all medicines out of reach of children. In case of accidental overdose, seek professional assistance or contact a poison control center immediately. As with any drug, if you are pregnant or nursing a baby, seek the advice of a health professional before using this product.
Store at controlled room temperature (59°–86°F.).

How Supplied: In consumer packages of 24 and 48 caplets. Also, Dispensary Packages of 792 caplets for industrial dispensaries and student health clinics only.

Shown in Product Identification Section, page 418

S.T.37®
Antiseptic Solution

Active Ingredients: Hexylresorcinol (0.1%), Glycerin (27.1%).

Inactive Ingredients: Edentate Disodium, Monobasic Sodium Phosphate, Phosphoric Acid, Water.

Indications: For use as a soothing antiseptic and anesthetic solution on minor cuts, abrasions, and burns.

For temporary relief of occasional minor irritation or pain associated with sore mouth or sore throat.
May also be used to cleanse cuts and scrapes.

Directions: Adults and children 2 years of age and older:
For external use: Use full strength. Apply liberally as often as necessary.
For the mouth: Use full strength. Gargle or rinse for about 15 seconds, then spit out. May be repeated up to 4 times daily, if necessary.

Warnings: Do not use S.T.37 to treat deep or puncture wounds, wild or domestic animal bites, or infections. Instead, consult your doctor immediately. If sore throat is severe or persists for more than 2 days, or worsens, is accompanied or followed by fever, headache, rash, nausea, or vomiting, consult your doctor promptly. If sore mouth symptoms do not improve in 7 days, see your dentist or doctor. Do not administer to children under 2 years of age, unless directed by your doctor. Avoid contact with the eyes. Keep this and all medicines out of the reach of children. As with any drug, if you are pregnant or nursing a baby, seek the advice of a health professional before using.

How Supplied:
5.5 and 12 fl. oz. bottles.

SERUTAN®
Toasted Granules
(brand of psyllium hydrophilic mucilloid)

Description: Serutan Toasted Granules is a psyllium based, bulk-forming fiber for gentle restoration and maintenance of regularity. Its unique, chewable granule form allows for easy and palatable dosing when sprinkled on foods such as cereals, salad, or desserts, and accompanied by 8 oz. of liquid. Serutan is formulated without chemical stimulants and is not habit-forming.

Action: Serutan Toasted Granules promotes normal elimination and regularity by increasing bulk volume and water content of the stool.

Indications: For the management of chronic constipation, irritable bowel syndrome and constipation due to pregnancy, convalescence or senility. Also for stool softening in hemorrhoid patients.

Dosage and Administration: Each heaping teaspoon provides 2.5 grams of psyllium. The recommended initial dosage for adults and children 12 and over is one heaping teaspoon, one to three times daily. Serutan Toasted Granules can be sprinkled on food, including cereal, salads, casseroles and ice cream. Each dose must be accompanied by at least 8 oz. (a full glass) of liquid. Serutan should always be put on food, not taken directly from a spoon. For children 6–12, use half the adult dose (½ teaspoon) with 8 oz. of liquid one to three times daily.
If needed, dosage can be increased to a maximum of three heaping teaspoons for adults (1½ teaspoons for children 6–12), four times daily. Do not exceed 12 teaspoons (30 grams psyllium) per day for adults, or 6 teaspoons per day for children 6–12.
It may require two to three days' therapy to produce full effectiveness.

Contraindications: Fecal impaction or intestinal obstruction.

Warning: Keep this and all medications out of reach of children. May cause allergic reaction in those individuals sensitive to psyllium.

Active Ingredient: 2.5 grams psyllium hydrophilic mucilloid per heaping teaspoon.

Inactive Ingredients: Acacia, BHA, calcium propionate, caramel color, carboxymethylcellulose sodium, citric acid, cornstarch, invert sugar, magnesium stearate, oat flour, propylene glycol, propyl gallate, sodium benzoate, sodium saccharin, wheat germ. Each teaspoon contains less than 0.03 grams sodium.

How Supplied: Available in 6 oz. and 18 oz. plastic jars. Serutan is also available in two other formulas: Regular Powder (in 7 oz., 14 oz. and 21 oz. sizes) and Fruit Flavored Powder (in 6 oz., 12 oz. and 18 oz. sizes).

Shown in Product Identification Section, page 418

THERMOTABS®
[ther 'mo-tabs]
Buffered Salt Tablets

Active Ingredients: Per tablet—Sodium chloride—450 mg.; Potassium chloride —30 mg.

Inactive Ingredients: Acacia, Calcium carbonate, Calcium stearate, Dextrose.

Indications: To minimize fatigue and prevent muscle cramps and heat prostration due to excessive perspiration.

Actions: Thermotabs are designed for tennis players, joggers, golfers and other athletes who experience excessive perspiration. Also for use in steel mills, industrial plants, kitchens, stores, or other locations where high temperatures cause heat fatigue, cramps or heat prostration.

Warnings: Keep out of reach of children. As with any drug, if you are pregnant or nursing a baby, seek the advice of a health professional before using this product.

Precaution: Individuals on a salt-restricted diet should use THERMOTABS only under the advice and supervision of a physician.

Symptoms and Treatment of Oral Overdosage: Signs of salt overdose include diarrhea and muscular twitching. If an overdose is suspected, contact a physician, the local poison control center, or call the Rocky Mt. Poison Control Center at 303-592-1710 (Collect), 24 hours a day.

Dosage and Administration: One tablet with a full glass of water, 5 to 10 times a day depending on temperature and conditions.

How Supplied: 100 tablet bottles.

TROPH-IRON®
Vitamins B_1, B_{12} and Iron

Indications: For deficiencies of vitamins B_1, B_{12} and iron.

Directions: Liquid—One teaspoonful daily, or as directed by physician. While its effectiveness is in no way affected, TROPH-IRON Liquid may darken as it ages.

TAMPER-RESISTANT PACKAGE FEATURE: Sealed, imprinted bottle cap; do not use if broken.

Warning: The treatment of any anemic condition should be under the advice and supervision of a physician. Since oral iron products interfere with absorption of oral tetracycline antibiotics, these products should not be taken within two hours of each other.
Iron-containing medications may occasionally cause gastrointestinal discomfort, such as nausea, constipation or diarrhea.
Keep this and all drugs out of reach of children. In case of accidental overdose, seek professional assistance or contact a poison control center immediately.
As with any drug, if you are pregnant or nursing a baby, seek the advice of a health professional before using this product.
Store at room temperature (59°–86°F).

Formula: Each 5 ml. (1 teaspoonful) contains Thiamine Hydrochloride (vitamin B_1), 10 mg.; Cyanocobalamin (vitamin B_{12}), 25 mcg.; Iron, 20 mg., present as soluble ferric pyrophosphate. **Inactive Ingredients (listed for individuals with specific allergies):** Citric Acid, FD&C Red 40, Flavor, Glucose, Glycerin, Methyl and Propyl Paraben, Saccharin Sodium, Sodium Citrate, Purified Water.

How Supplied: Liquid—in 4 fl. oz. (118 ml) bottles.

TROPHITE®
Vitamins B_1 and B_{12}

Indications: For deficiencies of vitamins B_1 and B_{12}.

Directions: One 5 ml. teaspoonful or as directed by physician.

Important: Dispense liquid only in original bottle or an amber bottle. This product is light-sensitive. Never dispense in a flint, green, or blue bottle.
Trophite Liquid may be mixed with water, milk, or fruit or vegetable juices immediately before taking.
Store at controlled room temperature (59°–86°F.).

TAMPER-RESISTANT PACKAGE FEATURE: Liquid—Sealed, imprinted bottle cap; do not use if broken.

Warning: Keep this and all drugs out of reach of children. In case of accidental

Continued on next page

Menley & James—Cont.

overdose, seek professional assistance or contact a poison control center immediately.
As with any drug, if you are pregnant or nursing a baby, seek the advice of a health professional before using this product.

Formula: Each 5 ml. (1 teaspoonful) contains Thiamine Hydrochloride (vitamin B_1), 10 mg.; and Cyanocobalamin (vitamin B_{12}), 25 mcg. **Inactive Ingredients (listed for individuals with specific allergies):** LIQUID—D&C Red 33, Yellow 10, Dextrose, FD&C Blue 1, Flavor, Glycerin, Methyl and Propyl Paraben, Sodium Tartrate, Tartaric Acid, Purified Water.

How Supplied: Liquid—4 fl. oz. (118 ml.) bottles.

Miles Inc.
P. O. BOX 340
ELKHART, IN 46515

ALKA-MINTS® Chewable Antacid Rich in Calcium

Active Ingredient: Each ALKA-MINTS Chewable Antacid tablet contains calcium carbonate 850 mg. (340 mg of elemental calcium). Each tablet contains less than .5 mg sodium per tablet, and is dietarily sodium free.

Inactive Ingredients: Dioctyl sodium sulfosuccinate, flavor, hydrolyzed cereal solids, polyethylene glycol, sugar (compressible), magnesium stearate, sorbitol.

Indications: ALKA-MINTS is an antacid for occasional use for relief of acid indigestion, heartburn and sour stomach.

Actions: ALKA-MINTS has a natural, clean, spearmint taste that leaves the mouth feeling refreshed. Measured by the in-vitro standard established by the Food and Drug Administration, one ALKA-MINTS tablet neutralizes 15.9 mEq of acid.

Warnings: Do not take more than 9 tablets in a 24 hour period, or use the maximum dosage of this product for more than 2 weeks, except under the advice and supervision of a physician. May cause constipation. As with any drug, if you are pregnant or nursing a baby, seek the advice of a health professional before using this product. Keep this and all drugs out of the reach of children.

Dosage and Administration: Chew 1 tablet every 2 hours or as directed by a physician.

How Supplied: Cartons of 30's. Each carton contains convenient pocket-sized packs with individually sealed tablets so ALKA-MINTS stay fresh wherever you go.

Product Identification Mark: ALKA-MINTS embossed on each tablet.

Shown in Product Identification Section, page 418

ALKA-SELTZER® ADVANCED FORMULA

Active Ingredients: Each tablet contains: acetaminophen 325 mg, calcium carbonate 280 mg, citric acid 900 mg, potassium bicarbonate 300 mg, heat-treated sodium bicarbonate 465 mg. Alka-Seltzer Advanced Formula in water contains principally the antacid citrates of sodium, potassium and calcium.

Inactive Ingredients: Each tablet contains: Aminoacetic acid, aspartame, calcium saccharin, flavors, hydrolyzed cereal solids, hydroxypropyl methylcellulose, lactose, sorbitol, tableting aids. Contains 75% less sodium per tablet than Original Alka-Seltzer.

Indications: For speedy relief of ACID INDIGESTION, SOUR STOMACH or HEARTBURN with HEADACHE, or BODY ACHES AND PAINS. Also for fast relief of UPSET STOMACH with HEADACHE from overindulgence in food and drink—especially recommended for taking before bedtime and again on arising. EFFECTIVE FOR PAIN RELIEF ALONE: HEADACHE or BODY and MUSCULAR ACHES and PAINS.

Warnings: Do not take more than 8 tablets in a 24-hour period or use the maximum dosage of this product for more than 10 days, except under the advice and supervision of a physician. May cause constipation. If symptoms persist or recur frequently or if you are on a sodium-restricted diet, do not take this product except under the supervision of a physician. As with any drug, if you are pregnant or nursing a baby, seek the advice of a health professional before using this product. Keep this and all drugs out of the reach of children. In case of accidental overdose, contact a physician or poison control center immediately. Each tablet contains 141 mg sodium.
PHENYLKETONURICS: Contains 4.2 mg Phenylalanine per tablet.

Directions: Adults: Take 2 tablets fully dissolved in water every 4 hours or as directed by a physician.

How Supplied: Tablets: Foil sealed; box of 36 tablets in 18 twin packs; box of 24 in 12 foil twin packs.

Shown in Product Identification Section, page 418

ALKA-SELTZER® Effervescent Antacid & Pain Reliever With Specially Buffered Aspirin

Active Ingredients: Each tablet contains: aspirin 325 mg., heat treated sodium bicarbonate 1916 mg., citric acid 1000 mg. ALKA-SELTZER® in water contains principally the antacid sodium citrate and the analgesic sodium acetylsalicylate. Buffered pH is between 6 and 7.

Inactive Ingredients: None.

Indications: ALKA-SELTZER® Effervescent Antacid & Pain Reliever is an analgesic and an antacid and is indicated for relief of sour stomach, acid indigestion or heartburn with headache or body aches and pains. Also for fast relief of upset stomach with headache from overindulgence in food and drink—especially recommended for taking before bed and again on arising. Effective for pain relief alone: headache or body and muscular aches and pains.

Actions: When the ALKA-SELTZER® Effervescent Antacid & Pain Reliever tablet is dissolved in water, the acetylsalicylate ion differs from acetylsalicylic acid chemically, physically and pharmacologically. Being fat insoluble, it is not absorbed by the gastric mucosal cells. Studies and observations in animals and man including radiochrome determinations of fecal blood loss, measurement of ion fluxes and direct visualization with gastrocamera, have shown that, as contrasted with acetylsalicylic acid, the acetylsalicylate ion delivered in the solution does not alter gastric mucosal permeability to permit back-diffusion of hydrogen ion, and gastric damage and acute gastric mucosal lesions are therefore not seen after administration of the product. ALKA-SELTZER® Effervescent Antacid & Pain Reliever has the capacity to neutralize gastric hydrochloric acid quickly and effectively. In-vitro, 154 ml. of 0.1 N hydrochloric acid are required to decrease the pH of one tablet of ALKA-SELTZER® Effervescent Antacid & Pain Reliever in solution to 4.0. Measured against the in vitro standard established by the Food and Drug Administration one tablet neutralizes 17.2 mEq of acid. In vivo, the antacid activity of two ALKA-SELTZER® Antacid & Pain Reliever tablets is comparable to that of 10 ml. of milk of magnesia. ALKA-SELTZER® Effervescent Antacid & Pain Reliever is able to resist pH changes caused by the continuing secretion of acid in the normal individual and to maintain an elevated pH until emptying occurs.
ALKA-SELTZER® Effervescent Antacid & Pain Reliever provides highly water soluble acetylsalicylate ions which are fat insoluble. Acetylsalicylate ions are not absorbed from the stomach. They empty from the stomach and thereby become available for absorption from the duodenum. Thus, fast drug absorption and high plasma acetylsalicylate levels are achieved. Plasma levels of salicylate following the administration of ALKA-SELTZER® Effervescent Antacid & Pain Reliever solution (acetylsalicylate ion equivalent to 648 mg. acetylsalicylic acid) can reach 29 mg./liter in 10 minutes and rise to peak levels as high as 55 mg./liter within 30 minutes.

Warnings: Children and teenagers should not use this medicine for chicken pox or flu symptoms before a doctor is

consulted about Reye Syndrome, a rare but serious illness reported to be associated with aspirin. As with any drug, if you are pregnant or nursing a baby, seek the advice of a health professional before using this product. IT IS ESPECIALLY IMPORTANT NOT TO USE ASPIRIN DURING THE LAST 3 MONTHS OF PREGNANCY UNLESS SPECIFICALLY DIRECTED TO DO SO BY A DOCTOR BECAUSE IT MAY CAUSE PROBLEMS IN THE UNBORN CHILD OR COMPLICATIONS DURING DELIVERY. Except under the advice and supervision of a physician, do not take more than, Adults: 8 tablets in a 24 hour period. (60 years of age or older: 4 tablets in a 24 hour period), or use the maximum dosage for more than 10 days. Do not use if you are allergic to aspirin or have asthma, if you have a coagulation (bleeding) disease, or if you are on a sodium restricted diet. Each tablet contains 567 mg. of sodium.
Keep this and all drugs out of the reach of children.

Dosage and Administration:
ALKA-SELTZER® must be dissolved in water before taking.
Adults: 2 tablets every 4 hours.
CAUTION: If symptoms persist or recur frequently, or if you are under treatment for ulcer, consult your physician.

Professional Labeling:

ASPIRIN FOR MYOCARDIAL INFARCTION

Indication: The Aspirin contained in ALKA-SELTZER® is indicated to reduce the risk of death and/or non-fatal myocardial infarction in patients with a previous infarction or unstable angina pectoris.

Clinical Trials: The indication is supported by the results of six, large, randomized multicenter, placebo-controlled studies[1–7] involving 10,816, predominantly male, post-myocardial infarction (MI) patients and one randomized placebo-controlled study of 1,266 men with unstable angina. Therapy with aspirin was begun at intervals after the onset of acute MI varying from less than 3 days to more than 5 years and continued for periods of from less than one year to four years. In the unstable angina study, treatment was started within 1 month after the onset of unstable angina and continued for 12 weeks and complicating conditions such as congestive heart failure were not included in the study.
Aspirin therapy in MI patients was associated with about a 20 percent reduction in the risk of subsequent death and/or non-fatal reinfarction, a median absolute decrease of 3 percent from the 12 to 22 percent event rates in the placebo groups. In aspirin-treated unstable angina patients the reduction in risk was about 50 percent, a reduction in event rate of 5 percent from the 10 percent rate in the placebo group over the 12 weeks of the study.
Daily dosage of aspirin in the post-myocardial infarction studies was 300 mg in one study and 900 to 1500 mg in five studies. A dose of 325 mg was used in the study of unstable angina.

Adverse Reactions: Gastrointestinal Reactions: Symptoms and signs of gastrointestinal irritation were not significantly increased in subjects treated for unstable angina with buffered aspirin in solution. (ALKA-SELZER®.) Doses of 1000 mg per day of aspirin tablets caused gastrointestinal symptoms and bleeding that in some cases were clinically significant. In the largest post-infarction study (the Aspirin Myocardial Infarction Study (AMIS) with 4,500 people), the percentage incidences of gastrointestinal symptoms for the aspirin (1000 mg of a standard, solid-tablet formulation) and placebo-treated subjects, respectively, were: stomach pain (14.5%; 4.4%); heartburn (11.9%; 4.8%); nausea and/or vomiting (7.6%; 2.1%); hospitalization for gastrointestinal disorder (4.9%; 3.5%). In the AMIS and other trials, aspirin treated patients had increased rates of gross gastrointestinal bleeding. As with all aspirin products ALKA-SELTZER is contraindicated in patients with aspirin sensitivity, with asthma, or with coagulation disease.

Cardiovascular and Biochemical: In the AMIS trial, the dosage of 1000 mg per day of aspirin was associated with small increases in systolic blood pressure (BP) (average 1.5 to 2.1 mm) and diastolic BP (0.5 to 0.6 mm), depending upon whether maximal or last available readings were used. Blood urea nitrogen and uric acid levels were also increased, but by less than 1.0 mg%. Subjects with marked hypertension or renal insufficiency had been excluded from the trial so that the clinical importance of these observations for such subjects or for any subjects treated over more prolonged periods is not known. It is recommended that patients placed on long-term aspirin treatment, even at doses of 300 mg per day, be seen at regular intervals to assess changes in these measurements.

Sodium in Buffered Aspirin for Solution Formulations: One tablet daily of buffered aspirin in solution adds 567 mg of sodium to that in the diet and may not be tolerated by patients with active sodium-retaining states such as congestive heart or renal failure. This amount of sodium adds about 30 percent to the 70 to 90 meq intake suggested as appropriate for dietary treatment of essential hypertension in the 1984 Report of the Joint National Committee on Detection, Evaluation, and Treatment of High Blood Pressure[8].

Dosage and Administration: Although most of the studies used dosages exceeding 300 mg, daily, two trials used only 300 mg and pharmacologic data indicate that this dose inhibits platelet function fully. Therefore, 300 mg or a conventional 325 mg aspirin dose daily is a reasonable, routine dose that would minimize gastrointestinal adverse reactions. This use of aspirin applies to both solid, oral dosage forms (buffered and plain aspirin) and buffered aspirin in solution.

References:

(1) Elwood, P. C., et al., A Randomized Controlled Trial of Acetysalicylic Acid in the Secondary Prevention of Mortality from Myocardial Infarction," *British Medical Journal* 1:436–440, 1974.
(2) The Coronary Drug Project Research Group, "Aspirin in Coronary Heart Disease," *Journal of Chronic Diseases,* 29:625–642, 1976.
(3) Breddin K., et al., "Secondary Prevention of Myocardial Infarction: A Comparison of Acetylsalicylic Acid, Phenprocoumon or Placebo," *International Congress Series* 470:263–268, 1979.
(4) Aspirin Myocardial Infarction Study Research Group, "A Randomized, Controlled Trial of Aspirin in Persons Recovered from Myocardial Infarction," *Journal American Medical Association* 245:661–669, 1980.
(5) Elwood, P. C., and P. M. Sweetnam, "Aspirin and Secondary Mortality after Myocardial Infarction," *Lancet* pp. 1313–1315, December 22–29, 1979.
(6) The Persantine-Aspirin Reinfarction Study Research Group, "Persantine and Aspirin in Coronary Heart Disease," *Circulation,* 62: 449–460, 1980.
(7) Lewis, H. D., et al., "Protective Effects of Aspirin Against Acute Myocardial Infarction and Death in Men with Unstable Angina, Results of a Veterans Administration Cooperative Study," *New England Journal of Medicine* 309:396–403, 1983.
(8) "1984 Report of the Joint National Committee on Detection, Evaluation, Treatment of High Blood Pressure," U.S. Department of Health and Human Services and United States Public Health Service, National Institutes of Health.

How Supplied: Tablets: foil sealed; box of 12 in 6 foil twin packs; box of 24 in 12 foil twin packs; box of 36 tablets in 18 foil twin packs; 100 tablets in 50 foil twin packs; carton of 72 tablets in 36 foil twin packs; 96's card in 48 foil twin packs. Product Identification Mark: "ALKA-SELTZER" embossed on each tablet.

Shown in Product Identification Section, page 418

Flavored ALKA-SELTZER® Effervescent Antacid & Pain Reliever

Active Ingredients: Each tablet contains: Aspirin 325 mg, heat treated sodium bicarbonate 1710 mg, citric acid 1220 mg. Alka-Seltzer in water contains principally the antacid sodium citrate and the analgesic sodium acetylsalicylate.

Inactive Ingredients: Flavors, Saccharin Sodium.

Indications: SPARKLING FRESH TASTE!

Continued on next page

Miles—Cont.

Flavored Alka-Seltzer®

For speedy relief of ACID INDIGESTION, SOUR STOMACH or HEARTBURN with HEADACHE, or BODY ACHES AND PAINS. Also for fast relief of UPSET STOMACH with HEADACHE from overindulgence in food and drink —especially recommended for taking before bed and again on arising. EFFECTIVE FOR PAIN RELIEF ALONE: HEADACHE or BODY and MUSCULAR ACHES and PAINS.

Warnings: Children and teenagers should not use this medicine for chicken pox or flu symptoms before a doctor is consulted about Reye Syndrome, a rare but serious illness reported to be associated with aspirin.

As with any drug, if you are pregnant or nursing a baby, seek the advice of a health professional before using this product. IT IS ESPECIALLY IMPORTANT NOT TO USE ASPIRIN DURING THE LAST 3 MONTHS OF PREGNANCY UNLESS SPECIFICALLY DIRECTED TO DO SO BY A DOCTOR BECAUSE IT MAY CAUSE PROBLEMS IN THE UNBORN CHILD OR COMPLICATIONS DURING DELIVERY.

Except under the advice and supervision of a physician: Do not take more than, ADULTS: 6 tablets in a 24-hour period, (60 years of age or older: 4 tablets in a 24-hour period), or use the daily maximum dosage for more than 10 days. Do not use if you are allergic to aspirin or have asthma, if you have a coagulation (bleeding) disease, or if you are on a sodium restricted diet. Each tablet contains 506 mg of sodium.

Keep this and all drugs out of the reach of children.

Directions: Alka-Seltzer must be dissolved in water before taking. ADULTS: 2 tablets every 4 hours. CAUTION: If symptoms persist or recur frequently or if you are under treatment for ulcer, consult your physician.

Professional Labeling:

ASPIRIN FOR MYOCARDIAL INFARCTION

Indication: The Aspirin contained in Alka-Seltzer is indicated to reduce the risk of death and/or non-fatal myocardial infarction in patients with a previous infarction or unstable angina pectoris.

Clinical Trials: The indication is supported by the results of six, large, randomized multicenter, placebo-controlled studies[1–7] involving 10,816, predominantly male, post-myocardial infarction (MI) patients and one randomized placebo-controlled study of 1,266 men with unstable angina. Therapy with aspirin was begun at intervals after the onset of acute MI varying from less than 3 days to more than 5 years and continued for periods of from less than one year to four years. In the unstable angina study, treatment was started within 1 month after the onset of unstable angina and continued for 12 weeks and complicating conditions such as congestive heart failure were not included in the study.

Aspirin therapy in MI patients was associated with about a 20 percent reduction in the risk of subsequent death and/or non-fatal reinfarction, a median absolute decrease of 3 percent from the 12 to 22 percent event rates in the placebo groups. In aspirin-treated unstable angina patients the reduction in risk was about 50 percent, a reduction in event rate of 5 percent from the 10 percent rate in the placebo group over the 12 weeks of the study.

Daily dosage of aspirin in the post-myocardial infarction studies was 300 mg in one study and 900 to 1500 mg in five studies. A dose of 325 mg was used in the study of unstable angina.

Adverse Reactions: Gastrointestinal Reactions: Symptoms and signs of gastrointestinal irritation were not significantly increased in subjects treated for unstable angina with buffered aspirin in solution (ALKA-SELZER®). Doses of 1000 mg per day of aspirin tablets caused gastrointestinal symptoms and bleeding that in some cases were clinically significant. In the largest post-infarction study (the Aspirin Myocardial Infarction Study (AMIS) with 4,500 people), the percentage incidences of gastrointestinal symptoms for the aspirin (1000 mg of a standard, solid-tablet formulation) and placebo-treated subjects, respectively, were: stomach pain (14.5%; 4.4%); heartburn (11.9%; 4.8%); nausea and/or vomiting (7.6%; 2.1%); hospitalization for gastrointestinal disorder (4.9%; 3.5%). In the AMIS and other trials, aspirin treated patients had increased rates of gross gastrointestinal bleeding. As with all aspirin products Alka-Seltzer is contraindicated in patients with aspirin sensitivity, with asthma, or with coagulation disease.

Cardiovascular and Biochemical: In the AMIS trial, the dosage of 1000 mg per day of aspirin was associated with small increases in systolic blood pressure (BP) (average 1.5 to 2.1 mm) and diastolic BP (0.5 to 0.6 mm), depending upon whether maximal or last available readings were used. Blood urea nitrogen and uric acid levels were also increased, but by less than 1.0 mg%. Subjects with marked hypertension or renal insufficiency had been excluded from the trial so that the clinical importance of these observations for such subjects or for any subjects treated over more prolonged periods is not known. It is recommended that patients placed on long-term aspirin treatment, even at doses of 300 mg per day, be seen at regular intervals to assess changes in these measurements.

Sodium in Buffered Aspirin for Solution Formulations: One tablet daily of flavored buffered aspirin in solution adds 506 mg of sodium to that in the diet and may not be tolerated by patients with active sodium-retaining states such as congestive heart or renal failure. This amount of sodium adds about 30 percent to the 70 to 90 meq intake suggested as appropriate for dietary treatment of essential hypertension in the 1984 Report of the Joint National Committee on Detection, Evaluation, and Treatment of High Blood Pressure[8].

Dosage and Administration: Although most of the studies used dosages exceeding 300 mg, daily, two trials used only 300 mg and pharmacologic data indicate that this dose inhibits platelet function fully. Therefore, 300 mg or a conventional 325 mg aspirin dose daily is a reasonable, routine dose that would minimize gastrointestinal adverse reactions. This use of aspirin applies to both solid, oral dosage forms (buffered and plain aspirin) and buffered aspirin in solution.

References:

(1) Elwood, P. C., et al., A Randomized Controlled Trial of Acetysalicylic Acid in the Secondary Prevention of Mortality from Myocardial Infarction," *British Medical Journal* 1:436–440, 1974.

(2) The Coronary Drug Project Research Group, "Aspirin in Coronary Heart Disease," *Journal of Chronic Diseases,* 29:625–642, 1976.

(3) Breddin K., et al., "Secondary Prevention of Myocardial Infarction: A Comparison of Acetylsalicylic Acid, Phenprocoumon or Placebo," *International Congress Series* 470:263–268, 1979.

(4) Aspirin Myocardial Infarction Study Research Group, "A Randomized, Controlled Trial of Aspirin in Persons Recovered from Myocardial Infarction," *Journal American Medical Association* 245:661–669, 1980.

(5) Elwood, P. C., and P. M. Sweetnam, "Aspirin and Secondary Mortality after Myocardial Infarction," *Lancet* pp. 1313–1315, December 22–29, 1979.

(6) The Persantine Aspirin Reinfarction Study Research Group, "Persantine and Aspirin in Coronary Heart Disease," *Circulation,* 62: 449–460, 1980.

(7) Lewis, H. D., et al., "Protective Effects of Aspirin Against Acute Myocardial Infarction and Death in Men with Unstable Angina, Results of a Veterans Administration Cooperative Study," *New England Journal of Medicine* 309:396–403, 1983.

(8) "1984 Report of the Joint National Committee on Detection, Evaluation, Treatment of High Blood Pressure," U.S. Department of Health and Human Services and United States Public Health Service, National Institutes of Health.

How Supplied: Foil sealed effervescent tablets in cartons of 12's in 6 foil twin packs; 24's in 12 foil twin packs; 36's in 18 foil twin packs.

Shown in Product Identification Section, page 418

ALKA-SELTZER® Effervescent Antacid

Active Ingredients: Each tablet contains heat treated sodium bicarbonate 958 mg., citric acid 832 mg., potassium bicarbonate 312 mg. ALKA-SELTZER® Effervescent Antacid in water contains principally the antacids sodium citrate and potassium citrate.

Inactive Ingredients: A tableting aid.

Indications: ALKA-SELTZER® Effervescent Antacid is indicated for relief of acid indigestion, sour stomach or heartburn.

Actions: The ALKA-SELTZER® Effervescent Antacid solution provides quick and effective neutralization of gastric acid. Measured by the in vitro standard established by the Food and Drug Administration one tablet will neutralize 10.6 mEq of acid.

Warnings: Except under the advice and supervision of a physician, do not take more than: Adults: 8 tablets in a 24 hour period (60 years of age or older: 7 tablets in a 24 hour period), Children: 4 tablets in a 24 hour period; or use the maximum dosage of this product for more than 2 weeks.
Do not use this product if you are on a sodium restricted diet. Each tablet contains 311 mg. of sodium.
Keep this and all drugs out of the reach of children. As with any drug, if you are pregnant or nursing a baby, seek the advice of a health professional before using this product.

Dosage and Administration: Adults: Take 1 or 2 tablets fully dissolved in water every 4 hours. Children: ½ the adult dosage.

How Supplied: Boxes of 20 tablets in 10 foil twin packs; 36 tablets in 18 foil twin packs.

Shown in Product Identification Section, page 418

ALKA-SELTZER® Extra Strength Antacid & Pain Reliever

Active Ingredients: Each tablet contains: Aspirin 500mg, heat treated sodium bicarbonate 1985mg, citric acid 1000mg. Alka-Seltzer in water contains principally the antacid sodium citrate and the analgesic sodium acetylsalicylate.

Inactive Ingredients: Flavors

Indications: For speedy relief of acid indigestion, sour stomach or heartburn with headache or body aches and pains. Also, for fast relief of upset stomach with headache from overindulgence in food and drink—especially recommended for taking before bed and again on arising. Effective for pain relief alone: headache or body and muscular aches and pains.

Warnings: Children and teenagers should not use this medicine for chicken pox or flu symptoms before a doctor is consulted about Reye Syndrome, a rare but serious illness reported to be associated with aspirin. As with any drug, if you are pregnant or nursing a baby, seek the advice of a health professional before using this product. IT IS ESPECIALLY IMPORTANT NOT TO USE ASPIRIN DURING THE LAST 3 MONTHS OF PREGNANCY UNLESS SPECIFICALLY DIRECTED TO DO SO BY A DOCTOR BECAUSE IT MAY CAUSE PROBLEMS IN THE UNBORN CHILD OR COMPLICATIONS DURING DELIVERY. Except under the advice and supervision of a physician, do not take more than, Adults: 7 tablets in a 24-hour period (60 years of age or older, 4 tablets in a 24-hour period), or use the daily maximum dosage for more than 10 days. Do not use if you are allergic to aspirin or have asthma, if you have a coagulation (bleeding) disease, or if you are on a sodium restricted diet. Each tablet contains 588mg of sodium. Keep this and all drugs out of the reach of children.

Dosage and Administration: Extra Strength Alka-Seltzer must be dissolved in water before taking. Adults: 2 tablets every 4 hours. Caution: If symptoms persist, or recur frequently, or if you are under treatment for ulcer, consult your physician.

How Supplied: Foil sealed effervescent tablets in cartons of 12's in 6 foil twin packs; 24's in 12 foil twin packs.

Shown in Product Identification Section, page 418

ALKA-SELTZER PLUS® Cold Medicine

Active Ingredients:
Each dry ALKA-SELTZER PLUS® Cold Tablet contains the following active ingredients: Phenylpropanolamine bitartrate 24.08 mg., chlorpheniramine maleate 2 mg., acetylsalicylic acid (aspirin) 325 mg. The product is dissolved in water prior to ingestion and the aspirin is converted into its soluble ionic form, sodium acetylsalicylate.

Inactive Ingredients: Citric acid, flavors, sodium bicarbonate.

Indications: For relief of the symptoms of common colds and flu.

Actions: Provides temporary relief of these major cold and flu symptoms: nasal and sinus congestion, runny nose, sneezing, headache, sore throat, fever, body aches and pains.

Warnings: Children and teenagers should not use this medicine for chicken pox or flu symptoms before a doctor is consulted about Reye Syndrome, a rare but serious illness reported to be associated with aspirin. Do not exceed recommended dosage because at higher doses nervousness, dizziness or sleeplessness may occur. May cause excitability, especially in children. Do not take this product if you are allergic to aspirin or have asthma, glaucoma, bleeding problems, emphysema, chronic pulmonary disease, shortness of breath, difficulty in breathing, heart disease, high blood pressure, thyroid disease, diabetes or difficulty in urination due to enlargement of the prostate gland or on a sodium-restricted diet unless directed by a doctor. Each tablet contains 506 mg of sodium. May cause drowsiness; alcohol, sedatives and tranquilizers may increase drowsiness effect. Avoid alcoholic beverages while taking this product. Do not take this product if you are taking sedatives or tranquilizers without first consulting your doctor. Use caution when driving a motor vehicle or operating machinery. If sore throat is severe, persists for more than 2 days, is accompanied by a high fever, headache, nausea or vomiting, consult a physician promptly. Do not take this product for more than 7 days. If symptoms do not improve or are accompanied by fever or if fever persists for more than 3 days, consult a doctor. As with any drug, if you are pregnant or nursing a baby, seek the advice of a health professional before using this product. IT IS ESPECIALLY IMPORTANT NOT TO USE ASPIRIN DURING THE LAST 3 MONTHS OF PREGNANCY UNLESS SPECIFICALLY DIRECTED TO DO SO BY A DOCTOR BECAUSE IT MAY CAUSE PROBLEMS IN THE UNBORN CHILD OR COMPLICATIONS DURING DELIVERY. Keep this and all drugs out of the reach of children.

Drug Interaction Precaution: Do not take this product if you are presently taking a prescription drug for anticoagulation (thinning the blood), high blood pressure or depression without first consulting your doctor.

Dosage and Administration:
ALKA-SELTZER PLUS® is taken in solution; approximately 4 ounces of water per tablet is sufficient. Adults: two tablets every 4 hours up to 8 tablets in 24 hours.

How Supplied: Tablets: carton of 12 tablets in 6 foil twin packs; 20 tablets in 10 foil twin packs; carton of 36 tablets in 18 foil twin packs; carton of 48 tablets in 24 foil twin packs.

Product Identification Mark:
"Alka-Seltzer Plus" embossed on each tablet.

Shown in Product Identification Section, page 418

ALKA-SELTZER PLUS® Night-Time Cold Medicine

Active Ingredients: Each tablet contains phenylpropanolamine bitartrate 24.08 mg, diphenhydramine citrate 38.33 mg, acetylsalicylic acid (aspirin) 325 mg. In water the aspirin is converted into its soluble ionic form, sodium acetylsalicylate.

Inactive Ingredients: Citric acid, flavors, heat-treated sodium bicarbonate, tableting aids.

Indications: For relief of the symptoms of common colds and flu, to help you get the rest you need.

Actions: Provides temporary relief of these major cold and flu symptoms: nasal and sinus congestion, runny nose, sneezing, headache, sore throat, fever, body aches and pains.

Warnings: Children and teenagers should not use this medicine for chicken

Continued on next page

Miles—Cont.

pox or flu symptoms before a doctor is consulted about Reye Syndrome, a rare but serious illness reported to be associated with aspirin. Do not exceed recommended dosage because at higher doses nervousness, dizziness or sleeplessness may occur. May cause excitability, especially in children. Do not take this product if you are allergic to aspirin or have asthma, glaucoma, bleeding problems, emphysema, chronic pulmonary disease, shortness of breath, difficulty in breathing, heart disease, high blood pressure, thyroid disease, diabetes or difficulty in urination due to enlargement of the prostate gland or on a sodium-restricted diet unless directed by a doctor. Each tablet contains 506 mg of sodium. May cause marked drowsiness; alcohol, sedatives and tranquilizers may increase drowsiness effect. Avoid alcoholic beverages while taking this product. Do not take this product if you are taking sedatives or tranquilizers without first consulting your doctor. Use caution when driving a motor vehicle or operating machinery. If sore throat is severe, persists for more than 2 days, is accompanied by high fever, headache, nausea or vomiting, consult a physician promptly. Do not take this product for more than 7 days. If symptoms do not improve or are accompanied by fever or if fever persists for more than 3 days, consult a doctor. As with any drug, if you are pregnant or nursing a baby, seek the advice of a health professional before using this product. IT IS ESPECIALLY IMPORTANT NOT TO USE ASPIRIN DURING THE LAST 3 MONTHS OF PREGNANCY UNLESS SPECIFICALLY DIRECTED TO DO SO BY A DOCTOR BECAUSE IT MAY CAUSE PROBLEMS IN THE UNBORN CHILD OR COMPLICATIONS DURING DELIVERY. Keep this and all drugs out of the reach of children.

Drug Interaction Precaution: Do not take this product if you are presently taking a prescription drug for anticoagulation (thinning the blood), high blood pressure or depression without first consulting your doctor.

Dosage and Administration: Adults: Take 2 tablets dissolved in 4 ounces of water every 4 to 6 hours, not to exceed 8 tablets daily.

How Supplied: Tablets: carton of 12 tablets in 6 child-resistant foil twin packs; carton of 20 tablets in 10 child-resistant foil twin packs; carton of 36 tablets in 18 child-resistant foil twin packs.

Product Identification Mark: "A/S PLUS NIGHT-TIME" etched on each tablet

Shown in Product Identification Section, page 418

ALKA-SELTZER PLUS®
Sinus Allergy Medicine

Active Ingredients: Phenylpropanolamine bitartrate 24.08 mg, brompheniramine maleate 2 mg, acetylsalicylic acid (aspirin) 500 mg. In water the aspirin is converted into its soluble ionic form, sodium acetylsalicylate.

Inactive Ingredients: Aspartame, citric acid, flavors, heat-treated sodium bicarbonate, tableting aids

Indications: For the temporary relief of nasal congestion, sinus pain and pressure headache, runny nose, sneezing and itchy, watery eyes due to sinusitis, allergic rhinitis, hay fever or other upper respiratory allergies.

Warnings: Children and teenagers should not use this medicine for chicken pox or flu symptoms before a doctor is consulted about Reye Syndrome, a rare but serious illness reported to be associated with aspirin. Do not exceed recommended dosage because at higher doses nervousness, dizziness or sleeplessness may occur. Adults: Do not take this product for more than 7 days. If symptoms do not improve or are accompanied by fever or if fever persists for more than 3 days, consult a doctor. May cause excitability, especially in children. Do not take this product if you have thyroid or heart disease, diabetes, high blood pressure, asthma, glaucoma, emphysema, chronic pulmonary disease, shortness of breath, difficulty in breathing, difficulty in urination due to enlargement of the prostate gland, bleeding problems, allergy to aspirin or are on a sodium restricted diet, unless directed by a doctor. Each tablet contains 506 mg of sodium. May cause drowsiness. Alcohol, sedatives and tranquilizers may increase the drowsiness effect. Avoid alcoholic beverages while taking this product. Do not take this product if you are taking sedatives or tranquilizers without first consulting your doctor. Use caution when driving a motor vehicle or operating machinery. As with any drug, if you are pregnant or nursing a baby, seek the advice of a health professional before using this product. IT IS ESPECIALLY IMPORTANT NOT TO USE ASPIRIN DURING THE LAST 3 MONTHS OF PREGNANCY UNLESS SPECIFICALLY DIRECTED TO DO SO BY A DOCTOR BECAUSE IT MAY CAUSE PROBLEMS IN THE UNBORN CHILD OR COMPLICATIONS DURING DELIVERY. Keep this and all drugs out of the reach of children.

Drug Interaction: Do not take this product if you are presently taking a prescription drug for anticoagulation (thinning of the blood), high blood pressure or depression without first consulting your doctor.

PHENYLKETONURICS: Contains 8.98 mg phenylalanine per tablet.

Directions: Adults: Take 2 tablets dissolved in approximately 4 ounces (½ glass) of water every 4 hours. Do not exceed 8 tablets in any 24-hour period.

How Supplied: Boxes of 32 tablets in 16 foil twin packs; 16 tablets in 8 foil twin packs

Shown in Product Identification Section, page 418

BACTINE® Antiseptic·Anesthetic First Aid Spray

Active Ingredients: Benzalkonium Chloride 0.13% w/w, Lidocaine HCl 2.5% w/w.
Aerosol ingredients are % w/w of concentrate.

Inactive Ingredients:
Liquid—Edetate Disodium, Fragrances, Octoxynol 9, Propylene Glycol, Purified Water, Alcohol 3.17% w/w.
Aerosol—Dimethyl Polysiloxane Fluid 1000, Edetic Acid, Fragrances, Isobutane, Malic Acid, Povidone, Propylene Glycol, Purified Water, Sorbitol, and Emulsifier System.

Indications: Antiseptic/anesthetic for helping prevent infection, cleanse wounds, and for the temporary relief of pain and itching due to insect bites, minor burns, sunburn, minor cuts and minor skin irritations.

Warnings: (Aerosol Spray and Liquid Spray)
For external use only. Do not use in large quantities, particularly over raw surfaces or blistered areas. Avoid spraying in eyes, mouth, ears or on sensitive areas of the body. This product is not for use on wild or domestic animal bites. If you have an animal bite or puncture wound, consult your physician immediately. If condition worsens or if symptoms persist for more than 7 days, discontinue use of this product and consult a physician. Do not bandage tightly. Keep this and all drugs out of reach of children. In case of accidental ingestion, seek professional assistance or contact a Poison Control Center immediately.
(Aerosol Only): Contents under pressure. Do not puncture or incinerate. Do not store at temperature above 120° F. Use only as directed. Intentional misuse by deliberately concentrating and inhaling the contents can be harmful or fatal.

Dosage and Administration: For adults and children 2 years of age or older. For superficial skin wounds, cuts, scratches, scrapes, cleanse affected area thoroughly.

Directions: (Liquid) First Aid Spray
To apply, hold bottle 2 to 3 inches from injured area and squeeze repeatedly. To aid in removing foreign particles, dab injured area with clean gauze saturated with product. For sunburn, minor burns, insect bites, and minor skin irritations, apply to affected area of skin for temporary relief. Product can be applied to affected area with clean gauze saturated with product.
(Aerosol First Aid Spray)
Shake well. For adults and children 2 years of age and older. For superficial skin wounds, cuts, scratches, scrapes, cleanse affected area thoroughly. Hold can upright 2 to 3 inches from injured area and spray until wet. To aid in removing foreign particles, dab injured area with clean gauze saturated with

product. For sunburn, minor burns, insect bites, and minor skin irritations, hold can upright 4 to 6 inches from injured area and spray until wet. Product can be applied to affected area with clean gauze saturated with product.

How Supplied: 2 oz., 4 oz. liquid spray, 16 oz. liquid, 3 oz. aerosol.

Shown in Product Identification Section, page 418

BACTINE® First Aid Antibiotic Plus Anesthetic Ointment

Active Ingredients: Each gram contains Polymyxin B Sulfate 5000 units; Bacitracin 400 units; Neomycin Sulfate 5 mg (equivalent to 3.5 mg Neomycin base); Diperodon HCl 10 mg (pain reliever).

Inactive Ingredients: Mineral Oil, White Petrolatum.

Indications: First aid to help prevent infection, guard against bacterial contamination, relieve pain and itching in minor cuts, scrapes and burns.

Warning: For external use only. Do not use in the eyes or apply over large areas of the body. In case of deep or puncture wounds, animal bites or serious burns, consult a physician. Stop use and consult a physician if the condition persists or gets worse. Do not use longer than one (1) week unless directed by a physician. Keep this and all medicines out of children's reach. In case of accidental ingestion, seek professional assistance or contact a Poison Control Center immediately.

Directions: Clean the affected area. Apply a small amount of this product (an amount equal to the surface area of the tip of a finger) one to three times daily. May be covered with a sterile bandage.

How Supplied: ½ oz. tube.

Shown in Product Identification Section, page 418

BACTINE® Brand Hydrocortisone Anti-Itch Cream

Active Ingredient: Hydrocortisone 0.5%.

Inactive Ingredients: Butylated Hydroxyanisole, Butylated Hydroxytoluene, Butylparaben, Carbomer, Cetyl Alcohol, Colloidal Silicon Dioxide, Corn oil (and) Gylceryl Oleate (and) Propylene Glycol (and) (BHA) (and) BHT (and) Propyl Gallate (and) Citric Acid, DEA-Oleth-3 Phosphate, Diisopropyl Sebacate, Edetate Disodium, Glycerin, Hydroxypropyl Methylcellulose 2906, Lanolin Alcohol, Methylparaben, Mineral Oil (and) Lanolin Alcohol, Propylene Glycol Stearate SE, Propylparaben, Purified Water.

Indications: For the temporary relief of minor skin irritations, itching, and rashes due to eczema, insect bites, poison ivy, poison oak, poison sumac, soaps, detergents, cosmetics, and jewelry.

Warnings: For external use only. Avoid contact with the eyes. If condition worsens or if symptoms persist for more than seven days, discontinue use and consult a physician.
Do not use on children under 2 years of age except under the advice and supervision of a physician.
Keep this and all drugs out of the reach of children. In case of accidental ingestion, seek professional assistance or contact a Poison Control Center immediately.

Directions: For adults and children 2 years of age and older. Gently massage into affected skin area not more than 3 or 4 times daily.

How Supplied: ½ oz. plastic tube.

Shown in Product Identification Section, page 418

BIOCAL® 500 mg Tablets Calcium Supplement

Each Tablet Contains: 1250 mg of calcium carbonate, U.S.P. which provides elemental calcium 500 mg.

Indications: Calcium supplementation.

Description: BIOCAL 500 mg Tablets are white, capsule-shaped tablets containing pure calcium carbonate. No sugar, salt, preservatives, artificial colors or flavors added.

Directions: Two tablets daily provide:

Elemental Calcium	For Adults % U.S. RDA	For Pregnant or Lactating Women % U.S. RDA
1000 mg	100%	77%

Take one or two tablets daily or as recommended by a physician.
Keep out of reach of children.

How Supplied: Bottles of 60 tablets in tamper-resistant package.

Shown in Product Identification Section, page 419

BUGS BUNNY™ Children's Chewable Vitamins (Sugar Free)
BUGS BUNNY™ Children's Chewable Vitamins Plus Iron (Sugar Free)
FLINTSTONES™ Children's Chewable Vitamins
FLINTSTONES™ Children's Chewable Vitamins Plus Iron

Vitamin Ingredients: Each multivitamin supplement with iron contains the ingredients listed in the chart below:
[See table above.]

BUGS BUNNY™ Children's Chewable Vitamins Plus Iron (Sugar Free)
FLINTSTONES™ Children's Chewable Vitamins Plus Iron

One Tablet Provides

Vitamins	Quantity	% of U.S. RDA For Children 2 to 4 Years of Age	% of U.S. RDA For Adults and Children over 4 Years of Age
Vitamin A (as acetate)	1250 I.U.	100	50
Vitamin A (as beta carotene)	1250 I.U.		
Vitamin D	400 I.U.	100	100
Vitamin E	15 I.U.	150	50
Vitamin C	60 mg.	150	100
Folic Acid	0.3 mg.	150	75
Thiamine	1.05 mg.	150	70
Riboflavin	1.20 mg.	150	70
Niacin	13.50 mg.	150	67
Vitamin B_6	1.05 mg.	150	52
Vitamin B_{12}	4.5 mcg.	150	75
Mineral:			
Iron (Elemental)	15 mg.	150	83

BUGS BUNNY™ Children's Chewable Vitamins and FLINTSTONES™ Children's Chewable Vitamins provide the same quantities of vitamins, but do not provide iron.

Indication: Dietary supplementation.

Dosage and Administration: One chewable tablet daily. For adults and children two years and older; tablet must be chewed.

Warning For Bugs Bunny Only: Phenylketonurics: Contains Phenylalanine.

Precaution:
IRON SUPPLEMENTS ONLY.
Contains iron, which can be harmful in large doses. Close tightly and keep out of reach of children. In case of overdose contact a Poison Control Center immediately.

How Supplied: Flintstones are supplied in bottles of 60 and 100, Bugs Bunny in bottles of 60 with child-resistant caps.

Shown in Product Identification Section, page 419

Continued on next page

Miles—Cont.

FLINTSTONES™ With Extra C
Children's Chewable Vitamins
BUGS BUNNY™ With Extra C
Children's Chewable Vitamins
(Sugar Free)

Vitamin Ingredients: Each multivitamin supplement contains the ingredients listed in the chart above:
[See table below.]

Indication: Dietary supplementation.

Dosage and Administration: One tablet daily for adults and children two years and older; tablet must be chewed.

Warning For Bugs Bunny Only: Phenylketonurics: Contains Phenylalanine.

How Supplied: Flintstones in bottles of 60's & 100's, Bugs Bunny in bottles of 60 with child-resistant caps.

Shown in Product Identification Section, page 419

FLINTSTONES™ COMPLETE
With Iron, Calcium & Minerals
Children's Chewable Vitamins
BUGS BUNNY™ Children's
Chewable Vitamins + Minerals
With Iron and Calcium
(Sugar Free)

Ingredients: Each supplement provides the ingredients listed in the chart below:
[See table above.]

Indication: Dietary Supplementation.

Dosage and Administration: 2–4 years of age: Chew one-half tablet daily. Over 4 years of age: Chew one tablet daily.

Warning: Phenylketonurics: Contains Phenylalanine.

Precaution: Contains iron, which can be harmful in large doses. Close tightly and keep out of reach of children. In case of overdose, contact a physician or Poison Control Center immediately.

How Supplied: Bottles of 60's with child-resistant caps.

Shown in Product Identification Section, page 419

FLINTSTONES® COMPLETE
Children's Chewable Vitamins
BUGS BUNNY™
Children's Chewable
Vitamins + Minerals
(Sugar Free)

Vitamins	Quantity Per Tablet	Percentage of U.S. Recommended Daily Allowance (U.S. RDA): For Children 2 to 4 Years of Age (½ tablet)	For Adults & Children Over 4 Years of Age (1 tablet)
Vitamin A (as acetate)	2500 I.U.	100	100
Vitamin A (as beta carotene)	2500 I.U.		
Vitamin D	400 I.U.	50	100
Vitamin E	30 I.U.	150	100
Vitamin C	60 mg.	75	100
Folic Acid	0.4 mg.	100	100
Vitamin B-1 (Thiamine)	1.5 mg.	107	100
Vitamin B-2 (Riboflavin)	1.7 mg.	106	100
Niacin	20 mg.	111	100
Vitamin B-6 (Pyridoxine)	2 mg.	143	100
Vitamin B-12 (Cyanocobalamin)	6 mcg.	100	100
Biotin	40 mcg.	13	13
Pantothenic Acid	10 mg.	100	100
Minerals	**Quantity**	**Percent U.S. RDA**	
Iron (elemental)	18 mg.	90	100
Calcium	100 mg.	6	10
Copper	2 mg.	100	100
Phosphorus	100 mg.	6	10
Iodine	150 mcg.	107	100
Magnesium	20 mg.	5	5
Zinc	15 mg.	94	100

BUGS BUNNY™ With Extra C
Children's Chewable Vitamins
(Sugar Free)
FLINTSTONES™ With Extra C
Children's Chewable Vitamins

One Tablet Provides: Vitamins		Quantity	% of U.S. RDA: For Children 2 To 4 Years of Age	For Adults and Children Over 4 Years of Age
Vitamin A (as acetate)	I.U.	1250	100	50
Vitamin A (as beta carotene)	I.U.	1250		
Vitamin D	I.U.	400	100	100
Vitamin E	I.U.	15	150	50
Vitamin C	mg.	250	625	417
Folic Acid	mg.	0.3	150	75
Thiamine	mg.	1.05	150	70
Riboflavin	mg.	1.20	150	70
Niacin	mg.	13.50	150	67
Vitamin B_6	mg.	1.05	150	52
Vitamin B_{12}	mcg.	4.5	150	75

DOMEBORO® Astringent Solution Powder Packets

Active Ingredients: Each powder packet contains aluminum sulfate 1191 mg and calcium acetate 938 mg. DOMEBORO in water contains principally, the astringent aluminum acetate buffered to an acid pH.

Inactive Ingredient: Dextrin

Indications: For temporary relief of minor skin irritations due to poison ivy, poison oak, poison sumac, insect bites, althlete's foot or rashes caused by soaps, detergents, cosmetics or jewelry.

Actions: DOMEBORO provides soothing, effective relief of minor skin irritations. For over 50 years, doctors have been recommending DOMEBORO ASTRINGENT SOLUTION to help relieve minor skin irritations.

Warnings: If condition worsens or symptoms persist for more than 7 days, discontinue use of the product and consult a doctor. For external use only. Avoid contact with the eyes. Do not cover compress or wet dressing with plastic to prevent evaporation. Keep this and all drugs out of the reach of children. In case of accidental ingestion, seek professional assistance or contact a Poison Control Center immediately.

Directions: One packet dissolved in 16 ounces of water makes a modified Burow's Solution approximately equivalent to a 1:40 dilution; two packets, a 1:20 dilution; and four packets, a 1:10 dilution. Dissolve one or two packets in water and stir the solution until fully dissolved. Do not strain or filter the solution. Can be used as a compress, wet dressing or as a soak. AS A COMPRESS OR WET DRESSING: Saturate a clean, soft, white cloth or gauze in the solution; gently squeeze and apply loosely to the affected area. Saturate the cloth in the solution every 15 to 30 minutes and apply to the affected area. Repeat as often as necessary. Discard remaining solution after use. AS A SOAK: Soak affected area in the solution for 15 to 30 minutes. Repeat 3 times a day. Discard remaining solution after use.

How Supplied: Boxes of 12 or 100 powder packets.

DOMEBORO® Astringent Solution Effervescent Tablets

Active Ingredients: Aluminum sulfate 878 mg and calcium acetate 604 mg. DOMEBORO in water contains principally the astringent aluminum acetate buffered to an acid pH.

Inactive Ingredients: Dextrin, polyethylene glycol, sodium bicarbonate

Indications: For temporary relief of minor skin irritations due to poison ivy, poison oak, poison sumac, insect bites, athlete's foot or rashes caused by soaps, detergents, cosmetics or jewelry.

Actions: DOMEBORO provides soothing, effective relief of minor skin irritations. For over 50 years doctors have been recommending DOMEBORO ASTRINGENT SOLUTION to help relieve minor skin irritations.

Warnings: If conditions worsens or symptoms persist for more than 7 days, discontinue use of the product and consult a doctor. For external use only. Avoid contact with the eyes. Do not cover compress or wet dressing with plastic to prevent evaporation. Keep this and all drugs out of the reach of children. In case of accidental ingestion, seek professional assistance or contact a Poison Control Center immediately.

Directions: One tablet dissolved in 12 ounces of water makes a modified Burow's Solution approximately equivalent to a 1:40 dilution; two tablets, a 1:20 dilution; and four tablets, a 1:10 dilution. Dissolve one or two tablets in water and stir the solution until fully dissolved. Do not strain or filter the solution. Can be used as a compress, wet dressing or as a soak. AS A COMPRESS OR WET DRESSING: Saturate a clean, soft, white cloth or gauze in the solution; gently squeeze and apply loosely to the affected area. Saturate the cloth in the solution every 15 to 30 minutes and apply to the affected area. Repeat as often as necessary. Discard remaining solution after use. AS A SOAK: Soak affected area in the solution for 15 to 30 minutes. Repeat 3 times a day. Discard remaining solution after use.

How Supplied: Boxes of 12 or 100 effervescent tablets

Shown in Product Identification Section, page 419

MILES® Nervine Nighttime Sleep–Aid

Active Ingredient: Each capsule-shaped tablet contains diphenhydramine HCl 25 mg.

Inactive Ingredients: Calcium Phosphate Dibasic, Calcium Sulfate, Carboxymethylcellulose Sodium, Corn Starch, Magnesium Stearate, Microcrystalline Cellulose.

Indications: Miles® Nervine helps you fall asleep and relieves occasional sleeplessness.

Actions: Antihistamines act on the central nervous system and produce drowsiness.

Warnings: Do not give to children under 12 years of age. Avoid alcoholic beverages while taking this product. Do not take this product if you are taking sedatives or tranquilizers without first consulting your doctor. If sleeplessness persists continuously for more than 2 weeks, consult your doctor. Insomnia may be a symptom of serious underlying medical illness. Do not take this product if you have asthma, glaucoma, emphysema, chronic pulmonary disease, shortness of breath, difficulty in breathing or difficulty in urination due to enlargement of the prostate gland unless directed by a doctor. As with any drug, if you are pregnant or nursing a baby, seek the advice of a health professional before using this product. Keep this and all drugs out of the reach of children. In case of accidental overdose, seek professional assistance or contact a poison control center immediately.

Dosage and Administration: Two tablets once daily at bedtime or as directed by a physician.

How Supplied: Blister pack 12's, bottle of 30's with a child-resistant cap.

Shown in Product Identification Section, page 419

ONE–A–DAY® Essential Vitamins 11 Essential Vitamins

Ingredients: One tablet daily of ONE-A-DAY® Essential provides:

Vitamins	Quantity	U.S. RDA
Vitamin A (as Acetate and Beta Carotene)	5000 I. U.	100
Vitamin C	60 mg.	100
Thiamine (B_1)	1.5 mg.	100
Riboflavin (B_2)	1.7 mg.	100
Niacin	20 mg.	100
Vitamin D	400 I.U.	100
Vitamin E	30 I.U.	100
Vitamin B_6	2 mg.	100
Folic Acid	0.4 mg.	100
Vitamin B_{12}	6 mcg.	100
Pantothenic Acid	10 mg.	100

Indication: Dietary supplementation.

Dosage and Administration: One tablet daily for adults and teens.

How Supplied: ONE-A-DAY® Essential, bottles of 60 and 100.

Shown in Product Identification Section, page 419

ONE-A-DAY® Maximum Formula Vitamins and Minerals Supplement for adults and teens The most complete ONE-A-DAY® brand.

Ingredients:
One tablet daily of ONE-A-DAY® Maximum Formula provides:

Vitamins	Quantity	% of U.S. RDA
Vitamin A Beta Carotene)	5000 I.U.	100
Vitamin A (as Acetate)	1500 I.U.	30
Vitamin C	60 mg.	100
Thiamine (B_1)	1.5 mg.	100
Riboflavin (B_2)	1.7 mg.	100
Niacin	20 mg.	100
Vitamin D	400 I.U.	100
Vitamin E	30 I.U.	100
Vitamin B_6	2 mg.	100
Folic Acid	0.4 mg.	100
Vitamin B_{12}	6 mcg.	100
Biotin	30 mcg.	10
Pantothenic Acid	10 mg.	100

Minerals	Quantity	% of U.S. RDA
Iron (Elemental)	18 mg.	100
Calcium	130 mg.	13
Phosphorus	100 mg.	10
Iodine	150 mcg.	100
Magnesium	100 mg.	25
Copper	2 mg.	100
Zinc	15 mg.	100
Chromium	10 mcg.	*
Selenium	10 mcg.	*
Molybdenum	10 mcg.	*
Manganese	2.5 mg.	*
Potassium	37.5 mg.	*
Chloride	34 mg.	*

*No U.S. RDA established

Indication: Dietary supplementation.

Dosage and Administration: One tablet daily for adults and teens.

Precaution: Contains iron, which can be harmful in large doses. Close tightly and keep out of reach of children. In case of overdose, contact a physician or Poison Control Center immediately.

How Supplied: Bottles of 30, 60, and 100 with child-resistant caps.

Shown in Product Identification Section, page 419

ONE-A-DAY® Plus Extra C Vitamins. For adults and teens.

Vitamin ingredients: One tablet daily of ONE-A-DAY® Plus Extra C provides:

Vitamins	Quantity	% of U.S. RDA
Vitamin A (as Beta Carotene)	2500 I.U.	100 (combined)
Vitamin A (as Acetate)	2500 I.U.	
Vitamin C	300 mg.	500
Thiamine (B_1)	1.5 mg.	100
Riboflavin (B_2)	1.7 mg.	100
Niacin	20 mg.	100
Vitamin D	400 I.U.	100
Vitamin E	30 I.U.	100
Vitamin B_6	2 mg.	100
Folic Acid	0.4 mg.	100
Vitamin B_{12}	6 mcg.	100
Pantothenic Acid	10 mg.	100

Indication: Dietary supplementation.

Dosage and Administration: One tablet daily.

How Supplied: Bottles of 60's with child resistant caps.

Shown in Product Identification Section, page 419

Continued on next page

Miles—Cont.

STRESSGARD®
High Potency B Complex and C plus A, D, E, Iron and Zinc
The most complete stress product.
Multivitamin/Multimineral Supplement For Adults

Ingredients:

Vitamins	Quantity	% of U.S. RDA
Vitamin A (as Beta Carotene)	2500 I.U.	100
Vitamin A (as Acetate)	2500 I.U.	
Vitamin C	600 mg.	1000
Thiamine (B_1)	15 mg.	1000
Riboflavin (B_2)	10 mg.	588
Niacin	100 mg.	500
Vitamin D	400 I.U.	100
Vitamin E	30 I.U.	100
Vitamin B_6	5 mg.	250
Folic Acid	400 mcg.	100
Vitamin B_{12}	12 mcg.	200
Pantothenic Acid	20 mg.	200

Minerals	Quantity	% of U.S. RDA
Iron (Elemental)	18 mg.	100
Zinc	15 mg.	100
Copper	2 mg.	100

Indication: Dietary supplementation.

Dosage and Administration: Adults—one tablet daily with food.

Precaution: Contains iron, which can be harmful in large doses. Close tightly and keep out of reach of children. In case of overdose, contact a physician or Poison Control Center immediately.

How Supplied: Bottles of 60 with child-resistant caps.

Shown in Product Identification Section, page 419

WITHIN® Women's Formula
Advanced Multivitamin Formula with Calcium, Extra Iron, Zinc and Beta Carotene.
Provides calcium and extra iron Plus the daily nutritional support of 11 essential vitamins.

Ingredients: One tablet daily of WITHIN® provides:

Vitamins	Quantity	% of U.S. RDA
Vitamin A (as Beta Carotene)	2500 I.U.	100
Vitamin A (as Acetate)	2500 I.U.	
Vitamin C	60 mg.	100
Thiamine (B_1)	1.5 mg.	100
Riboflavin (B_2)	1.7 mg.	100
Niacin	20 mg.	100
Vitamin D	400 I.U.	100
Vitamin E	30 I.U.	100
Vitamin B_6	2 mg.	100
Folic Acid	0.4 mg.	100
Vitamin B_{12}	6 mcg.	100
Pantothenic Acid	10 mg.	100

Mineral	Quantity	% of U.S. RDA
Iron (Elemental)	27 mg.	150
Calcium (Elemental)	450 mg.	45
Zinc	15 mg.	100

Indication: Dietary supplementation.

Dosage and Administration: One tablet daily.

Precaution: Contains iron, which can be harmful in large doses. Close tightly and keep out of reach of children. In case of overdose, contact a physician or Poison Control Center immediately.

How Supplied: Bottles of 60 and 100 with child-resistant caps.

Shown in Product Identification Section, page 419

More Direct Health Products

6351-E YARROW DRIVE
CARLSBAD, CA 92009

CigArrest™
Smoking Deterrent Tablets

Active Ingredient: Lobeline sulfate 2 mg.

Indications: A temporary aid to breaking the cigarette habit. The effectiveness of the tablet is directly related to the user's motivation to stop smoking.

Use: Lobeline sulfate resembles nicotine both chemically and pharmacologically which aids the smoker in developing a sense of satiety for smoking almost identical to that obtained from tobacco. Not habit forming.

Warnings: As with any drug, if you are pregnant or nursing a baby, seek the advice of a health professional before using CigArrest.™ Keep this and all drugs out of the reach of children.

Symptoms and Treatment of Overdosage: In case of accidental overdose, seek the advice of a physician immediately.

Dosage and Administration: Take 1 (one) tablet at or after each meal, 3 (three) tablets per day. Recommended usage not to exceed six weeks.

How Supplied: Consumer packages of 15 (fifteen) blister packed tablets.

IDENTIFICATION PROBLEM?
Consult the
Product Identification Section
where you'll find
products pictured
in full color.

Muro Pharmaceutical, Inc.

890 EAST STREET
TEWKSBURY, MA 01876-9987

BROMFED® SYRUP
Antihistamine-Decongestant
(alcohol free)
ORANGE-LEMON FLAVOR

Each 5 mL (1 teaspoonful) contains: 2 mg brompheniramine maleate and 30 mg pseudoephedrine hydrochloride; also contains citric acid, FD & C Yellow #6, flavor, glycerin, methyl paraben, sodium benzoate, sodium citrate, sodium saccharin, sorbitol, sucrose, purified water.

Indications: For temporary relief of nasal congestion, sneezing, itchy and watery eyes and running nose due to common cold, hay fever or other upper respiratory allergies.

Directions: Adults and children 12 years of age and over: 2 teaspoonfuls every 4–6 hours. Children 6 to 12 years of age: 1 teaspoonful every 4–6 hours. Do not exceed 4 doses in 24 hours. Children under 6 years of age, consult a physician.

Warnings: If symptoms do not improve within 7 days or are accompanied by high fever, consult a physician before continuing use. May cause drowsiness. May cause excitability especially in children. DO NOT exceed recommended daily dosage because at higher doses nervousness, dizziness, or sleeplessness may occur. **Except under the advice and supervision of a physician:** DO NOT give this product to children under 6 years. DO NOT take this product if you have asthma, glaucoma, difficulty in urination due to enlargement of the prostate gland, high blood pressure, heart disease, diabetes, or thyroid disease. As with any drug, if you are pregnant or nursing a baby, seek the advice of a health professional before using this product.

Caution: Avoid operating a motor vehicle or heavy machinery and alcoholic beverages while taking this product. Keep this and all drugs out of the reach of children.

Drug Interaction Precaution: Do not take this product if you are presently taking a prescription antihypertensive or antidepressant drug containing a monoamine oxidase inhibitor except under the advice and supervision of a physician.

Overdosage: In case of accidental overdose, seek professional assistance or contact a Poison Control Center immediately.

Store between 15° and 30°C (59° and 86°F). Dispense in tight, light resistant containers as defined in USP.

How Supplied: NDC 0451-4201-16—16 fl. oz. (480 mL), NDC 0451-4201-04—4 fl. oz. (120 mL).

GUAIFED® SYRUP
Expectorant/Decongestant

GUAIFED® SYRUP: A red colored syrup

Each 5mL (teaspoonful) contains:

Pseudoephedrine HCl	30mg
Guaifenesin	200mg

CONTAINS NO ANTIHISTAMINE which may cause drowsiness or excessive drying.

Guaifed® Syrup also contains inactive ingredients:
Benzoic Acid, Berry Citrus Flavor, Citric Acid, FD&C Red #40, Glycerin, Propylene Glycol, Purified Water, Saccharin Sodium, Sorbitol, Sucrose. "ALCOHOL FREE"

Indications: For the temporary relief of nasal congestion associated with the common cold, sinusitis, hay fever or other upper respiratory allergies. Also helps loosen phlegm (sputum) and thin bronchial secretions to rid the bronchial passageways of bothersome mucus, drain bronchial tubes, and make coughs more productive.

Warnings: Do not exceed recommended dosage because at higher doses nervousness, dizziness or sleeplessness may occur. Do not use if you have high blood pressure, heart disease, diabetes, thyroid disease or a persistent chronic cough, except under the advice and supervision of a physician. Do not take this product for persistent or chronic cough such as occurs with smoking, asthma, chronic bronchitis, or emphysema, or where cough is accompanied by excessive phlegm (sputum) unless directed by a doctor. A persistent cough may be a sign of a serious condition. If cough persists for more than 1 week, tends to recur, or is accompanied by a fever, rash or persistent headache, consult a doctor.

Geriatrics: Pseudoephedrine should be used with caution in the elderly because they may be more sensitive to the effect of the sympathomimetics.
In the case of accidental overdose, seek professional assistance or contact a Poison Control Center immediately. As with any drug, if you are pregnant or nursing a baby, seek the advice of a health professional before using this product.

Contraindications: Hypersensitivity to guaifenesin or sympathomimetic amines; marked hypertension, hyperthyroidism; or in patients receiving monoamine oxidase (MAO) inhibitors.

Adverse Reactions: Possible side effects include nausea, vomiting, nervousness, restlessness, rash (including urticaria), headache, or dry mouth.

Note: Guaifenesin has been shown to produce a color interference with certain clinical laboratory determinations of 5-hydroxyindoleacetic acid (5-HIAA) and vanillylmandelic acid (VMA).

DRUG INTERACTION PRECAUTIONS: Do not take this medication if you are presently taking a prescription antihypertensive or antidepressant drug containing a monoamine oxidase inhibitor except under the advice and supervision of a physician.

Directions: Guaifed Syrup—Adults and Children 12 years of age and over: Two teaspoonfuls every 4–6 hours, not to exceed eight teaspoonfuls in 24 hours. Children 6 to under 12 years of age: One teaspoonful every 4–6 hours, not to exceed four teaspoonfuls in 24 hours. Children 2 to under 6 years of age: ½ teaspoonful every 4–6 hours, not to exceed two teaspoonfuls in 24 hours. Children under 2 years of age: consult a physician.

How Supplied: Guaifed® Syrup is a red colored, berry citrus flavored syrup supplied in 16 fl. oz. bottles (NDC# 0451-2600-16) and 4 fl. oz. bottles (NDC# 0451-2600-04).
Store at controlled room temperature between 15°C and 30°C (59°F and 86°F).
Dispense in Child Resistant, tight and light resistant containers.
KEEP THIS AND ALL DRUGS OUT OF REACH FROM CHILDREN.

SALINEX NASAL MIST AND DROPS
Buffered Isotonic Saline Solutions

Ingredients: Sodium Chloride 0.4%. Also contains disodium phosphate, edetate disodium, hydroxypropyl methylcellulose, monosodium phosphate, polyethylene glycol, propylene glycol and purified water. Preservative used is benzalkonium chloride 0.01%.

Indications: Rhinitis Medicamentosa and Rhinitis Sicca. For relief of nasal congestion associated with overuse of nasal sprays, drops and inhalers.
To alleviate crusting due to nose bleeds; to compensate for nasal stuffiness and dryness due to lack of humidity.

Directions: Squeeze twice in each nostril as needed.

How Supplied: SPRAY: 50 ml plastic spray bottle. DROPS: 15 ml plastic dropper bottle.

Nature's Bounty, Inc.
90 ORVILLE DRIVE
BOHEMIA, NY 11716

ENER–B®
Vitamin B-12 Nasal Gel
Dietary Supplement

Description: ENER-B™ is the first intra-nasal application for Vitamin B-12. Each delivery supplies 400 mcg. of Vitamin B-12. This method of delivery provides the highest Vitamin B-12 blood levels that can be obtained without a prescription. Clinical tests show that ENER-B produced 8.4 to 10 times more Vitamin B-12 in the blood than tablets.

Clinical Tests results are available by writing Nature's Bounty.

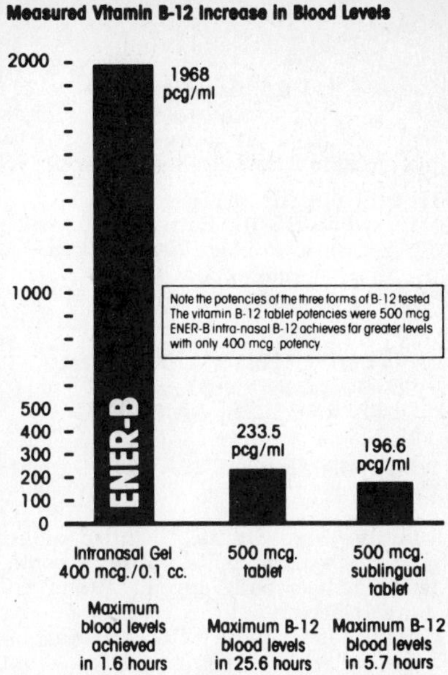

Potency and Administration: Each nasal applicator delivers $\frac{1}{10}$ cc of gel into the nose which adheres to the mucous membranes providing 400 mcg. of Vitamin B-12. Odorless and non-irritating to the nose.

Directions: As a dietary supplement, one unit every two to three days.

How Supplied: Packages of 12 unit doses. Supplies 400 mcg. of B-12 each.
Shown in Product Identification Section, page 419

Neutrin Drug, Inc.
1800 NORTH CHARLES STREET
BALTIMORE, MD 21201

ANTICON

Active Ingredients:

Docusate Sodium	100 mg.
Casanthranol	30 mg.

Inactive Ingredients: Gelatin, Polyethylene Glycol, Glycerin, Propylene Glycol, Titanium Dioxide, Methyl Paraben, FD&C Red #40, FD&C Red #3, D&C Red #33, Propyl Paraben.
Useful in the management of chronic constipation.

Indications: Anticon is a combination of the mild stimulant laxative casanthranol and the stool softener Docusate Sodium. Bowel movement is induced gently—usually overnight or in 8 to 12 hours.

Warnings: Not to be taken in case of nausea, vomiting, or abdominal pain. Frequent or continued use of this preparation may result in dependence on laxatives. As with any drug, if you are pregnant or nursing a baby, seek the advice of a health professional before using this product.

Continued on next page

Neutrin—Cont.

Dosage and Administration: Adults—1 or 2 capsules at bed time, or as indicated. In severe cases, dosage may be increased to 2 capsules two times daily.

How Supplied: Anticon capsule NDC 57655-315-01 Bottles of 60

Shown in Product Identification Section, page 419

Neutrogena Corporation

5760 W. 96TH ST.
LOS ANGELES, CA 90045

NEUTROGENA® CLEANSING WASH

Inactive Ingredients: Purified water, glycerin, sodium oleate, sodium cocoate, lauroamphocarboxyl glycinate (and) sodium trideceth sulfate, cocamidopropyl betaine, lauramide DEA, triethanolamine, BHA, BHT, citric acid, trisodium HEDTA.

Indications: A mild-lather cleanser especially formulated for dry, sensitive skin, for skin irritated by drying medications, or for use in conjunction with dermabrasions, chemical peels or facial surgery.

Actions: Neutrogena Cleansing Wash is a gentle, glycerin-enriched formula designed to effectively cleanse skin, extremely sensitive skin or skin made hyperirritable by drying medications or facial procedures. It is residue-free so as not to interfere with skin treatments. It is fragrance-free, contains no color and is noncomedogenic.

Dosage and Administration: Use twice daily, or as directed by physician. Mix with water, work Neutrogena Cleansing Wash into a creamy lather and apply to face. Gently massage in a circular motion. Rinse completely.

How Supplied: Available in 6 oz pump dispenser bottle.

Shown in Product Identification Section, page 419

NEUTROGENA MOISTURE®

Active Ingredient: Octyl methoxycinnamate (SPF 5).

Inactive Ingredients: Purified water, glycerin, glyceryl stearate and PEG-100 stearate, petrolatum, isopropyl isostearate, octyl palmitate, soya sterol, cetyl alcohol, PEG-10 soya sterol, carbomer 954, methylparaben, imidazolidinyl urea, sodium hydroxide, tetrasodium EDTA, propylparaben, tocopherol.

Actions: Neutrogena Moisture is an extremely effective facial moisturizer for even the most fragile complexions. It is noncomedogenic, fragrance-free, and contains no color. Hypoallergenic. Provides an SPF 5 protection for the skin.

Dosage and Administration: Apply Neutrogena Moisture over face and throat morning and night, after thoroughly cleansing the skin.

How Supplied: 2 oz and 4 oz bottle.

Shown in Product Identification Section, page 419

NEUTROGENA MOISTURE® SPF 15 UNTINTED

Active Ingredients: Octyl methoxycinnamate and benzophenone-3.

Inactive Ingredients: Purified water, PPG-1 isoceteth-3 acetate, glycerin, emulsifying wax NF, glyceryl stearate, PEG-100 stearate, dimethicone, PEG-6000 monostearate, triethanolamine, methylparaben, diazolidinyl urea, carbomer 954, ethylparaben, propylparaben.

Actions: Effective 8 hours' moisturization with maximum sunblock protection (SPF 15) in a noncomedogenic facial moisturizer. Fragrance-free, hypoallergenic.

Dosage and Administration: Use daily after thorough cleansing of skin, alone or under makeup.

How Supplied: 4 oz bottle.

Shown in Product Identification Section, page 419

NEUTROGENA MOISTURE® SPF 15 WITH SHEER TINT

Active Ingredients: Octyl methoxycinnamate and benzophenone-3.

Inactive Ingredients: Purified water, PPG-1 Isoceteth-3 acetate, glycerin, emulsifying wax NF, glyceryl stearate, PEG-100 stearate, dimethicone, PEG-6000 monostearate, triethanolamine, methylparaben, diazolidinyl urea, carbomer 954, ethylparaben, propylparaben, iron oxides.

Actions: A PABA-free, noncomedogenic facial moisturizer that provides maximum sunblock protection (SPF 15). Fragrance-free, hypoallergenic. Moisturizes for 8 hours with just a hint of color.

Dosage and Administration: Use during the day with or without makeup.

How Supplied: 4 oz bottle.

Shown in Product Identification Section, page 419

NEUTROGENA® SUNBLOCK

Active Ingredients: Octyl methoxycinnamate, Octyl salicylate, and Menthyl anthranilate (SPF 15).

Inactive Ingredients: Mineral oil, aluminum starch octenylsuccinate, silica, PVP/eicosene copolymer, glyceryl tribenate and calcium behenate, phenyltrimethicone, cyclomethicone and dimethiconol, titanium dioxide, C_{18}–C_{36} acid triglyceride, propylparaben.

Indications: Neutrogena Sunblock provides broad spectrum protection (UVA/UVB/IR) from the damaging rays of the sun.

Actions: Provides broad spectrum protection with a SPF 15 effective in preventing sun damage. Liberal and regular use of Neutrogena Sunblock may help reduce the chance of premature aging of the skin and protects against the cancer-causing rays of the sun.

Waterproof: Stays on the skin even after long exposure in the water. Excellent for children above the age of 6 months. Remove with soap and water.

Rubproof/Sweatproof: Abrasion-resistant. Stays on even after rubbing or towel drying. Lower potential to run into eyes and cause stinging.

PABA-Free/Noncomedogenic: Suitable for those sensitive to PABA and its related compounds; won't clog pores. Fragrance-free. Hypoallergenic.

Warnings: For external use only, not to be swallowed. Avoid contact with eyes. Discontinue use if irritation or rash develops.

Dosage and Administration: For best results, apply to face and body 15 minutes before sun exposure. Reapply after rigorous swimming or exercise.

How Supplied: 2¼ oz tube.

Shown in Product Identification Section, page 420

Numark Laboratories, Inc.

P.O. BOX 6321
EDISON, NJ 08818

CERTAIN DRI® ANTIPERSPIRANT

Active Ingredient: Aluminum Chloride

Actions: Antiperspirant protection—helps solve, control and lessen underarm perspiration.

Warnings: Do not apply after shaving, on broken skin, or immediately after bathing. If rash develops, discontinue use. Keep out of reach of children.

Directions: Must be applied sparingly on dry skin at bedtime only. Recommended for underarm use only.

How Supplied: 1.5 oz. unscented roll-on. For more information contact NUMARK Laboratories, Inc., PO Box 6321, Edison, NJ 08818 for a free booklet, "Important Facts About Perspiration Problems." Call 1-800-331-0221.

Shown in Product Identification Section, page 420

IDENTIFICATION PROBLEM?
Consult the
Product Identification Section
where you'll find
products pictured
in full color.

Ohm Laboratories, Inc.
P. O. BOX 279
FRANKLIN PARK, NJ 08823

IBUPROHM®
Ibuprofen Tablets, USP
Ibuprofen Caplets, USP

Active Ingredient: Each tablet contains Ibuprofen USP, 200 mg.

Warning: ASPIRIN SENSITIVE PATIENTS: Do not take this product if you have had a severe allergic reaction to aspirin, e.g., asthma, swelling, shock or hives, because even though this product contains no aspirin or salicylates, cross-reactions may occur in patients allergic to aspirin.

Indications: For the temporary relief of minor aches and pains associated with the common cold, headache, toothache, muscular aches, backache, for the minor pain of arthritis, for the pain of menstrual cramps, and for reduction of fever.

Directions: *Adults:* Take 1 tablet every 4 to 6 hours while symptoms persist. If pain or fever does not respond to 1 tablet, 2 tablets may be used but do not exceed 6 tablets in 24 hours, unless directed by a doctor. The smallest effective dose should be used. Take with food or milk if occasional and mild heartburn, upset stomach, or stomach pain occurs with use. Consult a doctor if these symptoms are more than mild or if they persist. Children: Do not give this product to children under 12 except under the advice and supervision of a doctor.

Warnings: Do not take for pain for more than 10 days or for fever for more than 3 days unless directed by a doctor. If pain or fever persists or gets worse, if new symptoms occur, or if the painful area is red or swollen, consult a doctor. These could be signs of serious illness. If you are under a doctor's care for any serious condition, consult a doctor before taking this product. As with aspirin and acetaminophen, if you have any condition which requires you to take prescription drugs or if you have had any problems or serious side effects from taking any nonprescription pain reliever, do not take this product without first discussing it with your doctor. If you experience any symptoms which are unusual or seem unrelated to the condition for which you took ibuprofen, consult a doctor before taking any more of it. Although ibuprofen is indicated for the same conditions as aspirin and acetaminophen, it should not be taken with them except under a doctor's direction. Do not combine the product with any other ibuprofen-containing product. As with any drug, if you are pregnant or nursing a baby, seek the advice of a health professional before using this product. IT IS ESPECIALLY IMPORTANT NOT TO USE IBUPROFEN DURING THE LAST 3 MONTHS OF PREGNANCY UNLESS SPECIFICALLY DIRECTED TO DO SO BY A DOCTOR BECAUSE IT MAY CAUSE PROBLEMS IN THE UNBORN CHILD OR COMPLICATIONS DURING DELIVERY. Keep this and all drugs out of the reach of children. In case of accidental overdose, seek professional assistance or contact a poison control center immediately.

How Supplied: Coated tablets in bottles of 24, 50, 100, 165, 250, 500 and 1000. Coated caplets in bottles of 24, 50, 100 and 250.

Storage: Store at room temperature; avoid excessive heat 40° (104°F).

Shown in Product Identification Section, page 420

Ortho Pharmaceutical Corporation
Advanced Care Products
RARITAN, NJ 08869

CONCEPTROL®
Contraceptive Gel/Inserts

Description: CONCEPTROL Contraceptive Gel: An unscented, unflavored, colorless, greaseless and non-staining gel in convenient, easy-to-use disposable plastic applicators. Each applicator is filled with a single, pre-measured dose containing the active spermicide Nonoxynol-9—4.0%, (100 mg per application) at pH 4.5.
CONCEPTROL Contraceptive Inserts: A non-foaming, single dose vaginal contraceptive containing the active spermicide Nonoxynol-9-8.34% (150 mg per insert).

Indication: Contraception.

Actions and Uses: Spermicidal products for use whenever control of conception is desirable.

Warning: Occasional burning and/or irritation of the vagina or penis have been reported. If this occurs, discontinue use and consult a physician as necessary. Not effective if taken orally. Keep out of reach of children. When pregnancy is contraindicated, the contraceptive program should be discussed with a health care professional.

Dosage and Administration:
CONCEPTROL Contraceptive Gel: One applicatorful of CONCEPTROL Contraceptive Gel should be inserted deeply into the vagina just before intercourse. An additional applicatorful is required each time intercourse is repeated.
CONCEPTROL Contraceptive Inserts: One insert should be placed into the vagina at least ten minutes prior to male penetration to insure proper dispersion. An additional insert is required each time intercourse is repeated.
CONCEPTROL Contraceptive Gel/Inserts:
If intercourse has not occurred within one hour after the application of CONCEPTROL, repeat application. Add a new application each time intercourse is repeated. Douching after use of CONCEPTROL is not recommended; however should you desire to do so, wait at least six hours to avoid interfering with contraceptive protection. CONCEPTROL is an effective method of contraception. While no method of birth control can provide an absolute guarantee against becoming pregnant, for maximum protection, CONCEPTROL must be used according to directions.

How Supplied:
CONCEPTROL Contraceptive Gel is available in packages of 6 or 10 easy-to-use single-dose applicators.
CONCEPTROL Contraceptive Inserts are available in packages containing 10 inserts.

Inactive Ingredients:
CONCEPTROL Contraceptive Gel:
Lactic Acid, Methylparaben, Povidone, Propylene Glycol, Purified Water, Sodium Carboxymethylcellulose, Sorbic Acid, Sorbitol Solution.
CONCEPTROL Contraceptive Inserts:
Lauroamphodiacetate Sodium Trideceth Sulfate, Polyethylene Glycol 1000, Polyethylene Glycol 1450, Povidone.

Storage: Avoid excessive heat (over 86°F or 30°C).

Shown in Product Identification Section, page 420

DELFEN®
Contraceptive Foam

Description: A contraceptive foam in an aerosol dosage formulation containing 12.5% Nonoxynol-9 (100 mg. per application) and buffered to normal vaginal pH 4.5.

Indication: Contraception.

Action and Uses: A spermicidal foam for intravaginal contraception.

Warning: Occasional burning and/or irritation of the vagina or penis have been reported. In such cases, the use of the product should be discontinued and a physician consulted as necessary. Not effective if taken orally. Keep out of reach of children.
When pregnancy is contraindicated, the contraceptive program should be discussed with a health care professional.

Dosage and Administration: Insert DELFEN Contraceptive Foam just prior to each act of intercourse. You may have intercourse any time up to one hour after you have inserted the foam. If you repeat intercourse, insert another applicatorful of DELFEN Foam. After shaking the can, remove cap and place can upright on a level surface. Place the measured-dose (5cc) applicator on top of the can, then press applicator down very gently to fill. Fill to the top of the ribbed section of the applicator. Remove applicator from can to stop flow of foam. Insert the filled applicator well into the vagina and depress the plunger. Remove the applicator with the plunger in depressed position. Douching is not recommended after using DELFEN Foam. However, if douching is desired for cleansing purposes, wait at least six hours after intercourse. Refer to direction circular in package for diagrams and detailed instructions. While

Continued on next page

Ortho Pharm.—Cont.

no method of contraception can provide an absolute guarantee against becoming pregnant, for maximum protection, DELFEN Foam must be used according to directions.

How Supplied: DELFEN Contraceptive Foam 0.60 oz. Starter can with applicator. Also 1.40 oz. refill can without applicator.

Inactive Ingredients: Benzoic Acid, Cetyl Alcohol, Cellulose Gum, Glacial Acetic Acid, Methylparaben, Perfume, Phosphoric Acid, Polyvinyl Alcohol, Propellant A-31, Propylene Glycol, Purified Water, Stearamidoethyl Diethylamine, Sorbic Acid, Stearic Acid.

Storage: Contents under pressure. Do not puncture or incinerate container. Do not expose to heat or store at temperatures above 120°F.

Shown in Product Identification Section, page 420

GYNOL II® Original Formula ORTHO-GYNOL® Contraceptive Jelly

Description:
GYNOL II Original Formula:
A colorless, unscented, unflavored, greaseless and non-staining contraceptive jelly containing the active spermicide Nonoxynol-9 (2%, 100 mg. per application) and having a pH of 4.5.
ORTHO-GYNOL: Is a water-dispersible spermicidal jelly having a pH of 4.5 and contains the active spermicide Octoxynol-9 (1%).

Indication: Contraception.

Actions and Uses: An aesthetically pleasing spermicidal vaginal jelly for use with a vaginal diaphragm whenever the control of conception is desired.

Warning: Occasional burning and/or irritation of the vagina or penis have been reported. In such cases, use of the product should be discontinued and a physician consulted as necessary. Not effective if taken orally. Keep out of reach of children. When pregnancy is contraindicated, the contraceptive program should be discussed with a health care professional.

Dosage and Administration: Used in conjunction with a vaginal diaphragm. Prior to insertion, put about a teaspoonful of contraceptive jelly into the cup of the dome of the diaphragm and spread a small amount around the edge with your fingertip. This will aid in insertion and provide protection.
It is also important to remember that if intercourse occurs more than six hours after insertion, or if repeated intercourse takes place, an additional application of contraceptive jelly is necessary. DO NOT REMOVE THE DIAPHRAGM—simply add more contraceptive jelly with the applicator provided in the applicator package, being careful not to dislodge the diaphragm. Remember, another application of contraceptive jelly is required each time intercourse is repeated, regardless of how little time has transpired since the diaphragm has been in place.
IMPORTANT—For contraceptive effectiveness, the diaphragm should remain in place for six hours after intercourse and should be removed as soon as possible thereafter. Continuous wearing of the diaphragm for more than 24 hours is not recommended. Retention of the diaphragm for prolonged periods may encourage the growth of certain bacteria in the vaginal tract. It has been suggested that under certain as yet unestablished conditions overgrowth of these bacteria may lead to symptoms of toxic shock syndrome (TSS). For further information, consult your physician.
If a douche is desired for cleansing purposes, wait at least six hours after intercourse. While no method of contraception can provide an absolute guarantee against becoming pregnant, for maximum protection, the contraceptive jelly must be used according to directions. Refer to direction circular enclosed in the package for diagrams and complete instructions.

Inactive Ingredients:
GYNOL II Original Formula:
Lactic Acid, Methylparaben, Povidone, Propylene Glycol, Purified Water, Sodium Carboxymethylcellulose, Sorbic acid, Sorbitol Solution.
ORTHO-GYNOL:
Benzoic Acid, Castor Oil, Fragrance, Glacial Acetic Acid, Methylparaben, Potassium Hydroxide, Propylene Glycol, Purified Water, Sodium Carboxymethylcellulose, Sorbic Acid.

How Supplied: 2.5 oz and 3.8 oz tube packages.

Storage: Should be stored at room temperature.

Shown in Product Identification Section, page 420

GYNOL II EXTRA STRENGTH CONTRACEPTIVE JELLY

Description: GYNOL II Extra Strength Contraceptive Jelly is a clear, unscented, water-soluble, greaseless gel. It is mildly lubricating and non-staining. Each applicatorful contains 150 mg of nonoxynol-9 (3%), a potent spermicide which provides effective protection against pregnancy when used with a diaphragm or a condom or alone. A diaphragm alone is not effective protection against pregnancy.

Indication: Contraception.

Actions and Uses: An aesthetically pleasing spermicidal jelly for use alone, with a condom or a diaphragm whenever control of contraception is desired.

Warning: Occasional burning and/or irritation of the vagina or penis have been reported. In such cases, the medication should be discontinued and a physician consulted as necessary. Not effective if taken orally. Keep out of reach of children. When pregnancy is contraindicated, the contraceptive program should be discussed with a health care professional.

Dosage and Administration: When used in conjunction with a vaginal diaphragm. Prior to insertion, put about a teaspoonful of GYNOL II Extra Strength Contraceptive Jelly into the cup of the dome of the diaphragm and spread a small amount around the edge with your fingertip then insert.
It is also important to remember that if intercourse occurs more than six hours after insertion, or if repeated intercourse takes place, an additional application of GYNOL II Extra Strength is necessary. DO NOT REMOVE THE DIAPHRAGM, simply add more GYNOL II Extra Strength with the applicator provided in the applicator package, being careful not to dislodge the diaphragm. Remember, another application of GYNOL II Extra Strength is required each time intercourse is repeated, regardless of how little time has transpired since the diaphragm has been in place.
IMPORTANT—For contraceptive effectiveness, the diaphragm should remain in place for six hours after intercourse and should be removed as soon as possible thereafter. Continuous wearing of the diaphragm for more than 24 hours is not recommended. Retention of the diaphragm for prolonged periods may encourage the growth of certain bacteria in the vaginal tract. It has been suggested that under certain as yet unestablished conditions overgrowth of these bacteria may lead to symptoms of toxic shock syndrome (TSS). For further information, consult your physician.

Dosage and Administration: For use with a condom or as a use-alone product. Insert an applicatorful of GYNOL II Extra Strength into the vagina as shown in the illustration. Intercourse should occur within one hour after GYNOL II Extra Strength has been inserted. An additional application must be used prior to each additional act of intercourse. This method of contraception must be used each and every time intercourse takes place, regardless of the time of the month.

Inactive Ingredients: Lactic Acid, Methylparaben, Povidone, Propylene Glycol, Purified Water, Sodium Carboxymethylcellulose, Sorbic Acid, Sorbitol Solution.

Shown in Product Identification Section, page 420

MICATIN®
[*'mī-kə-tin*]
Antifungal For Athlete's Foot

Description: An antifungal containing the active ingredient miconazole nitrate 2%, clinically proven to cure athlete's foot, jock itch and ringworm.

Indications: Athlete's foot (tinea pedis), jock itch (tinea cruris), and ringworm (tinea corporis).

Actions and Uses: Proven clinically effective in the treatment of athlete's foot (tinea pedis), jock itch (tinea cruris), and ringworm (tinea corporis). For effective relief of the itching, scaling, burning and discomfort that can accompany these conditions.

Directions: Cleanse skin with soap and water and dry thoroughly. Apply a thin layer of MICATIN over affected area morning and night or as directed by a doctor. For athlete's foot, pay special attention to the spaces between the toes. It is also helpful to wear well-fitting, ventilated shoes and to change shoes and socks at least once daily. Best results in athlete's foot and ringworm are usually obtained with 4 weeks' use of this product and in jock itch with 2 weeks' use. If satisfactory results have not occurred within these times, consult a doctor or pharmacist. Children under 12 years of age should be supervised in the use of this product. This product is not effective on the scalp or nails.

Do not use on children under 2 years of age except under the advice and supervision of a doctor. For external use only. If irritation occurs, or if there is no improvement within 4 weeks (for athlete's foot or ringworm) or within 2 weeks (for jock itch), discontinue use and consult a doctor or pharmacist. Keep this and all drugs out of the reach of children. In case of accidental ingestion, seek professional assistance or contact a Poison Control Center immediately.

How Supplied:
MICATIN® Antifungal Cream is available in a 0.5 oz. tube and a 1.0 oz. tube.
MICATIN Antifungal Spray Powder is available in a 3.0 oz. aerosol can.
MICATIN Antifungal Deodorant Spray Powder is available in a 3.0 oz. aerosol can.
MICATIN Antifungal Powder is available in a 3.0 oz. plastic bottle.
MICATIN Antifungal Spray Liquid is available in a 3.5 oz. aerosol can.

Inactive Ingredients:
MICATIN Antifungal Cream: Benzoic Acid, BHA, Mineral Oil, Peglicol 5 Oleate, Pegoxol 7 Stearate, Purified Water.
MICATIN Antifungal Spray Powder: Alcohol, Propellant A-46, Sorbitan Sesquioleate, Stearalkonium Hectorite, Talc.
MICATIN Antifungal Deodorant Spray Powder: Alcohol, Propellant A-46, Talc, Stearalkonium Hectorite, Sorbitan Sesquioleate, Fragrance.
MICATIN Antifungal Powder: Talc.
MICATIN Antifungal Spray Liquid: Alcohol, Benzyl Alcohol, Cocamide DEA, Propellant A-46, Sorbitan Sesquioleate, Tocopherol.

Storage: Store at room temerature.

Shown in Product Identification Section, page 420

MICATIN®
['mī-kə-tin]
Antifungal For Jock Itch

Description: An antifungal containing the active ingredient miconazole nitrate 2%, clinically proven to cure jock itch.

Indications: Jock itch (tinea cruris).

Actions and Uses: Proven clinically effective in the treatment of jock itch (tinea cruris). For effective relief of the itching, scaling, burning and discomfort that can accompany this condition.

Directions: Cleanse skin with soap and water and dry thoroughly. Apply a thin layer of product over affected area morning and night or as directed by a doctor. Best results are usually obtained within 2 weeks' use of this product. If satisfactory results have not occurred within this time, consult a doctor or pharmacist. Children under 12 years of age should be supervised in the use of this product. This product is not effective on the scalp or nails.

Warnings: Do not use on children under 2 years of age except under the advice and supervision of a doctor. For external use only. If irritation occurs, or if there is no improvement of jock itch within 2 weeks, discontinue use and consult a doctor or pharmacist. Keep this and all drugs out of the reach of children. In case of accidental ingestion, seek professional assistance or contact a Poison Control Center immediately.

How Supplied:
MICATIN® Jock Itch Cream is available in a 0.5 oz. tube.
MICATIN Jock Itch Spray Powder is available in a 3.0 oz. aerosol can.

Inactive Ingredients:
MICATIN Jock Itch Cream: Benzoic Acid, BHA, Mineral Oil, Peglicol 5 Oleate, Pegoxol 7 Stearate, Purified Water.
MICATIN Jock Itch Spray Powder: Alcohol, Propellant A-46, Sorbitan Sesquioleate, Stearalkonium Hectorite, Talc.

Storage: Store at room temperature.

P & S Laboratories
210 WEST 131st STREET
LOS ANGELES, CA 90061

See Standard Homeopathic Company.

Paddock Laboratories, Inc.
3101 LOUISIANA AVE. NORTH
MINNEAPOLIS, MN 55427

ACTIDOSE-AQUA
(Highly Activated Charcoal Suspension)

Supplied in bottles containing 25 grams per 120ml, 50 grams per 240ml, and 15 grams per 72 ml highly activated charcoal suspension. Each milliliter contains 208mg (0.208 grams) highly activated charcoal in aqueous suspension. Detailed blue color-coded attached package insert.

ACTIDOSE with SORBITOL
(Highly Activated Charcoal Suspension with Sorbitol)

Supplied in bottles containing 25 grams per 120ml and 50 grams per 240ml highly activated charcoal suspension. Each milliliter contains 208mg (0.208 grams) highly activated charcoal and 400mg (0.4 grams) sorbitol. Detailed red color-coded attached package insert.

EMULSOIL®
[ē-muls-oil]
Castor Oil

Emulsoil is a self-emulsifying, flavored castor oil formulated to instantly mix with any beverage.

Active Ingredient: Each 2-ounce bottle contains 95% w/w Castor Oil, USP with self-emulsifying and natural sugarless flavoring agents.

Indications: Emulsoil is used in the preparation of the small and large bowel for radiography, colonoscopy, surgery, proctologic procedures and exploratory IVP use. Can also be used for isolated bouts of constipation.

Warnings: Not to be used when abdominal pain, nausea, vomiting or other symptoms of appendicitis are present. Frequent or prolonged use may result in dependence on laxatives. Do not use during pregnancy except under competent advice.

Dosage and Administration: Adults: 1–4 tablespoonfuls. Children: 1–2 teaspoonfuls.

How Supplied: Available in 2-ounce bottles. Packaged 12 and 48 bottles per case.

GLUTOSE®
[glū-tose]
Dextrose Gel

Active Ingredient: Dextrose 40%, Each 80-gram bottle contains 32 grams dextrose in a dye free jel base.

Indications: Glutose is a concentrated glucose (40% Dextrose) used for insulin reactions and hypoglycemic states.

Dosage and Administration: Usual dose is 25 grams (10 grams of dextrose) orally, which can be repeated in 10 minutes if necessary. Response should be noticed in 10 minutes. The physician should then be notified when a hypoglycemic reaction occurs so that the insulin dose can be accurately adjusted. Glutose should not be given to children under 2 years of age unless otherwise directed by physician.

How Supplied: 80-gram squeeze bottle, 6 bottles/case. 25-gram unit-dose tube, 3 tubes/box.

IPECAC SYRUP
[ĭp-ĕ-kak]

Active Ingredients: Ipecac Syrup, USP contains in each 30 ml, not less than

Continued on next page

Paddock—Cont.

36.9 mg and not more than 47.1 mg of the total ether soluble alkaloids of ipecac. The content of emetine and cephaeline together is not less than 90.0% of the amount of the total ether-soluble alkaloids.

Indications: Ipecac Syrup is indicated for emergency use to cause vomiting in poisoning.

Warnings: Do not use in unconscious persons. Ordinarily, this drug should not be used if strychnine, corrosives such as alkalies, lye and strong acids, or petroleum distillates such as kerosene, gasoline, coal oil, fuel oil, paint thinners, or cleaning fluids have been ingested.

Dosage and Administration: Usual Dosage: One tablespoonful (15 ml) followed by one to two glasses of water, in persons over 1 year of age. Repeat dosage in 20 minutes if vomiting does not occur.

How Supplied: Available in 1-ounce bottles. Packaged 12 bottles per case.

Parke-Davis

Consumer Health Products Group
Division of Warner-Lambert Company
201 TABOR ROAD
MORRIS PLAINS, NJ 07950
(See also Warner-Lambert)

AGORAL® Plain
[ă 'gō-răl "]
AGORAL® Raspberry
AGORAL® Marshmallow

Description: Each tablespoonful (15 mL) of Agoral Plain contains 4.2 grams mineral oil in a thoroughly homogenized emulsion.
Also contains acacia; agar; benzoic acid; egg albumin; flavors; glycerin; sodium benzoate; tragacanth; citric acid or sodium hydroxide to adjust pH; water.
Each tablespoonful (15 mL) of Agoral Raspberry (pink) or of Agoral Marshmallow (white) contains 4.2 grams mineral oil and 0.2 gram phenolphthalein in a thoroughly homogenized emulsion.
Also contains acacia; agar; benzoic acid; egg albumin; flavors; glycerin; saccharin sodium; sodium benzoate; tragacanth; citric acid or sodium hydroxide to adjust pH; water. Agoral Raspberry Flavor also contains D&C Red No. 30 Lake.

Actions: Agoral, containing mineral oil, facilitates defecation by lubricating the fecal mass and softening the stool. More effective than nonemulsified oil in penetrating the feces, Agoral thereby greatly reduces the possibility of oil leakage at the anal sphincter. Phenolphthalein gently stimulates motor activity of the lower intestinal tract. Agoral's combined lubricating-softening and peristaltic actions can help to restore a normal pattern of evacuation.

Indications: Relief of constipation. Agoral may be especially required when straining at stool is a hazard, as in hernia, cardiac, or hypertensive patients; during convalescence from surgery; before and after surgery for hemorrhoids or other painful anorectal disorders; for patients confined to bed.
The management of chronic constipation should also include attention to fluid intake, diet and bowel habits.

Contraindication: Sensitivity to phenolphthalein.

Warning: Do not use laxative products when abdominal pain, nausea, or vomiting are present unless directed by a physician. If you have noticed a sudden change in bowel habits that persists over a period of 2 weeks, consult a physician before using a laxative. Laxative products should not be used for a period longer than 1 week unless directed by a physician. Rectal bleeding or failure to have a bowel movement after use of a laxative may indicate a serious condition. Discontinue use and consult your physician. Do not administer to children under 6 years of age, to pregnant women, to bedridden patients or to persons with difficulty swallowing. As with any drug, if you are nursing a baby, seek the advice of a health professional before using this product. Do not take with meals. If skin rash appears, do not use this product or any other preparation containing phenolphthalein. Keep this and all drugs out of the reach of children. In case of accidental overdose, seek professional assistance or contact a Poison Control Center immediately. Drug interaction precaution: Do not take this product if you are presently taking a stool softener laxative.

Dosage: Agoral Plain—Adults—1 to 2 tablespoonfuls at bedtime only, unless other time is advised by physician. Children—Over 6 years, 2 to 4 teaspoonfuls at bedtime only, unless other time is advised by physician.
Agoral Raspberry and Marshmallow—Adults—½ to 1 tablespoonful at bedtime only, unless other time is advised by physician. Children—Over 6 years, ½ to ¾ teaspoonfuls at bedtime only, unless other time is advised by physician. This product generally produces bowel movement in 6 to 8 hours.

Supplied: Agoral Plain (without phenolphthalein), plastic bottles of 16 fl oz. Agoral (raspberry flavor), plastic bottles of 16 fl oz. Agoral (marshmallow flavor), plastic bottles of 16 fl oz.

Store between 15°–30° C (59°–86° F). Keep this and all drugs out of the reach of children.

In case of accidental overdose, seek professional assistance or contact a Poison Control Center immediately.

ANUSOL®
[ă 'nū-sōl "]
Suppositories/Ointment

Description:

	Anusol Suppositories each contains	Anusol Ointment each gram
Bismuth subgallate	2.25%	—
Bismuth Resorcin Compound	1.75%	—
Benzyl Benzoate	1.2 %	12 mg
Peruvian Balsam	1.8 %	18 mg
Zinc Oxide	11.0 %	110 mg
Analgine™ (pramoxine hydrochloride)	—	10 mg
	Also contains the following inactive ingredients: calcium phosphate dibasic; coconut oil base, FD&C Blue No. 2 Lake and Red No. 40 Lake, hydrogenated fatty acid in a bland hydrogenated vegetable oil base.	Also contains the following inactive ingredients: calcium phosphate dibasic; cocoa butter; glyceryl monooleate; glyceryl monostearate; kaolin; mineral oil; polyethylene wax; Peruvian balsam.

Actions: Anusol Suppositories and Anusol Ointment help to relieve pain, itching and discomfort arising from irritated anorectal tissues. They have a soothing, lubricant action on mucous membranes. Analgine (pramoxine hydrochloride) in Anusol Ointment is a rapidly acting local anesthetic for the skin and mucous membranes of the anus and rectum. Analgine is also chemically distinct from procaine, cocaine, and dibucaine and can often be used in the patient previously sensitized to other surface anesthetics. Surface analgesia lasts for several hours.

Indications: For prompt, temporary symptomatic relief of minor pain, itching, burning and soreness of hemorrhoids and other simple anorectal irritation.

Contraindications: Anusol Suppositories and Anusol Ointment are contraindicated in those patients with a history of hypersensitivity to any of the components of the preparations.

Precautions: Symptomatic relief should not delay definitive diagnoses or treatment.
If irritation develops, these preparations should be discontinued. In case of rectal bleeding or persistence of the condition, consult your physician. Keep this and all drugs out of the reach of children. In case of accidental ingestion seek professional assistance or contact a Poison Control Center immediately. Do not use in the eyes or nose.

Adverse Reactions: Upon application of Anusol Ointment, which contains Analgine (pramoxine HCl), a patient may occasionally experience burning, especially if the anoderm is not intact. Sensitivity reactions have been rare; discontinue medication if suspected.

Dosage and Administration: Anusol Suppositories—Adults: Remove foil wrapper and insert suppository into the anus. Insert one suppository in the morning and one at bedtime, and one immediately following each evacuation.
Anusol Ointment—Adults: After gentle bathing and drying of the anal area, remove tube cap and apply freely to the exterior surface and gently rub in. Ointment should be applied every 3 or 4 hours.
NOTE: If staining from either of the above products occurs, the stain may be removed from fabric by hand or machine washing with household detergent.

How Supplied: Anusol Suppositories—boxes of 12, 24 and 48; in silver foil strips. Anusol Ointment—1-oz tubes and 2-oz tubes with plastic applicator.
Store between 15° and 30°C (59° and 86°F).

Shown in Product Identification Section, page 420

BENADRYL Anti-Itch Cream

Active Ingredients: BENADRYL® (diphenhydramine hydrochloride USP) 1%.

Inactive Ingredients: Cetyl Alcohol, Methylparaben, Polyethylene Glycol Monostearate, Propylene Glycol and Water, Purified.

Indications: For the temporary relief of ITCHING and PAIN associated with minor skin irritations, allergic itches, rashes, insect bites and sunburn.

Actions: Benadryl, the most prescribed topical antihistamine, in a soothing, greaseless cream, is easily absorbed into the skin. It provides safe, effective, temporary relief from many different types of itching.

Warnings: For external use only. Do not apply to blistered, raw or oozing areas of the skin. Do not use on chicken pox or measles unless supervised by a physician. Do not use on extensive areas of the skin or for longer than 7 days except as directed by a physician. Avoid contact with the eyes or other mucous membranes. If condition worsens, or if symptoms persist for more than 7 days, or clear up and occur again within a few days, discontinue use of this product and consult a physician. Do not use any other drugs containing diphenhydramine while using this product. KEEP THIS AND ALL DRUGS OUT OF THE REACH OF CHILDREN. In case of accidental ingestion, seek professional assistance or contact a Poison Control Center immediately.

Dosage and Administration: Regular Strength 1%—For adults and children 6 years of age and older: Apply to affected area not more than three to four times daily, or as directed by a physician. For children under 6 years of age: consult a physician.
Maximum Strength 2%—For adults and children 12 years of age and older: Apply to affected area not more than three to four times daily, or as directed by a physician. For children under 12 years of age: consult a physician.

How Supplied: Benadryl Anti-Itch Cream is available in ½ oz. Regular Strength and ½ oz. Maximum Strength tubes.

Shown in Product Identification Section, page 420

BENADRYL®

[bĕ'nă-drĭl]

Decongestant Elixir

Description: Each teaspoonful (5 mL) contains: Benadryl (diphenhydramine hydrochloride) 12.5 mg; pseudoephedrine hydrochloride 30 mg; alcohol 5%. Also contains: FD&C Yellow No. 6; glucose, liquid; glycerin, USP; flavors; menthol, USP; saccharin sodium, USP; sodium citrate, USP; sucrose, NF; water, purified, USP.

Indications: Temporarily relieves nasal congestion, runny nose, sneezing, itching of the nose or throat, itchy, watery eyes due to hay fever or other upper respiratory allergies, and runny nose, sneezing and nasal congestion of the common cold.

Warnings: Do not exceed recommended dosage because at higher doses nervousness, dizziness, or sleeplessness may occur. Do not take this product for more than 7 days. If symptoms do not improve or are accompanied by fever, consult a physician. Do not take this product if you have high blood pressure, heart disease, diabetes, thyroid disease, asthma, glaucoma, emphysema, chronic pulmonary disease, shortness of breath, difficulty in breathing or difficulty in urination due to enlargement of the prostate gland unless directed by a physician. May cause excitability, especially in children. May cause marked drowsiness: alcohol may increase the drowsiness effect. Avoid alcoholic beverages while taking this product. Use caution when driving a motor vehicle or operating machinery. As with any drug, if you are pregnant or nursing a baby seek the advice of a health professional before using this product. Keep this and all drugs out of the reach of children. In case of accidental overdose, seek professional assistance or contact a poison control center immediately.

Drug Interaction Precaution: Do not take this product if you are presently taking a prescription drug for high blood pressure or depression without first consulting your physician.

Directions: Children 6 to under 12 years oral dosage is one teaspoonful every 4 to 6 hours not to exceed 4 teaspoonfuls in 24 hours, or as directed by a physician. For children under 6 years of age, consult a physician. Adult oral dosage is two teaspoonfuls every 4 to 6 hours not to exceed 8 teaspoonfuls in 24 hours, or as directed by a physician.

How Supplied: Benadryl Decongestant Elixir is supplied in 4-oz bottles. Store below 30° C (86°F). Protect from freezing.

Shown in Product Identification Section, page 421

BENADRYL® Decongestant

[bĕ'nă-drĭl]

Decongestant Tablets and Kapseals®

Active Ingredients: Each tablet/Kapseal® contains: Benadryl® (diphenhydramine hydrochloride USP) 25 mg. and pseudoephedrine hydrochloride 60 mg.

Inactive Ingredients: Each tablet contains: Corn Starch, Croscarmelose Sodium, Dibasic Calcium Phosphate Dihydrate, FD&C Blue No. 1 Aluminum Lake, Hydroxypropyl Methylcellulose, Microcrystalline Cellulose, Polyethylene Glycol, Polysorbate 80, Stearic Acid, Titanium Dioxide and Zinc Stearate.
Each Kapseals® capsule contains: Calcium Stearate, Lactose (Hydrous), Syloid Silica Gel. The Kapseals® capsule shell contains: D&C Red No. 28, FD&C Blue No. 1 and Red No. 3, Gelatin, Glyceryl Monooleate, PEG-200 Ricinoleate and Titanium Dioxide.

Indications: Temporarily relieves nasal congestion, runny nose, sneezing, itching of the nose or throat, itchy, watery eyes due to hay fever or other upper respiratory allergies, and runny nose, sneezing and nasal congestion of the common cold.

Warning: Do not exceed recommended dosage because at higher doses nervousness, dizziness, or sleeplessness may occur. Do not take this product for more than 7 days. If symptoms do not improve or are accompanied by fever, consult a physician. Do not take this product if you have high blood pressure, heart disease, diabetes, thyroid disease, asthma, glaucoma, emphysema, chronic pulmonary disease, shortness of breath, difficulty in breathing or difficulty in urination due to enlargement of the prostate gland unless directed by a physician. May cause excitability, especially in children. May cause marked drowsiness: alcohol may increase the drowsiness effect. Avoid alcoholic beverages while taking this product. Use caution when driving a motor vehicle or operating machinery. Do not give this product to children under 12 years except under the advice and supervision of a physician. As with any drug, if you are pregnant or nursing a baby seek the advice of a health professional before using this product. Keep this and all

Continued on next page

This product information was prepared in November 1990. On these and other Parke-Davis Products, detailed information may be obtained by addressing PARKE-DAVIS, Consumer Health Products Group, Division of Warner-Lambert Company, Morris Plains, NJ 07950.

Parke-Davis—Cont.

drugs out of the reach of children. In case of accidental overdose, seek professional assistance or contact a poison control center immediately.

Drug Interaction Precaution: Do not take this product if you are presently taking a prescription drug for high blood pressure or depression without first consulting your physician.

Directions: Adults and children over 12 years of age: 1 tablet/Kapseal® every 4 to 6 hours not to exceed 4 tablets/Kapseals® in 24 hours. Benadryl Decongestant is not recommended for children under 12 years of age.

How Supplied: Benadryl Decongestant Tablets and Kapseals® are supplied in boxes of 24.
Store at room temperature 15°–30° C (59°–86° F).
Protect from moisture.

Shown in Product Identification Section, page 420

BENADRYL® Elixir

Active Ingredients: Each teaspoonful (5 mL) contains: Benadryl® (diphenhydramine hydrochloride USP) 12.5 mg. and Alcohol 5.6%.

Inactive Ingredients: Also contains: Citric Acid, D&C Red No. 33, EDTA, FD&C Red No. 40, Flavors, Glycerin, Mono Ammonium Glycyrrhizinate, Propyl Gallate, Sodium Citrate, Sodium Saccharin, Sugar, Water, purified.

Indications: Temporarily relieves runny nose, sneezing, itching of the nose or throat and itchy, watery eyes due to hay fever or other upper respiratory allergies and runny nose and sneezing associated with the common cold.

Warnings: Do not take this product if you have asthma, glaucoma, emphysema, chronic pulmonary disease, shortness of breath, difficulty in breathing or difficulty in urination due to enlargement of the prostate gland unless directed by a physician. May cause excitability especially in children. May cause marked drowsiness; alcohol may increase the drowsiness effect. Avoid alcoholic beverages while taking this product. Use caution when driving a motor vehicle or operating machinery. As with any drug if you are pregnant or nursing a baby seek the advice of a healthy professional before using this product. Keep this and all drugs out of the reach of children. In case of accidental overdose, seek professional assistance or contact a Poison Control Center immediately.

Dosage and Administration: Children 6 to under 12 years of age oral dosage is 12.5 to 25 mg. (1 to 2 teaspoonfuls) every 4 to 6 hours not to exceed 12 teaspoonfuls in 24 hours, or as directed by a physician. For children under 6 years your physician should be contacted for the recommended dosage. Adult oral dosage is 25 mg. (2 teaspoonfuls) to 50 mg. (4 teaspoonfuls) every 4 to 6 hours not to exceed 24 teaspoonfuls in 24 hours, or as directed by a physician.

How Supplied: Benadryl Elixir is supplied in 4 oz. and 8 oz. bottles.

Shown in Product Identification Section, page 421

BENADRYL® 25

[*bĕ 'nă-drĭl*]

Tablets and Kapseals®

Active Ingredient: Each tablet/Kapseal® contains: Benadryl® (diphenhydramine hydrochloride USP) 25 mg.

Inactive Ingredients: Each tablet contains: Corn Starch, Croscarmellose Sodium, Dibasic Calcium Phosphate Dihydrate, D&C Red No. 27 Aluminum Lake, Hydroxypropyl Methylcellulose, Microcrystalline Cellulose, Polyethylene Glycol, Polysorbate 80, Stearic Acid, Titanium Dioxide and Zinc Stearate. Each Kapseal capsule contains: Lactose (Hydrous) and Magnesium Stearate. The Kapseal capsule shell contains: Artificial Colors, Gelatin, Glyceryl Mono-oleate, PEG-200 Ricinolcate and Titanium Dioxide.

Indications: Temporarily relieves runny nose, sneezing, itching of the nose or throat, itchy, watery eyes due to hay fever or other upper respiratory allergies and runny nose and sneezing of the common cold.

Warnings: Do not take this product if you have asthma, glaucoma, emphysema, chronic pulmonary disease, shortness of breath, difficulty in breathing or difficulty in urination due to enlargement of the prostate gland unless directed by physician. May cause excitability, especially in children. May cause marked drowsiness: alcohol may increase the drowsiness effect. Avoid alcoholic beverages while taking this product. Use caution when driving a motor vehicle or operating machinery. As with any drug if you are pregnant or nursing a baby seek the advice of a health professional before using this product. Keep this and all drugs out of the reach of children. In case of accidental overdose, seek professional assistance or contact a poison control center immediately.

Directions: Adult oral dosage is 25–50 mg (1 to 2 tablets/Kapseals®) every 4 to 6 hours not to exceed 12 tablets/Kapseals® in 24 hours, or as directed by a physician. Children 6 to under 12 years oral dosage is 12.5 mg to 25 mg (1 tablet/-Kapseal®) every 4 to 6 hours, not to exceed 6 tablets/Kapseals® in 24 hours, or as directed by a physician. For children under 6 years your physician should be contacted for the recommended dosage.

How Supplied: Benadryl 25 Tablets and Kapseals® are supplied in boxes of 24 and 48.
Store at room temperature 15°–30° C (59°–86° F). Protect from moisture.

Shown in Product Identification Section, page 421

BENADRYL PLUS®
Tablets

Active Ingredients: Each tablet contains: Benadryl® (diphenhydramine hydrochloride USP) 12.5 mg., pseudoephedrine hydrochloride 30 mg., and acetaminophen 500 mg.

Inactive Ingredients: Each tablet contains: Carboxymethylcellulose, Croscarmellose Sodium, Hydroxypropyl Cellulose, Hydroxypropyl Methylcellulose, Magnesium Stearate, Microcrystalline Cellulose, Polyethylene Glycol, Propylene Glycol, Starch, Stearic Acid, Titanium Dioxide, and Zinc Stearate.

Indications: Temporarily relieves sneezing, running nose, nasal and sinus congestion, fever, minor sore throat pain, headache, sinus pressure, body aches and pain due to the common cold, and sneezing, runny nose, itching of the nose or throat, and itchy, watery eyes due to hay fever or other upper respiratory allergies.

Warnings: Do not exceed recommended dosage because at higher doses nervousness, dizziness, or sleeplessness may occur. Do not take this product if you have high blood pressure, heart disease, diabetes, thyroid disease, asthma, glaucoma, emphysema, chronic pulmonary disease, shortness of breath, difficulty in breathing, or difficulty in urination due to enlargement of the prostate gland unless directed by a physician. May cause excitability especially in children. May cause marked drowsiness; alcohol may increase the drowsiness effect. Avoid alcoholic beverages while taking this product. Use caution when driving a motor vehicle or operating machinery. If fever persists for more than 3 days (72 hours) or recurs, consult your physician. If sore throat persists for more than 2 days, is accompanied or followed by fever, headache, rash, nausea or vomiting, consult a physician promptly. As with any drug if you are pregnant or nursing a baby seek the advice of a health professional before using this product. Keep this and all drugs out of the reach of children. In case of accidental overdose, seek professional assistance or contact a Poison Control Center immediately. Do not give this product to children under 12 years except under the advice and supervision of a physician.

Drug Interaction Precaution: Do not take this product if you are presently taking a prescription drug for high blood pressure or depression without consulting your physician.

Directions: Adults (12 years and over): Two tablets every 6 hours, not to exceed 8 tablets in a 24-hour period. Benadryl Plus is not recommended for children under 12 years of age.

How Supplied: Benadryl Plus Tablets are supplied in boxes of 24 and 48.
Store at room temperature 15°–30°C (59°–86°F). Protect from moisture.

Shown in Product Identification Section, page 421

BENADRYL® PLUS NIGHTTIME

Active Ingredients: Each fluid ounce or 2 tablespoons contains: Acetaminophen 1000 mg., diphenhydramine hydrochloride 50 mg., and pseudoephedrine hydrochloride 60 mg.

Inactive Ingredients: Alcohol 10%, citric acid, D&C Yellow No. 10, FD&C Red No. 40, FD&C Green No. 3, disodium edetate, flavoring, glycerin, polyethylene glycol, potassium sorbate, propyl gallate, propylene glycol, sodium benzoate, sodium citrate, sodium saccharin and purified water.

Indications: Benadryl Plus Nighttime provides temporary relief of nasal congestion, runny nose, sneezing, itching of the nose or throat, itchy watery eyes due to hay fever or other upper respiratory allergies and runny nose, sneezing and nasal congestion of the common cold, and fever, headache, sore throat pain, and body aches and pains associated with these conditions.

Warnings: Do not exceed recommended dosage because at higher doses nervousness, dizziness, or sleeplessness may occur. Do not take this product for more than 7 days. If symptoms do not improve or are accompanied by fever, consult a physician. Do not take this product if you have high blood pressure, heart disease, diabetes, thyroid disease, asthma, glaucoma, emphysema, chronic pulmonary disease, shortness of breath, difficulty in breathing, or difficulty in urination due to enlargement of the prostate gland unless directed by a physician. If fever persists for more than 3 days (72 hours) or recurs, consult your physician. If sore throat is severe, persists for more than 2 days, is accompanied or followed by fever, headache, rash, nausea or vomiting, consult a physician promptly. As with any drug if you are pregnant or nursing a baby seek the advice of a health professional before using this product. Keep this and all drugs out of the reach of children. In case of accidental ingestion, seek professional assistance or contact a Poison Control Center immediately. May cause marked drowsiness; alcohol may increase the drowsiness effect. Do not give this product to children under 12 years except under the advice of a physician.

Caution: Avoid alcoholic beverages while taking this product. Use caution when driving a motor vehicle or operating heavy machinery.

Drug Interaction Precaution: Do not take this product if you are presently taking a prescription drug for high blood pressure or depression without first consulting your physician.

Directions for Use: Adults take one fluid ounce using dosage cup or two (2) tablespoons at bedtime for nighttime relief. Dosage may be repeated every six (6) hours or as directed by a physician. Do not exceed 4 fluid ounces or eight (8) tablespoons in any 24-hour period. Children under 12 should use only as directed by a physician.

How Supplied: Benadryl Plus Nighttime is supplied in 6 ounce and 10 ounce bottles. Store at room temperature, 15°–30°C (59°–86°F).

Questions about Benadryl® Plus Nighttime?
Call us toll free 8 AM to 5 PM EST. Weekdays at 1-800-524-2624. In New Jersey call 1-800-338-0326.

Shown in Product Identification Section, page 421

BENADRYL® Spray Regular Strength 1%
BENADRYL® Spray Maximum Strength 2%

Active Ingredients: Regular Strength contains Benadryl® (diphenhydramine hydrochloride USP) 1% and alcohol 90%; Maximum Strength contains Benadryl® (diphenhydramine hydrochloride USP) 2% and alcohol 90%.

Inactive Ingredients: Glycerin, Povidone, Tromethamine, and Water, Purified.

Indications: For the temporary relief of ITCHING and PAIN associated with insect bites, rashes, poison oak, poison sumac, allergic itches, and minor skin irritations.

Actions: Benadryl Spray forms a clear, anti-itch "bandage" to protect and relieve affected areas. Benadryl stops the itch at the source by blocking the action of histamine that causes the itch. Benadryl also provides an anesthetic action to soothe the pain. The spray feature allows soothing relief without touching or rubbing the affected area. Benadryl spray is clear, won't stain clothing and won't rinse off (can be easily removed with soap and water).

Warnings: FOR EXTERNAL USE ONLY. Do not apply to blistered, raw or oozing areas of the skin. Do not use on chicken pox or measles unless supervised by a physician. Do not use on extensive areas of the skin for longer than 7 days except as directed by a physician. Avoid contact with the eyes or other mucous membranes. If condition worsens or if symptoms persist for more than 7 days or clear up and occur again within a few days, discontinue use of this product and consult a physician. Do not use any other drugs containing diphenhydramine while using this product. KEEP THIS AND ALL DRUGS OUT OF THE REACH OF CHILDREN. In case of accidental ingestion, seek professional assistance or contact a Poison Control Center immediately. Flammable, keep away from fire or flame.

Dosage and Administration: Regular Strength 1%—For adults and children 6 years of age and older: Spray on affected area not more than three to four times daily, or as directed by a physician. For children under 6 years of age: consult a physician. **Maximum Strength 2%**—For adults and children 12 years of age or older: Spray on affected area not more than three to four times daily, or as directed by a physician. For children under 12 years of age: consult a physician.

How Supplied: Benadryl® Spray is available in a 2 oz. pump spray bottle.

Shown in Product Identification Section, page 420

BENYLIN®
Cough Syrup

Description: Each teaspoonful (5 ml) contains:

Diphenhydramine Hydrochloride	12.5 mg

Also contains: Alcohol 5%; Ammonium Chloride; Caramel; Citric Acid; D&C Red No. 33; FD&C Red No. 40; Flavor; Glucose Liquid; Glycerin; Menthol; Purified Water; Sodium Citrate; Sodium Saccharin; Sucrose.

Indications: For the temporary relief of cough due to minor throat and bronchial irritation as may occur with the common cold or with inhaled irritants.

Warnings: A persistent cough may be a sign of a serious condition. Do not take this product for persistent or chronic cough such as occurs with smoking, asthma, emphysema, or when cough is accompanied by excessive phlegm (mucus). If cough persists for more than (1) week, tends to recur, or is accompanied by fever, rash, or persistent headache, consult a physician. May cause excitability, especially in children. Do not take this product if you have glaucoma, or difficulty in urination due to enlargement of the prostate gland except under the advice of a physician. May cause marked drowsiness. Avoid driving a motor vehicle or operating heavy machinery, or drinking alcoholic beverages. Do not give to children under six (6) years of age except under the advice and supervision of a physician. Keep this and all drugs out of the reach of children. In case of accidental overdose, seek professional assistance or contact a Poison Control Center immediately. As with any drug, if you are pregnant or nursing a baby, seek the advice of a health professional before using this product.

Directions for Use:
Adults: (12 years and older): Take 2 teaspoonfuls every 4 hours. Do not exceed 12 teaspoonfuls in 24 hours.
Children (6–12 years): Take 1 teaspoonful every 4 hours. Do not exceed 6 teaspoonfuls in 24 hours.
Children (under 6 years): Consult physician for recommended dosage.

Continued on next page

This product information was prepared in November 1990. On these and other Parke-Davis Products, detailed information may be obtained by addressing PARKE-DAVIS, Consumer Health Products Group, Division of Warner-Lambert Company, Morris Plains, NJ 07950.

Parke-Davis—Cont.

How Supplied: Benylin Cough Syrup is supplied in 4-oz and 8-oz bottles. Store at 59°–86°F.

Shown in Product Identification Section, page 421

BENYLIN® DM® dextromethorphan cough syrup

Description: Each teaspoonful (5 ml) contains:

Dextromethorphan Hydrobromide	10 mg

Also contains: Alcohol 5%; Ammonium Chloride; Caramel; Citric Acid; D&C Red No. 33; Flavor; Glucose Liquid; Glycerin; Menthol; Purified Water; Sodium Citrate; Sucrose.

Indications: Nonnarcotic cough suppressant for the temporary relief of coughs due to minor bronchial irritation as may occur with the common cold or inhaled irritants.

Warnings: A persistent cough may be a sign of a serious condition. If cough persists for more than one week, tends to recur, or is accompanied by fever, rash, or persistent headache, consult a physician. Do not take this product for persistent or chronic cough such as occurs with smoking, asthma, emphysema, or if cough is accompanied by excessive phlegm (mucus) unless directed by a physician. As with any drug, if you are pregnant or nursing a baby, seek the advice of a health professional before using this product. Keep this and all drugs out of reach of children. In case of accidental overdose, seek professional assistance or contact a Poison Control Center immediately.

Directions for Use:
Adults (12 years and older): Take 1 to 2 teaspoonfuls every 4 hours or 3 teaspoonfuls every 6 to 8 hours. Do not exceed 12 teaspoonfuls in 24 hours.
Children (6–12 years): Take ½–1 teaspoonful every 4 hours or 1½ teaspoonfuls every 6 to 8 hours. Do not exceed 6 teaspoonfuls in 24 hours.
Children (2–6 years): Take ¼ to ½ teaspoonful every 4 hours or ¾ teaspoonful every 6 to 8 hours. Do not exceed 3 teaspoonfuls in 24 hours.
Children (under 2 years): Consult physician for recommended dosage.

How Supplied: 4-oz bottles. Store at 59°–86°F.

Shown in Product Identification Section, page 421

BENYLIN® Decongestant

Description: Each teaspoonful (5 ml) contains:

Diphenhydramine Hydrochloride	12.5 mg
Pseudoephedrine Hydrochloride	30.0 mg

Also contains: Alcohol 5%; FD&C Yellow No. 6 (Sunset Yellow); Flavors; Glucose Liquid; Glycerin; Menthol; Purified Water; Saccharin Sodium; Sodium Citrate; Sucrose.

Indications: For the temporary relief of cough due to minor throat and bronchial irritations as may occur with the common cold or with inhaled irritants; and nasal congestion due to the common cold, hay fever, or other upper respiratory allergies.

Warnings: A persistent cough may be a sign of a serious condition. Do not take this product for persistent or chronic cough such as occurs with smoking, asthma, emphysema, or when cough is accompanied by excessive phlegm (mucus). If cough persists for more than one (1) week, tends to recur, or is accompanied by fever, rash, or persistent headache, consult a physician. May cause excitability, especially in children. Do not take this product if you have high blood pressure, heart disease, diabetes, thyroid disease, glaucoma, or difficulty in urination due to enlargement of the prostate gland except under the advice and supervision of a physician. Do not exceed recommended dosage because at higher doses nervousness, dizziness, or sleeplessness may occur. Do not give to children under six (6) years of age except under the advice and supervision of a physician. May cause marked drowsiness. Avoid driving a motor vehicle or operating heavy machinery, or drinking alcoholic beverages. Keep this and all drugs out of the reach of children. In case of accidental overdose, seek professional assistance or contact a Poison Control Center immediately. As with any drug, if you are pregnant or nursing a baby, seek the advice of a health professional before using this product.

Drug Interaction Precaution: Do not take this product if you are presently taking a prescription drug for high blood pressure or depression without first consulting your doctor.

Directions for Use:
Adults (12 years and older): Take 2 teaspoonfuls every 4 hours. Do not exceed 8 teaspoonfuls in 24 hours.
Children (6–12 years): Take 1 teaspoonful every 4 hours. Do not exceed 4 teaspoonfuls in 24 hours.
Children (under 6 years): Consult physician for recommended dosage.

How Supplied: 4-oz. bottles. Store at 59°–86°F.

Shown in Product Identification Section, page 421

BENYLIN® Expectorant

Description: Each teaspoonful (5 ml) contains:

Dextromethorphan Hydrobromide	5.0 mg
Guaifenesin	100.0 mg

Also contains: Alcohol 5%; Citric Acid; FD&C Red No. 40; Flavors; Glycerin; Purified Water; Saccharin Sodium, Sodium Benzoate, Sodium Citrate; Sucrose.

Indications: Nonnarcotic cough suppressant for the temporary relief of coughs plus an expectorant to relieve upper chest congestion due to minor bronchial irritations as may occur with the common cold, or inhaled irritants. Helps loosen phlegm (sputum) and thin bronchial secretions to rid the bronchial passageways of bothersome mucus.

Warnings: Do not take this product for persistent or chronic cough such as occurs with smoking, asthma, chronic bronchitis, or emphysema, or where cough is accompanied by excessive phlegm (mucus or sputum) unless directed by a physician. A persistent cough may be a sign of a serious condition. If cough persists for more than one week, tends to recur, or is accompanied by fever, rash, or persistent headache, consult a physician. Do not give to children under 2 years of age unless directed by a physician. As with any drug, if you are pregnant or nursing a baby, seek the advice of a health professional before using this product. Keep this and all drugs out of the reach of children. In case of accidental overdose, seek professional assistance or contact a Poison Control Center immediately.

Directions for Use:
Adults (12 years and older): Take 2–4 teaspoonfuls every 4 hours (or fill dosage cup to the corresponding teaspoon level indicated). Do not exceed 24 teaspoonfuls in 24 hours.
Children (6–12 years): Take 1–2 teaspoonfuls every 4 hours (or fill dosage cup to the corresponding teaspoon level indicated). Do not exceed 12 teaspoonfuls in 24 hours.
Children (2–6 years): Take ½–1 teaspoonful every 4 hours (or fill dosage cup to the corresponding teaspoon level indicated). Do not exceed 6 teaspoonfuls in 24 hours.
Children (under 2 years): Consult your physician for recommended dosage.

How Supplied: Benylin Expectorant is supplied in 4-oz and 8-oz bottles. Store at 59°–86°F.

Shown in Product Identification Section, page 421

CALADRYL® Lotion
[*că 'lă drĭl "*]
CALADRYL Cream
CALADRYL Spray

Description: Caladryl Lotion—A drying, calamine-antihistamine lotion containing Calamine 8%, Benadryl® (diphenhydramine hydrochloride), 1%. Also contains: Alcohol 2%; Camphor; Fragrances; Glycerin; Sodium Carboxymethylcellulose; and Water, Purified.
Caladryl Cream—Calamine 8%, Benadryl (diphenhydramine hydrochloride) 1%. Also contains: Camphor; Cetyl Alcohol; Cresin White; Fragrance; Propylene Glycol; Proplyparaben; Polysorbate 60; Sorbitan Stearate; Water, Purified.
Caladryl Spray—Calamine 8%, Benadryl (diphenhydramine hydrochloride) 1%. Also contains: Alcohol 9%, Campor, FD&C Red #40, Fragrance, Isobutane, Quarternium-18 Hectorite, Sorbitan Sesquioleate, and Talc.

Indications: For relief of itching due to mild poison ivy or oak, insect bites, or other minor skin irritations.

Warnings: For external use only. Do not apply to blistered, raw or oozing areas of the skin. Do not use on chicken pox or measles, unless supervised by a doctor. Do not use on extensive areas of the skin or for longer than 7 days except as directed by a doctor. Avoid contact with the eyes or other mucous membranes. Discontinue use if burning sensation or rash develops or condition persists. Remove by washing with soap and water. Do not use any other drugs containing diphenhydramine while using this product. Additional spray warnings: Flammable. Do not use while smoking or near an open flame. Contents under pressure. Do not puncture or incinerate. Do not store at temperatures above 120°F. Intentional misuse by deliberately concentrating and inhaling the contents can be harmful or fatal.
KEEP THIS AND ALL DRUGS OUT OF THE REACH OF CHILDREN. In case of accidental ingestion seek professional assistance or contact a Poison Control Center immediately.

Directions: For adults and children 6 years of age and older: Apply sparingly to the affected area three to four times daily. Before each application cleanse skin with soap and water and dry affected area. Children under 6 years of age: Consult a doctor.

How Supplied: Caladryl Cream; 1½-oz tubes.
Caladryl Lotion—2½ fl.-oz. (75 ml) squeeze bottles and 6 fl.-oz. bottles.
Caladryl spray—4 oz. can.

Shown in Product Identification Section, page 421

GELUSIL®
[*jĕl'ū-sĭl"*]
Antacid–Anti-gas Liquid/Tablets Sodium Free

Each teaspoonful (5 ml) or tablet contains:
200 mg aluminum hydroxide
200 mg magnesium hydroxide
25 mg simethicone
Also contains: Liquid: Citric Acid; Flavors; Hydroxypropyl Methylcellulose; Methylparaben; Propylparaben; Sodium Carboxymethyl Cellulose; Sodium Saccharin; Sorbitol Solution; Water; Xanthan Gum.
Tablets: Flavors; Magnesium Stearate; Mannitol; Sorbitol; Sugar.

Advantages:

- High acid-neutralizing capacity
- Sodium free
- Simethicone for antiflatulent activity
- Good taste for better patient compliance
- Fast dissolution of chewed tablets for prompt relief

Indications: For the relief of heartburn, sour stomach, acid indigestion and to relieve symptoms of gas.

Dosage and Administration: Two or more teaspoonfuls or tablets one hour after meals and at bedtime, or as directed by a physician.
Tablets should be chewed.

Warnings: Do not take more than 12 tablets or teaspoonfuls in a 24-hour period, or use this maximum dosage for more than two weeks, or use this product if you have kidney disease, except under the advice and supervision of a physician.
Keep this and all drugs out of the reach of children.

Professional Warnings: Prolonged use of aluminum-containing antacids in patients with renal failure may result in or worsen dialysis osteomalacia. Elevated tissue aluminum levels contribute to the development of the dialysis encephalopathy and osteomalacia syndromes. Small amounts of aluminum are absorbed from the gastrointestinal tract and renal excretion of aluminum is impaired in renal failure. Aluminum is not well removed by dialysis because it is bound to albumin and transferrin, which do not cross dialysis membranes. As a result, aluminum is deposited in bone, and dialysis osteomalacia may develop when large amounts of aluminum are ingested orally by patients with impaired renal function. Aluminum forms insoluble complexes with phosphate in the gastrointestinal tract, thus decreasing phosphate absorption. Prolonged use of aluminum-containing antacids by normophosphatemic patients may result in hypophosphatemia if phosphate intake is not adequate. In its more severe forms, hypophosphatemia can lead to anorexia, malaise, muscle weakness, and osteomalacia.

Drug Interaction Precaution: Do not take this product if you are presently taking a prescription antibiotic drug containing any form of tetracycline.

How Supplied:
Liquid—In plastic bottles of 12 fl oz.
Tablets—White, embossed Gelusil P-D 034—individual strips of 10 in boxes of 50 and 100.
Store at 59°–86°F (15°–30°C).

Shown in Product Identification Section, page 421

GERIPLEX-FS® KAPSEALS®
[*jĕ'rĭ-plĕx"*]

Composition: Each Kapseal represents:
Vitamin A ....(1.5 mg) 5,000 IU*
(acetate)
Vitamin C........ 50 mg
(ascorbic acid)†
Vitamin B_1........ 5 mg
(thiamine mononitrate)
Vitamin B_2........ 5 mg
(riboflavin)
Vitamin B_{12}, crystalline
(cyanocobalamin)........ 2 mcg
Choline dihydrogen
citrate........ 20 mg
Nicotinamide........ 15 mg
(niacinamide)
Vitamin E (*dl*-alpha-tocopheryl acetate) .... (5 mg) 5 IU*
Iron‡........ 6 mg
Copper sulfate........ 4 mg
Manganese sulfate
(monohydrate)........ 4 mg
Zinc sulfate........ 2 mg
Calcium phosphate, dibasic
(anhydrous)........ 200 mg
Taka-Diastase® (*Aspergillus oryzae* enzymes)........ 2½ gr
Docusate sodium........ 100 mg
Also contains magnesium stearate, NF.

*International Units
†Supplied as sodium ascorbate
‡Supplied as dried ferrous sulfate equivalent to the labeled amount of elemental iron

The capsule shell contains FD&C Blue No. 1, FD&C Red No. 3 and Gelatin.

Action and Uses: A preparation containing vitamins, minerals, and a fecal softener for middle-aged and older individuals. The fecal softening agent, docusate sodium, acts to soften stools and make bowel movements easier.

Administration and Dosage: USUAL DOSAGE—One capsule daily, with or immediately after a meal.

How Supplied: Bottles of 100.
Store at controlled room temperature 15°–30°C (59° to 86°F). Protect from light and moisture.

GERIPLEX-FS®
[*jĕ'rĭ-plĕx"*]
LIQUID
Geriatric Vitamin Formula with Iron and a Fecal Softener

Composition: Each 30 ml represents vitamin B_1 (thiamine hydrochloride), 1.2 mg; vitamin B_2 (as riboflavin-5'-phosphate sodium), 1.7 mg; vitamin B_6 (pyridoxine hydrochloride), 1 mg; vitamin B_{12} (cyanocobalamin) crystalline, 5 mcg; niacinamide, 15 mg; iron (as ferric ammonium citrate, green), 15 mg; Pluronic® F-68,* 200 mg; alcohol, 18%.
Also contains: Brandy, Caramel NF, Citric Acid Anhydrous NF, D&C Red No. 33, Flavors, FD&C Red No. 40, Glucono Delta Lactone, Glucose Liquid USP, Glycerin USP, Sodium Citrate USP, Sodium Saccharin NF, Sorbitol Solution USP, Sugar, Water Purified.

Administration and Dosage: USUAL ADULT DOSAGE—Two tablespoonfuls (30 ml) daily or as recommended by the physician.

*Pluronic is a registered trademark of BASF Wyandotte Corporation for polymers of ethylene oxide and propylene oxide.

Continued on next page

This product information was prepared in November 1990. On these and other Parke-Davis Products, detailed information may be obtained by addressing PARKE-DAVIS, Consumer Health Products Group, Division of Warner-Lambert Company, Morris Plains, NJ 07950.

Parke-Davis—Cont.

How Supplied: 16-oz bottles.
Store below 30° (86°F). Protect from light and freezing.

MEDI-FLU™ Caplet, Liquid

Composition:
Each Caplet contains: **Active Ingredients**—Pseudoephedrine Hydrochloride 30mg., Chlorpheniramine Maleate 2mg., Dextromethorphan Hydrobromide 15mg., Acetaminophen 500mg. **Inactive Ingredients**—Cellulose derivatives, croscarmellose sodium, magnesium stearate, mauba wax, polyethylene glycol, starch, stearic acid.
Each fluid ounce contains: **Active Ingredients**—Acetaminophen 1000mg., Chlorpheniramine Maleate 4mg., Dextromethorphan Hydrobromide 30mg., and Pseudoephedrine Hydrochloride 60mg. **Inactive Ingredients**—Alcohol (19%), Citric Acid, D&C Red No. 33, FD&C Red No. 40, Flavors, Glycerin, Propylene Glycol, Sodium Citrate, Sodium Chloride, Sodium Saccharin, Sorbitol Solution, Sugar and Water.

Actions: Medi-Flu provides temporary relief of these flu symptoms: Fever, body aches & pains, nasal congestion, runny nose, minor sore throat pain, coughing, sneezing, headache and watery eyes.

Warnings: Do not exceed recommended dosage because at higher doses nervousness, dizziness or sleeplessness may occur. Do not take this product for more than 7 days. If symptoms do not improve or are accompanied by fever for more than 3 days or if fever recurs after 3 days consult a doctor. Do not take this product if you have high blood pressure, heart disease, diabetes, thyroid disease, asthma, glaucoma, emphysema, chronic pulmonary disease, shortness of breath, difficulty in breathing, or difficulty in urination due to an enlargement of the prostate gland unless directed by a doctor. Do not take this product for persistent or chronic cough such as occurs with smoking, or if cough is accompanied by excessive phlegm (mucus) unless directed by a doctor. A persistent cough may be a sign of a serious condition. If cough persists for more than one week, tends to recur, or is accompanied or followed by fever, headache, rash, nausea, or vomiting consult a doctor promptly. May cause drowsiness: alcohol, sedatives, and tranquilizers may increase drowsiness effect. Avoid alcoholic beverages while taking this product. May cause excitability. Do not take this product if you are taking sedatives or tranquilizers without first consulting your doctor. Use caution when driving a motor vehicle or operating machinery. As with any drug if you are pregnant or nursing a baby, seek the advise of a health professional before using this product. KEEP THIS AND ALL DRUGS OUT OF THE REACH OF CHILDREN. In case of accidental overdose, seek professional assistance or contact a Poison Control Center immediately. Do not give this product to children under 12 years of age except under the advice and supervision of a doctor.

Drug Interaction Precaution: Do not take this product if you are presently taking a prescription drug for high blood pressure or depression without first consulting your doctor.

Dosage and Administration:
Caplets: Adults—two caplets every 6 hours, as needed, not to exceed 8 caplets in 24 hours. Under 12 consult a physician.
Liquid: 1 fluid ounce (2 tablespoonfuls) every 6 hours as needed, not to exceed 4 fluid ounces in 24 hours. Under 12 consult a physician.

How Supplied: 16 caplets or 6 fl. oz. liquid

Shown in Product Identification Section, page 421

MYADEC ®
High Potency Multivitamin Multimineral Formula

Each Tablet Represents:		% of US Recommended Daily Allowances (US RDA)
Vitamins		
Vitamin A	9,000 IU*	180%
Vitamin D	400 IU	100%
Vitamin E	30 IU	100%
Vitamin C (ascorbic acid)	90 mg	150%
Folic Acid	0.4 mg	100%
Thiamine (vitamin B_1)	10 mg	667%
Riboflavin (vitamin B_2)	10 mg	588%
Niacin**	20 mg	100%
Vitamin B_6	5 mg	250%
Vitamin B_{12}	10 mcg	167%
Pantothenic Acid	20 mg	200%
Vitamin K	25 mcg	***
Biotin	45 mcg	15%
Minerals		
Iodine	150 mcg	100%
Iron	30 mg	167%
Magnesium	100 mg	25%
Copper	3 mg	150%
Zinc	15 mg	100%
Manganese	7.5 mg	***
Calcium	70 mg	7%
Phosphorus	54 mg	5%
Potassium	8 mg	***
Selenium	15 mcg	***
Molybdenum	15 mcg	***
Chromium	15 mcg	***

* International Units
** Supplied as niacinamide
*** No US Recommended Daily Allowance (US RDA) has been established for this nutrient.

Ingredients: Dicalcium phosphate, magnesium oxide, niacinamide ascorbate, ferrous fumarate, *dl*-alpha-tocopheryl acetate, zinc sulfate, ascorbic acid, calcium pantothenate, Vitamin A acetate, manganese sulfate, potassium chloride, hydroxypropyl methylcellulose, povidone, microcrystalline cellulose, calcium sulfate, artificial colors (including FD&C Yellow No. 6), thiamine mononitrate, riboflavin, magnesium stearate, silica gel, cupric sulfate, croscarmellose sodium, Vitamin D, pyridoxine hydrochloride, phytonadione, polyethylene glycol, methylparaben (preservative), folic acid, candelilla wax, hydroxypropyl cellulose, polysorbate 80, vanillin, potassium iodide, propylparaben (preservative), chromium chloride, biotin, sodium molybdate, sodium selenate, cyanocobalamin.

Actions and Uses: High potency vitamin supplement with minerals for adults.

Dosage: One tablet daily with a full meal.

How Supplied: In bottles of 130. Store below 30°C (86°F). Protect from moisture.

Shown in Product Identification Section, page 421

NATABEC® KAPSEALS®

Each capsule represents:

Vitamins	
Vitamin A	4,000 IU*
Vitamin D	400 IU
Vitamin C	50 mg
Vitamin B_1	3 mg
Vitamin B_2	2.0 mg
Nicotinamide†	10 mg
Vitamin B_6	3 mg
Vitamin B_{12}	5 mcg
Minerals	
Precipitated Calcium carbonate	600 mg
Iron	30 mg

*IU = International Units
†Supplied as niacinamide

Action and Uses: A multivitamin and mineral supplement for use during pregnancy and lactation.

Dosage: One capsule daily, or as directed by physician.

How Supplied: In bottles of 100.
The color combination of the banded capsule is a Warner-Lambert trademark.

SINUTAB® Allergy Formula Sustained Action Tablets

Active Ingredients: Each sustained action tablet contains: Dexbrompheniramine maleate 6 mg., pseudoephedrine sulfate 120 mg.

Inactive Ingredients: Acacia, calcium carbonate, carnauba wax, confectioner's sugar, D&C yellow No. 10, FD&C blue No. 1, FD&C yellow No. 6, gelatin, hydrogenated castor oil, magnesium stearate, methylparaben, povidone, propylparaben, shellac, sodium benzoate, sucrose, talc, titanium dioxide.

Indications: For temporary relief of nasal congestion due to the common cold, hay fever or other upper respiratory allergies and associated with sinusitis. Combines a nasal decongestant with an antihistamine in a special continuous-acting, timed-release tablet to provide temporary relief from nasal congestion, running nose, and sneezing.

Actions: Sinutab Allergy Formula Sustained Action Tablets contain an antihistamine (dexbrompheniramine maleate) to help control upper respiratory allergic symptoms and a decongestant (pseudoephedrine sulfate) to reduce congestion of the nasopharyngeal mucosa. Half of the medication is released after the tablet is swallowed, and the remaining amount of medication is released hours later, providing continuous long-lasting relief for 12 hours.

Dexbrompheniramine maleate is an antihistamine incorporated to alleviate runny nose, sneezing, itching of the nose or throat, and itchy watery eyes as may occur in allergic rhinitis (such as hay fever). Pseudoephedrine sulfate, a sympathomimetic drug, provides vasoconstriction of the nasopharyngeal mucosa, resulting in a nasal decongestant effect (decongests sinus openings and passages, reduces swelling of nasal passages, shrinks swollen membranes, and temporarily restores free breathing through the nose).

Warnings: If symptoms do not improve within 7 days or are accompanied by high fever, consult a physician before continuing use. May cause drowsiness; alcohol may increase the drowsiness effect. May cause excitability, especially in children. Do not exceed recommended dosage because at higher doses nervousness, dizziness, or sleeplessness may occur. Do not give this product to children under 12 years except under the advice and supervision of a physician. Do not take this product if you have emphysema, chronic pulmonary disease, shortness of breath and difficulty in breathing, asthma, glaucoma, difficulty in urination due to enlargement of the prostate gland, high blood pressure, heart disease, diabetes, or thyroid disease except under the advice and supervision of a physician. As with any drug, if you are pregnant or nursing a baby, seek the advice of a health professional before using this product.

Caution: Avoid driving a motor vehicle or operating heavy machinery. Avoid alcoholic beverages while taking this product.

Drug Interaction: Do not take this product if you are presently taking a prescription antihypertensive or antidepressant drug containing a monoamine oxidase inhibitor except under the advice and supervision of a physician.

Precaution: Keep this and all drugs out of the reach of children.

Symptoms and Treatment of Oral Overdosage: In case of accidental overdose, seek professional assistance or contact a Poison Control Center immediately.

Dosage and Administration: Adults and children 12 years and over—1 tablet, every 12 hours. Do not exceed two tablets in 24 hours.

How Supplied: Sinutab Allergy Formula Sustained Action Tablets are green and coated. They are supplied in easy-to-open blister packs of 10 and 20 tablets.

Shown in Product Identification Section, page 422

SINUTAB® Regular Strength Without Drowsiness Formula Tablets

Active Ingredients: Each tablet contains: Acetaminophen 325 mg., pseudoephedrine hydrochloride 30 mg.

Inactive Ingredients: Cellulose microcrystalline, croscarmellose sodium, D&C red No. 33, FD&C red No. 40, hydroxypropyl cellulose, hydroxypropyl methylcellulose, magnesium stearate, propylene glycol, simethicone, starch pregelatinized, titanium dioxide, zinc stearate.

Indications: For temporary relief of sinus symptoms due to colds, flu, allergy and hay fever. Contains a nonaspirin analgesic to relieve headache pain and a decongestant to ease pressure and congestion.

Actions: Sinutab® Regular Strength Without Drowsiness Formula Tablets contain an analgesic (acetaminophen) to relieve pain and a decongestant (pseudoephedrine hydrochloride) to reduce congestion of the nasopharyngeal mucosa.

Acetaminophen is both analgesic and antipyretic. Because acetaminophen is not a salicylate, Sinutab® Regular Strength Without Drowsiness Formula Tablets can be used by patients who are allergic to aspirin.

Pseudoephedrine hydrochloride, a sympathomimetic drug, provides vasoconstriction of the nasopharyngeal mucosa resulting in a nasal decongestant effect. The absence of antihistamine in the formula provides the added benefit of reduced likelihood of drowsiness side effects.

Warnings: Do not exceed recommended dosage. If symptoms persist, do not improve within 7 days, or are accompanied by high fever, or if new symptoms occur, see your doctor before continuing use. Do not take this product if you have high blood pressure, heart disease, diabetes, thyroid disease, or difficulty in urination due to an enlarged prostate except under doctor's supervision. Do not take this product for more than 10 days. As with any drug, if you are pregnant or nursing a baby, seek the advice of a health professional before using this product.

Drug Interaction: Do not take this product if you are presently taking a prescription drug for high blood pressure or depression without first consulting your doctor.

Precaution: Keep this and all drugs out of the reach of children.

Symptoms and Treatment of Oral Overdosage: In case of accidental overdose, seek professional help or contact a Poison Control Center immediately.

Dosage and Administration: Adults 2 tablets every 4 hours, not to exceed 8 tablets in 24 hours, or as directed by physician. Children under 12 should use only as directed by physician.

How Supplied: Sinutab® Regular Strength Without Drowsiness Formula Tablets are pink, coated and scored so that tablets may be split in half. They are supplied in child-resistant blister packs in boxes of 12 tablets and in easy-to-open (exempt) blister packs of 24 tablets, and in bottles of 100 tablets with child-resistant caps.

Shown in Product Identification Section, page 421

SINUTAB® Maximum Strength Formula Tablets and Caplets

Active Ingredients: Each tablet/caplet contains: Acetaminophen 500 mg., chlorpheniramine maleate 2 mg., pseudoephedrine hydrochloride 30 mg.

Inactive Ingredients:
Tablets contain: Carboxymethyl starch, cellulose, corn starch, croscarmellose sodium, hydroxypropyl cellulose, stearic acid, zinc stearate, D&C yellow No. 10 aluminum lake and FD&C yellow No. 6 aluminum lake.

Caplets contain: Cellulose, corn starch, croscarmellose sodium, hydroxypropyl cellulose, hydroxypropyl methylcellulose, magnesium stearate, polyethylene glycol, sodium starch glycolate, stearic acid, titanium dioxide, zinc stearate, D&C yellow No. 10 aluminum lake, and FD&C yellow No. 6 aluminum lake.

Indications: For temporary relief of sinus symptoms due to colds, flu, allergy and hay fever. Contains a nonaspirin analgesic to relieve headache pain, a decongestant to ease pressure and congestion and an antihistamine to dry up runny nose, watery eyes.

Actions: Sinutab® Maximum Strength Formula Tablets and Caplets contain an analgesic (acetaminophen) to relieve pain, a decongestant (pseudoephedrine hydrochloride) to reduce congestion of the nasopharyngeal mucosa, and an antihistamine (chlorpheniramine maleate) to help control allergic symptoms.

Acetaminophen is both analgesic and antipyretic. Because acetaminophen is not a salicylate, Sinutab® Maximum

Continued on next page

This product information was prepared in November 1990. On these and other Parke-Davis Products, detailed information may be obtained by addressing PARKE-DAVIS, Consumer Health Products Group, Division of Warner-Lambert Company, Morris Plains, NJ 07950.

Parke-Davis—Cont.

Strength Formula Tablets and Caplets can be used by patients who are allergic to aspirin.
Pseudoephedrine hydrochloride, a sympathomimetic drug, provides vasoconstriction of the nasopharyngeal mucosa resulting in a nasal decongestant effect.
Chlorpheniramine maleate is an antihistamine incorporated to provide relief of running nose, sneezing, itching of the nose or throat, and itchy and watery eyes as may occur in allergic rhinitis.

Warnings: Do not exceed recommended dosage. If symptoms persist, do not improve within 7 days, or are accompanied by high fever, or if new symptoms occur, see your doctor before continuing use. Do not take this product if you have high blood pressure, heart disease, diabetes, thyroid disease, asthma, glaucoma, or difficulty in urination due to an enlarged prostate except under doctor's supervision. Do not take this product for more than 10 days. As with any drug, if you are pregnant or nursing a baby, seek the advice of a health professional before using this product. This product may cause drowsiness. Avoid driving a motor vehicle or operating heavy machinery and avoid alcoholic beverages while taking this product.

Drug Interaction: Do not take this product if you are presently taking a prescription drug for high blood pressure or depression without first consulting your doctor.

Precaution: Keep this and all drugs out of the reach of children.

Symptoms and Treatment of Oral Overdosage: In case of accidental overdose, seek professional help or contact a Poison Control Center immediately.

Dosage and Administration: Adults 2 tablets or caplets every 6 hours, not to exceed 8 tablets or caplets in 24 hours, or as directed by physician. Children under 12 should use only as directed by physician.

How Supplied: Sinutab® Maximum Strength Formula Caplets are yellow and coated. The Tablets are yellow and uncoated. They are supplied in child-resistant blister packs in boxes of 24 tablets or caplets.

Shown in Product Identification Section, page 421

SINUTAB® Maximum Strength Without Drowsiness Formula Tablets and Caplets

Active Ingredients: Each tablet/caplet contains: Acetaminophen 500 mg., pseudoephedrine hydrochloride 30 mg.

Inactive Ingredients:
Tablets contain: Carboxymethyl starch, cellulose, corn starch, croscarmellose sodium, hydroxypropyl cellulose, stearic acid, zinc stearate, D&C yellow No. 10 aluminum lake and FD&C yellow No. 6 aluminum lake.
Caplets contain: Cellulose, corn starch, croscarmellose sodium, hydroxypropyl cellulose, hydroxypropyl methylcellulose, magnesium stearate, polyethylene glycol, sodium starch glycolate, stearic acid, titanium dioxide, zinc stearate, D&C yellow No. 10 aluminum lake and FD&C yellow No. 6 aluminum lake.

Indications: For temporary relief of sinus symptoms due to colds, flu, allergy and hay fever. Contains a nonaspirin analgesic to relieve headache pain and a decongestant to ease pressure and congestion.

Actions: Sinutab® Maximum Strength Without Drowsiness Formula Tablets and Caplets contain an analgesic (acetaminophen) to relieve pain, and a decongestant (pseudoephedrine hydrochloride) to reduce congestion of the nasopharyngeal mucosa.
Acetaminophen is both analgesic and antipyretic. Because acetaminophen is not a salicylate, Sinutab® Maximum Strength Without Drowsiness Formula can be used by patients who are allergic to aspirin.
Pseudoephedrine hydrochloride, a sympathomimetic drug, provides vasoconstriction of the nasopharyngeal mucosa resulting in a nasal decongestant effect.
The absence of antihistamine in the formula provides the added benefit of reduced likelihood of drowsiness side effects.

Warnings: Do not exceed recommended dosage. If symptoms persist, do not improve within seven days, or are accompanied by high fever, or if new symptoms occur, see your doctor before continuing use. Do not take this product if you have high blood pressure, heart disease, diabetes, thyroid disease, or difficulty in urination due to an enlarged prostate except under doctor's supervision. Do not take this product for more than 10 days. As with any drug, if you are pregnant or nursing a baby, seek the advice of a health professional before using this product.

Drug Interaction: Do not take this product if you are presently taking a prescription drug for high blood pressure or depression without first consulting your doctor.

Precaution: Keep this and all drugs out of the reach of children.

Symptoms and Treatment of Oral Overdosage: In case of accidental overdose, seek professional help or contact a Poison Control Center immediately.

Dosage and Administration: Adults 2 tablets every 6 hours, not to exceed 8 tablets in 24 hours or as directed by physician. Children under 12 should use only as directed by physician.

How Supplied: Sinutab® Maximum Strength Without Drowsiness Formula Caplets are orange and coated. The Tablets are orange and uncoated. They are supplied in child-resistant blister packs in boxes of 24 tablets or caplets and in bottles of 50 tablets with child-resistant caps.

Shown in Product Identification Section, page 422

THERA-COMBEX H-P®
High-Potency Vitamin B Complex with 500 mg Vitamin C

Composition: Each Kapseal contains:

Ascorbic acid (vitamin C)	500 mg
Thiamine (vitamin B_1) mononitrate	25 mg
Riboflavin (vitamin B_2)	15 mg
Pyridoxine hydrochloride (vitamin B_6)	10 mg
Vitamin B_{12} (cyanocobalamin)	5 mcg
Niacinamide	100 mg
dl-Panthenol	20 mg

Uses: For the prevention or treatment of vitamin B complex and vitamin C deficiencies.

Dosage: One or two capsules daily

How Supplied: Bottles of 100.

TUCKS®
Pre-moistened Hemorrhoidal/Vaginal Pads

Indications: For prompt, temporary relief of minor external itching, burning and irritation associated with hemorrhoids, rectal or vaginal surgical stitches and other minor rectal or vaginal irritation.
—Soothe, cool, and comfort itching, burning, and irritation of sensitive rectal and outer vaginal areas.
—As a compress, to help relieve discomfort from rectal/vaginal surgical stitches.
—Effective hygienic wipe to cleanse rectal area of irritation-causing residue.
—Solution buffered to help prevent further irritation.

Directions: For external use only. Use as a wipe following bowel movement, during menstruation, or after napkin or tampon change. Or, as a compress, apply to affected area 10 to 15 minutes as needed.

Warnings: In case of rectal bleeding, consult physician promptly. In case of continued irritation, discontinue use and consult a physician. Keep this and all medication out of the reach of children. In case of accidental ingestion seek professional assistance or contact a Poison Control Center immediately.

Contains: Soft pads pre-moistened with a solution containing 50% Witch Hazel; 10% Glycerin USP; also contains: Benzalkonium Chloride NF 0.003%, Citric acid, USP ; Methylparaben NF 0.1%; sodium citrate, USP; water, purified USP. Buffered to acid pH.

How Supplied: Jars of 40 and 100. Also available as Tucks Take-Alongs®, individual, foil-wrapped, nonwoven wipes, 12 per box.

Shown in Product Identification Section, page 422

TUCKS® CREAM

Composition: Tucks Cream contains a specially formulated aqueous phase of 50% Witch Hazel (hamamelis water). Tucks Cream also contains: alcohol 7%; arlacel; benzethonium chloride; cetyl alcohol; lanolin anhydrous; polyethylene stearate; polysorbate; sorbitol solution; and white petrolatum.

Action and Uses: Nonstaining Tucks Cream exerts a temporary soothing, cooling, mildly astringent effect on such superficial irritations as simple hemorrhoids, vaginal and rectal area itch, postepisiotomy discomfort and anorectal surgical wounds. The Cream does not contain steroids.

Warning: If itching or irritation continues, discontinue use and consult your physician. In case of rectal bleeding, consult physician promptly. Keep this and all drugs out of the reach of children. In case of accidental ingestion seek professional assistance or contact a Poison Contol Center immediately.

Directions: Apply locally 3 or 4 times daily to temporarily soothe anal or outer vaginal irritation and itching, hemorrhoids, postepisiotomy and posthemorrhoidectomy discomfort.

How Supplied: Tucks Cream (water-washable) in 40-g tube with rectal applicator.

ZIRADRYL® Lotion

[*zĭ'ră-drĭl*]

Description: A zinc oxide-antihistaminic lotion of 1% Benadryl® (diphenhydramine hydrochloride) and 2% zinc oxide; contains 2% alcohol. Also contains: camphor; chlorophylline sodium polysorbate; fragrances; glycerin; methocel; and water, purified.

Indications: For relief of itching due to mild poison ivy, poison oak or insect bites.

Directions: SHAKE WELL. For adults and children 6 years of age and older: Apply to the affected area not more than three to four times daily or as directed by your physician. Before each application, cleanse skin with soap and water and dry affected area. Temporary stinging sensation may follow application. Discontinue use if stinging persists. Removes easily with water. Children under 6 years of age: consult a physician.

Warnings: For external use only. Do not apply to blistered, raw or oozing areas of the skin. Do not use on chicken pox or measles unless supervised by a physician. Do not use on extensive areas of the skin or for longer than 7 days except as directed by a physician. Avoid contact with the eyes or other mucous membranes. If condition worsens or if symptoms persist for more than 7 days or clear up and occur again within a few days or if burning sensation or rash develops discontinue use of this product and consult a physician. KEEP THIS AND ALL DRUGS OUT OF REACH OF CHILDREN. In case of accidental ingestion, seek professional assistance or contact a Poison Control Center immediately.

How Supplied: 6-oz bottles. Protect from freezing.

Shown in Product Identification Section, page 422

Pfizer Consumer Health Care Division

Division of Pfizer Inc.
140 JEFFERSON ROAD
PARSIPPANY, NJ 07054

BEN-GAY® External Analgesic Products

Description: Ben-Gay is a combination of methyl salicylate and menthol in a suitable base for topical application. In addition to the Original Ointment (methyl salicylate, 18.3%; menthol, 16%), Ben-Gay is offered as a Greaseless/Stainless Ointment (methyl salicylate, 15%; menthol, 10%), an Extra Strength Arthritis Rub (methyl salicylate, 30%; menthol, 8%), a Lotion and a Clear Gel (both of which contain methyl salicylate, 15%; menthol, 7%) and Ben-Gay Warming Ice (2.5% menthol in an alcohol base gel). Ben-Gay Sports-Gel (3.0% menthol in an alcohol base gel) and Extra Strength Ben-Gay Sports-Balm (methyl salicylate 28%; menthol 10%) are available for use before and after exercise.

Action and Uses: Methyl salicylate and menthol are external analgesics which stimulate sensory receptors of warmth and cold. This produces a counter-irritant response which provides temporary relief of minor aches and pains of muscles and joints associated with simple backache, arthritis, strains, bruises and sprains.

Several double-blind clinical studies of Ben-Gay products have shown the effectiveness of the menthol-methyl salicylate combination in counteracting minor pain of skeletal muscle stress and arthritis.

Three studies involving a total of 102 normal subjects in which muscle soreness was experimentally induced showed statistically significant beneficial results from use of the active product vs. placebo for lowered Muscle Action Potential (spasms), greater rise in threshold of muscular pain and greater reduction in perceived muscular pain.

Six clinical studies of a total of 207 subjects suffering from minor pain and skeletal muscular spasms due to osteoarthritis and rheumatoid arthritis showed the active product to give statistically significant beneficial results vs. placebo for lowered Muscle Action Potential (spasm), greater relief of perceived pain, increased range of motion of the affected joints and increased digital dexterity.

In two studies designed to measure the effect of topically applied Ben-Gay vs. Placebo on muscular endurance, discomfort, onset of exercise pain and fatigue, and cardiovascular efficiency, 30 subjects performed a submaximal three-hour run and another 30 subjects performed a maximal treadmill run. Ben-Gay was found to significantly decrease the discomfort during the submaximal and maximal run, and increase the time before onset of fatigue during the maximal run. It did not improve cardiovascular function or affect recovery. Applied before workouts, Ben-Gay exercise rubs relax tight muscles and increase circulation to make exercising more comfortable, longer.

To help reduce muscle ache and soreness after exercise, a Ben-Gay exercise rub can be applied and allowed to work before taking a shower.

Directions: Rub generously into painful area, then massage gently until Ben-Gay disappears. Repeat as necessary.

Warning: Use only as directed. Do not use with a heating pad. Keep away from children to avoid accidental poisoning. Do not swallow. In case of accidental ingestion, seek professional assistance or contact a Poison Control Center immediately. Keep away from eyes, mucous membrane, broken or irritated skin. If skin irritation develops, pain lasts 10 days or more, redness is present, or with arthritis-like conditions in children under 12, call a physician.

BONINE®
(meclizine hydrochloride)
Chewable Tablets

Action: BONINE (meclizine) is an H_1 histamine receptor blocker of the piperazine side chain group. It exhibits its action by an effect on the Central Nervous System (CNS), possibly by its ability to block muscarinic receptors in the brain.

Indications: BONINE is effective in the management of nausea, vomiting and dizziness associated with motion sickness.

Contraindications: Asthma, glaucoma, emphysema, chronic pulmonary disease, shortness of breath, difficulty in breathing, or difficulty in urination due to enlargement of the prostate gland unless directed by a doctor.

Warnings: May cause drowsiness; alcohol, sedatives and tranquilizers may increase the drowsiness effect. Avoid alcoholic beverages while taking this product. Do not take this product if you are taking sedatives or tranquilizers without first consulting your doctor. Do not drive or operate dangerous machinery while taking this medication.

Usage in Children: Clinical studies establishing safety and effectiveness in children have not been done; therefore,

Continued on next page

Pfizer Consumer—Cont.

usage is not recommended in children under 12 years of age.
Usage in Pregnancy: As with any drug, if you are pregnant or nursing a baby, seek advice of a health care professional before taking this product.

Adverse Reactions: Drowsiness, dry mouth, and on rare occasions, blurred vision have been reported.

Dosage and Administration: For motion sickness, take one or two tablets of Bonine once daily, one hour before travel starts, for up to 24 hours of protection against motion sickness. The tablet can be chewed with or without water or swallowed whole with water. Thereafter, the dose may be repeated every 24 hours for the duration of the travel.

How Supplied: BONINE (meclizine HCl) is available in convenient packets of 8 chewable tablets of 25 mg. meclizine HCl.

Inactive Ingredients: Cornstarch, FD&C Red #40, Lactose, Magnesium Stearate, Purified Siliceous Earth, Raspberry Flavor, Sodium Saccharin, Talc.

DESITIN® OINTMENT

Description: Desitin Ointment combines Zinc Oxide (40%) with Cod Liver Oil (high in Vitamins A & D), and Talc in a petrolatum-lanolin base suitable for topical application.

Actions and Uses: Desitin Ointment is designed to provide relief of diaper rash, superficial wounds and burns, and other minor skin irritations. It helps prevent incidence of diaper rash, protects against urine and other irritants, soothes chafed skin and promotes healing.
Relief and protection is afforded by Zinc Oxide, Cod Liver Oil, Lanolin and Petrolatum. They provide a physical barrier by forming a protective coating over skin or mucous membrane which serves to reduce further effects of irritants on the affected area and relieves burning, pain or itch produced by them. In addition to its protective properties, Zinc Oxide acts as an astringent that helps heal local irritation and inflammation by lessening the flow of mucus and other secretions.
Several studies have shown the effectiveness of Desitin Ointment in the relief and prevention of diaper rash.
Two clinical studies involving 90 infants demonstrated the effectiveness of Desitin Ointment in curing diaper rash. The diaper rash area was treated with Desitin Ointment at each diaper change for a period of 24 hours, while the untreated site served as controls. A significant reduction was noted in the severity and area of diaper dermatitis on the treated area.
Ninety-seven (97) babies participated in a 12-week study to show that Desitin Ointment helps prevent diaper rash. Approximately half of the infants (49) were treated with Desitin Ointment on a regular daily basis. The other half (48) received the ointment as necessary to treat any diaper rash which occurred. The incidence as well as the severity of diaper rash was significantly less among the babies using the ointment on a regular daily basis.
In a comparative study of the efficacy of Desitin Ointment vs. a baby powder, forty-five babies were observed for a total of eight weeks. Results support the conclusion that Desitin Ointment is a better prophylactic against diaper rash than the baby powder.
In another study, Desitin was found to be dramatically more effective in reducing the severity of medically diagnosed diaper rash than a commercially available diaper rash product in which only anhydrous lanolin and petrolatum are listed as ingredients. Fifty infants participated in the study, half of whom were treated with Desitin and half with the other product. In the group (25) treated with Desitin, seventeen infants showed significant improvement within 10 hours which increased to twenty-three improved infants within 24 hours. Of the group (25) treated with the other product, only three showed improvement at ten hours with a total of four improved within twenty-four hours. These results are statistically valid to conclude that Desitin Ointment reduces severity of diaper rash within ten hours.
Several other studies show that Desitin Ointment helps relieve other skin disorders, such as contact dermatitis.

Directions: Prevention: To prevent diaper rash, apply Desitin Ointment to the diaper area—especially at bedtime when exposure to wet diapers may be prolonged.
Treatment: If diaper rash is present, or at the first sign of redness, minor skin irritation or chafing, simply apply Desitin Ointment three or four times daily as needed. In superficial noninfected surface wounds and minor burns, apply a thin layer of Desitin Ointment, using a gauze dressing, if necessary. For external use only.

How Supplied: Desitin Ointment is available in 1 ounce (28g), 2 ounce (57g), 4 ounce (114g), 8 ounce (227g) tubes, and 9 ounce (255g), 1 lb. (454g) jar.

Shown in Product Identification Section, page 422

RHEABAN® Maximum Strength TABLETS
[*rē'ăban*]
(attapulgite)

Description: Maximum Strength Rheaban is an anti-diarrheal medication containing activated attapulgite and is offered in tablet form.
Each white Rheaban tablet contains 750 mg. of colloidal activated attapulgite. Rheaban provides the maximum level of medication when taken as directed.
Rheaban contains no narcotics, opiates or other habit-forming drugs.

Actions and Uses: Rheaban is indicated for relief of diarrhea and the cramps and pains associated with it. Attapulgite, which has been activated by thermal treatment, is a highly sorptive substance which absorbs nutrients and digestive enzymes as well as noxious gases, irritants, toxins and some bacteria and viruses that are common causes of diarrhea.
In clinical studies to show the effectiveness in relieving diarrhea and its symptoms, 100 subjects suffering from acute gastroenteritis with diarrhea participated in a double-blind comparison of Rheaban to a placebo. Patients treated with the attapulgite product showed significantly improved relief of diarrhea and its symptoms vs. the placebo.

Dosage and Administration:
TABLETS
Adults—2 tablets after initial bowel movement, 2 tablets after each subsequent bowel movement. For a maximum of 12 tablets in 24 hours.
Children 6 to 12 years—1 tablet after initial bowel movement, 1 tablet after each subsequent bowel movement. For a maximum of 6 tablets in 24 hours, or as directed by a physician.

Warnings: Do not exceed 12 tablets in 24 hours. Swallow tablets with water, do not chew. Do not use for more than two days, or in the presence of high fever. Tablets should not be used for infants or children under 6 years of age unless directed by physician. If diarrhea persists consult a physician.

How Supplied:
Tablets—Boxes of 12 tablets.

Inactive Ingredients: Colloidal Silicon Dioxide, Croscarmellose Sodium, Ethylcellulose, Hydroxypropyl Methylcellulose 2910, Pectin, Pharmaceutical Glaze, Sucrose, Talc, Titanium Dioxide, Zinc Stearate.

RID® Spray
Lice Control Spray

THIS PRODUCT IS NOT FOR USE ON HUMANS OR ANIMALS

Active Ingredient:

*Permethrin	0.50%
INERT INGREDIENTS	99.50%
	100.00%

*(3-phenoxyphenyl) methyl (±) cis,trans 3-(2,2-dichloroethenyl) 2,2-dimethylcyclopropanecarboxylate. Cis, trans ratio: min. 35% (±) cis and max. 65% (±) trans

Actions: A highly active synthetic pyrethroid for the control of lice and louse eggs on garments, bedding, furniture and other inanimate objects.

Warnings: Harmful if swallowed. May be absorbed through skin. Avoid inhalation of spray mist. Avoid contact with skin, eyes or clothing. Wash thoroughly after handling and before smoking or eating. Avoid contamination of feed and foodstuffs. Remove pets and birds and cover fish aquaria before space spraying or surface applications. *This product is not for use on humans or animals.* If lice infestation should occur on humans, use Rid Lice Killing Shampoo. Vacate room after treatment and ventilate before reoccupying. Do not allow children or pets to contact treated areas until surfaces are dry.

Physical and Chemical Hazards: Contents under pressure. Do not use or store near heat or open flame. Do not puncture or incinerate container. Exposure to temperatures above 130° F may cause bursting.
CAUTION: Avoid spraying in eyes. Avoid breathing spray mist. Use only in well ventilated areas. Avoid contact with skin. In case of contact wash immediately with soap and water. Vacate room after treatment and ventilate before reoccupying.
Statement of Practical Treatment: If inhaled: Remove affected person to fresh air. Apply artificial respiration if indicated.
If in eyes: Flush with plenty of water. Contact physician if irritation persists.
If on skin: Wash affected areas immediately with soap and water.

Direction For Use: It is a violation of Federal law to use this product in a manner inconsistent with its labeling.
Shake well before each use. Remove protective cap. Aim spray opening away from person. Push button to spray.
To kill lice and louse eggs: Spray in an inconspicuous area to test for possible staining or discoloration. Inspect again after drying, then proceed to spray entire area to be treated.
Hold container upright with nozzle away from you. Depress valve and spray from a distance of 8 to 10 inches.
Spray each square foot for 3 seconds. Spray only those garments, parts of bedding, including mattresses and furniture that cannot be either laundered or dry cleaned.
Allow all sprayed articles to dry thoroughly before use. Repeat treatment as necessary.
Buyer assumes all risks of use, storage or handling of this material not in strict accordance with direction given herewith.
STORAGE AND DISPOSAL
Store in cool, dry area. Do not store below 32°F.
Wrap container in several layers of newspaper and dispose of in trash. Do not incinerate or puncture.

How Supplied: 5 oz. aerosol can.
Also available in combination with RID® Lice Treatment Kit as the RID® Lice Elimination System.

RID®
Lice Killing Shampoo

Description: Rid contains a liquid pediculicide whose active ingredients are: pyrethrins 0.3% and piperonyl butoxide, technical 3.00%, equivalent to 2.4% (butylcarbityl) (6-propylpiperonyl) ether and to 0.6% related compounds. Also contains petroleum distillate 1.20% and benzyl alcohol 2.4%. Inert ingredients 93.1%.

Actions: RID kills head lice *(Pediculus humanus capitis)*, body lice *(Pediculus humanus humanus)*, and pubic or crab lice *(Phthirus pubis)*, and removes their eggs.
The pyrethrins act as a contact poison and affect the parasite's nervous system, resulting in paralysis and death. The efficacy of the pyrethrins is enhanced by the synergist, piperonyl butoxide. Rid rinses out completely after treatment and is not designed to leave long-acting residues.
The active ingredients in RID are poorly absorbed through the skin. Of the relatively minor amounts that are absorbed, they are rapidly metabolized to water-soluble compounds and eliminated from the body without ill effects.

Indications: RID is indicated for the treatment of infestations of head lice, body lice and pubic (crab) lice, and their eggs.

Warning: RID should be used with caution by ragweed sensitized persons.

Precautions: This product is for external use only. It is harmful if swallowed. If accidentally swallowed, call a physician or Poison Control Center immediately. It should not be inhaled. It should be kept out of the eyes and contact with mucous membranes should be avoided. If accidental contact with eyes occur, flush eyes immediately with plenty of water. Call a physician if irritation persists. In the case of infection or skin irritation, discontinue use and consult a physician. Consult a physician if infestation of eyebrows or eyelashes occurs. Avoid contamination of feed or foodstuffs.

Storage and Disposal: Do not store below 32°F (0°C). Do not reuse empty container. Wrap in several layers of newspaper and discard in trash.

Dosage and Administration: (1) Shake well. Apply undiluted RID to dry hair and scalp or to any other infested area until entirely wet. Do not use on eyelashes or eyebrows. (2) Allow RID to remain on area for 10 minutes but no longer. (3) Wash thoroughly with warm water and soap or shampoo. (4) Dead lice and eggs should be removed with the special nit comb provided. (5) Repeat treatment in 7 to 10 days to kill any newly hatched lice. Do not exceed two consecutive applications within 24 hours.
Since lice infestations are spread by contact, each family member should be examined carefully. If infested, he or she should be treated promptly to avoid spread or reinfestation of previously treated individuals. Contaminated clothing and other articles, such as hats, etc. should be dry cleaned, boiled or otherwise treated until decontaminated to prevent reinfestation or spread.

How Supplied: In 2, 4 and 8 fl. oz. plastic bottles. Exclusive nit removal comb that removes all the nits and patient instruction booklet (English and Spanish) are included in each package of RID.
Also available in combination with RID Lice Control Spray as the RID Lice Elimination System.

UNISOM DUAL RELIEF®
Nighttime Sleep Aid and Pain Reliever

Description: Unisom Dual Relief® is a pale blue, capsule-shaped, coated tablet.

Active ingredients: 650 mg. acetaminophen and 50 mg. diphenhydramine HCl per tablet.

Inactive Ingredients: Corn starch, FD&C Blue #1, FD&C Blue #2, hydroxypropyl methylcellulose, magnesium stearate, polyethylene glycol, polysorbate 80, polyvinylpyrrolidone, stearic acid, titanium dioxide.

Indications: Unisom Dual Relief (diphenhydramine sleep aid formula) is indicated to help reduce difficulty in falling asleep while relieving accompanying minor aches and pains such as headache, muscle ache or menstrual discomfort. If there is difficulty in falling asleep, but pain is not being experienced at the same time, regular Unisom sleep aid is indicated which contains doxylamine succinate as its active ingredient.

Administration and Dosage: One tablet 30 minutes before retiring. Take once daily or as directed by a physician.

Warnings: DO NOT TAKE THIS PRODUCT IF YOU HAVE ASTHMA, GLAUCOMA OR ENLARGEMENT OF THE PROSTATE GLAND EXCEPT UNDER THE ADVICE AND SUPERVISION OF A PHYSICIAN.
Do not take this product for treatment of arthritis except under the advice and supervision of a physician. Do not exceed recommended dosage because severe liver damage may occur. If symptoms persist continuously for more than ten days, consult your physician. Insomnia may be a symptom of serious underlying medical illness. Take this product with caution if alcohol is being consumed. Do not take this product if pregnant or nursing a baby. For adults only. Do not give to children under 12 years of age. Keep this and all medications out of reach of children. IN CASE OF ACCIDENTAL OVERDOSE SEEK PROFESSIONAL ADVICE OR CONTACT A POISON CONTROL CENTER IMMEDIATELY.

Caution: This product contains an antihistamine and will cause drowsiness. It should be used only at bedtime.

Drug Interaction: Monoamine oxidase (MAO) inhibitors prolong and intensify the anticholinergic effects of antihistamines. The CNS depressant effect is heightened by alcohol and other CNS depressant drugs.

Attention: Use only if tablet blister seals are unbroken. Child resistant packaging.

How Supplied: Boxes of 8 and 16 tablets in child resistant blisters.

Continued on next page

Pfizer Consumer—Cont.

UNISOM® NIGHTTIME SLEEP AID
[*yu 'na-som*]
(doxylamine succinate)

Description: Pale blue oval scored tablets containing 25 mg. of doxylamine succinate, 2-[α-(2-dimethylaminoethoxy)α-methylbenzyl] pyridine succinate.

Action and Uses: Doxylamine succinate is an antihistamine of the ethanolamine class, which characteristically shows a high incidence of sedation. In a comparative clinical study of over 20 antihistamines on more than 3000 subjects, doxylamine succinate 25 mg. was one of the three most sedating antihistamines, producing a significantly reduced latency to end of wakefulness and comparing favorably with established hypnotic drugs such as secobarbital and pentobarbital in sedation activity. It was chosen as the antihistamine, based on dosage, causing the earliest onset of sleep. In another clinical study, doxylamine succinate 25 mg. scored better than secobarbital 100 mg. as a nighttime hypnotic. Two additional, identical clinical studies involving a total of 121 subjects demonstrated that doxylamine succinate 25 mg. reduced the sleep latency period by a third, compared to placebo. Duration of sleep was 26.6% longer with doxylamine succinate, and the quality of sleep was rated higher with the drug than with placebo. An EEG study of 6 subjects confirmed the results of these studies. In yet another study, no statistically significant difference was found between doxylamine succinate and flurazepam in the average time required for 200 patients with mild to moderate insomnia to fall asleep over 5 nights following a nightly dose of doxylamine succinate 25 mg. or flurazepam 30 mg., nor was any statistically significant difference found in the total time the 200 patients slept. Patients on doxylamine succinate awoke an average of 1.2 times per night while those on flurazepam awoke an average of 0.9 times per night. In either case the patients awoke rested the following morning. On a rating scale of 1 to 5, doxylamine succinate was given a 3.0, flurazepam a 3.4 by patients rating the degree of restfulness provided by their medication (5 represents "very well rested"). Although statistically significant, the difference between doxylamine succinate 25 mg. and flurazepam 30 mg. in the number of awakenings and degree of restfulness is clinically insignificant.

Administration and Dosage: One tablet 30 minutes before retiring. Not for children under 12 years of age.

Side Effects: Occasional anticholinergic effects may be seen.

Precautions: Unisom® should be taken only at bedtime.

Contraindications: This product should not be taken by pregnant women, or those who are nursing a baby. This product is also contraindicated for asthma, glaucoma, enlargement of the prostate gland.

Warnings: Should be taken with caution if alcohol is being consumed. Product should not be taken if patient is concurrently on any other drug, without prior consultation with physician. Should not be taken for longer than two weeks unless approved by physician.

How Supplied: Boxes of 8, 32 or 48 tablets in child resistant blisters, and in boxes of 16 with non–child resistant packaging.

Inactive Ingredients: Dibasic Calcium Phosphate, FD&C Blue #1 Aluminum Lake, Magnesium Stearate, Microcrystalline Cellulose, Sodium Starch Glycolate.

VISINE®
Tetrahydrozoline Hydrochloride Redness Reliever Eye Drops

Description: Visine is a sterile, isotonic, buffered ophthalmic solution containing tetrahydrozoline hydrochloride 0.05%, boric acid, sodium borate, sodium chloride and water. It is preserved with benzalkonium chloride 0.01% and edetate disodium 0.1%. Visine is a decongestant ophthalmic solution designed to provide symptomatic relief of conjunctival edema and hyperemia secondary to minor irritations, due to conditions such as smoke, dust, other airborne pollutants, swimming etc. and so-called nonspecific or catarrhal conjunctivitis. Relief is afforded by tetrahydrozoline hydrochloride, a sympathomimetic agent, which brings about decongestion by vasoconstriction. Reddened eyes are rapidly whitened by this effective vasoconstrictor, which limits the local vascular response by constricting the small blood vessels. The onset of vasoconstriction becomes apparent within minutes.
The effectiveness of Visine in relieving conjunctival hyperemia has been demonstrated by numerous clinicals, including several double-blind studies, involving more than 2,000 subjects suffering from acute or chronic hyperemia induced by a variety of conditions. Visine was found to be efficacious in providing relief from conjunctival hyperemia.

Indications: Relieves redness of the eye due to minor eye irritations.

Directions: Place 1 to 2 drops in the affected eye(s) up to four times daily.

Warning: To avoid contamination, do not touch tip of container to any surface. Replace cap after using. If you experience eye pain, changes in vision, continued redness or irritation of the eye, or if the condition worsens or persists for more than 72 hours, discontinue use and consult a doctor. If you have glaucoma, do not use this product except under the advice and supervision of a doctor. Overuse of this product may produce increased redness of the eye. If solution changes color or becomes cloudy, do not use. Remove contact lenses before using.

Parents: Before using with children under 6 years of age, consult your physician. Keep this and all other medications out of the reach of children. In case of accidental ingestion, seek professional assistance or contact a poison control center immediately.

How Supplied: In 0.5 fl. oz., 0.75 fl. oz., and 1.0 fl. oz. plastic dispenser bottle and 0.5 fl. oz. plastic bottle with dropper.

Shown in Product Identification Section, page 422

VISINE A.C.®
Astringent/Redness Reliever Eye Drops

Description: Visine A.C. is a sterile, isotonic, buffered ophthalmic solution containing tetrahydrozoline hydrochloride 0.05%, zinc sulfate 0.25%, boric acid, sodium chloride, sodium citrate and purified water. It is preserved with benzalkonium chloride 0.01% and edetate disodium 0.1%. Visine A.C. is an ophthalmic solution combining the effects of the vasoconstrictor tetrahydrozoline hydrochloride with the astringent effects of zinc sulfate. The vasoconstrictor provides symptomatic relief of conjunctival edema and hyperemia secondary to minor irritation due to conditions such as dust and airborne pollutants as well as so-called nonspecific or catarrhal conjunctivitis, while zinc sulfate provides relief from burning and itching, symptoms often associated with hay fever, allergies, etc. Beneficial effects include amelioration of burning, irritation, pruritis, and removal of mucus from the eye. Relief is afforded by both ingredients, tetrahydrozoline hydrochloride and zinc sulfate.
Tetrahydrozoline hydrochloride is a sympathomimetic agent, which brings about decongestion by vasoconstriction. Reddened eyes are rapidly whitened by this effective vasoconstrictor, which limits the local vascular response by constricting the small blood vessels. The onset of vasoconstriction becomes apparent within minutes. Zinc sulfate is an ocular astringent which, by precipitating protein, helps to clear mucus from the outer surface of the eye.
The effectiveness of Visine A.C. in relieving conjunctival hyperemia and associated symptoms induced by allergies has been clinically demonstrated. In one double-blind study allergy sufferers experienced acute episodes of minor eye irritation. Visine A.C. produced statistically significant beneficial results versus a placebo of normal saline solution in relieving irritation of bulbar conjunctiva, irritation of palpebral conjunctiva, and mucous build-up. Treatment with Visine A.C. containing zinc sulfate also significantly improved burning and itching symptoms.

Indications: For temporary relief of discomfort and redness due to minor eye irritations.

Directions: Place 1 to 2 drops in the affected eye(s) up to 4 times daily.

Warning: To avoid contamination, do not touch tip of container to any surface. Replace cap after using. If you experience eye pain, changes in vision, continued redness or irritation of the eye, or if the condition worsens or persists for more than 72 hours, discontinue use and consult a doctor. If you have glaucoma, do not use this product except under the advice and supervision of a doctor. Overuse of this product may produce increased redness of the eye. If solution changes color or becomes cloudy, do not use. Remove contact lenses before using.

Parents: Before using with children under 6 years of age, consult your physician. Keep this and all other medications out of the reach of children. In case of accidental ingestion, seek professional assistance or contact a poison control center immediately.

How Supplied: In 0.5 fl. oz. and 1.0 fl. oz. plastic dispenser bottle.

Shown in Product Identification Section, page 422

VISINE EXTRA®
Redness Reliever/Lubricant Eye Drops

Description: Visine Extra is a sterile, isotonic, buffered ophthalmic solution containing tetrahydrozoline hydrochloride 0.05%, polyethylene glycol 400 1.0%, boric acid, sodium borate, sodium chloride and water. It is preserved with benzalkonium chloride 0.013% and edetate disodium 0.1%.

Visine Extra is an ophthalmic solution combining the effects of the decongestant tetrahydrozoline hydrochloride with the demulcent effects of polyethylene glycol. It provides symptomatic relief of conjunctival edema and hyperemia secondary to ocular allergies, minor irritations and so-called nonspecific or catarrhal conjunctivitis. Tetrahydrozoline hydrochloride is a sympathomimetic agent, which brings about decongestion by vasoconstriction. Reddened eyes are rapidly whitened by this effective vasoconstrictor, which limits the local vascular response by constricting the small blood vessels. The onset of vasoconstriction becomes apparent within minutes. Additional effects include amelioration of burning, irritation, pruritus, soreness, and excessive lacrimation. Relief is afforded by polyethylene glycol.

Polyethylene glycol is an ophthalmic demulcent which has been shown to be effective for the temporary relief of discomfort of minor irritations of the eye due to exposure to wind or sun. It is effective as a protectant and lubricant against further irritation or to relieve dryness of the eye.

The effectiveness of tetrahydrozoline hydrochloride in relieving conjunctival hyperemia and associated symptoms has been demonstrated by numerous clinicals, including several double-blind studies, involving more than 2000 subjects suffering from acute or chronic hyperemia induced by a variety of conditions. Visine Extra is a product that combines the redness relieving effects of a vasoconstrictor and the soothing moisturizing and protective effects of a demulcent.

Indications: Relieves redness of the eye due to minor eye irritations. For use as a protectant against further irritation or to relieve dryness.

Directions: Place 1 to 2 drops in the affected eye(s) up to 4 times daily.

Warning: To avoid contamination, do not touch tip of container to any surface. Replace cap after using. If you experience eye pain, changes in vision, continued redness or irritation of the eye, or if the condition worsens or persists for more than 72 hours, discontinue use and consult a doctor. If you have glaucoma, do not use this product except under the advice and supervision of a doctor. Overuse of this product may produce increased redness of the eye. If solution changes color or becomes cloudy, do not use. Remove contact lenses before using.

Parents: Before using with children under 6 years of age, consult your physician. Keep this and all other medications out of the reach of children. In case of accidental ingestion, seek professional assistance or contact a poison control center immediately.

How Supplied: In 0.5 fl. oz. and 1.0 fl. oz. plastic dispenser bottle.

Shown in Product Identification Section, page 422

VISINE L. R.™ EYE DROPS
(oxymetazoline hydrochloride)

Description: Visine L. R. is a sterile, isotonic, buffered ophthalmic solution containing oxymetazoline hydrochloride 0.025%, boric acid, sodium borate, sodium chloride and water. It is preserved with benzalkonium chloride 0.01% and edetate disodium 0.1%.

Visine L. R. is produced by a process that assures sterility.

Indications: Visine L. R. is a decongestant ophthalmic solution designed for the relief of redness of the eye due to minor eye irritations. Visine L. R. is specially formulated to relieve redness of the eye in minutes with effective relief that lasts up to 6 hours.

Directions: *Adults and children 6 years of age and older*—Place 1 or 2 drops in the affected eye(s). This may be repeated as needed every 6 hours or as directed by a physician.

Warning: If you experience eye pain, changes in vision, continued redness or irritation of the eye, or if the condition worsens or persists for more than 72 hours, discontinue use and consult a physician. If you have glaucoma, do not use this product except under the advice and supervision of a physician. As with any medication, if you are pregnant seek the advice of a physician before using this product. Overuse of this product may produce increased redness of the eye. If solution changes color or becomes cloudy, do not use. To avoid contamination of this product, do not touch tip of container to any surface. Replace cap after using. Remove contact lenses before using this product.

Parents: Before using with children under 6 years of age, consult your physician. Keep this and all other medications out of the reach of children. In case of accidental ingestion, seek professional assistance or contact a poison control center immediately.

Caution: Should not be used if Visine-imprinted neckband on bottle is broken or missing.

Storage: Store between 2° and 30°C (36° and 86°F).

How Supplied: In 0.5 fl. oz. and 1 fl. oz. plastic dispenser bottle.

Shown in Product Identification Section, page 422

WART-OFF®
Liquid

Active Ingredient: Salicylic Acid, U.S.P., 17%.

Inactive Ingredients: Alcohol, 18.1%, Camphor, Castor Oil, Ether 47.7%, Lactic Acid, Pyroxylin.

Indications: Removal of Warts

Warnings: Keep this and all medications out of reach of children to avoid accidental poisoning.

Flammable—Do not use near fire or flame. For external use only. In case of accidental ingestion, contact a physician or a Poison Control Center immediately. Do not use near eyes or on mucous membranes. Diabetics or other people with impaired circulation should not use Wart-Off®. Do not use on moles, birthmarks or unusual warts with hair growing from them. If wart persists, see your physician. If pain should develop, consult your physician. **Do not apply to surrounding skin.**

Instructions For Use: Read warning and enclosed instructional brochure. Apply Wart-Off® to warts only. Do not apply to surrounding skin. Make sure that surrounding skin is protected from accidental application. Before applying, soak affected area in hot water for several minutes. If any tissue has been loosened, remove by rubbing surface of wart gently with cleaning brush enclosed in Wart-Off® package. Dry thoroughly. Warts are contagious, so don't share your towel. Apply once or twice daily. Using pinpoint applicator attached to cap, apply one drop at a time until entire wart is covered. Lightly cover with small adhesive bandage. Replace cap tightly to avoid evaporation. This treatment may be used daily for three to four weeks if necessary.

How Supplied: 0.5 fluid ounce bottle with special pinpoint plastic applicator, cleaning brush and instructional brochure.

Procter & Gamble
P. O. BOX 5516
CINCINNATI, OH 45201

DENQUEL® Sensitive Teeth Toothpaste
Desensitizing Dentifrice

Description: Each tube contains potassium nitrate (5%) in a low-abrasion, pleasant mint-flavored dentifrice.
Dentinal hypersensitivity is a condition in which pain or discomfort arises when various stimuli, such as hot, cold, sweet, sour or touch contact exposed dentin. Exposure of dentin often occurs as a result of either gingival recession or periodontal surgery.
Daily use of Denquel can provide, within the first 2 weeks of regular brushing, a significant decrease in hypersensitivity. See a dentist if tooth sensitivity is not reduced after 4 weeks of regular use, as this may indicate a dental condition other than hypersensitivity. The Council on Dental Therapeutics of the American Dental Association has given Denquel the ADA Seal of Acceptance as an effective desensitizing dentifrice for teeth sensitive to hot, cold or pressure (tactile) in otherwise normal teeth.

Dosage: Use twice a day or as directed by a dentist.

How Supplied: Denquel Sensitive Teeth Toothpaste is supplied in tubes containing 1.6, 3.0, or 4.5 ounces.

HEAD & SHOULDERS®
Antidandruff Shampoo

Head & Shoulders Shampoo offers effective dandruff control and beautiful hair in a formula that is pleasant to use. Independently conducted clinical testing (double-blind and dermatologist-graded) has proved that Head & Shoulders reduces dandruff flaking. Head & Shoulders is also gentle enough to use every day for clean, manageable hair.

Active Ingredient: 1.0% pyrithione zinc suspended in an anionic detergent system. Cosmetic ingredients are also included.

Indications: For effective control of typical dandruff and seborrheic dermatitis of the scalp.

Actions: Pyrithione zinc is substantive to the scalp and remains after rinsing. Its mechanism of action has not been fully established, but it is believed to control the microorganisms associated with dandruff flaking and itching.

Precautions: Not to be taken internally. Keep out of children's reach. Avoid getting shampoo in eyes—if this happens, rinse eyes with water.

Dosage and Administration: For best results in controlling dandruff, Head & Shoulders should be used regularly. It is gentle enough to use for every shampoo. In treating seborrheic dermatitis, a minimum of four shampooings are needed to achieve full effectiveness.

Composition:
Lotion—Normal to Oily Formula: Pyrithione zinc in a shampoo base of water, ammonium laureth sulfate, ammonium lauryl sulfate, cocamide MEA, glycol distearate, ammonium xylenesulfonate, fragrance, citric acid, methylchloroisothiazolinone, methylisothiazolinone, and FD&C Blue No. 1.
Lotion—Normal to Dry Formula: Pyrithione zinc in a shampoo base of water, ammonium laureth sulfate, ammonium lauryl sulfate, cocamide MEA, glycol distearate, ammonium xylenesulfonate, propylene glycol, fragrance, citric acid, methylchloroisothiazolinone, methylisothiazolinone, and FD&C Blue No. 1.
Cream—Normal to Oily Formula: Pyrithione zinc in a shampoo base of water, sodium cocoglyceryl ether sulfonate, sodium chloride, sodium lauroyl sarcosinate, cocamide DEA, cocoyl sarcosine, fragrance, and FD&C Blue No. 1.
Cream—Normal to Dry Formula: Pyrithione zinc in a shampoo base of water, sodium cocoglyceryl ether sulfonate, sodium chloride, sodium lauroyl sarcosinate, cocamide DEA, propylene glycol, cocoyl sarcosine, fragrance, and FD&C Blue No. 1.

How Supplied: Lotion available in 4.0, 7.0, 11.0, and 15.0 fl. oz. unbreakable plastic bottles. Concentrate cream available in 5.5 oz. tube. Both lotion and concentrate are available in formulas for "Normal to Oily" and "Normal to Dry" hair.

Shown in Product Identification Section, page 422

HEAD & SHOULDERS® DRY SCALP SHAMPOO

Head & Shoulders Dry Scalp Shampoo offers effective control of irritating itching and flaking due to dry scalp. Dry Scalp Shampoo is gentle enough to use every day for clean, manageable hair.

Active Ingredient: 1.0% pyrithione zinc suspended in a mild surfactant base. Shampoo also includes mild conditioning agents.

Indications: For effective control of dry scalp and dry scalp symptoms.

Actions: Mild surfactants' gentle action reduces insult to the scalp, allowing the scalp to maintain its natural moisture balance. Pyrithione zinc is substantive to the scalp, and remains after rinsing.

Precautions: Not to be taken internally. Keep out of children's reach. Avoid getting shampoo in eyes—if this happens, rinse eyes with water.

Dosage and Administration: For best results in controlling dry scalp and dry scalp symptoms, Head & Shoulders Dry Scalp Shampoo should be used regularly. It is gentle enough to use for every shampoo.

Composition:
Lotion-Dry Scalp Regular Formula: Pyrithione zinc in a shampoo base of water, ammonium laureth sulfate, ammonium lauryl sulfate, cocamide MEA, glycol distearate, dimethicone, ammonium xylenesulfonate, fragrance, tricetylmonium chloride, cetyl alcohol, stearyl alcohol, DMDM hydantoin, sodium chloride, FD&C blue no. 1.
Lotion-Dry Scalp Conditioning Formula: Pyrithione zinc in a shampoo base of water, ammonium laureth sulfate, ammonium lauryl sulfate, cocamide MEA, glycol distearate, dimethicone, ammonium xylenesulfonate, fragrance, tricetylmonium chloride, cetyl alcohol, DMDM hydantoin, sodium chloride FD&C blue no. 1.

How Supplied: Lotion is available in 7.0, 11.0, and 15.0 fl. oz. unbreakable plastic bottles. All sizes are available in two formulas: Regular and Conditioning.

Shown in Product Identification Section, page 422

HEAD & SHOULDERS® INTENSIVE TREATMENT DANDRUFF SHAMPOO

Head & Shoulders Intensive Treatment Dandruff Shampoo offers effective control of persistent dandruff, and beautiful hair from a pleasant-to-use formula. Double-blind and expert-graded testing have proven that Intensive Treatment Dandruff Shampoo reduces persistent dandruff. It is also gentle enough to use every day for clean, manageable hair.

Active Ingredient: 1% selenium sulfide suspended in a mild surfactant base. Shampoo also includes mild conditioning agents.

Indications: For effective control of seborrheic dermatitis and persistent dandruff of the scalp.

Actions: Selenium sulfide is substantive to the scalp and remains after rinsing. Its mechanism is believed to be an antihyperproliferative, and to also control the microorganisms associated with persistent dandruff flaking and itching.

Warnings: For external use only. Avoid contact with eyes—if this happens, rinse thoroughly with water. If condition worsens, or does not improve, consult a doctor. Keep out of reach of children.

Caution: If used on bleached, tinted, or permanent waved hair, rinse for 5 minutes.

Dosage and Administration: For best results in controlling persistent dandruff, Head & Shoulders Intensive Treatment Dandruff Shampoo should be used regularly. It is gentle enough to use for every shampoo.

Composition:
Lotion—Intensive Treatment Regular Formula: Ingredients: Selenium sulfide in a shampoo base of water, ammonium laureth sulfate, ammonium lauryl sulfate, cocamide MEA, glycol distearate, ammonium xylenesulfonate, dimethicone, fragrance, tricetylmonium chloride, cetyl alcohol, DMDM hydantoin, sodium chloride, stearyl alcohol, hydroxypropyl methylcellulose, FD&C Red no. 4.

Lotion—Intensive Treatment Conditioning Formula: Ingredients: Selenium sulfide in a shampoo base of water ammonium laureth sulfate, ammonium lauryl sulfate, cocamide MEA, glycol distearate, ammonium xylenesulfonate, dimethicone, fragrance, tricetylmonium chloride, cetyl alcohol, DMDM hydantoin, sodium chloride, stearyl alcohol, hydroxypropyl methylcellulose, FD&C Red no. 4.

How Supplied: Lotion is available in 4.0, 7.0, and 11.0 fl. oz. unbreakable plastic bottles. All sizes are available in two formulas: Regular and Conditioning.

Shown in Product Identification Section, page 422

PEPTO-BISMOL® ORIGINAL LIQUID AND ORIGINAL AND CHERRY TABLETS

For diarrhea, heartburn, indigestion, upset stomach and nausea.

Description: Each Pepto-Bismol Tablet contains 262 mg bismuth subsalicylate and each tablespoonful (15 ml) of Pepto-Bismol Liquid contains 262 mg bismuth subsalicylate. Each tablet contains 102 mg salicylate (99 mg salicylate for Cherry) and each tablespoonful of liquid contains 130 mg salicylate. Liquid and tablets contain no sugar. Tablets are sodium-free (less than 2 mg/tablet) and Liquid is low in sodium (5 mg/tablespoonful). Inactive ingredients include (Tablets): adipic acid (in Cherry only), calcium carbonate, D&C Red No. 27, D&C Red No. 40 (in Cherry only), flavors, magnesium stearate, mannitol, povidone, saccharin sodium and talc; (Liquid): benzoic acid, D&C Red No. 22, D&C Red No. 28, flavor, magnesium aluminum silicate, methylcellulose, saccharin sodium, salicylic acid, sodium salicylate, sorbic acid and water.

Indications: Pepto-Bismol controls diarrhea within 24 hours, relieving associated abdominal cramps; soothes heartburn and indigestion without constipating; and relieves nausea and upset stomach.

Caution: This product contains salicylates. If taken with aspirin and ringing of the ears occurs, discontinue use. This product does not contain aspirin, but should not be administered to those patients who have a known allergy to aspirin or salicylates. Caution is advised in the administration to patients taking medication for anticoagulation, diabetes and gout.

Warning: Children and teenagers who have or are recovering from chicken pox or flu should NOT use this medicine to treat vomiting. If vomiting is present, consult a doctor because this could be an early sign of Reye's Syndrome, a rare but serious illness. As with any drug, caution is advised in the administration to pregnant or nursing women.

Note: This medication may cause a temporary and harmless darkening of the tongue and/or stool. Stool darkening should not be confused with melena.

Dosage and Administration:

Tablets:

Adults—Two tablets
Children (according to age)—
9–12 yr 1 tablet
6–9 yr ⅔ tablet
3–6 yr ⅓ tablet

Chew or dissolve in mouth. Repeat every ½ to 1 hour as needed, to a maximum of 8 doses in a 24-hour period.

Liquid: Shake well before using.

Adults—2 tablespoonfuls
Children (according to age)—
9–12 yr 1 tablespoonful
6–9 yr 2 teaspoonfuls
3–6 yr 1 teaspoonful

Repeat dosage every ½ to 1 hour, if needed, to a maximum of 8 doses in a 24-hour period.

For children under 3 years, dose according to weight.

18–28 lb 1 teaspoonful
14–18 lb ½ teaspoonful

Repeat every 4 hours, if needed, to a maximum of 6 doses in a 24-hour period.

How Supplied:
Pepto-Bismol Liquid is available in: 4 fl oz bottle, 8 fl oz bottle, 12 fl oz bottle, 16 fl oz bottle

Pepto-Bismol Tablets are pink, round, chewable, tablets imprinted with "Pepto-Bismol" on one side. Tablets are available in: box of 30, box of 42, and roll pack of 12 (cherry only).

Shown in Product Identification Section, page 422

PEPTO-BISMOL® MAXIMUM STRENGTH LIQUID

For diarrhea, heartburn, indigestion, upset stomach and nausea.

Description: Each tablespoonful (15 ml) of Maximum Strength Pepto-Bismol Liquid contains 525 mg bismuth subsalicylate (236 mg salicylate). Maximum Strength Pepto-Bismol Liquid contains no sugar and is low in sodium (less than 5 mg/tablespoonful). Inactive ingredients include: benzoic acid, D&C Red No. 22, D&C Red No. 28, flavor, magnesium aluminum silicate, methylcellulose, saccharin sodium, salicylic acid, sodium salicylate, sorbic acid, and water.

Indications: Maximum Strength Pepto-Bismol controls diarrhea within 24 hours, relieving associated abdominal cramps; soothes heartburn and indigestion without constipating; and relieves nausea and upset stomach.

Caution: This product contains salicylates. If taken with aspirin and ringing of the ears occurs, discontinue use. This product does not contain aspirin, but should not be administered to those patients who have a known allergy to aspirin or salicylates. Caution is advised in the administration to patients taking medication for anticoagulation, diabetes, and gout.

Warning: Children and teenagers who have or are recovering from chicken pox or flu should NOT use this medicine to treat vomiting. If vomiting is present, consult a doctor because this could be an early sign of Reye's Syndrome, a rare but serious illness. As with any drug, caution is advised in the administration to pregnant or nursing women.

Note: This medication may cause a temporary and harmless darkening of the tongue and/or stool. Stool darkening should not be confused with melena.

Dosage and Administration: Shake well before using.

Adults—2 tablespoonfuls
Children (according to age)—
9–12 yr 1 tablespoonful
6–9 yr 2 teaspoonfuls
3–6 yr 1 teaspoonful

Repeat dosage every hour, if needed, to a maximum of 4 doses in a 24-hour period.

How Supplied:
Maximum Strength Pepto-Bismol is available in:

4 fl oz bottle
8 fl oz bottle
12 fl oz bottle

Shown in Product Identification Section, page 422

METAMUCIL®

[met'uh-mū'sil]

(psyllium hydrophilic mucilloid)

Description: Metamucil is a bulk forming natural therapeutic fiber for restoring and maintaining regularity. It contains hydrophilic mucilloid, a highly efficient dietary fiber derived from the husk of the psyllium seed (*Plantago ovata*). Metamucil contains no chemical stimulants and is nonaddictive. Each dose contains approximately 3.4 grams of psyllium hydrophilic mucilloid. Inactive ingredients, sodium, potassium, calories, and carbohydrate content are shown in Table 1 for all forms and flavors. Sugar-free forms contain NutraSweet®* brand sweetener (aspartame). Metamucil is gluten-free.

[See table on next page.]

Actions: Metamucil provides bulk that promotes normal elimination. The product is uniform, instantly miscible, palatable, and nonirritative in the gastrointestinal tract.

Indications: Metamucil is indicated in the management of chronic constipation, in irritable bowel syndrome, as adjunctive therapy in the constipation of diverticular disease, in the bowel management of patients with hemorrhoids, and for constipation during pregnancy, convalescence, and senility.

Contraindications: Intestinal obstruction, fecal impaction.

Warning: Phenylketonurics should be aware that Sugar Free forms of Metamucil contain phenylalanine (see Table 1).

Precaution: May cause allergic reaction in people sensitive to inhaled or ingested psyllium powder. Notice to Health Care

Continued on next page

Procter & Gamble—Cont.

Professionals: To minimize the potential for allergic reaction, health care professionals who frequently dispense powdered psyllium products should avoid inhaling airborne dust while dispensing these products. Handling and Dispensing: To minimize generating airborne dust, spoon product from the canister into a glass according to label directions.

Dosage and Administration: The usual adult dosage is one rounded teaspoonful or tablespoonful, depending on the flavor, stirred into a standard 8-oz glass of cool water, fruit juice, milk or other beverage. See Table 1. With effervescent forms, the contents of a packet are poured into an 8-oz glass and the glass is slowly filled with liquid. Metamucil can be taken orally one to three times a day, depending on the need and response. It may require continued use for 2 to 3 days to provide optimal benefit. An additional glass of liquid after each dose is helpful. For children (6 to 12 years old), use ½ the adult dose in 8-oz of liquid, 1 to 3 times daily.

New Users: Medical research shows that high fiber intake is important for good digestive health. To help the body adjust and avoid the minor gas and bloat-

Table 1 — METAMUCIL

Forms/ Flavors	Inactive Ingredients	Sodium* mg/dose	Potassium mg/dose	Calories per dose	Carbohydrate content g/dose	Phenylalanine mg/dose	Dosage 1–3 times daily. Each dose contains 3.4 g of psyllium hydrophilic Mucilloid	How Supplied
Regular Flavor METAMUCIL Powder	Dextrose	<10	31	14	3.5	—	1 rounded teaspoonful 7 g	Canisters: 7, 14, 21, and 32 ozs. (OTC); Cartons: 30 single-dose packets (OTC), 100 single-dose packets (Institutional)
Sugar-Free Regular Flavor METAMUCIL Powder	Aspartame, Maltodextrin	<10	31	1	0.3	6	1 rounded teaspoonful 3.7 g	Canisters: 3.7, 7.4, 11.1, and 16.9 ozs. (OTC); Cartons: 100 single-dose packets (Institutional)
Sugar-Free Orange Flavor METAMUCIL Powder	Aspartame, Citric acid, FD&C Yellow No. 6, Flavoring, Maltodextrin, Silicon dioxide	<10	31	5	1.4	30	1 rounded teaspoonful 5.2 g	Canisters: 4.7, 8.7, 12.9, and 20.7 ozs. (OTC)
Orange Flavor METAMUCIL Powder	Citric acid, FD&C Yellow No. 6, Flavoring, Sucrose (a carbohydrate)	<10	31	30	7.1	—	1 rounded tablespoonful 11 g	Canisters: 7, 14, 21 and 32 ozs. (OTC); Cartons: 30 single-dose packets (OTC)
Strawberry Flavor METAMUCIL Powder	Citric acid FD&C Red No. 40, Flavoring, Sucrose	<10	31	30	7.1	—	1 rounded tablespoonful 11 g	Canisters: 7, 14, and 21 ozs. (OTC)
Sugar-Free Lemon-Lime Flavor METAMUCIL Effervescent Powder	Aspartame, Calcium carbonate, Citric acid, Flavoring, Potassium bicarbonate, Silicon dioxide, Sodium bicarbonate	<10	290	1	—	30	1 packet 0.19 oz.	Cartons: 30 single-dose packets (OTC): 100 single-dose packets (Institutional)
Sugar-Free Orange Flavor METAMUCIL Effervescent Powder	Aspartame, Citric acid FD&C Yellow No. 6, Flavoring, Potassium bicarbonate, Silicon dioxide, Sodium bicarbonate	<10	310	1	—	30	1 packet 0.18 oz.	Cartons: 30 single-dose packets (OTC)

*Each dose of Metamucil contains less than 10 mg of sodium.

ing sometimes associated with high fiber intake, it may be necessary to increase fiber intake gradually. Begin taking one dose of Metamucil per day. If minor gas or bloating occurs, reduce the amount for several days. Gradually increase to 3 doses per day if needed.

How Supplied: Canisters (OTC); and cartons of single-dose packets (OTC and Institutional). (See Table 1.)

*NutraSweet® is a registered trademark of the NutraSweet Company.

Shown in Product Identification Section, page 422

EDUCATIONAL MATERIAL

Journal Reprints for Physicians

Reprints of published journal articles illustrating the effectiveness of bismuth subsalicylate (Pepto-Bismol) for the treatment of diarrhea.

Reed & Carnrick
1 NEW ENGLAND AVENUE
PISCATAWAY, NJ 08855-9998

PHAZYME® and PHAZYME®-95
[fay-zime]
Tablets

Description: Contains (simethicone/antigas), an antiflatulent to alleviate or relieve the symptoms of gas.

Actions: Simethicone minimizes gas formation and relieves gas entrapment in both the stomach and the lower G.I. tract. This action helps combat the painful sensation due to gastrointestinal gas. Also, for relief of gas distress associated with other functional or organic conditions such as: diverticulitis, spastic colitis, hyperacidity, postcholecystectomy syndrome and chronic cholecystitis.

Indications: PHAZYME is indicated for the relief of occasional or chronic discomfort caused by gas entrapped in the stomach or in the lower gastrointestinal tract—resulting from aerophagia, dyspepsia and food intolerance.

Contraindications: A known sensitivity to any ingredient.

Warnings: Keep this and all drugs out of the reach of children.

PHAZYME®

Active Ingredient: specially activated simethicone 60 mg.

Inactive Ingredients: acacia, calcium sulfate, carnauba wax, crospovidone, FD&C red No. 7 lake, FD&C blue No. 1 lake, gelatin, lactose, microcrystalline cellulose, polyoxyl-40 stearate, povidone, pregelatinized starch, rice starch, sodium benzoate, sucrose, talc, titanium dioxide, white wax.

Dosage: One or two tablets with each meal and at bedtime as needed except under the advice and supervision of a physician.
Maximum daily dose: 500 mg.

How Supplied: Pink coated tablet in bottles of 100, NDC #0021-1400-01

PHAZYME® 95

Active Ingredient: simethicone 95 mg.

Inactive Ingredients: acacia, calcium sulfate, carnauba wax, crospovidone, FD&C yellow No. 6 lake, FD&C red No. 40 lake, gelatin, lactose, microcrystalline cellulose, polyoxyl-40 stearate, povidone, pregelatinized starch, rice starch, sodium benzoate, sucrose, talc, titanium dioxide, white wax.

Dosage: One tablet with each meal and at bedtime or as needed except under the advice and supervision of a physician.
Maximum daily dose: 500 mg.

How Supplied: Red coated tablet in
10 pack, NDC #0021-0450-10
50's NDC #0021-0450-50
100's, NDC #0021-0450-01

Shown in Product Identification Section, page 422

PHAZYME® DROPS
[fay-zime]

Description:
Active Ingredients: Each 0.6 mL contains 40 mg. simethicone.
Inactive Ingredients: carbomer 934 P, citric acid, methylcellulose, natural orange flavor, polyoxyethylene 8 stearate, potassium citrate, potassium sorbate, sodium saccharin.

Actions: Simethicone minimizes gas formation and relieves gas entrapment in both the stomach and the lower G.I. tract. This action combats the painful sensation due to gastrointestinal gas. Also, for relief of gas distress associated with other functional or organic conditions such as diverticulitis, spastic colitis, hyperacidity, post-cholecystectomy syndrome and chronic cholecystitis.

Indications: PHAZYME® Drops are useful for relief of the painful symptoms of excess gas associated with such conditions as colic or air swallowing.

Contraindications: A known sensitivity to any ingredient.

Warnings: Keep this and all drugs out of the reach of children.

Dosage: Adults and children: 0.6 mL four times daily after meals and at bedtime or as needed. Shake well before using.
Infants (under 2 years): Initally, 0.3 mL four times daily, after meals and at bedtime, except under the advice and supervision of a physician. The dosage can also be mixed with 1 oz. of cool water, infant formula, or other suitable liquids to ease administration.
Dosage should not exceed 12 doses per day.
Maximum Daily Dose: 500 mg

How Supplied: Dropper bottles of 30 mL (1 fl oz).

NDC-0021-4300-17

Shown in Product Identification Section, page 423

Maximum Strength PHAZYME®-125 Capsules

Description: A red softgel containing the highest dose of simethicone available in a single capsule.
Active Ingredients: simethicone 125 mg.
Inactive Ingredients: soybean oil, gelatin, glycerin, vegetable shortening, polysorbate 80, purified water, hydrogenated soybean oil, yellow wax, lecithin, titanium dioxide, FD&C red #40, methylparaben, propylparaben.

Actions: Simethicone minimizes gas formation and relieves gas entrapment in both the stomach and the lower G.I. tract. This action combats the painful sensation due to gastrointestinal gas. Also, for relief of gas distress associated with other functional or organic conditions such as diverticulitis, spastic colitis, hyperacidity, post-cholecystectomy syndrome and chronic cholecystitis.

Indications: PHAZYME-125 is indicated for the relief of acute severe lower intestinal discomfort due to gas—resulting from aerophagia, dyspepsia and food intolerance.

Contraindications: A known sensitivity to any ingredient.

Warnings: Keep this and all drugs out of the reach of children.

Dosage: One capsule with each meal and at bedtime, or as needed except under the advice and supervision of a physician.

How Supplied: Red capsule in bottles of 50, NDC #0021-0450-50 and 10 pack, NDC #0021-0450-02.

Shown in Product Identification Section, page 423

proctoFoam®/non-steroid (pramoxine HCl 1%)

Composition: Active Ingredients: pramoxine hydrochloride 1%.
Inactive Ingredients: butane, cetyl alcohol, emulsifying wax, methylparaben, mineral oil, polysorbate 60, propane, propylparaben, sorbitan sesquioleate, trolamine, water.

Indications: Temporary relief of anorectal itching and pain associated with hemorrhoids.

Warnings: Do not exceed the recommended daily dosage unless directed by a physician. If condition worsens or does not improve within 7 days, consult a physician. In case of bleeding, consult a physician promptly. Do not put this product into the rectum by using fingers or any mechanical device or applicator. Certain persons can develop allergic reactions to ingredients in this product. If the symptom being treated does not subside or if redness, irritation, swelling, pain or

Continued on next page

Reed & Carnrick—Cont.

other symptoms develop or increase, discontinue use and consult a physician.

Caution: Do not insert any part of the aerosol container into the anus. Contents of the container are under pressure, but not flammable. Do not burn or puncture the aerosol container. Store at room temperature, 57°–86°F (15–30°C).
SHAKE WELL BEFORE USE. DO NOT REFRIGERATE.
EXPLOSIVE — AVOID EXCESSIVE HEAT.
The contents of this can are under pressure. Do not puncture or throw into a fire or incinerator. Exposure to high temperatures may cause bursting. Keep out of the reach of children.

Directions: Adults: Cleanse the affected area with mild soap and warm water and rinse thoroughly. Gently dry by patting or blotting with toilet tissue or a soft cloth before application of proctoFoam. Children under 12 years of age: consult a physician.
Shake cannister well before each use. Dispense proctoFoam onto a clean tissue or pad and apply externally to the affected area up to 5 times daily.

How Supplied: Available in 15 g aerosol container.

Shown in Product Identification Section, page 423

R&C® SHAMPOO
Shampoo Pediculicide

Description: R&C SHAMPOO is a one-step pediculicide shampoo available without a prescription.

Active Ingredients:

Pyrethrins	0.30%
Piperonyl Butoxide Technical*	3.00%
Inert Ingredients	96.70%

C-13-14 Isoparaffin, Fragrance, Isocetyl Alcohol, Isopropyl Alcohol, Lauramine Oxide, Laureth-4, Laureth-23, Petroleum Distillate, TEA-Lauryl Sulfate, Water.

TOTAL	100.00%

*Equivalent to 2.40% (butylcarbityl) (6-propylpiperonyl) ether and 0.60% related compounds.

Action: R&C SHAMPOO kills head lice (pediculus capitis), crab lice (phthirus pubis) and body lice (pediculus corporis) and their eggs.

Indications: R&C SHAMPOO is indicated for the treatment of infestations with head lice, crab lice and body lice.

Precaution: For external use only.

Warning: Should not be used by ragweed-sensitized persons.

Caution: Harmful if swallowed. Do not inhale. Avoid contact with eyes and mucous membranes. If case of accidental eye contact, flush immediately with water. In case of infection or skin irritation, discontinue use and consult a physician. Consult a physician if lice infestation of eyebrows and eyelashes occurs. Avoid contamination of feed or foodstuffs.

Storage and Disposal:
Storage: Store below 120°F.
Disposal: Do not reuse container. Rinse thoroughly before discarding in trash.

KEEP OUT OF REACH OF CHILDREN.
CAUTION: FOR EXTERNAL USE ONLY.

Directions for Use: (Package also has Spanish instructions)
Do not use on eyelashes or eyebrows.

1. Begin with DRY hair—do not wet hair prior to using R&C Shampoo.
2. SHAKE WELL. Apply enough R&C Shampoo to saturate the hair, paying particular attention to the infested and adjacent hairy areas.
3. Allow undiluted shampoo to remain on the area for ten minutes.
4. Then add small amounts of water, working the shampoo into the hair and skin until a lather forms. Rinse thoroughly.
5. Treatment should be repeated in 7–10 days if needed. Do not apply R&C Shampoo more than twice within 24 hours.

Conditioning Rinse and Special Comb
To help remove dead lice and eggs apply enclosed conditioning rinse, leaving on the area for one minute. Rinse thoroughly.
Remove dead lice and eggs with the specially designed fine-tooth comb. Illustrated combing instructions are enclosed.
NOTE: TO AVOID REINFESTATION, wash or dry clean all clothing and linens of the infested person at time of treatment. Items that cannot be cleaned in this way, such as bedding, furniture and carpeting, should be treated with R&C Spray Lice Control Insecticide.

How Supplied: In 2 and 4 fl oz. plastic bottles with pourable cap. Fine-tooth comb, a special conditioning rinse to aid in removal of dead lice and nits, and patient booklet are included in each package of R&C SHAMPOO.

Literature Available: For free patient information brochures and filmstrips, please call 1-800-KIL-LICE. A Reed & Carnrick health consultant will be glad to assist you.

Shown in Product Identification Section, page 423

R&C® SPRAY III Lice Control Insecticide

Description: Active ingredients: 3-Phenoxybenzyl d-cis and trans 2,2-dimethyl-3-(2-methylpropenyl)

cyclopropanecarboxylate	0.382%
Other Isomers	0.018%
Petroleum Distillates	4.255%
Inert Ingredients:	95.345%
	100.000%

Actions: R&C SPRAY is specially formulated to kill lice and their nits on inanimate objects.

Indications: R&C SPRAY is recommended for use only on bedding, mattresses, furniture and other objects infested or possibly infested with lice which cannot be laundered or dry cleaned.

Warnings: Contents under pressure. Do not use or store near heat or open flame. Do not puncture or incinerate container. Exposure to temperatures above 130°F may cause bursting. It is a violation of Federal law to use this product in a manner inconsistent with its labeling. NOT FOR USE ON HUMANS OR ANIMALS.

Caution: Avoid spraying in eyes. Avoid breathing spray mist. Avoid contact with the skin. May be absorbed through the skin. In case of contact, wash immediately with soap and water. Harmful if swallowed. Vacate room after treatment and ventilate before reoccupying. Avoid contamination of feed and foodstuffs. Remove pets, birds and cover fish aquariums before spraying.

Directions: SHAKE WELL BEFORE AND OCCASIONALLY DURING USE. Spray on an inconspicuous area to test for possible staining or discoloration. Inspect after drying, then proceed to spray entire area to be treated.
Hold container upright with nozzle away from you. Depress valve and spray from a distance of 8 to 10 inches.
Spray each square foot for about three seconds. For mattresses, furniture, or similar objects (that cannot be laundered or dry cleaned): Spray thoroughly. Do not use article until spray is dry. Repeat treatment as necessary. Do not use in commercial food processing, preparation, storage or serving areas.

Storage and Disposal:
Storage: Store in a cool area away from heat or open flame.
Disposal: Wrap container and put in trash.

How Supplied: In 5 oz. and 10 oz. aerosol container.

Literature Available: For free patient information brochures and filmstrips, please call 1-800-KIL-LICE. A Reed & Carnrick health consultant will be glad to assist you.

Shown in Product Identification Section, page 423

EDUCATIONAL MATERIAL

Brochures
Questions and Answers About Head Lice
Available in English and Spanish to physicians, pharmacists and patients.

Products are indexed by generic and chemical names in the **YELLOW SECTION**

The Reese Chemical Co.
10617 FRANK AVENUE
CLEVELAND, OHIO 44106

COLICON® DROPS

Active Ingredient: Simethicone.

Inactive Ingredients: Citric Acid, Carbomer 934P, Hydroxypropyl Methylcellulose, Sodium Benzoate, Sodium Saccharin, deionized water and flavor.

Indications: For relief of the painful symptoms of excess gas in the digestive tract.
The defoaming action of Colicon relieves flatulence by dispersing and preventing the formation of mucus-surrounded gas pockets in the gastrointestintal tract. Infants: Colicon drops are also useful for relief of the painful symptoms of excess gas associated with such conditions as colic, lactose intolerance or air swallowing.

Warnings: Keep this and all drugs out of the reach of children. In case of accidental overdose consult a physician immediately.

Dosage and Administration: Adults and children 0.6cc four times a day after meals and at bedtime or as directed by a physician. Infants (under two years) 0.3cc four times a day after meals and at bedtime, or as directed by a physician.

How Supplied: 1 Fl. oz. (30cc) plastic dropper enclosed.
NDC 10956-639-01

Shown in Product Identification Section, page 423

REESE'S PINWORM MEDICINE
Pyrantel Pamoate

Active Ingredient: Pyrantel pamoate, 144 mg/cc (the equivalent of 50 mg pyrantel base per cc).

Indications: For the treatment of enterobiasis (pinworm infection) and ascariasis (common roundworm infection).

Warnings: Keep this and all drugs out of the reach of children. In case of accidental overdose, seek professional assistance or contact a poison control center immediately.

Precaution: If you are pregnant or have liver disease, do not take this product unless directed by a doctor.

Dosage and Administration: Adults, children 12 years of age and over, and children 2 years to under 12 years of age —Oral dosage is a single dose of 5 mg of pyrantel pamoate base per pound of body weight, not to exceed 1 gram.
Read package insert before taking this medicine. Do not administer to children under 2 years of age.

How Supplied: Reese's Pinworm Medicine is available in one-ounce bottles as a pleasant-tasting suspension which contains the equivalent of 50 mg pyrantel base per cc. It is supplied with English and Spanish label copy and directions.

Shown in Product Identification Section, page 423

SLEEP-ETTES-D

Active Ingredient: Diphenhydramine HCl USP 50mg.

Indications: For relief of occasional sleeplessness.

Warnings: Do not give to children under 12 years of age. If sleeplessness persists continuously for more than 2 weeks, consult your doctor. Insomnia may be a symptom of serious underlying medical illness. Do not take this product if you have asthma, glaucoma, emphysema, chronic pulmonary disease, shortness of breath, difficulty in breathing, or difficulty in urination due to enlargement of the prostate gland unless directed by a doctor. Avoid alcoholic beverages while taking this product. Do not take this product if you are taking sedatives or tranquilizers, without first consulting your doctor. As with any drug, if you are nursing a baby, seek the advice of a health professional before using this product. Keep this and all drugs out of the reach of children. In case of accidental overdose, seek professional assistance or contact a poison control center immediately.

Dosage and Administration: Adults and children 12 years of age and over: one tablet at bedtime if needed or as directed by a doctor.

How Supplied: Sleep-ettes-D is strip packed in cartons or sealed in bottles of 24 and 48 tablets.

Shown in Product Identification Section, page 423

Requa, Inc.
BOX 4008
1 SENECA PLACE
GREENWICH, CT 06830

CHARCOAID
Poison Adsorbent, liquid has sweet, pleasant taste and feel; especially good for young patients.

Active Ingredient: Activated vegetable charcoal U.S.P., 30g per bottle, suspended in 70% sorbitol solution U.S.P., 110 g.

Indication: For the emergency treatment of acute poisoning.

Action: Adsorbent

Warnings: Before using call a poison control center, emergency room, or a physician for advice. If the patient has been given Ipecac Syrup, do not give activated charcoal until after patient has vomited. Do not use in a semi-conscious or unconscious person.

Precaution: May cause laxation. Careful attention to fluids and electrolytes is important, especially with young children and multiple dose therapy.

Dosage and Administration: Adults: Shake well and drink entire contents (add water if too sweet). To insure a full dose, rinse bottle with water and drink. For children, refer to Poison Control Center.

Professional Labeling: Some dilution may be necessary for administration via lavage tube. Add a small amount of water to bottle and shake.

How Supplied: 5 fl. oz. unit dose bottle, 30g activated charcoal U.S.P., suspended in 70% sorbitol solution U.S.P., 110 g.
U.S. Patent #4,122,169

CHARCOCAPS®
Activated Charcoal Capsules

Active Ingredient: Activated vegetable charcoal U.S.P., 260 mg per capsule.

Indications: Relief of intestinal gas, diarrhea, gastrointestinal distress associated with indigestion. Also to aid in the prevention of non-specific pruritus associated with kidney dialysis treatment.

Actions: Adsorbent, detoxicant, soothing agent. Reduces the volume of intestinal gas and allays related discomfort.

Warnings: As with all anti-diarrheals—not for children under 3 unless directed by physician. If diarrhea persists more than two days or is accompanied by high fever, consult physician.

Drug Interaction: Activated Charcoal USP can adsorb medication while they are in the digestive tract.

Precaution: **General Guidelines—** Take two hours before or one hour after medication including oral contraceptives.

Symptoms and Treatment of Oral Overdosage: Overdosage has not been encountered. Medical evidence indicates that high dosage or prolonged use does not cause side effect or harm the nutritional state of the patient.

Dosage and Administration: Two capsules after meals or at first sign of discomfort. Repeat as needed up to eight doses (16 capsules) per day.

Professional Labeling: None.

How Supplied: Bottles of 8, 36, 100 capsules

EDUCATIONAL MATERIAL

Questions & Answers
Brochure with questions and answers about the use of activated charcoal.

Trial Size
Professional sample of Charcocaps, which includes coupon for regular size for the patient.

Rhone-Poulenc Rorer Pharmaceuticals Inc.
Consumer Pharmaceutical Products
500 VIRGINIA DRIVE
FORT WASHINGTON, PA 19034

Regular Strength
ASCRIPTIN®
[*ă"skrĭp'tin*]
Analgesic
Aspirin buffered with Maalox®

Active Ingredients: Each coated tablet contains Aspirin (325 mg) and Maalox (Magnesium Hydroxide 50 mg, Dried Aluminum Hydroxide Gel 50 mg), buffered with Calcium Carbonate.

Inactive Ingredients: Hydroxypropyl Methylcellulose, Magnesium Stearate, Microcrystalline Cellulose, Starch, Talc, Titanium Dioxide, and other ingredients.

Description: Ascriptin is an excellent analgesic, antipyretic, and anti-inflammatory agent for general use, particularly where there is concern over aspirin-induced gastric distress. When large doses are used, as in arthritis and rheumatic disorders, gastric discomfort is rare. Coated tablets make swallowing easy.

Indications: As an analgesic for the relief of pain in such conditions as headache, neuralgia, minor injuries, and dysmenorrhea. As an analgesic and antipyretic in colds and fever. As an analgesic and anti-inflammatory agent in arthritis and other rheumatic diseases. As an inhibitor of platelet aggregation, see MI's and TIA's indications.

Usual Adult Dose: Two or three tablets, four times daily. Do not exceed 12 tablets in a 24-hour period. For children under twelve, consult a doctor.
WARNINGS: Children and teenagers should not use this medicine for chicken pox or flu symptoms before a doctor is consulted about Reye syndrome, a rare but serious illness reported to be associated with aspirin. Keep this and all medicines out of children's reach. If pain persists more than 10 days, redness or swelling is present, fever persists more than 3 days, or symptoms worsen, consult a doctor immediately. If you are under medical care or have a history of stomach, kidney, or bleeding disorders or asthma, consult a doctor before using. Do not use if allergic to aspirin. As with any drug, if you are pregnant or nursing a baby, consult a doctor before using. **IT IS ESPECIALLY IMPORTANT NOT TO USE ASPIRIN DURING THE LAST 3 MONTHS OF PREGNANCY UNLESS SPECIFICALLY DIRECTED TO DO SO BY A DOCTOR BECAUSE IT MAY CAUSE PROBLEMS IN THE UNBORN CHILD OR COMPLICATIONS DURING DELIVERY. If ringing in the ears or loss of hearing occurs, consult a doctor before taking any more of this product. In case of accidental overdose, contact a doctor immediately.**

Drug Interaction Precaution: Do not use if taking a prescription drug for anticoagulation (blood thinning), diabetes, gout or arthritis, or a tetracycline antibiotic unless directed by a doctor.

Professional Labeling:
Aspirin for Myocardial Infarction
Indication: Aspirin is indicated to reduce the risk of death and/or non-fatal myocardial infarction in patients with a previous infarction or unstable angina pectoris.

Dosage and Administration: Although most of the studies used dosages exceeding 300 mg, two trials used only 300 mg, and pharmacologic data indicate that this dose inhibits platelet function fully. Therefore, 300 mg or a conventional 325-mg aspirin dose is a reasonable, routine dose that would minimize gastrointestinal adverse reactions. This use of aspirin applies to both solid, oral dosage forms (buffered and plain aspirin), and buffered aspirin in solution. *Note:* Complete information and references available.
RECURRENT TIA's IN MEN
Indications: For reducing the risk of recurrent transient ischemic attacks (TIA's) or stroke in men who have had transient ischemia of the brain due to fibrin platelet emboli. There is inadequate evidence that aspirin or buffered aspirin is effective in reducing TIA's in women at the recommended dosage. There is no evidence that aspirin or buffered aspirin is of benefit in the treatment of completed strokes in men or women.

Precautions: (1) Patients presenting with signs and symptoms of TIA's should have a complete medical and neurologic evaluation. Consideration should be given to other disorders which resemble TIA's. **(2)** Attention should be given to risk factors; it is important to evaluate and treat, if appropriate, other diseases associated with TIA's and stroke such as hypertension, diabetes, CHD and PVD. **(3)** Concurrent administration of absorbable antacids at therapeutic doses may increase the clearance of salicylates in some individuals. The concurrent administration of nonabsorbable antacids may alter the rate of absorption of aspirin, thereby resulting in a decreased acetylsalicylic acid/salicylate ratio in plasma. The clinical significance on TIA's of these decreases in available aspirin is unknown. Low-dose aspirin may be associated with an increase in uric acid levels.

Dosage: 1300 mg a day, in divided doses of 650 mg twice a day or 325 mg four times a day.

How Supplied: Bottles of 50 tablets (NDC 0067-0145-50), 100 tablets (NDC 0067-0145-68), and 225 tablets (NDC 0067-0145-77) with child-resistant caps. Bottles of 500 tablets (NDC 0067-0145-74) without child-resistant closures (for arthritic patients). Military Stock #NSN 6505-00-135-2783 V.A. Stock #6505-00-890-1979 (bottles of 500).

Shown in Product Identification Section, page 423

ASCRIPTIN® A/D for arthritis pain
Analgesic
Aspirin buffered with Maalox®

Aspirin for arthritis pain relief buffered with extra Maalox for extra stomach comfort.

Active Ingredients: Each coated caplet contains Aspirin (325 mg) and Maalox (Magnesium Hydroxide 75 mg, Dried Aluminum Hydroxide Gel 75 mg), buffered with Calcium Carbonate.

Inactive Ingredients: Hydroxypropyl Methylcellulose, Magnesium Stearate, Microcrystalline Cellulose, Starch, Talc, Titanium Dioxide, and other ingredients.

Description: Ascriptin A/D is a highly buffered analgesic, anti-inflammatory, and antipyretic agent for use in the treatment of rheumatoid arthritis, osteoarthritis, and other arthritic conditions. It is formulated with extra Maalox to provide increased neutralization of gastric acid thus improving the likelihood of GI tolerance when large antiarthritic doses of aspirin are used. Coated caplets make swallowing easy.

Indications: As an analgesic, anti-inflammatory, and antipyretic agent in rheumatoid arthritis, osteoarthritis, and other arthritic conditions.

Usual Adult Dose: Two or three caplets, four times daily, or as directed by the physician for arthritis therapy. For children under twelve, at the discretion of the physician.
WARNINGS: Children and teenagers should not use this medicine for chicken pox or flu symptoms before a doctor is consulted about Reye syndrome, a rare but serious illness reported to be associated with aspirin. Keep this and all medicines out of children's reach. If pain persists more than 10 days, redness or swelling is present, fever persists more than 3 days, or symptoms worsen, consult a doctor immediately. If you are under medical care or have a history of stomach, kidney, or bleeding disorders or asthma, consult a doctor before using. Do not use if allergic to aspirin. As with any drug, if you are pregnant or nursing a baby, consult a doctor before using. **IT IS ESPECIALLY IMPORTANT NOT TO USE ASPIRIN DURING THE LAST 3 MONTHS OF PREGNANCY UNLESS SPECIFICALLY DIRECTED TO DO SO BY A DOCTOR BECAUSE IT MAY CAUSE PROBLEMS IN THE UNBORN CHILD OR COMPLICATIONS DURING DELIVERY. If ringing in the ears or loss of hearing occurs, consult a doctor before taking any more of this product. In case of accidental overdose, contact a doctor immediately.**

Drug Interaction Precaution: Do not use if taking a prescription drug for anticoagulation (blood thinning), diabetes, gout or arthritis, or a tetracycline antibiotic unless directed by a doctor.

How Supplied: Available in bottles of 100 caplets (NDC 0067-0147-68), and 225 caplets (NDC 0067-0147-77) with child-resistant caps and in special bottles of 500 caplets (without child-resistant closures) for arthritic patients (NDC 0067-0147-74).

Shown in Product Identification Section, page 423

EXTRA STRENGTH MAALOX® Plus (Reformulated Maalox Plus)
Alumina, Magnesia and Simethicone Oral Suspension and Tablets, Rorer
Antacid/Anti-Gas

- ☐ **Lemon Swiss creme**
  Cherry creme
  Mint creme
  ... the flavors preferred by the physician and patient.
- ☐ **Physician-proven Maalox® formula for antacid effectiveness.**
- ☐ **Simethicone, at a recognized clinical dose, for antiflatulent action.**

Description: Extra Strength Maalox® Plus, a balanced combination of magnesium and aluminum hydroxides plus simethicone, is a non-constipating antacid/anti-gas product to provide symptomatic relief of hyperacidity plus alleviation of gas symptoms. Available in cherry creme, mint creme or lemon swiss creme flavors.

Composition: To provide symptomatic relief of hyperacidity plus alleviation of gas symptoms, each teaspoonful/tablet contains:

Active Ingredients	Extra Strength Maalox® Plus Per Tsp. (5 mL)	Maalox® Plus Per Tablet
Magnesium Hydroxide	450 mg	200 mg
Aluminum Hydroxide (equivalent to dried gel, USP)	500 mg	200 mg
Simethicone	40 mg	25 mg

Inactive Ingredients: Extra Strength Maalox® Plus Suspension: Citric acid, flavors, methylparaben, propylparaben, purified water, saccharin sodium, sorbitol, and other ingredients.
Maalox® Plus Tablets: Citric acid, confectioners' sugar, D&C red No. 30, D&C yellow No. 10, dextrose, flavors, glycerin, magnesium stearate, mannitol, saccharin sodium, sorbitol solution, starch, talc.
To aid in establishing proper dosage schedules, the following information is provided:

Minimum Recommended Dosage:	Per 2 Tsp. (10 mL)	Per Tablet
Acid neutralizing capacity	58.1 mEq	11.4 mEq
Sodium content*	2.3 mg	0.8 mg
Sugar content	None	0.55 g
Lactose content	None	None

Indications: As an antacid for symptomatic relief of hyperacidity associated with the diagnosis of peptic ulcer, gastritis, peptic esophagitis, gastric hyperacidity, heartburn, or hiatal hernia. As an antiflatulent to alleviate the symptoms of gas, including postoperative gas pain.

Advantages: Among antacids, Extra Strength Maalox® Plus Suspension and Maalox® Plus Tablets are uniquely palatable—an important feature which encourages patients to follow your dosage directions. Extra Strength Maalox® Plus Suspension and Maalox® Plus Tablets have the time-proven, nonconstipating, sodium-free* Maalox® formula —useful for those patients suffering from the problems associated with hyperacidity. Additionally, Extra Strength Maalox® Plus Suspension and Maalox® Plus Tablets contain simethicone to alleviate discomfort associated with entrapped gas.

*Dietetically insignificant. Contains approximately 0.05 mEq sodium per teaspoonful of Suspension. Each Maalox® Plus Tablet contains approximately 0.03 mEq sodium per Tablet.

Directions for Use:
Extra Strength Maalox® Plus Suspension: Two to four teaspoonfuls, four times a day, taken twenty minutes to one hour after meals and at bedtime, or as directed by a physician.

Professional Labeling

Warnings:
(i) Prolonged use of aluminum-containing antacids in patients with renal failure may result in or worsen dialysis osteomalacia. Elevated tissue aluminum levels contribute to the development of the dialysis encephalopathy and osteomalacia syndromes. Small amounts of aluminum are absorbed from the gastrointestinal tract and renal excretion of aluminum is impaired in renal failure. Aluminum is not well removed by dialysis because it is bound to albumin and transferrin, which do not cross dialysis membranes. As a result, aluminum is deposited in bone, and dialysis osteomalacia may develop when large amounts of aluminum are ingested orally by patients with impaired renal function.
(ii) Aluminum forms insoluble complexes with phosphate in the gastrointestinal tract, thus decreasing phosphate absorption. Prolonged use of aluminum-containing antacids by normophosphatemic patients may result in hypophosphatemia if phosphate intake is not adequate. In its more severe forms, hypophosphatemia can lead to anorexia, malaise, muscle weakness, and osteomalacia.

Patient Warnings: Do not take more than 12 teaspoonfuls in a 24-hour period or use the maximum dosage for more than 2 weeks or use if you have kidney disease except under the advice and supervision of a physician.
Maalox® Plus Tablets: One to four tablets, well chewed, four times a day, taken twenty minutes to one hour after meals and at bedtime, or as directed by a physician.

Patient Warnings: Do not take more than 16 tablets in a 24-hour period or use the maximum dosage for more than two weeks or use if you have kidney disease except under the advice and supervision of a physician.

Drug Interaction Precaution: Do not use with patients taking a prescription antibiotic containing any form of tetracycline. As with all aluminum-containing antacids, Maalox® Plus may prevent the proper absorption of the tetracycline.
Keep this and all drugs out of the reach of children.

How Supplied:
Extra Strength Maalox® Plus Suspension is available in plastic bottles of 5 fl oz (148 mL) (NDC 0067-0333-62), 12 fl oz (355 mL) (NDC 0067-0333-71), and 26 fl oz (769 mL) (NDC 0067-0333-44) in lemon Swiss creme; 12 fl oz in cherry creme (NDC 0067-0336-71); and 12 fl oz in mint creme (NDC 0067-0338-71).
Maalox® Plus Tablets are available in bottles of 50 tablets (NDC 0067-0339-50) and 100 tablets (NDC 0067-0339-67), convenience packs of 12 tablets (NDC 0067-0339-19), Roll Packs of 12 tablets (NDC 0067-0339-23), and 36 tablets (NDC 0067-0339-33).

Shown in Product Identification Section, page 423

PERDIEM®
[*pĕr"dē'ŭm*]

Indication: For relief of constipation.

Actions: Perdiem®, with its 100% natural, gentle action provides comfortable relief from constipation. Perdiem® is a unique combination of bulk-forming fiber and natural stimulant. The vegetable mucilages of Perdiem® soften the stool and provide pain-free evacuation of the bowel with no chemical stimulants. Perdiem® is effective as an aid to elimination for the hemorrhoid or fissure patient prior to and following surgery.

Composition: Perdiem® contains as its active ingredients, 82% psyllium (Plantago Hydrocolloid) and 18% senna (Cassia Pod Concentrate) which are natural vegetable derivatives. Each rounded teaspoonful (6.0 g) contains 3.25 g psyllium, 0.74 g senna, 1.8 mg of sodium, 35.5 mg of potassium, and 4 calories. Perdiem® is "Dye-Free" and contains no artificial sweeteners.

Inactive Ingredients: Acacia, iron oxides, natural flavors, paraffin, sucrose, talc.

Patient Warning: Should not be used in the presence of undiagnosed abdomi-

Continued on next page

Rhone-Poulenc Rorer—Cont.

nal pain. Frequent or prolonged use without the direction of a physician is not recommended, as it may lead to laxative dependence. Do not use in patients with a history of psyllium allergy. Psyllium allergy is rare but can be severe. If an allergic reaction occurs, discontinue use and contact your physician.
Bulk-forming agents have the potential to obstruct the esophagus, particularly in the presence of esophageal narrowing or when consumed with insufficient fluid. Patients should be made aware of the symptoms of esophageal obstruction, including chest pain/pressure, regurgitation, and difficulty swallowing. Patients experiencing these symptoms should seek immediate medical attention. Patients with esophageal narrowing or dysphagia should not use Perdiem®.
As with any drug, if you are pregnant or nursing a baby, seek the advice of a physician before using this product. Keep this and all drugs out of the reach of children. In case of accidental overdose, seek professional assistance or contact a poison control center immediately.

Directions for Use—Adults: In the evening and/or before breakfast, 1–2 rounded teaspoonfuls of Perdiem® granules (in single or partial teaspoon doses) should be placed in the mouth and swallowed with at least 8 fl oz of cool beverage. Additional liquid would be helpful. Perdiem® granules should not be chewed.
Perdiem® generally takes effect within 12 hours. Subsequent doses may be adjusted after adequate laxation is obtained.

Note: It is extremely important that Perdiem® be taken with at least 8 fl oz of cool liquid and should not be chewed.

In Severe Cases of Constipation: Perdiem® may be taken more frequently, up to 2 rounded teaspoonfuls every 6 hours not to exceed 5 teaspoonfuls in a 24-hour period. In severe cases, 24 to 72 hours may be required for optimal relief. However, a physician should be consulted in cases of severe constipation.

For Patients Habituated to Strong Purgatives: Two rounded teaspoonfuls of Perdiem® in the morning and evening may be required along with half the usual dose of the purgative being used. The purgative should be discontinued as soon as possible and the dosage of Perdiem® granules reduced when and if bowel tone shows lessened laxative dependence.

For Colostomy Patients: To ensure formed stools, give one to two rounded teaspoonfuls of Perdiem® in the evening.

For Clinical Regulation: For patients confined to bed, for those of inactive habits, and in the presence of cardiovascular disease where straining must be avoided, one rounded teaspoonful of Perdiem® taken once or twice daily will provide regular bowel habits.

For Children: From age 7–11 years, give one rounded teaspoonful one to two times daily. From age 12 and older, give adult dosage.

How Supplied: Granules: 100-gram (3.5 oz) (NDC 0067-0690-68) and 250-gram (8.8 oz) (NDC 0067-0690-70) canisters.

Shown in Product Identification Section, page 423

PERDIEM® FIBER

[pĕr″dē′ŭm]

Indications: Perdiem® Fiber provides gentle relief from simple, chronic, and spastic constipation. In addition, it relieves constipation associated with convalescence, pregnancy, and advanced age. Perdiem® Fiber is also indicated for use in special diets lacking in residue fiber to aid regularity and in the management of constipation associated with irritable bowel syndrome, diverticular disease, hemorrhoids, and anal fissures.

Action: Perdiem® Fiber, is a 100% natural bulk-forming fiber that gently helps maintain regularity and prevents constipation. Perdiem® Fiber's unique form is easy to swallow and requires no mixing but must be followed by at least 8 ounces of cool liquid. Perdiem® Fiber's 100% natural psyllium formulation can safely be taken for prolonged periods as a source of fiber under the direction of a physician.

Composition: Perdiem® Fiber contains as its active ingredient 100% psyllium (Plantago Hydrocolloid), a natural vegetable derivative. Each rounded teaspoonful (6.0 g) contains 4.03 g of psyllium, 1.8 mg of sodium, 36.1 mg of potassium and 4 calories. Perdiem® Fiber is "Dye-Free" and contains no artificial sweeteners.

Inactive Ingredients: Acacia, iron oxides, natural flavors, paraffin, sucrose, talc, titanium dioxide.

Patient Warning: Should not be used in the presence of undiagnosed abdominal pain. Frequent or prolonged use without the direction of a physician is not recommended.
Do not use in patients with a history of psyllium allergy. Psyllium allergy is rare but can be severe. If an allergic reaction occurs, discontinue use.
Bulk-forming agents have the potential to obstruct the esophagus, particularly in the presence of esophageal narrowing or when consumed with insufficient fluid. Patients should be made aware of the symptoms of esophageal obstruction, including chest pain/pressure, regurgitation, and difficulty swallowing. Patients experiencing these symptoms should seek immediate medical attention. Patients with esophageal narrowing or dysphagia should not use Perdiem® Fiber.
Keep this and all drugs out of the reach of children. In case of accidental overdose, seek professional assistance or contact a poison control center immediately.

Directions for Use—Adults: In the evening and/or before breakfast, 1 to 2 rounded teaspoonfuls (6.0 to 12.0 g) of Perdiem® Fiber granules (in full or partial teaspoon doses) should be placed in the mouth and swallowed with at least 8 fl oz of cool beverage. Additional liquid would be helpful. Perdiem® Fiber granules should not be chewed. Children: For children age 7–11, give 1 rounded teaspoonful 1–2 times daily. Age 12 and older, give adult dosage.

Note: It is extremely important that Perdiem® Fiber be taken with at least 8 fl oz of cool liquid.

In Severe Cases of Constipation: Perdiem® Fiber may be taken more frequently, up to 2 rounded teaspoonfuls every 6 hours depending upon need and response not to exceed 5 teaspoonfuls in a 24-hour period. In obstinate cases, 48 to 72 hours may be required to provide optimal benefit.

After Rectal Surgery: The vegetable mucilages of Perdiem® Fiber soften the stool and provide pain-free evacuation of the bowel. Perdiem® Fiber is effective as an aid to elimination for the hemorrhoid or fissure patient prior to and following surgery.

For Clinical Regulation: For patients confined to bed—after an operation for example—and for those of inactive habits, 1 rounded teaspoonful of Perdiem® Fiber taken 1–2 times daily will contribute to regular bowel habits.

During Pregnancy: Because of its natural ingredient and bulking action, Perdiem® Fiber is effective for expectant mothers when used under a physician's care. In most cases 1–2 rounded teaspoonfuls taken each evening is sufficient.

How Supplied: Granules: 100-gram (3.5 oz) (NDC 0067-0795-68) and 250-gram (8.8 oz) (NDC 0067-0795-70) canisters.

Shown in Product Identification Section, page 424

Richardson-Vicks Inc.
ONE FAR MILL CROSSING
SHELTON, CT 06484

CHILDREN'S CHLORASEPTIC® LOZENGES

Active Ingredients: Benzocaine 5 mg per lozenge.

Inactive Ingredients: Corn syrup, FD&C Blue No. 1, FD&C Red No. 40, flavor, sucrose.

Indications: For temporary relief of occasional minor sore throat, pain and irritation. Also for temporary relief of pain associated with canker sores.

Directions: Adults and children 2 years of age and older: Allow lozenge to dissolve slowly in mouth. May be repeated every 2 hours as needed or as directed by a doctor or dentist. Children under 2 years of age: Consult a doctor or a dentist.

Warning: If sore throat is severe, or is accompanied by difficulty in breathing, or persists for more than two days, do not use, and consult a doctor promptly. If sore throat is accompanied or followed by fever, headache, rash, nausea, or vomiting, consult a doctor promptly. If sore mouth symptoms do not improve in 7 days, see your doctor or dentist promptly. KEEP THIS AND ALL DRUGS OUT OF THE REACH OF CHILDREN. In case of accidental overdose seek professional assistance or contact a poison control center immediately. As with any drug if you are pregnant or nursing a baby, seek the advice of a health professional before using this product.
Store at room temperature.

How Supplied: Cartons of 18.
Shown in Product Identification Section, page 424

CHLORASEPTIC® LIQUID
(oral anesthetic, antiseptic)
Cherry, Menthol and Cool Mint Flavors

Active Ingredients: Phenol 1.4%.

Inactive Ingredients:
Menthol Liquid: Citric acid, D&C Yellow No. 10, FD&C Green No. 3, flavor, glycerin, menthol, propylene glycol, purified water, sodium citrate, saccharin sodium, and sorbitol. Alcohol (12.5%).
Menthol Aerosol Spray: D&C Yellow No. 10, FD&C Green No. 3, flavor, glycerin, purified water and saccharin sodium.
Cherry Liquid: Citric acid, FD&C Red No. 40, flavor, glycerin, propylene glycol, sodium citrate, saccharin sodium and sorbitol. Alcohol (12.5%).
Cherry Aerosol Spray: FD&C Red No. 40, flavor, glycerin, purified water and saccharin sodium.
Cool Mint Liquid: Citric acid, FD&C Blue No. 1, flavor, glycerin, menthol, propylene glycol, purified water, sodium citrate, saccharin sodium and sorbitol. Alcohol (12.5%).

Indications: For temporary relief of occasional minor irritations, pain, sore mouth, sore throat and pain associated with canker sores. Also for the temporary relief of pain associated with tonsillitis, pharyngitis and throat infections.

Administration and Dosage:
Chloraseptic Spray (Pump): Spray 5 times (Children 2–12 years of age, 3 times) and swallow. Repeat every 2 hours or as directed by a doctor or dentist. Children under 2 years: consult a doctor or dentist.
Chloraseptic Gargle: Adults and children 12 years of age and older: Gargle or swish around the mouth for at least 15 seconds and then spit out. Use every 2 hours or as directed by a doctor or dentist. Children 6 to 12 years: Apply 2 teaspoons to the affected area and gargle or swish around in mouth for at least 15 seconds and then spit out. Use every 2 hours or as directed by a doctor or dentist. Children under 12 years should be supervised in product use. Children under 6 years: Consult a doctor or dentist.
Chloraseptic Aerosol Spray: Adults—Spray for 2 seconds directly on affected area (children 2 to 12 years, spray for 1 second) and swallow. Use every 2 hours or as directed by a doctor or dentist. Children under 12 years of age should be supervised in the use of this product. Children under 2 years of age: Consult a doctor or dentist.

Warning: If sore throat is severe, or is accompanied by difficulty in breathing, or persists for more than two days, do not use, and consult a doctor promptly. If sore throat is accompanied or followed by fever, headache, rash, nausea, or vomiting, consult a doctor promptly. If sore mouth symptoms do not improve in 7 days, see your doctor or dentist promptly. KEEP THIS AND ALL DRUGS OUT OF THE REACH OF CHILDREN. In case of accidental overdose, seek professional assistance or contact a poison control center immediately. As with any drug, if you are pregnant or nursing a baby, seek the advice of a health professional before using this product. Do not administer to children under 2 years of age unless directed by a physician or dentist.
For 1.5 oz. Aerosol Spray—Avoid spraying in eyes. Contents under pressure. Do not puncture or incinerate. Do not store at temperature above 120°F.
Store at room temperature.

How Supplied: Available in Menthol, Cherry, and Cool Mint flavors in 6 fl. oz. plastic bottles with sprayer. Menthol and Cherry Flavors also available in 12 fl. oz. gargle and 1.5 oz. nitrogen-propelled aerosol sprays.
Shown in Product Identification Section, page 424

CHLORASEPTIC® LOZENGES
Cherry, Menthol, and Cool Mint Flavor

Active Ingredients:
Cherry and Cool Mint: Benzocaine (6.0 mg./lozenge) and Menthol (10 mg./lozenge).
Menthol: Phenol (32.5 mg./lozenge).

Inactive Ingredients:
Menthol: Corn syrup, D&C Yellow No. 10, FD&C Blue No. 1, FD&C Yellow No. 6, flavor and sucrose.
Cherry: Corn syrup, FD&C Blue No. 1, FD&C Red No. 40, flavor, and sucrose.
Cool Mint: Corn syrup, FD&C Blue No. 1, flavor and sucrose.

Indications: For temporary relief of occasional minor sore throat, pain and irritation. Also, for temporary relief of pain associated with sore mouth, canker sores, tonsillitis, pharyngitis and throat infections.

Directions:
Cherry and Cool Mint
Adults and children 2 years of age and older: Allow lozenge to dissolve slowly in mouth. May be repeated every 2 hours as needed or as directed by a doctor or dentist. Children under 2 years of Age: Consult a doctor or a dentist.
Menthol
Adults and children 12 years of age and older: Allow lozenge to dissolve slowly in mouth. May be repeated every two hours or as directed by a dentist or doctor. Children 6 to under 12 years of age: Allow lozenge to dissolve slowly in mouth. May be repeated every two hours, not to exceed 9 lozenges per day. Children under 6 years of age: Consult a dentist or a doctor.

Warning: If sore throat is severe, or is accompanied by difficulty in breathing, or persists for more than two days, do not use, and consult a doctor promptly. If sore throat is accompanied or followed by fever, headache, rash, nausea, or vomiting, consult a doctor promptly. If sore mouth symptoms do not improve in 7 days, see your doctor or dentist promptly. KEEP THIS AND ALL DRUGS OUT OF THE REACH OF CHILDREN. In case of accidental overdose seek professional assistance or contact a Poison Control Center immediately. As with any drug if you are pregnant or nursing a baby, seek the advice of a health professional before using this product.

How Supplied: Available in Menthol and Cherry flavors in packages of 18 and 36. Also available in Cool Mint flavor in packages of 18.
Shown in Product Identification Section, page 424

CLEARASIL® Adult Care—Medicated Blemish Cream

Active Ingredient: Sulfur, Resorcinol (alcohol 10%) in a cream base which contains water, bentonite, glyceryl stearate SE, propylene glycol, isopropyl myristate, sodium bisulfite, dimethicone, methylparaben, propylparaben, fragrance, iron oxides.

Indications: For the topical treatment of acne in adults or persons demonstrating sensitivity to benzoyl peroxide.

Actions: CLEARASIL Adult Care—Medicated Blemish Cream is an acne medication specifically suited for adult usage since it dries acne lesions without over-drying or irritating the skin the way many benzoyl peroxide-containing products can. The product contains sulfur and resorcinol to help heal acne pimples.

Warnings: FOR EXTERNAL USE ONLY. USING OTHER TOPICAL ACNE MEDICATIONS AT THE SAME TIME OR IMMEDIATELY FOLLOWING USE OF THIS PRODUCT MAY INCREASE DRYNESS OR IRRITATION OF THE SKIN. IF THIS OCCURS, ONLY ONE MEDICATION SHOULD BE USED UNLESS DIRECTED BY A DOCTOR. DO NOT GET INTO EYES. IF EXCESSIVE SKIN IRRITATION DEVELOPS OR INCREASES, DISCONTINUE USE AND CONSULT A DOCTOR. APPLY TO AFFECTED AREAS ONLY. DO NOT USE ON BROKEN SKIN OR APPLY TO LARGE AREAS OF THE BODY.

Continued on next page

Richardson-Vicks—Cont.

KEEP THIS AND ALL MEDICINE OUT OF REACH OF CHILDREN.

Symptoms and Treatment of Ingestion: These symptoms are based upon medical judgement, not on actual experience. Theoretically, ingestion of very large amounts may cause nausea, vomiting, abdominal discomfort and diarrhea. Treatment is symptomatic, with bed rest and observation.

Directions for Use:
1. Cleanse skin thoroughly before applying medication.
2. Apply Clearasil Adult Care directly on and around the affected area two or three times daily.
3. To prevent new pimples, apply to oily areas of the face.

How Supplied: Available in a .6 oz. tube.

Shown in Product Identification Section, page 425

CLEARASIL DOUBLE TEXTURED PADS—Maximum Strength and Regular Strength

Active Ingredients: *Regular Strength:* Salicylic Acid 1.25%, (Alcohol 40%) *Maximum Strength:* Salicylic Acid 2.00% (Alcohol 40%). Also contains water, witch hazel distillate, sodium methyl cocoyl taurate, quaternium-22, aloe vera gel, menthol, fragrance.

Indications: Topical skin cleanser for the treatment of acne vulgaris.

Actions: Clearasil Double Textured Pads contain a comedolytic agent that penetrates to clean out oil and dead skin cells that may lead to clogged pores and pimples.

Warnings: FOR EXTERNAL USE ONLY. IF IRRITATION OR DRYNESS OCCURS, REDUCE FREQUENCY OF USE. IF EXCESSIVE ITCHING, REDNESS, BURNING OR SWELLING OCCURS, DISCONTINUE USE. IF SYMPTOMS PERSIST, CONSULT A PHYSICIAN PROMPTLY. MAY IRRITATE EYES. IF CONTACT OCCURS, FLUSH THOROUGHLY WITH WATER. KEEP AWAY FROM EXTREME HEAT OR OPEN FLAME.

KEEP THIS AND ALL MEDICINE OUT OF THE REACH OF CHILDREN.

Symptoms and Treatment of Ingestion: Product contains Ethyl Alcohol and Salicylic Acid. If large amounts are ingested, nausea, vomiting, gastrointestinal irritation and lethargy may develop and should be treated symptomatically.

Directions for Use:
1. Wash face thoroughly.
2. Use rough side to deep clean.
3. Use smooth side to deliver pimple fighting medicine.
4. For maximum effectiveness do not rinse.
5. Use morning or night or whenever you wash your face.

How Supplied: Both Maximum and Regular Strength are supplied in 8 ounce jars containing 32 pads.

Shown in Product Identification Section, page 425

CLEARASIL® 10% BENZOYL PEROXIDE ACNE MEDICATION CREAM—Vanishing and Tinted

Active Ingredient: Benzoyl Peroxide 10% in an odorless, greaseless cream base, containing water, propylene glycol, aluminum hydroxide, bentonite, glyceryl stearate SE, PEG-12, isopropyl myristate, potassium carbomer, methylparaben, and propylparaben. The tinted formula also contains dimethicone, titanium dioxide and iron oxides.

Indications: For the topical treatment of acne vulgaris.

Actions: Clearasil Cream contains 10% Benzoyl Peroxide. The product:

1) **Clears existing pimples**—Clearasil's micronized benzoyl peroxide penetrates clogged pores to help dry and clear up existing pimples and blackheads.
2) **Helps prevent new pimples**—Clearasil Cream continues to keep skin clearer by killing acne bacteria. Its medicine works to help stop new pimples before they appear.

Additional Benefits: Clearasil Cream is available in two forms: tinted and vanishing. Tinted covers up pimples while the vanishing formula blends invisibly into the skin. Clearasil Cream also contains two oil-absorbing ingredients that soak up excess oil all day long, giving cleaner, clearer looking skin.

Warnings: FOR EXTERNAL USE ONLY. USING OTHER TOPICAL ACNE MEDICATIONS AT THE SAME TIME OR IMMEDIATELY FOLLOWING USE OF THIS PRODUCT MAY INCREASE DRYNESS OR IRRITATION OF THE SKIN. IF THIS OCCURS, ONLY ONE MEDICATION SHOULD BE USED UNLESS DIRECTED BY A DOCTOR. DO NOT USE THIS MEDICATION IF YOU HAVE VERY SENSITIVE SKIN OR IF YOU ARE SENSITIVE TO BENZOYL PEROXIDE. THIS PRODUCT MAY CAUSE IRRITATION, CHARACTERIZED BY REDNESS, BURNING, ITCHING, PEELING OR POSSIBLY SWELLING. MORE FREQUENT USE OR HIGHER CONCENTRATIONS MAY AGGRAVATE SUCH IRRITATION. MILD IRRITATION MAY BE REDUCED BY USING THE PRODUCT LESS FREQUENTLY OR IN A LOWER CONCENTRATION. IF IRRITATION BECOMES SEVERE, DISCONTINUE USE. IF IRRITATION STILL CONTINUES, CONSULT A DOCTOR. KEEP AWAY FROM EYES, LIPS AND MOUTH. AVOID CONTACT WITH HAIR, FABRICS, INCLUDING CARPET, AND CLOTHING WHICH MAY BE BLEACHED BY THE BENZOYL PEROXIDE IN THIS PRODUCT.

KEEP THIS AND ALL MEDICINE OUT OF THE REACH OF CHILDREN.

Symptoms and Treatment of Ingestion: These symptoms are based upon medical judgement, not on actual experience. Theoretically, ingestion of very large amounts may cause nausea, vomiting, abdominal discomfort and diarrhea. Treatment is symptomatic, with bed rest and observation.

Directions for Use:
1. Wash thoroughly.
2. Apply Clearasil Cream wherever pimples and oily skin occur.
3. Apply extra Clearasil Cream on existing pimples.

How Supplied: Available in both Vanishing and Tinted formulas in 1 oz. and .65 oz. squeeze tubes.

Shown in Product Identification Section, page 425

CLEARASIL® 10% BENZOYL PEROXIDE ACNE MEDICATION VANISHING LOTION

Active Ingredient: Benzoyl Peroxide 10% in a colorless, greaseless lotion which contains water, aluminum hydroxide, isopropyl stearate, PEG-100 stearate, glyceryl stearate, cetyl alcohol, glycereth-26, isocetyl stearate, glycerin, dimethicone copolyol, sodium citrate, citric acid, methylparaben, propylparaben, fragrance.

Indications: For the topical treatment of acne vulgaris.

Actions: Clearasil Lotion contains 10% Benzoyl Peroxide. The product:

1) **Clears existing pimples**—Clearasil's micronized benzoyl peroxide penetrates clogged pores to help dry and clear up existing pimples and blackheads.
2) **Helps prevent new pimples**—Clearasil Lotion continues to keep skin clearer by killing acne bacteria. Its medicine works to help stop new pimples before they appear.

Additional Benefits: Clearasil Lotion contains two special oil-absorbing ingredients that soak up oil all day long, giving cleaner, clearer looking skin.

Warnings: FOR EXTERNAL USE ONLY. USING OTHER TOPICAL ACNE MEDICATIONS AT THE SAME TIME OR IMMEDIATELY FOLLOWING USE OF THIS PRODUCT MAY INCREASE DRYNESS OR IRRITATION OF THE SKIN. IF THIS OCCURS, ONLY ONE MEDICATION SHOULD BE USED UNLESS DIRECTED BY A DOCTOR. DO NOT USE THIS MEDICATION IF YOU HAVE VERY SENSITIVE SKIN OR IF YOU ARE SENSITIVE TO BENZOYL PEROXIDE. THIS PRODUCT MAY CAUSE IRRITATION, CHARACTERIZED BY REDNESS, BURNING, ITCHING, PEELING OR POSSIBLY SWELLING. MORE FREQUENT USE OR HIGHER CONCENTRATIONS MAY AGGRAVATE SUCH IRRITATION. MILD IRRITATION MAY BE REDUCED BY USING THE PRODUCT LESS FREQUENTLY OR IN A LOWER CONCENTRATION. IF IRRI-

TATION BECOMES SEVERE. DISCONTINUE USE. IF IRRITATION STILL CONTINUES, CONSULT A DOCTOR. KEEP AWAY FROM EYES, LIPS AND MOUTH. AVOID CONTACT WITH HAIR, FABRICS, INCLUDING CARPET, AND CLOTHING WHICH MAY BE BLEACHED BY THE BENZOYL PEROXIDE IN THIS PRODUCT.
KEEP THIS AND ALL MEDICINE OUT OF THE REACH OF CHILDREN.

Symptoms and Treatment of Ingestion: These symptoms are based upon medical judgement, not on actual experience. Theoretically, ingestion of very large amounts may cause nausea, vomiting, abdominal discomfort and diarrhea. Treatment is symptomatic, with bed rest and observation.

Directions for Use:
1. Wash thoroughly.
2. Apply Clearasil Lotion wherever pimples and oily skin occur.
3. Apply extra Clearasil Lotion on existing pimples.

How Supplied: Available in a 1 fl. oz. squeeze bottle.

DRAMAMINE® Liquid
[*dram 'uh-meen*]
(dimenhydrinate syrup USP)
DRAMAMINE® Tablets
(dimenhydrinate USP)
DRAMAMINE® Chewable Tablets
(dimenhydrinate USP)

Description: Dimenhydrinate is the chlorotheophylline salt of the antihistaminic agent diphenhydramine. Dimenhydrinate contains not less than 53% and not more than 56% of diphenhydramine, and not less than 44% and not more than 47% of 8-chlorotheophylline, calculated on the dried basis.

Active Ingredients:
Dramamine Tablets and Chewable Tablets: Dimenhydrinate 50 mg.
Dramamine Liquid: Dimenhydrinate 12.5 mg. per 5 ml, Ethyl Alcohol 5%.

Inactive Ingredients:
Dramamine Tablets: Acacia, Carboxymethylcellulose Sodium, Corn Starch, Magnesium Stearate, and Sodium Sulfate.
Dramamine Liquid: FD&C Red No. 40, Flavor, Glycerin, Methylparaben, Sucrose, and Water. Ethyl Alcohol 5%.
Dramamine Chewable Tablets: Aspartame, Citric Acid, FD&C Yellow No. 6, Flavor, Magnesium Stearate, Methacrylic Acid Copolymer, Sorbitol.
Phenylketonurics: Contains Phenylalanine 1.5 mg per tablet.
Contains FD&C Yellow No. 5 (tartrazine) as a color additive.

Actions: While the precise mode of action of dimenhydrinate is not known, it has a depressant action on hyperstimulated labyrinthine function.

Indications: For the prevention and treatment of the nausea, vomiting, or dizziness associated with motion sickness.

Directions:
Dramamine Tablets and Chewable Tablets: To prevent motion sickness, the first dose should be taken one half to one hour before starting activity.
ADULTS: 1 to 2 tablets every 4 to 6 hours, not to exceed 8 tablets in 24 hours or as directed by a doctor.
CHILDREN 6 TO UNDER 12: ½ to 1 tablet every 6 to 8 hours, not to exceed 3 tablets in 24 hours or as directed by a doctor.
CHILDREN 2 to UNDER 6: ¼ to ½ tablet every 6 to 8 hours not to exceed 1½ tablets in 24 hours or as directed by a doctor.
Children may also be given Dramamine Cherry Flavored Liquid in accordance with directions for use.
Dramamine Liquid: To prevent motion sickness, the first dose should be taken one half to one hour before starting activity. ADULTS: 4 to 8 teaspoons (5 ml per teaspoonful) every 4 to 6 hours, not to exceed 32 teaspoonfuls in 24 hours or as directed by a doctor. CHILDREN 6 TO UNDER 12: 2 to 4 teaspoonfuls every 6 to 8 hours, not to exceed 12 teaspoonfuls in 24 hours or as directed by a doctor. CHILDREN 2 TO UNDER 6: 1 to 2 teaspoonfuls every 6 to 8 hours not to exceed 6 teaspoonfuls in 24 hours or as directed by a doctor. Use of a measuring device is recommended for all liquid medication.

Warnings: Do not take this product if you have asthma, glaucoma, emphysema, chronic pulmonary disease, shortness of breath, difficulty in breathing, or difficulty in urination due to enlargement of the prostate gland unless directed by a doctor. Do not give to children under 2 years of age unless directed by a doctor. May cause marked drowsiness; alcohol, sedatives, and tranquilizers may increase the drowsiness effect. Avoid alcoholic beverages while taking this product. Do not take this product if you are taking sedatives or tranquilizers, without first consulting your doctor. Use caution when driving a motor vehicle or operating machinery. Not for frequent or prolonged use except on advice of a doctor. Do not exceed recommended dosage. Keep this and all drugs out of the reach of children. In case of accidental overdose, seek professional assistance or contact a poison control center immediately. As with any drug, if you are pregnant or nursing a baby, seek the advice of a health professional before using this product.

How Supplied: *Tablets* —scored, white tablets available in packets of 12 and 36 and bottles of 100 (OTC); *Liquid* —Available in bottles of 3 fl oz (OTC); *Chewables* —scored, orange tablets available in packets of 8 and 24 (OTC).

Shown in Product Identification Section, page 424

ICY HOT® Balm
[*ī 'see hot*]
(topical analgesic balm)
ICY HOT® Cream
(topical analgesic cream)
ICY HOT® Stick
(topical analgesic stick)

Active Ingredients: Icy Hot Balm contains methyl salicylate 29%, menthol 7.6%. Icy Hot Cream contains methyl salicylate 30%, menthol 10%. Icy Hot Stick contains methyl salicylate 30%, menthol 10%.
Inactive ingredients of Icy Hot Balm include paraffin and white petrolatum. Inactive ingredients of Icy Hot Cream include carbomer, cetyl esters wax, emulsifying wax, oleth-3 phosphate, stearic acid, trolamine, and water. Inactive ingredients of Icy Hot Stick include ceresin, cyclomethicone, hydrogenated castor oil, microcrystalline wax, paraffin, PEG-150 distearate, propylene glycol, stearic acid, and stearyl alcohol.

Description: Icy Hot Balm, Icy Hot Cream, and Icy Hot Stick are topically applied analgesics containing two active ingredients, methyl salicylate and menthol. It is the particular concentration of these ingredients, in combination with inert ingredients, that results in the distinct, combined heating/cooling sensation of Icy Hot.

Actions: Icy Hot is classified as a counterirritant which, when rubbed into the intact skin, provides relief of deep-seated pain through a counterirritant action rather than through a direct analgesic effect. In acting as a counterirritant, Icy Hot replaces the perception of pain with another sensation that blocks deep pain temporarily by its action on or near the skin surface.

Indications: For the temporary relief of minor aches and pains of muscles and joints associated with arthritis, simple backache, strains, bruises, and sprains.

Directions: Adults and children 2 years of age and older: Apply to affected area not more than 3 to 4 times daily. Children under 2 years of age: Do not use, consult a doctor.
Stick: Twist base to raise Icy Hot approximately one-quarter inch above container.
Adults and children 2 years of age and older: Apply to affected area not more than 3 to 4 times daily. Children under 2 years of age: Do not use, consult a doctor.

Warnings: For external use only. Do not use otherwise than as directed. Keep this an all drugs out of the reach of children. In case of accidental ingestion, seek professional assistance or contact a poison control center immediately. Avoid contact with eyes. Avoid contact with mouth, genitalia, and mucous membranes, irritated, or very sensitive skin. If you have diabetes or impaired circulation, use Icy Hot only upon the advice of a physician. Do not apply to wounds or damaged skin, Do not bandage tightly.

Continued on next page

Richardson-Vicks—Cont.

Do not apply external heat or hot water. If condition worsens, or if symptoms persist for more than 7 days or clear up and occur again within a few days, discontinue use of this product and consult a doctor.
CAUTION: Discontinue use if excessive irritation of the skin develops.

Adverse Reactions: The most common adverse reactions that may occur with Icy Hot use are skin irritation and blistering. The most serious adverse reaction is severe toxicity that occurs if the product is ingested.

How Supplied: Icy Hot Balm is available in a 3½ oz jar. Icy Hot Cream is available in tubes in two sizes, 1¼ oz and 3 oz. Icy Hot Stick is available as a 1¾ oz stick.

Shown in Product Identification Section, page 424

PERCOGESIC®
[*pĕrkō-jē 'zĭk*]
Analgesic Tablets

Description: Each tablet contains:
Acetaminophen .... 325 mg
Phenyltoloxamine citrate .... 30 mg

Inactive Ingredients: Cellulose, Flavor, FD&C Yellow No. 6, Hydroxypropyl Methylcellulose, Magnesium Stearate, Polyethylene Glycol, Povidone, Silica Gel, Starch, Stearic Acid, Sucrose.

Indications: For temporary relief of minor aches and pains associated with headache, backache, muscular aches, the premenstrual and menstrual periods, the common cold and flu, toothache, and for the minor pain from arthritis, and to reduce fever.

Dosage and Administration: *Adults* (12 years and over)—1 or 2 tablets every four hours. Maximum daily dose—8 tablets
Children (6–12 years)—one tablet every 4 hours. Maximum daily dose—4 tablets. Children under 6 years of age consult a doctor.

Warning: May cause excitability especially in children. Do not take this product if you have asthma, glaucoma, emphysema, chronic pulmonary disease, shortness of breath, difficulty in breathing, or difficulty in urination due to enlargement of the prostate gland unless directed by a doctor. May cause drowsiness; alcohol, sedatives, and tranquilizers may increase the drowsiness effect. Avoid alcoholic beverages while taking this product. Do not take this product if you are taking sedatives or tranquilizers, without first consulting your doctor. Use caution when driving a motor vehicle or operating machinery. Do not take this product for pain for more than 10 days (adults) or 5 days (children), and do not take for fever for more than 3 days unless directed by a doctor. If pain or fever persists or gets worse, if new symptoms occur, or if redness or swelling is present, consult a doctor because these could be signs of a serious condition. Do not give this product to children for the pain of arthritis unless directed by a doctor. Keep this and all drugs out of the reach of children. In case of accidental overdose, seek professional assistance or contact a poison control center immediately. Prompt medical attention is critical for adults as well as for children even if you do not notice any signs or symptoms. As with any drug, if you are pregnant or nursing a baby, seek the advice of a health professional before using this product.

How Supplied: Child-resistant bottles of 24 and 90 tablets, and bottles of 50 tablets.

Shown in Product Identification Section, page 424

VICKS® CHILDREN'S COUGH SYRUP
Cough Suppressant • Expectorant

Active Ingredients per tsp. (5 ml.): Dextromethorphan Hydrobromide 3.5 mg., Guaifenesin 50 mg.

Inactive Ingredients: Citric Acid, FD&C Green No. 3, FD&C Red No. 40, Flavor, Methylparaben, Propylene Glycol, Purified Water, Sodium Citrate, Sodium Saccharin, Sucrose.

Indications: Temporarily reduces cough due to a cold or inhaled irritants. Helps loosen phlegm (sputum) and thin bronchial secretions to drain bronchial tubes to make coughs more productive.

Actions: VICKS Children's COUGH SYRUP is an alcohol-free antitussive and expectorant. It calms, quiets coughs of colds; loosens phlegm, promotes drainage of bronchial tubes; and coats and soothes a cough irritated throat.

Directions:
12 years and over: 4 teaspoonfuls
6–under 12 years: 2 teaspoonfuls
2–under 6 years: 1 teaspoonful
Repeat every 4 hours as needed.

Warning: A persistent cough may be a sign of a serious condition. If cough persists for more than 1 week, tends to recur, or is accompanied by fever, rash, or persistent headache, consult a doctor. Do not take this product for persistent or chronic cough such as occurs with smoking, asthma, chronic bronchitis, or emphysema, or where cough is accompanied by excessive phlegm (sputum) unless directed by a doctor. KEEP THIS AND ALL DRUGS OUT OF THE REACH OF CHILDREN. In case of accidental overdose, seek professional assistance or contact a poison control center immediately. As with any drug, if you are pregnant or nursing a baby, seek the advice of a health professional before using this product.

How Supplied: Available in 4 fl. oz. bottles.

VICKS® COUGH SILENCERS
Cough Drops

Active Ingredients per drop: Dextromethorphan (expressed as Dextromethorphan Hydrobromide) 2.5 mg., Benzocaine 1 mg.

Inactive Ingredients: Corn Syrup, FD&C Blue No. 1, Flavor, Silicon Dioxide, Sodium Chloride, Sucrose.
Contains FD&C Yellow No. 5 (tartrazine) as a color additive.

Indications: Temporarily relieves cough due to minor throat and bronchial irritations as may occur with a cold. Also for temporary relief of occasional minor irritation and sore throat.

Directions for Use: Age 12 and over: 4 drops every four hours. Dissolve in mouth one at a time. Do not exceed 48 drops in 24 hours or as directed by a doctor. Ages 6 to under 12: 2 to 4 drops every four hours. Dissolve in mouth one at a time. Do not exceed 24 drops in 24 hours or as directed by a doctor. Ages 3 to under 6: 2 drops every four hours. Dissolve in mouth one at a time. Do not exceed 12 drops in 24 hours or as directed by a doctor. Children under 3, consult doctor.

Warning: A persistent cough may be a sign of a serious condition. If cough persists for more than one week, tends to recur, or is accompanied by fever, rash, or persistent headache, consult a doctor. Do not take this product for persistent chronic cough such as occurs with smoking, asthma, emphysema, or if cough is accompanied by excessive phlegm (mucus) unless directed by a doctor. If sore throat is severe, or is accompanied by difficulty in breathing, or persists for more than two days, do not use, and consult a doctor promptly. If sore throat is accompanied or followed by fever, headache, rash, nausea, or vomiting, consult a doctor promptly. If sore mouth symptoms do not improve in 7 days, see your doctor or dentist promptly. KEEP THIS AND ALL DRUGS OUT OF THE REACH OF CHILDREN. In case of accidental overdose, seek professional assistance or contact a poison control center immediately. As with any drug, if you are pregnant or nursing a baby, seek the advice of a health professional before using this product.

How Supplied: Available in boxes of 14's.

VICKS DAYCARE® LIQUID
VICKS DAYCARE® CAPLETS
Multi-Symptom Colds Medicine

Active Ingredients: LIQUID — per fluid ounce (2 Tbs.) or **CAPLET** — per **two** caplets, contains Acetaminophen 650 mg., Dextromethorphan Hydrobromide 20 mg., Pseudoephedrine Hydrochloride 60 mg., Guaifenesin 200 mg.

Inactive Ingredients:
Liquid: Citric Acid, FD&C Yellow No. 6, Flavor, Glycerin, Propylene Glycol, Purified Water, Saccharin, Sodium Benzoate, Sodium Citrate, Sucrose. Also contains Alcohol 10%.

Caplets: Cellulose, Croscarmellose Sodium, FD&C Yellow No. 6, Magnesium Stearate, Povidone, Starch, Stearic acid.

Indications: For the temporary relief of minor aches, pains, headache, muscular aches, and fever associated with a cold, sore throat, or flu. Temporarily relieves nasal congestion and coughing due to a cold. Helps make coughs more productive by loosening phlegm (sputum) and draining bronchial tubes.

Actions: VICKS DAYCARE is a decongestant, antitussive, expectorant, analgesic and antipyretic. It helps clear stuffy nose, congested sinus openings. Calms, quiets coughing. Eases headache pain and the ache-all-over feeling. Reduces fever due to colds and flu. It relieves these symptoms without drowsiness. DAYCARE LIQUID also soothes a cough-irritated throat.

Directions: Take as directed.
Adults 12 years and over: one fluid ounce in medicine cup (2 tablespoons), or 2 caplets.
Children 6 to under 12 years of age: one half fluid ounce in medicine cup (1 tablespoon), or 1 caplet.
Children 2 to under 6 years of age: 1½ teaspoons.
Children under 2 years of age: Consult a doctor.
Repeat every 4 hours, not to exceed 4 doses per day, or as directed by a doctor.

Warning: Do not exceed recommended dosage because at higher doses, nervousness, dizziness, or sleeplessness may occur. Do not take this product if you have heart disease, high blood pressure, thyroid disease, diabetes, or difficulty in urination due to enlargement of the prostate gland unless directed by a doctor. DRUG INTERACTION PRECAUTION: Do not take this product if you are presently taking a prescription drug for high blood pressure or depression, without first consulting your doctor. Do not take this product for persistent or chronic cough such as occurs with smoking, asthma, chronic bronchitis, or emphysema, or where a cough is accompanied by excessive phlegm (sputum) unless directed by a doctor. Do not take this product for more than 7 days (for adults) or 5 days (for children). A persistent cough may be a sign of serious condition. If cough persists for more than 7 days, tends to recur, or is accompanied by rash, or persistent headache, consult a doctor. If symptoms do not improve or are accompanied by fever that lasts for more than 3 days, or if new symptoms occur, consult a doctor. If sore throat is severe, persists for more than 2 days, is accompanied or followed by fever, headache, rash, nausea, or vomiting, consult a doctor promptly. Keep this and all drugs out of the reach of children. In case of accidental overdose, seek professional assistance or contact a poison control center immediately. Prompt medical attention is critical for adults as well as for children even if you do not notice any signs or symptoms. As with any drug, if you are pregnant or nursing a baby, seek the advice of a health professional before using this product.
TAKE ONLY AS DIRECTED.

How Supplied: Available in: **LIQUID** with child-resistant, tamper-evident cap—6 and 10 fl. oz. plastic bottles.
CAPLET in child-resistant packages—20.

Shown in Product Identification Section, page 424

VICKS FORMULA 44® COUGH CONTROL DISCS

Active Ingredients per disc: Dextromethorphan (expressed as Dextromethorphan Hydrobromide) 5 mg., Benzocaine 1.25 mg., Menthol 4.3 mg.

Inactive Ingredients: Corn Syrup, Flavor, Silicon Dioxide, Sodium Chloride, Sucrose.

Indications: Temporarily relieves cough due to minor throat and bronchial irritation associated with a cold. Also for occasional minor sore throat.

Actions: VICKS FORMULA 44 COUGH CONTROL DISCS have antitussive and local-anesthetic actions in a solid disc form. They calm, quiet coughs and help coat and soothe irritated throats.

Directions:
Adults 12 years and over:
Dissolve two discs in mouth, one at a time. Repeat every 4 hours not to exceed 12 discs in 24 hours or as directed by doctor.
Children 2 to under 12 years:
Dissolve one disc in mouth. Repeat every 4 hours not to exceed 6 discs in 24 hours or as directed by doctor.
Children under 2 years, consult a doctor.

Warnings: A persistent cough may be a sign of a serious condition. If cough persists for more than 1 week, tends to recur, or is accompanied by fever, rash, or persistent headache, consult a doctor. Do not take this product for persistent or chronic cough such as occurs with smoking, asthma, emphysema, or if cough is accompanied by excessive phlegm (mucus) unless directed by a doctor. If sore throat is severe, or is accompanied by difficulty in breathing, or persists for more than two days, do not use, and consult a doctor promptly. If sore throat is accompanied or followed by fever, headache, rash, nausea or vomiting, consult a doctor promptly. If sore mouth symptoms do not improve in 7 days, see your doctor or dentist promptly. KEEP THIS AND ALL DRUGS OUT OF THE REACH OF CHILDREN. In case of accidental overdose, seek professional assistance or contact a poison control center immediately. As with any drug, if you are pregnant or nursing a baby, seek the advice of a health professional before using this product.

How Supplied: Available as individual foil-wrapped portable packets in boxes of 24.

VICKS FORMULA 44® COUGH MEDICINE

Active Ingredients per 2 tsp. (10 mL.): Dextromethorphan Hydrobromide 30 mg., Chlorpheniramine Maleate 4 mg.

Inactive Ingredients: Caramel, citric acid, flavor, FD&C Red #40, Propylene Glycol, Povidone, Purified water, Sodium Citrate, Invert Sugar. Also contains Alcohol 10%.

Indications: Formula 44 provides temporary relief of coughs due to a common cold, or minor throat or bronchial irritations. Also dries a runny nose due to a cold.

Actions: VICKS FORMULA 44 COUGH MIXTURE is a cough suppressant, and an antihistamine. It calms and quiets coughs. Reduces sneezing and sniffling.

Directions:
Adults: 12 years and over—2 teaspoonfuls
Children: 6 to under 12 years: 1 teaspoonful
Children under 6 consult a doctor.
Repeat every 6 hours as needed.
No more than 4 doses per day.

Warning: A persistent cough may be a sign of a serious condition. If cough persists for more than 1 week, tends to recur, or is accompanied by fever, rash, or persistent headache, consult a doctor. Do not take this product for persistent or chronic cough such as occurs with smoking, asthma, emphysema, or if cough is accompanied by excessive phlegm (mucus) unless directed by a doctor. May cause excitablility especially in children. Do not take this product if you have asthma, glaucoma, emphysema, chronic pulmonary disease, shortness of breath, difficulty in breathing or difficulty in urination due to enlargement of the prostate gland unless directed by a doctor. May cause marked drowsiness; alcohol, sedatives, and tranquilizers may increase the drowsiness effect. Avoid alcoholic beverages while taking this product. Do not take this product if you are taking sedatives or tranquilizers, without first consulting your doctor. Use caution when driving a motor vehicle or operating machinery. KEEP THIS AND ALL DRUGS OUT OF THE REACH OF CHILDREN. In case of accidental overdose, seek professional assistance or contact a poison control center immediately. As with any drug, if you are pregnant or nursing a baby, seek the advice of a health professional before using this product.

How Supplied: Available in 4 fl. oz. and 8 fl. oz. bottles.

Shown in Product Identification Section, page 424

Continued on next page

Richardson-Vicks—Cont.

VICKS FORMULA 44D® DECONGESTANT COUGH MEDICINE

Active Ingredients per 3 tsp. (15 ml.): Dextromethorphan Hydrobromide 30 mg., Pseudoephedrine Hydrochloride 60 mg.

Inactive Ingredients: Citric Acid, FD&C Red No. 40, Flavor, Propylene Glycol, Purified Water, Sodium Benzoate, Sodium Citrate, Sodium Saccharin, Sucrose. Contains Alcohol 10%.

Indications: Formula 44D provides temporary relief of coughs and nasal congestion due to a common cold.

Actions: VICKS FORMULA 44D is an antitussive and a nasal decongestant. It calms, quiets coughs; relieves nasal congestion; coats and soothes a cough-irritated throat.

Dosage:

ADULT DOSE	12 years and over— 3 teaspoonfuls
CHILD DOSE	6–12 years— 1½ teaspoonfuls
	2–6 years— ¾ teaspoonful.

Repeat ever 6 hours as needed, no more than 4 doses per day.

Warning: A persistent cough may be a sign of a serious condition. If cough persists for more than 1 week, tends to recur, or is accompanied by fever, rash, or persistent headache, consult a doctor. Do not take this product for persistent or chronic cough such as occurs with smoking, asthma, emphysema, or if cough is accompanied by excessive phlegm (mucus) unless directed by a doctor. Do not exceed recommended dosage because at higher doses nervousness, dizziness, or sleeplessness may occur. Do not take this product for more than 7 days. If symptoms do not improve or are accompanied by fever, consult a doctor. Do not take this product if you have heart disease, high blood pressure, thyroid disease, diabetes, or difficulty in urination due to enlargement of the prostate gland unless directed by a doctor. *Drug Interaction Precaution.* Do not take this product if you are presently taking a prescription drug for high blood pressure or depression, without first consulting your doctor. KEEP THIS AND ALL DRUGS OUT OF THE REACH OF CHILDREN. In case of accidental overdose, seek professional assistance or contact a poison control center immediately. As with any drug, if you are pregnant, or nursing a baby, seek the advice of a health professional before using this product.

How Supplied: Available in 4 fl. oz., 8 fl. oz. and 12 fl. oz. bottles.

Shown in Product Identification Section, page 424

VICKS FORMULA 44M® MULTI-SYMPTOM COUGH MEDICINE

Active Ingredients per 4 tsp. (20 ml.): Dextromethorphan Hydrobromide 30 mg., Pseudoephedrine Hydrochloride 60 mg., Chlorpheniramine Maleate 4 mg., Acetaminophen 500 mg.

Inactive Ingredients: Citric Acid, FD&C Blue No. 1, FD&C Red No. 40, Flavor, Glycerin, Purified Water, Sodium Benzoate, Sodium Citrate, Sodium Saccharin, Sucrose. Also contains alcohol 20%.

Indications: VICKS FORMULA 44M provides temporary relief of coughing, nasal congestion, runny nose and sneezing due to a cold. Also for temporary relief of headache, fever and muscular aches due to a cold or flu.

Actions: VICKS FORMULA 44M is a cough suppressant, nasal decongestant, antihistamine and analgesic. It calms, quiets coughs; relieves nasal congestion; runny nose, sneezing and coats, soothes and eases the pain of a cough-irritated throat.

Directions: 12 years and over—4 teaspoonfuls
6–12 years—2 teaspoonfuls
Repeat every 6 hours as needed. No more than 4 doses per day.

Warning: Do not take this product for persistent or chronic cough such as occurs with smoking, asthma, or emphysema, or if cough is accompanied by excessive phlegm (mucus) unless directed by a doctor. Do not exceed recommended dosage because at higher doses nervousness, dizziness, or sleeplessness may occur. Do not take this product if you have heart disease, high blood pressure, thyroid disease, diabetes, or difficulty in urination due to enlargement of the prostate gland unless directed by a doctor. *Drug Interaction Precaution.* Do not take this product if you are presently taking a prescription drug for high blood pressure or depression, without first consulting your doctor. May cause excitability especially in children. Do not take this product if you have asthma, glaucoma, emphysema, chronic pulmonary disease, shortness of breath, or difficulty in breathing unless directed by a doctor. May cause marked drowsiness; alcohol, sedatives, and tranquilizers may increase the drowsiness effect. Avoid alcoholic beverages while taking this product. Do not take this product if you are taking sedatives or tranquilizers, without first consulting your doctor. Use caution when driving a motor vehicle or operating machinery. Do not take this product for more than 7 days (for adults) or 5 days (for children). A persistent cough may be a sign of a serious condition. If cough persists for more than 7 days, tends to recur, or is accompanied by rash, persistent headache, fever that lasts for more than 3 days, or if new symptoms occur, consult a doctor. If symptoms do not improve or are accompanied by fever that lasts for more than 3 days, or if new symptoms occur, consult a doctor. KEEP THIS AND ALL DRUGS OUT OF THE REACH OF CHILDREN. In case of accidental overdose, seek professional assistance or contact a poison control center immediately. Prompt medical attention is critical for adults as well as for children, even if you do not notice any signs or symptoms. As with any drug, if you are pregnant or nursing a baby, seek the advice of a health professional before using this product.

How Supplied: Available in 4 fl. oz. and 8 fl. oz. bottles.

Shown in Product Identification Section, page 424

VICKS® PEDIATRIC FORMULA 44® COUGH MEDICINE

Active Ingredient per 1 Tbs. (15 ml.): Dextromethorphan Hydrobromide USP 15 mg.

Inactive Ingredients: Carboxymethylcellulose Sodium, Cellulose, Citric Acid, FD&C Red No. 40, Flavor, Glycerin, Polysorbate 80, Potassium Sorbate, Propylene Glycol, Purified Water, Sodium Citrate, Sorbitol, Sucrose.

Indications: For the temporary relief of coughs due to the common cold or minor throat and bronchial irritation.

Administration and Dosage:
Directions for Use: SHAKE WELL BEFORE USING

Squeeze bottle to accurately dispense medicine into dosage cup provided.

(CUP INSIDE)

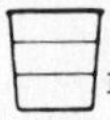

1 Tbs.
½ Tbs.

Dosage:

Age, yr.	Weight, lb.	Dose
Under 2	Under 28	Consult physician*
2–5	28–47	Fill cup to ½ Tbs.
6–11	48–95	Fill cup to 1 Tbs.
12 and over	96 and over	2 Tbs. or Try one of the Adult Formula 44® Medicines

Repeat every 6–8 hours as needed, not to exceed 4 doses in 24 hours.
*Suggested doses for children under 2 years are:

Professional Dosage:

Age, mo.	Weight, lb.	Dose
6–11	17–21	1 tsp. (5 ml.)
12–23	22–27	1¼ tsp. (6.25 ml.)

Repeat every 6–8 hours, not to exceed 4 doses in 24 hours or as directed by doctor.
*Based on extrapolation from studies on the safety and efficacy of active ingredients conducted among older children and adults. Use caution in treating children under 2 years of age who were born prematurely.

Warning: A persistent cough may be a sign of a serious condition. If cough persists for more than 1 week, tends to recur, or is accompanied by fever, rash, or persistent headache, consult a doctor. Do not take this product for persistent or chronic cough such as occurs with smoking, asthma, emphysema, or if cough is accompanied by excessive phlegm (mucus) unless directed by a doctor. KEEP THIS AND ALL DRUGS OUT OF THE REACH OF CHILDREN. In case of accidental overdose, seek professional assistance or contact a poison control center immediately. As with any drug, if you are nursing a baby, seek the advice of a health professional before using this product.

STORE AT ROOM TEMPERATURE. AVOID EXCESSIVE HEAT.

How Supplied: 4 fl. oz. squeeze bottles with VicksAccuTip™ Dispenser for clean, easy, accurate dosing. Calibrated dose cup accompanies each bottle.

Shown in Product Identification Section, page 424

VICKS® PEDIATRIC FORMULA 44® COUGH & COLD MEDICINE

Active Ingredients: Per 1 Tbs. (15 ml.): Dextromethorphan Hydrobromide USP 15 mg., Pseudoephedrine Hydrochloride USP 30 mg., Chlorpheniramine Maleate USP 2 mg.

Inactive Ingredients: Carboxymethylcellulose Sodium, Cellulose, Citric Acid, FD&C Red No. 40, Flavor, Glycerin, Polysorbate 80, Potassium Sorbate, Propylene Glycol, Purified Water, Sodium Citrate, Sorbitol, Sucrose.

Indications: For the temporary relief of coughs, nasal congestion, runny nose and sneezing due to the common cold or upper respiratory allergies.

Administration and Dosage:
DIRECTIONS FOR USE: SHAKE WELL BEFORE USING
Squeeze bottle to accurately dispense medicine into dosage cup provided

(CUP INSIDE)
1 Tbs.
½Tbs.

Dosage:

Age, yr.	Weight, lb.	Dose
Under 6	Under 48	Consult physician*
6–11	48–95	Fill cup to 1 Tbs.
12 and over	96 and over	2 Tbs. or try one of the Adult Formula 44® Medicines

*Physicians: Suggested doses for children under 6 years of age:

Age, Mo.	Weight, lb.	Dose
6–11	17–21	1 tsp. (5 ml.)
12–23	22–27	1½ tsp. (6.25 ml.)
2–5 yrs.	28–47	½ tbsp. (7.5 ml.)

Repeat every 6 hours, not to exceed 4 doses in 24 hours, or as directed by doctor.

*Based on extrapolation from studies on the safety and efficacy of active ingredients conducted among older children and adults. Use caution in treating children under 2 years of age who were born prematurely.

Warning: A persistent cough may be a sign of a serious condition. If cough persists for more than 1 week, tends to recur, or is accompanied by fever, rash, or persistent headache, consult a doctor. Do not take this product for persistent or chronic cough such as occurs with smoking, asthma, emphysema, or if cough is accompanied by excessive phlegm (mucus) unless directed by a doctor. Do not exceed recommended dosage because at higher doses nervousness, dizziness, or sleeplessness may occur. Do not take this product for more than 7 days. If symptoms do not improve or are accompanied by fever, consult a doctor. Do not take this product if you have heart disease, high blood pressure, thyroid disease, diabetes, or difficulty in urination due to enlargement of the prostate gland unless directed by a doctor. *Drug Interaction Precaution.* Do not take this product if you are presently taking a prescription drug for high blood pressure or depression, without first consulting your doctor. May cause excitability especially in children. Do not take this product if you have asthma, glaucoma, emphysema, chronic pulmonary disease, shortness of breath, or difficulty in breathing unless directed by a doctor. May cause marked drowsiness; alcohol, sedatives, and tranquilizers may increase the drowsiness effect. Avoid alcoholic beverages while taking this product. Do not take this product if you are taking sedatives or tranquilizers, without first consulting your doctor. Use caution when driving a motor vehicle or operating machinery. KEEP THIS AND ALL DRUGS OUT OF THE REACH OF CHILDREN. In case of accidental overdose, seek professional assistance or contact a poison control center immediately. As with any drug, if you are pregnant or nursing a baby, seek the advice of a health professional before using this product.

STORE AT ROOM TEMPERATURE. AVOID EXCESSIVE HEAT.

How Supplied: 4 fl. oz. squeeze bottles with VicksAccuTip™ Dispenser for clean, easy, accurate dosing. Calibrated dose cup accompanies each bottle.

Shown in Product Identification Section, page 424

VICKS® PEDIATRIC FORMULA 44® COUGH & CONGESTION MEDICINE

Active Ingredients: Per 1 Tbs. (15 ml.): Dextromethorphan Hydrobromide USP 15 mg., Pseudoephedrine Hydrochloride USP 30 mg.

Inactive Ingredients: Carboxymethylcellulose Sodium, Cellulose, Citric Acid, FD&C Red No. 40, Flavor, Glycerin, Polysorbate 80, Potassium Sorbate, Propylene Glycol, Purified Water, Sodium Citrate, Sorbitol, Sucrose.

Indications: For the temporary relief of coughs and nasal congestion due to the common cold or upper respiratory allergies.

Administration and Dosage:
DIRECTIONS FOR USE: SHAKE WELL BEFORE USING
Squeeze bottle to accurately dispense medicine into dosage cup provided

(CUP INSIDE)
1 Tbs.
½ Tbs.

Dosage:

Age, yr.	Weight, lb.	Dose
Under 2	Under 28	Consult physician
2–5	28–47	Fill cup to ½ Tbs.
6–11	48–95	Fill cup to 1 Tbs.
12 and over	96 and over	2 Tbs.

Repeat every 6 hours, not to exceed 4 doses in 24 hours.

Physicians: Suggested dose for children under 2 years**

Age, mo.	Weight, lb.	Dose
6–11	17–21	1 tsp. (5ml)
12–23	22–27	1¼ tsp. (6.25ml)

**Based on extrapolation from studies on the safety and efficacy of active ingredients conducted among older children and adults. Use caution in treating children under 2 years who were born prematurely.

Warning: A persistent cough may be a sign of a serious condition. If cough persists for more than 1 week, tends to recur, or is accompanied by fever, rash, or persistent headache, consult a doctor. Do not take this product for persistent or chronic cough such as occurs with smoking, asthma, emphysema, or if cough is accompanied by excessive phlegm (mucus) unless directed by a doctor. Do not exceed recommended dosage because at higher doses nervousness, dizziness, or sleeplessness may occur. Do not take this product for more than 7 days. If symptoms do not improve or are accompanied by fever, consult a doctor. Do not take this product if you have heart disease, high blood pressure, thyroid disease, diabetes, or difficulty in urination due to enlargement of the prostate gland unless directed by a doctor. *Drug Interaction Precaution.* Do not take this product if you are presently taking a prescription drug for high blood pressure or depression, without first consulting your doctor. KEEP THIS AND ALL DRUGS OUT OF THE REACH OF CHILDREN. In case of accidental overdose, seek profes-

Continued on next page

Richardson-Vicks—Cont.

sional assistance or contact a poison control center immediately. As with any drug, if you are pregnant or nursing a baby, seek the advice of a health professional before using this product.

STORE AT ROOM TEMPERATURE. AVOID EXCESSIVE HEAT.

How Supplied: 4 fl. oz. squeeze bottles with VicksAccuTip™ Dispenser for clean, easy, accurate dosing. Calibrated dose cup accompanies each bottle.

Shown in Product Identification Section, page 424

VICKS® INHALER
with decongestant action

Active Ingredient per inhaler: l Desoxyephedrine 50 mg.

Inactive Ingredients: Special Vicks Vapors (bornyl acetate, camphor, lavender oil, menthol).

Indications: For the temporary relief of nasal congestion due to the common cold, hay fever, upper respiratory allergies or sinusitis.

Actions: VICKS INHALER contains a volatile decongestant which, when inhaled, shrinks swollen membranes and provides fast relief from a stuffy nose.

Directions: Adults: 2 inhalations in each nostril not more often than every 2 hours. Children 6 to under 12 years of age (with adult supervision): 1 inhalation in each nostril not more often than every 2 hours. Children under 6 years of age: consult a doctor.

Warnings: Do not exceed recommended dosage because burning, stinging, sneezing, or increase of nasal discharge may occur. The use of this container by more than one person may spread infection. Do not use this product for more than 7 days. If symptoms persist, consult a doctor. Keep out of the reach of children.
In case of accidental ingestion, seek professional assistance or contact a Poison Control Center immediately.

VICKS INHALER is effective for a minimum of 3 months after first use.

How Supplied: Available as a cylindrical plastic nasal inhaler (net weight: 0.007 oz.).

VICKS CHILDREN'S NYQUIL®

Children's NyQuil was specially formulated with the maximum allowable nonprescription levels of three effective ingredients to relieve nighttime cough, nasal congestion, and runny nose so children can rest. Children's NyQuil is alcohol free and analgesic free and has a pleasant cherry flavor.

Active Ingredients: Each ½ oz dose (1 tbs) Chlorpheniramine Maleate 2 mg, Pseudoephedrine HCl 30 mg, Dextromethorphan Hydrobromide 15 mg.

Inactive Ingredients: Citric Acid, Flavor, FD&C Red No. 40, Grape Juice, Potassium Sorbate, Propylene Glycol, Purified Water, Sodium Citrate, Sucrose.

Indications: For temporary relief of nasal congestion, runny nose, sneezing, and coughing due to a cold.

Directions: Take at bedtime as directed. Use medicine cup provided.
If cold symptoms keep your child confined to bed or at home, a total of 4 doses may be taken per day, each 6 hours apart or use as directed by a doctor.

Age, yr.	Weight, lb.	Dose
Under 2	Under 28	Consult physician**
2–5	28–47	Fill cup to ½ Tbs.
6–11	48–95	Fill cup to 1 Tbs.
12 and over*	96 and over	2 Tbs. or Try one of the Adult Formula 44® Medicines

Repeat every 6–8 hours as needed, not to exceed 4 doses in 24 hours.
*Or use NyQuil Adult Nighttime Cold Medicine as directed. Available in original or cherry flavors.
**Suggested doses for children under 2 years are:

Professional Dosage

Age, mo.	Weight, lb.	Dose
6–11	17–21	1 tsp. (5 ml.)
12–23	22–27	1¼ tsp. (6.25 ml.)

Repeat every 6–8 hours, not to exceed 4 doses in 24 hours or as directed by doctor.
**Based on extrapolation from studies on the safety and efficacy of active ingredients conducted among older children and adults. Use caution in treating children under 2 years of age who were born prematurely.

Warning: Do not exceed recommended dosage, because at higher doses nervousness, dizziness or sleeplessness may occur. Do not take this product for more than 7 days. If symptoms do not improve or are accompanied by fever, consult a doctor. Do not take this product if you have heart disease, high blood pressure, thyroid disease, diabetes, or difficulty in urination due to enlargement of the prostate gland unless directed by a doctor. A persistent cough may be a sign of a serious condition. If cough persists for more than one week, tends to recur, or is accompanied by fever, rash, or persistent headache, consult a doctor. Do not take this product for persistent or chronic cough such as occurs with smoking, asthma, emphysema, or cough is accompanied by excessive phlegm (mucus) unless directed by a doctor. May cause excitability especially in children. Do not take this product if you have asthma, glaucoma, emphysema, chronic pulmonary disease, shortness of breath or difficulty in breathing unless directed by a doctor. May cause marked drowsiness; alcohol, sedatives, and tranquilizers may increase the drowsiness effect. Avoid alcoholic beverages while taking this product. Do not take this product if you are taking sedatives or tranquilizers, without first consulting your doctor. Use caution when driving a motor vehicle or operating machinery. In case of accidental overdose, seek professional assistance or contact a poison control center immediately. If you are pregnant or nursing a baby, seek the advice of a health professional before using this product.

Drug Interaction Precaution: Do not take this product if you are presently taking a prescription drug for high blood pressure or depression without first consulting your doctor.
KEEP OUT OF THE REACH OF CHILDREN.
Store at room temperature.

How Supplied: 4 fl. oz. and 8 fl. oz. bottles with child-resistant, tamper-evident cap, and a dosage cup.

Shown in Product Identification Section, page 424

VICKS NYQUIL®
[*nī'quĭl*]
Adult Nighttime Colds Medicine in oral liquid form.
Original and Cherry Flavor

Active Ingredients per fluid oz. (2 Tbs.): Acetaminophen 1000 mg., Doxylamine Succinate 7.5 mg., Pseudoephedrine HCl 60 mg, and Dextromethorphan Hydrobromide 30 mg.

Inactive Ingredients: Original Flavor: Citric Acid, FD&C Blue No. 1, Flavor, Glycerin, Purified Water, Sodium Benzoate, Sodium Citrate, Sucrose.
Contains FD&C Yellow No. 5 (tartrazine) as a color additive.
Contains alcohol 25%.
Cherry Flavor: Citric Acid, FD&C Blue No. 1, FD&C Red No. 40, Flavor, Glycerin, Purified Water, Sodium Citrate, Sodium Saccharin, Sucrose.
Contains alcohol 25%.

Indications: For the temporary relief of minor aches, pains, headache, muscular aches, sore throat, and fever associated with a cold or flu. Temporarily relieves nasal congestion, cough due to minor throat and bronchial irritations, runny nose and sneezing associated with the common cold.

Actions: Decongestant, antipyretic, antihistaminic, antitussive, analgesic. Helps decongest nasal passages and sinus openings, relieves sniffles and sneezing, eases aches and pains, reduces fever, relieves headache, minor sore throat pain, and quiets coughing due to a cold. By relieving these symptoms, also helps patient to sleep and get the rest he needs.

Dosage and Dosage Form: A plastic measuring cup with 2 tablespoonful gradation is supplied.

Directions:
ADULTS (12 and over): One fluid ounce in medicine cup (2 tablespoonfuls) at bedtime.
Not recommended for children.
If confined to bed or at home, a total of 4 doses may be taken per day, each 6 hours apart.

Warning: Do not exceed recommended dosage because at higher doses nervousness, dizziness or sleeplessness may occur. Do not take this product if you have heart disease, high blood pressure, thyroid disease, diabetes, or difficulty in urination due to enlargement of the prostate gland unless directed by a doctor. Do not take this product for persistent or chronic cough such as occurs with smoking, asthma, emphysema, or if cough is accompanied by excessive phlegm (mucus) unless directed by a doctor. Do not take this product for more than 7 days. A persistent cough may be a sign of a serious condition. If cough persists for more than 7 days, tends to recur or is accompanied by rash, persistent headache, fever that lasts for more than 3 days, or if new symptoms occur, consult a doctor. May cause excitability especially in children. Do not take this product if you have asthma, glaucoma, emphysema, chronic pulmonary disease, shortness of breath, or difficulty in breathing unless directed by a doctor. May cause marked drowsiness; alcohol, sedatives, and tranquilizers may increase the drowsiness effect. Avoid alcoholic beverages while taking this product. Do not take this product if you are taking sedatives or tranquilizers, without first consulting your doctor. Use caution when driving a motor vehicle or operating machinery. If symptoms do not improve or are accompanied by fever that lasts for more than 3 days, or if new symptoms occur, consult a doctor. If sore throat is severe, persists for more than 2 days, is accompanied or followed by fever, headache, rash, nausea, or vomiting, consult a doctor promptly. In case of accidental overdose, seek professional assistance or contact a poison control center immediately. Prompt medical attention is critical for adults as well as for children even if you do not notice any signs or symptoms. As with any drug, if you are pregnant or nursing a baby, seek the advice of a health professional before using this product.
KEEP OUT OF THE REACH OF CHILDREN.
TAKE ONLY AS DIRECTED.

How Supplied: Available in 6, 10, and 14 fl. oz. plastic bottles with child-resistant, tamper-evident cap.
Shown in Product Identification Section, page 424

VICKS SINEX™
[*sī′nĕx*]
Decongestant Nasal Spray and Ultra Fine Mist

Active Ingredient: Phenylephrine Hydrochloride 0.5%.

Inactive Ingredients: Aromatic Vapors (Camphor, Eucalyptol, Menthol), Cetylpyridinium Chloride, Potassium Phosphate, Purified Water, Sodium Chloride, Sodium Phosphate, Tyloxapol. Preservative: Thimerosal 0.001%.

Indications: For temporary relief of nasal congestion due to colds, hay fever, upper respiratory allergies or sinusitis.

Actions: *Provides fast decongestant relief*—Sinex gives fast relief of nasal stuffiness that often accompanies colds and hay fever. A strong decongestant shrinks swollen nasal membranes and relieves sinus pressure so you can breathe more freely.

Dosage and Administration: Keep head and dispenser upright. May be used every 4 hours as needed.
Ultra Fine Mist: Remove protective cap. Hold atomizer with thumb at base and nozzle between first and second fingers. Without tilting head, insert nozzle into nostril. Fully depress rim with a firm even stroke and sniff deeply. *Adults:* 2 or 3 sprays in each nostril not more often than every 4 hours. Not for use by children under 12 years of age unless directed by a doctor.
Squeeze Bottle: *Adults:* 2 or 3 sprays in each nostril not more often than every 4 hours. Not for use by children under 12 years of age unless directed by a doctor.

Warning: Do not exceed recommended dosage because burning, stinging, sneezing or increase of nasal discharge may occur. Do not use this product for more than 3 days. If symptoms persist, consult a physician. Do not take this product if you have heart disease, high blood pressure, thyroid disease, diabetes, or difficulty in urination due to enlargement of the prostate gland unless directed by a doctor. The use of this dispenser by more than one person may spread infection. KEEP THIS AND ALL DRUGS OUT OF THE REACH OF CHILDREN.

Accidental Ingestion: In case of accidental ingestion, seek professional assistance or contact a Poison Control Center immediately.

How Supplied: Available in ½ fl. oz. and 1 fl. oz. plastic squeeze bottles and ½ fl. oz. measured dose atomizer.
Shown in Product Identification Section, page 424

VICKS SINEX™ LONG-ACTING
[*sī′nĕx*]
12-hour Formula Decongestant Nasal Spray and Ultra Fine Mist

Active Ingredient: Oxymetazoline Hydrochloride 0.05%.

Inactive Ingredients: Aromatic Vapors (Camphor, Eucalyptol, Menthol), Potassium Phosphate, Purified Water, Sodium Chloride, Sodium Phosphate, Tyloxapol. Preservative: Thimerosal 0.001%.

Indications: For temporary relief of nasal congestion due to colds, hay fever, upper respiratory allergies or sinusitis.

Actions: Oxymetazoline constricts the arterioles of the nasal passages—resulting in a nasal decongestant effect which lasts up to 12 hours, restoring freer breathing through the nose. SINEX LONG-ACTING helps decongest sinus openings and sinus passages, thus promoting sinus drainage.

- *Quickly helps you breathe more freely:* Shrinks swollen nasal membranes and opens up nasal passages.
- *Works effectively up to 12 hours:* Contains the strongest topical decongestant available to provide longer-lasting relief.
- *Provides special extra feeling of relief:* Unique Vicks vapors provide a cool, soothing feeling of relief.

Warning: Do not exceed recommended dosage because burning, stinging, sneezing or increase of nasal discharge may occur. Do not use this product for more than 3 days. If symptoms persist, consult a physician. Do not take this product if you have heart disease, high blood pressure, thyroid disease, diabetes, or difficulty in urination due to enlargement of the prostate gland unless directed by a doctor. The use of this dispenser by more than one person may spread infection. KEEP THIS AND ALL MEDICINES OUT OF THE REACH OF CHILDREN.

Accidental Ingestion: In case of accidental ingestion, seek professional assistance or contact a Poison Control Center immediately.

Dosage and Administration: Keep head and dispenser upright. May be used twice daily (morning and evening) or as directed by a physician.
Ultra Fine Mist: Remove protective cap. Hold atomizer with thumb at base and nozzle between first and second fingers. Without tilting head, insert nozzle into nostril. Fully depress rim with a firm even stroke and sniff deeply. *Adults, and children 6 to under 12 years of age (with adult supervision):* 2 or 3 sprays in each nostril not more often than every 10 to 12 hours. Do not exceed 2 applications in any 24-hour period. Children under 6 years of age: consult a doctor.
Squeeze Bottle: *Adults, and children 6 to under 12 years of age (with adult supervision):* 2 or 3 sprays in each nostril not more often than every 10 to 12 hours. Do not exceed 2 applications in any 24-hour period. Children under 6 years of age: consult a doctor.

How Supplied: Available in ½ fl. oz. and 1 fl. oz. plastic squeeze bottles and ½ fl. oz. measured-dose atomizer.
Shown in Product Identification Section, page 425

VICKS® THROAT LOZENGES

Active Ingredient per lozenge: Benzocaine 5 mg.

Inactive Ingedients: Cetylpyridinium chloride, D&C Red No. 27, D&C Red No.

Continued on next page

Richardson-Vicks—Cont.

30, Flavor, Polyethylene Glycol, Sodium Citrate, Sucrose, Talc.

Indications: For temporary relief of occasional minor sore throat, pain, sore mouth and irritation. Also for the temporary relief of pain associated with canker sores.

Actions: Fast acting local anesthetic action to help temporarily soothe minor throat irritations... ease pain. Relieves irritation and dryness of the mouth and throat.

Directions: *Adults and Children 2 years of age and older:* allow lozenge to dissolve slowly in mouth. May be repeated every 2 hours as needed or as directed by a dentist or doctor. Children under 2 years of age: Consult a dentist or doctor.

Warning: If sore throat is severe, or is accompanied by difficulty in breathing, or persists for more than two days, do not use and consult a doctor promptly. If sore throat is accompanied or followed by fever, headache, rash, nausea, or vomiting, consult a doctor promptly. If sore mouth symptoms do not improve in 7 days, see your dentist or doctor promptly. KEEP THIS AND ALL DRUGS OUT OF THE REACH OF CHILDREN. In case of accidental overdose, seek professional assistance or contact a poison control center immediately. As with any drug, if you are pregnant or nursing a baby, seek the advice of a health professional before using this product.

How Supplied: Box of 12's.

VICKS® VAPORUB®

[*vā 'pō-rub*]

Nasal Decongestant/Cough Suppressant

Active Ingredients: Menthol 2.6%, Camphor 4.7%, Eucalyptus Oil 1.2%.

Inactive Ingredients: Cedarleaf Oil, Mineral Oil, Nutmeg Oil, Petrolatum, Thymol, Spirits of Turpentine.

Indications: For the temporary relief of nasal congestion and coughing associated with a cold to help you rest.

Actions: The inhaled vapors of VICKS VAPORUB have a decongestant and antitussive effect.

Directions: Adults and children over 2 years of age: Rub a thick layer of Vicks VapoRub on chest and throat. If desired, cover with a dry, warm cloth, but keep clothing loose to let vapors rise to the nose and mouth. Repeat up to three times daily, especially at bedtime, or as directed by a doctor. Children under two years of age, consult a doctor.

Warning: A persistent cough may be a sign of a serious condition. If cough persists for more than 1 week, tends to recur, or is accompanied by fever, rash, or persistent headache, consult a doctor. Do not use this product for persistent or chronic cough such as occurs with smoking, asthma, emphysema, or if cough is accompanied by excessive phlegm (mucus) unless directed by a doctor. For external use only. Do not take by mouth or place in nostrils. Never expose VapoRub to flame or place in boiling water. Keep this and all drugs out of the reach of children. In case of accidental ingestion, seek professional assistance or contact a poison control center immediately.

How Supplied: Available in 1.5 oz., 3.0 oz. and 6.0 oz. plastic jars and 2.0 oz. tubes.

Shown in Product Identification Section, page 425

VICKS VAPOSTEAM®

[*vā 'pō "stēm*]

Liquid Medication for Hot Steam Vaporizers.

Active Ingredients: Menthol 3.2%, Camphor 6.2%, Eucalyptus Oil 1.5%.

Inactive Ingredients: Cedarleaf Oil, Nutmeg Oil, Poloxamer 124, Polyoxyethylene Dodecanol, Silicone.
Alcohol 74%.

Indications: For temporary relief of nasal congestion due to a cold, hay fever or other respiratory allergies. Temporarily relieves cough occurring with a cold.

Actions: VAPOSTEAM increases the action of steam to help relieve colds symptoms in the following ways: relieves coughs of colds, eases nasal congestion, and moistens dry, irritated breathing passages.

Directions: In Hot Steam Vaporizers: VAPOSTEAM is formulated for use in HOT STEAM VAPORIZERS. Follow directions for use carefully.
Adults and children 2 years and older: Add 1 tablespoon of VAPOSTEAM for each quart of water directly to the water in a hot steam vaporizer, bowl or wash basin, or add 1½ teaspoonfuls of solution for each pint of water to an open container of boiling water. Breathe in medicated vapors. May be repeated up to three times daily or as directed by a doctor.
Children under 2 years of age: consult a doctor.

Warning: For hot steam medication only. Do not use in cold steam vaporizers/humidifiers. Not to be taken by mouth. Keep away from open flame or extreme heat. Do not direct steam from vaporizer towards face. A persistent cough may be a sign of a serious condition. If cough persists for more than a week, tends to recur or is accompanied by fever, rash or persistent headache, consult a doctor. Do not use this product for persistent or chronic cough such as occurs with smoking, asthma, or emphysema, or if cough is accompanied by excessive phlegm (mucus) unless directed by a doctor.
KEEP OUT OF THE REACH OF CHILDREN.

Accidental Ingestion: In case of accidental ingestion, seek professional assistance or contact a Poison Control Center immediately.

Consumer Information: For best performance, vaporizer should be thoroughly cleaned after each use according to manufacturer's instructions. In soft water areas, it may be necessary to add salt or other steaming aid to promote boiling. Follow directions of vaporizer manufacturer for best results.

How Supplied: Available in 4 fl. oz. and 6 fl. oz. bottles.

VICKS VATRONOL®

[*vātrōnŏl*]

Nose Drops

Active Ingredients: Ephedrine Sulfate 0.5%.

Inactive Ingredients: Camphor, Cedarleaf Oil, Eucalyptol, Menthol, Nutmeg Oil, Potassium Phosphate, Purified Water, Sodium Chloride, Sodium Phosphate, Tyloxapol.
Preservative: Thimerosal 0.001%.

Indications: For temporary relief of nasal congestion due to a cold, hay fever or other respiratory allergies.

Actions: VICKS VATRONOL helps restore freer breathing by relieving nasal stuffiness. Relieves sinus pressure.

Dosage: *Adults:* Fill dropper to upper mark. *Children (6–12 years):* Fill dropper to lower mark. *Children under 6 years of age:* consult a doctor.
Apply up one nostril, repeat in other nostril.
Repeat not more than every four hours as needed.

Warning: Do not exceed recommended dosage because burning, stinging, sneezing, or increase of nasal discharge may occur. The use of this container by more than one person may spread infection. Do not take this product for more than 3 days. If symptoms persist, consult a doctor. Do not use this product if you have heart disease, high blood pressure, thyroid disease, diabetes, or difficulty in urination due to enlargement of the prostate gland unless directed by a doctor. Keep this and all drugs out of the reach of children. In case of accidental ingestion, seek professional assistance or contact a poison control center immediately.

How Supplied: Available in ½ fl. oz. and 1 fl. oz. dropper bottles.

IDENTIFICATION PROBLEM?
Consult the
Product Identification Section
where you'll find
products pictured
in full color.

Roberts Pharmaceutical Corporation

6-G INDUSTRIAL WAY WEST
EATONTOWN, NJ 07724

CHERACOL® Nasal Spray Pump Cherry Scented

Description: CHERACOL® NASAL SPRAY PUMP is a cherry scented long acting topical nasal decongestant. One application lasts up to 12 hours.

Indications: For the temporary relief of a nasal congestion associated with colds ("flu"), hay fever, and sinusitis.

Active Ingredients: Oxymetazoline hydrochloride USP 0.05% (0.5 mg/ml).

Inactive Ingredients: Benzalkonium chloride, glycine, phenylmercuric acetate (0.02 mg/ml), sorbitol, cherry flavor, and purified water.

Dosage and Administration: CHERACOL Nasal Spray has a long duration of action lasting up to 12 hours with each topical application. One application mornings and at bedtime is usually sufficient for round-the-clock action. For adults and children 6 years of age and over: Two or three sprays in each nostril twice daily—morning and bedtime. Remove protective cap. Hold bottle with thumb at base and nozzle between first and second fingers. With head upright, insert metered pump spray nozzle in nostril. Depress pump 2 or 3 times all the way down with a firm even stroke and sniff deeply. Repeat in other nostril. Do not tilt head backward while spraying. Wipe tip clean after each use. Before using the first time, remove the protective cap from the tip and prime the metered pump by depressing pump firmly several times.

Warning: Do not give this product to children under 6 years of age except under the advice and supervision of a physician. Do not exceed recommended dosage because symptoms may occur such as burning, stinging, sneezing or increase of nasal discharge. Do not use this product for more than 3 days. If symptoms persist, consult a physician. The use of this dispenser by more than one person may spread infection. Store at room temperature. Keep this and all medicines out of children's reach. In case of accidental ingestion contact a physician or poison control center immediately.

Overdosage: For overdose treatment, contact a regional poison control center.

How Supplied: Available in 1 fluid ounce bottles fitted with a metered pump (NDC 54092-0880-30).

CHERACOL® Sore Throat Spray Anesthetic/Antiseptic Liquid

Description: A pleasant tasting cherry flavored liquid spray with anesthetic and antiseptic properties.

Indications: For the temporary relief of occasional minor sore throat pain and irritation. Also for temporary relief of pain associated with sore mouth, canker sores, tonsillitis, pharnyngitis and throat infections.

Active Ingredients: Phenol 1.4%.

Inactive Ingredients: Alcohol 12.5%, citric acid, FD&C Red No. 40, flavor, glycerin, propylene glycol, sodium citrate, sodium saccharin, sorbitol and purified water.

Directions For Use: Mouthwash and gargle: Irritated throat: Spray 5 times (children 2–12 years of age, 3 times) and swallow. May be used as a gargle. Repeat every 2 hours or as directed by physician or dentist. Children under 12 years of age should be supervised in the use of this product.

Warning: If sore throat is severe, persists for more than 2 days, is accompanied or followed by fever, headache, rash, nausea or vomiting, consult a doctor promptly. If sore mouth symptoms do not improve in 7 days, see your doctor or dentist promptly. In case of accidental overdosage, seek professional assistance or contact poison control center immediately. As with any drug, if you are pregnant or nursing a baby, seek the advice of a health professional before using this product. Do not administer to children under 2 years unless directed by a physician or dentist. Keep this and all medicines out of the reach of children.

How Supplied: Available in 12 fluid ounce spray pump bottle (NDC 54092-0340-06).

CHERACOL-D® Cough Formula Maximum Strength Cough Formula

Description: CHERACOL-D® is a non-narcotic cough formula which combines two important medicines in one safe, fast-acting pleasant tasting liquid:

- The highest level of cough suppressant available without prescription.
- A clinically proven expectorant to help loosen phlegm and drain bronchial tubes.

Indications: CHERACOL-D® cough formula helps quiet dry, hacking coughs, and helps loosen phlegm and mucus. Recommended for adults and children 2 years of age and older.

Active Ingredients: Each teaspoonful (5 ml) contains dextromethorphan hydrobromide, 10 mg; guaifenesin, 100 mg; alcohol, 4.75%. Also contains benzoic acid, FD&C Red #40, flavors, fragrances, fructose, glycerin, propylene glycol, sodium chloride, sucrose, and purified water.

Dosage and Administration: Adults and children 12 years of age and over: 2 teaspoonfuls. Children 6 to 12 years: 1 teaspoonful. Children 2 to 6 years: ½ teaspoonful. May be repeated every 4 hours if necessary. Children under 2 years, consult a physician.

Warnings: Keep this and all drugs out of the reach of children. In case of accidental overdose, seek professional assistance or contact a poison control center immediately. Do not give this product to children under 2 years of age except under the advice and supervision of a physician. Do not use this product for persistent or chronic cough such as occurs with smoking, asthma, or emphysema or where cough is accompanied by excessive secretions except under the advice and supervision of a physician. As with any drug, if you are pregnant or nursing a baby, seek the advice of a health professional before using this product.

Caution: A persistent cough may be a sign of a serious condition. If cough persists for more than 1 week, tends to recur or is accompanied by high fever, rash or persistent headache, consult a physician.

How Supplied: Available in 2 oz bottle (NDC 54092-0400-60), 4 oz bottle (NDC 54092-0400-04), and 6 oz bottle (NDC 54092-0400-06).

Shown in Product Identification Section, page 425

CHERACOL PLUS® Cough Syrup Multisymptom cough/cold formula

Description: CHERACOL PLUS® Cough Syrup is a pleasant tasting 3-ingredient non-narcotic liquid formulation.

Indications: Cheracol Plus syrup is an effective 3-ingredient, maximum strength formula for the temporary relief of head cold symptoms and cough (without narcotic side effects).

Active Ingredients: Each tablespoonful (15ml) contains phenylpropanolamine, 25 mg; dextromethorphan hydrobromide, 20 mg; chlorpheniramine maleate, 4 mg; and alcohol, 8%.

Inactive Ingredients: Flavors, glycerin, methylparaben, propylene glycol, propylparaben, FD&C Red No. 40, sodium chloride, sorbitol solution, and purified water.

Dosage and Administration: Adults and children over 12 years of age: 1 tablespoonful (15ml) every 4 hours or as directed by a physician. Do not take more than 6 tablespoonfuls in a 24 hour period. Do not administer to children under 12 years of age.

Uses: Cheracol Plus® multisymptom head cold/cough formula provides cough suppressant and decongestant activity and controls runny nose associated with the common cold ("flu").

Warnings: Do not take this product for persistent or chronic cough such as occurs with smoking, asthma, or emphysema or where cough is accompanied by excessive secretions or if you have high blood pressure, heart or thyroid disease, diabetes, asthma, glaucoma, or difficulty in urination due to enlargement of the prostate gland except under the advice and supervision of a physician. If symptoms do not improve within 7 days or are accompanied by high fever, consult a physician before continuing use. May cause excitability, especially in children.

Continued on next page

Roberts—Cont.

Do not give this product to children under 12 years except under the advice and supervision of a physician. As with any drug, if you are pregnant or nursing a baby consult a health professional before using this product.

Drug Interaction Precaution: Do not take this product if you are presently taking antihypertensive or antidepressant medication containing a monoamine oxidase inhibitor except under the advice and supervision of a physician.

How Supplied: Available in 4 oz bottle (NDC 54092-0401-04), 6 oz bottle (54092-0401-06).

Shown in Product Identification Section, page 425

CITROCARBONATE® Antacid

Active Ingredients: When dissolved, each 3.9 grams (1 teaspoonful) contains approximately: sodium bicarbonate, 0.78 gram and sodium citrate, 1.82 grams. **As derived from (per teaspoonful):** sodium bicarbonate 2.34 gram; citric acid anhydrous, 1.19 gram; sodium citrate hydrous, 254 mg; calcium lactate pentahydrate, 151 mg; sodium chloride, 79 mg; monobasic sodium phosphate anhydrous, 44 mg; and, magnesium sulfate dried, 42 mg. Each 3.9 grams (teaspoonful) contains 30.46 mEq (700.6 mg) of sodium.

Indications: For the relief of heartburn, acid indigestion, and sour stomach; and upset stomach associated with these symptoms.

Dosage and Administration: Adults: 1 to 2 teaspoonfuls (not to exceed 5 level teaspoonfuls per day) in a glass of cold water after meals. Persons 60 years or older; ½ to 1 teaspoonful after meals. Children 6 to 12 years: ¼ to ½ teaspoonful. For children under 6 years: Consult physician.

How Supplied: Available in 5 oz (NDC 54092-0900-05) and 10 oz (NDC 54092-0900-10) bottles.

CLOCREAM®
Skin Protectant Cream

Description: CLOCREAM® skin protectant cream contains Vitamins A and D in a greaseless vanishing cream base that leaves no residue. Also contains cetylpalmitate, cottonseed oil, glyceryl monostearate, fragrance, methylparaben, mineral oil, potassium stearate, propylparaben, sodium citrate, and purified oil. Each ounce of CLOCREAM® contains Vitamins A and D equivalent to 1 ounce of cod liver oil.

Indications: CLOCREAM® is indicated for the temporary relief of chapped skin, diaper rash, wind burn and sunburn; and minor non-infected skin irritations. CLOCREAM® promotes epithelialization.

Uses: CLOCREAM® may be particularly useful for health care personnel or others who frequently wash their hands and for general patient care to reduce dermal excoriation and breakdown from prolonged bed rest, bedwetting and abrasions. The vanishing action of CLOCREAM skin protectant cream makes it cosmetically acceptable when the skin treated is on an exposed part of the body such as the hands or arms.

Warnings: CLOCREAM® skin protectant cream is for external use only. Avoid contact with the eyes. If condition worsens or if symptoms persist for more than 7 days, discontinue use of this product and consult a physician. Keep this and all medications out of the reach of children. In case of accidental ingestion seek professional assistance or contact a poison control center immediately.

Dosage and Administration: Gently massage or apply liberally to unbroken skin or abraded skin where promotion of epitheliazation is denied. Use as often as desired.

How Supplied: Available in 1 ounce tubes (NDC 54092-0300-30).

HALTRAN® Tablets
Ibuprofen/Analgesic
MENSTRUAL CRAMP RELIEVER

WARNING: ASPIRIN SENSITIVE PATIENTS. Do not take this product if you have had a severe allergic reaction to aspirin, eg—asthma, swelling, shock or hives, because even though this product contains no aspirin or salicylates cross-reactions may occur in patients allergic to aspirin.

Indications: For the pain of menstrual cramps and also the temporary relief of minor aches and pains associated with the common cold, headache, toothache, muscular aches, backache, for the minor pain of arthritis and for reduction of fever.

Directions: *Adults:* Take 1 tablet every 4 to 6 hours while symptoms persist. If pain or fever does not respond to 1 tablet, 2 tablets may be used, but do not exceed 6 tablets in 24 hours, unless directed by a doctor. The smallest effective dose should be used. Take with food or milk if occasional and mild heartburn, upset stomach, or stomach pain occurs with use. Consult a doctor if these symptoms are more than mild or if they persist. *Children:* Do not give this product to children under 12 except under the advice and supervision of a doctor.

Warnings: Do not take for pain for more than 10 days or for fever for more than 3 days unless directed by a doctor. If pain or fever persists or gets worse, if new symptoms occur, or if the painful area is red or swollen, consult a doctor. These could be signs of serious illness. If you are under a doctor's care for any serious condition, consult a doctor before taking this product. As with aspirin and acetaminophen, if you have any condition which requires you to take prescription drugs or if you have had any problems or serious side effects from taking any non-prescription pain reliever, do not take HALTRAN Tablets (ibuprofen) without first discussing it with your doctor. If you experience any symptoms which are unusual or seem unrelated to the condition for which you took ibuprofen, consult a doctor before taking any more of it. Although ibuprofen is indicated for the same conditions as aspirin and acetaminophen, it should not be taken with them except under a doctor's direction. Before using any drug, including HALTRAN, you should seek the advice of a health professional if you are pregnant or nursing a baby. IT IS ESPECIALLY IMPORTANT NOT TO USE IBUPROFEN DURING THE LAST 3 MONTHS OF PREGNANCY UNLESS SPECIFICALLY DIRECTED TO DO SO BY A DOCTOR BECAUSE IT MAY CAUSE PROBLEMS IN THE UNBORN CHILD OR COMPLICATIONS DURING DELIVERY. Keep this and all drugs out of the reach of children. In case of accidental overdose, seek professional assistance or contact a poison control center immediately.

Active Ingredient: Each tablet contains ibuprofen USP 200 mg.

Other Ingredients: Carnauba wax, cornstarch, hydroxypropyl methylcellulose, propylene glycol, silicon dioxide, pregelatinized starch, stearic acid, and titanium dioxide.
Store at room temperature. Avoid excessive heat 40°C (104°F).

How Supplied: Available in bottles of 30 (NDC 54092-0020-30).

Shown in Product Identification Section, page 425

ORTHOXICOL® Cough Syrup
Multisymptom cough/cold formula

Description: ORTHOXICOL® Cough Syrup is a pleasant tasting 3-ingredient non-narcotic liquid formulation.

Indications: Orthoxicol syrup is an effective 3-ingredient, maximum strength formula for the temporary relief of head cold symptoms and cough (without narcotic side effects).

Active Ingredients: Each tablespoonful (15 ml) contains phenylpropanolamine, 25 mg; dextromethorphan hydrobromide, 20 mg; chlorpheniramine, 4 mg; and alcohol, 8%.

Inactive Ingredients: Flavors, glycerin, methylparaben, propylene glycol, propylparaben, FD&C Red No. 40, sodium chloride, sorbitol solution, and purified water.

Dosage and Administration: Adults and children over 12 years of age: 1 tablespoonful (15 ml) every 4 hours or as directed by a physician. Do not take more than 6 tablespoonfuls in a 24 hour period. Do not administer to children under 12 years of age.

Uses: Orthoxicol multisymptom head cold/cough formula provides cough suppressant and decongestant activity and controls runny nose associated with the common cold ("flu").

Warnings: Do not take this product for persistent or chronic cough such as occurs with smoking, asthma, or emphysema or where cough is accompanied by excessive secretions or if you have high blood pressure, heart or thyroid disease, diabetes, asthma, glaucoma, or difficulty in urination due to enlargement of the prostate gland except under the advice and supervision of a physician. If symptoms do not improve within 7 days or are accompanied by high fever, consult a physician before continuing use. May cause excitability, especially in children. Do not give this product to children under 12 years except under the advice and supervision of a physician. As with any drug, if you are pregnant or nursing a baby consult a health professional before using this product.

Drug Interaction Precaution: Do not take this product if you are presently taking antihypertensive or antidepressant medication containing a monoamine oxidase inhibitor except under the advice and supervision of a physician.

How Supplied: Available in 2 oz bottle (NDC 54092-0410-60), 4 oz bottle (NDC 54092-0410-04), 16 oz bottle (NDC 54092-0410-16).

P-A-C® Analgesic Tablets

Description: A combination tablet formulation providing more pain-relieving ingredients per tablet than conventional tablets.

Indications: P-A-C® tablets are indicated for the temporary relief of occasional minor aches, pains, headache and the reduction of fever.

Active Ingredients: Each tablet contains: aspirin; caffeine anhydrous, 32 mg. Contains non-standard strength of 400 mg (6.17 gr) aspirin per tablet compared to the established standard of 325 mg (5 gr) aspirin per tablet.

Inactive Ingredients: Cellulose, corn starch, croscarmellose sodium, FD&C Blue No. 2, FD&C Yellow No. 5 (tartrazine), sucrose.

Directions For Use: (except under the advice and supervision of a physician): Adults—1 or 2 tablets every 4 hours while symptoms persist not to exceed 10 tablets in 24 hours for not more than 10 days, or in the presence of fever for more than 3 days (72 hours). Children (see warnings)—9 to 12 years: 1 tablet every 4 hours while symptoms persist not to exceed 5 single doses in 24 hours for not more than 5 days, or in the presence of fever for not more than 3 days (72 hours). Do not use in children under 9 years.

Warnings: Children and teenagers should not use this product for chickenpox or flu symptoms before a physician is consulted about Reye Syndrome, a rare but serious illness reported to be associated with aspirin. Do not take this product if you are allergic to aspirin or if you have asthma. As with any drug, if you are pregnant or nursing a baby seek the advice of a health professional before you use this product. Do not exceed recommended dosage.

Cautions: (except under the advice and supervision of a physician): Do not take this product if you have stomach distress, ulcers, bleeding problems, are presently taking a prescription drug for anticoagulation (thinning of the blood), diabetes, gout, arthritis, or for the treatment of arthritis. Stop taking this product if ringing of the ears or other symptoms occur. In case of accidental overdose seek professional assistance or contact a poison control center immediately.

How Supplied: Available in bottles of 100 (NDC 54092-0010-01), and 1000 (NDC 54092-0010-10) tablets.

Shown in Product Identification Shown, page 425

PYRROXATE® Capsules
Extra Strength Decongestant/Antihistamine/ Analgesic Capsules

Description: *Pyrroxate®* provides single-capsule, multisymptom relief for colds, allergies, nasal/sinus congestion, runny nose, sneezing, and watery eyes. Because it contains the non-aspirin analgesic **acetaminophen,** *Pyrroxate* gives temporary relief of occasional minor aches, pains, headache, and helps in the reduction of fever. *Pyrroxate* is caffeine and aspirin-free.

Ingredients: Each *Pyrroxate* Capsule contains: chlorpheniramine maleate, 4 mg; phenylpropanolamine HCl, 25 mg; acetaminophen, 500 mg. The 500 mg (7.69 gr) strength of acetaminophen per capsule is non-standard, as compared to the established standard of 325 mg (5 gr) acetaminophen per capsule. Also contains benzyl alcohol, butylparaben, D&C yellow No. 10, erythrosine sodium, FD&C blue No. 1, FD&C yellow No. 6 (sunset yellow) as a color additive, gelatin, glycerin, magnesium stearate, methylparaben, propylparaben, sodium lauryl sulfate, sodium propionate, starch, and talc.

Indications: *Pyrroxate* Capsules are for the temporary relief of runny nose, sneezing, itching of the nose or throat; for the temporary relief of nasal congestion due to the common cold, allergies (hay fever), and sinus congestion; for the temporary relief of occasional minor aches, pains, headache, and for the reduction of fever.

Actions: Chlorpheniramine maleate is an antihistamine effective in controlling runny nose, sneezing, watery eyes, and itching of the nose and throat. Phenylpropanolamine HCl is an oral nasal decongestant effective in relieving nasal/sinus congestion due to the common cold or allergies (hay fever). Acetaminophen is a clinically effective analgesic and antipyretic without aspirin side effects.

Warnings: Do not take this product for more than 7 days. If symptoms persist, do not improve, or new ones occur, or if fever persists for more than 3 days, discontinue use and consult your physician. Do not take this product if you have asthma, glaucoma, difficulty in urination due to the enlargement of the prostate gland, high blood pressure, diabetes, thyroid disease, or if you are presently taking a prescription antihypertensive or antidepressant drug containing a monamine oxidase inhibitor, except under the advice and supervision of a physician. As with any drug, if you are pregnant or nursing a baby, seek the advice of a health professional before using this product. Do not exceed recommended dosage because severe liver damage may occur and at higher doses, nervousness, dizziness or sleeplessness may occur. Do not take this product for the treatment of arthritis except under the advice and supervision of a physician.

Cautions: Avoid alcoholic beverages, driving a motor vehicle, or operating heavy machinery while taking this product. This product may cause drowsiness or excitability, especially in children. Keep this and all drugs out of the reach of children. In case of accidental overdose, seek professional assistance or contact a poison control center immediately.

Dosage and Administration: Take 1 capsule every 4 hours or as directed by a physician. Do not take more than 6 capsules in a 24-hour period. Do not administer to children under 12 years of age.

How Supplied: Black/yellow capsules available in bottles of 24 (NDC 54092-0040-24) and 500 (NDC 54092-0040-05).

Shown in Product Identification Section, page 425

SIGTAB® Tablets
High Potency Vitamin Supplement

Each tablet contains:		% U.S. RDA*
Vitamin A	5000 IU	100
Vitamin D	400 IU	100
Vitamin E	15 IU	50
Vitamin C	333 mg	555
Folic Acid	0.4 mg	100
Thiamine	10.3 mg	686
Riboflavin	10 mg	588
Niacin	100 mg	500
Vitamin B_6	6 mg	300
Vitamin B_{12}	18 mcg	300
Pantothenic Acid	20 mg	200

*Percentage of U.S. Recommended Daily Allowance.

Recommended Dosage: 1 tablet daily

Ingredient List: Sucrose, Sodium Ascorbate (Vit. C), Calcium Sulfate, Niacinamide, Vitamin E Acetate, Calcium Pantothenate, Vitamin A Acetate, Thiamine Mononitrate (B-1), Riboflavin (B-2), Gelatin, Pyridoxine HCl (B-6), Povidone, Lacca, Magnesium Stearate, Silica, Artificial Color, Sodium Benzoate, Folic Acid, Polyethylene Glycol, Cholecalciferol (Vit. D), Carnauba Wax, Cyanocobalamin (B-12), Medical Antifoam.

Continued on next page

Roberts—Cont.

How Supplied: Available in bottles of 90 (NDC 54092-0033-90) and 500 (NDC 54092-0033-05).

Shown in Product Identification Section, page 425

ZYMACAP® Capsules
High Potency Vitamin Supplement

Description: Dietary multivitamin supplement providing 150% of the RDA for Vitamin B and Vitamin C plus 100% of the RDA for Vitamins A and D.

Each Capsule Contains:		% US RDA*
Vitamin A	5,000 IU	100
Vitamin D	400 IU	100
Vitamin E	15 IU	50
Vitamin C	90 mg	150
Folic Acid	400 mcg	100
Thiamine	2.25 mg	150
Riboflavin	2.6 mg	150
Niacin	30 mg	150
Vitamin B-6	3 mg	150
Vitamin B-12	9 mcg	150
Pantothenic Acid	15 mg	150

*Percentage of U.S. recommended daily allowance.

Recommended Dosage: 1 Capsule daily.

Ingredient List: Soybean oil, ascorbic acid (Vitamin C), gelatin, glycerin, niacinamide, calcium pantothenate, Vitamin E acetate, lecithin, pyridoxine hydrochloride (Vitamin B-6), yellow wax, thiamine mononitrate (Vitamin B-1), riboflavin (Vitamin B-2), Vitamin A palmitate, corn oil, FD&C Red No. 40, folic acid, titanium dioxide, ethyl vanillin, vanilla enhancer, cholecalciferol (Vitamin D), cyanocobalamin (Vitamin B-12).

How Supplied: Available in bottles of 90 capsules (NDC 54092-0030-90).

A. H. Robins Company, Inc.

Subsidiary of American Home Products Corporation
CONSUMER PRODUCTS DIVISION
3800 CUTSHAW AVENUE
RICHMOND, VIRGINIA 23230

ALLBEE® C-800 TABLETS
[*all-be'*]
ALLBEE® C-800
plus IRON TABLETS

Allbee C-800

One tablet daily provides:	Percentage of U.S. Recommended Daily Allowances (U.S. RDA)	
Vitamin E	150	45 I.U.
Vitamin C	1333	800 mg
Thiamine (Vitamin B_1)	1000	15 mg
Riboflavin (Vitamin B_2)	1000	17 mg
Niacin	500	100 mg
Vitamin B_6	1250	25 mg
Vitamin B_{12}	200	12 mcg
Pantothenic Acid	250	25 mg

Ingredients: Ascorbic Acid, Niacinamide Ascorbate, Modified Starch, Vitamin E Acetate, Hydrolyzed Protein, Calcium Pantothenate, Hydroxypropyl Methylcellulose, Pyridoxine Hydrochloride, Riboflavin, Stearic Acid, Thiamine Mononitrate, Artificial Color, Silicon Dioxide, Lactose, Magnesium Stearate, Povidone, Polyethylene Glycol 400 or 4000, Vanillin, Gelatin, Polysorbate 20 or 80, Sorbic Acid, Sodium Benzoate, Cyanocobalamin. May also contain: Hydroxypropylcellulose and Propylene Glycol.

Allbee C-800 plus Iron

One tablet daily provides: Vitamin Composition	Percentage of U.S. Recommended Daily Allowances (U.S. RDA)	
Vitamin E	150	45.0 I.U.
Vitamin C	1333	800.0 mg
Folic Acid	100	0.4 mg
Thiamine (Vitamin B_1)	1000	15.0 mg
Riboflavin (Vitamin B_2)	1000	17.0 mg
Niacin	500	100.0 mg
Vitamin B_6	1250	25.0 mg
Vitamin B_{12}	200	12.0 mcg
Pantothenic Acid	250	25.0 mg
Mineral Composition		
Iron	150	27.0 mg

Ingredients: Ascorbic Acid, Niacinamide Ascorbate, Ferrous Fumarate, Modified Starch, Vitamin E Acetate, Hydrolyzed Protein, Calcium Pantothenate, Hydroxypropyl Methylcellulose, Pyridoxine Hydrochloride, Riboflavin, Stearic Acid, Thiamine Mononitrate, Povidone, Silicon Dioxide, Artificial Color, Lactose, Magnesium Stearate, Polyethylene Glycol 400 or 4000, Vanillin, Gelatin, Folic Acid, Polysorbate 20 or 80, Sorbic Acid, Sodium Benzoate, Cyanocobalamin. May also contain: Hydroxypropylcellulose and Propylene Glycol.

Actions and Uses: The components of Allbee C-800 have important roles in general nutrition, healing of wounds, and prevention of hemorrhage. Allbee C-800 is recommended for nutritional supplementation of these components in conditions such as febrile diseases, chronic or acute infections, burns, fractures, surgery, physiologic stress, alcoholism, prolonged exposure to high temperature, geriatrics, gastritis, peptic ulcer, and colitis; and in weight-reduction and other special diets.
In dentistry, Allbee C-800 is recommended for nutritional supplementation of its components in conditions such as herpetic stomatitis, aphthous stomatitis, cheilosis, herpangina and gingivitis.
In addition, Allbee C-800 Plus Iron is recommended as a nutritional source of iron. The iron is present as ferrous fumarate, a well-tolerated salt. The ascorbic acid in the formulation enhances the absorption of iron.

Precautions: Do not take Allbee C-800 Plus Iron within two hours of oral tetracycline antibiotics, since oral iron products interfere with absorption of tetracycline. Not intended for treatment of iron-deficiency anemia.

Adverse Reactions: Iron-containing medications may occasionally cause gastrointestinal discomfort, nausea, constipation or diarrhea.

Dosage: The recommended OTC dosage for adults and children twelve or more years of age is one tablet daily. Under the direction and supervision of a physician, the dose and frequency of administration may be increased in accordance with the patient's requirements.

How Supplied: Allbee C-800—orange, film-coated, elliptically-shaped tablets engraved AHR on one side and 0677 on the other in bottles of 60 (NDC 0031-0677-62). Allbee C-800 Plus Iron—red, film-coated, elliptically-shaped tablets engraved AHR on one side and 0678 on the other in bottles of 60 (NDC 0031-0678-62).

ALLBEE® WITH C CAPLETS
[*all-be'*]

One caplet daily provides:	Percentage of U.S. Recommended Daily Allowance (U.S. RDA)	
Vitamin C	500	300.0 mg
Thiamine (Vitamin B_1)	1000	15.0 mg
Riboflavin (Vitamin B_2)	600	10.2 mg
Niacin	250	50.0 mg
Vitamin B_6	250	5.0 mg
Pantothenic Acid	100	10.0 mg

Ingredients: Niacinamide Ascorbate; Ascorbic Acid; Microcrystalline Cellulose; Corn Starch; Thiamine Mononitrate; Calcium Pantothenate; Riboflavin; Hydroxypropyl Methylcellulose; Pyridoxine Hydrochloride; Magnesium Stearate; Silicon Dioxide; Propylene Glycol; Lactose; Methacrylic Acid Copolymer; Triethyl Citrate; Titanium Dioxide; Polysorbate 20; Artificial Flavor; Saccharin Sodium; Sodium Sorbate.

Action and Uses: Allbee with C is a high-potency formulation of B and C vitamins. Its components have important roles in general nutrition, healing of wounds, and prevention of hemorrhage. It is recommended for deficiencies of B-vitamins and ascorbic acid in conditions such as febrile diseases, chronic or acute infections, burns, fractures, surgery, toxic conditions, physiologic stress, alcoholism, prolonged exposure to high temperature, geriatrics, gastritis, peptic ulcer, and colitis; and in conditions involving special diets and weight-reduction diets.
In dentistry, Allbee with C is recommended for deficiencies of B-vitamins and ascorbic acid in conditions such as herpetic stomatitis, aphthous stomatitis, cheilosis, herpangina, gingivitis.

Dosage: The recommended OTC dosage for adults and children twelve or more years of age, is one caplet daily. Under the direction and supervision of a physician, the dose and frequency of administration may be increased in accordance with the patient's requirements.

How Supplied: Yellow, capsule-shaped, film-coated tablets engraved AHR on one side and Allbee C on the other in bottles of 130 (NDC 0031-0673-66), 1,000 caplets (NDC 0031-0673-74), and in Dis-Co® Unit Dose Packs of 100 (NDC 0031-0673-64).

CHAP STICK® Lip Balm

Active Ingredients: 44% Petrolatums, 1.5% Padimate O (2-ethyl-hexyl *p*-dimethylaminobenzoate, 1% Lanolin, 1% Isopropyl Myristate, 0.5% Cetyl Alcohol.

Inactive Ingredients:
Regular: Arachadyl Propionate, Camphor, Carnauba Wax, D&C Red 6 Barium Lake, FD&C Yellow 5 Aluminum Lake, Fragrance, Isopropyl Lanolate, Methylparaben, Mineral Oil, 2-Octyl Dodecanol, Oleyl Alcohol, Polyphenylmethylsiloxane 556, Propylparaben, Titanium Dioxide, Wax Paraffin, White Wax.
Cherry: Arachadyl Propionate, Camphor, Carnauba Wax, D&C Red 6 Barium Lake, Flavors, Isopropyl Lanolate, Methylparaben, Mineral Oil, 2-Octyl Dodecanol, Polyphenylmethylsiloxane 556, Propylparaben, Saccharin, Wax Paraffin, White Wax.
Mint: Arachadyl Propionate, Carnauba Wax, FD&C Blue 1 Aluminum Lake, FD&C Yellow 5 Lake, Flavors, Isopropyl Lanolate, Methylparaben, Mineral Oil, 2-Octyl Dodecanol, Polyphenylmethylsiloxane 556, Propylparaben, Saccharin, Wax Paraffin, White Wax.
Orange: Arachadyl Propionate, Carnauba Wax, FD&C Yellow 6 Aluminum Lake, Flavors, Isopropyl Lanolate, Methylparaben, Mineral Oil, 2-Octyl Dodecanol, Polyphenylmethylsiloxane 556, Propylparaben, Saccharin, Wax Paraffin, White Wax.
Strawberry: Arachadyl Propionate, Camphor, Carnauba Wax, D&C Red 6 Barium Lake, Flavors, Isopropyl Lanolate, Methylparaben, Mineral Oil, 2-Octyl Dodecanol, Polyphenylmethylsiloxane 556, Propylparaben, Saccharin, Wax Paraffin, White Wax.

Indications: Helps prevention and healing of dry, chapped, sun and windburned lips.

Actions: A specially designed lipid complex hydrophobic base containing Padimate O which forms a barrier to prevent moisture loss and protect lips from the drying effects of cold weather, wind and sun which cause chapping. The special emollients soften the skin by forming an occlusive film thus inducing hydration, restoring suppleness to the lips, and preventing drying from evaporation of water that diffuses to the surface from the underlying layers of tissue. Chap Stick also protects the skin from the external environment and its sunscreen offers protection from exposure to the sun.

Warning: Discontinue use if signs of irritation appear.

Symptoms and Treatment of Oral Ingestion: The oral LD_{50} in rats is greater than 5 gm/kg. There have been no reported overdoses in humans. There are no known symptoms of overdosage.

Dosage and Treatment: For dry, chapped lips apply as needed. To help prevent dry, chapped sun or windburned lips, apply to lips as needed before, during and following exposure to sun, wind, water and cold weather.

Professional Labeling: None.

How Supplied: Available in 4.25 gm tubes in Regular, Mint, Cherry, Orange, and Strawberry flavors.

Shown in Product Identification Section, page 425

CHAP STICK® SUNBLOCK 15 Lip Balm

Active Ingredients: 44% Petrolatums, 7% Padimate O, 3% Oxybenzone, 0.5% Lanolin, 0.5% Isopropyl Myristate, 0.5% Cetyl Alcohol.

Inactive Ingredients: Camphor, Carnauba Wax, D&C Red 6 Barium Lake, FD&C Yellow 5 Aluminum Lake, Fragrance, Isopropyl Lanolate, Methylparaben, Mineral Oil, Propylparaben, Titanium Dioxide, Wax Paraffin, White Wax.

Indications: Ultra Sunscreen Protection (SPF-15). Helps prevention and healing of dry, chapped, sun and windburned lips. Overexposure to sun may lead to premature aging of skin and lip cancer. Liberal and regular use may help reduce the sun's harmful effects.

Actions: Ultra sunscreen protection for the lips, plus the attributes of Chap Stick® Lip Balm. The emollients in the specially designed lipid complex hydrophobic base soften the lips by forming an occlusive film while the two sunscreens have specific ultraviolet absorption ranges which overlap to offer ultra sunscreen protection (SPF-15).

Warning: Discontinue use if signs of irritation appear.

Symptoms and Treatment of Oral Ingestion: Toxicity studies indicate this product to be extremely safe. The oral LD_{50} in rats is greater than 5 gm./kg. There are no known symptoms of overdosage.

Dosage and Treatment: For ultra sunscreen protection, apply evenly and liberally to lips before exposure to sun. Reapply as needed. For dry, chapped lips, apply as needed. To help prevent dry, chapped, sun, and windburned lips, apply to lips as needed before, during, and following exposure to sun, wind, water, and cold weather.

How Supplied: 4.25 gm. tube.

Shown in Product Identification Section, page 425

CHAP STICK® PETROLEUM JELLY PLUS

REGULAR:

Active Ingredients: 99% White Petrolatum, USP

Other Ingredients: Aloe, Butylated Hydroxytoluene, Flavor, Lanolin, Phenonip.

CHERRY:

Active Ingredients: 98.85% White Petrolatum, USP.

Other Ingredients: Aloe, Butylated Hydroxytoluene, D&C Red 6 Barium Lake, Flavors, Lanolin, Phenonip, and Saccharin.

Indications: Helps prevent and protect against dry, chapped, sun and windburned lips.

Actions: White Petrolatum, USP forms a barrier to prevent moisture loss and protect lips from the drying effects of cold weather, wind and sun which cause chapping. White Petrolatum, USP helps soften the skin by forming an occlusive film for inducing hydration, restoring suppleness to the lips and preventing drying from evaporation of water that diffuses to the surface from the underlying layers of tissue.

Warning: If condition worsens or does not improve within 7 days, consult a doctor.

Dosage and Treatment: To help prevent dry, chapped, sun or wind-burned lips, apply to lips as needed before, during and following exposure to sun, wind, water and cold weather.

How Supplied: Regular and Cherry flavored available in 0.35 oz. (10 grams) polyethylene tube.

Shown in Product Identification Section page 425

CHAP STICK® PETROLEUM JELLY PLUS WITH SUNBLOCK 15

Active Ingredients: 89% White Petrolatum, USP, 7% Padimate O, 3% Oxybenzone.

Other Ingredients: Aloe, Butylated Hydroxytoluene, Flavor, Lanolin, Phenonip.

Indications: Ultra Sunscreen Protection (SPF-15). Helps prevent and protect against dry, chapped, sun and windburned lips. Overexposure to sun may lead to premature aging of skin and skin cancer. Liberal and regular use may help reduce the sun's harmful effects.

Continued on next page

Prescribing information on A.H. Robins products listed here is based on official labeling in effect November 1, 1990 with Indications, Contraindications, Warnings, Precautions, Adverse Reactions, and Dosage stated in full.

Robins—Cont.

Actions: Ultra sunscreen protection for the lips, plus the attributes of Chap Stick® Petroleum Jelly Plus. White Petrolatum, USP forms a barrier to prevent moisture loss and protect lips from the drying effects of wind and sun while two sunscreens, which have specific ultra violet absorption ranges, overlap to provide ultra sunscreen protection (SPF-15).

Warning: For external use only. Avoid contact with eyes. Discontinue use if signs of irritation or rash occur.

Dosage and Treatment: For ultra sunscreen protection, apply evenly and liberally to lips before exposure to sun. Reapply as needed. For dry chapped lips, apply as needed. To help prevent dry, chapped, sun and windburned lips, apply to lips as needed before, during and following exposure to sun, wind, water and cold weather.

How Supplied: Available in 0.35 oz (10 grams) polyethylene tube.

Shown in Product Identification Section, page 425

DIMACOL® Caplets

[*di 'mă-col*]

Description: Each caplet contains:

Guaifenesin, USP ....100 mg
Pseudoephedrine Hydrochloride, USP ....30 mg
Dextromethorphan Hydrobromide, USP ....10 mg

Inactive Ingredients: D&C Yellow 10 Aluminum Lake, FD&C Yellow 6 Aluminum Lake, Flavor, Hydroxypropyl Methylcellulose, Magnesium Stearate, Methacrylic Acid Copolymer, Methylparaben, Microcrystalline Cellulose, Polysorbate 20, Potassium Sorbate, Povidone, Propylene Glycol, Propylparaben, Saccharin Sodium, Silicon Dioxide, Titanium Dioxide, Triethyl Citrate, Xanthan Gum.

Indications: Temporarily relieves cough due to minor throat and bronchial irritation and nasal congestion as may occur with a cold. Expectorant action to help loosen phlegm and thin bronchial secretions to make coughs more productive.

Warnings: A persistent cough may be a sign of a serious condition. If cough persists for more than 1 week, tends to recur, or is accompanied by fever, rash, or persistent headache, patients should consult a doctor. Patients are advised not to take this product for persistent or chronic cough such as occurs with smoking, asthma, chronic bronchitis, emphysema, or if cough is accompanied by excessive phlegm (mucus) unless directed by a doctor. Likewise, persons with high blood pressure, heart disease, diabetes, thyroid disease or difficulty in urination due to enlargement of the prostate gland, are advised to use this product only as directed by a doctor. The recommended dosage should not be exceeded because at higher doses nervousness, dizziness, or sleeplessness may occur. As with any drug, women who are pregnant or nursing a baby should seek the advice of a health professional before using this product.

Contraindications: Hypersensitivity to any of the ingredients; marked hypertension, hyperthyroidism or in patients who are receiving monoamine oxidase inhibitors (MAOIs).

Adverse Reactions: The following adverse reactions may possibly occur: nausea, vomiting, dry mouth, nervousness, insomnia and rash (including urticaria).

NOTE: Guaifenesin has been shown to produce a color interference with certain clinical laboratory determinations of 5-hydroxyindoleacetic acid (5-HIAA) and vanillylmandelic acid (VMA).

Drug Interaction Precautions: Concomitant administration of pseudoephedrine with other sympathomimetic agents may produce additive effects and increased toxicity; with MAOIs may produce a hypertensive crisis; with certain antihypertensive agents may diminish their antihypertensive effect. Serious toxicity may result if dextromethorphan is used with MAOIs.

Directions: Adults and children 12 years and over, 2 caplets every 4 hours; children 6 to under 12 years of age, 1 caplet every 4 hours; children under 6 years—consult a doctor. DO NOT EXCEED 4 DOSES IN A 24-HOUR PERIOD.

How Supplied: Orange, film-coated caplets engraved AHR on one side and DIMACOL on the other in bottles of 100 (NDC 0031-1653-63), and 500 (NDC 0031-1653-70) and consumer packages of 12 (NDC 0031-1653-46), and 24 (NDC 0031-1653-54) (individually packaged).
Store at Controlled Room Temperature, between 15°C and 30°C (59°F and 86°F).

DIMETANE®

[*dī' mĕ-tāne*]

brand of Brompheniramine Maleate, USP
Tablets—4 mg
Elixir—2 mg/5 mL (Alcohol, 3%)
Extentabs®—8 mg and 12 mg

Family Description: Dimetane® is Robins brand name for Brompheniramine Maleate, USP, an antihistamine. It comes in several oral dosage forms (tablets, elixir and Extentabs®) and can be used when an antihistamine is indicated.

Inactive Ingredients:
Tablets: Corn Starch, D&C Yellow 10 Aluminum Lake, Dibasic Calcium Phosphate, FD&C Yellow 6 Aluminum Lake, Lactose, Magnesium Stearate, Polyethylene Glycol.
Elixir: Citric Acid, FD&C Yellow 6, Flavors, Glucose, Saccharin Sodium, Sodium Benzoate, Water.
Extentabs® 8 mg: Acacia, Acetylated Monoglycerides, Calcium Carbonate, Calcium Sulfate, Carnauba Wax, Cellulose Acetate Phthalate, Corn Starch, Diethyl Phthalate, Edible Ink, FD&C Blue 2 Aluminum Lake, FD&C Red 3, Gelatin, Guar Gum, Magnesium Stearate, Pharmaceutical Glaze, Polysorbates, Stearic Acid, Sucrose, Titanium Dioxide, Wheat Flour, White Wax and other ingredients, one of which is a corn derivative. May contain FD&C Red 40 and FD&C Yellow 6 Aluminum Lakes.
Extentabs® 12 mg: Acacia, Acetylated Monoglycerides, Calcium Carbonate, Calcium Sulfate, Carnauba Wax, Cellulose Acetate Phthalate, Corn Starch, Diethyl Phthalate, Edible Ink, FD&C Blue 2 Aluminum Lake, FD&C Red 3, FD&C Yellow 6, Gelatin, Guar Gum, Magnesium Stearate, Pharmaceutical Glaze, Polysorbates, Stearic Acid, Sucrose, Titanium Dioxide, Wheat Flour, White Wax and other ingredients, one of which is a corn derivative. May contain FD&C Red 40 and FD&C Yellow 6 Aluminum Lakes.

Indications: For temporary relief of running nose, sneezing, itching of the nose or throat; and itchy, watery eyes as may occur in allergic rhinitis (such as hay fever).

Warnings: May cause drowsiness. May cause excitability, especially in children. This product should not be taken by patients who have asthma, glaucoma or difficulty in urination due to enlargement of the prostate gland. The tablets and liquid should not be given to children under six years, except under the advice and supervision of a physician. The Extentabs should not be given to children under 12 years, except under the advice and supervision of a physician. Should not be taken if hypersensitivity to any of the ingredients exists. As with any drug, women who are pregnant or nursing a baby should seek the advice of a health professional before using these products.

Cautions: Patients should be warned to avoid driving a motor vehicle, operating heavy machinery, or consuming alcoholic beverages while taking this product.

Directions: Tablets and Liquid—The recommended OTC dosage is: Adults and children 12 years of age and over: 1 tablet or 2 teaspoonfuls every four to six hours, not to exceed 6 tablets or 12 teaspoonfuls in 24 hours. Children 6 to under 12 years: ½ tablet or 1 teaspoonful every four to six hours, not to exceed 3 whole tablets or 6 teaspoonfuls in 24 hours.
Professional Labeling: Children under 6 years: Use only as directed by a physician. The suggested dosage for children age 2 to under 6 years, only when the child is under the care of a physician, is ½ teaspoonful every 4 to 6 hours, not to exceed 6 doses in a 24-hour period. The dosage for a child under 2 years should be determined by the physician on the basis of the patient's weight, physical condition, or other appropriate consideration. Dimetane Elixir is contraindicated in neonates (children under the age of one month).
Extentabs®—The recommended OTC dosage is: Adults and children 12 years of age and over:

8 mg Extentab: One tablet every eight to twelve hours, NOT TO EXCEED 1 TABLET EVERY 8 HOURS OR 3 TABLETS IN A 24-HOUR PERIOD.
12 mg Extentab: One tablet every twelve hours, NOT TO EXCEED 1 TABLET EVERY 12 HOURS OR 2 TABLETS IN A 24-HOUR PERIOD.
Children under 12 years of age should use only as directed by a physician.

How Supplied: [See table .]
Store at Controlled Room Temperature, between 15°C and 30°C (59°F and 86°F).

Shown in Product Identification Section, page 425

Product Name	Form	Strength	Package Size	Package Type	NDC 0031-
Dimetane Tablets	Peach-colored, compressed scored tablet	4 mg tablet	24	Blister Unit	1857-54
			100	Bottles	1857-63
Dimetane Elixir	Peach-colored liquid	2 mg/ 5 mL	4 fl. oz.	Bottles	1807-12
			1 Pint	Bottles	1807-25
Dimetane Extentabs 8 mg	Persian rose-colored, tablets	8 mg tablet	12	Blister Unit	1868-46
			100	Bottles	1868-63
Dimetane Extentabs 12 mg	Peach-colored, coated tablets	12 mg tablet	12	Blister Unit	1843-46
			100	Bottles	1843-63

DIMETANE® DECONGESTANT ELIXIR

[*dī' mĕ-tāne*]

DIMETANE® DECONGESTANT CAPLETS

Elixir:
Each 5 mL (1 teaspoonful) contains:
Phenylephrine Hydrochloride, USP ....5 mg
Brompheniramine Maleate, USP ....2 mg
Alcohol 2.3%

Inactive Ingredients: Citric Acid, FD&C Blue 1, FD&C Red 40, Flavors, Sodium Benzoate, Sorbitol, Water.

Caplets:
Each caplet contains:
Phenylephrine Hydrochloride, USP ....10 mg
Brompheniramine Maleate, USP ....4 mg

Inactive Ingredients: Corn Starch, FD&C Blue 1 Aluminum Lake, Magnesium Stearate, Microcrystalline Cellulose.

Indications: For temporary relief of nasal congestion due to the common cold, sinusitis, hay fever or other upper respiratory allergies; runny nose, sneezing, itching of the nose or throat and itchy and watery eyes as may occur in allergic rhinitis (such as hay fever). Temporarily restores freer breathing through the nose.

Warnings: These products may cause excitability, especially in children. These products should not be taken by patients with asthma, glaucoma, difficulty in urination due to enlargement of the prostate gland, high blood pressure, heart disease, diabetes or thyroid disease except under the advice and supervision of a physician. Should not be taken by persons hypersensitive to any of the ingredients. May cause drowsiness. Doses in excess of the recommended dosage may cause nervousness, dizziness or sleeplessness. If symptoms do not improve within 7 days or are accompanied by fever, a physician should be consulted before continuing use. As with any drug, women who are pregnant or nursing a baby should seek the advice of a health professional before using this product.

Drug Interaction Precautions: Concomitant administration of phenylephrine with other sympathomimetic agents may produce additive effects and increased toxicity: with monoamine oxidase inhibitors (MAOIs) may produce a hypertensive crisis; with certain antihypertensive agents may diminish their antihypertensive effect.

Cautions: Patients should be warned to avoid driving a motor vehicle, operating heavy machinery, or consuming alcoholic beverages while taking this product.

Directions: ***Caplets:*** Adults and children 12 years of age and over: 1 caplet every 4 hours, not to exceed 6 caplets in a 24-hour period; children 6 to under 12 years: ½ caplet every 4 hours, not to exceed 3 caplets in a 24-hour period; children under 6 years: use only as directed by a physician.
Elixir: Adults and children 12 years of age and over: 2 teaspoonfuls every 4 hours, not to exceed 12 teaspoonfuls in a 24-hour period; children 6 to under 12 years: 1 teaspoonful every 4 hours, not to exceed 6 teaspoonfuls in a 24-hour period. Children under 6 years: use only as directed by a physician.
Professional Labeling: The suggested dosage for children age 2 to under 6 years, only when the child is under the care of a physician, is ½ teaspoonful every 4 hours, not to exceed 6 doses in a 24-hour period. The dosage for a child under 2 years should be determined by the physician on the basis of the patient's weight, physical condition, or other appropriate consideration. Dimetane Decongestant is contraindicated in neonates (children under the age of one month).

How Supplied: ***Caplets***—light blue, capsule-shaped, compressed tablets engraved AHR on one side and scored and engraved 2117 on the other, in cartons of 24 (NDC 0031-2117-54) and 48 (NDC 0031-2117-59) individually packaged blister units.
Elixir—red-colored, grape-flavored liquid in 4 fl oz bottle (NDC 0031-2127-12).
Store at Controlled Room Temperature, between 15°C and 30°C (59°F and 86°F).

Shown in Product Identification Section, page 425

DIMETAPP® Elixir

[*dī' mĕ-tap*]

Description: Each 5 mL (1 teaspoonful) contains:
Brompheniramine Maleate, USP ....2 mg
Phenylpropanolamine Hydrochloride, USP ....12.5 mg
Alcohol 2.3%

Inactive Ingredients: Citric Acid, FD&C Blue 1, FD&C Red 40, Flavor, Saccharin Sodium, Sodium Benzoate, Sorbitol, Water.

Indications: For temporary relief of nasal congestion due to the common cold, hay fever or other upper respiratory allergies and associated with sinusitis; temporarily relieves runny nose, sneezing, and itchy and watery eyes as may occur in allergic rhinitis (such as hay fever). Temporarily restores freer breathing through the nose.

Warnings: This product may cause excitability, especially in children. This product should not be taken by patients with high blood pressure, heart disease, diabetes, thyroid disease, asthma, glaucoma or difficulty in urination due to enlargement of the prostate gland, except under the advice and supervision of a physician. May cause drowsiness. Doses in excess of the recommended dosage may cause nervousness, dizziness, or sleeplessness. If symptoms do not improve within 7 days or are accompanied by high fever, a physician should be consulted before continuing use. Should not

Continued on next page

Prescribing information on A.H. Robins products listed here is based on official labeling in effect November 1, 1990 with Indications, Contraindications, Warnings, Precautions, Adverse Reactions, and Dosage stated in full.

Robins—Cont.

be taken by persons hypersensitive to any of the ingredients. As with any drug, women who are pregnant or nursing a baby should seek the advice of a health professional before using this product.

Caution: Patients should be warned to avoid driving a motor vehicle, operating heavy machinery or consuming alcoholic beverages while taking this product.

Drug Interaction Precaution: Concomitant administration of phenylpropanolamine with other sympathomimetic agents may produce additive effects and increased toxicity; with monamine oxidase inhibitors (MAOIs) may produce a hypertensive crisis; with certain antihypertensive agents may diminish their antihypertensive effect.

Directions: Adults and children 12 years of age and over: 2 teaspoonfuls every 4 hours; children 6 to under 12 years: 1 teaspoonful every 4 hours; DO NOT EXCEED 6 DOSES IN A 24-HOUR PERIOD. Children under 6 years: use only as directed by a physician.

Professional Labeling: The suggested dosage for children age 2 to under 6 years, only when the child is under the care of a physician, is ½ teaspoonful every 4 hours, not to exceed 6 doses in a 24-hour period. The dosage for children under 2 years should be determined by the physician on the basis of the patients' weight, physical condition, or other appropriate consideration. Dimetapp Elixir is contraindicated in neonates (children under the age of one month).

How Supplied: Purple, grape-flavored liquid in bottles of 4 fl. oz. (NDC 0031-2230-12), 8 fl. oz. (NDC 0031-2230-18), 12 fl. oz. (NDC 0031-2230-22), pints (NDC 0031-2230-25), gallons (NDC 0031-2230-29), and 5 mL Dis-Co® Unit Dose Packs (10 × 10s) (NDC 0031-2230-23).
Store at Controlled Room Temperature, between 15°C and 30°C (59°F and 86°F).

Shown in Product Identification Section, page 425

DIMETAPP® DM ELIXIR

[*dī'mĕ-tap*]

Description: Each 5 mL (1 teaspoonful) contains:
Brompheniramine Maleate, USP .... 2 mg
Phenylpropanolamine Hydrochloride, USP .... 12.5 mg
Dextromethorphan Hydrobromide, USP .... 10.0 mg
Alcohol 2.3%

Inactive Ingredients: Citric Acid, FD&C Blue 1, FD&C Red 40, Flavors, Glycerin, Propylene Glycol, Saccharin Sodium, Sodium Benzoate, Sorbitol, Water.

Indications: Temporarily relieves cough due to minor throat and bronchial irritation as may occur with a cold. For temporary relief of nasal congestion due to the common cold, hay fever or other upper respiratory allergies and associated with sinusitis; temporarily relieves runny nose, sneezing, and itchy and watery eyes as may occur in allergic rhinitis (such as hay fever). Temporarily restores freer breathing through the nose.

Warnings: This product may cause excitability, especially in children. This product should not be taken by patients with high blood pressure, heart disease, diabetes, thyroid disease, asthma, glaucoma or difficulty in urination due to enlargement of the prostate gland, except under the advice and supervision of a physician. May cause drowsiness. Doses in excess of the recommended dosage may cause nervousness, dizziness, or sleeplessness. A persistent cough may be a sign of a serious condition. If cough or other symptoms do not improve within 7 days, tend to recur, or are accompanied by fever, rash or persistent headache, patients should consult a physician. Patients are advised not to take this product for persistent or chronic cough such as occurs with smoking, asthma, emphysema, or if cough is accompanied by excessive phlegm (mucus) unless directed by a physician. Patients who are hypersensitive to any of the ingredients should not take this drug. As with any drug, women who are pregnant or nursing a baby should seek the advice of a health professional before using this product.

Caution: Patients should be warned to avoid driving a motor vehicle, operating heavy machinery or consuming alcoholic beverages while taking this product.

Drug Interaction Precautions: Concomitant administration of phenylpropanolamine with other sympathomimetic agents may produce additive effects and increased toxicity; with monamine oxidase inhibitors (MAOIs) may produce a hypertensive crisis; with certain antihypertensive agents may diminish their antihypertensive effect. Serious toxicity may result if dextromethorphan is used with MAOIs.

Directions: Adults and children 12 years of age and over: Two teaspoonfuls every 4 hours; children 6 to under 12 years: one teaspoonful every 4 hours. **DO NOT EXCEED 6 DOSES IN A 24-HOUR PERIOD.** Children under 6 years: use only as directed by a physician.

Professional Labeling: The suggested dosage for children age 2 to under 6 years, only when the child is under the care of a physician, is ½ teaspoonful every 4 hours, not to exceed 6 doses in a 24-hour period. The dosage for children under 2 years should be determined by the physician on the basis of the patients' weight, physical condition, or other appropriate consideration. Dimetapp DM Elixir is contraindicated in neonates (children under the age of one month).

How Supplied: Red, grape-flavored liquid in bottles of 4 and 8 fl. oz.
Store at Room Temperature.

Shown in Product Identification Section, page 426

DIMETAPP® Extentabs®

[*dī'mĕ-tap*]

Description: Each **Dimetapp Extentabs®** Tablet contains:
Brompheniramine Maleate, USP .... 12 mg
Phenylpropanolamine Hydrochloride, USP .... 75 mg

Inactive Ingredients: Acacia, Acetylated Monoglycerides, Calcium Sulfate, Carnauba Wax, Castor Wax or Oil, Citric Acid, Edible Ink, FD&C Blue 1 and FD&C Blue 2 Aluminum Lake, Gelatin, Magnesium Stearate, Magnesium Trisilicate, Pharmaceutical Glaze, Polysorbates, Povidone, Silicon Dioxide, Stearyl Alcohol, Sucrose, Titanium Dioxide, Wheat Flour, White Wax. May contain FD&C Red 40 and FD&C Yellow 6 Aluminum Lakes.

Indications: For temporary relief of nasal congestion due to the common cold, hay fever or other upper respiratory allergies and associated with sinusitis; temporarily relieves runny nose, sneezing, and itchy and watery eyes as may occur in allergic rhinitis (such as hay fever). Temporarily restores freer breathing through the nose.

Warnings: This product may cause excitability, especially in children. This product should not be taken by patients with high blood pressure, heart disease, diabetes, thyroid disease, asthma, glaucoma or difficulty in urination due to enlargement of the prostate gland, except under the advice and supervision of a physician. This product should not be given to children under 12 years except under the advice and supervision of a physician. May cause drowsiness. Doses in excess of the recommended dosage may cause nervousness, dizziness, or sleeplessness. If symptoms do not improve within 7 days or are accompanied by high fever, a physician should be consulted before continuing use. Should not be taken by persons hypersensitive to any of the ingredients. As with any drug, women who are pregnant or nursing a baby should seek the advice of a health professional before using this product.

Caution: Patients should be warned to avoid driving a motor vehicle, operating heavy machinery or consuming alcoholic beverages while taking this product.

Drug Interaction Precaution: Concomitant administration of phenylpropanolamine with other sympathomimetic agents may produce additive effects and increased toxicity; with monoamine oxidase inhibitors (MAOIs) may produce a hypertensive crisis; with certain antihypertensive agents may diminish their antihypertensive effect.

Directions: Adults and children 12 years of age and over: one tablet every 12 hours. DO NOT EXCEED 1 TABLET EVERY 12 HOURS OR 2 TABLETS IN A 24-HOUR PERIOD.

How Supplied: Pale blue sugar-coated tablets monogrammed DIMETAPP AHR in bottles of 100 (NDC 0031-2277-63), 500

(NDC 0031-2277-70); Dis-Co® Unit Dose Packs of 100 (NDC 0031-2277-64); and consumer packages of 12 tablets (NDC 0031-2277-46), and 24 tablets (NDC 0031-2277-54) and 48 tablets (NDC 0031-2277-59) (individually packaged).
Store at Controlled Room Temperature, between 15°C and 30°C (59°F and 86°F).
Dimetapp Extentabs® Tablets are the A. H. Robins Company's uniquely constructed extended action tablets.

Shown in Product Identification Section, page 426

DIMETAPP® Tablets

[*dī' mĕ-tap*]

Description: Each **Dimetapp** Tablet contains:
Brompheniramine Maleate, USP ....4 mg
Phenylpropanolamine Hydrochloride, USP ....25 mg

Inactive Ingredients: Corn Starch, FD&C Blue 1 Aluminum Lake, Magnesium Stearate, Microcrystalline Cellulose.

Indications: For temporary relief of nasal congestion due to the common cold, hay fever or other upper respiratory allergies and associated with sinusitis; temporarily relieves runny nose, sneezing, and itchy and watery eyes as may occur in allergic rhinitis (such as hay fever). Temporarily restores freer breathing through the nose.

Warnings: This product may cause excitability, especially in children. This product should not be taken by patients with high blood pressure, heart disease, diabetes, thyroid disease, asthma, glaucoma or difficulty in urination due to enlargement of the prostate gland, except under the advice and supervision of a physician. May cause drowsiness. Doses in excess of the recommended dosage may cause nervousness, dizziness, or sleeplessness. If symptoms do not improve within 7 days or are accompanied by high fever, a physician should be consulted before continuing use. Should not be taken by persons hypersensitive to any of the ingredients. As with any drug, women who are pregnant or nursing a baby should seek the advice of a health professional before using this product.

Caution: Patients should be warned to avoid driving a motor vehicle, operating heavy machinery or consuming alcoholic beverages while taking this product.

Drug Interaction Precaution: Concomitant administration of phenylpropanolamine with other sympathomimetic agents may produce additive effects and increased toxicity; with monoamine oxidase inhibitors (MAOIs) may produce a hypertensive crisis; with certain antihypertensive agents may diminish their antihypertensive effect.

Directions: Adults and children 12 years of age and over: one tablet every 4 hours. Children 6 to under 12 years: one-half tablet every 4 hours. DO NOT EXCEED 6 DOSES IN A 24-HOUR PERIOD. Children under 6 years: Use only as directed by a physician.

How Supplied: Blue, scored compressed tablets engraved AHR and 2254 in consumer packages of 24 (NDC 0031-2254-54) (individually packaged).
Store at Controlled Room Temperature, between 15°C and 30°C (59°F and 86°F).

Shown in Product Identification Section, page 426

DIMETAPP PLUS® CAPLETS

[*dī' mĕ-tap*]

Description: Each **Dimetapp PLUS® Caplet** contains:
Acetaminophen, USP ....500 mg
Phenylpropanolamine Hydrochloride, USP ....12.5 mg
Brompheniramine Maleate, USP ...2 mg

Inactive Ingredients: Corn Starch, FD&C Blue 2 Aluminum Lake, Hydroxypropyl Methylcellulose, Magnesium Stearate, Microcrystalline Cellulose, Polysorbate 20, Povidone, Propylene Glycol, Stearic Acid, Titanium Dioxide. May also contain Calcium Phosphate, Hydroxypropyl Cellulose, Methylparaben, Propylparaben.

Indications: For the temporary relief of minor aches, pains, and headache; for the reduction of fever; for the relief of nasal congestion due to the common cold or associated with sinusitis; and for the relief of runny nose, sneezing, itching of the nose or throat and itchy and watery eyes as may occur in allergic rhinitis (such as hay fever). Temporarily restores freer breathing through the nose.

Warnings: May cause drowsiness. May cause excitability, especially in children. If symptoms do not improve within 7 days or are accompanied by high fever, a physician should be consulted before continuing use. Patients who have asthma, glaucoma, heart disease, high blood pressure, thyroid disease, diabetes, emphysema, chronic pulmonary disease, shortness of breath, difficulty in urination due to enlargement of the prostate gland should not take this product unless directed by a physician. Recommended dosage should not be exceeded because at higher dosages severe liver damage, nervousness, dizziness, or sleeplessness may occur. As with any drug, women who are pregnant or nursing a baby should seek the advice of a health professional before using this product.

Caution: Patients should be warned to avoid driving a motor vehicle, operating heavy machinery or consuming alcoholic beverages while taking this product.

Drug Interaction Precaution: Concomitant administration of phenylpropanolamine with other sympathomimetic agents may produce additive effects and increased toxicity; with monoamine oxidase inhibitors (MAOIs) may produce a hypertensive crisis; with certain antihypertensive agents may diminish their antihypertensive effect.

Directions: Adults and children (12 years and over): Two caplets every 6 hours. DO NOT EXCEED 8 CAPLETS IN A 24-HOUR PERIOD.
Not recommended for children under 12 years of age.

How Supplied: Dimetapp Plus® Caplets are supplied as blue capsule-shaped film-coated tablets engraved AHR on one side and 2278 on the other in consumer packages of 24 (NDC 0031-2278-54), and 48 (NDC 0031-2278-59) (individually packaged).
Store at Controlled Room Temperature, between 15°C and 30°C (59°F and 86°F).

Shown in Product Identification Section, page 426

DONNAGEL®

[*don 'nă-jel*]

Each 30 mL (1 fl. oz.) contains:
Kaolin, USP (90 gr) ....6.0 g
Pectin, USP (2 gr)....142.8 mg
Hyoscyamine Sulfate, USP.....0.1037 mg
Atropine Sulfate, USP....0.0194 mg
Scopolamine Hydrobromide, USP ....0.0065 mg
Sodium Benzoate, NF (preservative) ....60 mg
Alcohol 3.8%

Inactive Ingredients: Citric Acid, D&C Yellow 10, FD&C Blue 1, Flavors, Sodium Carboxymethylcellulose, Sodium Chloride, Sorbitol, Water.

Indications: Donnagel is indicated in the treatment of diarrhea and associated cramping.

Description: Donnagel combines the adsorbent and detoxifying effects of kaolin and pectin with the antispasmodic efficacy of the natural belladonna alkaloids. The latter, present in a specific, fixed ratio, help control hypermotility and hypersecretion in the gastrointestinal tract.

Contraindications: Glaucoma or increased ocular pressure, advanced renal or hepatic disease or hypersensitivity to any of the ingredients.

Warnings: As with any drug, women who are pregnant or nursing a baby should seek the advice of a health professional before taking this product.

Precautions: As with all preparations containing belladonna alkaloids, Donnagel must be administered cautiously to patients with incipient glaucoma or urinary bladder neck obstruction as in prostatic hypertrophy. Use with caution in elderly patients (where undiagnosed glaucoma or excessive pressure occurs most frequently).

Adverse Reactions: Blurred vision, dry mouth, difficult urination, flushing

Continued on next page

Prescribing information on A.H. Robins products listed here is based on official labeling in effect November 1, 1990 with Indications, Contraindications, Warnings, Precautions, Adverse Reactions, and Dosage stated in full.

Robins—Cont.

and dryness of the skin, dizziness or tachycardia may occur at higher dosage levels, rarely at the usual dose.

Dosage and Administration:
[See table.]
Do not take more than 4 doses in any 24-hour period.

How Supplied: Donnagel (light green, aromatic suspension) in 4 fl. oz. (NDC 0031-3016-12), 8 fl. oz. (NDC 0031-3016-18), and pint (NDC 0031-3016-25).
Store at Controlled Room Temperature, between 15°C and 30°C (59°F and 86°F).

Shown in Product Identification Section, page 426

	Initial	Every 3 Hours
Adults	2 tablespoonfuls (1 fl. oz.)	1 tablespoonful
Children:		
Over 12 Years:	2 tablespoonfuls	1 tablespoonful
6–12 Years:	2 teaspoonfuls	1–2 teaspoonfuls

ROBITUSSIN®
(Guaifenesin Syrup, USP)
[ro "bĭ-tuss 'ĭn]

Active Ingredients per teaspoonful (5 mL)—Guaifenesin, USP 100 mg in pleasant tasting syrup with alcohol 3.5%.

Inactive Ingredients: Caramel, Citric Acid, FD&C Red 40, Flavors, Glucose, Glycerin, High Fructose Corn Syrup, Saccharin Sodium, Sodium Benzoate, Water.

Indications: Expectorant action to help loosen phlegm and thin bronchial secretions to make coughs more productive.

Professional Labeling: Helps loosen phlegm and thin bronchial secretions in patients with stable chronic bronchitis.

Warnings: A persistent cough may be a sign of a serious condition. If cough persists for more than 1 week, tends to recur, or is accompanied by fever, rash, or persistent headache, patients should consult a doctor. Patients are advised not to take this product for persistent or chronic cough such as occurs with smoking, asthma, chronic bronchitis, emphysema, or if cough is accompanied by excessive phlegm (mucus) unless directed by a doctor. As with any drug, women who are pregnant or nursing a baby should seek the advice of a health professional before using this product.

Contraindications: Hypersensitivity to any of the ingredients.

Adverse Reactions: Guaifenesin is well tolerated and has a wide margin of safety. Nausea and vomiting are the side effects that occur most commonly, and other reported adverse reactions have included dizziness, headache, and rash (including urticaria).

Note: Guaifenesin has been shown to produce a color interference with certain clinical laboratory determinations of 5-hydroxyindoleacetic acid (5-HIAA) and vanillylmandelic acid (VMA).

Directions: Adults and children 12 years and over: 2–4 teaspoonfuls every 4 hours; children 6 years to under 12 years: 1–2 teaspoonfuls every 4 hours. Children 2 years to under 6 years: ½–1 teaspoonful every 4 hours; children under 2 years—consult your doctor. DO NOT EXCEED RECOMMENDED DOSAGE.

How Supplied: Robitussin (wine-colored) in bottles of 4 fl. oz. (NDC 0031-8624-12), 8 fl. oz. (NDC 0031-8624-18), pint (NDC 0031-8624-25) and gallon (NDC 0031-8624-29).
Robitussin also available in 1 fl. oz. bottles (4 × 25's) (NDC 0031-8624-02) and Dis-Co® Unit Dose Packs of 10 × 10's in 5 mL (NDC 0031-8624-23), 10 mL (NDC 0031-8624-26) and 15 mL (NDC 0031-8624-28).
Store at Controlled Room Temperature, between 15°C and 30°C (59°F and 86°F).

Shown in Product Identification Section, page 426

ROBITUSSIN-CF®
[ro "bĭ-tuss 'ĭn]

Active Ingredients per teaspoonful (5 mL)—Guaifenesin, USP 100 mg; Phenylpropanolamine Hydrochloride, USP 12.5 mg and Dextromethorphan Hydrobromide, USP 10 mg in pleasant-tasting syrup with alcohol 4.75%.

Inactive Ingredients: Citric Acid, FD&C Red 40, Flavors, Glycerin, Propylene Glycol, Saccharin Sodium, Sodium Benzoate, Sorbitol, Water.

Indications: Temporarily relieves coughs due to minor throat and bronchial irritation and nasal congestion as may occur with a cold. Expectorant action to help loosen phlegm and thin bronchial secretions to make coughs more productive.

Warnings: A persistent cough may be a sign of a serious condition. If cough persists for more than 1 week, tends to recur, or is accompanied by fever, rash, or persistent headache, patients should consult a doctor. Patients are advised not to take this product for persistent or chronic cough such as occurs with smoking, asthma, chronic bronchitis, emphysema, or if cough is accompanied by excessive phlegm (mucus) unless directed by a doctor. Likewise, persons with high blood pressure, heart disease, diabetes, thyroid disease or difficulty in urination due to enlargement of the prostate gland are advised to use this product only as directed by a doctor. The recommended dosage should not be exceeded because at higher doses nervousness, dizziness, or sleeplessness may occur. As with any drug, women who are pregnant or nursing a baby should seek the advice of a health professional before using this product.

Contraindications: Hypersensitivity to any of the ingredients; marked hypertension; hyperthyroidism; patients who are receiving monoamine oxidase inhibitors (MAOIs).

Adverse Reactions: The following adverse reactions may occur: nausea, vomiting, dizziness, dry mouth, nervousness, insomnia, restlessness, headache, or rash (including urticaria).

Note: Guaifenesin has been shown to produce a color interference with certain clinical laboratory determinations of 5-hydroxyindoleacetic acid (5-HIAA) and vanillylmandelic acid (VMA).

Drug Interaction Precautions: Concomitant administration of phenylpropanolamine with other sympathomimetic agents may produce additive effects and increased toxicity; with MAOIs may produce a hypertensive crisis; with certain antihypertensive agents may diminish their antihypertensive effect. Serious toxicity may result if dextromethorphan is used with MAOIs.

Directions: Adults and children 12 years and over, 2 teaspoonfuls every 4 hours; children 6 years to under 12 years, 1 teaspoonful every 4 hours; children 2 years to under 6 years, ½ teaspoonful every 4 hours; children under 2 years —as directed by a physician. DO NOT EXCEED 6 DOSES IN A 24-HOUR PERIOD.

How Supplied: Robitussin-CF (red-colored) in bottles of 4 fl. oz. (NDC 0031-8677-12), 8 fl. oz. (NDC 0031-8677-18), 12 fl. oz. (NDC 0031-8677-22), and one pint (NDC 0031-8677-25).
Store at Controlled Room Temperature, between 15°C and 30°C (59°F and 86°F).

Shown in Product Identification Section, page 426

ROBITUSSIN-DM®
[ro "bĭ-tuss 'ĭn]

Active Ingredients per teaspoonful (5 mL)—Guaifenesin, USP 100 mg and Dextromethorphan Hydrobromide, USP 10 mg in pleasant-tasting syrup.

Inactive Ingredients: Citric Acid, FD&C Red 40, Flavors, Glucose, Glycerin, High Fructose Corn Syrup, Saccharin Sodium, Sodium Benzoate, Water.

Indications: Temporarily relieves coughs due to minor throat and bronchial irritation as may occur with a cold. Expectorant action to help loosen phlegm and thin bronchial secretions to make coughs more productive.

Warnings: A persistent cough may be a sign of a serious condition. If cough persists for more than 1 week, tends to recur, or is accompanied by fever, rash, or persistent headache, patients should consult a doctor. Patients are advised not to take this product for persistent or chronic cough such as occurs with smoking, asthma, chronic bronchitis, emphysema, or if cough is accompanied by excessive phlegm (mucus), unless directed by a doctor. As with any drug, women who are pregnant or nursing a baby should seek the advice of a health professional before using this product.

Contraindications: Hypersensitivity to any of the ingredients, or in patients who are receiving monoamine oxidase inhibitors (MAOIs).

Adverse Reactions: The incidence of side effects is low. Reported side effects include nausea and vomiting, as well as diarrhea, drowsiness, and rash (including urticaria).
Overdose: Symptoms may include ataxia, respiratory depression and convulsions in children, whereas adults may exhibit altered sensory perception, ataxia, slurred speech and dysphoria.
Note: Guaifenesin has been shown to produce a color interference with certain clinical laboratory determinations of 5-hydroxyindoleacetic acid (5-HIAA) and vanillylmandelic acid (VMA).

Drug Interaction Precaution: Serious toxicity may result if dextromethorphan is used with MAOIs.

Directions: Adults and children 12 years and over, 2 teaspoonfuls every 4 hours; children 6 years to under 12 years, 1 teaspoonful every 4 hours; children 2 years to under 6 years, ½ teaspoonful every 4 hours; children under 2 years—consult your doctor. DO NOT EXCEED 6 DOSES IN A 24-HOUR PERIOD.

How Supplied: Robitussin-DM (cherry-colored) in bottles of 4 fl. oz. (NDC 0031-8685-12), 8 fl. oz. (NDC 0031-8685-18), 12 fl. oz. (NDC 0031-8685-22), single doses: 6 premeasured doses—⅓ fl. oz. each (NDC 0031-8685-06), pint (NDC 0031-8685-25), and gallon (NDC 0031-8685-29).
Robitussin-DM also available in Dis-Co® Unit Dose Packs of 10 × 10's in 5 mL (NDC 0031-8685-23) and 10 mL (NDC 0031-8685-26).
Store at Controlled Room Temperature, between 15°C and 30°C (59°F and 86°F).

Shown in Product Identification Section, page 426

ROBITUSSIN-PE®
[ro″bĭ-tuss′ĭn]

Active Ingredients per teaspoonful (5 mL)—Guaifenesin, USP 100 mg and Pseudoephedrine Hydrochloride, USP 30 mg in pleasant tasting syrup with alcohol 1.4%.

Inactive Ingredients: Citric Acid, FD&C Red 40, Flavors, Glucose, Glycerin, High Fructose Corn Syrup, Saccharin Sodium, Sodium Benzoate, Water.

Indications: Temporarily relieves nasal congestion as may occur with a cold. Expectorant action to help loosen phlegm and thin bronchial secretions to make coughs more productive.

Warnings: A persistent cough may be a sign of a serious condition. If cough persists for more than 1 week, tends to recur, or is accompanied by fever, rash, or persistent headache, patients should consult a doctor. Patients are advised not to take this product for persistent or chronic cough such as occurs with smoking, asthma, chronic bronchitis, emphysema, or if cough is accompanied by excessive phlegm (mucus) unless directed by a doctor. Likewise, persons with high blood pressure, heart disease, diabetes, thyroid disease or difficulty in urination due to enlargement of the prostate gland are advised to use this product only as directed by a doctor. The recommended dosage should not be exceeded because at higher doses nervousness, dizziness, or sleeplessness may occur. As with any drug, women who are pregnant or nursing a baby should seek the advice of a health professional before using this product.

Contraindications: Hypersensitivity to any of the ingredients; marked hypertension; hyperthyroidism; or in patients who are receiving monoamine oxidase inhibitors (MAOIs).

Adverse Reactions: Possible side effects include nausea, vomiting, nervousness, restlessness, rash (including urticaria), headache, or dry mouth.
Note: Guaifenesin has been shown to produce a color interference with certain clinical laboratory determinations of 5-hydroxyindoleacetic acid (5-HIAA) and vanillylmandelic acid (VMA).

Drug Interaction Precautions: Concomitant administration of pseudoephedrine with other sympathomimetic agents may produce additive effects and increased toxicity; with MAOIs may produce a hypertensive crisis; with certain antihypertensive agents may diminish their antihypertensive effect.

Directions: Adults and children 12 years and over, 2 teaspoonfuls every 4 hours; children 6 years to under 12 years, 1 teaspoonful every 4 hours; children 2 years to under 6 years, ½ teaspoonful every 4 hours; children under 2 years —as directed by physician. DO NOT EXCEED 4 DOSES IN A 24-HOUR PERIOD.

How Supplied: Robitussin-PE (orange-red) in bottles of 4 fl. oz. (NDC 0031-8695-12), 8 fl. oz. (NDC 0031-8695-18) and pint (NDC 0031-8695-25).
Store at Controlled Room Temperature, between 15°C and 30°C (59°F and 86°F).

Shown in Product Identification Section, page 426

ROBITUSSIN COUGH CALMERS®
[ro″bi-tuss′in]

Description: Each lozenge contains:
Dextromethorphan
Hydrobromide, USP ....5 mg

Inactive Ingredients: Corn Syrup, FD&C Red 40, flavors, glycerin, gum acacia, sucrose.

Indications: Temporarily relieves coughs due to minor throat and bronchial irritation as may occur with a cold.

Warnings: A persistent cough may be a sign of a serious condition. If cough persists for more than 1 week, tends to recur, or is accompanied by fever, rash, or persistent headache, patients should consult a doctor. Patients are advised not to take this product for persistent or chronic cough such as occurs with smoking, asthma, emphysema, or if cough is accompanied by excessive phlegm (mucus) unless directed by a doctor. As with any drug, women who are pregnant or nursing a baby should seek the advice of a health professional before using this product.

Contraindications: Hypersensitivity to any of the ingredients, or in patients who are receiving monoamine oxidase inhibitors (MAOIs).

Adverse Reactions: Side effects may include nausea.

Overdose: Symptoms may include ataxia, respiratory depression and convulsions in children; whereas, adults may exhibit altered sensory perception, ataxia, slurred speech and dysphoria.

Drug Interaction Precaution: Serious toxicity may result if dextromethorphan is used with MAOIs.

Directions: Adults and children 12 years and over: Dissolve 2–4 lozenges in mouth every 4 hours as needed.
Children 6 to under 12 years: Dissolve 1–2 lozenges in mouth every 4 hours or as directed by a doctor.
Children 4 to under 6 years: Dissolve one lozenge in mouth every 4 hours or as directed by a doctor.
Do not exceed recommended dosage.

How Supplied: Square, red cherry-flavored lozenge engraved AHR on both sides. Each consumer carton contains 8 tandem-joined pouches containing 2 lozenges each (16 lozenges total).
Store at Controlled Room Temperature, between 15°C and 30°C (59°F and 86°F).

Shown in Product Identification Section, page 426

ROBITUSSIN NIGHT RELIEF®
[ro″bĭ-tuss′ĭn]
COLDS FORMULA

Composition:
Each fluid ounce contains:
Acetaminophen, USP ....650 mg
Phenylephrine HCl, USP ....10 mg
Pyrilamine Maleate, USP ....50 mg
Dextromethorphan
Hydrobromide, USP ....30 mg

Inactive Ingredients: Citric Acid, FD&C Blue 1, FD&C Red 40, Flavors, Glycerin, Propylene Glycol, Saccharin Sodium, Sodium Benzoate, Sorbitol, Water.

Continued on next page

Prescribing information on A.H. Robins products listed here is based on official labeling in effect November 1, 1990 with Indications, Contraindications, Warnings, Precautions, Adverse Reactions, and Dosage stated in full.

Robins—Cont.

Indications: Temporarily relieves cough, runny nose, sneezing and nasal congestion as may occur with a cold. Also relieves fever, headache, minor sore throat pain, and body aches and pains as may occur with a cold.

Warnings: This preparation may cause drowsiness. Patients should be warned not to drive or operate machinery or consume alcoholic beverages while taking this medication. This product should not be given to children under 6 years of age, except under the advice and supervision of a physician. Patients are cautioned not to use the product for more than 10 days. Persons with asthma, glaucoma, high blood pressure, diabetes, heart or thyroid disease or difficulty in urination due to enlargement of the prostate gland should use only as directed by a doctor. Dosage should be reduced if nervousness, restlessness or sleeplessness occurs. Since a persistent cough may be a sign of a serious condition, patients are advised to consult a physician if cough persists for more than 1 week, tends to recur, or is accompanied by high fever, rash or persistent headache. Likewise, patients are warned not to take this product for persistent or chronic cough such as occurs with smoking, asthma, chronic bronchitis, emphysema, or if cough is accompanied by excessive phlegm (mucus) unless directed by a doctor. As with any drug, women who are pregnant or nursing a baby should seek the advice of a health professional before using this product.

Contraindications: Hypersensitivity to any of the ingredients; marked hypertension; hyperthyroidism; patients who are receiving monoamine oxidase inhibitors (MAOIs).

Adverse Effects: The following adverse reactions may possibly occur: nausea, vomiting, dizziness, diarrhea, nervousness, insomnia and drowsiness.

Drug Interaction Precautions: Concomitant administration of phenylephrine with other sympathomimetic agents may produce additive effects and increased toxicity; with MAOIs may produce a hypertensive crisis; with certain antihypertensive agents may diminish their antihypertensive effect. Serious toxicity may result if dextromethorphan is used with MAOIs.

Dosage: If cold keeps the patient confined to bed or at home, one dose should be taken every 6 hours, not to exceed 4 doses in a 24-hour period.
Adults (and children 12 years and over): one fluid ounce in medicine cup at bedtime (2 tablespoons). Children (6 years to under 12 years): ½ fluid ounce in medicine cup at bedtime (1 tablespoon). Under 6 years—consult your doctor.

How Supplied: Bottles of 4 fl. oz. (NDC 0031-8641-12) and 8 fl. oz. (NDC 0031-8641-18).
Store at Controlled Room Temperature, between 15°C and 30°C (59°F and 86°F).

Shown in Product Identification Section, page 426

ROBITUSSIN PEDIATRIC™

[ro "bi-tuss 'in]

Description: Each 5 mL (1 teaspoonful) contains:
Dextromethorphan Hydrobromide, USP ....7.5 mg
in a pleasant tasting nonalcoholic liquid.

Inactive Ingredients: Citric Acid, FD&C Red 40, Flavors, Glycerin, Propylene Glycol, Saccharin Sodium, Sodium Benzoate, Sorbitol, Water.

Indications: Temporarily relieves coughs due to minor throat and bronchial irritation as may occur with a cold.

Warnings: A persistent cough may be a sign of a serious condition. If cough persists for more than one week, tends to recur, or is accompanied by fever, rash, or persistent headache, patients should consult a doctor. Patients are advised not to take this product for persistent or chronic cough such as occurs with smoking, asthma, emphysema, or if cough is accompanied by excessive phlegm (mucus), unless directed by a doctor. As with any drug, women who are pregnant or nursing a baby should seek the advice of a health professional before using this product.

Contraindications: Hypersensitivity to any of the ingredients, or in patients who are receiving monoamine oxidase inhibitors (MAOIs).

Adverse Reactions: Side effects may include nausea.

Overdose: Symptoms may include ataxia, respiratory depression and convulsions in children, whereas adults may exhibit altered sensory perception, ataxia, slurred speech and dysphoria.

Drug Interaction Precaution: Serious toxicity may result if dextromethorphan is used with MAOIs.

Directions: Patients are instructed to follow recommendations on the bottle or carton (see below) or to use as directed by a physician. Doses may be repeated every 6–8 hours, not to exceed 4 doses in a 24-hour period. Dosage should be chosen by weight, if known; if weight is not known, choose by age. [See table below.]

How Supplied: Robitussin Pediatric (cherry-colored) in bottles of 4 fl. oz. (NDC 0031-8610-12) and 8 fl. oz. (NDC 0031-8610-18).
Store at Controlled Room Temperature, between 15°C and 30°C (59°F and 86°F).

Shown in Product Identification Section, page 426

Age	Weight	Dose
Under 2 yrs.	Under 24. lbs.	As directed by physician.
2 to under 6 yrs.	24–27 lbs.	1 Teaspoonful
6 to under 12 yrs.	48–95 lbs.	2 Teaspoonfuls
12 yrs. and older	96 lbs. and over	4 Teaspoonfuls

Z-BEC® Tablets

[zē 'bĕk]

One tablet daily provides:

Vitamin Composition	Percentage of U.S. Recommended Daily Allowance (U.S. RDA)	
Vitamin E	150	45.0 I.U.
Vitamin C	1000	600.0 mg
Thiamine (Vitamin B_1)	1000	15.0 mg
Riboflavin (Vitamin B_2)	600	10.2 mg
Niacin	500	100.0 mg
Vitamin B_6	500	10.0 mg
Vitamin B_{12}	100	6.0 mcg
Pantothenic Acid	250	25.0 mg
Mineral Composition		
Zinc	150	22.5 mg*

*22.5 mg zinc (equivalent to zinc content in 100 mg zinc sulfate, USP)

Ingredients: Niacinamide Ascorbate; Ascorbic Acid; Microcrystalline Cellulose; Zinc Sulfate; Vitamin E Acetate; Calcium Pantothenate; Food Starch—Modified; Hydroxypropyl Methylcellulose; Thiamine Mononitrate; Stearic Acid; Pyridoxine Hydrochloride; Riboflavin; Silicon Dioxide; Polysorbate 20; Magnesium Stearate; Lactose; Polyvinylpyrrolidone; Propylene Glycol; Artificial Color; Vanillin; Hydroxypropyl Cellulose; Gelatin; Sorbic Acid; Sodium Benzoate; Cyanocobalamin.

Actions and Uses: Z-BEC is a high potency formulation. Its components have important roles in general nutrition, healing of wounds, and prevention of hemorrhage. It is recommended for deficiencies of these components in conditions such as febrile diseases, chronic or acute infections, burns, fractures, surgery, leg ulcers, toxic conditions, physiologic stress, alcoholism, prolonged exposure to high temperature, geriatrics, gastritis, peptic ulcer, and colitis; and in conditions involving special diets and weight-reduction diets.
In dentistry, Z-BEC is recommended for deficiencies of its components in conditions such as herpetic stomatitis, aphthous stomatitis, cheilosis, herpangina and gingivitis.

Precaution: Not intended for the treatment of pernicious anemia.

Dosage: The recommended OTC dosage for adults and children 12 or more years of age is one tablet daily with food or after meals. Under the direction and supervision of a physician, the dose and frequency of administration may be increased in accordance with the patient's requirements.

How Supplied: Green film-coated, capsule-shaped tablets engraved AHR on one side and Z-BEC on the other in bottles of 60 (NDC 0031-0689-62), 500 (NDC 0031-0689-70), and Dis-Co® Unit Dose Packs of 100 (NDC 0031-0689-64).

Ross Laboratories
COLUMBUS, OH 43216

PEDIATRIC NUTRITIONAL PRODUCTS

Alimentum® Protein Hydrolysate Formula With Iron

Isomil® Soy Protein Formula With Iron

Isomil® SF Sucrose-Free Soy Protein Formula With Iron

PediaSure® Liquid Nutrition for Children

RCF® Ross Carbohydrate Free Low-Iron Soy Protein Formula Base

Similac® Low-Iron Infant Formula

Similac® PM 60/40 Low-Iron Infant Formula

Similac® Special Care® With Iron 24 Premature Infant Formula

Similac® With Iron Infant Formula

For most current information, refer to product labels.

CLEAR® EYES
[klēr īz]
Lubricating Eye Redness Reliever

Description: Clear Eyes is a sterile, isotonic buffered solution containing the active ingredients naphazoline hydrochloride (0.012%) and glycerin (0.2%). It also contains boric acid, purified water and sodium borate. Edetate disodium (0.1%) and benzalkonium chloride (0.01%) are added as preservatives. Clear Eyes is a lubricating, decongestant ophthalmic solution specially designed for temporary relief of redness and drying due to minor eye irritation caused by dust, smoke, smog, sun glare, wearing contact lenses, colds, allergies, swimming, reading, driving, TV or close work. Clear Eyes contains laboratory tested and scientifically blended ingredients, including an effective vasoconstrictor which narrows swollen blood vessels and rapidly whitens reddened eyes in a formulation which also contains a lubricant and produces a refreshing, soothing effect. Clear Eyes is a sterile, isotonic solution compatible with the natural fluids of the eye.

Indications: For the temporary relief of redness due to minor eye irritation AND for protection against further irritation or dryness of the eye.

Warnings: To avoid contamination, do not touch tip of container to any surface. Replace cap after using. If you experience eye pain, changes in vision, continued redness or irritation of the eye, or if the condition worsens or persists for more than 72 hours, discontinue use and consult a doctor. If you have glaucoma, do not use this product except under the advice and supervision of a physician. Overuse of this product may produce increased redness of the eye. If solution changes color or becomes cloudy, do not use. Keep this and all drugs out of the reach of children. **Remove contact lenses before using.**

Directions: Instill 1 or 2 drops in the affected eye(s), up to four times daily.

How Supplied: In 0.5-fl-oz and 1.0-fl-oz plastic dropper bottles.

Shown in Product Identification Section, page 426

(FAN 2222-03)

EAR DROPS BY MURINE®
[myūr 'ēn]
See Murine Ear Wax Removal System/Murine Ear Drops.

MURINE® EAR WAX REMOVAL SYSTEM/MURINE® EAR DROPS
[myūr 'ēn]
Carbamide Peroxide
Ear Wax Removal Aid

Description: MURINE EAR DROPS contains the active ingredient carbamide peroxide, 6.5%. It also contains alcohol (6.3%), glycerin, polysorbate 20 and other ingredients. The MURINE EAR WAX REMOVAL SYSTEM includes a 1.0-fl-oz soft bulb ear syringe. This system is a complete medically approved system to safely remove ear wax. Application of carbamide peroxide drops followed by warm-water irrigation is an effective, medically recommended way to help loosen excessive and/or hardened ear wax.

Actions: The carbamide peroxide formula in MURINE EAR DROPS is an aid in the removal of wax from the ear canal. Anhydrous glycerin penetrates and softens wax while the release of oxygen from carbamide peroxide provides a mechanical action resulting in the loosening of the softened wax accumulation. It is usually necessary to remove the loosened wax by gently flushing the ear with warm water using the soft bulb ear syringe provided.

Indications: The MURINE EAR WAX REMOVAL SYSTEM is indicated for occasional use as an aid to soften, loosen and remove excessive ear wax.

Warning: DO NOT USE if you have ear drainage or discharge, ear pain, irritation, or rash in the ear or are dizzy; consult a doctor. DO NOT USE if you have an injury or perforation (hole) of the eardrum or after ear surgery, unless directed by a doctor.
DO NOT USE for more than 4 days; if excessive ear wax remains after use of this product, consult a doctor. Avoid contact with the eyes. KEEP THIS AND ALL MEDICINES OUT OF THE REACH OF CHILDREN.

Directions: FOR USE IN THE EAR ONLY. Adults and children over 12 years of age: Tilt head sideways and place 5 to 10 drops in ear. Tip of applicator should not enter ear canal. Keep drops in ear for several minutes by keeping head tilted or placing cotton in the ear. Use twice daily for up to 4 days if needed, or as directed by a doctor. Any wax remaining after treatment may be removed by gently flushing the ear with warm water, using a soft bulb ear syringe. Children under 12 years, consult a doctor.

Note: When the ear canal is irrigated, the tip of the ear syringe should not obstruct the flow of water leaving the ear canal.

How Supplied: The MURINE EAR WAX REMOVAL SYSTEM contains 0.5-fl-oz drops and a 1.0-fl-oz soft bulb ear syringe.
Also available in 0.5-fl-oz drops only, MURINE EAR DROPS.

Shown in Product Identification Section, page 426

(FAN 2273)

MURINE®
[myūr 'ēn]
Eye Lubricant

Description: Murine eye lubricant is a sterile buffered solution containing the active ingredients 1.4% polyvinyl alcohol and 0.6% povidone. Also contains benzalkonium chloride, dextrose, disodium edetate, potassium chloride, purified water, sodium bicarbonate, sodium chloride, sodium citrate and sodium phosphate (mono- and dibasic). Murine is a clear solution formulated to more closely match the natural tear fluid of the eye for gentle, soothing relief from minor eye irritation while moisturizing and relieving dryness. Use as desired to temporarily relieve minor eye irritation, dryness and burning due to dust, smoke, smog, sun glare, wearing contact lenses, colds, allergies, swimming, reading, driving, TV or close work.

Indications: For the temporary relief or prevention of further discomfort due to minor eye irritations and symptoms related to dry eyes.

Warning: To avoid contamination, do not touch tip of container to any surface. Replace cap after using. If you experience eye pain, changes in vision, continued redness or irritation of the eye, or if the condition worsens or persists for more than 72 hours, discontinue use and consult a doctor. If solution changes color or becomes cloudy, do not use. Keep this and all drugs out of the reach of children. **Remove contact lenses before using.**

Directions: Instill 1 or 2 drops in the affected eye(s) as needed.

How Supplied: In 0.5-fl-oz and 1.0-fl-oz plastic dropper bottles.

Shown in Product Identification Section, page 426

(FAN 2202-04)

Continued on next page

If desired, additional information on any Ross Product will be provided upon request to Ross Laboratories.

Ross—Cont.

MURINE® PLUS

[myūr 'ēn]

Lubricating Eye Redness Reliever

Description: Murine Plus is a sterile, non-staining buffered solution containing the active ingredients 1.4% polyvinyl alcohol, 0.6% povidone and 0.05% tetrahydrozoline hydrochloride. Also contains benzalkonium chloride, dextrose, disodium edetate, potassium chloride, purified water, sodium bicarbonate, sodium chloride, sodium citrate and sodium phosphate (mono- and dibasic). Murine Plus is an isotonic, sterile ophthalmic solution, formulated to more closely match the natural tear fluid of the eye. Its contains demulcents for gentle, soothing relief from minor eye irritation as well as the sympathomimetic agent, tetrahydrozoline hydrochloride, which produces local vasoconstriction in the eye. Thus, the drug effectively narrows swollen blood vessels locally and provides symptomatic relief of edema and hyperemia of conjunctival tissues due to eye allergies, minor local irritations and conjunctivitis. Use up to 4 times daily, to remove redness due to minor eye irritation caused by dust, smoke, smog, sun glare, wearing contact lenses, colds, allergies, swimming, reading, driving, TV or close work. The effect of Murine Plus is prompt (apparent within minutes) and sustained.

Indications: For the temporary relief or prevention of further discomfort due to minor eye irritations and symptoms related to dry eyes PLUS removal of redness.

Warning: To avoid contamination, do not touch tip of container to any surface. Replace cap after using. If you experience eye pain, changes in vision, continued redness or irritation of the eye, or if the condition worsens or persists for more than 72 hours, discontinue use and consult a doctor. If you have glaucoma, do not use this product except under the advice and supervision of a physician. Overuse of this product may produce increased redness of the eye. If solution changes color or becomes cloudy, do not use. Keep this and all drugs out of the reach of children. **Remove contact lenses before using.**

Directions: Instill 1 or 2 drops in the affected eye(s), up to four times daily.

How Supplied: In 0.5-fl-oz and 1.0-fl-oz plastic dropper bottle.

Shown in Product Identification Section, page 426

(FAN 2202-04)

Pedialyte, Rehydralyte Administration Guide

For Infants and Young Children

Age	2 Weeks	3	6 Months	9	1	1½	2	2½ Years	3	3½	4
Approximate Weight[2]											
(lb)	7	13	17	20	23	25	28	30	32	35	38
(kg)	3.2	6.0	7.8	9.2	10.2	11.4	12.6	13.6	14.6	16.0	17.0
PEDIALYTE UNFLAVORED or FRUIT-FLAVORED fl oz/day for maintenance*	13 to 16	28 to 32	34 to 40	38 to 44	41 to 46	45 to 50	48 to 53	51 to 56	54 to 58	56 to 60	57 to 62
REHYDRALYTE fl oz/day for Replacement for 5% Dehydration (including maintenance)*	18 to 21	38 to 42	47 to 53	53 to 59	58 to 63	64 to 69	69 to 74	74 to 79	78 to 82	83 to 87	85 to 90
REHYDRALYTE fl oz/day for Replacement for 10% Dehydration (including maintenance)*	23 to 26	48 to 52	60 to 66	68 to 74	75 to 80	83 to 88	90 to 95	97 to 102	102 to 106	110 to 114	113 to 118

Administration Guide does not apply to infants less than 1 week of age. For children over 4 years, maintenance intakes may exceed 2 qt daily.

1. Extrapolated from Barness L: Nutrition and nutritional disorders, in Behrman RE, Vaughan VC III: *Nelson Textbook of Pediatrics,* ed 12. Philadelphia, WB Saunders Co, 1983, pp 136-138.
2. Weight based on the 50th percentile of weight for age of the National Center for Health Statistics (NCHS) reference data. Hamill PVV, Drizd TA, Johnson CL, et al: Physical growth: National Center for Health Statistics percentiles. *Am J Clin Nutr* 1979; 32:607-629.

* Fluid intakes do not take into account ongoing stool losses. Fluid loss in the stool should be replaced by consumption of an extra amount of Pedialyte or Rehydralyte equal to stool losses in addition to the amounts given in this Administration Guide.

PEDIALYTE®

[pē 'dē-ah-līt "]

Oral Electrolyte Maintenance Solution

Usage: To restore fluid and minerals lost in diarrhea and vomiting by infants and children; to maintain water and electrolytes following corrective parenteral therapy for severe diarrhea.

Features:

- Ready To Use—no mixing or dilution necessary.
- Balanced electrolytes to replace usual stool losses and provide maintenance requirements.
- Provides glucose to promote sodium and water absorption.
- Fruit-flavored form available to enhance compliance in older infants and children.
- Plastic quart bottles are resealable, easy to pour and easy to measure.
- No coloring added.
- Widely available in grocery, drug and convenience stores.

Availability:

32-fl-oz plastic bottles; 8 per case; Unflavored, No. 336—NDC 0074-6470-32; Fruit-flavored, No. 365—NDC 0074-6471-32.

8-fl-oz bottles; 4 six-packs per case; Unflavored, No. 160—NDC 0074-6470-08. For hospital use, Pedialyte is available in the Ross Hospital Formula System.

Dosage: See Administration Guide to restore fluid and minerals lost in diarrhea and vomiting (Pedialyte Unflavored or Fruit-Flavored) and to manage mild to moderate dehydration secondary to moderate to severe diarrhea (Rehydralyte® Oral Electrolyte Rehydration Solution). Pedialyte (Unflavored or Fruit-Flavored) or Rehydralyte should be offered frequently in amounts tolerated. Total daily intake should be adjusted to meet individual needs, based on thirst and response to therapy. The suggested intakes for maintenance are based on water requirements for ordinary energy expenditure.[1] The suggested intakes for replacement are based on fluid losses of 5% or 10% of body weight, including maintenance requirement.

[See table .]

Composition: Unflavored Pedialyte (Fruit-Flavored Pedialyte has similar composition and nutrient value. For specific information, see product label.)

Ingredients: (Pareve, Ⓤ) Water, dextrose, potassium citrate, sodium chloride and sodium citrate.

Provides:	Per 8 Fl Oz	Per Liter	Per 32 Fl Oz
Sodium (mEq)	10.6	45	42.4
Potassium (mEq)	4.7	20	18.8
Chloride (mEq)	8.3	35	33.2
Citrate (mEq)	7.1	30	28.4
Dextrose (g)	5.9	25	23.6
Calories	24	100	96

(FAN 718-01)

REHYDRALYTE®

[*rē-hī ′drə-līt ″*]

Oral Electrolyte Rehydration Solution

Usage: For replacement of water and electrolytes lost during moderate to severe diarrhea.

Features:

- Ready To Use—no mixing or dilution necessary.
- Safe, economical alternative to IV therapy.
- 75 mEq of sodium per liter for effective replacement of fluid deficits.
- 2½% glucose solution to promote sodium and water absorption and provide energy.
- Widely available in pharmacies.

Availability: 8-fl-oz bottles; 4 six-packs per case; No. 162; NDC 0074-0162-01.

Dosage: (See Administration Guide under Pedialyte.)

Ingredients: (Pareve, ⓤ) Water, dextrose, sodium chloride, potassium citrate and sodium citrate.

Provides:	Per 8 Fl Oz	Per Liter
Sodium (mEq)	17.7	75
Potassium (mEq)	4.7	20
Chloride (mEq)	15.4	65
Citrate (mEq)	7.1	30
Dextrose (g)	5.9	25
Calories	24	100

(FAN 437-01)

SELSUN BLUE®

[*sel ′sən blü*]

Dandruff Shampoo (selenium sulfide lotion, 1%)

Selsun Blue is a non-prescription antidandruff shampoo containing the active ingredient selenium sulfide, 1%, in a freshly scented, pH balanced formula to leave hair clean and manageable. Available in Dry, Oily, Regular, Extra Conditioning and Extra Medicated formulas (also contains 0.5% menthol).

Inactive ingredients:

Dry formula —Acetylated lanolin alcohol, ammonium laureth sulfate, ammonium lauryl sulfate, cetyl acetate, citric acid, cocamide DEA, cocamidopropyl betaine, DMDM hydantoin, FD&C blue No. 1, fragrance, hydroxypropyl methylcellulose, magnesium aluminum silicate, polysorbate 80, sodium chloride, titanium dioxide, water and other ingredients.

Regular formula —Ammonium laureth sulfate, ammonium lauryl sulfate, citric acid, cocamide DEA, cocamidopropyl betaine, DMDM hydantoin, FD&C blue No. 1, fragrance, hydroxypropyl methylcellulose, magnesium aluminum silicate, sodium chloride, titanium dioxide, water and other ingredients.

Oily formula —Ammonium laureth sulfate, ammonium lauryl sulfate, citric acid, cocamide DEA, cocamidopropyl betaine, DMDM hydantoin, FD&C blue No. 1, fragrance, hydroxypropyl methylcellulose, magnesium aluminum silicate, sodium chloride, titanium dioxide, water and other ingredients.

Extra Conditioning formula —Acetylated lanolin alcohol, aloe, ammonium laureth sulfate, ammonium lauryl sulfate, cetyl acetate, citric acid, cocamide DEA, cocamidopropyl betaine, DMDM hydantoin, FD&C blue No. 1, fragrance, glycol distearate, hydroxypropyl methylcellulose, magnesium aluminum silicate, polysorbate 80, propylene glycol, sodium chloride, TEA-lauryl sulfate, titanium dioxide, water and other ingredients.

Extra Medicated formula —Ammonium laureth sulfate, ammonium lauryl sulfate, citric acid, cocamide DEA, cocamidopropyl betaine, DMDM hydantoin, D&C red No. 33, FD&C blue No. 1, fragrance, hydroxypropyl methylcellulose, magnesium aluminum silicate, sodium chloride, TEA-lauryl sulfate, water and other ingredients.

Clinical testing has shown Selsun Blue to be as safe and effective as other leading shampoos in helping control dandruff symptoms with regular use.

Directions: Shake well before using. Lather, rinse thoroughly and repeat. For best results, use at least twice a week, or as directed by doctor.

Warnings: For external use only. Avoid contact with eyes—if this happens, rinse thoroughly with water. If condition worsens or does not improve, consult doctor. Keep out of the reach of children. **Caution:** If used on bleached, tinted, or permanent-waved hair, rinse for 5 minutes.

How Supplied: 4-, 7- and 11-fl-oz plastic bottles.

Shown in Product Identification Section, page 427

(FAN 2260-02)

TRONOLANE®

[*tron ′ə-lān*]

Anesthetic Cream for Hemorrhoids
Anesthetic Suppositories for Hemorrhoids

Description: The active ingredient in Tronolane is a topical anesthetic agent (Cream: pramoxine hydrochloride 1%; Suppositories: pramoxine 1% as pramoxine and pramoxine HCl), chemically unrelated to the benzoate esters of the "caine" type, which is chemically designated as a 4-n-butoxyphenyl gammamorpholinopropyl-ether hydrochloride. The cream contains the following inactive ingredients: A nongreasy zinc oxide cream base containing beeswax, cetyl alcohol, cetyl esters wax, glycerin, methylparaben, propylparaben, sodium lauryl sulfate, water and zinc oxide. The suppository contains the following inactive ingredients: A base containing hydrogenated cocoa glycerides and zinc oxide.

Indications: Tronolane is a topical anesthetic indicated for the temporary relief of the pain, burning, itching and discomfort that accompany hemorrhoids. It has a soothing, lubricating action on mucous membranes.

Tronolane contains a rapidly acting topical anesthetic producing analgesia that lasts up to 5 hours. Because the drug is chemically unrelated to other anesthetics, cross-sensitization is unlikely. Patients who are already sensitized to the "caine" anesthetics can generally use Tronolane.

The emollient/emulsion base of Tronolane cream provides soothing lubrication, making bowel movements more comfortable. Tronolane cream is in a nondrying base that is nongreasy and nonstaining to undergarments.

Warnings: If bleeding is present, consult physician. Certain persons can develop allergic reactions to ingredients in this product. During treatment, if condition worsens or persists 7 days, consult physician. For children under 12 years, use only as directed by physician. Keep out of the reach of children. As with any drug, if you are pregnant or nursing a baby, we recommend that you seek the advice of a health care professional before using this product.

Dosage and Administration: CREAM: Apply up to five times daily, especially morning, night, and after bowel movements, or as directed by physician. *External* —Apply liberally to affected area. *Intrarectal* —Remove cap from tube and attach clean applicator. Remove protective cover from clean applicator. Squeeze tube to fill applicator and lubricate tip with cream. Gently insert applicator into rectum and squeeze tube again. Thoroughly cleanse applicator after use. SUPPOSITORIES: Use up to five times daily, especially morning, night, and after bowel movements, or as directed by physician. Detach one suppository from pack. Separate foil at rounded end and peel apart until suppository is exposed. Insert suppository into the rectum, rounded end first.

How Supplied: Tronolane is available in 1-oz and 2-oz cream tubes and 10- and 20-count suppository boxes.

Shown in Product Identification Section, page 427

(FAN 2093-03)

If desired, additional information on any Ross Product will be provided upon request to Ross Laboratories.

Products are indexed by generic and chemical names in the
YELLOW SECTION

Russ Pharmaceuticals, Inc.
22 INVERNESS CENTER PARKWAY
BIRMINGHAM, AL 35238-0188

AMESEC®
[*am 'ah-sec*]
Aminophylline Compound Antiasthmatic

Description: Each capsule contains:

Aminophylline	130 mg
(equivalent to 104 mg theophylline)	
Ephedrine hydrochloride	25 mg

Each capsule also contains colloidal silicon dioxide, FD&C Blue No. 2, FD&C Red No. 3, FD&C Yellow No. 6, gelatin, iron oxide black, and starch.

Indications: For temporary relief of bronchial asthma.

Warnings: Do not take this product unless a diagnosis of asthma has been made by a physician.
As with any drug, if you are pregnant or nursing a baby, seek the advice of a health professional before using this product.
Keep this and all drugs out of the reach of children. In case of accidental overdose, seek professional assistance or contact a Poison Control Center immediately.

Drug Interaction Precaution: Do not take this product if you are presently taking a prescription antihypertensive or antidepressant drug containing a monoamine oxidase inhibitor.

Caution: Do not continue to take this product but seek medical assistance immediately if symptoms are not relieved within one hour or become worse. Do not take this product if you are presently taking a drug or suppository containing any form of theophylline or give to children under 12 years or exceed recommended dosage except under the advice and supervision of a physician. Excessive use may cause toxic effects and even death in children. Do not take this product if you have heart disease, high blood pressure, thyroid disease, diabetes, or difficulty in urination due to enlargement of the prostate gland, or if nausea, vomiting, or restlessness occurs. Nervousness, tremor, sleeplessness, nausea, and loss of appetite may occur.

Usual Adult Dosage: One capsule every six hours not to exceed five capsules a day or as directed by a physician.

How Supplied: Bottles of 100 capsules.

CORTICAINE®
[*kort 'ah-kān "*]
(hydrocortisone acetate)

Description: The active ingredient in Corticaine® is hydrocortisone acetate 0.5%. Corticaine also contains esters of mixed saturated fatty acids, stearyl alcohol, glycerin, polysorbate 40, menthol, BHA, BHT, disodium EDTA, and purified water with methylparaben and propylparaben as preservatives.
Store at controlled room temperature 15° to 30°C (59° to 86°F). Keep tube well closed.

Indications: For the temporary relief of itching associated with external anal inflammation.

Warnings: For External Use Only. Avoid contact with the eyes. In case of accidental ingestion, seek professional assistance or contact a Poison Control Center immediately. If condition worsens or symptoms persist for more than 7 days, discontinue use of this product and consult a physician. Do not use on children under the age of 3 years unless under the advice and supervision of a physician. Keep this and all drugs out of the reach of children.

Dosage and Administration: For adults and children 3 years of age and older, apply to the affected area from one to four times daily. For children under 3 years of age, use only under the advice and supervision of a physician.

How Supplied: Corticaine® (hydrocortisone acetate) is supplied in 1 ounce tubes.

Shown in Product Identification Section, page 427

VICON–C® Capsules
[*vī 'kon*]
(Therapeutic Vitamins and Minerals)

Description: Each yellow and orange capsule contains:

Ascorbic acid	300 mg
Niacinamide	100 mg
Zinc sulfate, USP*	80 mg
Magnesium sulfate, USP**	70 mg
Thiamine mononitrate	20 mg
d-Calcium pantothenate	20 mg
Riboflavin	10 mg
Pyridoxine hydrochloride	5 mg

*As 50 mg dried zinc sulfate.
**As 50 mg dried magnesium sulfate.

Each capsule also contains D&C Yellow No. 10, FD&C Yellow No. 6, gelatin, microcrystalline cellulose, soybean oil, stearic acid, talc, sodium propionate, and titanium dioxide.

Indications and Usage: VICON-C® is indicated in the treatment of patients with deficiencies of, or increased requirements for, Vitamin C, B-complex vitamins, zinc, and/or magnesium. The components of VICON-C have important roles in nutrition, tissue growth and repair, and the prevention of hemorrhage. Tissue injury resulting from trauma, burns, or surgery may rapidly deplete the body stores of Vitamin C, the B-Complex vitamins, and zinc. Patients maintained on parenteral fluids for extended periods or patients with burns, wounds, or diarrhea often develop deficiencies of Vitamin C, the B-Complex vitamins, and zinc.
VICON-C is recommended for deficiencies or the prevention of deficiencies of Vitamin C, the B-Complex vitamins, magnesium, and/or zinc in conditions such as febrile diseases, chronic or acute infections, burns, fractures, surgery, toxic conditions, physiologic stress, alcoholism, pregnancy, lactation, geriatrics, peptic ulcer, colitis, and in conditions involving special diets and weight-reduction diets. It is also recommended in dentistry for these deficiencies in conditions such as herpetic stomatitis, aphthous stomatitis, cheilosis, herpangina, gingivitis, and states involving oral surgery.

Dosage and Administration: One capsule two or three times daily or as directed by a physician for treatment of deficiencies.

How Supplied: Bottles of 60 capsules and unit dose pack of 100 capsules.

Shown in Product Identification Section, page 427

VICON® PLUS Capsules
[*vī 'kon*]
(Therapeutic Vitamins and Minerals)

Description: Each red and beige capsule contains:

Vitamin A	4,000 IU
Vitamin E	50 IU
Ascorbic Acid	150 mg
Zinc sulfate, USP*	80 mg
Magnesium sulfate, USP**	70 mg
Niacinamide	25 mg
Thiamine mononitrate	10 mg
d-Calcium pantothenate	10 mg
Riboflavin	5 mg
Magnanese chloride	4 mg
Pyridoxine hydrochloride	2 mg

*As 50 mg dried zinc sulfate.
**As 50 mg dried magnesium sulfate.

Each capsule also contains D&C Yellow No. 10, FD&C Blue No. 1, FD&C Red No. 40, FD&C Yellow No. 6, gelatin, lactose, magnesium stearate, talc, and titanium dioxide.
VICON® PLUS is an extended range vitamin-mineral supplement formulated to aid patient recovery by helping to meet increased nutritional demands.

Indications and Usage: For nutritional supplementation of the patient undergoing physiologic stress due to surgery, burns, trauma, febrile illnesses, or poor nutrition.

Dosage and Administration: One capsule twice daily or as prescribed by a physician for treatment of deficiencies. Dosage should not exceed eight capsules daily due to the possible toxicity of large doses of vitamin A.

How Supplied: Bottles of 60 capsules.

Shown in Product Identification Section, page 427

VI–ZAC® Capsules
[*vī-zak*]
(Therapeutic Vitamin-Mineral)

Description: Each orange capsule contains:

Vitamin A	5,000 IU
Absorbic acid	500 mg
Vitamin E	50 IU
Zinc sulfate, USP*	80 mg

*As 50 mg dried zinc sulfate

Each capsule also contains methylcellulose, FD&C Yellow No. 6, FD&C Yellow No. 10, gelatin, lactose, magnesium stearate, and titanium dioxide.

Indications and Usage: VI-ZAC® is indicated in the treatment of patients with deficiencies of, or increased requirements for, Vitamins A, C, and E and zinc. The VI-ZAC formulation is a limited vitamin-mineral formulation designed to meet special needs. It is particularly indicated where there is no requirement for supplemental amounts of the B-Complex vitamins and their attendant appetite stimulation. The formulation is also designed for patients who cannot tolerate magnesium supplements but do need supplemental amounts of zinc.

Precautions: Although rarely encountered, vitamin A in large doses daily for several months or longer may cause toxicity.

Dosage and Administration: One or two capsules daily or as directed by the physician for the treatment of deficiencies.

How Supplied: Bottles of 60.
Shown in Product Identification Section, page 427

Rydelle Laboratories

Division of S. C. Johnson & Son, Inc.
1525 HOWE STREET
RACINE, WI 53403

AVEENO® ANTI-ITCH
[ah-ve 'no]
CREAM
(External analgesic/Skin protectant)

Aveeno® Anti-Itch Cream provides fast temporary relief of the itching and pain associated with many minor skin irritations such as chicken pox rash, poison ivy/oak/sumac, and insect bites. Unlike hydrocortisone products, Aveeno Anti-Itch Cream contains calamine to dry up weepy rashes, help control further spreading and promote healing. Aveeno's soothing oatmeal-enriched formula is non-greasy and invisible when rubbed into the skin.

Directions: Adults and children 2 years and older: Apply no more than 4 times daily. Children under 2: Consult a physician.

Warnings: For external use only. Avoid contact with eyes. If condition does not improve or recurs within 7 days, discontinue use and consult a physician. Keep out of children's reach. If ingested, contact a physician or poison control center. Store at 59°–86°F.

Active Ingredients: CALAMINE 3.0%, PRAMOXINE HCl 1.0%, CAMPHOR 0.3% IN A BASE OF WATER, GLYCERIN, DISTEARYLDIMONIUM CHLORIDE, PETROLATUM, OATMEAL FLOUR, ISOPROPYL PALMITATE, CETYL ALCOHOL, DIMETHICONE, SODIUM CHLORIDE.

How Supplied: 1 oz. tube.
Shown in Product Identification Section, page 427

AVEENO® ANTI-ITCH
[ah-ve 'no]
CONCENTRATED LOTION
(External analgesic/Skin protectant)

Aveeno® Anti-Itch Concentrated Lotion provides fast, temporary relief of the itching and pain associated with minor skin irritations such as chicken pox rash, poison ivy/oak/sumac, and insect bites. Unlike hydrocortisone products, Aveeno Anti-Itch Lotion contains calamine to dry up weepy rashes, help control further spreading and promote healing. But Aveeno's thick, creamy formula is concentrated—with less water and more emollients—so it won't run or drip. It's non-greasy and invisible when rubbed into skin.
Can be used in between Aveeno Bath Treatments for on-the-spot itch relief.

Directions: Adults and children 2 years and older: Apply no more than 4 times daily. Children under 2: Consult a physician.

Warnings: For external use only. Avoid contact with eyes. If condition does not improve or recurs within 7 days, discontinue use and consult a physician. Keep out of children's reach. If ingested, contact a physician or poison control center. Store at 59°–86°F.

Active Ingredients: CALAMINE 3.0%, PRAMOXINE HCl 1.0%, CAMPHOR 0.3% IN A BASE OF WATER, GLYCERIN, DISTEARYLDIMONIUM CHLORIDE, PETROLATUM, OATMEAL FLOUR, ISOPROPYL PALMITATE, CETYL ALCOHOL, DIMETHICONE, SODIUM CHLORIDE.

How Supplied: 4 oz bottle.
Shown in Product Identification Section, page 427

AVEENO® BATH TREATMENTS
[ah-ve 'no]
REGULAR FORMULA AND OILATED FOR DRY SKIN

AVEENO® BATH TREATMENTS contain colloidal oatmeal, a natural oat derivative developed especially for soothing and cleaning itchy, sore, sensitive skin.
AVEENO® BATH TREATMENTS contain no soaps or synthetic detergents that may be harmful to the skin. They cleanse naturally because of their unique adsorptive properties.
AVEENO BATH TREATMENTS can be used in the care of itch due to dry skin, rashes, psoriasis, hemorrhoidal and genital irritations, poison ivy/oak, and sunburn. They are safe for use on children and can be used in the treatment of chicken pox, diaper rash, prickly heat and hives.

Ingredients: Aveeno Bath Regular: 100% colloidal oatmeal; Aveeno Bath Oilated: 43% colloidal oatmeal, mineral oil.
Shown in Product Identification Section, page 427

AVEENO® CLEANSING BAR
[ah-ve 'no]
FOR NORMAL TO OILY SKIN

AVEENO® Cleansing Bar For Normal To Oily Skin is made especially for itchy, sensitive skin that is irritated by ordinary soaps.
More than 50% of this mild skin cleanser is colloidal oatmeal, noted for its soothing and protective qualities.
Aveeno® Cleansing Bar is completely soap-free. It leaves no harsh alkaline film to irritate delicate skin, and it leaves skin feeling soft and comfortable.

Ingredients: Aveeno® Colloidal Oatmeal, 51%; in a sudsing soap-free base containing a mild surfactant.
Shown in Product Identification Section, page 427

AVEENO® CLEANSING BAR
[ah-ve 'no]
FOR ACNE

AVEENO® Cleansing Bar For Acne is a unique soap-free cleanser. It combines colloidal oatmeal, a long recognized, natural anti-itch treatment and gentle adsorbing cleanser, with special medication to eliminate most blackheads or acne pimples.

Ingredients: Aveeno® Colloidal Oatmeal, 51%; salicylic acid 2%; in a sudsing soap-free base containing a mild surfactant.
Shown in Product Identification Section, page 427

AVEENO® CLEANSING BAR
[ah-ve 'no]
FOR DRY SKIN

AVEENO® Cleansing Bar For Dry Skin is a unique, soap-free cleanser for itchy, dry, sensitive skin that is irritated by ordinary soaps. It contains over 15% skin-softening emollients to help replace natural skin oils and 51% colloidal oatmeal, recommended for its soothing and protective qualities.

Ingredients: Aveeno® Colloidal Oatmeal, 51%, in a sudsing soap-free base containing vegetable oils, glycerine, and a mild surfactant.
Shown in Product Identification Section, page 427

AVEENO® MOISTURIZING LOTION
[ah-ve 'no]
FOR RELIEF OF DRY, ITCHY SKIN

AVEENO® Moisturizing Lotion has been clinically proven to relieve dry skin. It contains natural colloidal oatmeal to relieve the itch often associated with dry skin. It is noncomedogenic and contains

Continued on next page

Rydelle—Cont.

no fragrance, parabens, or lanolin which can cause allergic reactions.

Active Ingredient: Colloidal oatmeal 1%.
Also Contains: Water, glycerin, distearyldimonium chloride, petrolatum, isopropyl palmitate, cetyl alcohol, dimethicone, sodium chloride, benzyl alcohol.

Shown in Product Identification Section, page 427

AVEENO® SHOWER AND BATH OIL
[*ah-ve 'no*]
FOR RELIEF OF DRY, ITCHY SKIN

AVEENO® Shower and Bath Oil combines the lubricating properties of mineral oil with the natural anti-itch benefits of colloidal oatmeal for the relief of dry, itchy skin. It contains no fragrance, parabens or lanolin which can cause allergic reactions.

Active Ingredient: Colloidal oatmeal 5%.
Also contains: Mineral oil, glyceryl stearate and PEG 100 stearate, laureth-4, benzyl alcohol, silica, benzaldehyde.

Shown in Product Identification Section, page 427

RHULICREAM®
(External analgesic/Skin protectant)

Rhulicream® works on contact to provide fast, soothing, temporary relief of the itching and pain associated with many minor skin irritations. Apply this non-greasy calamine formula after exposure to poison ivy/oak/sumac to dry oozing and weeping, help to control further spreading and promote healing.

Directions: Adults and children 2 years and older: Apply to affected area no more than 4 times daily. Children under 2: Consult a physician.

Warnings: For external use only. Avoid contact with eyes. If condition does not improve or recurs within 7 days, discontinue use and consult a physician. Keep out of children's reach. If ingested contact a physician or poison control center. Store at 59°–86°F.

Active Ingredients: Benzocaine 5.0%, Calamine 3.0%, Camphor 0.3% in a base of Water, Glycerin, Distearyldimonium Chloride, Petrolatum, Isopropyl Palmitate, Cetyl Alcohol, Dimethicone, Sodium Chloride.

How Supplied: 2 oz. tube.

Shown in Product Identification Section, page 427

RHULIGEL®
(External analgesic)

Rhuligel® provides fast, cooling, temporary relief of the itching and pain associated with many minor skin irritations, including poison ivy/oak/sumac, insect bites, and sunburn. Clear Rhuligel is non-greasy and invisible on the skin. Won't stain clothing.

Directions: Adults and children 2 years and older: Apply to affected area no more than 4 times daily. Children under 2: Consult a physician.

Warnings: For external use only. Avoid contact with eyes. If condition does not improve or recurs within 7 days, discontinue use and consult a physician. Keep out of children's reach. If ingested contact a physician or poison control center. Store at 59°–86°F.

Active Ingredients: Benzyl Alcohol 2%, Menthol 0.3%, Camphor 0.3% in a base of SD Alcohol 23A 31% w/w, Purified Water, Propylene Glycol, Carbomer 940, Triethanolamine, Benzophenone-4, EDTA.

How Supplied: 2 oz. tube.

Shown in Product Identification Section, page 427

RHULISPRAY®
(External analgesic/Skin protectant)

Rhulispray® works on contact to provide fast, cooling, temporary relief of the itching and pain associated with many minor skin irritations. Calamine-based formula dries the oozing and weeping of poison ivy/oak/sumac. Convenient spray action eliminates the need to touch delicate inflamed skin.

Directions: Shake well before use. Adults and children 2 years and older: Apply to affected area no more than 4 times daily. Children under 2: Consult a physician.

Warnings: For external use only. Avoid contact with eyes. If condition does not improve or recurs within 7 days, discontinue use and consult a physician. Keep out of children's reach. If ingested contact a physician or poison control center. Store at 59°–86°F.

Caution: Flammable. Contents under pressure. Do not puncture or incinerate. Intentional misuse by deliberately concentrating and inhaling the contents can be harmful or fatal. Do not use near an open flame. May burst at temperatures above 120°F.

Active Ingredients (in concentrate): Calamine 13.8%, Benzocaine 5.0%, Camphor 0.7% in a base of Benzyl Alcohol, Hydrated Silica, Isobutane, Isopropyl Alcohol 70% w/w (concentrate), Oleyl Alcohol, Sorbitan Trioleate.

How Supplied: 4 oz. aerosol.

Shown in Product Identification Section, page 427

Products are indexed alphabetically in the **PINK SECTION**

Sandoz Pharmaceuticals/ Consumer Division
59 ROUTE 10
EAST HANOVER, NJ 07936

ACID MANTLE® CREME
[*ă 'sĭd-mănt 'l*]
Acid pH

Description: A greaseless, water-miscible preparation containing buffered aluminum acetate. Other ingredients: aluminum sulfate, calcium acetate, cetearyl alcohol, glycerin, light mineral oil, methylparaben, purified water, sodium lauryl sulfate, synthetic beeswax, white petrolatum, white potato dextrin. May also contain: ammonium hydroxide, citric acid.

Indications: A vehicle for compatible topical drugs. Restores and maintains protective acidity of the skin. Provides relief of mildly irritated skin due to exposure to soaps, detergents, chemicals, alkalis. Aids in the treatment of bath dermatitis, athlete's foot, anogenital pruritis, acne, winter eczema and dry, rough, scaly skin of varied causes.

Caution: Limited compatibility and stability with Vitamin A, neomycin and other water-sensitive antibiotics. For external use only. Not for ophthalmic use.

Warnings: Keep this and all drugs out of the reach of children. In case of accidental ingestion, seek professional assistance or contact a Poison Control Center immediately.

Directions: Apply several times daily, especially after wet work.

How Supplied: 1 oz tubes; 4 oz and 1 lb jars.

BiCOZENE® Creme External Analgesic
[*bī-cō-zēn*]

Active Ingredients: Benzocaine 6%, resorcinol 1.67% in a specially prepared cream base.

Inactive Ingredients: Castor Oil, Chlorothymol, Ethanolamine Stearates, Glycerin, Glyceryl Borate, Glyceryl Stearates, Parachlorometaxylenol, Polysorbate 80, Sodium Stearate, Triglycerol Diisostearate, Perfume.

Indications: For the temporary relief of pain and itching associated with minor burns, sunburn, minor cuts, scrapes, insect bites or minor skin irritations.

Actions: Benzocaine is a topical anesthetic and resorcinol is a topical antipruritic, at the concentrations used in BiCozene Creme. Both exert their actions by depressing cutaneous sensory receptors.

Warnings: Do not apply over large areas of the body. Caution: Use only as directed. Keep away from the eyes. Not for prolonged use. If the symptoms persist for more than seven days or clear up and reoccur within a few days, or if a rash or irritation develops, discontinue use and consult a physician. For external use only. **KEEP ALL MEDICINES OUT OF THE REACH OF CHILDREN.** In case of accidental ingestion, seek professional assistance or contact a Poison Control Center immediately.

Drug Interaction Precautions: No known drug interaction.

Dosage and Administration: Adults and children 2 years of age and older: apply to affected area not more than 3 to 4 times daily. Children under 2 years of age: consult a physician. Apply liberally to affected area as needed, several times a day.

How Supplied: BiCozene Creme is available in 1-ounce tubes.

Shown in Product Identification Section, page 427

CAMA® ARTHRITIS PAIN RELIEVER

[*kă 'măh*]

Description: Each CAMA Inlay-Tab® contains: Active ingredients: aspirin, USP, 500 mg (7.7 grains); magnesium oxide, USP, 150 mg; dried aluminum hydroxide gel, USP, 150 mg. Other ingredients: colloidal silicon dioxide, croscarmellose sodium, hydrogenated vegetable oil, methylcellulose, methylparaben, microcrystalline cellulose, polyethylene glycol, povidone, pregelatinized starch, starch, Yellow 6, Yellow 10.

Indications: For the temporary relief of minor arthritic pain.

Warnings: If redness or swelling is present, consult a doctor because these could be signs of a serious condition. Do not take this drug if you have asthma unless directed by a doctor. Do not take this product if you have stomach problems (such as heartburn, upset stomach, or stomach pain) that persists or recurs, or if you have ulcers or bleeding problems, unless directed by a doctor. Children and teenagers should not use this medicine for chicken pox or flu symptoms before a doctor is consulted about Reye syndrome, a rare but serious illness reported to be associated with aspirin. If pain persists for more than 10 days, consult a physician immediately. As with any drug, if you are pregnant or nursing a baby, seek the advice of a health professional before using this product. **IT IS ESPECIALLY IMPORTANT NOT TO USE ASPIRIN DURING THE LAST 3 MONTHS OF PREGNANCY UNLESS SPECIFICALLY DIRECTED TO DO SO BY A DOCTOR BECAUSE IT MAY CAUSE PROBLEMS IN THE UNBORN CHILD OR COMPLICATIONS DURING DELIVERY.** If ringing in the ears or a loss of hearing occurs, consult a doctor before taking any more of this product. Stop taking this product if dizziness occurs. Do not take this product if you are presently taking a prescription drug for anticoagulation (thinning the blood), gout or if you have an aspirin allergy. Do not take this product if you are taking a prescription drug for diabetes unless directed by a doctor. **Keep this and all medicines out of the reach of children. In case of accidental overdose, contact a physician immediately.**

Directions For Use: Adults—2 tablets with a full glass of water every 6 hours. Not to exceed 8 tablets in 24 hours unless directed by a physician. Do not use in children under 12 years of age except under the advice and supervision of a physician.

How Supplied: CAMA Arthritis Pain Reliever Tablets (white with salmon inlay), imprinted "Cama 500" on one side, "Dorsey" on the other, in bottles of 100 and 250.

DORCOL® CHILDREN'S COUGH SYRUP

[*door 'call*]

Description: Each teaspoonful (5 ml) of DORCOL Children's Cough Syrup contains pseudoephedrine hydrochloride 15 mg, guaifenesin 50 mg, dextromethorphan hydrobromide 5 mg. Other ingredients: benzoic acid, Blue 1, edetate disodium, flavors, glycerin, propylene glycol, purified water, Red 40, sodium hydroxide, sucrose, tartaric acid.

Indications: Temporarily relieves your child's cough due to minor throat and bronchial irritation as may occur with the common cold. Helps loosen phlegm (mucus) and thin bronchial secretions to rid the bronchial passageways of bothersome mucus. Helps drain bronchial tubes and makes coughs more productive. Temporarily relieves nasal stuffiness due to the common cold and promotes nasal and/or sinus drainage.

Warnings: Do Not give your child more than the recommended dosage because at higher doses nervousness, dizziness or sleeplessness may occur. Do Not give this preparation if your child has high blood pressure, heart disease, diabetes or thyroid disease. Do Not give this product for persistent or chronic cough such as occurs with asthma or where cough is accompanied by excessive secretions. Keep this and all drugs out of the reach of children. In case of accidental overdose, seek professional assistance or contact a Poison Control Center immediately. A persistent cough may be a sign of a serious condition. If cough or other symptoms persist for more than one week, tend to recur or are accompanied by high fever, rash or persistent headache, consult a physician before continuing use. *Drug Interaction Precaution:* Do not give this product if your child is presently taking a prescription antihypertensive or antidepressant drug containing a monoamine oxidase inhibitor except under the advice and supervision of a physician.

Directions For Use: Children under 2 years—consult physician.

By age:

Children 2 to under 6 years: 1 teaspoonful every 4 hours.

Children 6 to under 12 years: 2 teaspoonfuls every 4 hours.

By weight:

Children 25 to 45 pounds: 1 teaspoonful every 4 hours.

Children 46 to 85 pounds: 2 teaspoonfuls every 4 hours.

Unless directed by a physician, do not exceed 4 doses in 24 hours.

Professional Labeling: The suggested dosage for pediatric patients is:

3–12 months	3 drops/Kg of body weight every 4 hours
12–24 months	7 drops (0.2 ml)/Kg of body weight every 4 hours

Maximum 4 doses in 24 hours.

How Supplied: DORCOL Children's Cough Syrup (grape colored), in 4 fl oz and 8 fl oz plastic bottles with tamper-evident band around child-resistant cap.

Shown in Product Identification Section, page 427

DORCOL® CHILDREN'S DECONGESTANT LIQUID

[*door 'call*]

Description: Each teaspoonful (5 ml) of DORCOL Children's Decongestant Liquid contains pseudoephedrine hydrochloride 15 mg. Other ingredients: benzoic acid, edetate disodium, flavors, purified water, sodium hydroxide, sorbitol, sucrose, Yellow 6, Yellow 10.

Indications: Provides temporary relief of nasal congestion due to the common cold, hay fever or other upper respiratory allergies, or associated with sinusitis. Reduces swelling of nasal passages; to restore freer breathing through the nose. Promotes nasal and sinus drainage; relieves sinus pressure.

Directions For Use: Children under 2 years—consult physician.

By age:

Children 2 to under 6 years: 1 teaspoonful every 4 to 6 hours.

Children 6 years and older: 2 teaspoonfuls every 4 to 6 hours.

By weight:

Children 25 to 45 pounds: 1 teaspoonful every 4 to 6 hours.

Children 46 to 85 pounds: 2 teaspoonfuls every 4 to 6 hours.

Unless directed by a physician, do not exceed 4 doses in 24 hours.

Professional Labeling: The suggested dosage for pediatric patients is:

3–12 months	3 drops/Kg of body weight every 4–6 hours
12–24 months	7 drops (0.2 ml)/Kg of body weight every 4–6 hours.

Maximum of 4 doses in 24 hours.

Warnings: Do not give your child more than the recommended dosage because at higher doses nervousness, dizziness, or sleeplessness may occur. If symptoms do not improve within seven days or are accompanied by high fever, consult a physician before continuing use. Do not give this preparation if your child has high blood pressure, heart disease, diabetes,

Continued on next page

Sandoz Pharm.—Cont.

or thyroid disease except under the advice and supervision of a physician. Keep this and all drugs out of the reach of children. In case of accidental overdose, seek professional assistance or contact a Poison Control Center immediately. *Drug Interaction Precaution:* Do not give this product if your child is presently taking a prescription antihypertensive or antidepressant drug containing a monoamine oxidase inhibitor except under the advice and supervision of a physician.

How Supplied: DORCOL Children's Decongestant Liquid (pale orange), in 4 fl oz bottles with tamper-evident band around child-resistant cap.

Shown in Product Identification Section, page 427

DORCOL® CHILDREN'S FEVER & PAIN REDUCER

[*door 'call*]

Description: Each teaspoonful (5 ml) of DORCOL Children's Fever & Pain Reducer contains acetaminophen 160 mg. Other ingredients: benzoic acid, edetate disodium, flavors, glycerin, polyethylene glycol, purified water, Red 40, sodium chloride, sucrose.

Indications: For temporary relief of your child's fever and occasional minor aches, pains and headache.

Directions For Use: Children under 2 years—consult physician.
By age:
Children 2 to under 4 years: 1 teaspoonful
Children 4 to under 6 years: 1½ teaspoonfuls
Children 6 years of age and older: 2 teaspoonfuls
By weight:
Children 25 to 35 pounds: 1 teaspoonful
Children 36 to 45 pounds: 1½ teaspoonfuls
Children 46 to 60 pounds: 2 teaspoonfuls
Give every 4 hours while symptoms persist or as directed by a physician. Unless directed by a physician do not exceed 5 doses in 24 hours.

Professional Labeling: The suggested dosage for pediatric patients is:

3–12 months	3 drops/Kg of body weight every 4 hours
12–24 months	7 drops (0.2 ml)/Kg of body weight every 4 hours

Maximum of 5 doses in 24 hours.

Warnings: Do not give this product to your child for more than 5 days. Consult your physician if symptoms persist, new ones occur, or if fever persists for more than 3 days (72 hours) or recurs. Do not exceed recommended dosage. Keep this and all drugs out of the reach of children. In case of accidental overdose, seek professional assistance or contact a Poison Control Center immediately.

How Supplied: DORCOL Children's Fever & Pain Reducer (red), in 4 fl oz bottles with tamper-evident band around child-resistant cap.

Shown in Product Identification Section, page 427

DORCOL® CHILDREN'S LIQUID COLD FORMULA

[*door 'call*]

Description: Each teaspoonful (5 ml) of DORCOL Children's Liquid Cold Formula contains: pseudoephedrine hydrochloride 15 mg and chlorpheniramine maleate 1 mg. Other ingredients: benzoic acid, Blue 1, flavors, purified water, Red 40, sorbitol, sucrose, Yellow 10. May also contain sodium hydroxide.

Indications: Provides temporary relief of nasal congestion, sneezing and rhinorrhea due to the common cold, hay fever or other upper respiratory allergies or associated with sinusitis. Reduces swelling of nasal passages and restores freer breathing. Promotes nasal and sinus drainage; relieves sinus pressure.

Directions For Use: Children under 6 years—consult physician.
By age:
Children 6 to under 12 years: 2 teaspoonfuls every 4 to 6 hours.
By weight:
Children 45 to 85 pounds: 2 teaspoonfuls every 4 to 6 hours.
Unless directed by a physician, do not exceed 4 doses in 24 hours.

Professional Labeling: The suggested dosage for pediatric patients is:

3–12 months	2 drops/Kg of body weight every 4–6 hours
12–24 months	5 drops (0.2 ml)/Kg of body weight every 4–6 hours
2–6 years	1 teaspoonful every 4–6 hours

Maximum of 4 doses in 24 hours.

Warnings: Do not give your child more than the recommended dosage because at higher doses nervousness, dizziness, or sleeplessness may occur. Do not give this preparation if your child has high blood pressure, heart disease, diabetes, thyroid disease, asthma, glaucoma, or difficulty in urination due to enlargement of the prostate gland except under the advice and supervision of a physician. If symptoms do not improve within 7 days or are accompanied by high fever, consult a physician before continuing use. May cause drowsiness. May cause excitability especially in children. Keep this and all drugs out of the reach of children. In case of accidental overdose, seek professional assistance or contact a Poison Control Center immediately. *Drug Interaction Precaution:* Do not give this product if your child is presently taking a prescription antihypertensive, sedatives, tranquilizers, or antidepressant drug containing a monoamine oxidase inhibitor except under the advice and supervision of a physician.

Caution: Avoid alcoholic beverages or operating a motor vehicle or heavy machinery while taking this product.

How Supplied: DORCOL Children's Liquid Cold Formula (light brown), in 4 fl oz bottles with tamper-evident band around child-resistant cap.

Shown in Product Identification Section, page 427

EX-LAX® Chocolated Laxative

Active Ingredient: Yellow phenolphthalein, 90 mg phenolphthalein per tablet.

Inactive Ingredients: Cocoa, Confectioners' Sugar, Hydrogenated Palm Kernel Oil, Lecithin, Nonfat Dry Milk, Vanillin.

Indication: For relief of occasional constipation (irregularity).

Caution: Do not take any laxative when abdominal pain, nausea, or vomiting are present. Frequent or prolonged use of this or any other laxative may result in dependence on laxatives. If skin rash appears, do not use this or any other preparation containing phenolphthalein.

Warnings: Keep this and all drugs out of the reach of children. In case of accidental overdose, seek professional assistance or contact a poison control center immediately. As with any drug, if you are pregnant or nursing a baby, seek the advice of a health care professional before using this product.

Drug Interaction Precautions: No known drug interaction.

Dosage and Administration: Adults: Chew 1 to 2 tablets, preferably at bedtime. Children over 6 years: Chew ½ to 1 tablet.

How Supplied: Available in boxes of 6, 18, 48, and 72 chewable chocolate-flavored tablets.

Shown in Product Identification Section, page 427

EX-LAX® Unflavored Laxative Pills

Active Ingredient: Yellow phenolphthalein, 90 mg phenolphthalein per pill.

Inactive Ingredients: Acacia, Alginic Acid, Carnauba Wax, Colloidal Silicon Dioxide, Dibasic Calcium Phosphate, Iron Oxides, Magnesium Stearate, Microcrystalline Cellulose, Sodium Benzoate, Sodium Lauryl Sulfate, Starch, Stearic Acid, Sucrose, Talc, Titanium Dioxide.

Indication: For relief of occasional constipation (irregularity).

Caution: Do not take any laxative when abdominal pain, nausea, or vomiting are present. Frequent or prolonged use of this or any other laxative may result in dependence on laxatives. If skin rash appears, do not use this or any other preparation containing phenolphthalein.

Warnings: Keep this and all drugs out of the reach of children. In case of accidental overdose, seek professional assistance or contact a poison control center immediately. As with any drug, if you are pregnant or nursing a baby, seek the advice of a health care professional before using this product.

Drug Interaction Precautions: No known drug interaction.

Dosage and Administration: Adults take 1 to 2 pills with a glass of water, preferably at bedtime. Children over 6 years: 1 pill.

How Supplied: Available in boxes of 8, 30, and 60 unflavored pills.

Shown in Product Identification Section, page 427

EXTRA GENTLE EX-LAX®

Active Ingredients: Docusate Sodium, 75 mg. and Yellow Phenolphthalein 65 mg. per tablet.

Inactive Ingredients: Acacia, Croscarmellose Sodium, Dibasic Calcium Phosphate, Colloidal Silicon Dioxide, Magnesium Stearate, Microcrystalline Cellulose, Red 7, Stearic Acid, Sucrose, Talc, Titanium Dioxide.

Indication: For relief of occasional constipation (irregularity).

Caution: Do not take any laxative when abdominal pain, nausea or vomiting are present. Frequent or prolonged use of this or any other laxative may result in dependence on laxatives. If skin rash appears, do not use this or any other preparation containing phenolphthalein. Do not use in conjunction with mineral oil or a prescription drug.

Warnings: Keep this and all drugs out of the reach of children. In case of accidental overdose, seek professional assistance or contact a Poison Control Center immediately. As with any drug, if you are pregnant or nursing a baby, seek the advice of a health care professional before using this product.

Drug Interaction Precautions: No known drug interaction.

Dosage and Administration: Adults take 1 or 2 pills with water, preferably at bedtime, or as directed by physician. Children over 6 years: 1 pill, as needed.

How Supplied: Available in boxes of 24 pills.

Shown in Product Identification Section, page 427

GAS-X® AND EXTRA STRENGTH GAS-X®
High-Capacity Antiflatulent

Active Ingredients: GAS-X®—Each tablet contains 80 mg. simethicone.
EXTRA STRENGTH GAS-X®—Each tablet contains 125 mg. simethicone.

Inactive Ingredients: calcium phosphates dibasic and tribasic, colloidal silicon dioxide, calcium silicate, microcrystalline cellulose, flavors, compressible sugar and talc. Extra strength Gas-X also contains Red 30 and Yellow 10.

Indications: For relief of the pain and pressure symptoms of excess gas in the digestive tract, which is often accompanied by complaints of bloating, distention, fullness, pressure, pain, cramps or excess anal flatus.

Actions: GAS-X acts in the stomach and intestines to disperse and reduce the formation of mucus-trapped gas bubbles. The GAS-X defoaming action reduces the surface tension of gas bubbles so that they are more easily eliminated.

Warning: Keep this and all medicines out of the reach of children.

Drug Interaction Precautions: No known drug interaction.

Dosage and Administration: Adults: Chew thoroughly and swallow one or two tablets as needed after meals and at bedtime. Do not exceed six GAS-X tablets or four EXTRA STRENGTH GAS-X tablets in 24 hours, except under the advice and supervision of a physician.

Professional Labeling: GAS-X may be useful in the alleviation of postoperative gas pain, and for use in endoscopic examination.

How Supplied: GAS-X is available in white, chewable, scored tablets in boxes of 36 tablets and convenience packages of 12 tablets.
EXTRA STRENGTH GAS-X is available in yellow, chewable, scored tablets in boxes of 18 tablets and 48 tablets.

Shown in Product Identification Section, page 427

GENTLE NATURE® NATURAL VEGETABLE LAXATIVE

Active Ingredients: 20 mg. Sennosides per tablet.

Inactive Ingredients: Alginic Acid, Calcium Phosphate Dibasic, Magnesium Stearate, Microcrystalline Cellulose, Silicon Dioxide, Sodium Lauryl Sulfate, Starch, Stearic Acid.

Indications: For short-term relief of constipation.

Actions: Sennosides is a highly purified form of senna. The purification process removes components found in senna concentrate which may cause griping and cramps.
Sennosides has no laxative effect until they are carried to the lower part of the alimentary system by the regular working of the digestive process. In the bowel, the active glycosides are freed by the natural bowel micro-organisms. The freed laxative agent then gently encourages the muscle wave action of elimination. The gentle, predictable working of the laxative in the bowel, usually in 8–10 hours, or overnight if taken at bedtime, is apt to produce a well-formed stool in a natural-feeling way.

Caution: Not to be used when abdominal pain, nausea, or vomiting are present. Take only as needed. Frequent or prolonged use may result in dependence on laxatives. Keep this and all medications out of reach of children. In case of accidental overdose, seek professional assistance or contact a Poison Control Center immediately.

Drug Interaction Precautions: No known drug interaction.

Warning: As with any drug, if you are pregnant or nursing a baby, seek the advice of a health professional before using this product.

Dosage and Administration: Adults—Take 1 or 2 tablets daily with water, preferably at bedtime, or as directed by your physician. Children over 6 years—1 tablet daily as required.

How Supplied: Available in boxes of 16 blister packed uncoated pills.

Shown in Product Identification Section, page 428

THERAFLU®
Flu and Cold Medicine
Flu, Cold & Cough Medicine

Description: Each packet of TheraFlu Flu and Cold Medicine contains: acetaminophen 500 mg, pseudoephedrine hydrochloride 60 mg, and chlorpheniramine maleate 4 mg. Each packet of TheraFlu Flu, Cold & Cough Medicine also contains dextromethorphan hydrobromide 20 mg. Other ingredients: ascorbic acid, citric acid, natural lemon flavors, sodium citrate, sucrose, titanium dioxide, tribasic calcium phosphate, pregelatinized starch, Yellow 6, and Yellow 10.

Indications: Provides temporary relief of the symptoms associated with flu, common cold and other upper respiratory infections including: headache, bodyaches, fever, minor sore throat pain, nasal and sinus congestion, runny nose and sneezing. TheraFlu Flu, Cold & Cough Medicine also suppresses coughs due to minor throat and bronchial irritation.

Warnings: Keep this and all drugs out of the reach of children. In case of accidental overdose, seek professional assistance or contact a Poison Control Center immediately. Unless directed by a doctor, do not take this product if you have heart disease, high blood pressure, thyroid disease, diabetes, asthma, glaucoma, difficulty in breathing, or difficulty in urination due to enlargement of the prostate gland or are taking a prescription drug for high blood pressure or depression or are taking sedatives or tranquilizers without first consulting your doctor. Do not exceed recommended dosage or take for more than 7 days. If symptoms persist or new ones occur, or if fever persists for more than 3 days or recurs, consult a doctor. May cause excitability, especially in children. May cause drowsiness. Avoid drinking alcohol, driving or operating machinery while taking this product. As with any drug, if you are pregnant or nursing a baby, seek the advice of a health professional before using this product. Do not take the cough formula if cough is accompanied by excessive secretions, for persistent cough such as occurs with smoking, asthma, or emphysema. A persistent cough may be sign of a serious condition. If cough recurs, or

Continued on next page

Sandoz Pharm.—Cont.

is accompanied by fever, rash or persistent headache, consult a doctor.

Dosage and Administration: Adults and children 12 years and over—dissolve one packet in 6 oz. cup of hot water. Sip while hot. Sweeten to taste, if desired. May repeat every 4 hours, but not to exceed 4 doses in 24 hours.

How Supplied: TheraFlu Flu and Cold Medicine powder in foil packets, 6 or 12 packets per carton. TheraFlu Flu, Cold & Cough Medicine powder in foil packets, 6 or 12 packets per carton.

Shown in Product Identification Section, page 428

TRIAMINIC® ALLERGY TABLETS

[*trī″ah-mĭn′ĭc*]

Description: Each TRIAMINIC Allergy Tablet contains: phenylpropanolamine hydrochloride 25 mg, chlorpheniramine maleate 4.0 mg. Other ingredients: calcium stearate, calcium sulfate, colloidal silicon dioxide, methylcellulose, methylparaben, microcrystalline cellulose, polyethylene glycol, povidone, pregelatinized starch, titanium dioxide, Yellow 10.

Indications: For the temporary relief of runny nose, nasal congestion, sneezing, itching of the eyes, nose or throat and watery eyes as may occur in hay fever or other upper respiratory allergies (allergic rhinitis).

Warnings: Do not exceed the recommended dosage because at higher doses nervousness, dizziness or sleeplessness may occur. This preparation may cause drowsiness; alcohol, sedatives and tranquilizers may increase the drowsiness effect. This preparation may cause excitability especially in children. Do not take this preparation if you have high blood pressure, heart disease, diabetes, thyroid disease or are presently taking a prescription antihypertensive, an antidepressant drug containing a monoamine oxidase inhibitor or a sedative or tranquilizer except under the advice and supervision of a physician. Do not give this preparation to children under 6 years except under the advice and supervision of a physician. Do not take this preparation if you have asthma, emphysema, chronic pulmonary disease, shortness of breath, glaucoma or difficulty in urination due to enlargement of the prostate gland except under the advice and supervision of a physician. Do not take for more than 7 days. If symptoms do not improve within 7 days or are accompanied by high fever, consult a physician before continuing use. As with any drug, if you are pregnant or nursing a baby, seek the advice of a health professional before using this product. Keep this and all drugs out of the reach of children. In case of accidental overdose, seek professional assistance or contact a Poison Control Center immediately.

Caution: Avoid alcoholic beverages, operating a motor vehicle or machinery while taking this product.

Dosage: Adults and children 12 and over—1 tablet every 4 hours. Children 6 to under 12 years—½ tablet every 4 hours. Unless directed by physician, do not exceed 6 doses in 24 hours or give to children under 6 years.

How Supplied: TRIAMINIC Allergy Tablets (yellow), scored, in blister packs of 24.

TRIAMINIC® CHEWABLES

[*trī″ah-mĭn′ĭc*]

Description: Each TRIAMINIC Chewable contains: phenylpropanolamine hydrochloride 6.25 mg, chlorpheniramine maleate 0.5 mg. Other ingredients: calcium stearate, citric acid, flavors, magnesium trisilicate, mannitol, microcrystalline cellulose, saccharin sodium, sucrose, Yellow 6, Yellow 10.

Indications: For the temporary relief of children's nasal congestion, runny nose, and sneezing due to the common cold or hay fever.

Warnings: Do not exceed recommended dosage because at higher doses nervousness, dizziness, or sleeplessness may occur. Do not give this product to children for more than 7 days. If symptoms do not improve or are accompanied by fever, consult a doctor. Do not give this product to children who have heart disease, high blood pressure, thyroid disease, diabetes, asthma, emphysema, shortness of breath, chronic pulmonary disease or glaucoma unless directed by a doctor. May cause drowsiness. Sedatives and tranquilizers may increase the drowsiness effect. May cause excitability.
Drug Interaction Precaution: Do not give this product to a child who is taking a prescription drug for high blood pressure or depression, without first consulting the child's doctor. Keep this and all drugs out of the reach of children. In case of accidental overdose, seek professional assistance or contact a Poison Control Center immediately.

Dosage: Children 6 to 12 years—2 tablets every 4 hours. Children under 6, consult your physician.

Professional Labeling: The suggested dosage for children 2 to 6 years is 1 tablet every 4 hours.

How Supplied: TRIAMINIC Chewables (hexagonal, yellow), in blister packs of 24.

TRIAMINIC® COLD TABLETS

[*trī″ah-mĭn′ĭc*]

Description: Each TRIAMINIC Cold Tablet contains: phenylpropanolamine hydrochloride 12.5 mg and chlorpheniramine maleate 2 mg. Other ingredients: calcium stearate, colloidal silicon dioxide, flavor, lactose, methylcellulose, methylparaben, microcrystalline cellulose, polyethylene glycol, povidone, pregelatinized starch, Red 40, saccharin sodium, titanium dioxide, Yellow 6.

Indications: Temporarily relieves runny nose, nasal congestion and sneezing due to colds and allergies. Also relieves itching nose or throat and itchy, watery eyes associated with allergies.

Warnings: Unless directed by a doctor, do not take this product if you have heart disease, high blood pressure, thyroid disease, diabetes, asthma, glaucoma, difficulty in breathing, emphysema, chronic pulmonary disease, shortness of breath, difficulty in urination due to enlargement of the prostate gland or are taking a prescription drug for high blood pressure or depression. Do not exceed recommended dosage because at higher doses nervousness, dizziness, or sleeplessness may occur, or take for more than 7 days. If symptoms persist or are accompanied by fever, consult a doctor. May cause excitability especially in children. May cause drowsiness; alcohol, sedatives, and tranquilizers may increase the drowsiness effect. Avoid drinking alcohol, driving or operating machinery while taking this product. Do not take this product if you are taking sedatives or tranquilizers without first consulting your doctor. As with any drug, if you are pregnant or nursing a baby, seek the advice of a health professional before using this product. Keep this and all drugs out of the reach of children. In case of accidental overdose, seek professional assistance or contact a Poison Control Center immediately.

Caution: Avoid alcoholic beverages, operating a motor vehicle or heavy machinery while taking this product.

Dosage and Administration: Adults and children 12 and over—2 tablets every 4 hours. Children 6 to under 12 years—1 tablet every 4 hours. Unless directed by physician, do not exceed 6 doses in 24 hours.

How Supplied: TRIAMINIC Cold Tablets (orange), imprinted "DORSEY" on one side, "TRIAMINIC" on the other, in blister packs of 24.

Shown in Product Identification Section, page 428

TRIAMINIC® EXPECTORANT

[*trī″ah-mĭn′ĭc*]

Description: Each teaspoonful (5 ml) of TRIAMINIC Expectorant contains: phenylpropanolamine hydrochloride 12.5 mg and guaifenesin 100 mg. Other ingredients: alcohol (5%), benzoic acid, edetate disodium, flavors, purified water, saccharin, saccharin sodium, sodium hydroxide, sorbitol, sucrose, Yellow 6, Yellow 10.

Indications: Provides prompt relief of nasal congestion due to the common cold. The expectorant component helps loosen bronchial secretions and rid the bronchial passageways of bothersome mucus. The decongestant and expectorant are provided in an antihistamine-free formula.

Warnings: Do not take this product: 1) if cough is accompanied by excessive secretions, 2) for persistent cough such as occurs with smoking, asthma or emphysema, or 3) if you have heart disease, high blood pressure, thyroid disease, diabetes, difficulty in urination due to enlargement of the prostate gland, or are taking a prescription drug for high blood pressure or depression, unless directed by a doctor. Do not: 1) give this product to children under two years of age, 2) exceed recommended dosage, or 3) take for more than 7 days, unless directed by a doctor. If symptoms persist, are accompanied by a fever, rash or persistent headache or if cough recurs, consult a doctor. As with any drug, if you are pregnant or nursing a baby, seek advice from a health professional before using this product. Keep this and all drugs out of the reach of children. In case of accidental overdose, seek professional assistance or contact a Poison Control Center immediately.

Dosage and Administration: Adults and children 12 and over (96+ lbs)—2 teaspoonfuls every 4 hours. Children 6 to under 12 years (48–95 lbs)—1 teaspoonful every 4 hours. Children 2 to under 6 years (24–47 lbs)—½ teaspoonful every 4 hours. Unless directed by physician, do not exceed 6 doses in 24 hours or give to children under 2 years of age.

Professional Labeling: The suggested dosage for pediatric patients is:

3–12 months (12–17 lbs)	.75 ml (⅛ tsp)* every 4 hours
12–24 months (18–23 lbs)	1.25 ml (¼ tsp) every 4 hours

*(⅛ tsp is appproximately .75 ml)

How Supplied: TRIAMINIC Expectorant (yellow), in 4 fl oz and 8 fl oz plastic bottles with tamper-evident band around child-resistant cap.

Shown in Product Identification Section, page 428

TRIAMINIC® NITE LIGHT™ Nighttime Cough and Cold Medicine for Children

[*tri "ah-min 'ic*]

Description: Each teaspoonful (5 ml) of Triaminic® Nite Light™ contains: Pseudoephedrine hydrochloride 15 mg, chlorpheniramine maleate 1 mg, dextromethorphan hydrobromide 7.5 mg in a palatable non-alcoholic vehicle. Other ingredients: benzoic acid, Blue 1, citric acid, flavors, propylene glycol, purified water, Red 33, dibasic sodium phosphate, sorbitol, sucrose.

Indications: Temporarily quiets your child's cough associated with the common cold. Also, provides temporary relief of nasal stuffiness, sneezing, runny nose, and itchy watery eyes caused by the common cold, hay fever or other upper respiratory allergies.

Warnings: Do not exceed recommended dosage or take for more than 7 days. A persistent cough may be a sign of a serious condition. If symptoms persist for more than one week, tend to recur, or are accompanied by fever, rash, or persistent headache, consult a physician. May cause excitability especially in children. Unless directed by a physician, do not take this product: 1) if cough is accompanied by excessive phlegm (mucus), 2) for persistent or chronic cough such as occurs with smoking, asthma or emphysema, or 3) if you or your child has heart disease, high blood pressure, thyroid disease, diabetes, asthma, glaucoma, difficulty in breathing, or difficulty in urination due to enlargement of the prostate gland. May cause marked drowsiness. Alcohol, sedatives, and tranquilizers may increase the drowsiness effect. Avoid alcoholic beverages while taking this product. Use caution when driving a motor vehicle or operating machinery. As with any drug, if you are pregnant or nursing a baby, seek the advice of a health professional before using this product. Keep this and all drugs out of the reach of children. In case of accidental overdose, seek professional assistance, or call a Poison Control Center immediately.

Drug Interaction Precaution: Do not take this product if you are taking a prescription drug for high blood pressure or depression, or if you are taking sedatives or tranquilizers, without first consulting your physician.

Dosage and Administration: Children 12 and over (96+ lbs.)—4 teaspoonfuls every 6–8 hours. Children 6 to under 12 years (48–95 lbs.)—2 teaspoonfuls every 6–8 hours. Unless directed by physician, do not exceed 4 doses in 24 hours. For convenience, a True-Dose™ dosage cup is provided with each 4 fl. oz. and 8 fl. oz. bottle.

Professional Labeling: The suggested dosage for pediatric patients is:

3 to under 12 months (12–17 lbs.)	¼ teaspoon or 1.25 ml
12 months to under 2 years (18–23 lbs.)	½ teaspoon or 2.5 ml
2 to under 6 years	1 teaspoonful or 5 ml

How Supplied: Triaminic® Nite Light™ Nighttime Cough and Cold Medicine for Children, in 4 fl. oz. and 8 fl. oz. plastic bottles packaged in cartons with tamper-evident band around child-resistant cap.

Shown in Product Identification Section, page 428

TRIAMINIC® SYRUP

[*trī "ah-mĭn 'ĭc*]

Description: Each teaspoonful (5 ml) of TRIAMINIC Syrup contains: phenylpropanolamine hydrochloride 12.5 mg and chlorpheniramine maleate 2 mg in a nonalcoholic vehicle. Other ingredients: benzoic acid, edetate disodium, flavors, purified water, sodium hydroxide, sorbitol, sucrose. Contains FD&C Yellow No. 6 as a color additive.

Indications: Provides temporary relief of nasal congestion, runny nose and sneezing that may occur with the common cold or with hay fever or other upper respiratory allergies. Relieves itching of the nose or throat and itchy, watery eyes.

Warnings: Do not take this product: 1) if you have heart disease, high blood pressure, thyroid disease, diabetes, asthma, glaucoma, difficulty in breathing, difficulty in urination due to enlargement of the prostate gland, or 2) if you are taking a prescription drug for high blood pressure or depression, or 3) if you are taking sedatives or tranquilizers, unless directed by a doctor. Do not exceed recommended dosage or take for more than 7 days. If symptoms persist or are accompanied by fever, consult a doctor. May cause excitability especially in children. May cause drowsiness. Alcohol, sedatives, or tranquilizers may increase drowsiness. Avoid driving or operating machinery while taking this product. As with any drug, if you are pregnant or nursing a baby, seek the advice of a health professional before using this product. Keep this and all drugs out of the reach of children. In case of accidental overdose, seek professional assistance or contact a Poison Control Center immediately.

Dosage and Administration: Adults and children 12 and over (96+ lbs)—2 teaspoonfuls every 4 hours. Children 6 to under 12 years (48–95 lbs)—1 teaspoonful every 4 hours. Unless directed by physician, do not exceed 6 doses in 24 hours. Consult physician for dosage under 6 years of age.

Professional Labeling: The suggested dosage for pediatric patients is:

3–12 months (12–17 lbs)	.75 ml (⅛ tsp)* every 4 hours
12–24 months (18–23 lbs)	1.25 ml (¼ tsp) every 4 hours
2–6 years (24–47 lbs)	2.5 ml (½ tsp) every 4 hours

*(⅛ tsp is approximately .75 ml)

How Supplied: TRIAMINIC Syrup (orange), in 4 fl oz and 8 fl oz plastic bottles with tamper-evident band around child-resistant cap.

Shown in Product Identification Section, page 428

TRIAMINIC-DM® SYRUP

[*trī "ah-mĭn 'ĭc*]

Description: Each teaspoonful (5 ml) of TRIAMINIC-DM Syrup contains: phenylpropanolamine hydrochloride 12.5 mg and dextromethorphan hydrobromide 10 mg in a nonalcoholic vehicle. Other ingredients: benzoic acid, Blue 1, flavors, propylene glycol, purified water, Red 40, sodium chloride, sorbitol, sucrose.

Indications: Provides relief of cough due to minor throat and bronchial irritation

Continued on next page

Sandoz Pharm.—Cont.

as may occur with the common cold or inhaled irritants. Promotes nasal and sinus drainage. The decongestant and antitussive are provided in an alcohol-free and antihistamine-free formula.

Warnings: Do not take this product: 1) if cough is accompanied by excessive secretions, 2) for persistent cough such as occurs with smoking, asthma or emphysema, or 3) if you have heart disease, high blood pressure, thyroid disease, diabetes, difficulty in urination due to enlargement of the prostate gland, or are taking a prescription drug for high blood pressure or depression, unless directed by a doctor. Do not exceed recommended dosage or take for more than 7 days. If symptoms persist, are accompanied by a fever, rash or persistent headache or if cough recurs, consult a doctor. As with any drug, if you are pregnant or nursing a baby, seek the advice from a health professional before using this product. Keep this and all drugs out of the reach of children. In case of accidental overdose, seek professional assistance or contact a Poison Control Center immediately.

Dosage and Administration: Adults and children 12 and over (96+ lbs)—2 teaspoonfuls every 4 hours. Children 6 to under 12 years (48–95 lbs)—1 teaspoonful every 4 hours. Children 2 to under 6 years (24–47 lbs)—½ teaspoonful every 4 hours. Unless directed by physician, do not exceed 6 doses in 24 hours or give to children under 2 years of age.

Professional Labeling: The suggested dosage for pediatric patients is:

3–12 months	.75 ml (⅛ tsp)*
(12–17 lbs)	every 4 hours
12–24 months	1.25 ml (¼ tsp)
(18–23 lbs)	every 4 hours

*(⅛ tsp is approximately .75 ml)

How Supplied: TRIAMINIC-DM Syrup (dark red), in 4 fl oz and 8 fl oz plastic bottles with tamper-evident band around child-resistant cap.

Shown in Product Identification Section, page 428

TRIAMINIC-12® TABLETS

[trī″ah-mĭn′ĭc]

Description: Each TRIAMINIC-12 Tablet contains: phenylpropanolamine hydrochloride 75 mg and chlorpheniramine maleate 12 mg. Other ingredients: carnauba wax, colloidal silicon dioxide, lactose, methylcellulose, polyethylene glycol, povidone, Red 30, stearic acid, titanium dioxide, Yellow 6.
TRIAMINIC-12 Tablets contain the nasal decongestant phenylpropanolamine, and the antihistamine chlorpheniramine, in a formulation providing 12 hours of symptomatic relief.

Indications: For the temporary relief of nasal congestion due to the common cold, hay fever or other upper respiratory allergies and associated with sinusitis. Helps decongest sinus openings, sinus passages; promotes nasal and/or sinus drainage; temporarily restores freer breathing through the nose. For temporary relief of running nose, sneezing, itching of the nose or throat and itchy and watery eyes as may occur in allergic rhinitis (such as hay fever).

Warnings: Do not give this product to children under 12 years except under the advice and supervision of a physician. Do not take this preparation if you have high blood pressure, heart disease, diabetes, thyroid disease, asthma, emphysema, chronic pulmonary disease, shortness of breath, glaucoma or difficulty in urination due to enlargement of the prostate gland except under the advice and supervision of a physician. Do not exceed the recommended dosage because at higher doses nervousness, dizziness, or sleeplessness may occur. This preparation may cause drowsiness; alcohol, sedatives, and tranquilizers may increase the drowsiness effect. This preparation may cause excitability, especially in children. Do not take for more than 7 days. If symptoms do not improve within seven days or are accompanied by high fever, consult a physician before continuing use. As with any drug, if you are pregnant or nursing a baby, seek the advice of a health professional before using this product.
Keep this and all drugs out of the reach of children. In case of accidental overdose, seek professional assistance or contact a Poison Control Center immediately.

Caution: Avoid driving a motor vehicle or operating heavy machinery. Avoid alcoholic beverages while taking this product.

Drug Interaction Precaution: Do not take this product if you are presently taking a prescription antihypertensive, an antidepressant drug containing a monoamine oxidase inhibitor or a sedative or tranquilizer except under the advice and supervision of a physician.

Directions: Adults and children over 12 years of age—1 tablet swallowed whole every 12 hours. Unless directed by physician, do not exceed 2 tablets in 24 hours.

Note: The nonactive portion of the tablet that supplies the active ingredients may occasionally appear in your stool as a soft mass.

How Supplied: TRIAMINIC-12 Tablets (orange), imprinted "DORSEY" on one side, "TRIAMINIC 12" on the other, in blister packs of 10 and 20.

Shown in Product Identification Section, page 428

TRIAMINICIN® TABLETS

[trī″ah-mĭn′ĭ-sĭn]

Description: Each TRIAMINICIN Tablet contains: phenylpropanolamine hydrochloride 25 mg, chlorpheniramine maleate 4 mg and acetaminophen 650 mg. Other ingredients: calcium stearate, colloidal silicon dioxide, croscarmellose sodium, lactose, methylcellulose, methylparaben, polyethylene glycol, povidone, pregelatinized starch, Red 40, titanium dioxide, Yellow 10.

Indications: Temporarily relieves runny nose, sneezing, itching of the nose or throat, and itchy, watery eyes due to hay fever (allergic rhinitis) or other upper respiratory allergies. For the temporary relief of nasal congestion due to hay fever or other upper respiratory allergies or associated with sinusitis. Temporarily relieves nasal congestion, runny nose and sneezing associated with the common cold. For the temporary relief of occasional minor aches, pains and headache associated with the common cold.

Warnings: Do not take this product if you have heart disease, high blood pressure, thyroid disease, diabetes, asthma, glaucoma, emphysema, chronic pulmonary disease, shortness of breath, difficulty in breathing, or difficulty in urination due to enlargement of the prostate gland unless directed by a doctor. Do not exceed recommended dosage because at higher doses nervousness, dizziness, or sleeplessness may occur. Do not take this product for more than 7 days. If symptoms do not improve, new ones occur, or if fever persists for more than three days (72 hours) or recurs, consult a doctor. May cause drowsiness; alcohol, sedatives and tranquilizers may increase the drowsiness effect. Avoid alcoholic beverages while taking this product. Do not take this product if you are taking sedatives or tranquilizers without first consulting your doctor. Use caution when driving a motor vehicle or operating machinery. May cause excitability especially in children. As with any drug, if you are pregnant or nursing a baby, seek the advice of a health professional before using this product. *Drug Interaction Precaution:* Do not take this product if you are presently taking a prescription drug for high blood pressure or depression or are taking sedatives or tranquilizers, without first consulting your doctor. Keep this and all drugs out of the reach of children. In case of accidental overdose, seek professional assistance or contact a Poison Control Center immediately. Prompt medical attention is critical for adults as well as for children even if you do not notice any signs or symptoms.

Dosage and Administration: Adults and children 12 years and older: Take 1 tablet every 4 hours while symptoms persist or as directed by a physician. Unless directed by a physician, do not exceed 6 doses in 24 hours or give to children under 12 years.

How Supplied: TRIAMINICIN Tablets (yellow), imprinted "DORSEY" on one side, "TRIAMINICIN" on the other, in blister packs of 12, 24 and 48, and bottles of 100 tablets.

Shown in Product Identification Section, page 428

TRIAMINICOL® MULTI-SYMPTOM COLD TABLETS
[*trī ″ah-mĭn ′ĭ-call*]

Description: Each TRIAMINICOL Multi-Symptom Cold Tablet contains: phenylpropanolamine hydrochloride 12.5 mg, chlorpheniramine maleate 2 mg, dextromethorphan hydrobromide 10 mg. Other ingredients: calcium stearate, colloidal silicon dioxide, lactose, methylcellulose, methylparaben, microcrystalline cellulose, polyethylene glycol, povidone, pregelatinized starch, Red 40, titanium dioxide.

Indications: Temporarily relieves coughs due to minor throat and bronchial irritation. Temporarily relieves runny nose, nasal congestion and sneezing due to colds and allergies. Also relieves itching nose or throat and itchy, watery eyes associated with allergies.

Warnings: Unless directed by a doctor, **DO NOT** take this product: **1)** if cough is accompanied by excessive secretions, **2)** for persistent cough such as occurs with smoking, asthma or emphysema, or **3)** if you have heart disease, high blood pressure, thyroid disease, diabetes, asthma, glaucoma, difficulty in breathing, emphysema, chronic pulmonary disease, shortness of breath, difficulty in urination due to enlargement of the prostate gland or are taking a prescription drug for high blood pressure or depression. Do not exceed recommended dosage because at higher doses nervousness, dizziness, or sleeplessness may occur, or take for more than 7 days. If symtoms persist, are accompanied by fever, rash or persistent headache or if cough recurs, consult a doctor. May cause excitability especially in children. May cause drowsiness; alcohol, sedatives, and tranquilizers may increase the drowsiness effect. Avoid drinking alcohol, driving or operating machinery while taking this product. Do not take this product if you are taking sedatives or tranquilizers without first consulting your doctor. Do not take this product if you are taking a prescription drug for high blood pressure or depression without first consulting your doctor. As with any drug, if you are pregnant or nursing a baby, seek the advice of a health professional before using this product. Keep this and all drugs out of the reach of children. In case of accidental overdose, seek professional assistance or contact a Poison Control Center immediately.

Dosage and Administration: Adults and children 12 and over—2 tablets every 4 hours. Children 6 to under 12 years—1 tablet every 4 hours. For nighttime cough relief, give the last dose at bedtime. Unless directed by physician, do not exceed 6 doses in 24 hours or give to children under 6 years.

How Supplied: TRIAMINICOL Multi-Symptom Cold Tablets (cherry pink), imprinted "DORSEY" on one side, "TRIAMINICOL" on the other, in blister packs of 24.

Shown in Product Identification Section, page 428

TRIAMINICOL® MULTI-SYMPTOM RELIEF
[*trī ″ah-mĭn ′ĭ-call*]

Description: Each teaspoonful (5 ml) of TRIAMINICOL Multi-Symptom Relief contains: phenylpropanolamine hydrochloride 12.5 mg, chlorpheniramine maleate 2 mg, dextromethorphan hydrobromide 10 mg in a palatable nonalcoholic vehicle. Other ingredients: benzoic acid, flavors, propylene glycol, purified water, Red 40, saccharin sodium, sodium chloride, sorbitol, sucrose.

Indications: Provides relief of runny nose, nasal congestion and sneezing that may occur with the common cold. Suppresses cough due to minor throat and bronchial irritation. Promotes nasal and sinus drainage.

Warnings: Do not take this product: 1) if cough is accompanied by excessive secretions, 2) for persistent cough such as occurs with smoking, asthma or emphysema, or 3) if you have heart disease, high blood pressure, thyroid disease, diabetes, asthma, glaucoma, difficulty in breathing, difficulty in urination due to enlargement of the prostate gland, or 4) if you are taking a prescription drug for high blood pressure or depression, or are taking sedatives or tranquilizers, unless directed by a doctor. Do not exceed recommended dosage or take for more than 7 days. If symptoms persist, are accompanied by a fever, rash or persistent headache, or if cough recurs, consult a doctor. May cause excitability especially in children. May cause marked drowsiness. Alcohol, sedatives or tranquilizers may increase drowsiness. Avoid driving or operating machinery while taking this product. As with any drug, if you are pregnant or nursing a baby, seek advice of a health professional before using this product. Keep this and all drugs out of the reach of children. In case of accidental overdose, seek professional assistance or contact a Poison Control Center immediately.

Dosage and Administration: Adults and children 12 and over (96+ lbs)—2 teaspoonfuls every 4 hours. Children 6 to under 12 years (48–95 lbs)—1 teaspoonful every 4 hours. Unless directed by physician, do not exceed 6 doses in 24 hours or give to children under 6 years of age.

Professional Labeling: The suggested dosage for pediatric patients is:

3–12 months (12–17 lbs)	.75 ml (1/8 tsp)* every 4 hours
12–24 months (18–23 lbs)	1.25 ml (1/4 tsp) every 4 hours
2–6 years (24–47 lbs)	2.5 ml (1/2 tsp) every 4 hours

*(1/8 tsp is approximately .75 ml)

How Supplied: TRIAMINICOL Multi-Symptom Relief (red), in 4 fl oz and 8 fl oz plastic bottles with tamper-evident band around child-resistant cap.

Shown in Product Identification Section, page 428

URSINUS® INLAY-TABS®
[*yur ″sīgn ′us*]

Description: Each URSINUS INLAY-TAB contains: pseudoephedrine hydrochloride 30 mg and aspirin 325 mg. Other ingredients: calcium stearate, lactose, microcrystalline cellulose, pregelatinized starch, sodium starch glycolate, starch, Yellow 6, Yellow 10.

Indications: For the temporary relief of nasal congestion due to the common cold, hay fever or associated with sinusitis. For the temporary relief of occasional minor aches, pains and headache.

Warnings: Children and teenagers should not use this medicine for chicken pox or flu symptoms before a doctor is consulted about Reye syndrome, a rare but serious illness reported to be associated with aspirin. Unless directed by a doctor: 1) Do not take this product if you are allergic to aspirin or if you have asthma; or if you have stomach distress, ulcers or bleeding problems; 2) Do not take this product if you have heart disease, high blood pressure, thyroid disease, diabetes, or difficulty in urination due to enlargement of the prostate gland, and 3) As with any drug, if you are pregnant or nursing a baby, seek the advice of a health professional before using this product. **IT IS ESPECIALLY IMPORTANT NOT TO USE ASPIRIN DURING THE LAST 3 MONTHS OF PREGNANCY UNLESS SPECIFICALLY DIRECTED TO DO SO BY A DOCTOR BECAUSE IT MAY CAUSE PROBLEMS IN THE UNBORN CHILD OR COMPLICATIONS DURING DELIVERY.** Do not exceed recommended dosage because at higher doses nervousness, dizziness, or sleeplessness may occur. Do not take this product for more than 7 days. If symptoms do not improve, are accompanied by fever, or new symptoms occur, consult a doctor. Stop taking this product if ringing in the ears or other symptoms occur.

Drug Interaction Precaution: Do not take this product if you are presently taking a prescription drug for high blood pressure or depression. Do not take this product if you are presently taking a prescription drug for anticoagulation (thinning the blood), diabetes, gout or arthritis without first consulting your doctor.

Warning—Keep this and all medicines out of the reach of children. In case of accidental overdose, contact a physician immediately.

Directions: Adults and children 12 years and older: 2 tablets every 4 hours while symptoms persist or as directed by a physician. Drink a full glass of water with each dose. Do not take more than 4 doses in 24 hours. For chicken pox or flu see Warnings.

Continued on next page

Sandoz Pharm.—Cont.

How Supplied: URSINUS INLAY-TABS (white with yellow inlay), in bottles of 24 and 100.

Schering-Plough HealthCare Products, Inc.

LIBERTY CORNER, NJ 07938

A and D Ointment
REG. T.M.

Description: An ointment containing the emollients, anhydrous lanolin and petrolatum. Also contains: Cholecalciferol, Fish Liver Oil, Fragrance, Mineral Oil, Paraffin.

Indications: *Diaper rash*—**A and D Ointment** provides prompt, soothing relief for diaper rash and helps heal baby's tender skin; forms a moisture-proof shield that helps protect against urine and detergent irritants; comforts baby's skin and helps prevent chafing.
Chafed Skin—**A and D Ointment** helps skin retain its vital natural moisture; quickly soothes chafed skin in adults and children and helps prevent abnormal dryness.
Abrasions and Minor Burns—**A and D Ointment** soothes and helps relieve the smarting and pain of abrasions and minor burns, encourages healing and prevents dressings from sticking to the injured area.

Warning: Keep this and all drugs out of the reach of children.

Overdosage: In case of accidental ingestion, seek professional assistance or contact a poison control center immediately.

Dosage and Administration: *Diaper Rash*—Simply apply a thin coating of **A and D Ointment** at each diaper change. A modest amount is all that is needed to provide protective and healing action.
Chafed Skin—Gently smooth a small quantity of **A and D Ointment** over the area to be treated.
Abrasions, Minor Burns—Wash with lukewarm water and mild soap. When dry, apply **A and D Ointment** liberally. When a sterile dressing is used, change the dressing daily and apply fresh **A and D Ointment**. If no improvement occurs after 48 to 72 hours or if condition worsens, consult your physician.

How Supplied: A and D Ointment is available in 1½-ounce (42.5 g) and 4-ounce (113 g) tubes and 1-pound (454 g) jars.
Store away from heat.

Shown in Product Identification Section, page 428

AFRIN®
[a 'frin]
Nasal Spray 0.05%
Nasal Spray Pump 0.05%
Cherry Scented Nasal Spray 0.05%
Menthol Nasal Spray 0.05%
Nose Drops 0.05%
Children's Strength Nose Drops 0.025%

Description: AFRIN products contain oxymetazoline hydrochloride, the longest acting topical nasal decongestant available. Each ml of AFRIN Nasal Spray, Nasal Spray Pump, and Nose Drops contains Oxymetazoline Hydrochloride, USP 0.5 mg (0.05%); Benzalkonium Chloride, Glycine, Phenylmercuric Acetate (0.02 mg/ml), Sorbitol, and Water.
Each ml of AFRIN Children's Strength Nose Drops contains Oxymetazoline Hydrochloride, USP 0.25 mg (0.025%); Benzalkonium Chloride, Glycine, Phenylmercuric Acetate (0.02 mg/ml), Sorbitol, and Water.
AFRIN Menthol Nasal Spray contains cooling aromatic vapors of menthol, eucalyptol and camphor and polysorbate, in addition to the ingredients of AFRIN Nasal Spray.
AFRIN Cherry Scented Nasal Spray contains artificial cherry flavor in addition to the ingredients in regular AFRIN.

Indications: For temporary relief of nasal congestion "associated with" colds, hay fever and sinusitis.

Actions: The sympathomimetic action of AFRIN products constricts the smaller arterioles of the nasal passages, producing a prolonged, gentle and predictable decongesting effect. In just a few minutes a single dose, as directed, provides prompt, temporary relief of nasal congestion that lasts up to 12 hours. AFRIN products last up to 3 or 4 times longer than most ordinary nasal sprays.
AFRIN products used at bedtime help restore freer nasal breathing through the night.

Warnings: Do not exceed recommended dosage because burning, stinging, sneezing or increase of nasal discharge may occur. Do not use these products for more than 3 days. If nasal congestion persists, consult a physician. The use of the dispensers by more than one person may spread infection. Keep these and all medicines out of the reach of children.

Overdosage: In case of accidental ingestion, seek professional assistance or contact a Poison Control Center immediately.

Dosage and Administration: Because AFRIN has a long duration of action, twice-a-day administration—in the morning and at bedtime—is usually adequate.
AFRIN Nasal Spray, Cherry Scented Nasal Spray and Menthol Nasal Spray, 0.05%—For adults and children 6 years of age and over: With head upright, spray 2 or 3 times into each nostril twice daily—morning and evening. To spray, squeeze bottle quickly and firmly. Do not tilt head backward while spraying. Wipe nozzle clean after use. Not recommended for children under six.
Afrin Nasal Spray Pump, 0.05%—For adults and children 6 years of age and over: Two or three sprays in each nostril twice daily—morning and bedtime. Remove protective cap. Hold bottle with thumb at base and nozzle between first and second fingers. With head upright, insert metered pump spray nozzle in nostril. Depress pump 2 or 3 times, all the way down, with a firm even stroke and sniff deeply. Repeat in other nostril. Do not tilt head backward while spraying. Wipe tip clean after each use. Before using the first time, remove the protective cap from the tip and prime the metered pump by depressing pump firmly several times.
AFRIN Nose Drops—For adults and children 6 years of age and over: Tilt head back, apply 2 or 3 drops into each nostril twice daily—morning and evening. Immediately bend head forward toward knees. Hold a few seconds, then return to upright position. Wipe dropper clean after each use. Not recommended for children under six.
AFRIN Children's Strength Nose Drops—Children 2 through 5 years of age: Tilt head back, apply 2 or 3 drops into each nostril twice daily—morning and evening. Promptly move head forward toward knees. Hold a few seconds, then return child to upright position. Wipe dropper clean after each use. For children under 2 years, use only as directed by a physician.

How Supplied: AFRIN Nasal Spray 0.05% (1:2000), 15 ml and 30 ml plastic squeeze bottles.
AFRIN Nasal Spray Pump 0.05% (1:2000), 15 ml spray pump bottles.
AFRIN Cherry Scented Nasal Spray 0.05% (1:2000), 15 ml plastic squeeze bottle.
AFRIN Menthol Nasal Spray 0.05% (1:2000), 15 ml plastic squeeze bottle.
AFRIN Nose Drops, 0.05% (1:2000), 20 ml dropper bottle.
AFRIN Children's Strength Nose Drops, 0.025% (1:4000), 20 ml dropper bottle.
Store all nasal sprays and nose drops between 2° and 30°C (36° and 86°F).

Shown in Product Identification Section, page 428

AFRIN™
[a 'frin]
Saline Mist

Ingredients: Water, Sodium Chloride, Disodium Phosphate, Sodium Phosphate, Benzalkonium Chloride, Phenyl Mercuric Acetate 0.002% (Preservative).

Indications: Provides soothing moisture to dry, inflamed nasal membranes due to colds, allergies, low humidity, and other minor nasal irritations. Afrin Saline Mist loosens and thins mucus secretions to aid removal of mucus from nose and sinuses. Afrin Saline Mist can be used as often as needed, and is safe to use with cold, allergy, and sinus medications.

Directions: For infants, children, and adults, 2 to 6 sprays/drops in each nostril as often as needed or as directed by a physician. For a fine mist, keep bottle upright; for nose drops, keep bottle upside down; for a stream, keep bottle horizontal. Wipe nozzle clean after use.

Keep out of the reach of children.
The use of this dispenser by more than one person may spread infection.

CONTAINS NO ALCOHOL
Shown in Product Identification Section, page 428

AFRIN Tablets
[a 'frin]

Active Ingredients: Each Extended Release Tablet contains: 120 mg pseudoephedrine sulfate. Each tablet also contains: Acacia, Butylparaben, Calcium Sulfate, Carnauba Wax, Corn Starch, FD&C Blue No. 1, Gelatin, Lactose, Magnesium Stearate, Neutral Soap, Oleic Acid, Povidone, Rosin, Sugar, Talc, White Wax, Zein. Half the dose (60 mg) is released after the tablet is swallowed and the other half is released hours later; continuous relief is provided for up to 12 hours . . . without drowsiness.

Indications: For temporary relief of nasal congestion due to the common cold, hay fever or other upper respiratory allergies, and nasal congestion associated with sinusitis.

Actions: Promotes nasal and/or sinus drainage, helps decongest sinus openings, sinus passages.

Warnings: Do not exceed recommended dosage because at higher doses nervousness, dizziness or sleeplessness may occur. Do not take this preparation if you have high blood pressure, heart disease, diabetes, or thyroid disease, except under the advice and supervision of a physician. If symptoms do not improve within 7 days or are accompanied by fever, consult a physician before continuing use. Keep this and all drugs out of the reach of children.
As with any drug, if you are pregnant or nursing a baby, seek the advice of a health professional before using this product.

Drug Interactions: Do not take this product if you are presently taking a prescription drug for high blood pressure or depression, without first consulting your physician.

Overdosage: In case of accidental overdose, seek professional assistance or contact a poison control center immediately.

Dosage and Administration: Adults and children 12 years and over—One tablet every 12 hours. AFRINOL is not recommended for children under 12 years of age.

How Supplied: AFRINOL Extended Release Tablets—Boxes of 12 and bottles of 100.

Store between 2° and 30°C (36° and 86° F). Protect from excessive moisture.
Shown in Product Identification Section, page 428

AFTATE® Antifungal
Aerosol Liquid
Aerosol Powder
Gel
Powder

Active Ingredient: Tolnaftate 1% (Also contains: Aerosol Spray Liquid-36% alcohol; Aerosol Spray Powder-14% alcohol.)

How Supplied:
AFTATE for Athlete's Foot
Sprinkle Powder—2.25 oz. bottle
Aerosol Spray Powder—3.5 oz can
Gel—.5 oz. tube.
Aerosol Spray Liquid—4 oz. can.
AFTATE for Jock Itch
Aerosol Spray Powder—3.5 oz. can
Sprinkle Powder—1.5 oz. bottle.
Gel—.5 oz. tube.
Shown in Product Identification Section, page 429

CHLOR-TRIMETON®
[klor-tri 'mĕ-ton]
Allergy Syrup
Allergy Tablets 4 mg
Long Acting Allergy REPETABS® Tablets 8 mg and 12 mg

Active Ingredients: Each Allergy Tablet contains: 4 mg CHLOR-TRIMETON (brand of chlorpheniramine maleate, USP); also contains: Corn Starch, D&C Yellow No. 10 Al Lake, Lactose, Magnesium Stearate. Each REPETABS® Tablet contains: 8 mg or 12 mg CHLOR-TRIMETON (brand of chlorpheniramine maleate); 8 mg Repetabs also contains: Acacia, Butylparaben, Calcium Phosphate, Calcium Sulfate, Carnauba Wax, Corn Starch, D&C Yellow No. 10 Al Lake, FD&C Yellow No.6 Al Lake, Lactose, Magnesium Stearate, Neutral Soap, Oleic Acid, Povidone, Rosin, Sugar, Talc, White Wax, Zein.
12 mg Repetabs also contains: Acacia, Butylparaben, Calcium Phosphate, Calcium Sulfate, Carnauba Wax, Corn Starch, D&C Yellow No. 10 Al Lake, FD&C Blue No. 2 Al Lake, FD&C Yellow No. 6, FD&C Yellow No. 6 Al Lake, Lactose, Magnesium Stearate, Neutral Soap, Oleic Acid, Potato Starch, Rosin, Sugar, Talc, White Wax, Zein. Half the dose is released after the tablet is swallowed, and the other half is released hours later; continuous relief is provided for up to 12 hours.
Each teaspoonful (5 ml) of Allergy Syrup contains: 2 mg CHLOR-TRIMETON (brand of chlorpheniramine maleate) in a pleasant-tasting syrup containing approximately 7% alcohol. Also contains: Benzaldehyde, FD&C Green No. 3, FD&C Yellow No. 6, Flavor, Glycerin, Menthol, Methylparaben, Propylene Glycol, Propylparaben, Sugar, Vanillin, Water.

Indications: For temporary relief of hay fever symptoms: sneezing; runny nose; watery, itchy eyes, itching of the nose or throat.

Actions: The active ingredient in CHLOR-TRIMETON is an antihistamine with anticholinergic (drying) and sedative side effects. Antihistamines appear to compete with histamine for cell receptor sites on effector cells.

Warnings: May cause excitability especially in children. Do not give the REPETABS Tablets to children under 12 years, or the Allergy Syrup and Tablets to children under 6 years except under the advice and supervision of a physician. Do not take this product if you have asthma, glaucoma, emphysema, chronic pulmonary disease, shortness of breath, difficulty in breathing, or difficulty in urination due to enlargement of the prostate gland unless directed by a physician. May cause drowsiness; alcohol may increase the drowsiness effect. Avoid alcoholic beverages while taking this product. Use caution when driving a motor vehicle or operating machinery. As with any drug, if you are pregnant or nursing a baby, seek the advice of a health professional before using this product. Keep this and all drugs out of the reach of children. In case of accidental overdose, seek professional assistance or contact a Poison Control Center immediately.

Dosage and Administration: Allergy Syrup—Adults and Children 12 years and over: Two teaspoonfuls (4 mg) every 4 to 6 hours, not to exceed 12 teaspoonfuls in 24 hours. Children 6 through 11 years: one teaspoonful (2 mg) every 4 to 6 hours, not to exceed 6 teaspoonfuls in 24 hours. For children under 6 years, consult a physician.
Allergy Tablets—Adults and Children 12 years and over: One tablet (4 mg) every 4 to 6 hours, not to exceed 6 tablets in 24 hours. Children 6 through 11 years: One half the adult dose (break tablet in half) every 4 to 6 hours, not to exceed 3 whole tablets in 24 hours. For children under 6 years, consult a physician.
Allergy REPETABS Tablets—Adults and Children 12 years and over: One tablet in the morning and one tablet in the evening, not to exceed 24 mg (3 tablets of 8 mg; 2 tablets of 12 mg) in 24 hours. For children under 12 years, consult a physician.

Professional Labeling: Dosage—Allergy Syrup: Children 2 through 5 years: ½ teaspoonful (1 mg) every 4 to 6 hours; Allergy Tablets: Children 2 through 5 years: one-quarter tablet (1 mg) every 4 to 6 hours.
Allergy REPETABS Tablets—Children 6 to 12 years: One tablet (8 mg) at bedtime or during the day, as indicated.

How Supplied: CHLOR-TRIMETON Allergy Tablets, 4 mg, yellow com-

Continued on next page

Information on Schering-Plough HealthCare Products appearing on these pages is effective as of November 1990.

Schering-Plough—Cont.

pressed, scored tablets impressed with the Schering trademark and product identification letters, TW or numbers, 080; box of 24, bottles of 100.
CHLOR-TRIMETON Allergy Syrup: 2 mg per 5 ml, blue-green-colored liquid; 4-fluid ounce (118 ml). Protect from light; however, if color fades potency will not be affected.
CHLOR-TRIMETON Allergy REPETABS Tablets, 8 mg, sugar-coated, yellow tablets branded in red with the Schering trademark and product identification letters, CC or numbers, 374; boxes of 24, 48, bottles of 100.
CHLOR-TRIMETON REPETABS Tablets, 12 mg, sugar coated orange tablets branded in black with Schering trademark and product identification letters AAE or numbers 009; boxes of 12 and 24, bottles of 100.
Store the tablets and syrup between 2° and 30°C (36° and 86°F).

Shown in Product Identification Section, page 429

CHLOR-TRIMETON®
[*klor 'tri 'mĕ-ton*]
Decongestant Tablets
Long Acting CHLOR-TRIMETON®
Decongestant REPETABS® Tablets

Active Ingredients: Each tablet contains: 4 mg CHLOR-TRIMETON (brand of chlorpheniramine maleate, USP) and 60 mg pseudoephedrine sulfate. Each tablet also contains: Corn Starch, FD&C Blue No. 1, Lactose, Magnesium Stearate, Povidone.
Each REPETABS Tablet contains: 8 mg CHLOR-TRIMETON (brand of chlorpheniramine maleate) and 120 mg pseudoephedrine sulfate. Each repetab also contains: Acacia, Butylparaben, Calcium Sulfate, Carnauba Wax, Corn Starch, D&C Yellow No. 10 Al Lake, FD&C Blue No. 1 Al Lake, FD&C Yellow No. 6 Al Lake, Gelatin, Lactose, Magnesium Stearate, Neutral Soap, Oleic Acid, Povidone, Rosin, Sugar, Talc, White Wax, Zein. Half the dose of each ingredient is released after the tablet is swallowed and the other half is released hours later providing continuous long-lasting relief up to 12 hours.

Indications: For temporary relief of hay fever symptoms (sneezing; running nose; watery, itchy eyes, itching of the nose or throat) and nasal congestion due to hay fever and associated with sinusitis.

Actions: The antihistamine, chlorpheniramine maleate, provides temporary relief of running nose, sneezing, itching of the nose or throat, and itchy and watery eyes as may occur in allergic rhinitis (such as hayfever). The decongestant, pseudoephedrine sulfate reduces swelling of nasal passages; shrinks swollen membranes; and temporarily restores freer breathing through the nose.

Warnings: If symptoms do not improve within 7 days or are accompanied by fever, consult a physician before continuing use. May cause excitability especially in children. Do not exceed recommended dosage because at higher doses nervousness, dizziness or sleeplessness may occur. Do not take this product if you have asthma, glaucoma, emphysema, chronic pulmonary disease, shortness of breath, difficulty in breathing, heart disease, high blood pressure, thyroid disease, diabetes, or difficulty in urination due to enlargement of the prostate gland. Do not give the Decongestant Tablets to children under 6 years or the REPETABS Tablets to children under 12 years unless directed by a physician. May cause drowsiness; alcohol may increase the drowsiness effect. Avoid alcoholic beverages while taking this product. Use caution when driving a motor vehicle or operating machinery. Keep this and all drugs out of the reach of children. In case of accidental overdose, seek professional assistance or contact a Poison Control Center immediately. As with any drug, if you are pregnant or nursing a baby, seek the advice of a health professional before using this product.

Drug Interaction Precaution: Do not take this product if you are presently taking a prescription drug for high blood pressure or depression, without first consulting your doctor.

Dosage and Administration: Tablets —ADULTS AND CHILDREN 12 YEARS AND OVER: One tablet every 4 to 6 hours, not to exceed 4 tablets in 24 hours. CHILDREN 6 THROUGH 11 YEARS —One half the adult dose (break tablet in half) every 4 to 6 hours not to exceed 2 whole tablets in 24 hours. For children under 6 years, consult a physician. REPETABS Tablets—ADULTS AND CHILDREN 12 YEARS AND OVER: one tablet every 12 hours.

Professional Labeling: Tablets—Children 2-5 years—one quarter the adult dose every 4 hours, not to exceed 1 tablet in 24 hours.

How Supplied: CHLOR-TRIMETON Decongestant Tablets—boxes of 24 and 48. Long Acting CHLOR-TRIMETON Decongestant REPETABS Tablets boxes of 12 and 36.
Store these CHLOR-TRIMETON Products between 2° and 30°C (36°and 86°F); and protect from excessive moisture.

Shown in Product Identification Section, page 429

COD LIVER OIL CONCENTRATE
[*kod liv 'er oyl kon-sen-trāt*]
Tablets
Capsules
Tablets with Vitamin C

Active Ingredients: Tablets—A pleasantly flavored concentrate of cod liver oil with Vitamins A & D added. Each tasty, chewable tablet provides: 4000 IU of vitamin A and 200 IU of cholecalciferol (vitamin D).
Capsules—A concentrate of cod liver oil with Vitamins A and D added. Each capsule provides: 10,000 IU of vitamin A and 400 IU of cholecalciferol (vitamin D).
Tablets with Vitamin C—A pleasantly-flavored concentrate of cod liver oil with Vitamins A, D and C added. Each tablet provides, 4000 IU of Vitamin A, 200 IU of cholecalciferol (vitamin D) and 50 mg of Vitamin C.
Tablets may be chewed or swallowed.

Inactive Ingredients: Capsules— Corn oil, gelatin, glycerin, vitamin E .
Tablets with Vitamin C—Acacia, Butylparaben, Carnauba Wax, Confectioners Glaze, FD&C Yellow No. 5 Aluminum Lake, FD&C Yellow No. 6 Aluminum Lake, Flavor, Gelatin, Magnesium Stearate, Sugar, Wheat Flour, White Wax.

Indications: Cod Liver Oil Concentrate Tablets and Capsules are recommended for prevention and treatment of diseases due to deficiencies in Vitamins A and D. The tablets with Vitamin C are recommended for prevention and treatment of diseases due to deficiencies of Vitamins A, D and C.

Warnings: Keep these and all drugs out of the reach of children.
As with any drug, if you are pregnant or nursing a baby, seek the advice of a health professional before using these products.

Precautions: Cod Liver Oil Concentrate Tablets and Tablets with Vitamin C contain FD&C Yellow No. 5 (tartrazine) as a color additive.
Persons sensitive to tartrazine or aspirin should consult a physician.

Overdosage: In case of accidental overdose, seek professional assistance or contact a Poison Control Center immediately.

Dosage and Administration: Tablets: Two tablets daily, or as prescribed by a physician, taken preferably before meals.
Capsules: One capsule daily, or as prescribed by a physician, taken preferably before meals.
Tablets with Vitamin C: Two tablets daily, taken preferably before meals.

How Supplied: Cod Liver Oil Concentrate Tablets: bottles of 100. Cod Liver Oil Concentrate Capsules: bottles of 40 and 100. Cod Liver Oil Concentrate Tablets with Vitamin C: bottles of 100 tablets.

COMPLEX 15®
Phospholipid Hand & Body Moisturizing Cream
Formulated For Mild To Severe Dry Skin

Ingredients: Water, Mineral Oil, Glycerin, Squalane, Caprylic/Capric Triglyceride, Dimethicone, Glyceryl Stearate, Glycol Stearate, PEG-50 Stearate, Stearic Acid, Cetyl Alcohol, Myristyl Myristate, Lecithin, Diazolidinyl Urea, Carbomer 934, Magnesium Aluminum Silicate, C10–30 Carboxylic Acid Sterol Ester, Sodium Hydroxide, Tetrasodium EDTA, BHT

COMPLEX 15® Hand and Body Cream is formulated for mild to severe dry skin with a system modeled from nature. It contains lecithin, a phospholipid water-binding agent found naturally in the skin. Each phospholipid molecule holds 15 molecules of water, restoring the natural moisture balance. COMPLEX 15 Hand and Body Cream is nongreasy and absorbs quickly into the skin. COMPLEX 15 Hand and Body Cream is unscented, contains no parabens or lanolin. COMPLEX 15 Hand and Body Cream is proven to be hypoallergenic and noncomedogenic.

Directions: Apply to the hands and body as needed or as directed by a physician. Avoid contact with eyes.

FOR EXTERNAL USE ONLY

How Supplied: COMPLEX 15® Hand & Body Moisturizing Cream is available in 4 ounce jars (0085-4151-04).

Shown in Product Identification Section, page 429

COMPLEX 15®
Phospholipid Hand & Body Moisturizing Lotion
Formulated For Mild To Severe Dry Skin

Ingredients: Water, Caprylic/Capric Triglyceride, Glycerin, Glyceryl Stearate, Dimethicone, PEG-50 Stearate, Squalane, Cetyl Alcohol, Glycol Stearate, Myristyl Myristate, Stearic Acid, Lecithin, C10–30 Carboxylic Acid Sterol Ester, Diazolidinyl Urea, Carbomer 934, Magnesium Aluminum Silicate, Sodium Hydroxide, BHT, Tetrasodium EDTA

COMPLEX 15® Hand and Body Lotion is formulated for mild to severe dry skin with a system modeled from nature. It contains lecithin, a phospholipid water-binding agent found naturally in the skin. Each phospholipid molecule holds 15 molecules of water, restoring the natural moisture balance. COMPLEX 15 Hand and Body Lotion is nongreasy and absorbs quickly into the skin. COMPLEX 15 Hand and Body Lotion is unscented, contains no parabens, lanolin, or mineral oil. COMPLEX 15 Hand and Body Lotion is proven to be hypoallergenic and noncomedogenic.

Directions: Apply to the hands and body as needed, or as directed by a physician. Avoid contact with eyes.

FOR EXTERNAL USE ONLY

How Supplied: COMPLEX 15® Hand and Body Moisturizing Lotion is available in 8 fluid ounce bottles (0085-4115-08).

Shown in Product Identification Section, page 429

COMPLEX 15®
Phospholipid Moisturizing Face Cream

Ingredients: Water, Caprylic/Capric Triglyceride, Glycerin, Squalane, Glyceryl Stearate, Propylene Glycol, PEG-50 Stearate, Cetyl Alcohol, Dimethicone, Glycol Stearate, Myristyl Myristate, Stearic Acid, Carbomer 934, Magnesium Aluminum Silicate, Diazolidinyl Urea, Lecithin, Sodium Hydroxide, C10–30 Carboxylic Acid Sterol Ester, BHT, Tetrasodium EDTA

COMPLEX 15® Face Cream is formulated for mild to severe dry skin with a system modeled from nature. It contains lecithin, a phospholipid water-binding agent found naturally in the skin. Each phospholipid molecule holds 15 molecules of water, restoring the natural moisture balance. COMPLEX 15 Face Cream is nongreasy and absorbs quickly into the skin. COMPLEX 15 Face Cream is unscented, contains no parabens, lanolin or mineral oil. COMPLEX 15 Face Cream is proven to be hypoallergenic and noncomedogenic.

Directions: Apply to the face as needed or as directed by a physician. Avoid contact with eyes.

FOR EXTERNAL USE ONLY

How Supplied: COMPLEX 15® Moisturizing Face Cream is available in 2.5 oz. tubes (0085-4100-25).

Shown in Product Identification Section, page 429

COPPERTONE® Waterproof Sunscreens
COPPERTONE® Sunscreen Lotion SPF 6
COPPERTONE® Sunscreen Lotion SPF 8
COPPERTONE® Sunblock Lotion SPF 15
COPPERTONE® Sunblock Lotion SPF 25
COPPERTONE® Sunblock Lotion SPF 30
COPPERTONE® Sunblock Lotion SPF 45

New PABA-Free ingredients:

SPF 6–15: Ethylhexyl-p-methoxycinnamate, oxybenzone

SPF 25, 30: Ethylhexyl-p-methoxycinnamate, 2-ethylhexyl salicylate, homosalate, oxybenzone

SPF 45: Ethylhexyl-p-methoxycinnamate, 2-ethylhexyl salicylate, octocrylene, oxybenzone

How Supplied: 4 fl. oz. Plastic Bottles

Shown in Product Identification Section, page 431

CORICIDIN® Tablets
[kor-a-see 'din]
CORICIDIN 'D'® Decongestant Tablets
CORICIDIN® Nasal Mist

Active Ingredients: CORICIDIN Tablets—2 mg CHLOR-TRIMETON® (brand of chlorpheniramine maleate, USP); 325 mg (5 gr) acetaminophen.

CORICIDIN 'D' Decongestant Tablets—2 mg chlorpheniramine maleate, USP; 12.5 mg phenylpropanolamine hydrochloride, USP; 325 mg (5 gr) acetaminophen.

CORICIDIN Nasal Mist—.05% oxymetazoline hydrochloride.

Inactive Ingredients: CORICIDIN Tablets—Acacia, Butylparaben, Calcium Sulfate, Carnauba Wax, Cellulose, Corn Starch, FD&C Red No. 40, FD&C Yellow No. 6 Aluminum Lake, Lactose, Magnesium Stearate, Povidone, Sugar, Titanium Dioxide, and White Wax. May also contain Talc.

CORICIDIN 'D' Decongestant Tablets—Acacia, Butylparaben, Calcium Sulfate, Carnauba Wax, Cellulose, Corn Starch, Magnesium Stearate, Povidone, Sugar, Titanium Dioxide, and White Wax. May also contain Talc.

CORICIDIN Nasal Mist—Benzalkonium Chloride, Glycine, Phenylmercuric Acetate (0.02 mg/ml), Sorbitol, and Water.

Indications: CORICIDIN Tablets—For effective, temporary relief of cold and flu symptoms.

CORICIDIN 'D' Decongestant Tablets—For effective, temporary relief of congested cold, flu and sinus symptoms.

CORICIDIN Nasal Mist—For temporary relief of nasal congestion associated with the common cold, hay fever or sinusitis.

Actions: CORICIDIN Tablets relieve annoying cold and flu symptoms such as minor aches and pains, fever, sneezing, running nose and watery/itchy eyes.

CORICIDIN 'D' Tablets relieve the same annoying cold and flu symptoms as well as stuffy nose, nasal membrane swelling and sinus headache.

CORICIDIN Nasal Mist is "symptom specific" and designed to shrink swollen nasal membranes promptly and help restore freer breathing through the nose.

Warnings: CORICIDIN Tablets: Do not take this product for pain for more than 10 days (for adults) or 5 days (for children 6 years through 11 years), and do not take for fever for more than 3 days unless directed by a physician. If pain or fever persists or gets worse, if new symptoms occur, or if redness or swelling is present, consult a physician because these could be signs of a serious condition. May cause excitability especially in children. Do not take this product if you have asthma, glaucoma, emphysema, chronic pulmonary disease, shortness of breath, difficulty in breathing, difficulty in urination due to enlargement of the prostate gland, or give this product to children under 6 years, unless directed by a physician. May cause drowsiness; alcohol, sedatives, and tranquilizers may increase the drowsiness effect. Avoid alcoholic beverages while taking this product. Do not take this product if you are taking sedatives or tranquilizers, without first consulting your physician. Use caution when driving a motor vehicle or operating machinery. Keep this and all drugs out of the reach of children. In case of accidental overdose, seek professional assistance or contact a Poison Control Center immedi-

Continued on next page

Information on Schering-Plough HealthCare Products appearing on these pages is effective as of November 1990.

Schering-Plough—Cont.

ately. Prompt medical attention is critical for adults as well as for children even if you do not notice any signs or symptoms. As with any drug, if you are pregnant or nursing a baby, seek the advice of a health professional before using this product.
CORICIDIN 'D' Decongestant Tablets: Do not take this product for pain or congestion for more than 7 days (adults) or 5 days (children 6 through 11 years), and do not take for fever for more than 3 days unless directed by a physician. If pain or fever persists or gets worse, if new symptoms occur, or if redness or swelling is present, consult your physician because these could be signs of a serious condition. May cause excitability, especially in children. Do not exceed recommended dosage because at higher doses nervousness, dizziness, or sleeplessness may occur. Do not take this product if you have asthma, glaucoma, emphysema, chronic pulmonary disease, shortness of breath, difficulty in breathing, heart disease, high blood pressure, thyroid disease, diabetes, difficulty in urination due to enlargement of the prostate gland, or give this product to children under 6 years unless directed by a physician. May cause drowsiness; alcohol, sedatives, and tranquilizers may increase the drowsiness effect. Avoid alcoholic beverages while taking this product. Use caution when driving a motor vehicle or operating machinery. Keep this and all drugs out of the reach of children. In case of accidental overdose, seek professional assistance or contact a Poison Control Center immediately. Proper medical attention is critical for adults and children even if you do not notice any signs or symptoms. As with any drug, if you are pregnant or nursing a baby, seek the advice of a health care professional before using this product. *Drug Interaction Precaution:* Do not take this product if you are presently taking a prescription drug for high blood pressure or depression, sedatives, tranquilizers or appetite-controlling medication containing phenylpropanolamine without first consulting your physician.
CORICIDIN Nasal Mist—Do not exceed recommended dosage because burning, stinging, sneezing, or increase of nasal discharge may occur. Do not use this product for more than 3 days. If nasal congestion persists, consult a physician. The use of this dispenser by more than one person may spread infection. For adult use only. Keep this and all medicines out of the reach of children.

Dosage and Administration: CORICIDIN Tablets—Adults and children 12 years and over—2 tablets every 4 hours not to exceed 12 tablets in 24 hours. Children 6 through 11 years: 1 tablet every 4 hours not to exceed 5 tablets in 24 hours.
CORICIDIN 'D' Decongestant Tablets—Adults and children 12 years and over: 2 tablets every 4 hours not to exceed 12 tablets in 24 hours. Children 6 through 11 years: 1 tablet every 4 hours not to exceed 5 tablets in 24 hours.
CORICIDIN Nasal Mist— For adults and children 6 years of age and over: With head upright spray two or three times in each nostril twice daily—morning and evening, to spray squeeze bottle quickly and firmly. Do not tilt head backward while spraying. Wipe nozzle clean after use. Not recommended for children under six.

How Supplied: CORICIDIN Tablets—bottles of 12, 24, 48, and 100.
CORICIDIN 'D' Decongestant Tablets—bottles of 12, 24, 48, and 100.
CORICIDIN Decongestant Nasal Mist—Plastic squeeze bottles of ½ fl. oz. (15 ml.)
Store the tablets, nasal mist, and syrup between 2° and 30°C (36° and 86°F).

Shown in Product Identification Section, page 429

CORICIDIN® DEMILETS®
[*kor-a-see 'din dem 'ē-lets*]
Tablets for Children

CORICIDIN DEMILETS Tablets—1.0 mg chlorpheniramine maleate, USP; 80 mg acetaminophen, USP; 6.25 mg phenylpropanolamine hydrochloride, USP.

Inactive Ingredients: Corn Starch, D&C Yellow No. 10 Al Lake, FD&C Yellow No. 6 Al Lake, Flavor, Lactose, Magnesium Stearate, Mannitol, Saccharin, Stearic Acid.

Indications: CORICIDIN DEMILETS Tablets—For temporary relief of children's congested cold, flu and sinus symptoms.

Actions: CORICIDIN DEMILETS Tablets provide relief of annoying cold, flu and sinus symptoms: running nose, stuffy nose, sneezing, watery/itchy eyes, minor aches, pains and fever.

Warnings: CORICIDIN DEMILETS Tablets—Give water with each dose. Do not give this product for more than 5 days, but if fever is present, persists or recurs, limit dosage to 3 days; if symptoms persist or new ones occur, consult a physician. This product may cause drowsiness, therefore, driving a motor vehicle or operating heavy machinery must be avoided while taking it. Alcoholic beverages must also be avoided while taking this product. It may cause excitability, especially in children. Do not exceed recommended dosage because at higher doses severe liver damage, nervousness, dizziness, elevation of blood pressure or sleeplessness is more likely to occur. Do not administer this product to persons who have asthma, glaucoma, difficulty in urination due to enlargement of the prostate gland, high blood pressure, heart disease, diabetes or thyroid disease, or give this product to children less than 6 years old, except under the advice and supervision of a physician. Keep this and all drugs out of the reach of children. As with any drug, if you are pregnant or nursing a baby, seek the advice of a health professional before using this product.

Drug Interactions: CORICIDIN DEMILETS Tablets—Do not give this product to persons who are presently taking a prescription antihypertensive or antidepressant medication containing a monoamine oxidase inhibitor or an appetite-controlling medication containing phenylpropanolamine except under the advice and supervision of a physician.

Overdosage: In case of accidental overdose, seek professional assistance or contact a Poison Control Center immediately.

Dosage and Administration: CORICIDIN DEMILETS Tablets—Under 6 years: As directed by a physician. 6 through 11 years: Two DEMILETS Tablets every 4 hours not to exceed 12 tablets in a 24-hour period, or as directed by a physician.

How Supplied: CORICIDIN DEMILETS Tablets—boxes of 36, individually wrapped in a child's protective pack.
Store the tablets between 2° and 30°C (36° and 86°F). Protect from excessive moisture.

Shown in Product Identification Section, page 429

CORRECTOL®
Laxative
Tablets

Active Ingredients: Tablets—Yellow phenolphthalein, 65 mg. and docusate sodium, 100 mg. per tablet.

Inactive Ingredients: Butylparaben, calcium gluconate, calcium sulfate, carnauba wax, D&C No. 7 calcium lake, gelatin, magnesium stearate, sugar, talc, titanium dioxide, wheat flour, white wax, and other ingredients.

Indications: For relief of occasional constipation or irregularity. CORRECTOL generally produces bowel movement in 6 to 8 hours.

Actions: Yellow phenolphthalein—stimulant laxative; docusate sodium—fecal softener.

Warnings: Not to be taken in case of nausea, vomiting, abdominal pain, or signs of appendicitis. Take only as needed —as frequent or continued use of laxatives may result in dependence on them. If skin rash appears, do not use this or any other preparation containing phenolphthalein. As with any drug, if you are pregnant or nursing a baby, seek the advice of a health professional before using this product.

Dosage and Administration
Dosage: Adults—1 or 2 tablets daily as needed, at bedtime or on arising.
Children over 6 years—1 tablet daily as needed.

How Supplied: Tablets—Individual foil-backed safety sealed blister packaging in boxes of 15, 30, 60 and 90 tablets.

Shown in Product Identification Section, page 429

DEMAZIN®
[dem 'a-zin]
Nasal Decongestant/Antihistamine
TIMED-RELEASE Tablets
Syrup

Description: Each **TIMED-RELEASE Tablet** contains: 25 mg phenylpropanolamine hydrochloride and 4 mg CHLOR-TRIMETON® (brand of chlorpheniramine maleate, USP). Half the dose is released after the tablet is swallowed and the other half is released hours later; continuous relief is provided for up to 8 hours.
Each **TIMED-RELEASE Tablet** also contains: Acacia, Butylparaben, Calcium Phosphate, Calcium Sulfate, Carnauba Wax, Corn Starch, Diatomaceous Earth, FD&C Blue No. 1, FD&C Blue No. 2 Al Lake, Kaolin, Lactose, Magnesium Stearate, Neutral Soap, Oleic Acid, Stearic Acid, Sugar, Talc, White Wax, and Zein.
Each teaspoonful (5 ml) of **Syrup** contains 12.5 mg phenylpropanolamine hydrochloride, USP and 2 mg CHLOR-TRIMETON® (brand of chlorpheniramine maleate, USP) in a pleasant-tasting syrup containing approximately 7.5% alcohol.
Each teaspoonful of **Syrup** also contains: Benzaldehyde, FD&C Blue No. 1, FD&C Green No. 3, FD&C Yellow No. 6, Flavor, Glycerin, Menthol, Methylparaben, Propylene Glycol, Propylparaben, Sugar, Vanillin, and Water.

Indications: For temporary relief of running nose, sneezing, itching of the nose or throat, and itchy and watery eyes as may occur in allergic rhinitis (such as hay fever); nasal congestion due to the common cold (cold), hay fever or other upper respiratory allergies, or associated with sinusitis.

Actions: Phenylpropanolamine hydrochloride is a sympathomimetic agent which acts as an upper respiratory and pulmonary decongestant and mild bronchodilator. It exerts desirable sympathomimetic action with relatively little central nervous system excitation, so that wakefulness and nervousness are reduced to a minimum. Chlorpheniramine maleate antagonizes many of the characteristic effects of histamine. It is of value clinically in the prevention and relief of many allergic manifestations.
The oral administration of phenylpropanolamine hydrochloride with chlorpheniramine maleate produces a complementary action on congestive conditions of the upper respiratory tract, thus often obviating the need for topical nasal therapy.

Warnings: If symptoms do not improve within 7 days or are accompanied by high fever, consult a physician before continuing use. May cause excitability especially in children. Do not exceed recommended dosage because at higher doses nervousness, dizziness, or sleeplessness may occur. Do not take this product if you have asthma, glaucoma, emphysema, chronic pulmonary disease, shortness of breath, difficulty in breathing, heart disease, high blood pressure, thyroid disease, diabetes, or difficulty in urination due to enlargement of the prostate gland or give this product to children under 6 years, unless directed by a physician. May cause drowsiness; alcohol may increase the drowsiness effect. Avoid alcoholic beverages while taking this product. Use caution when driving a motor vehicle or operating machinery. Keep this and all drugs out of reach of children. In case of accidental overdose, seek professional assistance or contact a Poison Control Center immediately. As with any drug, if you are pregnant or nursing a baby, seek the advice of a health professional before using this product.

Drug Interaction Precaution: Do not take this product if you are presently taking a prescription drug for high blood pressure or depression or an appetite-controlling medication containing phenylpropanolamine without first consulting your doctor.

Dosage and Administration: TIMED-RELEASE Tablets—Adults and children 12 years and older: 2 tablets every 8 hours not to exceed 6 tablets in 24 hours. **Children 6 through 11 years:** 1 tablet every 8 hours not to exceed 3 tablets in 24 hours. For children under 6 years, consult a physician. **Syrup—Adults and children 12 years and older:** Two teaspoonfuls every 4–6 hours not to exceed 12 teaspoonfuls in 24 hours, or as directed by a physician. **Children 6 through 11 years:** One teaspoonful every 4 hours not to exceed 6 teaspoonfuls in 24 hours or as directed by a physician. For children under 6 years, consult a physician.

How Supplied: DEMAZIN TIMED-RELEASE Tablets, blue, sugar-coated tablets branded in red with the Schering trademark and product identification number 751; box of 24 and bottle of 100.
DEMAZIN Syrup, blue-colored liquid, bottles of 4 fluid ounces (118 ml).
Store DEMAZIN TIMED-RELEASE Tablets and Syrup between 2° and 30°C (36° and 86°F).

DERMOLATE® Anti-Itch Cream
[dur 'mō-lāt]

Active Ingredients: DERMOLATE Anti-Itch Cream contains hydrocortisone 0.5% in a greaseless, vanishing cream. It also contains: Ceteareth-30, Cetearyl Alcohol, Mineral Oil, Petrolatum, Propylene Glycol, Sodium Phosphate, Water.

Indications: For the temporary relief of minor skin irritations, itching and rashes due to eczema, dermatitis, insect bites, poison ivy, poison oak, poison sumac, soaps, detergents, cosmetics and jewelry.

Actions: DERMOLATE Anti-Itch Cream provides temporary relief of itching and minor skin irritation.

Warnings: DERMOLATE Anti-Itch Cream is for external use only. Avoid contact with the eyes. Discontinue use and consult a physician if condition worsens or if symptoms persist for more than seven days.
Do not use on children under 2 years of age except under the advice and supervision of physician. Keep these and all drugs out of the reach of children.

Overdosage: In case of accidental ingestion, seek professional assistance or contact a Poison Control Center immediately.

Dosage and Administration: *For adults and children 2 years of age and older:* Gently massage into affected skin area not more than 3 or 4 times daily. *For children under 2 years of age,* there is no recommended dosage except under the advice and supervision of a physician.

How Supplied: DERMOLATE Anti-Itch Cream—30 g (1.0 oz.) tube, and 15 g (½ oz) tubes.
Store between 2° and 30°C (36° and 86°F).

DI-GEL®
Antacid · Anti-Gas
Tablets/Liquid

DI-GEL Tablets: Active Ingredients: (Per Tablet)—Simethicone 20 mg., Calcium Carbonate 280 mg., Magnesium Hydroxide 128 mg. **Inactive Ingredients:** D & C yellow No. 10 aluminum lake, dextrin, FD&C yellow No. 6 aluminum lake, flavor, magnesium stearate, mannitol, polyvinyl-pyrrolidone, stearic acid, sucrose, talc.
Dietetically sodium free, calcium rich.

DI-GEL Liquid: Active Ingredients—per teaspoonful (5 ml): Simethicone 20 mg., aluminum hydroxide (equivalent to aluminum hydroxide dried gel USP) 200 mg., magnesium hydroxide 200 mg. **Also contains:** Flavor, methylcellulose, methylparaben, propylparaben, sodium saccharin, sorbitol, water.
Dietetically sodium free.

Indications: For fast, temporary relief of acid indigestion, heartburn, sour stomach and accompanying painful gas symptoms.

Actions: The antacid system in DI-GEL relieves and soothes acid indigestion, heartburn and sour stomach. At the same time, the simethicone "defoamers" eliminate gas.
When air becomes entrapped in the stomach, heartburn and acid indigestion can result, along with sensations of fullness, pressure and bloating.

Warnings: Do not take more than 20 teaspoonfuls or 24 tablets in a 24 hour period, or use the maximum dosage of this product for more than 2 weeks, except under the advice and supervision of a physician. If you have kidney disease do not use this product except under the advice and supervision of a physician.

Continued on next page

Information on Schering-Plough HealthCare Products appearing on these pages is effective as of November 1990.

Schering-Plough—Cont.

May cause constipation or have a laxative effect.

Drug Interaction: (Liquid Only) This product should not be taken if patient is presently taking a prescription antibiotic drug containing any form of tetracycline.

Dosage and Administration: Two teaspoonfuls or tablets every 2 hours, or after or between meals and at bedtime, not to exceed 20 teaspoonfuls or 24 tablets per day, or as directed by a physician.

How Supplied:
DI-GEL Liquid in Mint and Lemon/Orange Flavors - 6 and 12 fl. oz. bottles, safety sealed.
DI-GEL Tablets in Mint and Lemon/Orange Flavors - In boxes of 30 and 90 in handy portable safety sealed blister packaging. Also available in Mint 3-roll (36 tablets) and in Mint 60-tablet bottles.

Shown in Product Identification Section, page 429

DISOPHROL® Chronotab®
[*dī'sō-frōl*]
Sustained-Action Tablets

Description: EACH DISOPHROL® Chronotab® SUSTAINED-ACTION TABLET CONTAINS: 120 mg of pseudoephedrine sulfate and 6 mg of dexbrompheniramine maleate. Half of the medication is released after the tablet is swallowed and the remaining amount of medication is released hours later providing continuous long-lasting relief for 12 hours. Also contains: Acacia, Butylparaben, Calcium Sulfate, Carnauba Wax, Corn Starch, FD&C Yellow No. 6 Al Lake, FD&C Red No. 40 Al Lake, Gelatin, Lactose, Magnesium Stearate, Neutral Soap, Oleic Acid, Povidone, Rosin, Sugar, Talc, White Wax, Zein.

Indications: For temporary relief of nasal congestion due to the common cold, hay fever, or other upper respiratory allergies, and associated with sinusitis. Helps decongest sinus openings, sinus passages. Reduces swelling of nasal passages; shrinks swollen membranes; and temporarily restores freer breathing through the nose. Alleviates running nose, sneezing, itching of the nose or throat, and itchy and watery eyes as may occur in allergic rhinitis (such as hay fever).

Warnings: If symptoms do not improve within 7 days or are accompanied by fever, consult a physician before continuing use. May cause excitability especially in children. Do not exceed recommended dosage because at higher doses nervousness, dizziness, or sleeplessness may occur. Do not take this product if you have asthma, glaucoma, emphysema, chronic pulmonary disease, shortness of breath, difficulty in breathing, heart disease, high blood pressure, thyroid disease, diabetes, or difficulty in urination due to enlargement of the prostate gland or give this product to children under 12 years, unless directed by a physician. May cause drowsiness; alcohol may increase the drowsiness effect. Avoid alcoholic beverages while taking this product. Use caution when driving a motor vehicle or operating machinery. Keep this and all drugs out of the reach of children. In case of accidental overdose, seek professional assistance or contact a Poison Control Center immediately. As with any drug, if you are pregnant or nursing a baby, seek the advice of a health professional before using this product.

Drug Interaction Precaution: Do not take this product if you are presently taking a prescription drug for high blood pressure or depression, without first consulting your physician.

Dosage and Administration: ADULTS AND CHILDREN 12 YEARS AND OVER—one tablet every 12 hours. Do not exceed two tablets in 24 hours.

How Supplied: DISOPHROL Chronotab Sustained-Action Tablets, sugar-coated, cherry-red tablets branded in black with either the product identification code 85-WMH or one of the Schering trademarks and the numbers, 231; bottle of 100.
Store between 2° and 30°C (36° and 86°F).

DRIXORAL®
[*dricks-or'al*]
Antihistamine/Nasal Decongestant Syrup

Description: Each 5 ml (1 teaspoonful) of DRIXORAL Syrup contains 2 mg brompheniramine maleate and 30 mg pseudoephedrine sulfate; also contains Citric Acid, D&C Red No. 33, FD&C Yellow No. 6, Flavor, Propylene Glycol, Sodium Benzoate, Sodium Citrate, Sorbitol, Sugar, Water. Drixoral Syrup is alcohol-free.

Indications: DRIXORAL Syrup contains a nasal decongestant with an antihistamine in a pleasant-tasting wild cherry flavor to provide temporary relief of nasal congestion due to the common cold, hay fever or other upper respiratory allergies. Helps decongest sinus openings, sinus passages. Alleviates running nose, sneezing, itching of the nose or throat, and itchy and watery eyes due to hay fever. DRIXORAL Syrup is ideal for adults and children who prefer a syrup instead of tablets or capsules.

Warnings: If symptoms do not improve within 7 days or are accompanied by fever, consult a physician before continuing use. May cause drowsiness. May cause excitability especially in children. Do not exceed recommended dosage because at higher doses nervousness, dizziness, or sleeplessness may occur. Do not give this product to children under 6 years except under the advice and supervision of a physician. Do not take this product if you have asthma, glaucoma, emphysema, chronic pulmonary disease, shortness of breath, difficulty in breathing, difficulty in urination due to enlargement of the prostate gland, high blood pressure, heart disease, diabetes, or thyroid disease except under the advice and supervision of a physician. As with any drug, if you are pregnant or nursing a baby, seek the advice of a health professional before using this product. CAUTION: Avoid driving a motor vehicle or operating heavy machinery. Avoid alcoholic beverages while taking this product. Keep this and all drugs out of the reach of children. In case of accidental overdose, seek professional assistance or contact a Poison Control Center immediately.

Drug Interaction Precaution: Do not take this product if you are presently taking a prescription drug for high blood pressure or depression, without first consulting your doctor.

Directions: Adults and children 12 years of age and over: two teaspoonfuls every 4–6 hours. Children 6 to under 12 years of age: 1 teaspoonful every 4–6 hours. Do not exceed 4 doses in 24 hours. Children under 6 years of age, consult a physician.
Store between 2° and 30°C (36° and 86°F).

Overdosage: In case of accidental overdose, seek professional assistance or contact a Poison Control Center immediately.

How Supplied: DRIXORAL Syrup is available in 4 fl. oz. (118 ml) bottles.

Shown in Product Identification Section, page 430

DRIXORAL®
[*dricks-or'al*]
Sustained-Action Tablets

Description: EACH DRIXORAL SUSTAINED-ACTION TABLET CONTAINS: 120 mg of pseudoephedrine sulfate and 6 mg of dexbrompheniramine maleate. Half of the medication is released after the tablet is swallowed and the remaining amount of medication is released hours later providing continuous long-lasting relief for 12 hours. Also contains: Acacia, Butylparaben, Calcium Sulfate, Carnauba Wax, Corn Starch, D&C Yellow No. 10 Al Lake, FD&C Blue No. 1 Al Lake, FD&C Yellow No. 6 Al Lake, Gelatin, Lactose, Magnesium Stearate, Neutral Soap, Oleic Acid, Povidone, Rosin, Sugar, Talc, White Wax, Zein.

Indications: For temporary relief of nasal congestion due to the common cold, hay fever, or other upper respiratory allergies, and associated with sinusitis. Helps decongest sinus openings, sinus passages. Reduces swelling of nasal passages; shrinks swollen membranes; and temporarily restores freer breathing through the nose. Alleviates running nose, sneezing, itching of the nose or throat, and itchy and watery eyes as may occur in allergic rhinitis (such as hay fever).

Actions: The antihistamine, dexbrompheniramine maleate, provides temporary relief of sneezing; watery, itchy eyes; running nose due to hay fever and other upper respiratory allergies. The decongestant, pseudoephedrine sulfate, temporarily restores freer breathing through the nose and promotes sinus drainage.

Warnings: If symptoms do not improve within 7 days or are accompanied by fever, consult a physician before continuing use. May cause excitability especially in children. Do not exceed recommended dosage because at higher doses nervousness, dizziness, or sleeplessness may occur. Do not take this product if you have asthma, glaucoma, emphysema, chronic pulmonary disease, high blood pressure, thyroid disease, diabetes, or difficulty in urination due to enlargement of the prostate gland or give this product to children under 12 years, unless directed by a physician. May cause drowsiness; alcohol may increase the drowsiness effect. Avoid alcoholic beverages while taking this product. Use caution when driving a motor vehicle or operating machinery. Keep this and all drugs out of the reach of children. In case of accidental overdose, seek professional assistance or contact a Poison Control Center immediately. As with any drug, if you are pregnant or nursing a baby, seek the advice of a health professional before using this product.

Drug Interaction Precaution: Do not take this product if you are presently taking a prescription drug for high blood pressure or depression, without first consulting your physician.

Dosage and Administration: ADULTS AND CHILDREN 12 YEARS AND OVER—one tablet every 12 hours. Do not exceed two tablets in 24 hours.

How Supplied: DRIXORAL Sustained-Action Tablets, green, sugar-coated tablets branded in black with the product name, boxes of 10, 20, and 40, bottle of 100.

Store between 2° and 30°C (36° and 86°F).

Shown in Product Identification Section, page 429

DRIXORAL® NON-DROWSY FORMULA

[*dricks-or 'al*]

Long-Acting Nasal Decongestant

DRIXORAL NON-DROWSY FORMULA Long-Acting Nasal Decongestant Tablets contain pseudoephedrine sulfate, a nasal decongestant, in a special timed-release tablet providing up to 12 hours of continuous relief . . . without drowsiness.

Indications: For temporary relief of nasal congestion due to the common cold, hay fever or other upper respiratory allergies, and nasal congestion associated with sinusitis. Helps decongest sinus openings and sinus passages.

Directions: Adults and Children 12 Years and Over—One tablet every 12 hours. DRIXORAL NON-DROWSY FORMULA is not recommended for children under 12 years of age.

Each Extended-Release Tablet Contains: 120 mg pseudoephedrine sulfate. Half the dose is released after the tablet is swallowed and the other half is released hours later, providing continuous relief for up to 12 hours.

Warnings: Do not exceed recommended dosage because at higher doses, nervousness, dizziness, or sleeplessness may occur. Do not take this product if you have heart disease, high blood pressure, thyroid disease, diabetes, difficulty in urination due to enlargement of the prostate gland, or give this product to children under 12 years unless directed by a physician. If symptoms do not improve within 7 days or are accompanied by fever, consult your physician before continuing use. Keep this and all drugs out of the reach of children. In case of accidental overdose, seek professional assistance or contact a Poison Control Center immediately. As with any drug, if you are pregnant or nursing a baby, seek the advice of a health professional before using this product.

Drug Interaction Precautions: Do not take this product if you are presently taking a prescription drug for high blood pressure or depression, without first consulting your physician.

Active Ingredients: Pseudoephedrine Sulfate

Also Contains: Acacia, Butylparaben, Calcium Sulfate, Carnauba Wax, Corn Starch, FD&C Blue No. 1, Gelatin, Lactose, Magnesium Stearate, Neutral Soap, Oleic Acid, Povidone, Rosin, Sugar, Talc, White Wax, Zein.

Store between 2° and 30°C (36° and 86°F).

Protect from excessive moisture.

Shown in Product Identification Section, page 430

DRIXORAL® PLUS

[*dricks-or 'al*]

Extended-Release Tablets

Active Ingredients: Acetaminophen, Dexbrompheniramine Maleate, Pseudoephedrine Sulfate.

Also Contains: Calcium Phosphate, Carnauba Wax, D&C Yellow No. 10 Al Lake, FD&C Blue No. 1 Al Lake, FD&C Yellow No. 6 Al Lake, Hydroxypropyl Methylcellulose, Magnesium Stearate, Methylparaben, PEG, Propylparaben, Stearic Acid.

DRIXORAL® *PLUS* Extended-Release Tablets combine a nasal decongestant and an antihistamine with a nonaspirin analgesic in a special 12-hour continuous-acting timed-release tablet.

Indications: The *decongestant* temporarily relieves nasal congestion due to the common cold, hay fever or other upper respiratory allergies, and associated with sinusitis. Reduces swelling of nasal passages; shrinks swollen membranes; and temporarily restores freer breathing through the nose. Also helps decongest sinus openings, sinus passages. The *nonaspirin analgesic* temporarily relieves occasional minor aches, pains, and headache and reduces fever due to the common cold. The *antihistamine* alleviates running nose, sneezing, itching of the nose or throat, and itchy and watery eyes as may occur in allergic rhinitis (such as hay fever).

EACH DRIXORAL PLUS EXTENDED-RELEASE TABLET CONTAINS: 60 mg of pseudoephedrine sulfate, 3 mg of dexbrompheniramine maleate and 500 mg of acetaminophen. These ingredients are released continuously, providing long-lasting relief for 12 hours.

Directions: ADULTS AND CHILDREN 12 YEARS AND OVER—two tablets every 12 hours. Do not exceed four tablets in 24 hours. Children under 12 years of age: consult a doctor.

Warnings: Do not take this product for more than 7 days. If symptoms do not improve, or are accompanied by fever that lasts for more than three days (72 hours) or recurs, or if new symptoms occur, consult a physician before continuing use. If pain or fever persists or gets worse, or if redness or swelling is present, consult a physician because these could be signs of a serious condition. May cause excitability especially in children. Do not exceed recommended dosage because at higher doses nervousness, dizziness, or sleeplessness may occur. Do not take this product if you have asthma, glaucoma, emphysema, chronic pulmonary disease, shortness of breath, difficulty in breathing, heart disease, high blood pressure, thyroid disease, difficulty in urination due to enlargement of the prostate gland, or give this product to children under 12 years unless directed by a physician. May cause drowsiness; alcohol, sedatives, and tranquilizers may increase the drowsiness effect. Avoid alcoholic beverages while taking this product. Use caution when driving a motor vehicle or operating machinery. Keep this and all drugs out of the reach of children. In case of accidental overdose, seek professional assistance or contact a Poison Control Center immediately. Prompt medical attention is critical for adults as well as for children even if you do not notice any signs or symptoms. As with any drug, if you are pregnant or nursing a baby, seek the advice of a health professional before using this product.

Drug Interaction Precaution: Do not take this product if you are presently taking a prescription drug for high blood pressure or depression, sedatives or tranquilizers, without first consulting your physician.

How Supplied: DRIXORAL PLUS Extended-Release Tablets are available in boxes of 12's and 24's and bottles of 48.

Store between 2° and 30°C (36° and 86°F).

Protect from excessive moisture.

Shown in Product Identification Section, page 430

Continued on next page

Information on Schering-Plough HealthCare Products appearing on these pages is effective as of November 1990.

Schering-Plough—Cont.

DRIXORAL® SINUS
[*dricks-or 'al*]
Nasal decongestant/Pain reliever/Antihistamine

DRIXORAL® SINUS Extended-Release Tablets combine a nasal decongestant, and a non-aspirin analgesic, with an antihistamine in a special 12-hour continuous-acting timed-release tablet.

Indications: The *decongestant* temporarily relieves nasal congestion due to sinusitis, the common cold, and hay fever or other upper respiratory allergies. Helps decongest sinus openings, sinus passages; relieves sinus pressure. Reduces swelling of nasal passages; shrinks swollen membranes; and temporarily restores freer breathing through the nose. The *non-aspirin analgesic* temporarily relieves occasional headaches, minor aches and pains, and reduces fever due to the common cold. The *antihistamine* alleviates runny nose, sneezing, itching of the nose or throat, and itchy and watery eyes as may occur in allergic rhinitis (such as hay fever).

Each Drixoral Sinus Extended-Release Tablet Contains: 60 mg of pseudoephedrine sulfate, 3 mg of dexbrompheniramine maleate, and 500 mg of acetaminophen. These ingredients are released continuously, providing long-lasting relief for 12 hours.

Directions: ADULTS AND CHILDREN 12 YEARS AND OVER—two tablets every 12 hours. Do not exceed four tablets in 24 hours. Children under 12 years of age: consult a physician.

Store between 2° and 26°C (36° and 77°F).
Protect from excessive moisture.

Warnings: Do not take this product for more than 7 days. If symptoms do not improve, or are accompanied by fever that lasts for more than three days (72 hours) or recurs, or if new symptoms occur, consult a physician before continuing use. If pain or fever persists or gets worse, or if redness or swelling is present, consult a physician because these could be signs of a serious condition. May cause excitability especially in children. Do not exceed recommended dosage because at higher doses nervousness, dizziness, or sleeplessness may occur. Do not take this product if you have asthma, glaucoma, emphysema, chronic pulmonary disease, shortness of breath, difficulty in breathing, heart disease, high blood pressure, thyroid disease, diabetes, difficulty in urination due to enlargement of the prostate gland, or give this product to children under 12 years unless directed by a physician. May cause drowsiness; alcohol, sedatives, and tranquilizers may increase the drowsiness effect. Avoid alcoholic beverages while taking this product. Use caution when driving a motor vehicle or operating machinery. Keep this and all drugs out of the reach of children. In case of accidental overdose, seek professional assistance or contact a Poison Control Center immediately. Prompt medical attention is critical for adults as well as for children even if you do not notice any signs or symptoms. As with any drug, if you are pregnant or nursing a baby, seek the advice of a health care professional before using this product.

Drug Interaction Precaution: Do not take this product if you are presently taking a prescription drug for high blood pressure or depression, sedatives, or tranquilizers, without first consulting your physician.

Shown in Product Identification, Section, page 430

DURATION®
12 Hour Nasal Spray
12 Hour Mentholated Nasal Spray
Topical Nasal Decongestant

Active Ingredient:
12 Hour Nasal Spray:
Oxymetazoline HCl 0.05%

Other Ingredients:
12 Hour Nasal Spray: Preservative Phenylmercuric Acetate (Mentholated Nasal Spray also contains the following aromatics: menthol, camphor, eucalyptol).

Indications: Immediate relief for up to 12 hours of nasal congestion due to colds, hay fever and sinusitis.

Actions: The sympathomimetic action of DURATION constricts the smaller arterioles of the nasal passages, producing a gentle and predictable decongesting effect.

Warnings: Do not exceed recommended dosage because symptoms may occur such as burning, stinging, sneezing, or increase of nasal discharge. Do not use this product for more than 3 days. If symptoms persist, consult a physician. The use of dispenser by more than one person may spread infection.

Dosage and Administration:
DURATION 12 Hour Nasal Spray—With head upright, spray 2 or 3 times in each nostril twice daily—morning and evening. To spray, squeeze bottle quickly and firmly. Not recommended for children under 6.

How Supplied:
DURATION 12 Hour Nasal Spray—½ and 1 fl. oz. plastic squeeze bottle.
DURATION 12 Hour Mentholated Nasal Spray—½ fl. oz. plastic squeeze bottle.
All bottles in safety sealed cartons.

Shown in Product Identification Section, page 430

DURATION®
12 Hour Nasal Spray Pump

Active Ingredients: Oxymetazoline Hydrochloride 0.05%

Inactive Ingredients: Aminoacetic Acid, Benzalkonium Chloride, Phenylmercuric Acetate (Preservative), Sorbitol, Water.

Indications: Delivers a measured dosage every time. Immediate relief of nasal congestion for up to 12 hours due to common cold, hay fever and sinusitis.

Warnings: Do not exceed recommended dosage because symptoms may occur such as burning, stinging, sneezing, or increase of nasal discharge. Do not use this product for more than 3 days. If symptoms persist, consult a physician. The use of dispenser by more than one person may spread infection. Keep this and all medications out of the reach of children.

Symptoms and Treatment of Oral Overdosage: In case of accidental ingestion, seek professional assistance or contact a Poison Control Center immediately.

Dosage and Administration: Before using first time, remove protective cap. Prime the metered pump by depressing several times. Hold bottle with thumb at base and nozzle between first and second fingers. With head upright (do not tilt backward), insert metered pump-spray nozzle in nostril. Depress pump completely 2 or 3 times. Sniff deeply. Repeat in other nostil. Wipe tip clean after each use.

How Supplied: Available in ½ fl. oz. pump spray.

Shown in Product Identification Section, page 430

EMKO® BECAUSE®
[*em 'ko bē-koz '*]
Vaginal Contraceptive Foam

Description: A non-hormonal, nonscented aerosol foam contraceptive in a portable applicator/foam unit containing six applications of an 8.0% concentration of the spermicide nonoxynol-9. Also contains: Benzethonium Chloride, Glyceryl Monostearate, PEG, Pluronic F-68 (Poloxamer 188), Quaternium-15, Stearic Acid, Triethanolamine, and Water.

Indications: Vaginal contraceptive intended for the prevention of pregnancy.
BECAUSE Foam provides effective protection alone or it may be used instead of spermicidal jelly or cream to give added protection with a diaphragm.
BECAUSE Foam also may be used to give added protection to other methods of contraception: with a condom; as a backup to the IUD or oral contraceptives during the first month of use; in the event more than one oral contraceptive pill is forgotten and extra protection is needed during that menstrual cycle.

Actions: Each applicatorful of BECAUSE Foam provides the correct amount of nonoxynol-9, the most widely used spermicide, to prevent pregnancy effectively. The foam covers the inside of the vagina and forms a layer of spermicidal material between the sperm and the cervix. The powerful spermicide prevents pregnancy by killing sperm after contact. BECAUSE Foam is effective immediately upon insertion. No waiting period is needed for effervescing or melting to take place since BECAUSE is introduced into the vagina as a foam.

Warnings: If vaginal or penile irritation occurs and continues, a physician should be consulted. Not effective orally. Where pregnancy is contraindicated, further individualization of the contraceptive program may be needed. Do not burn, incinerate or puncture container. Keep this and all drugs out of the reach of children and in case of accidental ingestion, call a Poison Control Center, emergency medical facility, or a doctor.

Dosage and Administration: Although no contraceptive can guarantee 100% effectiveness, for reliable protection against pregnancy follow directions. One applicatorful of BECAUSE Contraceptive Foam must be inserted before each act of sexual intercourse. BECAUSE Foam can be inserted immediately or up to one hour before intercourse. If more than one hour has passed before intercourse or if intercourse is repeated, another applicatorful of BECAUSE Foam must be inserted.

Directions for Use: The BECAUSE CONTRACEPTOR has a foam container attached to an applicator barrel.
With the container pushed all the way into the barrel, shake well. Pull the container upward until it stops. Tilt container to side to release foam into barrel. Allow foam to fill barrel to about one inch from end and return container to straight position. Foam will expand to fill remainder of barrel.
Hold contraceptor at top of the barrel part and gently insert applicator barrel deep into the vagina (close to the cervix). For ease of insertion, lie on your back with knees bent. With applicator barrel in place, push container all the way into the barrel. This deposits the foam properly. Remove the Contraceptor with the container still pushed all the way in the applicator barrel to avoid withdrawing any of the foam. No waiting period is needed before intercourse. BECAUSE Contraceptive Foam is effective immediately after proper insertion.
As with other vaginal contraceptive foam, cream and jelly products, douching is *not* recommended after using BECAUSE Foam. However, if douching is desired for cleansing purposes, you *must* wait at least six hours following your last act of sexual intercourse to allow BECAUSE Foam's full spermicidal activity to take place. Refer to package insert directions and diagrams for further details and applicator cleansing instructions.
How to Use the BECAUSE CONTRACEPTOR with a Diaphragm.
Insert one applicatorful of BECAUSE Foam directly into the vagina according to above directions and then insert diaphragm. After insertion, BECAUSE Foam is effective immediately and remains effective up to one hour before intercourse. If more than one hour has passed or you are going to repeat intercourse, insert another applicatorful of BECAUSE Foam *without removing your diaphragm.*

Storage: Contents under pressure. Do not burn, incinerate, or puncture the applicator. Store at normal room temperature. Do not expose to extreme heat or open flame or store at temperatures above 120°F. If stored at temperatures below 60°F, warm to room temperature before using.

How Supplied: Disposable 10 gm CONTRACEPTOR containing six applications of BECAUSE Contraceptive Foam. This foam is also available in the original form of EMKO® Foam with the regular applicator.

Shown in Product Identification Section, page 430

EMKO®
[em 'kō]
Vaginal Contraceptive Foam

Description: A non-hormonal, non-scented aerosol foam contraceptive containing an 8.0% concentration of the spermicide nonoxynol-9. Also contains: Benzethonium Chloride, Glyceryl Monostearate, PEG, Pluronic F-68 (Poloxamer 188), Quaternium-15, Stearic Acid, Triethanolamine, and Water.

Indications: Vaginal contraceptive intended for the prevention of pregnancy. EMKO Foam provides effective protection alone or it may be used instead of spermicidal jelly or cream to give added protection with a diaphragm.
EMKO Foam also may be used to give added protection to other methods of contraception: with a condom; as a backup to the IUD or oral contraceptives during the first month of use; in the event more than one oral contraceptive pill is forgotten and extra protection is needed during that menstrual cycle.

Actions: Each applicatorful of EMKO Foam provides the correct amount of nonoxynol-9, the most widely used spermicide, to prevent pregnancy effectively. The foam covers the inside of the vagina and forms a layer of spermicidal material between the sperm and the cervix. The powerful spermicide prevents pregnancy by killing sperm after contact. EMKO Foam is effective immediately upon insertion. No waiting period is needed for effervescing or melting to take place since EMKO is introduced into the vagina as a foam.

Warnings: If vaginal or penile irritation occurs and continues, a physician should be consulted. Where pregnancy is contraindicated, further individualization of the contraceptive program may be needed. Do not burn, incinerate or puncture can. Keep this and all drugs out of the reach of children and in case of accidental ingestion, call a Poison Control Center, emergency medical facility, or a doctor.

Dosage and Administration: Although no contraceptive can guarantee 100% effectiveness, for reliable protection against pregnancy read and follow directions carefully. One applicatorful of EMKO Contraceptive Foam must be inserted before each act of sexual intercourse. EMKO Foam can be inserted immediately or up to one hour before intercourse. If more than one hour has passed before intercourse or if intercourse is repeated, another applicatorful of EMKO Foam must be inserted.

Directions for Use:
Check Foam Supply with Weigh Cap.
With the cap on the can, hold the can in midair by the white button. As long as the black is showing, a full dose of foam is available. When the black begins to disappear, purchase a new can of EMKO Foam. USE *only if black is showing* to assure a full application. SHAKE CAN WELL before filling applicator. *Remove cap and place the can in an upright position on a level surface.* Place the EMKO regular applicator in an upright position over valve on top of can. Press down on the applicator gently. Allow foam to fill to the ridge in applicator barrel. The plunger will rise up as the foam fills the applicator. Remove the filled applicator from the can to stop flow. Hold the filled applicator by the barrel and gently insert deep into the vagina (close to the cervix). For ease of insertion, lie on your back with knees bent. With the applicator in place, push plunger into applicator until it stops. This deposits the foam properly. Remove the applicator with the plunger still pushed all the way in to avoid withdrawing any of the foam. No waiting period is needed before intercourse. EMKO Contraceptive Foam is effective immediately after proper insertion. As with other vaginal contraceptive foam, cream, and jelly products, douching is *not* recommended after using EMKO Foam. However, if douching is desired for cleansing purposes, you *must* wait at least six hours following your last act of sexual intercourse to allow EMKO Foam's full spermicidal activity to take place. Refer to package insert directions and diagrams for further details and applicator cleansing instructions.
How to Use EMKO with a Diaphragm.
Insert one applicatorful of EMKO Foam directly into the vagina according to above directions and then insert your diaphragm. After insertion, EMKO Foam is effective immediately and remains effective up to one hour before intercourse. If more than one hour has passed or you are going to repeat intercourse, insert another applicatorful of EMKO Foam *without removing your diaphragm.*

Continued on next page

Information on Schering-Plough HealthCare Products appearing on these pages is effective as of November 1990.

Schering-Plough—Cont.

Storage: Contents under pressure. Do not burn, incinerate or puncture can. Store at normal room temperature. Do not expose to extreme heat or open flame or store at temperatures above 120°F. If stored at temperatures below 60°F, warm to room temperature before using.

How Supplied: EMKO Contraceptive Foam, 40 gm can with applicator and storage purse. Refill cans without applicator and purse available in 40 gm and 90 gm sizes. All sizes feature a unique weighing cap that indicates when a new foam supply is needed. EMKO Foam also comes in the convenient BECAUSE® CONTRACEPTOR®, a portable six-use, combination foam/applicator unit.

Shown in Product Identification Section, page 430

FEEN-A-MINT®
Laxative Gum/Pills

Active Ingredients: Gum—yellow phenolphthalein 97.2 mg. per tablet. Pills—yellow phenolphthalein, 65 mg., and docusate sodium 100 mg. per pill. Chocolated—yellow phenolphthalein, 65 mg.

Indications: For relief of occasional constipation or irregularity. FEEN-A-MINT generally produces bowel movement in 6 to 8 hours.

Inactive Ingredients: Gum—Acacia, butylated hydroxyanisole, gelatin, glycerin, glucose, gum base, peppermint oil, sodium benzoate, starch, sugar, talc, water.
Pills—Butylparaben, calcium gluconate, calcium slufate, carnauba wax, gelatin, magnesium stearate, sugar, talc, titanium dioxide, wheat flour, white wax and other ingredients.
Chocolated—Cocoa, partially hydrogenated cottonseed and palm kernel oils, peppermint oil (flavor), salt, soya lecithin, sugar, vanillin (flavor).

How Supplied: Gum—Individual foil-backed safety sealed blister packaging in boxes of 5, 16, and 40 tablets.
Pills—Safety sealed boxes of 15, 30, and 60 tablets.
Chocolated—Safety sealed boxes of 4, 18 and 36 tablets.

Shown in Product Identification Section, page 430

GYNE-LOTRIMIN®
Clotrimazole
Vaginal Cream
Antifungal

Active Ingredient: Clotrimazole 1%

Inactive Ingredients: Benzyl alcohol, cetearyl alcohol, cetyl esters wax, octyldodecanol, polysorbate 60, purified water, sorbitan monostearate.

Indications: Gyne-Lotrimin® will cure most recurrent vaginal yeast (Candida) infections. Gyne-Lotrimin® usually starts to relieve the itching and other symptoms of vaginal yeast infection within 3 days. If the patient does not improve in 3 days or if the patient does not get well in 7 days, a condition other than yeast infection may exist. The patient should discontinue use of the product and consult a doctor. Also, if symptoms recur within a 2-month period, patient should consult a doctor.

Important: In order to kill the yeast completely, GYNE-LOTRIMIN must be used the full seven days, even if symptoms are relieved sooner.

WARNINGS:
- Do not use if you have abdominal pain, fever, or a foul-smelling vaginal discharge. You may have a condition which is more serious than a yeast infection. Contact your doctor immediately.
- Do not use if this is your first experience with vaginal itch and discomfort. See your doctor.
- If there is no improvement within 3 days, you may have a condition other than a yeast infection. Stop using this product and see your doctor.
- If symptoms recur within a 2-month period, contact your doctor.
- Do not use during pregnancy except under the advice and supervision of a doctor.
- This medication is for vaginal use only. It is not for use in the mouth or the eyes. In case accidentally swallowed, seek professional assistance or contact a Poison Control Center immediately.
- Keep this and all drugs out of reach of children. This product is not to be used on children less than 12 years of age.

Dosage: Fill the applicator with the cream and then insert one applicatorful of cream into the vagina every day, preferably at bedtime. Repeat this procedure for seven consecutive days.

Shown in Product Identification Section, page 428

GYNE-LOTRIMIN®
Clotrimazole
Vaginal Inserts
Antifungal

Active Ingredient: Each insert contains Clotrimazole 100 mg.

Inactive Ingredients: Corn starch, lactose, magnesium stearate, povidone.

Indications: Gyne-Lotrimin® will cure most vaginal yeast (Candida) infections. Gyne-Lotrimin® usually starts to relieve the itching and other symptoms of vaginal yeast infection within 3 days. If the patient does not improve in 3 days or if the patient does not get well in 7 days, a condition other than yeast infection may exist. The patient should discontinue use of the product and consult a doctor. Also, if symptoms recur within a 2-month period, patient should consult a doctor.

Important: In order to kill the yeast completely, GYNE-LOTRIMIN must be used the full seven days, even if symptoms are relieved sooner.

WARNINGS:
- Do not use if you have abdominal pain, fever, or a foul-smelling vaginal discharge. You may have a condition which is more serious than a yeast infection. Contact your doctor immediately.
- Do not use if this is your first experience with vaginal itch and discomfort. See your doctor.
- If there is no improvement within 3 days, you may have a condition other than a yeast infection. Stop using this product and see your doctor.
- If symptoms recur within a 2-month period, contact your doctor.
- Do not use during pregnancy except under the advice and supervision of a doctor.
- This medication is for vaginal use only. It is not for use in the mouth or the eyes. In case accidentally swallowed, seek professional assistance or contact a Poison Control Center immediately.
- Keep this and all drugs out of reach of children. This product is not to be used on children less than 12 years of age.

Dosage: Using the applicator, place one insert into the vagina, preferably at bedtime. Repeat this procedure for seven consecutive days.

Shown in Product Identification Section, page 428

LOTRIMIN® AF ANTIFUNGAL
[*lo-tre-min*]
Cream 1%
Solution 1%
Lotion 1%

Description: Lotrimin® AF Cream 1% is a white fully vanishing homogeneous cream containing 1% clotrimazole. The cream contains no sensitizing parabens and is totally grease free and nonstaining.
Lotrimin® AF Solution 1% is a nonaqueous liquid, containing polyethylene glycol.
Lotrimin® AF Lotion 1% is light penetrating buffered emulsion also containing no common sensitizing agents and is greaseless and nonstaining.

Indications: Lotrimin® AF Cream, Solution and Lotion contain 1% clotrimazole, a synthetic broad-spectrum antifungal agent. Clotrimazole is used for the treatment of dermal infections caused by a variety of pathogenic dermatophytes, yeasts and *Malassezia furfur*. The primary action of clotrimazole is against dividing and growing organisms. Lotrimin® AF was first made available as an over-the-counter drug in 1990 and is indicated for superficial dermatophyte infections; athlete's foot (tinea pedis), jock itch (tinea cruris) and ringworm (tinea corporis). Lotrimin® remains on prescription for candidiasis due to *Candida albicans* and tinea versicolor due to *Malassezia furfur*.

Directions: Cleanse skin with soap and water and dry thoroughly. Apply a thin layer over affected area morning and evening or as directed by a physician. For athlete's foot, pay special attention to the spaces between the toes. It is also helpful to wear well-fitting, ventilated shoes and to change shoes and socks at least once daily. Best results in athlete's foot and ringworm are usually obtained with 4 weeks' use of this product, and in jock itch, with 2 weeks' use. If satisfactory results have not occurred within these times, consult a physician or pharmacist. Children under 12 years of age should be supervised in the use of this product. This product is not effective on the scalp or nails.

How Supplied: Lotrimin® AF Antifungal Cream is available in a 0.42 oz. tube (12 grams) and a 0.84 oz. tube (24 grams).
Inactive ingredients include: benzyl alcohol, cetearyl alcohol, cetyl esters wax, octyldodecanol, polysorbate, sorbitan monostearate and water.
Lotrimin® AF Antifungal Solution is available in a 0.33 fl. oz. (10 milliliters) bottle. Inactive ingredients include polyethylene glycol.
Lotrimin® AF Antifungal Lotion is available in a 0.66 fl. oz. (20 milliliters) bottle. Inactive ingredients include benzyl alcohol, ceteryl alcohol, cetyl esters wax, octyldodecanol, polysorbate, sodium phosphate, sorbitan monostearate and water.

Storage: Keep Lotrimin® AF products between 2° and 30°C (36° and 86°F).

Shown in Product Identification Section, page 430

MOL-IRON®
[mōl-i 'ern]
Tablets
Tablets with Vitamin C

Active Ingredients: MOL-IRON products are highly effective and unusually well tolerated even by children and pregnant women.
Tablets: Each tablet contains 195 mg ferrous sulfate, USP (39 mg elemental iron).
Tablets with Vitamin C: Each tablet contains 195 mg ferrous sulfate (39 mg elemental iron) and 75 mg ascorbic acid.

Inactive Ingredients: Each MOL-IRON Tablet contains Acacia, Butylparaben, Calcium Sulfate, Carnauba Wax, FD&C Blue No. 1 Aluminum Lake, FD&C Red No. 40 Aluminum Lake, Magnesium Stearate, Povidone, Stearic Acid, Sugar, Talc, Titanium Dioxide, White Wax.
In addition to the above ingredients, MOL-IRON Tablets with Vitamin C contain confectioners glaze.

Indications: For the prevention and treatment of iron-deficiency anemias.

Warnings: Keep these and all drugs out of the reach of children. In case of accidental overdose, seek professional assistance or contact a Poison Control Center immediately. As with any drug, if you are pregnant or nursing a baby, seek the advice of a health professional before using this product.

Dosage and Administration: Tablets—(Taken preferably after meals): Adults and Children 12 years and older—1 or 2 tablets 3 times daily; Children 6 through 11 years—1 tablet 3 times daily; or as prescribed by a physician.
Tablets with Vitamin C—(Taken preferably after meals): Adults and Children 12 years and older—1 or 2 tablets 3 times daily; Children 6 through 11 years—1 tablet 3 times daily; or as prescribed by a physician.

How Supplied: MOL-IRON Tablets—brownish colored tablets, bottles of 100; MOL-IRON Tablets with Vitamin C—bottles of 100.
Store between 2° and 30°C (36° and 86°F).

REGUTOL®
Stool Softener Tablets

Active Ingredient: Each tablet contains 100 mg. docusate sodium.

Inactive Ingredients: Acacia, butylparaben, calcium sulfate, carnauba wax, D&C yellow No. 10 aluminum lake, FD&C yellow No. 6 aluminum lake, gelatin, lactose, magnesium stearate, povidone, sugar, talc, titanium dioxide, white wax.

How Supplied: REGUTOL tablets in boxes of 30, 60 and 90 individually safety sealed blister packaging.

Shown in Product Identification Section, page 430

ST. JOSEPH®
ADULT CHEWABLE ASPIRIN
Low Strength Caplets (81 mg. each)

Active Ingredient: Each St. Joseph Adult Chewable Aspirin caplet contains 81 mg. (1.25 grains) aspirin in a chewable, pleasant citrus-flavored form.

Inactive Ingredients: D&C yellow No. 10 aluminum lake, FD&C yellow No. 6 aluminum lake, flavor, hydrogenated vegetable oil, maltodextrin, mannitol, saccharin, starch.

Indications: For safe, effective, temporary relief from: headache, muscular aches, minor aches and pain associated with overexertion, sprains, menstrual cramps, neuralgia, bursitis, and discomforts of fever due to colds.

Actions: Analgesic/Antipyretic.

Warnings: Children and teenagers should not use this medicine for chicken pox or flu symptoms before a doctor is consulted about Reye syndrome, a rare but serious illness reported to be associated with aspirin. As with any drug, if you are pregnant or nursing a baby, seek the advice of a health professional before using this product. Keep out of reach of children. In case of an accidental overdose, seek professional assistance or contact a poison control center immediately.

Dosage and Administration: Adult Dose—Analgesic/Antipyretic Indication: Take from 4 to 8 caplets (325 mg. to 650 mg.) every 4 hours as needed. Do not exceed 48 caplets in 24 hours. For professional dosage see below.

IN MYOCARDIAL INFARCTION PROPHYLAXIS

Indication: Aspirin is indicated to reduce the risk of death and/or nonfatal myocardial infarction in patients with a previous infarction or unstable angina pectoris.

Advantages of Product Form: Four St. Joseph Adult Chewable Aspirin caplets give patients the appropriate dosage (325 mg.) of aspirin to help prevent secondary MI. Because they're chewable, they can be taken anytime and anyplace. And they have a pleasant-tasting citrus flavor.

Clinical Trials: The indication is supported by the results of six, large, randomized, multicenter, placebo-controlled studies[1–7] involving 10,816, predominantly male, post-myocardial infarction (MI) patients and one randomized placebo-controlled study of 1,266 men with unstable angina. Therapy with aspirin was begun at intervals after the onset of acute MI varying from less than 3 days to more than 5 years and continued for periods of from less than 1 year to 4 years. In the unstable angina study, treatment was started within 1 month after the onset of unstable angina and continued for 12 weeks; complicating conditions, such as congestive heart failure were not included in the study.
Aspirin therapy in MI patients was associated with about a 20% reduction in the risk of subsequent death and/or nonfatal reinfarction, a median absolute decrease of 3% from the 12 to 22% event rates in the placebo groups. In aspirin-treated unstable angina patients the reduction in risk was about 50%, a reduction in event rate of 5% from the 10% rate in the placebo group over the 12 weeks of the study.
Daily dosage of aspirin in the post-myocardial infarction studies was 300 mg. in one study and 900 to 1500 mg. in five studies. A dose of 325 mg. was used in the study of unstable angina.

Adverse Reactions: Gastrointestinal Reactions—Doses of 1000 mg. per day of aspirin caused gastrointestinal symptoms and bleeding that in some cases were clinically significant. In the largest postinfarction study, the Aspirin Myocardial Infarction Study (AMIS) trial with 4,500 people, the percentage incidences of gastrointestinal symptoms for the aspirin (1000 mg. of a standard, solid-tablet formulation) and placebo-treated subjects, respectively, were: stomach pain (14.3%; 4.4%); heartburn (11.9%; 4.3%); nausea and/or vomiting (7.3%; 2.1%); hospitalization for GI disorder (4.9%; 3.3%). In the AMIS and other trials, aspirin-treated patients had increased rates of gross gastrointestinal bleeding.

Continued on next page

Information on Schering-Plough HealthCare Products appearing on these pages is effective as of November 1990.

Schering-Plough—Cont.

Cardiovascular and Biochemical: In the AMIS trial, the dosage of 1000 mg. per day of aspirin was associated with small increases in systolic blood pressure (BP) (average 1.5 to 2.1 mm) and diastolic BP (0.5 to 0.6 mm), depending upon whether maximal or last available readings were used. Blood urea nitrogen and uric acid levels were also increased, but by less than 1.0 mg.%. Subjects with marked hypertension or renal insufficiency had been excluded from the trial so that the clinical importance of these observations for such subjects or for any subjects treated over more prolonged periods is not known. It is recommended that patients placed on long-term aspirin treatment, even at doses of 300 mg. per day, be seen at regular intervals to assess changes in these measurements.

Dosage and Administration: Although most of the studies used dosages exceeding 300 mg., two trials used only 300 mg. daily, and pharmacologic data indicate that this dose inhibits platelet function fully. Therefore, 300 mg. or a conventional 325 mg. aspirin dose daily is a reasonable routine dose that would minimize gastrointestinal adverse reactions.

How Supplied: Chewable citrus-flavored caplets in plastic bottles of 36 caplets each.

References: (1) Elwood, P.C., et al.: A Randomized Controlled Trial of Acetylsalicylic Acid in the Secondary Prevention of Mortality from Myocardial Infarction, *British Medical Journal,* 1:436–440, 1974. (2) The Coronary Drug Project Research Group: "Aspirin in Coronary Heart Disease," *Journal of Chronic Disease,* 29:625–642, 1976. (3) Breddin, K., et al.: "Secondary Prevention of Myocardial Infarction: A Comparison of Acetylsalicylic Acid, Placebo and Phenprocoumon, *Homeostasis,* 9:325–344, 1980. (4) Aspirin Myocardial Infarction Study Research Group, "A Randomized, Controlled Trial of Aspirin in Persons Recovered from Myocardial Infarction," *Journal American Medical Association,* 245:661–669, 1980. (5) Elwood, P.C., and Sweetnam, P.M., "Aspirin and Secondary Mortality After Myocardial Infarction," *Lancet,* pp. 1313–1315, December 22–29, 1979. (6) The Persantine-Aspirin Reinfarction Study Research Group, "Persantine and Aspirin in Coronary Heart Disease," *Circulation,* 62: 449–460, 1980. (7) Lewis, H.D., et al., "Protective Effects of Aspirin Against Acute Myocardial Infarction and Death in Men with Unstable Angina. Results of a Veterans Administration Cooperative Study," *New England Journal of Medicine,* 309:396–403, 1983.

Shown in Product Identification Section, page 430

ST. JOSEPH® Aspirin–Free Fever Reducer for Children Chewable Tablets, Liquid, Drops

Active Ingredient: Each Children's St. Joseph Aspirin-Free Chewable Tablet contains 80 mg. acetaminophen in a fruit-flavored tablet. Children's St. Joseph Aspirin-Free Liquid is stable, cherry flavored, red in color and alcohol-free and sugar-free. Each 5 ml. contains 160 mg. acetaminophen. Infant's St. Joseph Aspirin-Free Drops are stable, fruit flavored, orange in color and alcohol-free and sugar-free. Each 0.8 ml. (one calibrated dropperful) contains 80 mg. acetaminophen.

Inactive Ingredients: Tablets: Cellulose, D&C red No. 7 calcium lake, D&C red No. 30 aluminum lake, flavor, mannitol, silicon dioxide, sodium saccharin, zinc stearate.
Liquid: FD&C yellow No. 6, flavor, glycerin, maltol, polyethylene glycol, propylene glycol, saccharin, sodium benzoate, sodium chloride, sodium saccharin, water.
Drops: FD&C yellow No. 6, flavor, glycerin, maltol, polyethylene glycol, propylene glycol, saccharin, sodium benzoate, sodium chloride, sodium saccharin, water.

Indications: For temporary reduction of fever, relief of minor aches and pains of colds and flu.

Actions: Analgesic/Antipyretic

Warnings: Do not administer this product for more than 5 days. If symptoms persist or new ones occur, consult physician. If fever persists for more than three days, or recurs, consult physician. When using St. Joseph Aspirin-Free products do not give other medications containing acetaminophen unless directed by your physician. NOTE: SEVERE OR PERSISTENT SORE THROAT, HIGH FEVER, HEADACHES, NAUSEA OR VOMITING MAY BE SERIOUS. DISCONTINUE USE AND CONSULT PHYSICIAN IF NOT RELIEVED IN 24 HOURS. Do not exceed recommended dosage because severe liver damage may occur. As with any drug, if you are pregnant or nursing a baby, seek the advice of a health professional before using this product.
[See table below.]

Dosage and Administration: [See table below.]
ST. JOSEPH Aspirin-Free Fever Reducer Tablets for Children may be given one of three ways. Always follow with ½ glass of water, milk or fruit juice.

1. Chewed, followed by liquid.
2. Crushed or dissolved in a teaspoon of liquid (for younger children).
3. Powdered for infant use, when so directed by physician.

How Supplied: Chewable fruit flavored tablets in plastic bottles of 30 tablets. Cherry tasting Liquid in 2 and 4 fl. oz. plastic bottles. Fruit flavored drops in ½ fl. oz. glass bottles, with calibrated plastic dropper.
All packages have child resistant safety caps and safety sealed packaging.

Shown in Product Identification Section, page 430

ST. JOSEPH® Cold Tablets for Children

Active Ingredients: Per tablet: Acetaminophen 80 mg and phenylpropanolamine hydrochloride 3.125 mg.

Inactive Ingredients: Cellulose, FD&C Yellow No. 6 aluminum lake, flavor, mannitol, silica, sodium saccharin, zinc stearate.

How Supplied: In bottle with 30 fruit flavored chewable tablets.

ST. JOSEPH CHILDREN'S DOSAGE CHART

Age	0–3 (months)	4–11 (months)	12–23 (months)	2–3 (years)	4–5 (years)	6–8 (years)	9–10 (years)	11 (years)	12+ (years)
Weight (lbs.)	7–12	13–21	22–26	27–35	36–45	46–65	66–76	77–83	84+
Dose of St. Joseph Acetaminophen Drops Dropperfuls	½	1	1½	2	3	4	5	—	—
Acetaminophen Liquid Teaspoonfuls	—	½	¾	1	1½	2	2½	3	4
Chewable Tablets Acetaminophen (80 mg. each)	—	—	1½	2	3	4	5	6	8

All dosages may be repeated every 4 hours, but do not exceed 5 dosages daily.
Note: Since St. Joseph pediatric products are available without prescription, parents are advised on the package label to consult a physician for use in children under two years.

ST. JOSEPH® Cough Suppressant for Children
Pediatric
Antitussive Suppressant

Active Ingredient: Dextromethorphan hydrobromide 7.5 mg. per 5 cc.

Inactive Ingredients: Caramel, citric acid, flavor, glycerin, methylparaben, propylparaben, sodium benzoate, sodium citrate, sucrose, water.

How Supplied: Alcohol-Free Cherry tasting suppressant in plastic bottle of 2 and 4 fl. ozs. In safety sealed packaging.

Shown in Product Identification Section, page 430

ST. JOSEPH® Nighttime Cold Medicine

Active Ingredients: Chlorpheniramine maleate, pseudoephedrine hydrochloride, acetaminophen, dextromethorphan hydrobromide

Inactive Ingredients: Citric acid, FD&C red No. 40, flavor, methylparaben, polyethylene glycol, propylene glycol, propylparaben, sodium benzoate, sodium citrate, sucrose, water

Indications: Temporary relief of major cold and flu symptoms

Actions: Antihistamine for relief of runny nose, sneezing, itchy watery eyes, scratchy throat and post-nasal drip; nasal decongestant for relief of nasal and sinus congestion; analgesic for aspirin-free relief to reduce fever of colds and flu and relieve body aches and pain; and cough suppressant to calm and quiet coughing.

Warning: For children under 6 years or 48 pounds, consult physician. Do not give this product to children for more than 5 days. If symptoms do not improve, or if new ones occur, or are accompanied by fever for over 3 days, consult physician. Do not exceed recommended dosage because at higher doses nervousness, dizziness, sleeplessness or severe liver damage may occur. May cause drowsiness or excitability. Keep this and all drugs out of reach of children.

Symptoms and Treatment of Oral Overdosage: In case of accidental overdose, seek professional assistance or contact a Poison Control Center immediately.

Dosage and Administration: One dose every 4 to 6 hours, not to exceed 3 times daily. Use the enclosed dosage cup to measure the right dose for your child.

Age/Weight Dosage Chart

AGE	WEIGHT	DOSE
Under 6 yrs.	Under 48 lbs.	Consult Physician
6–8 yrs.	48–65 lbs.	2 tsp.
9–10 yrs.	66–76 lbs.	2½ tsp.
11–12 yrs.	77–85 lbs.	3 tsp.

How Supplied: Alcohol-Free Cherry tasting syrup in plastic 4 oz. bottle. In safety sealed packaging.

Shown in Product Identification Section, page 430

SHADE® UVA/UVB Sunscreens

SHADE® Sunblock Lotion SPF 15
SHADE® Sunblock Lotion SPF 30
SHADE® Sunblock Lotion SPF 45
SHADE® Oil-Free Gel SPF 15
SHADE® Oil-Free Gel SPF 25
SHADE® Sunblock Stick SPF 30

Active Ingredients:
Lotions:
SPF 15—Ethylhexyl p-methoxycinnamate, oxybenzone
SPF 30—Ethylhexyl p-methoxycinnamate, oxybenzone, 2-ethylhexyl salicyylate
SPF 45—Ethylhexyl p-methoxycinnamate, oxybenzone, 2-ethylhexyl salicylate, octocrylene
Gels:
SPF 15, 25—Ethylhexyl p-methoxycinnamate, octyl salicylate, homosalate, oxybenzone
Shade Stick
SPF 30—Ethylhexyl p-methoxycinnamate, oxybenzone, 2-ethylhexyl salicylate, homosalate

Indications: Waterproof Paba-free sunscreens to help prevent harmful effects from the sun. SHADE screens both UVB and burning UVA rays. SHADE Protection Formulas provide 15, 25, 30, and 45 times your natural sunburn protection. Liberal and regular use may help reduce the chances of premature aging and wrinkling of skin, due to overexposure to the sun. All strengths are waterproof, maintaining sun protection for 80 minutes in water. Excellent for use on children.

Actions: Sunscreen

Warnings: For external use only. Avoid contact with eyes. Discontinue use if signs of irritation or rash appear.

Dosage and Administration: Apply evenly and liberally to all exposed skin. Reapply after prolonged swimming or excessive perspiration.

How Supplied: 4 fl. oz. Plastic Bottles

Shown in Product Identification Section, page 431

SOLARCAINE®
Antiseptic·Topical Anesthetic
Lotion/Cream/Aerosol Spray Liquid

Active Ingredients:
SOLARCAINE Aloe Aerosol Spray—.5% lidocaine.
Also contains aloe vera and Vitamin E. Non-stinging and alcohol/fragrance free.
SOLARCAINE Aerosol Spray—to deliver benzocaine 20% (w/w), triclosan 0.13% (w/w). Also contains SD alcohol 40 (35% w/w) in total contents.
SOLARCAINE Lotion—Benzocaine and triclosan.
SOLARCAINE ALOE EXTRA™ Gel and Mist—Lidocaine HCl
SOLARCAINE Medicated Cream—Lidocaine

Indications: Medicated first aid to provide fast temporary relief of sunburn pain, minor burns, cuts, scrapes, chapping and skin injuries, poison ivy, detergent hands, insect bites (non-venomous). Aloe aerosol spray provides longer lasting/more cooling relief.

Actions: Lidocaine and benzocaine provide local anesthetic action to relieve itching and pain. Triclosan provides antimicrobial activity.

Caution: Not for use in eyes. Not for deep or puncture wounds or serious burns, nor for prolonged use. If condition persists, or infection, rash or irritation develops, discontinue use. Sunburns can be serious. In cases where skin is blistered or raw surfaces exist, do not use this product.

Warnings: For Aerosol Spray—Flammable—Do not spray while smoking or near fire. Do not spray into eyes or mouth. Avoid inhalation. Contents under pressure. For external use only.

Dosage and Administration:
Lotion —Apply freely as needed.
Sprays—Hold 3 to 5 inches from injured area. Spray until wet. To apply to face, spray on palm of hand. Use often for antiseptic protection.

How Supplied:
SOLARCAINE Aloe Aerosol Spray—4.5-oz. can.
SOLARCAINE Aerosol Spray—3- and 5-oz. cans.
SOLARCAINE Lotion—3 oz. bottles.
SOLARCAINE Aloe Extra™ Gel—4- and 8-oz. bottles.
SOLARCAINE Aloe Extra™ Mist—3.75-fl. oz. bottle.
SOLARCAINE Aloe Cream—4 oz. jar.

Shown in Product Identification Section, page 430

WATER BABIES® BY COPPERTONE

Water Babies® Sunblock Lotion SPF 15
Water Babies® Sunblock Cream SPF 25
Water Babies® Sunblock Lotion SPF 30
Water Babies® Sunblock Lotion SPF 45
Water Babies Little Licks™ SPF 30 Sunblock Lip Balm

Active Ingredients:
SPF 15: Ethylhexyl *p*-methoxycinnamate, oxybenzone
SPF 25: Ethylhexyl *p*-methoxycinnamate, oxybenzone, 2-ethylhexyl salicylate, homosalate
SPF 30: Ethylhexyl *p*-methoxycinnamate, 2-ethylhexyl salicylate, homosalate, oxybenzone

Continued on next page

Information on Schering-Plough HealthCare Products appearing on these pages is effective as of November 1990.

Schering-Plough—Cont.

SPF 45: Ethylhexyl *p*-methoxycinnamate, 2-ethylhexyl salicylate, octocrylene, oxybenzone
Little Licks: Ethylhexyl *p*-methoxycinnamate, oxybenzone, 2-ethylhexyl salicylate

How Supplied: SPF 15, SPF 30, SPF 45—In plastic bottles of 4.0 fl oz.
SPF 25—In plastic tube (in carton) of 3.0 fl oz.
Little Licks—In 0.15 oz plastic tube (in blister pack).

Shown in Product Identification Section, page 431

TINACTIN® Antifungal
[*tin-ak'tin*]
Cream 1%
Solution 1%
Powder 1%
Powder (1%) Aerosol
Liquid (1%) Aerosol
Jock Itch Cream 1%
Jock Itch Spray Powder 1%

Description: TINACTIN Cream 1% is a white homogeneous, nonaqueous preparation containing the highly active synthetic fungicidal agent, tolnaftate. Each gram contains 10 mg tolnaftate solubilized in BHT, Carbomer 934 P, Monoamylamine, PEG, Propylene Glycol, and Titanium Dioxide.
TINACTIN Jock Itch Cream 1% is a smooth white homogeneous cream containing the highly active synthetic fungicidal agent, tolnaftate. Each gram contains 10 mg tolnaftate finely dispersed in a water-washable emulsion containing: Cetearyl Alcohol, Ceteareth-30, Chlorocresol, Mineral Oil, Petrolatum, Propylene Glycol, Sodium Phosphate and Water. Phosphoric acid and sodium hydroxide used to adjust pH.
TINACTIN Solution 1% contains in each ml tolnaftate 10 mg, BHT, and PEG. The solution solidifies at low temperatures but liquefies readily when warmed, retaining its potency.
TINACTIN Liquid Aerosol contains 91 mg tolnaftate in a vehicle of Alcohol SD-40-2 (36% w/w), BHT and PPG-12 Buteth-16. The spray deposits solution containing a concentration of 1% tolnaftate.
Each gram of **TINACTIN Powder 1%** contains tolnaftate 10 mg in a vehicle of corn starch and talc.
TINACTIN Powder Aerosol contains 91 mg tolnaftate in a vehicle of Alcohol SD-40-2 (14% w/w), BHT, Hydrocarbon Propellant, PPG-12 Buteth-16 and Talc. The spray deposits a white clinging powder containing a concentration of 1% tolnaftate.
TINACTIN Jock Itch Spray Powder contains 91 mg tolnaftate in a vehicle of Alcohol SD-40-2 (14% w/w), BHT, Hydrocarbon Propellant, PPG-12 Buteth-16, Talc. The spray deposits a white clinging powder containing a concentration of 1% tolnaftate.

Indications: TINACTIN Cream, Solution, Liquid Aerosol and **TINACTIN Jock Itch Cream** are highly active antifungal agents that are effective in killing superficial fungi of the skin which cause tinea pedis (athlete's foot), tinea cruris (jock itch) and tinea corporis (body ringworm).
TINACTIN Powder, Powder Aerosol and **TINACTIN Jock Itch Spray Powder** are effective in killing superficial fungi of the skin which cause tinea cruris (jock itch) and tinea pedis (athlete's foot). All forms begin to relieve burning, itching and soreness within 24 hours. The powder and powder aerosol forms aid the drying of naturally moist areas.

Actions: The active ingredient in TINACTIN, tolnaftate, is a highly active synthetic fungicidal agent that is effective in the treatment of superficial fungous infections of the skin. It is inactive systemically, virtually nonsensitizing, and does not ordinarily sting or irritate intact or broken skin, even in the presence of acute inflammatory reactions.
TINACTIN products are odorless, greaseless, and do not stain or discolor the skin, hair, or nails.

Warnings: Keep these and all drugs out of the reach of children. Do not use in children under 2 years of age except under the advice and supervision of a physician.
TINACTIN Powder Aerosol and **Liquid Aerosol:** Avoid spraying in eyes. Contents under pressure. Do not puncture or incinerate. Flammable mixture, do not use or store near heat or open flame. Exposure to temperatures above 120°F may cause bursting. Never throw container into fire or incinerator. Use only as directed. Intentional misuse by deliberately concentrating and inhaling the contents can be harmful or fatal.

Precautions: If irritation occurs or symptoms do not improve within 10 days, discontinue use and consult your physician or podiatrist.
TINACTIN products are for external use only. Keep out of eyes.
TINACTIN is not effective on nail or scalp infections.

Overdosage: In case of accidental ingestion, seek professional assistance or contact a Poison Control Center immediately.

Dosage and Administration: Children under 12 years of age should be supervised in the use of TINACTIN.
TINACTIN Cream and **TINACTIN Jock Itch Cream**—Wash and dry infected area. Then apply one-half inch ribbon of cream and rub gently on infected area morning and evening or as directed by a doctor. Spread evenly. Best results in athlete's foot and body ringworm are usually obtained with 4 weeks' use of this product and in jock itch, with 2 weeks' use. To help prevent recurrence of athlete's foot, continue treatment for two weeks after disappearance of all symptoms.
TINACTIN Solution—Wash and dry infected area. Then apply two or three drops morning and evening or as directed by a doctor, and massage gently to cover the infected area. Best results in athlete's foot and body ringworm are usually obtained with 4 weeks' use of this product and in jock itch, with 2 weeks' use. To help prevent recurrence of athlete's foot, continue treatment for two weeks after disappearance of all symptoms.
TINACTIN Liquid Aerosol—Wash and dry infected area. Spray from a distance of 6 to 10 inches morning and evening or as directed by a doctor. For athlete's foot, spray between toes and on feet. For jock itch, spray infected area. Best results in athlete's foot are usually obtained with 4 weeks' use of this product and in jock itch, with 2 weeks' use. Continue treatment for two weeks after symptoms disappear. To help prevent reinfection of athlete's foot, bathe daily, dry carefully and apply **TINACTIN Powder** daily.
TINACTIN Powder—Wash and dry infected area. Sprinkle powder liberally on all areas of infection and in shoes or socks morning and evening or as directed by a doctor. Best results in athlete's foot are usually obtained with 4 weeks' use of this product and in jock itch, with 2 weeks' use. Continue treatment for two weeks after symptoms disappear. To prevent recurrence of athlete's foot, bathe daily, dry carefully and apply **TINACTIN Powder.**
TINACTIN Powder Aerosol and **TINACTIN Jock Itch Spray Powder**—Wash and dry infected area. Shake container well before using. Spray liberally from a distance of 6 to 10 inches onto affected area morning and night or as directed by a doctor. Best results in athlete's foot are usually obtained with 4 weeks' use of this product and in jock itch, with 2 weeks' use. To help prevent recurrence of athlete's foot, bathe daily, dry carefully and apply **TINACTIN Powder Aerosol.**

How Supplied: TINACTIN Antifungal Cream 1%, 15 g (½ oz) and 30 g (1 oz) collapsible tube with dispensing tip. **TINACTIN Antifungal Solution 1%,** 10 ml (⅓ oz) plastic squeeze bottle. **TINACTIN Antifungal Liquid (1%) Aerosol,** 113 g (4 oz) spray can. **TINACTIN Antifungal Powder 1%,** 45 g (1.5 oz) and 90 g (3.0 oz) plastic containers. **TINACTIN Antifungal Powder (1%) Aerosol,** 100 g (3.5 oz) and 150 g (5.0 oz) spray containers. **TINACTIN Antifungal Jock Itch Cream 1%,** 15 g (½ oz) collapsible tube with dispensing tip. **TINACTIN Antifungal Jock Itch Spray Powder (1%),** 100 g (3.5 oz) spray can.
Store TINACTIN products between 36° and 86°F (2° and 30°C).

Shown in Product Identification Section, page 431

Products are indexed by generic and chemical names in the **YELLOW SECTION**

Schwarz Pharma

Kremers Urban Company
P.O. BOX 2038
MILWAUKEE, WI 53201

LACTRASE® Capsules

[*lăk 'trās*]
(lactase)

Description: Each LACTRASE® Capsule contains 250 mg of standardized lactase dispersed in a lactose-free base.
Inactive Ingredients: gelatin, magnesium stearate, maltodextrin, red iron oxide, titanium dioxide, yellow iron oxide, and other ingredients.

Indications: LACTRASE is indicated for individuals exhibiting symptoms of lactose intolerance or lactase insufficiency as identified by a lactose tolerance test or by exhibiting gastrointestinal disturbances after consumption of milk or dairy products.

Action: Though lactase is normally present in adequate quantities in infants, in many populations its concentration naturally declines starting at about 4–5 years of age and is low in a substantial number of individuals by their teens or early 20s. Within certain geographic and ethnic groups, especially in adult Blacks, Orientals, American Indians, and Eastern European Jews, the lactase activity may be low even earlier. Although many of them can easily digest smaller quantities of lactose in milk, after consumption of an excessive volume of milk or dairy products, they may exhibit symptoms of lactose intolerance.
Lactose is a nonabsorbable disaccharide found as a common constituent in most dairy products. Under normal conditions, dietary lactose is hydrolyzed in the jejunum and proximal ileum by beta-D-galactosidase or lactase. Lactase is produced in the brush border of the columnar epithelial cells of the intestinal villi. Lactase hydrolyzes lactose into two monosaccharides, glucose and galactose, that are readily absorbed by the intestine.
When available lactase is insufficient to split the lactose, the unabsorbable sugar remains in the small intestine for an extended period, presenting an osmotic load that increases and retains intraluminal fluid and intensifies intestinal motility; thus the individual reports a bloated feeling and cramps. The undigested lactose is decomposed by the intestinal flora in the lower intestine and excessive carbon dioxide and hydrogen is produced. These gases contribute to flatulence and increased abdominal discomfort. The lactic acid and other short-chain acids raise the osmolality, hinder fluid reabsorption and decrease transit time of the contents of the colon, leading to diarrhea. Often hydrogen is noticed in the expired breath of a lactase-deficient patient.

Precautions: It should be noted that in diabetic persons who use LACTRASE, the milk sugar will be metabolically available and may result in increased blood glucose levels. Individuals with galactosemia may not have milk in any form, lactose enzyme modified or not.

Directions: Generally, one or two LACTRASE Capsules swallowed **with** milk or dairy products is all that is necessary to digest the milk sugar contained in a normal serving. If the individual is severely intolerant to lactose, additional capsules may be taken until a satisfactory response is achieved as recognized by resolution of the symptoms. LACTRASE Capsules are safe to take and higher quantities in severe cases will be well-tolerated.
If the individual cannot swallow capsules, the contents of the capsules may be sprinkled onto dairy products before consuming. LACTRASE will not alter the taste of the dairy product when used in this manner.
Milk may also be pretreated with LACTRASE; simply add the contents from one or two capsules to each quart of milk, shake gently, and store the milk in the refrigerator for 24 hours. LACTRASE will break down milk sugars to digestible simple sugars. LACTRASE powder will not alter the appearance of milk; however the taste may be slightly sweeter than untreated milk.

How Supplied: LACTRASE Capsules are opaque orange and opaque white and are imprinted "KREMERS URBAN" and "505". They are supplied in blister packs containing 10 capsules (NDC 0091-3505-10) or 30 capsules (NDC 0091-3505-03) and in bottles containing 100 capsules (NDC 0091-3505-01).
Store at controlled room temperature 15°–30°C (59°–86°F).

Shown in Product Identification Section, page 431

EDUCATIONAL MATERIAL

Good News For People Who Can't Digest Milk
For people who cannot digest dairy products because they lack the enzyme necessary for the digestion of milk sugar, this pamphlet explains how the problem comes about, its symptoms and how it can be treated with Lactrase®, an enzyme supplement. A table addressing the lactose content of food is included.
When Your Doctor Says You Have Irritable Bowel Syndrome
Written for patients with IBS, this pamphlet explains the normal function of the digestive system and the symptomatic changes that occur in IBS. General aspects of dietary, fiber and drug treatment are discussed.
FREE TO HEALTH PROFESSIONALS AND CONSUMERS

Products are
indexed alphabetically
in the
PINK SECTION

Slim•Fast Foods Company

919 THIRD AVENUE
NEW YORK, NY 10022

ULTRA SLIM•FAST®
Nutritional Meal Replacement Drink—Part of the Ultra Slim·Fast Program

Description: A precisely portioned, nutritionally balanced liquid meal replacement to be used in conjunction with whole-food meals for weight loss or weight-loss maintenance. Unlike "fasting" diets, the ULTRA Slim·Fast program is a minimum of 1200 calories per day and provides a combination of convenient, palatable meal replacements and whole-food meals in an integrated program that makes it pleasant to lose weight and keep it off. The delicious, thick ULTRA Slim·Fast "milkshake" provides a nutritious, low-calorie answer to cravings for "sweet" food, while the high fiber content promotes feelings of satiety. The ULTRA Slim·Fast Program, scientifically developed with the help of physicians and dietitians, includes a complete diet plan with menu suggestions. The Program encourages both exercise and behavior modification to aid in the life-style changes that can make weight reduction succeed permanently.

Uses: The ULTRA Slim·Fast program is recommended to help the moderately obese patient (up to 30 pounds overweight) to achieve safe weight loss. It is also indicated for the patient who wishes to maintain weight loss, or to control or reverse modest weight gains.

Professional Supplementary Materials: Physicians and dietitians may also send for patient samples and free support materials. Write to Ultra SlimFast Medical Program, Slim·Fast Foods Company, PO Box 5047, FDR Station, NY, NY 10150.

Nutritional Information: ULTRA Slim·Fast provides an exceptionally safe, nutritious weight-loss regimen. One ULTRA Slim·Fast "shake" made with protein-fortified skim milk includes 35% of the U.S. RDA of 18 essential nutrients. It is an excellent source of dietary fiber (4–6 grams), calcium (50% of adult RDA), and protein (15 grams, largely from casein, providing 27% of total calories). And it is low in fat (less than 1 gram, 5% of calories).
[See table on next page.]
Ingredients: Sucrose, Whey Powder, Cocoa (Processed with Alkali), Calcium Caseinate, Corn Bran, Purified Cellulose, Soy Protein Isolate, Nonfat Dry Milk, Fructose, Carrageenan, Natural and Artificial Flavors, Maltodextrins, Lecithin, Guar or DL-Methionine, **Aspartame, and the following Vitamins and Minerals: Magnesium Carbonate, Calcium Phosphate, Sodium Phosphate, Potas-

**Phenylketonurics: Contains phenylalanine.

Continued on next page

Slim·Fast Foods—Cont.

sium Chloride, Calcium Carbonate, Ferric Orthophosphate, Vitamin E Acetate, Ascorbic Acid, Niacinamide, Zinc Oxide, Vitamin A Palmitate, Manganese Sulfate, Calcium Pantothenate, Copper Sulfate, Pyridoxine Hydrochloride, Thiamine Mononitrate, Vitamin D, Riboflavin, Biotin, Folic Acid, Potassium Iodide, Vitamin B_{12}.
Nutritional information and ingredient disclosure may vary slightly in Chocolate Royale and French Vanilla flavors.
FOR WEIGHT LOSS: Enjoy a rich, delicious and satisfying Ultra Slim·Fast shake for breakfast, one for lunch and another in the afternoon as a snack; then have a sensible, low-fat, well-balanced dinner. Three highly nutritious Ultra Slim·Fast shakes provide 12–18 grams of dietary fiber depending on flavor and 100% of the U.S. recommended daily allowance of high quality protein plus 18 essential vitamins and minerals, including iron and calcium. The Ultra Slim·Fast program is nutritionally balanced to help you feel great as you lose weight.

Directions USE A SHAKER OR BLENDER. Simply add 1 rounded measuring scoop (inside can) of ULTRA Slim·Fast to 8 oz. of protein-fortified skim milk. (For best taste, add ice.) SHAKE or BLEND for 30 seconds. Wait one minute as the shake thickens into a rich, delicious drink.
FOR WEIGHT MAINTENANCE AND GOOD HEALTH:

- Enjoy an ULTRA Slim·Fast shake as a delicious, healthy breakfast or snack everyday.

The Ultra Slim·Fast® Medical Program ...

... is NOT ...	***... IS ...***
•**A fasting program** requiring abstinence from solid foods.	•**A combination** of meal replacements and low-fat "real" foods.
•**A fad diet** with questionable nutritional balance.	•**A precisely proportioned, highly nutritious food** low in calories and fat.
•**An inconvenient diet** requiring complex preparation.	•**Convenient and readily available** (without prescription).
•**An unappealing diet** with unappetizing ingredients.	•**Palatable, delicious** "milkshake" meals plus tasty solid-food meals.
•**A "miracle" diet** promising unhealthy, overly rapid weight loss, with no follow-through.	•**An aid to behavior modification** vital for achieving and maintaining weight loss.
•**Expensive** (as some clinic- or hospital-based programs are)	•**Economical** (usually less costly than the meal or snack it replaces).

- When at your ideal weight, weigh yourself regularly. Anytime you gain 2 or 3 pounds, DON'T WAIT, go back to the Ultra Slim·Fast Weight Loss Program and get those pounds off.
- Get regular exercise and eat low-fat, high fiber food.
- Drink 6–8 glasses of water a day.

Warnings: Phenylketonurics—Contains phenylalanine.
IMPORTANT: Anyone who is pregnant or nursing, has a health problem, is under the age of 18, or wants to lose more than 30 pounds or more than 15% of their starting body weight should consult a physician before starting any weight-loss program. If after the first week weight loss exceeds 2 pounds a week, increase your calorie intake. Very rapid weight loss can cause health problems.

Ultra Slim·Fast should not be used as your sole source of nutrition; eat at least one well-balanced meal daily.

How Supplied: Flavors: Chocolate Royale, French Vanilla, Strawberry Supreme, Cafe Mocha. Available in 15 oz. cans (425 grams, 13 servings)—including measuring scoop and diet plan suggestions.
[See table above.]
Shown in Product Identification Section, page 431

Ultra Slim·Fast Chocolate Royale
Serving Size: 1.16 oz. Servings per container: 13

Each Serving Provides:	**One Serving**	**With 8 Fl. Oz. Vitamin A&D Protein-Fortified Skim Milk**
Calories	100	190
Protein	5 grams	15 grams
Carbohydrate	20 grams	33 grams
Fat	less than 1 gram	1 gram
Sodium	130 mg.	220 mg.
Potassium	220 mg.	790 mg.
Fiber (Dietary)	5 grams	5 grams
Percentage of Adult U.S. Recommended Daily Allowance (U.S. RDA):		
Protein	10%	35%
Vitamin A	25%	35%
Vitamin C (Ascorbic Acid)	30%	35%
Thiamine (Vitamin B_1)	30%	35%
Riboflavin (Vitamin B_2)	10%	35%
Niacin	35%	35%
Calcium	15%	50%
Iron	35%	35%
Vitamin D	10%	35%
Vitamin E	35%	35%
Vitamin B_6	30%	35%
Folic Acid	25%	30%
Vitamin B_{12}	20%	35%
Phosphorus	15%	40%
Iodine	10%	35%
Magnesium	25%	35%
Zinc	30%	35%
Copper	35%	35%
Biotin	35%	35%
Pantothenic Acid	25%	35%
Manganese	1 mg.*	1 mg.*

*No U.S. RDA established.

SmithKline Beecham Consumer Brands

Unit of SmithKline Beecham Inc.
POST OFFICE BOX 1467
PITTSBURGH, PA 15230

A-200® Pediculicide Shampoo Concentrate
A-200® Pediculicide Gel Concentrate

Description: Active ingredients: Pyrethrins 0.33%, Piperonyl butoxide technical 4.00% – Equivalent to 3.2% (butylcarbityl) (6-propylpiperonyl) ether and 0.8% related compounds. **Inactive Ingredients:** Shampoo—Benzyl alcohol, Butyl Stearate, Fragrance, Mineral Spirits, Octoxynol 9, Oleic Acid, Oleoresin Parsley Seed and Water. Gel—Benzyl alcohol, Butyl Stearate, Carbomer 940, Fragrance, Mineral Spirits, Octoxynol 9, Oleic Acid, Oleoresin Parsley Seed, Triisopropanolamine, and Water.

Inert ingredients: 95.67%.

Indications: A-200 is indicated for the treatment of human pediculosis—head lice, body lice and pubic lice, and their eggs. A-200 Gel is specially formulated for pubic lice and head lice in children, where control of application is desirable.

Actions: A-200 is an effective pediculicide for control of head lice (*Pediculus humanus capitis*), pubic lice (*Phthirus pubis*) and body lice (*Pediculus humanus corporis*), and their nits.

Warnings: May cause eye injury. Do not get in eyes or permit contact with mucous membranes. Harmful if swallowed. Wash thoroughly after handling.

Do not leave children unattended with product on their heads.

Drug Interaction: **NOT TO BE USED BY PERSONS ALLERGIC TO RAGWEED.** If skin irritation or infection is present or develops, discontinue use and consult a physician.

Precaution: If in Eyes: Flush with plenty of water. Get medical attention.

Symptoms and Treatment of Oral Overdosage: If swallowed: Call a physician, local Poison Control Center, or the Rocky Mountain Poison Control Center at 303-592-1710 (Collect) 24 hours a day. Drink 1 or 2 glasses of water and induce vomiting by touching the back of throat with finger. Do not induce vomiting or give anything by mouth to an unconscious person.

Dosage and Administration: It is a violation of Federal law to use this product in a manner inconsistent with its labeling.

Directions for Use: 1. Apply A-200 Shampoo to **dry** hair and scalp or other infested areas. Use enough to completely wet area being treated. Massage in. (For head lice, avoid getting product into eyes. Helpful hint: When shampooing a child's head, place towel across forehead.) 2. Allow product to remain for 10 minutes, but no longer. 3. Add small quantities of water, and work rich lather into hair and scalp. 4. Rinse thoroughly with warm water. Towel dry. 5. Comb hair with special A-200 precision comb to remove dead lice and eggs. (See left side panel for combing suggestions.) Repeat treatment in 7–10 days or earlier if reinfestation has occurred. Do not use more than 2 applications of A-200 Shampoo in 24 hours. When used on children, adult supervision is recommended.

Additional Control Measures: At time of shampoo treatment, all infested clothing, bed linen and other articles should be laundered in hot water or dry cleaned. Carpets, upholstery and mattresses should be vacuumed thoroughly. Combs and brushes should be soaked in hot water (above 130°) for 5 to 10 minutes.

Storage and Disposal: Store at room temperature. Do not reuse empty bottle. Wrap and put in trash.

How Supplied: A-200 Shampoo Concentrate in 2 and 4 fl. oz. unbreakable plastic bottles and A-200 Gel Concentrate in 1 oz. tubes, all with special comb and bilingual patient insert.

Literature Available: Additional patient literature available upon request.

Shown in Product Identification Section, page 431

CLEAR BY DESIGN®
Medicated Acne Gel for Sensitive Skin

Product Information: CLEAR BY DESIGN contains benzoyl peroxide, an effective anti-acne agent available without a prescription in a lower 2.5% strength. CLEAR BY DESIGN is as effective as 10% benzoyl peroxide but with less of the irritation and redness that you may get with the higher strengths. Greaseless, colorless CLEAR BY DESIGN is invisible while it works fast. Helps prevent new acne pimples and blackheads from forming.

Directions: Wash problem areas thoroughly but gently and dry well. Using fingertip, apply CLEAR BY DESIGN to all affected and surrounding areas of face, neck, and body. Apply one or two times a day as directed by a physician.

Warning: Persons with a known allergy to benzoyl peroxide should not use this medication. To test for an allergy, apply CLEAR BY DESIGN on a small affected area once a day for two days. If discomforting irritation or undue dryness occurs during treatment, reduce frequency of use or amount. If excessive itching, redness, burning, swelling, irritation or dryness occurs, discontinue use and consult a physician. Avoid contact with eyes, lips and mouth. May bleach hair or dyed fabrics. Keep tightly closed. Keep this and all drugs out of reach of children. Store at controlled room temperature (59°–86°F.); avoid excessive heat.
FOR EXTERNAL USE ONLY

Formula: Benzoyl Peroxide, 2.5% in a gel base. Also contains: Purified water, carbomer 940, dioctyl sodium sulfosuccinate, sodium hydroxide, and edetate disodium.

How Supplied: Available in 1.5 oz. tubes.

Shown in Product Identification Section, page 431

CLEAR BY DESIGN®
Medicated Cleansing Pads for Sensitive Skin

Product Information: CLEAR BY DESIGN Medicated Pads for sensitive skin are specially formulated to be less irritating. The pads clean deep down to remove the dirt and oil that can clog pores, clear up existing pimples and blackheads and prevent new acne pimples and blackheads from forming.

Directions: Cleanse the skin thoroughly. Use the pad to wipe face and neck thoroughly. Use one to three times daily. Do not rinse.

Warnings: Persons with a known allergy to salicylic acid should not use this medication. If discomforting irritation or undue dryness occurs during treatment, reduce frequency of use. If excessive itching, redness, burning, swelling, irritation or dryness occurs, discontinue use and consult a physician promptly. Using other topical acne medications at the same time or immediately following use of this product may increase dryness or irritation of the skin. If this occurs, only one medication should be used unless directed by a doctor. Avoid contact with eyes, lips and mouth. Keep jar tightly closed. Keep this and all drugs out of reach of children. In case of accidental ingestion, seek professional assistance or contact a poison control center immediately. Store at controlled room temperature (59°–86°F.). Avoid excessive heat.
FOR EXTERNAL USE ONLY

Contains: Active Ingredient: Salicylic Acid 1%. **Inactive Ingredients:** Water, SD Alcohol 40B 16% (w/w), Disodium Laurethsulfosuccinate, Dimethicone Copolyol, Citric Acid, Fragrance, Cocoamphodiacetate, Sodium Carbonate.

How Supplied: Available in Jars containing 60 pads.

Shown in Product Identification Section, page 431

CONTAC®
MAXIMUM STRENGTH
Continuous Action Nasal Decongestant/Antihistamine Caplets

Composition: [See table on page 711]

Product Information: Each CONTAC Maximum Strength continuous action caplet provides up to 12 hours of relief. Part of the caplet goes to work right away for fast relief; the rest is released gradually to provide up to 12 hours of prolonged relief. With just *one* caplet in the morning and *one* at bedtime, you feel better all day, sleep better at night, breathing freely without congestion. CONTAC Maximum Strength provides:

- A NASAL DECONGESTANT which helps clear nasal passages, shrinks swollen membranes and helps decongest sinus openings.
- AN ANTIHISTAMINE at the maximum level to help relieve itchy, watery eyes, sneezing, and runny nose.

Indications: For temporary relief of nasal congestion due to the common cold, hay fever or other upper respiratory allergies, and nasal congestion associated with sinusitis.

Directions: One caplet every 12 hours. Do not exceed 2 caplets in 24 hours.

NOTE: The nonactive portion of the caplet that supplies the active ingredients may occasionally appear in your stool as a soft mass.

TAMPER-RESISTANT PACKAGING FEATURES FOR YOUR PROTECTION:

- Each caplet is encased in a plastic cell with a foil back; do not use if cell or foil is broken.
- The name CONTAC appears on each caplet; do not use this product if the CONTAC name is missing.

Warnings: Do not give this product to children under 12 years except under the advice and supervision of a physician. Do not exceed recommended dosage because at higher doses nervousness, dizziness, or sleeplessness may occur. Do not take this product if you have high blood pressure, heart disease, diabetes or thyroid disease except under the advice and supervision

Continued on next page

SmithKline Beecham—Cont.

of a physician. If symptoms do not improve within 7 days or are accompanied by high fever, consult a physician before continuing use. Do not take this product if you have asthma, glaucoma or difficulty in urination due to enlargement of the prostate gland except under the advice and supervision of a physician. Do not take this product if you are taking another medication containing phenylpropanolamine. Avoid alcoholic beverages while taking this product. Do not drive or operate heavy machinery. May cause drowsiness. May cause excitability, especially in children. Keep this and all drugs out of reach of children. In case of accidental overdose, seek professional assistance or contact a poison control center immediately. As with any drug, if you are pregnant or nursing a baby, seek the advice of a health professional before using this product. Store at controlled room temperature (59°–86°F.).

Drug Interaction Precaution: Do not take this product if you are presently taking a prescription antihypertensive or antidepressant drug containing monoamine oxidase inhibitor except under the advice and supervision of a physician.

Formula: Active Ingredients: Each Maximum Strength caplet contains Phenylpropanolamine Hydrochloride 75 mg.; Chlorpheniramine Maleate 12 mg. (which is a higher dose of antihistamine than CONTAC capsules). **Inactive Ingredients (listed for individuals with specific allergies):** Acetylated Monoglycerides, Carnauba Wax, Colloidal Silicon Dioxide, Ethylcellulose, Hydroxypropyl Methylcellulose, Lactose, Stearic Acid, Titanium Dioxide.

How Supplied: Consumer packages of 10, 20 and 40 caplets.

Note: There are other CONTAC products. Make sure this is the one you are interested in.

Shown in Product Identification Section, page 431

CONTAC®
MAXIMUM STRENGTH SINUS
Caplets/Tablets
Non-Drowsy Formula
Decongestant • Analgesic

[See table on next page]

Product Information: Two caplets/tablets every 6 hours to help relieve the discomforts of sinusitis symptoms.

Product Benefits: CONTAC SINUS contains a decongestant and a non-aspirin analgesic. These safe and effective ingredients provide temporary relief from these major sinusitis symptoms: sinus pressure, nasal congestion, headache and pain.

NO ANTIHISTAMINE DROWSINESS

Directions: Two caplets/tablets every 6 hours, not to exceed 8 caplets/tablets in any 24-hour period. Children under 12 should use only as directed by physician.

TAMPER-RESISTANT PACKAGING FEATURES FOR YOUR PROTECTION:

- Two caplets/tablets (one dose) are encased in a clear plastic cell with a foil back; do not use if cell or foil is broken.
- The name CONTAC-S appears on each caplet; do not use this product if the CONTAC-S name is missing.
  The letters C-S appear on each tablet; do not use the product if these letters are missing.

Warnings: Do not exceed recommended dosage. If symptoms do not improve within 7 days, or worsen, consult a physician before continuing use. Individuals being treated for depression, high blood pressure, heart disease, diabetes, thyroid disease, or difficulty in urination due to enlargement of the prostate gland should use only as directed by a physician. Stop use if dizziness, sleeplessness or nervousness occurs. Keep this and all drugs out of reach of children. In case of accidental overdose, seek professional assistance or contact a poison control center immediately. As with any drug, if you are pregnant or nursing a baby, seek the advice of a health professional before using this product. Store at controlled room temperature (59°–86°F.).

Formula: Active Ingredients: Each caplet/tablet contains Decongestant—Pseudoephedrine Hydrochloride 30 mg., Analgesic and Fever Reducer—Acetaminophen 500 mg. (500 mg. is a non-standard dosage of acetaminophen, as compared to the standard of 325 mg.). **Inactive Ingredients (listed for individuals with specific allergies):** Cellulose, Crospovidone, Red 30, Hydroxypropyl Methylcellulose, Magnesium Stearate, Polyethylene Glycol, Polysorbate 80, Povidone, Starch, Titanium Dioxide and trace amounts of other inactive ingredients.

How Supplied: Consumer packages of 24 caplets or 24 tablets.

Note: There are other CONTAC products. Make sure this is the one you are interested in.

Shown in Product Identification Section, page 431

CONTAC®
Continuous Action Nasal Decongestant/Antihistamine Capsules

Composition:
[See table on next page.]

Product Information: Each CONTAC continuous action capsule contains over 600 "tiny time pills." Some go to work right away. The rest are scientifically timed to dissolve slowly to give up to 12 hours of relief. With just *one* capsule in the morning and *one* at bedtime, you feel better all day, sleep better at night, breathing freely without congestion. CONTAC provides:

- A NASAL DECONGESTANT which helps clear nasal passages, shrinks swollen membranes and helps decongest sinus openings.
- AN ANTIHISTAMINE to help relieve itchy, watery eyes, sneezing, and runny nose.

Indications: For temporary relief of nasal congestion due to the common cold, hay fever or other upper respiratory allergies, and nasal congestion associated with sinusitis.

Directions: One capsule every 12 hours. Do not exceed 2 capsules in 24 hours.

TAMPER-RESISTANT PACKAGING FEATURES FOR YOUR PROTECTION:

- Each capsule is encased in a plastic cell with a foil back; do not use if cell or foil is broken.
- Each CONTAC capsule is protected by a red Perma-Seal™ band which bonds the two capsule halves together; do not use if capsule or band is broken.

Warnings: Do not give this product to children under 12 years except under the advice and supervision of a physician. Do not exceed recommended dosage because at higher doses nervousness, dizziness, or sleeplessness may occur. Do not take this product if you have high blood pressure, heart disease, diabetes or thyroid disease except under the advice and supervision of a physician. If symptoms do not improve within 7 days or are accompanied by a high fever, consult a physician before continuing use. Do not take this product if you have asthma, glaucoma or difficulty in urination due to enlargement of the prostate gland except under the advice and supervision of a physician. Do not take this product if you are taking another medication containing phenylpropanolamine. Avoid alcoholic beverages while taking this product. Do not drive or operate heavy machinery. May cause drowsiness. May cause excitability, especially in children. Keep this and all drugs out of reach of children. In case of accidental overdose, seek professional assistance or contact a poison control center immediately. As with any drug, if you are pregnant or nursing a baby, seek the advice of a health professional before using this product. Store at controlled room temperature (59°–86°F.).

Drug Interaction Precaution: Do not take this product if you are presently taking a prescription antihypertensive or antidepressant drug containing monoamine oxidase inhibitor except under the advice and supervision of a physician.

Formula: Active Ingredients: Each capsule contains Phenylpropanolamine Hydrochloride 75 mg.; Chlorpheniramine Maleate 8 mg. **Inactive Ingredients (listed for individuals with specific allergies):** Benzyl Alcohol, Cetylpyridinium Chloride, Red 3, 27, 30, 40, Yel-

CONTAC	CONTAC Maximum Strength Continuous Action Decongestant Caplets	CONTAC Continuous Action Decongestant Capsules	CONTAC Severe Cold and Flu Formula Caplets (each 2 caplet dose)	CONTAC Sinus Non-Drowsy Formula Caplets (each 2 caplet dose)	CONTAC Sinus Non-Drowsy Formula Tablets (each 2 tablet dose)
Phenylpropanolamine HCl	75.0 mg	75.0 mg	25.0 mg	—	—
Chlorpheniramine Maleate	12.0 mg	8.0 mg	4.0 mg	—	—
Pseudoephedrine HCl				60.0 mg	60.0 mg
Acetaminophen	—	—	1000.0 mg	1000.0 mg	1000.0 mg
Dextromethorphan Hydrobromide	—	—	30.0 mg	—	—

low 6, 10, Gelatin, Glyceryl Distearate, Microcrystalline Wax, Silicon Dioxide, Sodium Lauryl Sulfate, Starch, Sucrose, and trace amounts of other inactive ingredients.

How Supplied: Consumer packages of 10, 20 and 40 capsules.

Note: There are other CONTAC products. Make sure this is the one you are interested in.

Shown in Product Identification Section, page 431

CONTAC®
Severe Cold and Flu Formula Caplets
Analgesic • Decongestant
Antihistamine • Cough Suppressant

Composition:
[See table above.]

Product Information: Two caplets every 6 hours to help relieve the discomforts of severe colds with flu-like symptoms.

Product Benefits: CONTAC Severe Cold and Flu Formula contains a non-aspirin analgesic, a decongestant, an antihistamine and a cough suppressant. These safe and effective ingredients provide temporary relief from these major cold symptoms: fever, body aches and pains, minor sore throat pain, headache, runny nose, postnasal drip, sneezing, itchy, watery eyes, nasal and sinus congestion, and temporarily relieves cough due to the common cold.

Directions: Two caplets every 6 hours, not to exceed 8 caplets in any 24 hour period. Children under 12 should use only as directed by physician.

TAMPER-RESISTANT PACKAGING FEATURES FOR YOUR PROTECTION:
- Each caplet is encased in a plastic cell with a foil back; do not use if cell or foil is broken.
- The letters SCF appear on each caplet; do not use this product if these letters are missing.

Warnings: Do not exceed recommended dosage. If symptoms do not improve within 7 days, or worsen, consult a physician before continuing use. Individuals being treated for depression, high blood pressure, asthma, heart disease, diabetes, thyroid disease, glaucoma or difficulty in urinating due to an enlarged prostate should use only as directed by a physician. Do not take this product if you are taking another medication containing phenylpropanolamine. Avoid alcoholic beverages while taking this product. Do not drive or operate heavy machinery. May cause drowsiness. Stop use if dizziness, sleeplessness or nervousness occurs. A persistent cough may be a sign of a serious condition. If cough persists for more than 1 week, tends to recur, or is accompanied by fever, rash or persistent headache, consult a doctor. Do not take this product for persistent or chronic cough such as occurs with smoking, asthma, emphysema, or if cough is accompanied by excessive phlegm (mucus), unless directed by a doctor. May cause excitability, especially in children. Keep this and all drugs out of reach of children. In case of accidental overdose, seek professional assistance or contact a poison control center immediately. As with any drug, if you are pregnant or nursing a baby, seek the advice of a health professional before using this product.

Store at controlled room temperature (59°–86°F.).

Drug Interaction Precaution: Do not take if you are presently taking a prescription antihypertensive or antidepressant drug containing monoamine oxidase inhibitor except under the advice and supervision of a physician.

Formula: Active Ingredients: Each caplet contains Acetaminophen, 500 mg. *(500 mg. is a non-standard dose of acetaminophen, as compared to the standard of 325 mg.);* Dextromethorphan Hydrobromide, 15 mg.; Phenylpropanolamine Hydrochloride, 12.5 mg.; Chlorpheniramine Maleate, 2 mg. **Inactive Ingredients (listed for individuals with specific allergies):** Cellulose, FD&C Blue 1, Hydroxypropyl Methylcellulose, Polyethylene Glycol, Polysorbate 80, Povidone, Sodium Starch Glycolate, Starch, Stearic Acid, Titanium Dioxide.

How Supplied: Consumer packages of 10, 20 and 40 caplets.

Note: There are other CONTAC products. Make sure this is the one you are interested in.

Shown in Product Identification Section, page 431

CONTAC® Cough Formula
Cough Suppressant and Expectorant

Composition: [See table on next page .]

Product Information: ALCOHOL-FREE, cherry flavored CONTAC Cough Formula provides temporary relief of coughs due to the common cold and chest congestion. It contains:
- A non-narcotic cough suppressant **to temporarily relieve your cough for 4 hours.**
- An expectorant to **help loosen phlegm (sputum)** and thin bronchial secretions to rid the bronchial passageways of bothersome mucus, drain bronchial tubes, and make coughs more productive.

Directions: Take every 4 hours.
ADULTS: Fill medicine cup provided to "ADULT DOSE" line (3 teaspoons). Do not exceed 6 doses (12 teaspoons) in 24 hours. CHILDREN 6–12: Fill medicine cup provided to "CHILDREN 6–12 DOSE" line (1½ teaspoons). Do not exceed 6 doses (6 teaspoons) in 24 hours.

TAMPER-RESISTANT PACKAGING FEATURES FOR YOUR PROTECTION:
- Imprinted seal around bottle cap. Do not use this product if the imprinted seal is missing or broken.

Warnings: Do not take this product for persistent or chronic cough such as occurs with smoking, asthma, chronic bronchitis, or emphysema, or where cough is accompanied by excessive phlegm (sputum), unless directed by a doctor. A persistent cough may be a sign of a serious condition. If cough persists for more than 1 week, tends to recur, or is accompanied by fever, rash or persistent headache, consult a doctor. Do not give this product to children under 6 years of age unless directed by a doctor. As with any drug, if you are pregnant or nursing a baby, seek the advice of a health professional before using this product. Keep this and all drugs out of the reach of children. In case of accidental overdose, seek professional assistance or contact a poison control center immediately.

Formula: Active Ingredients: Each Adult Dose (1 Tablespoon) contains: Dextromethorphan Hydrobromide 20 mg., Guaifenesin 200 mg.

Inactive Ingredients: Citric Acid, Flavors, Menthol, Methylparaben, Polyethylene Glycol, Propylene Glycol, Propyl-

Continued on next page

SmithKline Beecham—Cont.

paraben, Red 40, Saccharin Sodium, Sodium Benzoate, Sodium Citrate, Sucrose, and Water.

Store at controlled room temperature (59°–86°F.).

How Supplied: In 4 fl. oz. bottles.
Note: There are other CONTAC products. Make sure this is the one you are interested in.

Shown in Product Identification Section, page 432

CONTAC® Cough & Sore Throat Formula
Cough Suppressant • Expectorant and Non-Aspirin Analgesic

Composition:
[See table below.]

Product Information: ALCOHOL-FREE, cherry flavored CONTAC Cough & Sore Throat Formula provides temporary relief of coughs due to the common cold, and chest congestion and minor sore throat pain and irritation. It contains:

- A non-narcotic cough suppressant to **temporarily relieve your cough,**
- An expectorant to **help loosen phlegm (sputum)** and thin bronchial secretions to rid the bronchial passageways of bothersome mucus, drain bronchial tubes, and make coughs more productive,
- A non-aspirin analgesic to **temporarily relieve minor aches and pains associated with a sore throat,** and
- A soothing liquid formulation to **coat a raw and irritated throat.**

Directions: Take every 4 hours as needed. ADULTS: Fill medicine cup provided to "ADULT DOSE" line (3 teaspoons). Do not exceed 6 doses (18 teaspoons) in 24 hours. CHILDREN 6–12: Fill medicine cup provided to "CHILDREN 6–12 DOSE" line (1½ teaspoons). Do not exceed 5 doses (7½ teaspoons) in 24 hours.

TAMPER-RESISTANT PACKAGING FEATURES FOR YOUR PROTECTION:

- Imprinted seal around bottle cap. Do not use this product if the imprinted seal is missing or broken.

Warnings: Do not take this product for persistent or chronic cough such as occurs with smoking, asthma, chronic bronchitis, or emphysema, or where cough is accompanied by excessive phlegm (sputum), unless directed by a doctor. A persistent cough may be a sign of a serious condition. If cough persists for more than 1 week, tends to recur, or is accompanied by fever, rash or persistent headache, consult a doctor. Do not give this product to children under 6 years of age unless directed by a doctor. Do not take this product for pain for more than 10 days (for adults) or 5 days (for children), and do not take for fever for more than 3 days unless directed by a doctor. If pain or fever persists or gets worse, if new symptoms occur, or if redness or swelling is present, consult a doctor because these could be signs of a serious condition. Do not give this product to children for the pain of arthritis unless directed by a doctor. If sore throat is severe, persists for more than 2 days, is accompanied or followed by fever, headache, rash, nausea, or vomiting, consult a doctor promptly. Do not exceed recommended dosage because severe liver damage may occur. Do not take additional pain relievers/fever reducers while using this product. As with any drug, if you are pregnant or nursing a baby, seek the advice of a health professional before using this product. Keep this and all drugs out of the reach of children. In case of accidental overdose, seek professional assistance or contact a poison control center immediately. Prompt medical attention is critical for adults as well as for children even if you do not notice any signs or symptoms.

Formula: Active ingredients: Each Adult Dose (1 Tablespoon) contains: Acetaminophen 650 mg., Dextromethorphan Hydrobromide 20 mg., Guaifenesin 200 mg.

Inactive ingredients: Citric Acid, Flavors, Methylparaben, Polyethylene Glycol, Propylene Glycol, Propylparaben, Red 33, Red 40, Saccharin Sodium, Sodium Benzoate, Sodium Citrate, Sucrose, and Water.

Store at controlled room temperature (59°–86°F.).

How Supplied: In 4 fl. oz. bottles.
Note: There are other CONTAC products. Make sure this is the one you are interested in.

Shown in Product Identification Section, page 432

CONTAC JR.®
Non-Drowsy Cold Liquid
Analgesic • Decongestant
Cough Suppressant

Composition:
[See table below.]

Product Information: For nasal and sinus congestion, coughing and body aches and pains due to colds. Relieves symptoms with these reliable medicines.
A gentle decongestant. For temporary relief of nasal and sinus congestion. Helps your child breathe more freely. A safe, sensible, non-narcotic cough quieter. Calms worrisome coughs due to colds.
A trusted, aspirin-free pain reliever and fever reducer. Provides temporary relief of muscular aches and pains, headaches and discomforts of fever due to colds and "flu."

Product Benefits: The good medicines in CONTAC Jr. were specially chosen to help gently relieve your child's nasal and sinus congestion, coughing, body aches and pains due to colds. DOES NOT CONTAIN ANTIHISTAMINES WHICH MAY CAUSE DROWSINESS.
Medical authorities know that for children, dose by weight—not age—means the dose you give is right for consistent, controlled relief. Use the CONTAC Jr. Accu-Measure Cup to select the right dose for your child's body weight.

Directions: Shake well before using. One dose every 4 to 6 hours, not to exceed 4 times daily. Use the CONTAC Jr. Accu-Measure Cup to measure the right dose for your child. For dose by teaspoon see bottle label.

TAMPER-RESISTANT PACKAGING FEATURES FOR YOUR PROTECTION:

- Imprinted seal around bottle-cap. Do not use this product if the imprinted seal is missing or broken.

Warning: Do not exceed recommended dosage for your child's body weight. For children under 31 lbs. or under 3 years of age, consult a physician. If symptoms persist for 7 days or are accompanied by high fever, severe or recurrent pain, or if child is being treated for depression, high blood pressure, diabetes, heart disease or thyroid disease, consult a physician. Stop use if dizziness, sleeplessness or nervousness occurs. Do not give this product for persistent or chronic cough such as occurs with asthma or if cough is accompa-

CONTAC Liquid	CONTAC Cough Formula (each adult dose)	CONTAC Cough & Sore Throat Formula (each adult dose)	CONTAC JR. (each 5cc)	CONTAC Nighttime Cold Medicine (each fluid ounce)
Pseudoephedrine Hydrochloride	—	—	15.0 mg	60.0 mg
Acetaminophen	—	650.0 mg	160.0 mg	1000.0 mg
Dextromethorphan Hydrobromide	20.0 mg	20.0 mg	5.0 mg	30.0 mg
Doxylamine Succinate	—	—	—	7.5 mg
Guaifenesin	200.0 mg	200.0 mg	—	—
Alcohol	—	—	—	25%

nied by excessive phlegm (mucus) unless directed by a doctor. Keep this and all drugs out of reach of children. In case of accidental overdose, seek professional assistance or contact a poison control center immediately.

Formula: Active ingredients: Each 5 ml. (average teaspoon) contains Acetaminophen 160 mg., Pseudoephedrine Hydrochloride 15 mg., Dextromethorphan Hydrobromide 5 mg.
Inactive ingredients: Citric Acid, Flavors, Methylparaben, Polyethylene Glycol, Propylene Glycol, Propylparaben, Red 33, Saccharin Sodium, Sodium Benzoate, Sodium Citrate, Sorbitol, Water and Yellow 6.

Store at controlled room temperature (59°–86°F.).

How Supplied: A clear red liquid in 4 oz. size bottle.
Note: There are other CONTAC products. Make sure this is the one you are interested in.

Shown in Product Identification Section, page 432

CONTAC®
Nighttime Cold Medicine
Antihistamine • Analgesic
Cough Suppressant • Nasal Decongestant

Composition:
[See table on preceding page]

Product Information: CONTAC Nighttime Cold Medicine:

- Provides temporary relief from nasal and sinus congestion, runny nose, coughing, postnasal drip, sneezing, itchy, watery eyes and minor aches and pains associated with the common cold, sore throat, and flu, so you can get the rest you need.
- Contains a non-aspirin analgesic and fever reducer, a cough suppressant, a nasal decongestant and an antihistamine.

In consumer testing, the soothing mint taste of CONTAC Nighttime Cold Medicine was preferred over the taste of original NYQUIL* Nighttime Colds Medicine.

Directions: ADULTS—Take 1 fluid ounce at bedtime in dosage cup provided. May be repeated every 6 hours as needed, not to exceed 4 fluid ounces in 24 hours. Children under 12 should use only as directed by physician.

TAMPER-RESISTANT PACKAGING FEATURES FOR YOUR PROTECTION:

- Imprinted seal around bottle cap. Do not use this product if the imprinted seal is missing or broken.

Warnings: Do not exceed recommended dosage. If symptoms do not improve or worsen within 7 days, or are accompanied by high fever, or difficulty in breathing, consult a doctor before continuing use. Do not take this product for pain for more than 10 days or for fever for more than 3 days unless directed by a doctor. If pain or fever persists or gets worse, if new symptoms occur, or if redness or swelling is present, consult a doctor because these could be signs of a serious condition. If sore throat is severe, persists for more than 2 days, is accompanied or followed by fever, headache, rash, nausea, or vomiting, consult a doctor promptly. A persistent cough may be a sign of a serious condition. If cough persists for more than one week, tends to recur or is accompanied by a high fever, a fever lasting more than 3 days, a rash, a persistent headache, shortness of breath or chest pain when breathing, consult a doctor. Stop use if dizziness, sleeplessness, or nervousness occurs. Individuals who have been or are being treated for depression, high blood pressure, glaucoma, diabetes, asthma, difficulty in urination due to enlarged prostate, heart disease or thyroid disease should use only as directed by a doctor. Avoid alcoholic beverages while taking this product. Do not drive or operate heavy machinery. May cause marked drowsiness. May cause excitability, especially in children. Keep this and all drugs out of reach of children. In case of accidental overdose, seek professional assistance or contact a poison control center immediately. Prompt medical attention is critical for adults as well as children even if you do not notice any signs or symptoms. As with any drug, if you are pregnant or nursing a baby, seek the advice of a health professional before using this product.

Formula: Active ingredients: Each dose (1 Ounce) contains: Acetaminophen 1000 mg., Pseudoephedrine Hydrochloride 60 mg., Dextromethorphan Hydrobromide 30 mg., Doxylamine Succinate 7.5 mg.
Alcohol content: 25% by volume.
Inactive ingredients: Alcohol, Citric Acid, Flavor, Green 3, Polyethylene Glycol, Saccharin Sodium, Sodium Benzoate, Sodium Citrate, Sorbitol, Sucrose, Water and Yellow 6.

Store at controlled room temperature (59°–86°F.).

How Supplied: In 6 fl. oz. bottles.
Note: There are other CONTAC products. Make sure this is the one you are interested in.
*NYQUIL is a registered trademark of Richardson-Vicks Inc.

Shown in Product Identification Section, page 432

ECOTRIN®
Enteric-Coated Aspirin
Antiarthritic, Antiplatelet

Description: 'Ecotrin' is enteric-coated aspirin (acetylsalicylic acid, ASA) available in tablet and caplet forms in 325 mg. and 500 mg. dosage units. *(500 mg. is a non-standard, maximum strength dosage of aspirin, as compared to the standard of 325 mg.)*
The enteric coating covers a core of aspirin and is designed to resist disintegration in the stomach, dissolving in the more neutral-to-alkaline environment of the duodenum. Such action helps to protect the stomach from damage that may result from ingestion of plain, buffered or highly buffered aspirin (see SAFETY).

Indications: 'Ecotrin' is indicated for:

- conditions requiring chronic or long-term aspirin therapy for pain and/or inflammation, e.g., rheumatoid arthritis, juvenile rheumatoid arthritis, systemic lupus erythematosus, osteoarthritis (degenerative joint disease), ankylosing spondylitis, psoriatic arthritis, Reiter's syndrome and fibrositis,
- antiplatelet indications of aspirin (see the ANTIPLATELET-EFFECT section) and
- situations in which compliance with aspirin therapy may be affected because of the gastrointestinal side effects of plain, i.e., non-enteric-coated, or buffered aspirin.

Dosage: For analgesic or anti-inflammatory indications, the OTC maximum dosage for aspirin is 4000 mg. per day in divided doses, i.e., 2 325 mg. tablets or caplets q4h or 3 325 mg. tablets or caplets or 2 500 mg. tablets or caplets q6h.
For antiplatelet effect dosage: see the ANTIPLATELET EFFECT section.
Under a physician's direction, the dosage can be increased or otherwise modified as appropriate to the clinical situation. When 'Ecotrin' is used for anti-inflammatory effect, the physician should be attentive to plasma salicylate levels, and may also caution the patient to be alert to the development of tinnitus as an indicator of elevated salicylate levels. It should be noted that patients with a high frequency hearing loss (such as may occur in older individuals) may have difficulty perceiving the tinnitus. Tinnitus would then not be a reliable indicator in such individuals.

Inactive Ingredients: Cellulose, Cellulose Acetate Phthalate, D&C Yellow 10, Diethyl Phthalate, FD&C Yellow 6, Silicon Dioxide, Sodium Starch Glycolate, Starch, Stearic Acid, Titanium Dioxide, and trace amounts of other inactive ingredients.

Bioavailability: The bioavailability of aspirin from 'Ecotrin' has been demonstrated in a number of salicylate excretion studies. The studies show levels of salicylate (and metabolites) in urine excreted over 48 hours for 'Ecotrin' do not differ statistically from plain, i.e., non-enteric-coated, aspirin.
Plasma studies, in which 'Ecotrin' has been compared with plain aspirin in steady-state studies over eight days, also demonstrate that 'Ecotrin' provides plasma salicylate levels not statistically different from plain aspirin.
Information regarding salicylate levels over a range of doses was generated in a study in which 24 healthy volunteers (12 male and 12 female) took daily (divided) doses of either 2600 mg., 3900 mg., or 5200 mg. of 'Ecotrin'. Plasma salicylate levels generally acknowledged to be anti-inflammatory (15 mg./dL.) were attained

Continued on next page

SmithKline Beecham—Cont.

at daily doses of 5200 mg., on Day 2 by females and Day 3 by males. At 3900 mg., anti-inflammatory levels were attained at Day 3 by females and Day 4 by males. Dissolution of the enteric coating occurs at a neutral-to-basic pH and is therefore dependent on gastric emptying into the duodenum. With continued dosing, appropriate plasma levels are maintained.

Safety: The safety of 'Ecotrin' has been demonstrated in a number of endoscopic studies comparing 'Ecotrin', plain aspirin, as well as plain, buffered and "arthritis-strength" buffered preparations. In these studies, all forms of aspirin were dosed to the OTC maximum (3900–4000 mg. per day) for up to 14 days. The normal healthy volunteers participating in these studies were gastroscoped before and after the courses of treatment, and 14-day drug-free periods followed active drug. Compared to all the other preparations, there was statistically significantly less gastric damage during the 'Ecotrin' courses. There was also statistically less duodenal damage when compared with the plain, i.e., non-enteric-coated, aspirin.

Details of studies demonstrating the safety and bioavailability of 'Ecotrin' are available to health care professionals. Write: Professional Services Department, SmithKline Beecham Consumer Brands, P.O. Box 1467, Pittsburgh, Pa. 15230.

Warning:

Consumer Warning: Children and teenagers should not use this medicine for chicken pox or flu symptoms before a doctor is consulted about Reye syndrome, a rare but serious illness. If pain persists for more than 10 days, or if redness is present, or in arthritic or rheumatic conditions affecting children under 12, consult a physician immediately. Discontinue use if dizziness, ringing in ears, or impaired hearing occurs. If you experience persistent or unexplained stomach upset, consult a physician. Keep this and all drugs out of children's reach. In case of accidental overdose, seek professional assistance or contact a poison control center immediately. As with any medicine, if you are pregnant or nursing a baby, seek the advice of a health professional before using this product. **IT IS ESPECIALLY IMPORTANT NOT TO USE ASPIRIN DURING THE LAST 3 MONTHS OF PREGNANCY UNLESS SPECIFICALLY DIRECTED TO DO SO BY A DOCTOR, BECAUSE IT MAY CAUSE PROBLEMS IN THE UNBORN CHILD OR COMPLICATIONS DURING DELIVERY.** Store at controlled room temperature (59°–86°F.).

Professional Warning: There have been occasional reports in the literature concerning individuals with impaired gastric emptying in whom there may be retention of one or more 'Ecotrin' tablets over time. This unusual phenomenon may occur as a result of outlet obstruction from ulcer disease alone or combined with hypotonic gastric peristalsis. Because of the integrity of the enteric coating in an acidic environment, these tablets may accumulate and form a bezoar in the stomach. Individuals with this condition may present with complaints of early satiety or of vague upper abdominal distress. Diagnosis may be made by endoscopy or by abdominal films which show opacities suggestive of a mass of small tablets *(Ref.: Bogacz, K. and Caldron, P.: Enteric-coated Aspirin Bezoar: Elevation of Serum Salicylate Level by Barium Study. Amer. J. Med. 1987:83, 783–6.).* Management may vary according to the condition of the patient. Options include: gastrotomy and alternating slightly basic and neutral lavage *(Ref.: Baum, J.: Enteric-Coated Aspirin and the Problem of Gastric Retention. J. Rheum., 1984:11, 250–1.).* While there have been no clinical reports, it has been suggested that such individuals may also be treated with parenteral cimetidine (to reduce acid secretion) and then given sips of slightly basic liquids to effect gradual dissolution of the enteric coating. Progress may be followed with plasma salicylate levels or via recognition of tinnitus by the patient.

It should be kept in mind that individuals with a history of partial or complete gastrectomy may produce reduced amounts of acid and therefore have less acidic gastric pH. Under these circumstances, the benefits offered by the acid-resistant enteric coating may not exist.

Antiplatelet Effect: FDA approved professional labeling permits the use of aspirin to reduce the risk of death and/or nonfatal myocardial infarction (MI) in patients with a previous infarction or unstable angina pectoris and its use in reducing the risk of transient ischemic attacks in men.

Labeling for both indications follows:

"ASPIRIN FOR MYOCARDIAL INFARCTION"

Indication: Aspirin is indicated to reduce the risk of death and/or nonfatal myocardial infarction in patients with a previous infarction or unstable angina pectoris.

Clinical Trials: The indication is supported by the results of six, large, randomized multicenter, placebo-controlled studies involving 10,816 predominantly male, post-myocardial infarction (MI) patients and one randomized placebo-controlled study of 1,266 men with unstable angina.[1–7] Therapy with aspirin was begun at intervals after the onset of acute MI varying from less than three days to more than five years and continued for periods of from less than one year to four years. In the unstable angina study, treatment was started within one month after the onset of unstable angina and continued for 12 weeks, and patients with complicating conditions such as congestive heart failure were not included in the study.

Aspirin therapy in MI patients was associated with about a 20 percent reduction in the risk of subsequent death and/or nonfatal reinfarction, a median absolute decrease of 3 percent from the 12 to 22 percent event rates in the placebo groups. In aspirin-treated unstable angina patients, the reduction in risk was about 50 percent, a reduction in event rate to 5% from the 10% in the placebo group over the 12 weeks of the study.

Daily dosage of aspirin in the post-myocardial infarction studies was 300 mg. in one study and 900 to 1500 mg. in five studies. A dose of 325 mg. was used in the study of unstable angina.

Adverse Reactions

Gastrointestinal Reactions: Doses of 1000 mg. per day of plain aspirin caused gastrointestinal symptoms and bleeding that in some cases were clinically significant. In the largest postinfarction study (the Aspirin Myocardial Infarction Study [AMIS] with 4,500 people), the percentage incidences of gastrointestinal symptoms of a standard, solid-tablet formulation and placebo-treated subjects, respectively, were: stomach pain (14.5%; 4.4%); heartburn (11.9%; 4.8%); nausea and/or vomiting (7.6%; 2.1%); hospitalization for gastrointestinal disorder (4.9%; 3.5%). In the AMIS and other trials, plain aspirin-treated patients had increased rates of gross gastrointestinal bleeding. Symptoms and signs of gastrointestinal irritation were not significantly increased in subjects treated for unstable angina with buffered aspirin in solution.

Cardiovascular and Biochemical: In the AMIS trial, the dosage of 1000 mg. per day of plain aspirin was associated with small increases in systolic blood pressure (BP) (average 1.5 to 2.1 mmHg) and diastolic BP (0.5 to 0.6 mmHg), depending upon whether maximal or last available readings were used. Blood urea nitrogen and uric acid levels were also increased, but by less than 1.0 mg.%. Subjects with marked hypertension or renal insufficiency had been excluded from the trial so that the clinical importance of these observations for such subjects or for any subjects treated over more prolonged periods is not known. It is recommended that patients placed on long-term aspirin treatment, even at doses of 300 mg. per day, be seen at regular intervals to assess changes in these measurements.

Sodium in Buffered Aspirin for Solution Formulations: One tablet daily of buffered aspirin in solution adds 553 mg. of sodium to that in the diet and may not be tolerated by patients with active sodium-retaining states such as congestive heart or renal failure. This amount of sodium adds about 30 percent to the 70 to 90 meq. intake suggested as appropriate for dietary treatment of essential hypertension in the 1984 Report of the Joint National Committee on Detection, Evaluation, and Treatment of High Blood Pressure.[8]

Dosage and Administration: Although most of the studies used dosages exceeding 300 mg. daily, two trials used only 300 mg. and pharmacologic data indicate that this dose inhibits platelet function fully. Therefore, 300 mg. or a conventional 325 mg. aspirin dose daily is a reasonable, routine dose that would minimize gastrointestinal adverse reactions for both solid oral dosage forms (buffered and plain aspirin) and buffered aspirin in solution.

References:

1. Elwood, P.C., et al.: A Randomized Controlled Trial of Acetylsalicylic Acid in the Secondary Prevention of Mortality from Myocardial Infarction, *Br. Med. J.* 1:436–440, 1974.
2. The Coronary Drug Project Research Group: Aspirin in Coronary Heart Disease, *J. Chronic Dis.* 29:625–642, 1976.
3. Breddin, K., et al.: Secondary Prevention of Myocardial Infarction: A Comparison of Acetylsalicylic Acid, Phenprocoumon or Placebo, *Homeostasis* 470:263–268, 1979.
4. Aspirin Myocardial Infarction Study Research Group: A Randomized Controlled Trial of Aspirin in Persons Recovered from Myocardial Infarction, *J.A.M.A.* 243:661–669, 1980.
5. Elwood, P.C., and Sweetnam, P.M.: Aspirin and Secondary Mortality After Myocardial Infarction, *Lancet* pp. 1313–1315, Dec. 22–29, 1979.
6. The Persantine-Aspirin Reinfarction Study Research Group, Persantine and Aspirin in Coronary Heart Disease, *Circulation* 62: 449–469, 1980.
7. Lewis, H.D., et al.: Protective Effects of Aspirin Against Acute Myocardial Infarction and Death in Men with Unstable Angina, Results of a Veterans Administration Cooperative Study, *N. Engl. J. Med.* 309:396–403, 1983.
8. 1984 Report of the Joint National Committee on Detection, Evaluation, and Treatment of High Blood Pressure, U.S. Department of Health and Human Services and U.S. Public Health Service, National Institutes of Health. NIH Pub. No. 84–1088.

Aspirin for Transient Ischemic Attacks

Indication: For reducing the risk of recurrent transient ischemic attacks (TIAs) or stroke in men who have had transient ischemia of the brain due to fibrin platelet emboli. There is inadequate evidence that aspirin or buffered aspirin is effective in reducing TIAs in women at the recommended dosage. There is no evidence that aspirin or buffered aspirin is of benefit in the treatment of completed strokes in men or women.

Clinical Trials: The indication is supported by the results of a Canadian study[1] in which 585 patients with threatened stroke were followed in a randomized clinical trial for an average of 26 months to determine whether aspirin or sulfinpyrazone, singly or in combination, was superior to placebo in preventing transient ischemic attacks, stroke or death. The study showed that, although sulfinpyrazone had no statistically significant effect, aspirin reduced the risk of continuing transient ischemic attacks, stroke or death by 19 percent and reduced the risk of stroke or death by 31 percent. Another aspirin study carried out in the United States with 178 patients showed a statistically significant number of "favorable outcomes," including reduced transient ischemic attacks, stroke and death.[2]

Precautions: Patients presenting with signs and/or symptoms of TIAs should have a complete medical and neurologic evaluation. Consideration should be given to other disorders that resemble TIAs. Attention should be given to risk factors: it is important to evaluate and treat, if appropriate, other diseases associated with TIAs and stroke, such as hypertension and diabetes.

Concurrent administration of absorbable antacids at therapeutic doses may increase the clearance of salicylates in some individuals. The concurrent administration of nonabsorbable antacids may alter the rate of absorption of aspirin, thereby resulting in a decreased acetylsalicylic acid/salicylate ratio in plasma. The clinical significance of these decreases in available aspirin is unknown.

Aspirin at dosages of 1,000 mg. per day has been associated with small increases in blood pressure, blood urea nitrogen, and serum uric acid levels. It is recommended that patients placed on long-term aspirin treatment be seen at regular intervals to assess changes in these measurements.

Adverse Reactions: At dosages of 1,000 mg. or higher of aspirin per day, gastrointestinal side effects include stomach pain, heartburn, nausea and/or vomiting, as well as increased rates of gross gastrointestinal bleeding.

Dosage and Administration: Adult dosage for men is 1,300 mg. a day, in divided doses of 650 mg. twice a day or 325 mg. four times a day.

References:

1. The Canadian Cooperative Study Group: Randomized Trial of Aspirin and Sulfinpyrazone in Threatened Stroke, *N. Engl. J. Med.* 299:53, 1978.
2. Fields, W. S., et al.: Controlled Trial of Aspirin in Cerebral Ischemia, *Stroke* 8:301–316, 1980.

Store at controlled room temperature (59°–86°F.).

Supplied:

'Ecotrin' Tablets
325 mg. in bottles of 100*, 250 and 1000.
500 mg. in bottles of 60* and 150.
'Ecotrin' Caplets
325 mg. in bottles of 100.
500 mg. in bottles of 60.
* Without child-resistant caps.

TAMPER-RESISTANT PACKAGE FEATURES:

- Bottle has imprinted seal under cap.
- The words ECOTRIN REG or ECOTRIN MAX appear on each tablet or caplet (see product illustration printed on carton).
- **DO NOT USE THIS PRODUCT IF ANY OF THESE TAMPER-RESISTANT FEATURES ARE MISSING OR BROKEN.**

Comments or Questions? Call Toll-Free 800-245-1040 weekdays.

Shown in Product Identification Section, page 432

ESOTÉRICA® MEDICATED FADE CREAM
Regular
Sunscreen Formula
Facial with Sunscreens and Moisturizers
Sensitive Skin Formula—Unscented

Description:

Regular:

Active Ingredient: Hydroquinone 2%.

Inactive Ingredients: BHA, ceresin, citric acid, dimethicone, fragrance, glyceryl stearate, isopropyl palmitate, laureth-23, methylparaben, mineral oil, PEG 6-32 stearate, poloxamer 188, propylene glycol, propylene glycol stearate, propylparaben, sodium bisulfite, sodium lauryl sulfate, steareth-20, stearyl alcohol, trisodium EDTA, water.

Sunscreen Formula:

Active Ingredients: Octyl dimethyl PABA 3.3%, benzophenone-3 2.5%, hydroquinone 2%. **Inactive Ingredients:** Allantoin ascorbate, BHA, ceresin, dimethicone, fragrance, glyceryl stearate, isopropyl palmitate, laureth-23, methylparaben, mineral oil, PEG 6-32 stearate, poloxamer 188, propylene glycol, propylparaben, sodium bisulfite, sodium lauryl sulfate, steareth-10, steareth-20, stearyl alcohol, trisodium EDTA, water.

Facial—With Sunscreens and Moisturizers:

Active Ingredients: Octyl dimethyl PABA 3.3%, benzophenone-3 2.5%, hydroquinone 2%. **Inactive Ingredients:** BHA, ceresin, ceteareth-3, citric acid, dimethicone, fragrance, glyceryl stearate, isopropyl myristate, methylparaben, poloxamer 188, propylene glycol, propylparaben, sodium bisulfite, sodium lauryl sulfate, steareth-20, stearyl alcohol, trisodium EDTA, water.

Sensitive Skin Formula—Unscented:

Active Ingredient: Hydroquinone 1.5%.

Inactive Ingredients: BHA, ceresin, citric acid, dimethicone, glyceryl stearate, isopropyl palmitate, laureth-23, methylparaben, mineral oil, PEG 6-32 stearate, poloxamer 188, propylene glycol , propylene glycol stearate, propylparaben, sodium bisulfite, sodium lauryl sulfate, steareth-20, stearyl alcohol, trisodium EDTA, water.

Fragrance in all except Sensitive Skin Formula.

Indications: Regular, Sunscreen Formula and Sensitive Skin Formula: Indicated for helping fade darkened skin areas including age spots, liver spots, freckles and melasma on the face, hands, legs and body and when used as directed helps prevent their recurrence. Facial with Sunscreen: Specially designed to help fade darkened skin areas including age spots, liver spots, freckles and melasma on the face and when used as directed helps prevent their recurrence. It has emollients to help moisturize while it lightens, so it makes an excellent night cream as well.

Actions: Esotérica Medicated helps bleach and lighten hyperpigmented skin.

Continued on next page

SmithKline Beecham—Cont.

Contraindications: Should not be used by persons with known sensitivity to hydroquinone.

Warnings: Do not use if skin is irritated. Some individuals may be sensitive to the active ingredient(s) in this cream. Discontinue use if irritation appears. Avoid contact with eyes. Excessive exposure to the sun should be avoided. For external use only.
Facial and Sunscreen Formula: Not for use in the prevention of sunburn.

Directions: Apply Esotérica to areas you wish to lighten and rub in well. Use cream in the morning and at bedtime for at least six weeks for maximum results. Esotérica is greaseless and may be used under makeup.

How Supplied: 3 oz. plastic jars.

FEOSOL® CAPSULES
Hematinic

Product Information: FEOSOL capsules provide the body with ferrous sulfate, iron in its most efficient form, for iron deficiency and iron-deficiency anemia when the need for such therapy has been determined by a physician.
The special targeted-release capsule is formulated to reduce stomach upset, a common problem with iron.

Directions: *Adults:* 1 or 2 capsules daily or as directed by a physician. *Children:* As directed by a physician.
TAMPER-RESISTANT PACKAGING FEATURES FOR YOUR PROTECTION:

- The carton is protected by a clear overwrap printed with "safety sealed"; do not use if overwrap is missing or broken.
- Each capsule is encased in a plastic cell with a foil back; do not use if cell or foil is broken.
- Each FEOSOL capsule is protected by a red Perma-Seal™ band which bonds the two capsule halves together; do not use if capsule is broken or band is missing or broken.
- A package insert is provided for information on tamper-resistant packaging.

Warnings: Do not exceed recommended dosage. The treatment of any anemic condition should be under the advice and supervision of a physician. Iron-containing medication may occasionally cause constipation or diarrhea. Since oral iron products interfere with absorption of oral tetracycline antibiotics, these products should not be taken within two hours of each other. This package is child-safe; however, keep this and all drugs out of reach of children. In case of accidental overdose, seek professional assistance or contact a poison control center immediately. As with any drug, if you are pregnant or nursing a baby, seek the advice of a health professional before using this product.
Store at controlled room temperature (59°–86°F.).

Formula: Active Ingredients: Each capsule contains 159 mg. of dried ferrous sulfate USP (50 mg. of elemental iron), equivalent to 250 mg. of ferrous sulfate USP. **Inactive Ingredients (listed for individuals with specific allergies):** Benzyl Alcohol, Cetylpyridinium Chloride, D&C Red 33, Yellow 10, FD&C Blue 1, D&C Red #7, Red 40, Gelatin, Glyceryl Stearates, Iron Oxide, Polyethylene Glycol, Povidone, Sodium Lauryl Sulfate, Starch, Sucrose, White Wax and trace amounts of other inactive ingredients.

How Supplied: Packages of 30 and 60 capsules, bottles of 500; in Single Unit Packages of 100 capsules (intended for institutional use only).
Also available in Tablets and Elixir.
Note: There are other FEOSOL products. Make sure this is the one you are interested in.

Shown in Product Identification Section, page 432

FEOSOL® ELIXIR
Hematinic

Product Information: FEOSOL Elixir, an unusually palatable iron elixir, provides the body with ferrous sulfate—iron in its most efficient form. The standard elixir for simple iron deficiency and iron-deficiency anemia when the need for such therapy has been determined by a physician.

Directions: Adults: 1 to 2 teaspoonfuls three times daily. Children: ½ to 1 teaspoonful three times daily preferably between meals. Infants: as directed by physician. Mix with water or fruit juice to avoid temporary staining of teeth; do not mix with milk or wine-based vehicles.

TAMPER-RESISTANT PACKAGE FEATURE: Imprinted seal around top of bottle; do not use if seal is missing.

Warning: The treatment of any anemic condition should be under the advice and supervision of a physician. Since oral iron products interfere with absorption of oral tetracycline antibiotics, these products should not be taken within two hours of each other. Occasional gastrointestinal discomfort (such as nausea) may be minimized by taking with meals and by beginning with one teaspoonful the first day, two the second, etc. until the recommended dosage is reached. Iron-containing medication may occasionally cause constipation or diarrhea, and liquids may cause temporary staining of the teeth (this is less likely when diluted). Keep this and all drugs out of reach of children. In case of accidental overdose, seek professional assistance or contact a poison control center immediately.
As with any drug, if you are pregnant or nursing a baby, seek the advice of a health professional before using this product.
Store at controlled room temperature (59°–86°F.).

Formula: Each 5 ml. (1 teaspoonful) contains ferrous sulfate USP, 220 mg. (44 mg. of elemental iron); alcohol, 5%. **Inactive Ingredients (listed for individuals with specific allergies):** Citric Acid, FD&C Yellow 6 (Sunset Yellow) as a color additive, Flavors, Glucose, Saccharin Sodium, Sucrose, Purified Water.

How Supplied: A clear orange liquid in 16 fl. oz. bottles.
Also available in Tablets and Capsules.

Note: There are other FEOSOL products. Make sure this is the one you are interested in.

Shown in Product Identification Section, page 432

FEOSOL® TABLETS
Hematinic

Product Information: FEOSOL Tablets provide the body with ferrous sulfate, iron in its most efficient form, for iron deficiency and iron-deficiency anemia when the need for such therapy has been determined by a physician. The distinctive triangular-shaped tablet has a coating to prevent oxidation and improve palatability.

Directions: *Adults*—one tablet 3 to 4 times daily after meals and upon retiring or as directed by a physician. *Children 6 to 12 years*—one tablet three times a day after meals. *Children under 6 and infants*—use Feosol® Elixir.
TAMPER-RESISTANT PACKAGE FEATURES FOR YOUR PROTECTION:

- The carton has been sealed at the factory with a clear overwrap printed with "safety sealed."
- Bottle has imprinted "SKCP" seal under cap.
- FEOSOL Tablets are triangular shaped (see product illustration printed on carton).
- **DO NOT USE THIS PRODUCT IF ANY OF THESE TAMPER-RESISTANT FEATURES ARE MISSING OR BROKEN.**

Comments or Questions? Call Toll-Free 800-245-1040 Weekdays.

Warning: Do not exceed recommended dosage. The treatment of any anemic condition should be under the advice and supervision of a physician. Since oral iron products interfere with absorption of oral tetracycline antibiotics, these products should not be taken within two hours of each other.
Occasional gastrointestinal discomfort (such as nausea) may be minimized by taking with meals and by beginning with one tablet the first day, two the second, etc. until the recommended dosage is reached. Iron-containing medication may occasionally cause constipation or diarrhea.
Keep this and all drugs out of reach of children. In case of accidental overdose, seek professional assistance or contact a poison control center immediately.
As with any drug, if you are pregnant or nursing a baby, seek the advice of a health professional before using this product.

Store at controlled room temperature (59°–86°F.).

Formula: Active Ingredients: Each tablet contains 200 mg. of dried ferrous sulfate USP (65 mg. of elemental iron), equivalent to 325 mg. (5 grains) of ferrous sulfate USP. **Inactive Ingredients (listed for individuals with specific allergies):** Calcium Sulfate, D&C Yellow 10, FD&C Blue 2, Glucose, Hydroxypropyl Methylcellulose, Mineral Oil, Polyethylene Glycol, Sodium Lauryl Sulfate, Starch, Stearic Acid, Talc, Titanium Dioxide, and trace amounts of other inactive ingredients.

How Supplied: Bottles of 100 and 1000 tablets; in Single Unit Packages of 100 tablets (intended for institutional use only).
Also available in Capsules and Elixir.

Note: There are other FEOSOL products. Make sure this is the one you are interested in.

Shown in Product Identification Section, page 432

GERITOL COMPLETE™ Tablets

[jer 'e-tol]

The High Iron Multi-Vitamin/Mineral

Active Ingredients (Per Tablet): Vitamin A (6000 IU as Beta Carotene); Vitamin E (30 IU); Vitamin C (60 mg.); Folic Acid (400 mcg.); Vitamin B_1 (1.5 mg.); Vitamin B_2 (1.7 mg.); Niacin (20 mg.); Vitamin B_6 (2 mg.); Vitamin B_{12} (6 mcg.); Vitamin D (400 IU); Biotin (45 mcg.); Pantothenic Acid (10 mg.); Vitamin K (25 mcg.); Calcium (162 mg.); Phosphorus (125 mg.); Iodine (150 mcg.); Iron (50 mg.); Magnesium (100 mg.); Copper (2 mg.); Manganese (2.5 mg.); Potassium (37.5 mg.); Chloride (34 mg.); Chromium (15 mcg.); Molybdenum (15 mcg.); Selenium (15 mcg.); Zinc (15 mg.); Nickel (5 mcg.); Silicon (80 mcg.); Tin (10 mcg); Vanadium (10 mcg).

Inactive Ingredients: Carnauba wax, Crospovidone, Flavors, Gelatin, Glycerides of Stearic and Palmitic acids, Hydroxypropyl cellulose, Hydroxypropyl methylcellulose, Magnesium stearate, Microcrystalline cellulose, Polyethylene glycol, Silicon dioxide, Stearic acid, White wax, FD&C Red #40, FD&C Blue #2, FD&C Yellow #6, Titanium dioxide.

Indications: For use as a dietary supplement.

Actions: Help treat and prevent iron deficiency.

Warnings: Keep out of reach of children.

Precaution: Alcoholics and individuals with chronic liver or pancreatic disease may have enhanced iron absorption with the potential for iron overload.
NOTE: Unabsorbed iron may cause some darkening of the stool.

Symptoms and Treatment of Oral Overdose: Toxicity and symptoms are primarily due to iron overdose. Abdominal pain, nausea, vomiting and diarrhea may occur, with possible subsequent acidosis and cardiovascular collapse with severe poisoning. If an overdose is suspected, immediately seek professional assistance by contacting your physician, the local poison control center, or the Rocky Mt. Poison Control Center at 303-592-1710 (Collect), 24 hours a day.

Dosage and Administration (Adults): One (1) tablet daily after mealtime.

How Supplied: Bottles of 14, 40, 100, and 180 tablets.

GERITOL EXTEND™ Tablets or Caplets

Nutritional Supplement

Active Ingredients (per tablet); Vitamin A (3333 IU, including 1250 IU from Beta Carotene); Vitamin D (200 IU); Vitamin E (15 IU); Vitamin C (60 mg); Folic Acid (0.2 mg); Vitamin B_1 (1.2 mg); Vitamin B_2 (1.4 mg); Niacin (15 mg); Vitamin B_6 (2.0 mg); Vitamin B_{12} (2 mcg); Vitamin K (80 mcg); Calcium (130 mg); Phosphorus (100 mg); Magnesium (35 mg); Zinc (15 mg); Iodine (150 mcg); Iron (10 mg); Selenium (70 mcg)

Inactive Ingredients: Carnauba Wax, Croscarmelose Sodium, Flavors, Gelatin, Glycerides of Stearic and Palmitic Acids, Hydroxypropyl Methylcellulose, Magnesium Stearate, Microcrystalline Cellulose, Polyethylene Glycol, Silicon Dioxide, Stearic Acid, White Wax, FD&C Red #40, FD&C Blue #2, Titanium Dioxide.

Indications: For use as a dietary supplement. Recommended for active adults over 50.

Actions: Help treat and prevent iron deficiency.

Warnings: Keep out of reach of children.

Precaution: Alcoholics and individuals with chronic liver or pancreatic disease may have enhanced iron absorption with the potential for iron overload.
NOTE: Unabsorbed iron may cause some darkening of the stool.

Symptoms and Treatment of Oral Overdose: Toxicity and symptoms are primarily due to iron overdose. Abdominal pain, nausea, vomiting, and diarrhea may occur with possible subsequent acidosis and cardiovascular collapse with severe poisoning. If an overdose is suspected, immediately seek professional assistance by contacting your physician, the local poison control center, or the Rocky Mountain Poison Control Center at 303-592-1710 (collect), 24 hours a day.

Dosage and Administration (Adults 50+): One (1) tablet/caplet daily after mealtime.

How Supplied: Bottles of 40 and 100 tablets or caplets in blister-pack cartons.

GERITOL® Liquid

[jer 'e-tol]

High Potency Iron & Vitamin Tonic

Active Ingredients Per Dose (½ fluid ounce): Iron (as ferric ammonium citrate) 50 mg; Thiamine (B_1) 2.5 mg; Riboflavin (B_2) 2.5 mg; Niacinamide 50 mg; Panthenol 2 mg; Pyridoxine (B_6) 0.5 mg; Cyanocobalamin (B_{12}) 0.75 mcg; Methionine 25 mg; Choline Bitartrate 50 mg.

Inactive Ingredients: Alcohol, Benzoic acid, Caramel color, Citric acid, Invert sugar, Sucrose, Water, Flavors.

Indications: For use as a dietary supplement.

Actions: Help treat and prevent iron deficiency.

Warnings: Keep out of reach of children.

Precaution: Alcohol accelerates absorption of ferric iron. Alcoholics and individuals with chronic liver or pancreatic disease may have enhanced iron absorption with the potential for iron overload.
NOTE: Unabsorbed iron may cause some darkening of the stool.

Symptoms and Treatment of Oral Overdose: Toxicity and symptoms are primarily due to iron overdose. Abdominal pain, nausea, vomiting and diarrhea may occur, with possible subsequent acidosis and cardiovascular collapse with severe poisoning. If an overdose is suspected, immediately seek professional assistance by contacting your physician, the local poison control center, or the Rocky Mt. Poison Control Center at 303-592-1710 (Collect), 24 hours a day.

Dosage and Administration (Adults): As an iron supplement and for normal menstrual needs: One (1) tablespoonful (0.5 fl. oz.) daily at mealtime. For iron deficiency: One (1) tablespoonful (0.5 fl. oz.) three times daily at mealtime or as directed by a physician.

How Supplied: Bottles of 4 oz., and 12 oz.

7001M
11/14/83

MASSENGILL®

Baby Powder Soft Cloth Towelette
Unscented Soft Cloth Towelette

Inactive Ingredients: Baby Powder: Water, Lactic Acid, Sodium Lactate, Potassium Sorbate, Octoxynol-9, Disodium EDTA, Cetylpyridinium Chloride, and Fragrance. Unscented: Water, Octoxynol-9, Lactic Acid, Sodium Lactate, Potassium Sorbate, Disodium EDTA, and Cetylpyridinium Chloride.

Indications: For cleansing and refreshing the external vaginal area.

Actions: Massengill Soft Cloth Towelettes safely cleanse the external vaginal area. The towelette delivery system makes the application soft and gentle.

Warnings: For external use only. Avoid contact with eyes.

Directions: Remove towelette from foil packet, unfold, and gently wipe.

Continued on next page

SmithKline Beecham—Cont.

Throw away towelette after it has been used once.

How Supplied: Sixteen individually wrapped, disposable towelettes per carton.

MASSENGILL®
Disposable Douches
MASSENGILL®
Liquid Concentrate
MASSENGILL® Powder

Ingredients:
DISPOSABLES: Vinegar & Water-Extra Mild—Water and Vinegar.
Vinegar & Water-Extra Cleansing—Water, Vinegar, Cetylpyridinium Chloride, Diazolidinyl Urea, Disodium EDTA.
Belle-Mai—Water, SD Alcohol 40, Lactic Acid, Sodium Lactate, Octoxynol-9, Cetylpyridinium Chloride, Propylene Glycol (and) Diazolidinyl Urea (and) Methyl Paraben (and) Propyl Paraben, Disodium EDTA, Fragrance, FD&C Blue #1.
Country Flowers—Water, SD Alcohol 40, Lactic Acid, Sodium Lactate, Octoxynol-9, Cetylpyridinium Chloride, Propylene Glycol (and) Diazolidinyl Urea (and) Methyl Paraben (and) Propyl Paraben, Disodium EDTA, Fragrance, D&C Red #28, FD&C Blue #1.
Fresh Mountain Breeze—Water, SD Alcohol 40, Lactic Acid, Sodium Lactate, Octoxynol-9, Cetylpyridinium Chloride, Propylene Glycol (and) Diazolidinyl Urea (and) Methyl Paraben (and) Propyl Paraben, Disodium EDTA, Fragrance, D&C Yellow #10, FD&C Blue #1.
Unscented—Water, SD Alcohol 40, Lactic Acid, Sodium Lactate, Octoxynol-9, Cetylpyridinium Chloride, Propylene Glycol (and) Diazolidinyl Urea (and) Methyl Paraben (and) Propyl Paraben, Disodium EDTA.
Baking Soda & Water—Sanitized Water, Sodium Bicarbonate (Baking Soda).
LIQUID CONCENTRATE: Water, SD Alcohol 40, Lactic Acid, Sodium Lactate, Octoxynol-9, Methyl Salicylate, Eucalyptol, Menthol, Thymol, D&C Yellow #10, FD&C Yellow #6.
POWDER: Sodium Chloride, Ammonium alum, PEG-8, Phenol, Methyl Salicylate, Eucalyptus Oil, Menthol, Thymol, D&C Yellow #10, FD&C Yellow #6.
FLORAL POWDER: Sodium Chloride, Ammonium Alum, Octoxynol-9, SD Alcohol 23-A, Fragrance, FD&C Yellow #6.

Indications: Recommended for routine cleansing at the end of menstruation, after use of contraceptive creams or jellies (check the contraceptive package instructions first) or to rinse out the residue of prescribed vaginal medication (as directed by physician).

Actions: The buffered acid solutions of Massengill Douches are valuable adjuncts to specific vaginal therapy following the prescribed use of vaginal medication or contraceptives and in feminine hygiene.

Directions:
DISPOSABLES: Twist off flat, wing-shaped tab from bottle containing premixed solution, attach nozzle supplied and use. After douching, simply throw away bottle and nozzle.
LIQUID CONCENTRATE: Fill cap 3/4 full and pour contents into douche bag containing 1 quart of warm water. Mix thoroughly.
POWDER: Dissolve two rounded teaspoonfuls in a douche bag containing 1 quart of warm water. Mix thoroughly.

Warning: Vaginal cleansing douches should not be used more than twice weekly except on the advice of a physician. If irritation occurs, discontinue use. Consult your physician if you are experiencing any of the following symptoms: unusual vaginal discharge, painful urination, lower abdominal pain, or you or your sex partner has genital sores. Do not douche during pregnancy except under the advice and supervision of your physician. Douching does not prevent pregnancy.
Keep out of reach of children. In case of accidental ingestion, seek professional assistance by contacting your physician, the local poison control center, or the Rocky Mt. Poison Control Center at 303-592-1710 (Collect), 24 hours a day.

How Supplied: Disposable—6 oz. disposable plastic bottle.
Liquid Concentrate—4 oz., 8 oz., plastic bottles.
Powder—4 oz., 8 oz., 16 oz., 22 oz. Packettes—10's, 12's.

MASSENGILL® Medicated Disposable Douche
MASSENGILL® Medicated Liquid Concentrate

Active Ingredient: Cepticin™ (0.30% povidone-iodine).

Indications: For symptomatic relief of minor irritation and itching associated with vaginitis due to *Candida albicans, Trichomonas vaginalis* and *Gardnerella vaginalis.*

Action: Povidone-iodine is widely recognized as an effective broad spectrum microbicide against both gram-negative and gram-positive bacteria, fungi, yeasts and protozoa. While remaining active in the presence of blood, serum or bodily secretions, it possesses virtually none of the irritating properties of iodine.

Warnings: If symptoms persist after seven days of use, or if redness, swelling or pain develop during treatment, consult a physician. Women with iodine-sensitivity should not use this product. Women may douche during menstruation if they douche gently. Do not douche during pregnancy, or while nursing, unless directed by a physician. Douching does not prevent pregnancy. Consult your physician if you are experiencing any of the following symptoms: unusual vaginal discharge, painful urination, lower abdominal pain, or you or your sex partner has genital sores. Keep out of reach of children. In case of accidental ingestion, seek professional assistance by contacting your physician, the local poison control center, or the Rocky Mt. Poison Control Center at 303-592-1710 (Collect), 24 hours a day.

Dosage and Administration: Disposables: Dosage is provided as a single-unit concentrate to be added to 6 oz. of sanitized water supplied in a disposable bottle. A specially designed nozzle is provided. After use, the unit is discarded. Use one bottle daily for seven days. Even if symptoms are relieved earlier, treatment should be continued for the full seven days. Liquid Concentrate: The product is provided in concentrate form, to be mixed with water and administered using a douche bag or bulb syringe.
Fill cap and pour contents into 1 quart of warm water. Mix thoroughly. Use once daily for five days, even though symptoms may be relieved earlier. For maximum relief, use for seven days.

How Supplied: Disposables: 6 oz. bottle of sanitized water with 0.17 oz. vial of povidone-iodine and nozzle. Liquid Concentrate: 4 oz., 8 oz., plastic bottles.

Shown in Product Identification Section, page 432

MASSENGILL®
Medicated Soft Cloth Towelette

Active Ingredient: Hydrocortisone 0.5%.

Inactive Ingredients: Diazolidinyl Urea, DMDM Hydantoin, Isopropyl Myristate, Methylparaben, Polysorbate 60, Propylene Glycol, Propylparaben, Sorbitan Stearate, Steareth-2, Water.

Indications: For temporary, soothing relief of minor external feminine itching or other itching associated with minor skin irritations, inflammation, and rashes.

Actions: Adults and Children two years of age and older—apply to the affected area not more than three to four times daily. Children under two years of age—consult a physician before using.

Warning: For external use only. Avoid contact with eyes. If condition worsens, symptoms persist for more than seven days, or symptoms recur within a few days, discontinue use and consult a physician. If experiencing a vaginal discharge, see a physician. Keep this and all drugs out of the reach of children. As with any drug, if you are pregnant or nursing a baby, seek the advice of a health professional before using this product. In case of accidental ingestion, seek professional assistance or contact a Poison Control Center immediately.

Directions: Remove towelette from foil packet, unfold, and gently wipe. Throw away towelette after it has been used once.

How Supplied: Ten individually wrapped, disposable towelettes per carton.

NATURE'S REMEDY®
Natural Vegetable Laxative

Active Ingredients: Cascara sagrada 150 mg, aloe 100 mg.

Inactive Ingredients: Calcium stearate, cellulose, lactose, coating, colors (contains FD&C Yellow No. 6).

Indications: For gentle, overnight relief of constipation.

Actions: Nature's Remedy has two natural active ingredients that give gentle, overnight relief of constipation. These ingredients, cascara sagrada and aloe, gently stimulate the body's natural function.

Warnings: Do not take any laxative when nausea, vomiting, abdominal pain, or other symptoms of appendicitis are present. Frequent or prolonged use of laxatives may result in dependence on them. If pregnant or nursing, consult your physician before using this or any medicine.

Symptoms and Treatment of Oral Overdosage: If an overdose is suspected, immediately seek professional assistance by contacting your physician, local poison control center, or the Rocky Mountain Poison Control Center at 303-592-1710 (Collect) 24 hours a day.

Dosage and Administration: Adults, swallow two tablets daily along with a full glass of water; children (8–15 yrs.), one tablet daily; or as directed by a physician.

How Supplied: Beige, film-coated tablets with foil-backed blister packaging in boxes of 12s, 30s and 60s.

Shown in Product Identification Section, page 432

N'ICE® Sugarless Vitamin C Drops
[nis]

Description: Lemon, Orange—One drop provides: Vitamin C 60 mg. (100% U.S. Recommended Daily Allowance). Grape—One drop provides: Vitamin C 45 mg. (100% Children's U.S. Recommended Dietary Allowance).

Ingredients: Lemon—Sorbitol, Ascorbic Acid, Citric Acid, Natural and Artificial Flavoring, Menthol, and Artificial Color (including Yellow 5). Orange—Sorbitol, Ascorbic Acid, Natural and Artificial Flavoring, Citric Acid, Sodium Citrate, Menthol, and Artificial Color (including Yellow 6). Grape—Sorbitol, Ascorbic Acid, Natural and Artificial Flavoring, Tartaric Acid, Propylene Glycol, Menthol, and Artificial Color.

Indication: Dietary Supplementation.

How Supplied: Available in packages of 2 and 16 drops.

Shown in Product Identification Section, page 432

N'ICE® Medicated Sugarless Sore Throat and Cough Lozenges
[nis]

Active Ingredient: Cherry—Each lozenge contains 5.0 mg. menthol in a sorbitol base. Citrus—Each lozenge contains 5.0 mg. menthol in a sorbitol base. Menthol Eucalyptus—Each lozenge contains 5.0 mg. menthol in a sorbitol base. Menthol Mint—Each lozenge contains 5.0 mg. menthol in a sorbitol base. Children's Berry—Each lozenge contains 3.0 mg. menthol in a sorbitol base.

Inactive Ingredients: Cherry—Flavors, Red 33, Sorbitol, Tartaric Acid, Yellow 6, Citrus—Citric Acid, Flavors, Saccharin Sodium, Sodium Citrate, Sorbitol, Yellow 10. Menthol Eucalyptus—Citric Acid, Flavors, Sorbitol. Menthol Mint—Blue 1, Flavor, Hydrogenated Glucose Syrup, Sorbitol, Yellow 10. Children's Berry—Citric Acid, Flavors, Red 33, Sodium Citrate, Sorbitol.

Indications: Temporarily suppresses cough due to minor throat and bronchial irritation associated with a cold or inhaled irritants. Temporarily relieves minor sore throat pain.

Warnings: Do not administer to children under six years of age unless directed by a physician. Severe or persistent sore throat or sore throat accompanied by high fever, headache, nausea, and vomiting may be serious. Consult a physician in such case, or if sore throat persists for more than two days. A persistent cough may be a sign of a serious condition. If cough persists for more than one week, tends to recur, or is accompanied by fever, rash, or persistent headache, consult a physician. Do not take this product for persistent or chronic cough such as occurs with smoking, asthma, emphysema, or if cough is accompanied by excessive phlegm, unless directed by a physician.
Keep this and all medicines out of the reach of children.

Drug Interaction: No known drug interaction.

Dosage and Administration: Cherry, Citrus, Menthol Eucalyptus, Menthol Mint—Let lozenge dissolve slowly in the mouth. Repeat as needed, up to 10 lozenges per day. Children's Berry—Take two lozenges. Let lozenges dissolve slowly in the mouth. Repeat as needed, up to 10 lozenges per day.

Professional Labeling: For the temporary relief of pain associated with tonsillitis, pharyngitis, throat infections or stomatitis.

How Supplied: Available in packages of 2, 8 and 16 lozenges.

Shown in Product Identification Section, page 432

N'ICE® Sore Throat Spray
[nis]

Active Ingredients: Menthol 0.12%, Glycerin 25%.

Inactive Ingredients: Alcohol, Blue 1, Flavors, Hydrogenated Glucose Syrup, Phosphoric Acid, Poloxamer 338, Saccharin Sodium, Sodium Phosphate Dibasic, Sorbitol, Water.

Indications: For temporary relief of minor pain and protection of irritated areas in sore throat and mouth.

Warnings: If sore throat is severe, persists for more than 2 days, is accompanied by fever, headache, rash, nausea or vomiting, consult a doctor promptly. If sore mouth symptoms do not improve in 7 days, see your dentist or doctor promptly. KEEP THIS AND ALL MEDICINES OUT OF THE REACH OF CHILDREN.

Drug Interaction: No known drug interaction.

Directions: Adults and children 2 years and older: Spray affected area four times. Repeat as needed or as directed by a doctor. Children under 12 should be supervised in the use of this product. Children under 2: consult a doctor.

Professional Labeling: For the temporary relief of pain associated with tonsillitis, pharyngitis, throat infections or stomatitis.

How Supplied: In 6 fl. oz. plastic bottles with sprayer.

OXY ACNE MEDICATIONS
OXY-5® and OXY-10® with SORBOXYL®
Benzoyl peroxide lotion 5% and 10% with silica oil absorber
Vanishing and Tinted Formulas

Description: Active Ingredient: Oxy-5: Benzoyl peroxide 5%. Oxy-10: Benzoyl peroxide 10%.

Inactive Ingredients: Oxy-5 Vanishing: Water, sodium PCA, cetyl alcohol, silica (Sorboxyl®), propylene glycol, citric acid, sodium lauryl sulfate, methylparaben, propylparaben.
Oxy-5 Tinted: Water, titanium dioxide, sodium PCA, cetyl alcohol, silica (Sorboxyl®), iron oxides, propylene glycol, citric acid, sodium lauryl sulfate, stearyl alcohol, methylparaben, propylparaben.
Oxy-10 Vanishing: Water, silica (Sorboxyl®), cetyl alcohol, propylene glycol, citric acid, sodium citrate, sodium lauryl sulfate, methylparaben and propylparaben.
Oxy-10 Tinted: Water, titanium dioxide, silica (Sorboxyl®), cetyl alcohol, glyceryl stearate, propylene glycol, stearic acid, iron oxides, sodium lauryl sulfate, citric acid, sodium citrate, methylparaben, propylparaben.

Indications: Topical medications for the treatment of acne vulgaris.

Action: Provides antibacterial activity against Propionibacterium acnes.

Additional Benefits: Absorbs excess skin oil up to 12 hours. Vanishing formulas are colorless, odorless, greaseless

Continued on next page

SmithKline Beecham—Cont.

lotions that vanish upon application. Tinted formulas are flesh tone, odorless, greaseless lotions that cover up acne pimples while they treat them.

Directions for Use: Wash skin thoroughly and dry well. Shake well before using. Dab on smoothing into oily acne pimple areas of face, neck and body (see Warning). Apply once a day initially, then two or three times a day, or as directed by a physician.

Warning: Those with known sensitivity to benzoyl peroxide or especially sensitive skin should not use this medication. Before using, determine if you are sensitive by applying to a small affected area once a day for two days. Follow label instructions and continue use if no discomfort occurs. If, during treatment, irritation, redness, burning, itching or excessive drying and peeling occur, reduce dosage or frequency of use. Discontinue if irritation is severe and if it persists, consult a doctor. Keep away from eyes, lips, and mouth. Using other topical acne medications at the same time or immediately following use of this product may increase dryness or irritation of the skin. If this occurs, only one medication should be used unless directed by a doctor. Keep this and all drugs out of the reach of children. This product may bleach hair or dyed fabrics. Keep tightly closed. Store at room temperature, avoid excessive heat. For external use only.

Symptoms and Treatment of Ingestion: These symptoms are based upon medical judgment, not on actual experience. Theoretically, ingestion of very large amounts may cause nausea, vomiting, abdominal discomfort, and diarrhea. If an oral overdose is suspected, contact a physician, the local poison control center, or the Rocky Mountain Poison Control Center at 303-592-1710 (Collect) 24 hours a day.

How Supplied: 1 fl. oz. plastic bottles.

Shown in Product Identification Section, page 432

OXY CLEAN®
Medicated Cleanser, Medicated Soap, and Lathering Facial Scrub

Active Ingredient: Oxy Clean® Medicated Cleanser: Salicylic Acid* 0.5%.
Oxy Clean® Medicated Soap: Triclosan 1.0%.
Oxy Clean® Lathering Facial Scrub: None.
*Salicylic Acid (2-Hydroxybenzoic Acid).

Inactive Ingredients:
Oxy Clean® Medicated Cleanser: Citric acid, menthol, propylene glycol, sodium lauryl sulfate, water. Also contains SD Alcohol 40B 40%.
Oxy Clean® Lathering Facial Scrub: Fragrance, glyceryl stearate (and) PEG-100 stearate, Oleth-20, potassium sorbate, potassium undecylenoyl hydrolyzed animal protein, silica, sodium borate, sodium lauryl sulfoacetate, sodium laureth sulfate, sodium methyl cocoyl taurate, triclosan, water.
Oxy Clean Medicated Soap: Bentonite, cocoamphodipropionate, fragrance, glycerin, iron oxides, magnesium silicate, sodium borohydride, sodium chloride, sodium cocoate, sodium tallowate, talc, tetrasodium EDTA, titanium dioxide.

Indications: These skin care products are useful for opening plugged pores and for removing excess dirt and oil. Also helps remove and prevent blackheads.

Additional Benefits: When used regularly cleanses acne-prone skin and removes dirt, grime and excess skin oil. For a complete anti-acne program, after using Oxy Clean® follow use with Oxy-5® Tinted and Vanishing, or Oxy-10® Tinted and Vanishing acne pimple medications.

Warning (Oxy Clean® Medicated Cleanser and Soap): For external use only. If skin irritation develops, discontinue use and consult a physician. May be irritating to eyes or mucous membranes. If contact occurs, flush thoroughly with water. Using other topical acne medications at the same time or immediately following use of this product may increase dryness or irritation of the skin. If this occurs, only one medication should be used unless directed by a doctor. Keep this and all drugs out of reach of children. Store at room temperature. Keep away from flame, fire and heat.

Warning (Oxy Clean Medicated Soap): Do not use this product on infants under six months of age.

Warning (Oxy Clean® Lathering Facial Scrub): Avoid contact with eyes. If particles get into eyes, flush thoroughly with water and avoid rubbing eyes. Discontinue use if skin irritation or excessive dryness develops. Not to be used on infants or children under 3 years of age. Do not use on inflamed skin. Keep out of reach of children.

Symptoms and Treatment of Ingestion: If large amounts are ingested, nausea, vomiting, or gastrointestinal irritation may develop. If an oral overdose is suspected, contact a physician, the local poison control center, or the Rocky Mountain Poison Control Center at 303-592-1710 (Collect) 24 hours a day.

Dosage and Administration: See labeling instructions for use.

How Supplied:
Medicated Liquid Cleanser—4 fl. oz.
Medicated Soap—3.25 oz. soap bar.
Lathering Facial Scrub—2.65 oz. Plastic Tube.

Shown in Product Identification Section, page 433

OXY CLEAN® MEDICATED PADS
Regular, Sensitive Skin, and Maximum Strength

Active Ingredient:
Oxy Clean® Medicated Pads Regular Strength: Salicylic Acid* 0.5%.
Oxy Clean® Medicated Pads Sensitive Skin: Salicylic Acid* 0.5%.
Oxy Clean® Medicated Pads Maximum Strength: Salicylic Acid* 2.0%.
*Salicylic Acid (2-Hydroxybenzoic Acid).

Inactive Ingredients:
Oxy Clean® Medicated Pads Regular Strength: Citric acid, fragrance, menthol, propylene glycol, sodium lauryl sulfate, water. Also contains SD Alcohol 40B 40%.
Oxy Clean® Medicated Pads Sensitive Skin: Dimethicone copolyol, disodium lauryl sulfosuccinate, fragrance, menthol, PEG-4, sodium lauroyl sarcosinate, sodium PCA, trisodium EDTA, water. Also contains SD Alcohol 40B 22%.
Oxy Clean® Medicated Pads Maximum Strength: Citric acid, fragrance, menthol, PEG-8, propylene glycol, sodium lauryl sulfate, water. Also contains SD Alcohol 40B 50%.

Indications: These medicated pad products are useful for opening plugged pores and for removing excess dirt and oil. Also helps remove and prevent blackheads.

Additional Benefits: When used regularly cleanses acne-prone skin and removes dirt, grime and excess skin oil. For a complete anti-acne program, after using Oxy Clean® follow use with Oxy-5® Tinted and Vanishing, or Oxy-10® Tinted and Vanishing acne pimple medications.

Warning: For external use only. If skin irritation develops, discontinue use and consult a physician. May be irritating to eyes or mucous membranes. If contact occurs, flush thoroughly with water. Using other topical acne medications at the same time or immediately following use of this product may increase dryness or irritation of the skin. If this occurs, only one medication should be used unless directed by a doctor. Keep this and all drugs out of reach of children. Store at room temperature. Keep away from flame, fire and heat.

Symptoms and Treatment of Ingestion: If large amounts are ingested, nausea, vomiting, or gastrointestinal irritation may develop. If an oral overdose is suspected, contact a physician, the local poison control center, or the Rocky Mountain Poison Control Center at 303-592-1710 (Collect) 24 hours a day.

Dosage and Administration: See labeling instructions for use.

How Supplied:
Medicated Pads Regular Strength—Plastic Jar/50 pads or 90 pads
Medicated Pads Sensitive Skin—Plastic Jar/50 pads or 90 pads
Medicated Pads Maximum Strength—Plastic Jar/50 pads or 90 pads

Shown in Product Identification Section, page 432

SINE-OFF

Each tablet/ caplet contains:	SINE-OFF Tablets-Aspirin Formula	SINE-OFF Maximum Strength Allergy/Sinus Formula Caplets	SINE-OFF Maximum Strength No Drowsiness Formula Caplets
Chlorpheniramine maleate	2.0 mg	2.0 mg	—
Phenylpropanolamine HCl	12.5 mg	—	—
Aspirin	325.0 mg	—	—
Acetaminophen	—	500.0 mg	500.0 mg
Pseudoephedrine HCl	—	30.0 mg	30.0 mg

OXY NIGHT WATCH™
Maximum Strength and Sensitive Skin Formulas

Active Ingredient:
Oxy Night Watch™ Maximum Strength: Salicylic Acid (2-Hydroxybenzoic Acid) 2.0%.
Oxy Night Watch™ Sensitive Skin: Salicylic Acid (2-Hydroxybenzoic Acid) 1.0%.

Inactive Ingredients:
Water, cetyl alcohol, silica (Sorboxyl®), propylene glycol, sodium lauryl sulfate, stearyl alcohol, methylparaben, disodium EDTA and propylparaben.

Indications: These medicated skin products help unplug clogged pores and penetrate pores to treat pimples and blackheads before they form.

Additional Benefits: Absorbs excess skin oil up to 12 hours. Stays on all night to treat and prevent pimples and blackheads.

Directions for Use: At bedtime, wash face gently using a non-abrasive soap. Rinse thoroughly and pat dry. Shake tube well. Squeeze out a small amount of lotion. Smooth a thin layer evenly over entire face, avoiding eyes, lips and mouth. Do not wash off. Oxy Night Watch™ works best when left on overnight. The next morning, wash face and pat dry. If you have dry skin, apply a non-oily moisturizer.

Warning: For external use only. If skin irritation develops, discontinue use and consult a physician. Using other topical acne medications at the same time or immediately following use of this product may increase dryness or irritation of the skin. If this occurs, only one medication should be used unless directed by a doctor.

How Supplied: 2.0 oz. plastic tubes.

Shown in Product Identification Section, page 433

OXY 10® DAILY FACE WASH

Active Ingredient: Benzoyl peroxide 10%.

Inactive Ingredients: Water, sodium cocoyl isethionate, cocamidopropyl betaine, xanthan gum, sodium lauroyl sarcosinate, sodium citrate, citric acid, diazolidinyl urea, methylparaben, propylparaben.

Indications: Antibacterial skin wash used as an aid in the treatment of acne vulgaris.

Actions: Promotes antibacterial activity against Propionibacterium acnes.

Additional Benefits: When used instead of regular soap, cleanses acne-prone skin and removes dirt, grime and excess skin oil.
For a complete anti-acne program, follow Oxy 10® Daily Face Wash with Oxy-5® acne-pimple medication. Or for stubborn acne, use Oxy-10® maximum strength acne-pimple medication.

Contraindications: Should not be used by persons with known sensitivity to benzoyl peroxide.

Warning: Persons with sensitive skin or known allergy to benzoyl peroxide should not use this medication. First test on a small affected area by applying this product as directed once a day for two days. If discomforting irritation or undue dryness occurs during treatment, reduce frequency of use or dosage. If excessive itching, redness, burning, swelling, irritation or dryness occurs, discontinue use and consult a physician. Using other topical acne medications at the same time or immediately following use of this product may increase dryness or irritation of the skin. If this occurs, only one medication should be used unless directed by a doctor. Avoid contact with eyes, lips and mouth. May bleach hair or dyed fabrics. **For external use only.**

Directions: Shake well. Wet area to be washed. Apply Oxy 10® Daily Face Wash massaging gently for 1 to 2 minutes. Rinse thoroughly. Use 2 to 3 times daily or as directed by physician.

Symptoms and Treatment of Ingestion: These symptoms are based upon medical judgment, not on actual experience. Theoretically, ingestion of very large amounts may cause nausea, vomiting, abdominal discomfort, and diarrhea. If an oral overdose is suspected, contact a physician, the local poison control center, or the Rocky Mountain Poison Control Center at 303-592-1710 (Collect) 24 hours a day.

How supplied: 4 fl. oz. plastic bottles.

Shown in Product Identification Section, page 433

SINE–OFF® Maximum Strength Allergy/Sinus Formula Caplets

Composition:
[See table above.]

Product Information: SINE-OFF Maximum Strength Allergy/Sinus Formula provides maximum strength relief from upper respiratory allergy, hay fever and sinusitis symptoms. This formula contains acetaminophen, a non-aspirin pain reliever.

Product Benefits: Relieves itchy, watery eyes, sneezing, runny nose and post-nasal drip • Eases headache pain and pressure • Promotes sinus drainage • Shrinks swollen membranes to relieve congestion.

Directions: Adults and children over 12 years of age: 2 caplets every 6 hours, not to exceed 8 caplets in any 24-hour period. Children under 12 should use only as directed by a physician.

TAMPER-RESISTANT PACKAGING FEATURES FOR YOUR PROTECTION:

- Each caplet is encased in a clear plastic cell with a foil back.
- The name SINE-OFF appears on each caplet (see product illustration on front of carton).
- **DO NOT USE THIS PRODUCT IF ANY OF THESE TAMPER-RESISTANT FEATURES ARE MISSING OR BROKEN.**

Comments or Questions? Call Toll-Free 800-245-1040 Weekdays.

Warnings: Do not exceed recommended dosage. If symptoms do not improve within 7 days, consult a physician before continuing use. Individuals being treated for depression, high blood pressure, asthma, heart disease, diabetes, thyroid disease, glaucoma or difficulty urinating due to an enlarged prostate gland should use only as directed by a physician. Do not take this product if you are taking sedatives or tranquilizers. Avoid alcoholic beverages while taking this product. Do not drive or operate heavy machinery. May cause drowsiness. Stop use if dizziness, sleeplessness or nervousness occurs. May cause excitability, especially in children. **This package is child-safe;** however, keep this and all drugs out of reach of children. In case of accidental overdose, seek professional assistance or contact a poison control center immediately. As with any drug, if you are pregnant or nursing a baby, seek the advice of a health professional before using this product.
Store at controlled room temperature (59°–86°F.).

Formula: Active Ingredients: Each caplet contains Chlorpheniramine Maleate 2 mg., Pseudoephedrine Hydrochloride 30 mg., Acetaminophen 500 mg. *(500 mg. is a non-standard dosage of acetaminophen as compared to the standard of 325 mg.).* **Inactive Ingredients (listed for individuals with specific aller-**

Continued on next page

SmithKline Beecham—Cont.

gies): Blue 2, Cellulose, Crospovidone, Hydroxypropyl Methylcellulose, Magnesium Stearate, Polyethylene Glycol, Povidone, Red 30, Starch, Titanium Dioxide, Yellow 10, and trace amounts of other inactive ingredients.

How Supplied: Consumer packages of 24 caplets.

Note: There are other SINE-OFF products. Make sure this is the one you are interested in.

Also Available: SINE-OFF® Sinus Medicine Tablets with Aspirin in 24's, 48's, 100's. SINE-OFF® Maximum Strength No Drowsiness Formula Caplets 24's.

Shown in Product Identification Section, page 433

SINE-OFF® Maximum Strength No Drowsiness Formula Caplets

Composition: [See table page 721]

Product Information: SINE-OFF Maximum Strength No Drowsiness Formula provides maximum strength relief from headache and sinus pain. Relieves pressure and congestion due to sinusitis, allergic sinusitis or the common cold. This formula contains acetaminophen, a non-aspirin pain reliever.

NO ANTIHISTAMINE DROWSINESS

Product Benefits: Eases headache, pain and pressure • Promotes sinus drainage • Shrinks swollen membranes to relieve congestion.

Directions: Adults and children over 12 years of age: 2 caplets every 6 hours, not to exceed 8 caplets in any 24-hour period. Children under 12 should use only as directed by physician.

TAMPER-RESISTANT PACKAGE FEATURES FOR YOUR PROTECTION:

- Each caplet is encased in a clear plastic cell with a foil back.
- The name SINE-OFF appears on each caplet (see product illustration on front of carton).
- **DO NOT USE THIS PRODUCT IF ANY OF THESE TAMPER-RESISTANT FEATURES ARE MISSING OR BROKEN.**

Comments or Questions? Call Toll-Free 800-245-1040 Weekdays.

Warnings: Do not exceed recommended dosage. If symptoms do not improve within 7 days, consult a physician before continuing use. Individuals being treated for depression, high blood pressure, heart disease, diabetes, thyroid disease, or difficulty in urination due to enlargement of the prostate gland should use only as directed by a physician. Stop use if dizziness, sleeplessness or nervousness occurs. This package is child-safe; however, keep this and all drugs out of reach of children. In case of accidental overdose, seek professional assistance or contact a poison control center immediately. As with any drug, if you are pregnant or nursing a baby, seek the advice of a health professional before using this product.

Store at controlled room temperature (59°–86°F.).

Formula: Active Ingredients: Each caplet contains: 30 mg. Pseudoephedrine Hydrochloride, 500 mg. Acetaminophen *(500 mg. is a non-standard dosage of acetaminophen, as compared to the standard of 325 mg.).* **Inactive Ingredients (listed for individuals with specific allergies):** Cellulose, Crospovidone, Hydroxypropyl Methylcellulose, Magnesium Stearate, Polyethylene Glycol, Polysorbate 80, Povidone, Red 3, Starch, Titanium Dioxide, Yellow 6 (Sunset Yellow) as a color additive, and trace amounts of other inactive ingredients.

How Supplied: Consumer packages of 24 caplets.

Note: There are other SINE-OFF products. Make sure this is the one you are interested in.

Also Available:
SINE-OFF® Tablets with Aspirin
SINE-OFF® Maximum Strength Allergy/Sinus Formula Caplets

Shown in Product Identification Section, page 433

SINE-OFF® Sinus Medicine Tablets-Aspirin Formula Relieves sinus headache and congestion.

Composition: [See table page 721]

Product Information: SINE-OFF relieves headache, pain, pressure and congestion due to sinusitis, allergic sinusitis, or the common cold.

Product Benefits: Eases headache, pain and pressure • Promotes sinus drainage • Shrinks swollen membranes to relieve congestion • Relieves postnasal drip.

Directions: Adults: 2 tablets every 4 hours, not to exceed 8 tablets in any 24-hour period. Children (6–12) one-half the adult dosage. Children under 6 years should use only as directed by a physician.

TAMPER-RESISTANT PACKAGE FEATURES FOR YOUR PROTECTION:

- Each tablet is encased in a clear plastic cell with a foil back.
- The name SINE-OFF appears on each tablet (see product illustration on front of carton).
- **DO NOT USE THIS PRODUCT IF ANY OF THESE TAMPER-RESISTANT FEATURES ARE MISSING OR BROKEN.**

Comments or Questions? Call Toll-Free 800-245-1040 Weekdays.

Warning: Children and teenagers should not use this medicine for chicken pox or flu symptoms before a doctor is consulted about Reye syndrome, a rare but serious illness reported to be associated with aspirin. Do not exceed recommended dosage. If symptoms do not improve within 7 days, consult a physician before continuing use. Individuals being treated for depression, high blood pressure, asthma, heart disease, diabetes, thyroid disease, glaucoma or enlarged prostate should use only as directed by a physician. Do not take this product if you are taking another medication containing phenylpropanolamine. ☐ Avoid alcoholic beverages while taking this product. Do not drive or operate heavy machinery as this preparation may cause drowsiness. ☐ Stop use if dizziness, sleeplessness or nervousness occurs. ☐ May cause excitability, especially in children. Keep this and all drugs out of reach of children. In case of accidental overdose, seek professional assistance or contact a poison control center immediately. As with any drug, if you are pregnant or nursing a baby, seek the advice of a health professional before using this product. IT IS ESPECIALLY IMPORTANT NOT TO USE ASPIRIN DURING THE LAST 3 MONTHS OF PREGNANCY UNLESS SPECIFICALLY DIRECTED TO DO SO BY A DOCTOR BECAUSE IT MAY CAUSE PROBLEMS IN THE UNBORN CHILD OR COMPLICATIONS DURING DELIVERY.

Store at controlled room temperature (59°–86°F.).

Formula: Active Ingredients: Chlorpheniramine Maleate 2 mg.; Phenylpropanolamine Hydrochloride 12.5 mg. Aspirin 325 mg. **Inactive Ingredients (listed for individuals with specific allergies):** Acacia, Calcium Sulfate, Ethylcellulose, Gelatin, Guar Gum, Polysorbate 80, Silicon Dioxide, Starch, Sucrose, Titanium Dioxide, Yellow 10, Yellow 6 (Sunset Yellow) as a color additive, and trace amounts of other inactive ingredients.

How Supplied: Consumer packages of 24, 48 and 100 tablets.

Note: There are other SINE-OFF products. Make sure this is the one you are interested in.

Also Available: SINE-OFF® Maximum Strength Allergy/Sinus Formula Caplets 24's. SINE-OFF® Maximum Strength No Drowsiness Formula Caplets 24's.

Shown in Product Identification Section, page 433

SOMINEX®

[som 'in-ex]

Active Ingredients: Each tablet contains Diphenhydramine HCl, 25 mg. Each caplet contains Diphenhydramine HCl, 50 mg.

Inactive Ingredients Tablets: Corn starch, dibasic calcium phosphate, magnesium stearate, microcrystalline cellulose, powdered cellulose, silicon dioxide, FD&C Blue #1.

Inactive Ingredients Caplets: Carnauba Wax, corn starch, crospovidone, dibasic calcium phosphate, hydroxypropyl methylcellulose, magnesium stearate, microcrystalline cellulose, polyethylene glycol, Polysorbate 80, powdered cellulose, silicon dioxide, titanium dioxide, white wax, FD&C Blue #1.

Indications: Helps to reduce difficulty falling asleep.

Action: An antihistamine with anticholinergic and sedative effects.

Warnings: Do not give to children under 12 years of age. If sleeplessness persists continuously for more than two weeks, consult your doctor. Insomnia may be a symptom of serious underlying medical illness. Avoid alcoholic beverages while taking this product. Do not take this product if you are taking sedatives or tranquilizers, without first consulting your doctor. Do not take this product if you have asthma, glaucoma, emphysema, chronic pulmonary disease, shortness of breath, difficulty in breathing, or difficulty in urination due to enlargement of the prostate gland unless directed by a doctor. As with any drug, if you are pregnant or nursing a baby, seek the advice of a health professional before using this product. Keep this and all drugs out of the reach of children. In case of accidental overdose, seek professional assistance or contact a poison control center immediately or the Rocky Mountain Poison Control Center at 303-592-1710 (Collect) 24 hours a day.

Drug Interaction: Monoamine oxidase (MAO) inhibitors prolong and intensify the anticholinergic effects of antihistamines. The CNS depressant effect is heightened by alcohol and other CNS depressant drugs.

Symptoms and Treatment of Oral Overdosage: Antihistamine overdosage reactions may vary from central nervous system depression to stimulation. Stimulation is particularly likely in children. Atropine-like signs and symptoms, such as dry mouth, fixed and dilated pupils, flushing, and gastrointestinal symptoms, may also occur.

Dosage and Administration: Take 2 tablets or 1 caplet thirty minutes before bedtime, or as directed by a physician.

How Supplied Tablets: Available in blister packs of 16, 32, and 72.

How Supplied Caplets: Available in blister packs of 8, 16, and 32.

Shown in Product Identification Section, page 433

SOMINEX® Liquid

[som 'in-ex]

Active Ingredients: Each fluid ounce (30 ml.) contains 50 mg. Diphenhydramine HCl. Also contains Alcohol, 10% by volume.

Inactive Ingredients: Citric Acid, Dibasic Sodium Phosphate, Flavors, FD&C Blue No. 1, Glycerin, Polyethylene Glycol, Sodium Saccharin, Sorbitol, Water, Xanthan Gum.

Indications: Helps to reduce difficulty falling asleep.

Actions: An antihistamine with anticholinergic and sedative effects.

Warnings: Do not give to children under 12 years of age. If sleeplessness persists continuously for more than two weeks, consult your doctor. Insomnia may be a symptom of serious underlying medical illness. Avoid alcoholic beverages while taking this product. Do not take this product if you are taking sedatives or tranquilizers, without first consulting your doctor. Do not take this product if you have asthma, glaucoma, emphysema, chronic pulmonary disease, shortness of breath, difficulty in breathing, or difficulty in urination due to enlargement of the prostate gland unless directed by a doctor. As with any drug, if you are pregnant or nursing a baby, seek the advice of a health professional before using this product. Keep this and all drugs out of the reach of children. In case of accidental overdose, seek professional assistance or contact a poison control center immediately or the Rocky Mountain Poison Control Center at 303-592-1710 (Collect) 24 hours a day.

Drug Interaction: Monoamine oxidase (MAO) inhibitors prolong and intensify the anticholinergic effects of antihistamines. The CNS depressant effect is heightened by alcohol and other CNS depressant drugs.

Symptoms and Treatment of Oral Overdosage: Antihistamine overdosage reactions may vary from central nervous system depression to stimulation. Stimulation is particularly likely in children. Atropine-like signs and symptoms, such as dry mouth, fixed and dilated pupils, flushing, and gastrointestinal symptoms, may also occur.

Dosage and Administration: Dosage is one fluid ounce (30 ml.) thirty minutes before bedtime, or as directed by a physician. Use dosage cup provided, or two (2) measured tablespoons.

How Supplied: Available in 6 oz. bottles.

SOMINEX® Pain Relief Formula

[som 'in-ex]

Active Ingredients: Each tablet contains 25 mg. diphenhydramine HCl and 500 mg. acetaminophen.

Inactive Ingredients: Corn starch, crospovidone, povidone, silicon dioxide, stearic acid, FD&C Blue #1.

Indications: For sleeplessness with accompanying occasional minor aches, pains, or headache.

Action: An antihistamine with sedative effects combined with an internal analgesic.

Warnings: Do not give to children under 12 years of age. If symptoms persist continuously for more than 10 days, or if new ones occur, consult your physician. Do not exceed recommended dosage because severe liver damage may occur. Insomnia may be a symptom of serious underlying medical illness. Take this product with caution if alcohol is being consumed. Do not take this product for the treatment of arthritis, except under the advice and supervision of a physician. As with any drug, if you are pregnant or nursing a baby, seek the advice of a health professional before using this product. Keep this and all drugs out of the reach of children. In case of accidental overdose, seek professional assistance by contacting your physician, the local poison control center, or the Rocky Mountain Poison Control Center at 303-592-1710 (Collect), 24 hours a day.

DO NOT TAKE THIS PRODUCT IF YOU HAVE ASTHMA, GLAUCOMA OR ENLARGEMENT OF THE PROSTATE GLAND, EXCEPT UNDER THE ADVICE AND SUPERVISION OF A PHYSICIAN.

Drug Interaction: Monoamine oxidase (MAO) inhibitors prolong and intensify the anticholinergic effects of antihistamines. The CNS depressant effect is heightened by alcohol and other CNS depressant drugs.

Symptoms and Treatment of Oral Overdosage: Antihistamine overdosage reactions may vary from central nervous system depression to stimulation. Stimulation is particularly likely in children. Atropine-like signs and symptoms, such as dry mouth, fixed and dilated pupils, flushing, and gastrointestinal symptoms, may also occur.

Dosage and Administration: Take two tablets thirty minutes before bedtime, or as directed by a physician.

How Supplied: Available in blister packs of 16 tablets and bottles of 32 tablets.

SUCRETS® (Original Mint and Mentholated Mint) Sore Throat Lozenges

[su 'krets]

Active Ingredient: Hexylresorcinol, 2.4 mg. per lozenge.

Inactive Ingredients: Citric acid (Mentholated only), Blue 1, Corn Syrup, Flavors, Sucrose, Yellow 10.

Indications: For temporary relief of occasional minor sore throat pain and mouth irritations.

Actions: Hexylresorcinol's soothing anesthetic action quickly relieves minor throat irritations.

Warnings: If sore throat is severe, persists more than 2 days, is accompanied or followed by fever, rash, nausea or vomiting, see a doctor promptly. If sore mouth symptoms do not improve in 7 days, see a doctor or dentist promptly. KEEP THIS AND ALL MEDICINES OUT OF THE REACH OF CHILDREN.

Drug Interaction: No known drug interaction.

Symptoms and Treatment of Oral Overdosage: Should a large overdose

Continued on next page

SmithKline Beecham—Cont.

of Sucrets (Original Mint or Mentholated Mint) be suspected, with symptoms of profuse sweating, nausea, vomiting and diarrhea, seek professional assistance. Call your physician, local poison control center or the Rocky Mountain Poison Control Center at 303-592-1710 (Collect) 24 hours a day.

Dosage and Administration: Adults and children 2 years of age and older: Dissolve slowly in the mouth. Repeat as needed.

Professional Labeling: For the temporary relief of pain associated with tonsillitis, pharyngitis, throat infections or stomatitis.

How Supplied:
Available in tins of 24 individually wrapped lozenges.

Shown in Product Identification Section, page 433

SUCRETS® Cold Formula
[*su 'krets*]
Lozenges

Active Ingredients: Each lozenge contains Hexylresorcinol 2.4 mg., Menthol 10 mg.

Inactive Ingredients: Blue 1, Corn Syrup, Flavors, Silicon Dioxide, Sucrose.

Indications: For temporary relief of occasional minor sore throat pain, cough, and nasal congestion associated with a cold.

Warnings: A persistent cough may be a sign of a serious condition. If sore throat, cough or congestion is severe, lasts more than 2 days, is accompanied or followed by fever, rash, nausea, vomiting or persistent headache, see a doctor promptly. Do not take this product for chronic cough such as occurs with smoking, asthma, emphysema, or if cough is accompanied by excessive phlegm, unless directed by a doctor. KEEP THIS AND ALL MEDICINES OUT OF THE REACH OF CHILDREN.

Drug Interaction: No known drug interaction.

Symptoms and Treatment of Oral Overdosage: Should a large overdose of Sucrets Cold Formula be suspected, with symptoms of profuse sweating, nausea, vomiting and diarrhea, seek professional assistance. Call your doctor, local poison control center, or the Rocky Mountain Poison Control Center at 303-592-1710 (collect) 24 hours a day.

Dosage and Administration: Adults and children 2 years of age and older: Dissolve slowly in the mouth. Repeat every two hours as needed. Do not administer to children under 2 years of age, unless directed by a doctor.

Professional Labeling: For the temporary relief of pain associated with tonsillitis, pharyngitis, throat infections or stomatitis.

How Supplied: Available in tins of 24 individually wrapped lozenges.

Shown in Product Identification Section, page 433

SUCRETS® Cough Control
[*su 'krets*]
Cough Control Lozenges

Active Ingredient: Dextromethorphan hydrobromide, 5.0 mg. per lozenge.

Inactive Ingredients: Blue 1, Corn Syrup, Flavors, Red 40, Sucrose, Vegetable Oil, Yellow 10, and other ingredients.

Indications: For temporary suppression of cough due to minor throat and bronchial irritation associated with a cold or inhaled irritants.

Actions: Dextromethorphan is the most widely used non-narcotic/non-habit forming antitussive. A 10-20 mg. dose in adults (5–10 mg. in children over 6, and 2.5–5 mg. in children 2–5) has been recognized as being effective in relieving the frequency and intensity of cough for up to 4 hours.

Warnings: A persistent cough may be a sign of a serious condition. If cough persists for more than 1 week, tends to recur, or is accompanied by fever, rash or persistent headache, consult a doctor. Do not take this product for persistent or chronic cough such as occurs with smoking, asthma, emphysema or if cough is accompanied by excessive phlegm unless directed by a doctor. As with any drug, if you are pregnant or nursing a baby, seek the advice of a health professional before using this product.
KEEP THIS AND ALL MEDICINES OUT OF THE REACH OF CHILDREN.

Drug Interaction: No known drug interaction.

Symptoms and Treatment of Oral Overdosage: Slowing of respiration is the principal symptom of dextromethorphan HBr overdose. Should a large overdose be suspected, seek professional assistance. Call your physician, the local poison control center, or the Rocky Mt. Poison Control Center at 303-592-1710 (Collect), 24 hours a day.

Dosage and Administration: Adults and children 12 years and older: Take 2 lozenges. Children 2 to under 12 years: Take 1 lozenge. Repeat every 4 hours as needed. Do not administer to children under 2 years of age unless directed by a doctor.

Professional Labeling: Same as those outlined under Indications.

How Supplied: Available in tins of 24 lozenges.

Shown in Product Identification Section, page 433

SUCRETS® Maximum Strength Wintergreen
SUCRETS® Wild Cherry Regular Strength
SUCRETS® Children's Cherry Flavored
Sore Throat Lozenges
[*su 'krets*]

Active Ingredient: Maximum Strength-Wintergreen: Dyclonine Hydrochloride 3.0 mg. per lozenge. Wild Cherry, Regular Strength: Dyclonine Hydrochloride 2.0 mg. per lozenge. Children's Cherry: Dyclonine Hydrochloride 1.2 mg. per lozenge.

Inactive Ingredients: Maximum Strength Wintergreen: Citric Acid, Corn Syrup, Silicon Dioxide, Sucrose, Yellow 10. Wild Cherry Regular Strength: Blue 1, Corn Syrup, Flavor, Red 40, Silicon Dioxide, Sucrose, Tartaric Acid. Children's Cherry: Blue 1, Citric Acid, Corn Syrup, Red 40, Silicon Dioxide, Sucrose.

Indications: For temporary relief of occasional minor sore throat pain and mouth irritations.

Actions: Dyclonine Hydrochloride's soothing anesthetic action relieves minor throat irritations.

Warnings: If sore throat is severe, persists more than 2 days, is accompanied or followed by fever, headache, rash, nausea, or vomiting, consult a doctor promptly. If sore mouth symptoms do not improve in 7 days, see your dentist or doctor promptly. KEEP THIS AND ALL MEDICINES OUT OF THE REACH OF CHILDREN.

Drug Interaction: No known drug interaction.

Symptoms and Treatment of Oral Overdosage: Reactions due to large overdosage are systemic and involve the central nervous system and cardiovascular system. Central nervous system reactions are characterized by excitation and/or depression. Nervousness, dizziness, blurred vision or tremors may occur. Reactions involving the cardiovascular system include depression of the myocardium, hypotension or bradycardia. Should a large overdose be suspected seek professional assistance. Call your physician, local poison control center or the Rocky Mountain Poison Control Center at 303-592-1710 (Collect), 24 hours a day.

Dosage and Administration: Adults and children 2 years of age or older: Allow to dissolve slowly in the mouth. Repeat every two hours as needed. Do not administer to children under 2 years of age unless directed by a doctor.

Professional Labeling: For the temporary relief of pain associated with tonsillitis, pharyngitis, throat infections or stomatitis.

How Supplied: Available in tins of 24 lozenges.

Shown in Product Identification Section, page 433

SUCRETS MAXIMUM STRENGTH SPRAYS
[*su 'krets*]

Active Ingredient: Dyclonine Hydrochloride 0.1%.

Inactive Ingredients: Cherry: Alcohol (10%), Dibasic Sodium Phosphate, Flavor, Glycerin, Monobasic Sodium Phosphate, Phosphoric Acid, Potassium Sorbate, Red 33, Sorbitol, Water, Yellow 6. Mint: Alcohol (8.9%), Blue 1, Flavor, Glycerin, Monobasic Sodium Phosphate, Phosphoric Acid, Sodium Benzoate, Sorbitol, Water, Yellow 10.

Indications: Temporary relief of occasional minor sore throat pain due to colds, throat irritations, and mouth and gum irritations.

Actions: Dyclonine Hydrochloride's soothing anesthetic action quickly relieves minor throat irritations.

Warnings: If sore throat is severe, persists for more than 2 days, is accompanied or followed by fever, headache, rash, nausea or vomiting, consult a doctor promptly. If sore mouth symptoms do not improve in 7 days, see your dentist or doctor promptly. KEEP THIS AND ALL MEDICINES OUT OF THE REACH OF CHILDREN.

Drug Interaction: No known drug interaction.

Symptoms and Treatment of Oral Overdosage: Reactions due to large overdosage are systemic and involve the central nervous system and cardiovascular system. Central nervous system reactions are characterized by excitation and/or depression. Nervousness, dizziness, blurred vision or tremors may occur. Reactions involving the cardiovascular system include depression of the myocardium, hypotension or bradycardia. Should a large overdose be suspected seek professional assistance. Call your physician, local poison control center or the Rocky Mountain Poison Control Center at 303-592-1710 (Collect), 24 hours a day.

Dosage and Administration: Adults and children 2 years of age and older: Spray four times and swallow. Gargle/rinse affected area for 15 seconds then spit out. Repeat up to 4 times daily, as needed. Do not administer to children under 2 years of age unless directed by a doctor.

Professional Labeling: For the temporary relief of pain associated with tonsillitis, pharyngitis, throat infections or stomatitis.

How Supplied: Available in 6 fl. oz. and 3 fl. oz. plastic bottle sprayers.

Shown in Product Identification Section, page 433

TELDRIN®
Chlorpheniramine Maleate
Timed-Release Allergy Capsules
Maximum Strength 12 mg.

Product Information: Hay fever and allergies are caused by grass and tree pollen, dust and pollution. TELDRIN provides up to 12 hours of relief from hay fever/upper respiratory allergy symptoms: sneezing, runny nose, itchy, watery eyes. TELDRIN is formulated to release some medication initially and the rest gradually over a prolonged period.

Directions: Adults and children over 12: Just one capsule in the morning, and one in the evening. Do not give to children under 12 without the advice and consent of a physician. Not to exceed 24 mg. (2 capsules) in 24 hours.

TAMPER-RESISTANT PACKAGING FEATURES FOR YOUR PROTECTION:

- The carton is protected by a clear overwrap printed with "safety sealed"; do not use if overwrap is missing or broken.
- Each capsule is encased in a plastic cell with a foil back; do not use if the cell or foil is broken.
- Each TELDRIN capsule is protected by a green PERMA-SEAL™ band which bonds the two capsule halves together; do not use if capsule or band is broken.
- A package insert is provided for information on tamper-resistant packaging.

Warning: Do not take this product if you have asthma, glaucoma, or difficulty in urination due to enlargement of the prostate gland, except under the advice and supervision of a physician. Do not drive or operate heavy machinery. May cause drowsiness. Avoid alcoholic beverages while taking this product. May cause excitability, especially in children. Keep this and all drugs out of the reach of children. In case of accidental overdose, seek professional assistance or contact a poison control center immediately. As with any drug, if you are pregnant or nursing a baby, seek the advice of a health professional before using this product.

Formula: Active Ingredient: Each capsule contains Chlorpheniramine Maleate, 12 mg. **Inactive Ingredients (listed for individuals with specific allergies):** Benzyl Alcohol, Cetylpyridinium Chloride, D&C Red 33, Ethylcellulose, FD&C Green 3, Red 3, Red 40, Yellow 6 (Sunset Yellow) as a color additive, Gelatin, Hydrogenated Castor Oil, Silicon Dioxide, Sodium Lauryl Sulfate, Starch, Sucrose, and trace amounts of other inactive ingredients.
Store at controlled room temperature (59°–86°F.).

How Supplied: Maximum Strength 12 mg. Timed-Release capsules in packages of 12, 24 and 48 capsules.

Shown in Product Identification Section, page 433

TUMS® Antacid Tablets
TUMS E-X® Antacid Tablets

Description: Tums: Active Ingredient: Calcium Carbonate, precipitated U.S.P. 500 mg.
Tums Original Flavor: Inactive Ingredients: Flavor, mineral oil, sodium polyphosphate, starch, sucrose, talc.
Tums Assorted Flavors: Inactive Ingredients: Adipic acid, colors (contains FD&C Yellow No. 6), flavors, mineral oil, sodium polyphosphate, starch, sucrose, talc.
An antacid composition providing liquid effectiveness in a low-cost, pleasant-tasting tablet. Tums tablets are free of the chalky aftertaste usually associated with calcium carbonate therapy and remain pleasant tasting even during long-term therapy. Each TUMS tablet contains not more than 2 mg of sodium and is considered to be dietetically sodium free. Non-laxative/non-constipating.
Tums E-X: Active Ingredient: Calcium Carbonate, 750 mg.
Tums E-X Wintergreen Flavor Inactive Ingredients: Colors (contains FD&C Yellow No. 6), flavor, mineral oil, sodium polyphosphate, starch, sucrose, talc.
Tums E-X Cherry Flavor Inactive Ingredients: Adipic acid, color, flavor, mineral oil, sodium polyphosphate, starch, sucrose, talc.
Tums E-X Peppermint Flavor Inactive Ingredients: Flavor, mineral oil, sodium polyphosphate, starch, sucrose, talc.
Tums E-X Assorted Flavors Inactive Ingredients: Adipic acid, colors (contains FD&C Yellow No. 6), flavors, mineral oil, sodium polyphosphate, starch, sucrose, talc.
Each tablet contains not more than 2 mg of sodium and is considered to be dietetically sodium free. Non-laxative/non-constipating.

Indications: For fast relief of acid indigestion, heartburn, sour stomach and upset stomach associated with these symptoms.

Actions: Tums lowers the upper limit of the pH range without affecting the innate antacid efficiency of calcium carbonate. One tablet, when tested *in vitro* according to the *Federal Register* procedure (*Fed. Reg.* 39-19862, June 4, 1974), neutralizes 10 mEq of 0.1N HCl. This high neutralization capacity combined with a rapid rate of reaction makes Tums an ideal antacid for management of conditions associated with hyperacidity. It effectively neutralizes free acid yet does not cause systemic alkalosis in the presence of normal renal function. A double-blind placebo-controlled clinical study demonstrated that calcium carbonate taken at a dosage of 16 Tums tablets daily for a two-week period was non-constipating/non-laxative.

Warnings: Tums: Do not take more than 16 tablets in a 24-hour period or use the maximum dosage of this product for

Continued on next page

SmithKline Beecham—Cont.

more than 2 weeks, except under the advice and supervision of a physician.
Tums E-X: Do not take more than 10 tablets in a 24-hour period or use the maximum dosage of this product for more than two weeks, except under the advice and supervision of a physician. Keep this and all drugs out of the reach of children.

Dosage and Administration: Chew 1 or 2 TUMS tablets as symptoms occur. Repeat hourly if symptoms return, or as directed by a physician. No water is required. Simulated Drip Method: The pleasant-tasting TUMS tablet may be kept between the gum and cheek and allowed to dissolve gradually by continuous sucking to prolong the effective relief time.

Important Dietary Information—As a Source of Extra Calcium—Chew 1 or 2 tablets after meals or as directed by a physician.
Tums Original and Assorted Flavors: The 500 mg of calcium carbonate in each tablet provide 200 mg of elemental calcium which is 20% of the adult U.S. RDA for calcium. Five tablets provide 100% of the daily calcium needs for adults.
Tums E-X: The 750 mg of calcium carbonate in each tablet provide 300 mg of elemental calcium which is 30% of the adult U.S. RDA for calcium. Four tablets provide 120% of the daily calcium needs for adults.

Professional Labeling: Indicated for the symptomatic relief of hyperacidity associated with the diagnosis of peptic ulcer, gastritis, peptic esophagitis, gastric hyperacidity, and hiatal hernia.

How Supplied: Tums: Peppermint and Assorted Flavors of Cherry, Lemon, Orange and Lime are available in 12-tablet rolls, 3-roll wraps, and bottles of 75 and 150 tablets. **Tums E-X Wintergreen, E-X Cherry, E-X Peppermint, and Assorted Flavors of Cherry, Lemon, Lime and Orange:** 8-tablet rolls, 3-roll wraps and bottles of 48 and 96 tablets.

Shown in Product Identification Section, page 433

TUMS® Liquid Extra-Strength Antacid
TUMS® Liquid Extra-Strength Antacid with Simethicone

Description: Tums Liquid and Tums Liquid with Simethicone is an extra-strength antacid with a fresh, minty flavor.

Tums Liquid Extra-Strength Antacid

Active Ingredient: 1,000 mg Calcium Carbonate per teaspoon.

Inactive Ingredients: Carboxymethylcellulose Sodium, Citric Acid, Glycerin, Magnesium Aluminum Silicate, Methylparaben, Peppermint Oil, Potassium Pyrophosphate, Propylparaben, Sorbitol, Sucrose, Water.

Indications: For the relief of acid indigestion, heartburn, sour stomach and the symptoms of upset stomach associated with these conditions.

Tums Liquid Extra-Strength Antacid with Simethicone

Active Ingredients: 1,000 mg Calcium Carbonate and 30 mg Simethicone per teaspoon.

Inactive Ingredients: Carboxymethylcellulose Sodium, Citric Acid, Glycerin, Magnesium Aluminum Silicate, Methylparaben, Peppermint Oil, Potassium Pyrophosphate, Propylparaben, Sorbitol, Sucrose, Water.

Indications: For the relief of acid indigestion, heartburn, sour stomach and the symptoms of upset stomach and gas associated with these conditions.

Sodium Content: Tums Liquid and Tums Liquid with Simethicone: Each teaspoonful contains less than 5 mg of sodium which is considered dietetically sodium free.
Calcium Rich: Tums Liquid and Tums Liquid with Simethicone: Each teaspoonful contains 400 mg of elemental calcium which is 40% of the adult U.S. RDA for calcium.
Acid Neutralizing Capacity: Tums Liquid and Tums Liquid with Simethicone: 20.0 mEq/5 ml.

Directions: Tums Liquid and Tums Liquid with Simethicone: Take one or two teaspoonfuls as symptoms occur. Repeat hourly if symptoms return, or as directed by a physician.

Warnings: Tums Liquid and Tums Liquid with Simethicone: Do not take more than 8 teaspoonfuls in a 24-hour period or the maximum dosage of this product for more than 2 weeks except under the advice and supervision of a physician. Store at room temperature. Keep this and all drugs out of the reach of children.

How Supplied: Tums Liquid and Tums Liquid with Simethicone are available in 12 oz. bottles.

Shown in Product Identification Section, page 433

VIVARIN® Stimulant Tablets and Caplets
[*vi 'va-rin*]

Active Ingredient: Each tablet/caplet contains 200 mg. caffeine alkaloid.

Inactive Ingredients Tablets: Dextrose, magnesium stearate, microcrystalline cellulose, powdered cellulose, silicon dioxide, starch, Yellow #6, Yellow #10.

Inactive Ingredients Caplets: Carnauba wax, dextrose, hydroxypropyl methylcellulose, magnesium stearate, microcrystalline cellulose, polyethylene glycol, polysorbate 80, powdered cellulose, silicon dioxide, starch, titanium dioxide, white wax, Yellow #6, Yellow #10.

Indications: Helps restore mental alertness or wakefulness when experiencing fatigue or drowsiness.

Actions: Stimulates cerebrocortical areas involved with active mental processes.

Warnings: The recommended dose of this product contains about as much caffeine as two cups of coffee. Limit the use of caffeine containing medications, foods, or beverages while taking this product because too much caffeine may cause nervousness, irritability, sleeplessness, and, occasionally, rapid heart beat. For occasional use only. Not intended for use as a substitute for sleep. If fatigue or drowsiness persists or continues to recur, consult a doctor. Do not give to children under 12 years of age. As with any drug, if you are pregnant or nursing a baby, seek the advice of a health professional before using this product. In case of accidental overdose, seek professional assistance or contact a poison control center immediately. Keep this and all drugs out of the reach of children.

Drug Interaction: Use of caffeine should be lowered or avoided if drugs are being used to treat cardiovascular ailments, psychological problems, or kidney trouble.

Precaution: Higher blood glucose levels may result from caffeine use.

Symptoms and Treatment of Oral Overdosage: Convulsions may occur if caffeine is consumed in doses larger than 10 g. Emesis should be induced to empty the stomach. In case of accidental overdose, seek professional assistance by contacting your physician, the local poison control center, or the Rocky Mt. Poison Control Center at 303-592-1710 (Collect), 24 hours a day.

Dosage and Administration: Adults and children 12 years of age and over: Oral dosage is 1 tablet or caplet (200 mg.) not more than every 3 to 4 hours.

How Supplied Tablets: Available in packages of 16, 40 and 80 tablets.

How Supplied Caplets: Available in packages of 24 and 48.

EDUCATIONAL MATERIAL

Feminine Hygiene and You (Film, Video)
This 14-minute color film begins with a simple explanation of how a woman's body works (reproductive system, menstrual cycle, and vaginal secretions), then explains douching. Free loan to physicians, pharmacists and clinics. Available in 16mm and VHS.
A Personal Guide to Feminine Freshness
A 16-page illustrated booklet on vaginal infections, feminine hygiene and douching. Free to physicians, pharmacists and patients in limited quantities. These items are available by writing SmithKline Beecham Consumer Brands or by calling 800-245-1040.

E.R. Squibb & Sons, Inc.
Apothecon
A Bristol-Myers Squibb Company
P.O. BOX 4000
PRINCETON, NJ 08543-4000

THERAGRAN® LIQUID
High Potency Vitamin Supplement

Each 5 ml. teaspoonful contains:

		Percent US RDA*
Vitamin A	10,000 IU	200
Vitamin D	400 IU	100
Vitamin C	200 mg	333
Thiamine	10 mg	667
Riboflavin	10 mg	588
Niacin	100 mg	500
Vitamin B_6	4.1 mg	205
Vitamin B_{12}	5 mcg	83
Pantothenic Acid	21.4 mg	214

*US Recommended Daily Allowance

Ingredients: water, sugar, glycerin, propylene glycol, sodium ascorbate, niacinamide, polysorbate 80, ascorbic acid, carboxymethylcellulose sodium, d-panthenol, riboflavin-5-phosphate sodium, thiamine hydrochloride, vitamin A palmitate, pyridoxine hydrochloride, (sodium benzoate and methylparaben as preservatives), ferric ammonium citrate, artificial and natural flavors, cholecalciferol, cyanocobalamin

Warning: KEEP OUT OF REACH OF CHILDREN.

Usage: For adults—1 teaspoonful daily or as directed by physician.

How Supplied: In bottles of 4 fl. oz.

Storage: Store at room temperature; avoid excessive heat.
(C0262D)

Shown in Product Identification Section, page 434

ADVANCED FORMULA THERAGRAN® TABLETS
(High Potency Multivitamin Formula)

FOR ADULTS—PERCENTAGE OF U.S. RECOMMENDED DAILY ALLOWANCE

Vitamins	Quantity	US RDA
Vitamin A	5000 IU	100%
(as Acetate and Beta Carotene)		
Vitamin B_1	3 mg	200%
Vitamin B_2	3.4 mg	200%
Vitamin B_6	3 mg	150%
Vitamin B_{12}	9 mcg	150%
Vitamin C	90 mg	150%
Vitamin D	400 I.U.	100%
Vitamin E	30 I.U.	100%
Niacin	20 mg	100%
Folic Acid	400 mcg	100%
Pantothenic Acid	10.0 mg	100%
Biotin	30 mcg	10%

Ingredients: Lactose, ascorbic acid, microcrystalline cellulose, gelatin, dl-alpha-tocopheryl acetate, niacinamide, starch, calcium pantothenate, sodium caseinate, hydroxypropyl methylcellulose, povidone, pyridoxine hydrochloride, riboflavin, silicon dioxide, magnesium stearate, thiamine mononitrate, vitamin A acetate, polyethylene glycol, triacetin, stearic acid, titanium dioxide, annatto, beta carotene, FD&C Red 40, folic acid, biotin, ergocalciferol, cyanocobalamin.

Warning: KEEP OUT OF REACH OF CHILDREN.

Usage: For adults—1 tablet daily or as directed by physician.

How Supplied: Packs of 130; and Unimatic® cartons of 100.

Storage: Store at room temperature; avoid excessive heat; keep tightly closed. UNIMATIC® is a trademark of E.R. Squibb & Sons, Inc.

Shown in Product Identification Section, page 433

ADVANCED FORMULA THERAGRAN-M® TABLETS
(High Potency Multivitamin Formula with Minerals)

TABLET CONTENTS: FOR ADULTS—PERCENTAGE OF U.S. RECOMMENDED DAILY ALLOWANCE

Vitamins	Quantity	US RDA
Vitamin A	5000 IU	100%
(as Acetate and Beta Carotene)		
Vitamin B_1	3 mg	200%
Vitamin B_2	3.4 mg	200%
Vitamin B_6	3 mg	150%
Vitamin B_{12}	9 mcg	150%
Vitamin C	90 mg	150%
Vitamin D	400 IU	100%
Vitamin E	30 IU	100%
Niacin	20 mg	100%
Folic Acid	400 mcg	100%
Pantothenic Acid	10.0 mg	100%
Biotin	30 mcg	10%
Minerals		
Iron	27.0 mg	150%
Copper	2.0 mg	100%
Iodine	150.0 mcg	100%
Zinc	15.0 mg	100%
Magnesium	100.0 mg	25%
Calcium	40.0 mg	4%
Phosphorus	31 mg	3%
Chromium	15 mcg	*
Molybdenum	15 mcg	*
Selenium	10 mcg	*
Manganese	5 mg	*
ELECTROLYTES		
Chloride	7.5 mg	*
Potassium	7.5 mg	*

*US RDA not established.

Ingredients: Lactose, dibasic calcium phosphate, magnesium oxide, ascorbic acid, ferrous fumarate, gelatin, dl-alpha-tocopheryl acetate, crospovidone, niacinamide, hydroxypropyl methylcellulose, zinc oxide, povidone, manganese sulfate, potassium chloride, starch, calcium pantothenate, sodium caseinate, cupric sulfate, magnesium stearate, silicon dioxide, sucrose, pyridoxine hydrochloride, stearic acid, riboflavin, polyethylene glycol, triacetin, thiamine mononitrate, Vitamin A acetate, beta carotene, potassium citrate, FD&C Red 40, folic acid, titanium dioxide, potassium iodide, chromic chloride, FD&C Blue 2, sodium molybdate, biotin, sodium selenate, ergocalciferol, cyanocobalamin.

Warning: KEEP OUT OF REACH OF CHILDREN.

Usage: For adults—1 tablet daily or as directed by physician.

How Supplied: Packs of 90, 130 and 240; and Unimatic® cartons of 100.

Storage: Store at room temperature; avoid excessive heat; keep tightly closed. UNIMATIC® is a trademark of E.R. Squibb & Sons, Inc.

Shown in Product Identification Section, page 433

THERAGRAN® STRESS FORMULA
High Potency Multivitamin Formula with Iron and Biotin

TABLET CONTENTS: For Adults—Percentage of US Recommended Daily Allowance

Ingredients	Quantity	US RDA
Vitamin B_1	15 mg	1000%
Vitamin B_2	15 mg	882%
Vitamin B_6	25 mg	1250%
Vitamin B_{12}	12 mcg	200%
Vitamin C	600 mg	1000%
Vitamin E	30 IU	100%
Niacin	100 mg	500%
Pantothenic Acid	20 mg	200%
Iron	27 mg	150%
Folic Acid	400 mcg	100%
Biotin	45 mcg	15%

Ingredients: Ascorbic acid, niacinamide, ferrous fumarate, microcrystalline cellulose, lactose, pyridoxine hydrochloride, starch, *dl*-alpha-tocopheryl acetate, gelatin, calcium pantothenate, croscarmellose sodium, hydroxypropyl methylcellulose, povidone, riboflavin, thiamine mononitrate, sodium caseinate, magnesium stearate, silicon dioxide, stearic acid, titanium dioxide, Red 40, Yellow 6, polyethylene glycol, triacetin, folic acid, biotin, cyanocobalamin.

Warning: KEEP OUT OF REACH OF CHILDREN.

Usage: For adults—1 tablet daily or as directed by physician.

How Supplied: Bottles of 75.

Storage: Store at room temperature; avoid excessive heat.
(C0584)

Shown in Product Identification Section, page 433

Standard Homeopathic Company

210 WEST 131st STREET
BOX 61067
LOS ANGELES, CA 90061

HYLAND'S BED WETTING TABLETS

Active Ingredients: *Equisetum hyemale* (Scouring Rush) 2X HPUS, *Rhus aromatica* (Fragrant Sumac) 3X HPUS, *Belladonna* 3X HPUS (0.0003% Alkaloids).

Inactive Ingredients: Lactose USP.

Indications: A homeopathic combination for the temporary relief of involuntary urination (common bed wetting) in children.

Directions: Children 3 to 12 years: 2 to 3 tablets before meals and at bedtime, or as directed by a licensed health care practitioner. Children over 12 years: double the above recommended dose.

Warnings: If symptoms persist for more than seven days or worsen, consult a Health Care Professional. As with any drug, if you are pregnant or nursing a baby, seek the advice of a health professional before using this product. Keep this and all medication out of the reach of children.

How Supplied: Bottles of 125—one grain sublingual tablets (NDC 54973-7501-01). Store at room temperature.

HYLAND'S CALMS FORTÉ TABLETS

Active Ingredients: *Passiflora* (Passion Flower) 1X triple strength HPUS, *Avena sativa* (Oat) 1X triple strength HPUS, *Humulus lupulus* (Hops) 1X double strength HPUS, *Chamomilla* (Chamomile) 2X HPUS, *Calcarea Phosphorica* (Calcium Phosphate) 3X HPUS, *Ferrum Phosphorica* (Iron Phosphate) 3X HPUS, *Kali Phosphoricum* (Potassium Phosphate) 3X HPUS, *Natrum Phosphoricum* (Sodium Phosphate) 3X HPUS, *Magnesia Phosphoricum* (Magnesium Phosphate) 3X HPUS.

Inactive Ingredients: Lactose USP.

Indications: Temporary symptomatic relief of simple nervous tension and insomnia.

Directions: Adults, As a relaxant: 1 to 2 tablets as needed or 3 times daily between meals. In insomnia: 1 to 3 tablets ½ to 1 hour before retiring. Repeat as needed without danger of side effects. Children, As a relaxant: 1 tablet as needed or 3 times daily before meals. In insomnia: 1 to 2 tablets 1 hour before retiring. Non-habit-forming.

Warnings: If symptoms persist for more than seven days or worsen, consult a Health Care Professional. As with any drug, if you are pregnant or nursing a baby, seek the advice of a health professional before using this product. Keep this and all medication out of the reach of children.

How Supplied: Bottles of 100 four grain tablets (NDC 54973-1121-02). Store at room temperature. Bottles of 50 four grain tablets (NDC 54973-1121-01). Store at room temperature.

HYLAND'S COLIC TABLETS

Active Ingredients: *Disocorea* (Wild Yam) 2X HPUS, *Chamomilla* (Chamomile) 3X HPUS, *Colocynth* (Bitter Apple) 3X HPUS.

Inactive Ingredients: Lactose USP.

Indications: A homeopathic combination for the temporary relief of colic and gas pains caused by irritating food, feeding too quickly, swallowing air and similar conditions during teething, colds and other minor upset periods in children.

Directions: For children to 2 years of age: administer 2 tablets dissolved in a teaspoon of water or on the tongue every 15 minutes until relieved; then every 2 hours as required. Children over 2 years: 3 tablets dissolved on the tongue as above; or as recommended by a licensed health care practitioner.

Warnings: If symptoms persist for more than seven days or worsen, consult a Health Care Professional. Keep this and all medication out of the reach of children.

How Supplied: Bottles of 125—one grain sublingual tablets (NDC 54973-7502-01). Store at room temperature.

HYLAND'S COUGH SYRUP WITH HONEY™

Active Ingredients: Each fluid ounce contains: *Ipecacuanha* (Ipecac) 3X HPUS, *Aconitum napellus* (Aconite) 3X HPUS, *Spongia Tosta* (Sponge) 3X HPUS, *Antimonium Tartaricum* (Potassium Antimony Tartrate) 6X HPUS.

Inactive Ingredients: Simple syrup and honey.

Indications: A homeopathic combination for the temporary relief of symptoms of simple, dry, tight or tickling coughs due to colds in children.

Directions: Children 1 to 12 years: 1 to 3 teaspoonfuls as required. Children over 12 years and adults: 3 to 4 teaspoonfuls as required. May be taken with or without water. Repeat as often as necessary to relieve symptoms. For children under 1 year of age, consult a licensed health care practitioner.

Warnings: Do not use this product for persistent or chronic cough such as occurs with asthma, smoking or emphysema; or if cough is accompanied with excessive mucus, unless directed by a licensed health care practitioner. If symptoms persist for more than seven days, tend to recur, or are accompanied by a high fever, rash, or persistent headache, consult a Health Care Professional. As with any drug, if you are pregnant or nursing a baby, seek the advice of a health professional before using this product. Keep this and all medication out of the reach of children.

How Supplied: Bottles of 4 fluid ounces (120 ml) (NDC 54973-7503-02). Store at room temperature.

HYLAND'S C–PLUS™ COLD TABLETS

Active Ingredients: *Eupatorium perfoliatum* (Boneset) 2X HPUS, *Euphrasia officinalis* (Eyebright) 2X HPUS, *Gelsemium sempervirens* (Yellow Jasmine) 3X HPUS, *Kali Iodatum* (Potassium Iodide) 3X HPUS.

Inactive Ingredients: Lactose USP, Natural Raspberry Flavor.

Indications: A homeopathic combination for the temporary relief of symptoms of runny nose and sneezing due to common head colds in children.

Directions: Children 1 to 3 years: 2 tablets every 15 minutes for 4 doses, then hourly until relieved. For children 3 to 6 years: 3 tablets as above; for children 6 and older: 6 tablets as above or as directed by a licensed health care practitioner.

Warnings: If symptoms persist for more than seven days or worsen, consult a Health Care Professional. As with any drug, if you are pregnant or nursing a baby, seek the advice of a health professional before using this product. Keep this and all medication out of the reach of children.

How Supplied: Bottles of 125—one grain sublingual tablets (NDC 54973-7505-01). Store at room temperature.

HYLAND'S TEETHING TABLETS

Active Ingredients: *Calcarea Phosphorica* (Calcium Phosphate) 3X HPUS, *Chamomilla* (Chamomile) 3X HPUS, *Coffea Cruda* (Coffee) 3X HPUS, *Belladonna* 3X HPUS (Alkaloids 0.0003%).

Inactive Ingredients: Lactose USP.

Indications: A homeopathic combination for the temporary relief of symptoms of simple restlessness and wakeful irritability due to cutting of teeth.

Directions: 2 to 3 tablets in a teaspoon of water or on the tongue, 4 times per day. If the child is restless or wakeful, 2 tablets every hour for 6 doses or as directed by a licensed health care practitioner.

Warnings: If symptoms persist for more than seven days or worsen, consult a Health Care Professional. As with any drug, if you are pregnant or nursing a baby, seek the advice of a health professional before using this product. Keep this and all medication out of the reach of children.

How Supplied: Bottles of 125—one grain sublingual tablets (NDC 54973-7504-01). Store at room temperature.

HYLAND'S VITAMIN C FOR CHILDREN™

Active Ingredients: 25 mg Vitamin C as Sodium Ascorbate (30 mg).

Inactive Ingredients: Lactose USP, Natural Lemon Flavor.

Indications: Each tablet provides children with 55% of the daily recommended requirement of Vitamin C. Sodium Ascorbate is preferred to Ascorbic Acid when gastric irritation may result from free acid.

Directions: Children 2 years and older: 1 to 2 tablets on the tongue or as directed by a licensed health care practitioner.

Warning: Keep this and all medication out of the reach of children.

How Supplied: Bottles of 125—one grain sublingual tablets (NDC 54973-7506-01). Store at room temperature. Tablets may turn brown in color with exposure to light. Color change does not affect potency.

EDUCATIONAL MATERIAL

Booklets—Brochures
"Homeopathy—What it is, How it Works," A Consumer's Guide to Homeopathic Medicine, Free

Stellar Pharmacal Corp.

Div./Star Pharmaceuticals, Inc.
1990 N.W. 44TH STREET
POMPANO BEACH, FL
33064-8712

STAR-OTIC®
Antibacterial, Antifungal, Nonaqueous Ear Solution
For Prevention of "Swimmer's Ear"

Active Ingredients: Acetic acid nonaqueous, Burow's solution, Boric acid, in a propylene glycol vehicle, with an acid pH and a low surface tension.

Indications: For the prevention of otitis externa, commonly called "Swimmer's Ear".

Actions: Star-Otic is antibacterial, antifungal, hydrophilic, has an acid pH and a low surface tension. Acetic acid and boric acid inhibit the rapid multiplication of microorganisms and help maintain the lining mantle of the ear canal in its normal acid state. Burow's solution (aluminum acetate) is a mild astringent. Propylene glycol reduces moisture in the ear canal.

Warning: Do not use in ear if tympanic membrane (ear drum) is perforated or punctured.

Symptoms and Treatment of Overdosage: Discontinue use if undue irritation or sensitivity occurs.

Dosage and Administration: Adults and Children: For the prevention of otitis externa (Swimmer's Ear). In susceptible persons, instill 2–3 drops of Star-Otic in each ear before and after swimming or bathing, or as directed by physician.

Professional Labeling: Same as those outlined under Indications.

How Supplied: Available in ½ oz measured drop, safety tip, plastic bottle.

Shown in Product Identification Section, page 434

EDUCATIONAL MATERIAL

First Aid Prevention for Swimmer's Ear
Public health information on cause and care of preventing swimmer's ear.
Star-Otic Patient Instruction Pads
Instructions for patients on use of Star-Otic to prevent swimmer's ear.

Stuart Pharmaceuticals

a business unit of
ICI Americas Inc.
WILMINGTON, DE 19897 USA

HIBICLENS® Antiseptic/ Antimicrobial
[*hibi-klenz*]
Skin Cleanser
(chlorhexidine gluconate)

Description: HIBICLENS is an antiseptic antimicrobial skin cleanser possessing bactericidal activities. HIBICLENS contains 4% w/v HIBITANE® (chlorhexidine gluconate), a chemically unique hexamethylenebis biguanide with inactive ingredients: fragrance, isopropyl alcohol 4%, purified water, Red 40, and other ingredients, in a mild, sudsing base adjusted to pH 5.0–6.5 for optimal activity and stability as well as compatability with the normal pH of the skin.

Action: HIBICLENS is bactericidal on contact. It has antiseptic activity and a persistent antimicrobial effect with rapid bactericidal activity against a wide range of microorganisms, including gram-positive bacteria, and gram-negative bacteria such as *Pseudomonas aeruginosa*. The effectiveness of HIBICLENS is not significantly reduced by the presence of organic matter, such as blood.[1]

In a study[2] simulating surgical use, the immediate bactericidal effect of HIBICLENS after a single six-minute scrub resulted in a 99.9% reduction in resident bacterial flora, with a reduction of 99.98% after the eleventh scrub. Reductions on surgically gloved hands were maintained over the six-hour test period.

HIBICLENS displays persistent antimicrobial action. In one study,[2] 93% of a radiolabeled formulation of HIBICLENS remained present on uncovered skin after five hours.

HIBICLENS prevents skin infection thereby reducing the risk of cross-infection.

Indications: HIBICLENS is indicated for use as a surgical scrub, as a healthcare personnel handwash, for patient preoperative showering and bathing, as a patient preoperative skin preparation, and as a skin wound cleanser and general skin cleanser.

Safety: The extensive use of chlorhexidine gluconate for over 20 years outside the United States has produced no evidence of absorption of the compound through intact skin. The potential for producing skin reactions is extremely low. HIBICLENS can be used many times a day without causing irritation, dryness, or discomfort. Experimental studies indicate that when used for cleaning superficial wounds, HIBICLENS will neither cause additional tissue injury nor delay healing.

WARNINGS: FOR EXTERNAL USE ONLY. KEEP OUT OF EYES, EARS AND MOUTH. HIBICLENS SHOULD NOT BE USED AS A PREOPERATIVE SKIN PREPARATION OF THE FACE OR HEAD. MISUSE OF HIBICLENS HAS BEEN REPORTED TO CAUSE SERIOUS AND PERMANENT EYE INJURY WHEN IT HAS BEEN PERMITTED TO ENTER AND REMAIN IN THE EYE DURING SURGICAL PROCEDURES. IF HIBICLENS SHOULD CONTACT THESE AREAS, RINSE OUT PROMPTLY AND THOROUGHLY WITH WATER. Avoid contact with meninges. HIBICLENS should not be used by persons who have a sensitivity to it or its components. Chlorhexidine gluconate has been reported to cause deafness when instilled in the middle ear through perforated ear drums. Irritation, sensitization and generalized allergic reactions have been reported with chlorhexidine-containing products, especially in the genital areas. If adverse reactions occur, discontinue use immediately and if severe, contact a physician. Keep this and all drugs out of the reach of children. In case of accidental ingestion, seek professional assistance or contact a Poison Control Center immediately.

Accidental ingestion: Chlorhexidine gluconate taken orally is poorly absorbed. Treat with gastric lavage using milk, egg white, gelatin or mild soap. Employ supportive measures as appropriate. Avoid excessive heat (above 104°F).

DIRECTIONS FOR USE:
Preoperative Skin Preparation:
Apply HIBICLENS liberally to surgical site and swab for at least two minutes. Dry with a sterile towel. Repeat procedure for an additional two minutes and dry with a sterile towel.

Preoperative showering and whole-body bathing
The patient should be instructed to wash the entire body, including the scalp, on two consecutive occasions immediately prior to surgery. Each procedure should

Continued on next page

Stuart—Cont.

consist of two consecutive thorough applications of HIBICLENS followed by thorough rinsing. If the patient's condition allows, showering is recommended for whole-body bathing. The recommended procedure is: Wet the body, including hair. Wash the hair using 25 mL of HIBICLENS and the body with another 25 mL of HIBICLENS. Rinse. Repeat. Rinse thoroughly after second application.

Skin Wound and General Skin Cleansing:
Wounds which involve more than the superficial layers of the skin should not be routinely treated with HIBICLENS. HIBICLENS should not be used for repeated general skin cleansing of large body areas except in those patients whose underlying condition makes it necessary to reduce the bacterial population of the skin. To use, thoroughly rinse the area to be cleansed with water. Apply the minimum amount of HIBICLENS necessary to cover the skin or wound area and wash gently. Rinse again thoroughly.

Health-care personnel use
Surgical Hand Scrub:
Directions for use of HIBICLENS Liquid: Wet hands and forearms to the elbows with warm water. (Avoid using very cold or very hot water.) Dispense about 5 mL of HIBICLENS into cupped hands. Spread over both hands. Scrub hands and forearms for 3 minutes without adding water, using a brush or sponge. (Avoid using extremely hard-bristled brushes.) While scrubbing, pay particular attention to fingernails, cuticles, and interdigital spaces. (Do not use excessive pressure to produce additional lather.) Rinse thoroughly with warm water. Dispense about 5 mL of HIBICLENS into cupped hands. Wash for an additional 3 minutes. (No need to use brush or sponge.) Then rinse thoroughly. Dry thoroughly.

Hand Wash:
Wet hands with water. (Avoid using very cold or very hot water.) Dispense about 5 mL of HIBICLENS into cupped hands. Wash for 15 seconds. (Do not use excessive pressure to produce additional lather.) Rinse thoroughly with warm water. Dry thoroughly.

Directions for use of HIBICLENS® Sponge/Brush: Open package and remove nail cleaner. Wet hands. Use nail cleaner under fingernails and to clean cuticles. Wet hands and forearms to the elbow with warm water. (Avoid using very cold or very hot water.) Wet sponge side of sponge/brush. Squeeze and pump immediately to work up adequate lather. Apply lather to hands and forearms using *sponge* side of the product. *Start 3 minute scrub* by using the brush side of the product to scrub *only* nails, cuticles, and interdigital areas. Use sponge side for scrubbing hands and forearms. (Avoid using brush on these more sensitive areas.) Rinse thoroughly with warm water. Scrub for an additional 3 minutes *using sponge side* only. To produce additional lather, add a small amount of water and pump the sponge. (While scrubbing, do not use excessive pressure to produce lather—a small amount of lather is all that is required to adequately cleanse skin with HIBICLENS.) Rinse and dry thoroughly, blotting hands and forearms with a soft sterile towel.

IMPORTANT LAUNDERING ADVICE FOR HOSPITAL STAFF AND OTHER USERS OF ANTISEPTIC PATIENT SKIN PREPARATIONS CONTAINING CHLORHEXIDINE GLUCONATE

Chlorhexidine gluconate is a unique agent that most closely fits the definition of an ideal antimicrobial agent, having (among others) one of the most important characteristics of persistent activity. This persistence is due to chlorhexidine gluconate binding to the protein of the skin and, thus, being available for residual activity over a relatively long period of time.

Chlorhexidine gluconate, however, binds not only to protein of the skin, but also to many fabrics, particularly cotton. Thus, special laundering procedures should be considered when such products contact these fabrics. As a result of such contact, chlorhexidine gluconate may become adsorbed onto the fabric and not be removed by washing. If sufficient available chlorine is present during the washing procedure, a fast brown stain may develop due to a chemical reaction between chlorhexidine gluconate and chlorine.

SUGGESTED LAUNDERING PROCEDURES TO LIMIT STAINING

1. **Not Aging.** Avoid allowing the product to age (set) on unwashed linens.
2. **Flushing and Washing.** A flush operation as the initial step in the wash process is helpful in the laundering of linen exposed to chlorhexidine gluconate. Such flushing is also important in the laundering of linen which contains organic materials such as blood or pus. For best results, warm water flushes (90°–100°F) are recommended. After a number of initial flushings followed by a washing with a low alkaline/nonchlorine detergent, most articles which come in contact with chlorhexidine gluconate should have an acceptable level of whiteness. If a rewash process using bleach is necessary to achieve a greater degree of whiteness, the bleach used should be a nonchlorine bleach.
3. **Not Using Chlorine Bleach.** Modern laundering methods often make the use of chlorine bleach unnecessary. It is worthwhile trying to wash without chlorine to ascertain if the resulting degree of whiteness is acceptable. Omission of chlorine from the laundering process can extend the useful life of cotton articles since oxidizing bleaches such as chlorine may cause some damage to cellulose even when used in low concentration.
4. **Changing to a Peroxide-Type Bleach, Such as Sodium Perborate, Sodium Percarbonate or Hydrogen Peroxide.** This should eliminate the reaction which could occur with the use of chlorine bleaches. If a chlorine bleach must be used, a concentration of less than 7 ppm available chlorine (1/10 the normal bleach level) is suggested to minimize possible staining.

A NOTE ON LAUNDERING OF PERSONAL CLOTHING

The laundering procedures set forth above using low alkaline, nonchlorinated laundry detergents are also applicable to laundering of uniforms and lab coats. Commerically available laundry detergents which do not contain chlorine include Borax, Borateem, Dreft, Oxydol, and Ivory Snow. These products, however, will not remove stains previously set into the fabric.

RECLAMATION OF STAINED LINENS

For those linens which previously have been stained due to the chemical reaction between chlorhexidine gluconate and chlorine, the following laundering procedure may be helpful in reducing the visible stain:
[See table.]

Operation	Water Level	Temperature	Time (Min)	Supplies/ 100 lb
Break	Low	180°F	20	1.5 lb oxalic acid
Flush	High	Cold	1	—
Emulsify	Low	160°F	5	18 oz emulsifier
Flush	High	Cold	1	—
Bleach	Low	180°F	20	2 lb alkali builder and 1 lb organic bleach
Rinse	High	Cold	1	—
Antichlor	High	Cold	2	4 oz antichlor
Rinse	High	Cold	1	—
Rinse	High	Cold	1	—
Sour	Low	Cold	4	2 oz rust removing sour

How Supplied: *For general handwashing locations:* pocket-size, 15 mL foil Packettes; plastic disposable bottles of 4 oz and 8 oz with dispenser caps; and 16 oz filled globes. *For surgical scrub areas:* disposable, unit-of-use 22 mL impregnated Sponge/Brushes with nail cleaner; plastic disposable bottles of 32 oz and 1 gal. The 32-oz bottle is designed for a special foot-operated wall dispenser. A hand-operated wall dispenser is available for the 16-oz globe. Hand pumps are available for 16 oz, 32 oz, and 1 gal sizes.

NDC 0038-0575 (liquid).
NDC 0038-0577 (sponge/brush).

References:

1. Lowbury EJL, and Lilly HA: The effect of blood on disinfection of surgeons' hands, Brit. J. Surg. 61:19–21 (Jan.) 1974.
2. Peterson AF, Rosenberg A, Alatary SD: Comparative evaluation of surgical scrub preparations, Surg. Gynecol. Obstet. 146:63–65 (Jan.) 1978.

Shown in Product Identification Section, page 434

HIBISTAT®
Germicidal Hand Rinse
HIBISTAT® TOWELETTE
Germicidal Hand Wipe
[*hi-bi-stat*]
(chlorhexidine gluconate)

Description: HIBISTAT is a germicidal hand rinse which provides rapid bactericidal action and has a persistent antimicrobial effect against a wide range of microorganisms. HIBISTAT is a clear, colorless liquid containing 0.5% w/w HIBITANE® (chlorhexidine gluconate) with inactive ingredients: emollients, isopropanol 70%, purified water.

Indications: HIBISTAT is indicated for health-care personnel use as a germicidal hand rinse. HIBISTAT is for hand hygiene on physically clean hands. It is used in those situations where hands are physically clean, but in need of degerming, when routine handwashing is not convenient or desirable. HIBISTAT provides rapid germicidal action and has a persistent effect.
HIBISTAT should be used in-between patients and procedures where there are no sinks available or continued return to the sink area is inconvenient. HIBISTAT can be used as an alternative to detergent-based products when hands are physically clean. Also, HIBISTAT is an effective germicidal hand rinse following a soap and water handwash.

Warning: Flammable. This product is alcohol-based. Alcohol is extremely flammable. It should be kept away from flame or devices which may generate an electrical spark.

WARNINGS: FOR EXTERNAL USE ONLY. KEEP OUT OF EYES, EARS AND MOUTH. HIBISTAT SHOULD NOT BE USED AS A PREOPERATIVE SKIN PREPARATION OF THE FACE OR HEAD. MISUSE OF CHLORHEXIDINE-CONTAINING PRODUCTS HAS BEEN REPORTED TO CAUSE SERIOUS AND PERMANENT EYE INJURY WHEN IT HAS BEEN PERMITTED TO ENTER AND REMAIN IN THE EYE DURING SURGICAL PROCEDURES. IF HIBISTAT SHOULD CONTACT THESE AREAS, RINSE OUT PROMPTLY AND THOROUGHLY WITH WATER. Avoid contact with meninges. HIBISTAT should not be used by persons who have a sensitivity to it or its components. Chlorhexidine gluconate has been reported to cause deafness when instilled in the middle ear through perforated ear drums. Irritation, sensitization and generalized allergic reactions have been reported with chlorhexidine-containing products, especially in the genital areas. If adverse reactions occur, discontinue use immediately and if severe, contact a physician. Keep this and all drugs out of the reach of children. In case of accidental ingestion, seek professional assistance or contact a Poison Control Center immediately.
Avoid excessive heat (above 104°F).
Accidental ingestion: Chlorhexidine gluconate taken orally is poorly absorbed. Treat with gastric lavage using milk, egg white, gelatin or mild soap avoiding pulmonary aspiration. Do not use apomorphine. Assist respiration if necessary and keep patient warm. Intravenous levulose can accelerate alcohol metabolism. In severe cases, hemodialysis or peritoneal dialysis may be appropriate.

DIRECTIONS FOR USE: HIBISTAT Towelette: Rub hands vigorously with the HIBISTAT Towelette for approximately 15 seconds, paying particular attention to nails and interdigital spaces. HIBISTAT dries rapidly in use. No water or towel drying is necessary. The emollients contained in the HIBISTAT Towelette protect the hands from the potential drying effect of alcohol.
HIBISTAT Liquid: Dispense about 5 mL of HIBISTAT into cupped hands and rub vigorously until dry (about 15 seconds), paying particular attention to nails and interdigital spaces. HIBISTAT dries rapidly in use. No water or toweling is necessary. The emollients contained in HIBISTAT protect the hands from the potential drying effect of alcohol.
Laundering: Chlorhexidine gluconate chemically reacts with chlorine to form a brown stain on fabric. Fabric which has come in contact with chlorhexidine gluconate should be rinsed well and washed without the addition of chlorine products. If bleach is desired, only nonchlorine bleach should be used. Full laundering instructions are packed with each case of HIBISTAT. (Please see HIBICLENS for full laundering instructions.)

How Supplied: In plastic disposable bottles of 4 oz and 8 oz with flip-top cap, and in disposable towelettes containing 5 mL, packaged 50 towelettes to a carton.
NDC 0038-0585 (bottles)
NDC 0038-0587 (towelettes)

STUART PRENATAL® Tablets
Multivitamin/Multimineral Supplement

One Tablet Daily Provides:

VITAMINS	RDA*	
A	100%	4,000 IU
D	100%	400 IU
E	100%	11 mg
C	100%	100 mg
Folic Acid	100%	0.8 mg
B_1 (thiamin)	100%	1.5 mg
B_2 (riboflavin)	100%	1.7 mg
Niacin	100%	18 mg
B_6 (pyridoxine hydrochloride)	100%	2.6 mg
B_{12} (cyanocobalamin)	100%	4 mcg

MINERALS	RDA*	
Calcium	17%	200 mg
Iron	330%**	60 mg
Zinc	100%	25 mg

*Recommended Dietary Allowances (Food and Nutrition Board, NAS/NRC-1980) for pregnant and/or lactating women.
**Recommended Dietary Allowances (Food and Nutrition Board, NAS/NRC-1980) for adults, not pregnant and/or lactating women.

Ingredients
Active: calcium sulfate, ferrous fumarate, ascorbic acid, dl-alpha tocopheryl acetate, zinc oxide, niacinamide, vitamin A acetate, pyridoxine hydrochloride, riboflavin, thiamin mononitrate, folic acid, cholecalciferol, cyanocobalamin. Inactive: croscarmellose sodium, hydroxypropyl methylcellulose, microcrystalline cellulose, pregelatinized starch, red iron oxide, titanium dioxide.

Indications: STUART PRENATAL is a nonprescription multivitamin/multimineral supplement for use before, during, and after pregnancy. It provides vitamins equal to 100% or more of the RDA for pregnant, lactating and nonlactating women, plus essential minerals, including 60 mg of elemental iron as well-tolerated ferrous fumarate, and 200 mg of elemental calcium (nonalkalizing and phosphorus-free), and 25 mg zinc. STUART PRENATAL also contains 0.8 mg folic acid.

Directions: Before, during and after pregnancy, one tablet daily, or as directed by a physician.

Warning: In case of accidental overdose, seek professional assistance or contact a Poison Control Center immediately. Keep out of the reach of children.

How Supplied: Bottles of 100 light pink tablets imprinted "STUART 071". A child-resistant safety cap is standard on 100 tablet bottles as a safeguard against accidental ingestion by children.
NDC 0038-0071.

Shown in Product Identification Section, page 434

Syntex Laboratories, Inc
3401 HILLVIEW AVENUE
PALO ALTO, CA 94304

CARMOL® 10
10% urea lotion for total body dry skin care.

Active Ingredient: Urea 10% in a scented lotion of purified water, carbomer 940, cetyl alcohol, isopropyl palmitate, PEG-8 dioleate, PEG-8 distearate, propylene glycol, propylene glycol dipelargonate, stearic acid, sodium laureth sulfate, trolamine, and xanthan gum.

Indications: For total body dry skin care.

Actions: Keratolytic CARMOL 10 is non-occlusive, contains no mineral oil or petrolatum. CARMOL 10 is hypoallergenic; contains no lanolin, parabens or other preservatives.

Precautions: For external use only. Discontinue use if irritation occurs. Keep out of the reach of children. In case of accidental ingestion, seek professional assistance or contact a poison control center immediately.

Dosage and Administration: Rub in gently on hands, face or body. Repeat as necessary.

How Supplied: 6 fl. oz. bottle.

CARMOL® 20
20% Urea Cream Extra strength for rough, dry skin

Active Ingredients: Urea 20% in a nonlipid vanishing cream containing carbomer 940, hypoallergenic fragrance, isopropyl myristate, isopropyl palmitate, propylene glycol, purified water, sodium laureth sulfate, stearic acid, trolamine, xanthan gum.

Indications: Especially useful on rough, dry skin of hands, elbows, knees and feet.

Actions: Keratolytic. Contains no parabens, lanolin or mineral oil.

Precautions: For external use only. Keep away from eyes. Use with caution on face or broken or inflamed skin; transient stinging may occur. Discontinue use if irritation occurs. Keep out of the reach of children. In case of accidental ingestion, seek professional assistance or contact a poison control center immediately.

Dosage and Administration: Apply once or twice daily or as directed. Rub in well.

How Supplied: 3 oz. tubes, 1 lb. jars.

Products are indexed by generic and chemical names in the **YELLOW SECTION**

Tec Laboratories, Inc.
P.O. BOX 1958
ALBANY, OR 97321

TECNU® POISON OAK-N-IVY CLEANSER

Active Ingredients: Mixed alkanes, alkylarypolyalkoxy alcohols, propylene glycol, wood pulp.

Indications: TECNU is 100% effective in removing the irritant of poison oak, ivy and sumac from skin and clothing. If TECNU is used to cleanse skin before an allergic reaction begins, then no rash will occur.

Dosage and Administration: To prevent rash apply to skin 2 to 8 hours after exposure for normally sensitive people. Hypersensitive persons should use as soon as possible after contact. If rash has started, apply to affected skin and rub in for 2 minutes (avoid breaking skin). Rinse off with cool water to remove poison oils and towel dry gently.

Warnings: TECNU is not considered toxic. Do not take internally or get into eyes. For eye contact, flush with water. If swallowed, treat as though treating for petroleum jelly ingestion. Keep this and all drugs out of the hands of children.

Shown in Product Identification Section, page 434

Thompson Medical Company, Inc.
222 LAKEVIEW AVENUE
WEST PALM BEACH
FLORIDA 33401

ASPERCREME®
[*ăs-per-crēme*]
External Analgesic Rub

Description: ASPERCREME® is available as an odor-free creme and lotion for use as a topical massage rub that temporarily relieves minor muscle aches and pains without stomach upset. Aspercreme does not contain aspirin.

Active Ingredients: Salycin® 10% (Thompson Medical's brand of Trolamine Salicylate).

Other Ingredients: Creme: Cetyl Alcohol, Glycerin, Methylparaben, Mineral Oil, Potassium Phosphate, Propylparaben, Stearic Acid, Triethanolamine, Water. Lotion: Cetyl Alcohol, Fragrance, Glyceryl Stearate, Isopropyl Palmitate, Lanolin, Methylparaben, Potassium Phosphate, Propylene Glycol, Propylparaben, Sodium Lauryl Sulfate, Stearic Acid, Water.

Actions: External analgesic rub.

Indications: Analgesic rub for temporary relief of minor aches and pains of muscles associated with simple strains and sprains. **Aspercreme contains no aspirin.**

Warnings: Use only as directed. If prone to allergic reaction from aspirin or salicylate, consult your doctor before using. If redness is present or condition worsens, or if pain persists for more than 7 days or clears up and occurs again within a few days, discontinue use and consult a doctor. Do not use on children under 10 years of age. Do not apply if skin is irritated or if irritation develops. As with any drug, if you are pregnant or nursing a baby, seek the advice of a health professional before using this product. For external use only. Avoid contact with eyes. Keep this and all medicines out of the reach of children. In case of accidental ingestion seek professional assistance or contact a Poison Control Center immediately.

Dosage and Administration: Apply generously directly to affected area. Massage into painful area until thoroughly absorbed into skin, repeat as necessary, especially before retiring but not more than 4 times daily.

How to Store: Protect from freezing and temperatures above 100°F. Close cap tightly after use.

How Supplied: Creme: 1¼ oz., 3 oz. and 5 oz. tubes. Lotion: 6 oz. bottle.

CORTIZONE–5®
Creme and Ointment Anti-itch (hydrocortisone)

Description: CORTIZONE-5® creme and ointment are topical anti-itch preparations.

Active Ingredient: Hydrocortisone 0.5%.

Other Ingredients: Creme: Aluminum Sulfate, Calcium Acetate, Glycerin, Light Mineral Oil, Methylparaben, Potato Dextrin, Purified Water, Sodium Lauryl Sulfate, White Petroleum. May Also Contain: Cetearyl Alcohol, Propylparaben, Sodium C_{12-15} Alcohols Sulfate, Synthetic Beeswax, White Wax. Ointment: White Petrolatum.

Indications: CORTIZONE-5® is recommended for the temporary relief of itching associated with minor skin irritations, inflammations and rashes due to: eczema, dermatitis, psoriasis, insect bites, poison ivy, oak, sumac, detergents, soaps, cosmetics, jewelry, external anal and genital itching.

Warnings: For external use only. Avoid contact with the eyes. If condition worsens, or if symptoms persist for more than 7 days or clear up and occur again within a few days, do not use this or any other hydrocortisone product unless you have consulted a doctor. Do not use in genital area if you have a vaginal discharge. Consult a doctor. Do not use for the treatment of diaper rash. Consult a doctor.
Warnings For External Anal Itch Users: Do not exceed the recommended daily dosage unless directed by a doctor. In case of bleeding, consult a doctor promptly. Do not put this product into the rectum by using fingers or any mechanical device or applicator.

KEEP THIS AND ALL MEDICINES OUT OF THE REACH OF CHILDREN. In case of accidental ingestion, seek professional assistance or contact a poison control center immediately.

Dosage and Administration: Adults and children 2 years of age and older: Apply to affected area not more than 3 to 4 times daily. Children under 2 years of age: Do not use, consult a doctor. Directions For External Anal Itching Users: Adults: When practical, cleanse the affected area with mild soap and warm water and rinse thoroughly. Gently dry by patting or blotting with toilet tissue or a soft cloth before application of this product. Children under 12 years of age: Consult a doctor.

How to Store: Store at room temperature.

How Supplied: CORTIZONE-5 creme: 1 oz, and 2 oz. tubes. CORTIZONE-5 ointment: 1 oz tube.

Shown in Product Identification Section, page 434

DEXATRIM® Capsules

[*dĕx-a-trĭm*]

Prolonged action anorectic for weight control contains

phenylpropanolamine HCl 50mg (time release)

DEXATRIM® Maximum Strength Plus Vitamin C/Caffeine-Free Capsules

phenylpropanolamine HCl 75mg (time release)

Vitamin C 180mg (immediate release)

DEXATRIM® Maximum Strength Caffeine-Free Capsules

phenylpropanolamine HCl 75mg (time release)

DEXATRIM® Maximum Strength Plus Vitamin C/Caffeine-Free Caplets

phenylpropanolamine HCl 75mg (time release)

Vitamin C 180mg (immediate release)

DEXATRIM® Maximum Strength Caffeine-Free Caplets

phenylpropanolamine HCl 75mg (time release)

DEXATRIM® Maximum Strength Pre-Meal Caplets

phenylpropanolamine HCl 25mg (immediate release)

Indication: DEXATRIM® is an appetite suppressant for use in conjunction with a calorie-restricted diet for weight loss. It is available in time release and immediate release dosage forms.

Caution: READ BEFORE USING. For adult use only. Do not give this product to children under 12 years of age. Persons between the ages of 12 and 18 or over 60 are advised to consult their doctor or pharmacist before using this or any drug. If nervousness, dizziness, headaches, rapid pulse, palpitations, sleeplessness, or other symptoms occur, stop using and consult your physician.

Warning: DO NOT EXCEED RECOMMENDED DOSAGE. Taking more of this or any drug than is recommended can cause untoward health complications. It is sensible to check your blood pressure regularly. Do not use if you have high blood pressure, diabetes, heart, thyroid, kidney, or other disease or are being treated for high blood pressure or depression except under the advice and supervision of a doctor. As with any drug if you are pregnant or nursing a baby, seek the advice of a health professional before using this product. Do not use continuously for more than 3 months. When you have reached your desired weight or are able to control your appetite by yourself, use DEXATRIM only as needed.

Drug Interaction Precaution: Do not take if you are presently taking another medication containing phenylpropanolamine, or any type of nasal decongestant, or a prescription drug for high blood pressure or depression, or any other type of prescription medication except under the advice and supervision of a doctor.

KEEP THIS AND ALL MEDICATION OUT OF THE REACH OF CHILDREN. In case of accidental overdose seek professional assistance or contact a Poison Control Center immediately.

Dosage and Administration:

Capsule Dosage Forms: DEXATRIM®, DEXATRIM® Maximum Strength Plus Vitamin C, DEXATRIM® Maximum Strength/Caffeine-Free.

Caplet Dosage Forms: DEXATRIM® Maximum Strength Plus Vitamin C, DEXATRIM® Maximum Strength/Caffeine-Free.

Administration: One capsule or caplet at midmorning (10 am) with a full glass of water.

Immediate Release Caplet Dosage Form: DEXATRIM® Maximum Strength Pre-Meal Caplets:

Administration: One caplet 30 minutes before each meal with one or two full glasses of water. Do not exceed 3 caplets in 24 hours.

How Supplied: All Dexatrim products are supplied in tamper-evident blister packages. Do not use if individual seals are broken.

DEXATRIM® Capsules: Packages of 28 with 1250 calorie DEXATRIM Diet Plan.

DEXATRIM® Maximum Strength Plus Vitamin C/Caffeine-Free Capsules: Packages of 10, 20 and 40 with 1250 calorie DEXATRIM Diet Plan.

DEXATRIM® Maximum Strength Capsules/Caffeine-Free: Packages of 10, 20 and 40 with 1250 calorie DEXATRIM Diet Plan.

DEXATRIM® Maximum Strength Plus Vitamin C/Caffeine-Free Caplets: Packages of 10, 20 and 40 with 1250 calorie DEXATRIM Diet Plan.

DEXATRIM® Maximum Strength Caplets/Caffeine-Free: Packages of 10, 20 and 40 with 1250 calorie DEXATRIM Diet Plan.

DEXATRIM® Maximum Strength Pre-Meal Caplets: Packages of 30 with 1250 calorie DEXATRIM Diet Plan.

References:
Altschuler, S., and Frazer, D.L., Double-Blind Clinical Evaluation of the Anorectic Activity of Phenylpropanolamine Hydrochloride Drops and Placebo Drops in the Treatment of Exogenous Obesity. *Current Therapeutic Research,* 40(1), 211–217, July 1986.

Altschuler, S., et. al., Three Controlled Trials of Weight Loss with Phenylpropanolamine, *Int J Obesity,* 1982;6:549–556.

Blackburn, G.L., et. al., Determinants of the Pressor Effect of Phenylpropanolamine in Healthy Subjects. *JAMA,* 1989; 261:3267–3272.

Morgan, J.P., et. al., Subjective Profile of Phenylpropanolamine: Absence of Stimulant or Euphorigenic Effects at Recommended Dose Levels. *J Clin Psychopharm,* 1989;9(1):33–38.

Lasagna, L., *Phenylpropanolamine—A Review,* New York, John Wiley and Sons, 1988.

All referenced materials available on request.

Shown in Product Identification Section, page 434

ENCARE®

[*en'kar*]

Vaginal Contraceptive Suppositories

Description: Encare is a safe and effective contraceptive in a convenient vaginal suppository form available without a prescription. Encare is reliable because it offers two-way protection: (1) Encare kills sperm on contact by releasing a precise dose of nonoxynol 9, the spermicide most recommended by doctors. (2) Encare gently disperses a physical barrier of protection against the cervix to help prevent pregnancy.

Encare is an effective contraceptive in vaginal suppository form.

Active Ingredient: Each Suppository contains 2.27% Nonoxynol 9.

Other Ingredients: Fragrance, Lactalbumin, Polyethylene Glycols, Potassium Coco-Hydrolyzed Animal Protein, Sodium Bicarbonate, Sodium Lauryl Sulfate, Sodium Tartrate, Tartaric Acid.

Indications: Encare is effective in the prevention of pregnancy.

Action: Encare is 100% free of hormones and free of the serious side effects associated with oral contraceptives.

Encare is convenient and easy to use. Women like Encare because each insert is individually wrapped and can be easily carried in a pocket or purse. There are other reasons why women use Encare. It is approximately as effective as vaginal foam contraceptives in actual use, yet there is no applicator, so there is nothing to fill, remove, or clean. In addition, women may find Encare convenient to use in place of a second application of jelly or cream in conjunction with a diaphragm.

Continued on next page

Thompson Medical—Cont.

Because Encare can be inserted as much as an hour before intercourse, it does not interfere with spontaneity or ruin the mood. Many men are not even aware a woman is using Encare. Encare has been used successfully by millions of women throughout Europe and America.

Special Warning: Spermicidal contraceptives should not be used during pregnancy. Some experts believe that there may be an increased risk of birth defects occurring in children whose mothers used a spermicidal contraceptive at the time of conception or during pregnancy. If you believe you may be pregnant, have a pregnancy test before using a spermicidal contraceptive. If you have used a spermicidal contraceptive after becoming pregnant, or used a spermicidal contraceptive when you became pregnant, discuss this issue with your physician.

Cautions: If your doctor has told you that you should not become pregnant, consult him as to which method, including Encare, is best for you.
If vaginal irritation occurs and continues, contact your physician.
Do not take orally. **KEEP THIS AND ALL DRUGS OUT OF THE REACH OF CHILDREN.** In case of accidental ingestion, call a Poison Control Center, emergency medical facility or a doctor immediately.
Encare should be kept away from excessive heat. Store at room temperature. Should the product inadvertently be exposed to higher temperatures, hold under cold water for two minutes before removing protective wrap.

Dosage and Administration: For best protection against pregnancy, it is essential to follow package instructions. At least 10 minutes before intercourse, place one Encare insert with your fingertip as far as possible into the vagina, towards the small of your back. Best protection will occur when Encare is placed deep into the vagina. You may feel a pleasant sensation of warmth as Encare effervesces and distributes the spermicide, nonoxynol 9, within the vagina. This is a natural attribute to the product. **IMPORTANT:** It is essential to insert Encare at least 10 minutes before intercourse. If one chooses, Encare can be inserted up to one hour before intercourse. If intercourse has not taken place within one hour after insertion, use a new Encare insert. Use a new Encare insert each time intercourse is repeated. Encare can be used safely as frequently as needed. Douching after use of Encare is not required; however, should you desire to do so, wait at least six hours after intercourse.

How Supplied: Boxes of 12.

References: Barwin, B., Encare Oval: A Clinical Study, *Contraceptive Delivery System*, 4, 331–334, 1983. Masters, W., In Vivo Evaluation of an Effervescent Intravaginal Contraceptive Inserted by Simulated Coital Activity, *Fertility and Sterility*, 32, 161–165, 1979.

NP-27®
Cream, Solution, Spray Powder and Powder
Antifungal
(tolnaftate)

Description: NP-27 contains the maximum strength available without a prescription of tolnaftate, a clinically proven ingredient which kills athlete's foot fungus and jock itch fungus on contact. It is available as a cream, solution, spray powder and powder.

Active Ingredients: Cream, Solution and Powder: Tolnaftate 1%.
Spray Powder: Tolnaftate 1%, contains: SD Alcohol 40 14.9%.

Other Ingredients: Cream: BHT, Polyethylene Glycol 400, Propylene Glycol, Titanium Dioxide. May also contain: *n*-Amylamine, Carbomer 934P, Carbomer 940, Diisopropanolamine. Solution: BHT, Polyethylene Glycol 400. May also contain: Propylene Glycol. Spray Powder: Isobutane, Isopropyl Myristate, Talc. Powder: Cornstarch, Talc.

Indications: An effective antifungal agent that kills athlete's foot fungus and jock itch fungus on contact and helps prevent reinfection. Provides quick relief of the itching, burning, scaling and discomfort that can accompany these conditions.

Warnings: For external use only. Do not use on children under 2 years of age except under the advice and supervision of a doctor. Children under 12 years of age should be supervised in the use of the product. If irritation occurs or if there is no improvement within 2 weeks, discontinue use and consult a doctor or pharmacist. Keep this and all medications out of the reach of children. In case of accidental ingestion, seek professional assistance or contact a Poison Control Center immediately. Avoid eye contact. Not effective on scalp or nails.

Dosage and Administration: Cleanse skin with soap and water and dry thoroughly. Apply a thin layer over affected area morning and night or as directed by a doctor. To help prevent recurrence, continue treatment for 2 weeks after disappearance of all symptoms. For athlete's foot pay special attention to the spaces between the toes.

How Supplied: Available in 0.5 oz. and 1 oz. cream; 0.5 oz. solution; 3.5 oz. spray powder; 1.5 oz powder.

How to Store: Store at room temperature.

Shown in Product Identification Section, page 434

SLEEPINAL®
Night-time Sleep Aid Capsules
(Diphenhydramine HCl)

Description: SLEEPINAL is a night-time sleep aid. When taken prior to bedtime, it helps to relieve sleeplessness and aids in falling asleep.

Active Ingredient: Diphenhydramine HCl 50 mg.

Other Ingredients: FD&C Blue No. 1, Gelatin, Lactose, Magnesium Stearate, Povidone, Talc.

Indications: For relief of occasional sleeplessness.

Action: SLEEPINAL is an antihistamine with anticholinergic and sedative action.

Warnings: Read before using. Do not exceed recommended dosage. Do not give to children under 12 years of age. If sleeplessness persists continuously for more than 2 weeks, consult a doctor. Insomnia may be a symptom of serious underlying medical illness. Do not take this product if you have asthma, glaucoma, emphysema, chronic pulmonary disease, shortness of breath, difficulty in breathing, or difficulty in urination due to enlargement of the prostate gland unless directed by a doctor. Avoid alcoholic beverages while taking this product. Do not take this product if you are taking sedatives or tranquilizers, without first consulting your doctor. As with any drug, if you are pregnant or nursing a baby, seek the advice of a health professional before using this product.
KEEP THIS AND ALL MEDICATIONS OUT OF THE REACH OF CHILDREN. In the case of accidental overdose, seek professional assistance or contact a Poison Control Center immediately.

Dosage and Administration: Adults and children 12 years of age and over: Oral dosage, one capsule at bedtime if needed, or as directed by a doctor.

How to Store: Store in a dry place at controlled room temperature 15° C–30° C (59° F–86° F).

How Supplied: Sleepinal is supplied in tamper-evident blister packages. Do not use if individual seals are broken. Packages of 16 and 32 capsules.

Shown in Product Identification Section, page 434

Triton Consumer Products, Inc.
561 W. GOLF ROAD
ARLINGTON HEIGHTS, IL 60005

MG 217® PSORIASIS MEDICATION
Skin Care: Ointment and Lotion
Hair/Scalp Care: Shampoo and Conditioner

Active Ingredients: OINTMENT—Coal Tar Solution USP 2%, Salicylic Acid 1.5% and Colloidal Sulfur 1.1%. **LOTION**—Coal Tar Solution USP 5% with Jojoba. **SHAMPOO**—Coal Tar Solution USP 5%, Salicylic Acid 2% and Colloidal Sulfur 1.5%. **CONDITIONER**—Coal Tar Solution USP 2%.

Action/Uses: Effective relief for itching, scaling and flaking of Psoriasis or Seborrhea.

Caution: For external use only. Keep out of the reach of children. Avoid contact with eyes. If undue skin irritation occurs, discontinue use. For shampoo/conditioner, in isolated cases, temporary discoloration of blond, bleached or tinted hair may occur.

Administration: OINTMENT or LOTION—Wash affected areas of skin with mild soap/water and dry. Rub MG 217 in well. Apply twice daily or as needed. Not for use on the scalp. **SHAMPOO**—Shake well before using. Wet hair, then massage liberal amount of MG 217 into scalp and leave on for 5–10 minutes. Use daily or as needed. **CONDITIONER**—After shampooing, massage liberal amount of MG 217 into scalp and leave on for several minutes. Rinse thoroughly. Use daily or as needed.

How Supplied: OINTMENT—3.8 oz. and 15.3 oz. plastic jars. **LOTION**—4 oz. plastic bottles. **SHAMPOO**—4 oz., 8 oz. and 16 oz. plastic bottles. **CONDITIONER**—4 oz. plastic bottles.

UAS Laboratories
9201 PENN AVENUE SOUTH #10
MINNEAPOLIS, MN 55431

DDS-ACIDOPHILUS
Capsule, Tablet & Powder free of dairy products, corn, soy, and preservatives

Description: **DDS-Acidophilus** is the source of a special strain of Lactobacillus acidophilus free of dairy products, corn, soy and preservatives. Each capsule or tablet contains one billion viable DDS-1 L.acidophilus at the time of manufacturing. One gram of powder contains two billion viable DDS-1 L.acidophilus.

Indications and Usages: An aid in implanting the gut with beneficial Lactobacillus acidophilus under conditions of digestive disorders, acne, yeast infections, and following antibiotic therapy.

Administration: One to two capsules or tablets twice daily before meals. One-fourth teaspoon powder can be substituted for two capsules or tablets.

How Supplied: Bottles of 100 capsules or tablets. 12 bottles per case. Powder is available in 2 oz. bottle; 12 bottles per case.

Storage: Keep refrigerated under 40°F.

EDUCATIONAL MATERIAL

DDS-Acidophilus
Booklet describing superior-strain Acidophilus without dairy products, corn, soy, or preservatives. Two billion viable DDS-L. acidophilus per gram.

The Upjohn Company
KALAMAZOO, MI 49001

BACIGUENT® Antibiotic Ointment

Description: *Baciguent* Ointment (each gram contains 500 units of bacitracin) is a non-stinging first aid ointment. Also contains anhydrous lanolin, mineral oil and white petrolatum.

Indications: First aid ointment to help prevent infection and aid in the healing of minor burns, cuts, nicks, scrapes, scratches and abrasions.

Warnings: For external use only. Do not use in the eyes or apply over large areas of the body. In case of deep or puncture wounds, animal bites, or serious burns, consult a physician. Stop use and consult a physician if the condition persists or gets worse. Do not use longer than 1 week unless directed by a physician. Keep this and all medications out of the reach of children. In case of accidental ingestion, seek professional assistance or contact a poison control center immediately.

Dosage and Administration: For adults and children (all ages): Clean the affected area. Apply a small amount of *Baciguent* (an amount equal to the surface area of the tip of a finger) on the area 1 to 3 times daily. May be covered with a sterile bandage.

How Supplied: Available in ½ oz and 1 oz tubes.

CORTAID® Cream with Aloe
CORTAID® Ointment with Aloe
CORTAID® Lotion
(hydrocortisone acetate)
CORTAID® Spray
(hydrocortisone)

Antipruritic

Description: *Cortaid* Cream with Aloe contains hydrocortisone acetate (equivalent to 0.5% hydrocortisone) in a greaseless, odorless, vanishing cream that leaves no residue. Also contains aloe vera, butylparaben, cetyl palmitate, glyceryl stearate, methylparaben, polyethylene glycol, stearamidoethyl diethylamine, and purified water.
Cortaid Ointment with Aloe contains hydrocortisone acetate (equivalent to 0.5% hydrocortisone) in a soothing, lubricating ointment. Also contains aloe vera, butylparaben, cholesterol, methylparaben, mineral oil, white petrolatum, and microcrystalline wax.
Cortaid Lotion contains hydrocortisone acetate (equivalent to 0.5% hydrocortisone) in a greaseless, odorless, vanishing lotion. Also contains butylparaben, cetyl palmitate, glyceryl monostearate, methylparaben, polysorbate 80, propylene glycol, stearamidoethyl diethylamine, and purified water.
Cortaid Spray contains 0.5% hydrocortisone in a quick-drying, nonstaining, nonaerosol, vanishing spray. Also contains alcohol (46%), glycerin, methylparaben, and purified water.

Indications: For the temporary relief of minor skin irritations, inflammation, itches and rashes due to dermatitis, insect bites, eczema, psoriasis, poison ivy, poison oak, poison sumac, soaps, detergents, cosmetics, jewelry, and external genital and anal itching.

Uses: The vanishing action of *Cortaid* Cream with Aloe makes it cosmetically acceptable when the skin rash treated is on exposed parts of the body, such as the hands or arms. *Cortaid* Ointment with Aloe is best used where protection, lubrication and soothing of dry and scaly lesions is required, and is also preferred for treating itchy genital and anal areas. *Cortaid* Lotion is thinner than the cream and is especially suitable for hairy body areas, such as the scalp or arms. *Cortaid* Spray is a quick-drying, nonstaining formulation suitable for covering hard-to-reach areas of the skin.

Warnings: For external use only. Avoid contact with the eyes. If condition worsens, or if symptoms persist for more than 7 days, discontinue use of this product and consult a physician. Do not use on children under 2 years of age except under the advice and supervision of a physician. Keep this and all drugs out of the reach of children. In case of accidental ingestion, seek professional assistance or contact a poison control center immediately.

Dosage and Administration: For adults and children 2 years of age and older: Apply to affected area not more than 3 to 4 times daily. For children under 2 years of age there is no recommended dosage except under the advice and supervision of a physician.

How Supplied: Cream with Aloe: ½ oz and 1 oz tubes; Ointment with Aloe: ½ oz and 1 oz tubes; Lotion: 1 oz bottle. Spray: 1.5 fluid oz pump spray bottle.

Shown in Product Identification Section, page 434

CORTEF® Feminine Itch Cream
(hydrocortisone acetate)
Antipruritic

Description: *Cortef* Feminine Itch Cream contains hydrocortisone acetate (equivalent to hydrocortisone 0.5%) in an odorless, vanishing cream base that quickly disappears into the skin to avoid staining of clothing. Also contains aloe vera, butylparaben, cetyl palmitate, glyceryl monostearate, methylparaben, polyethylene glycol, stearamidoethyl diethylamine, and purified water.

Indications: For effective temporary relief of minor skin irritations and external genital itching. It relieves the itch and takes the redness out of the skin to break the annoying itch/scratch cycle.

Warnings: For external use only. Avoid contact with eyes. If condition worsens, or if symptoms persist for more than 7 days, discontinue use of this prod-

Continued on next page

Upjohn—Cont.

uct and consult a physician. Do not use on children under 2 years of age except under the advice and supervision of a physician. Keep this and all drugs out of the reach of children. In case of accidental ingestion, seek professional assistance or contact a poison control center immediately.

Dosage and Administration: Apply to affected area not more than 3 to 4 times daily.

How Supplied: Available in ½ oz tube.

DOXIDAN® Capsules
Stimulant/Stool Softener Laxative

Active Ingredients: Each soft gelatin capsule contains 65 mg yellow phenolphthalein and 60 mg docusate calcium.

Inactive Ingredients: Alcohol up to 1.5% (w/w), corn oil, FD&C Blue #1 and Red #40, gelatin, glycerin, hydrogenated vegetable oil, lecithin, parabens, sorbitol, titanium dioxide, vegetable shortening, yellow wax, and other ingredients.

Indications: DOXIDAN is a safe, reliable laxative for the relief of occasional constipation. The combination of a stimulant/stool softener laxative allows positive laxative action on a softened stool for gentle evacuation without straining. DOXIDAN generally produces a bowel movement in 6 to 12 hours.

Dosage and Administration: Adults and children 12 years of age and over: one or two capsules by mouth daily. For use in children under 12, consult a physician.

Warnings: Do not use laxative products when abdominal pain, nausea, or vomiting are present unless directed by a doctor. If you have noticed a sudden change in bowel habits that persists over a period of 2 weeks, consult a doctor before using a laxative. Laxative products should not be used for a period longer than 1 week unless directed by a doctor. Rectal bleeding or failure to have a bowel movement after use of a laxative may indicate a serious condition. Discontinue use and consult your doctor. If skin rash appears, do not use this product or any other preparation containing phenolphthalein. Keep this and all drugs out of the reach of children. In case of accidental overdose, seek professional assistance or contact a poison control center immediately. As with any drug, if you are pregnant or nursing a baby, seek the advice of a health professional before using this product.

How Supplied: Packages of 10, 30, 100 and 1,000 maroon soft gelatin capsules, and Unit Dose 100s (10 × 10 strips).
Store at controlled room temperature (59–86° F) in a dry place.

Shown in Product Identification Section, page 434

KAOPECTATE®
Concentrated Anti-Diarrheal, Peppermint Flavor and Regular Flavor

Active Ingredient: Each tablespoon contains 600 mg attapulgite.

Inactive Ingredients: Flavors, glucono-delta-lactone, magnesium aluminum silicate, methylparaben, sorbic acid, sucrose, titanium dioxide, xanthan gum and purified water; Peppermint flavor contains FD&C Red #40.

Indications: For the fast relief of diarrhea and cramping.

Dosage and Administration: For best results, take full recommended dose at first sign of diarrhea and after each subsequent bowel movement. (Maximum 7 times in 24 hours.) Adults and children 12 years of age and over: 2 tablespoons. Children 6 to under 12 years of age: 1 tablespoon. Children 3 to under 6 years of age: ½ tablespoon.

Warnings: Unless directed by a physician, do not use in infants and children under 3 years of age or for more than two days or in the presence of high fever. Keep this and all drugs out of the reach of children. In case of accidental overdose, seek professional assistance or contact a poison control center immediately.

How Supplied: Regular flavor available in 3 oz, 8 oz, 12 oz and 16 oz bottles. Peppermint flavor available in 8 oz and 12 oz bottles.

Shown in Product Identification Section, page 434

KAOPECTATE® Children's Chewable Tablets, Anti-Diarrheal

Active Ingredient: Each tablet contains 300 mg attapulgite.

Inactive Ingredients: Cornstarch, dextrins, dextrose, D&C Red #27, D&C Red #30, flavor, magnesium stearate, sucrose and titanium dioxide.

Indications: For the fast relief of diarrhea and cramping; in a good-tasting, easy-to-take form. Especially formulated to meet the needs of children age 3 and up.

Dosage and Administration: Chew tablets thoroughly and swallow. For best results, take full recommended dose at first sign of diarrhea and after each subsequent bowel movement (maximum 7 times in 24 hours). Children 3 to under 6 years of age: 1 tablet; Children 6 to under 12 years of age: 2 tablets; Children (and adults) 12 years of age and over: 4 tablets.

Warnings: Unless directed by a physician, do not use in infants and children under 3 years of age or for more than two days or in the presence of high fever. Keep this and all drugs out of the reach of children. In case of accidental overdose, seek professional assistance or contact a poison control center immediately.

How Supplied: Available in blister packs of 16 chewable tablets.

Shown in Product Identification Section, page 434

KAOPECTATE® Maximum Strength Caplets
Anti-Diarrheal

Active Ingredient: Each tablet contains 750 mg attapulgite.

Inactive Ingredients: Croscarmellose sodium, hydroxypropyl cellulose, hydroxypropyl methylcellulose, methylparaben, pectin, propylene glycol, propylparaben, sucrose, titanium dioxide and zinc stearate.

Indications: For the fast relief of diarrhea and cramping.

Dosage and Administration: Swallow whole caplets with water; do not chew. For best results, take full recommended dose.
Adults: Take 2 caplets after the initial bowel movement and 2 caplets after each subsequent bowel movement, not to exceed 12 caplets in 24 hours. Children 6 to 12 years of age: Take 1 caplet after the initial bowel movement and 1 caplet after each subsequent bowel movement, not to exceed 6 caplets in 24 hours.
Children 3 to under 6 years of age: Use Advanced Formula *Kaopectate* Concentrated Anti-Diarrheal, Regular or Peppermint Flavor, or *Kaopectate* Children's Chewable Caplets.

Warnings: Unless directed by a physician, do not use in infants and children under 6 years of age or for more than two days or in the presence of high fever. Keep this and all drugs out of the reach of children. In case of accidental overdose, seek professional assistance or contact a poison control center immediately.

How Supplied: Available in blister packs of 12 and 20 caplets.

Shown in Product Identification Section, page 434

MOTRIN® IB
Caplets or Tablets (ibuprofen, USP)
Pain Reliever/Fever Reducer

WARNING: ASPIRIN-SENSITIVE PATIENTS. Do not take this product if you have had a severe allergic reaction to aspirin, eg—asthma, swelling, shock or hives because even though this product contains no aspirin or salicylates, cross-reactions may occur in patients allergic to aspirin.

Indications: For the temporary relief of headache, muscular aches, minor pain of arthritis, toothache, backache, minor aches and pains associated with the common cold, pain of menstrual cramps, and for reduction of fever.

Directions: Adults: Take 1 caplet or tablet every 4 to 6 hours while symptoms persist. If pain or fever does not respond to 1 caplet or tablet, 2 caplets or tablets may be used, but do not exceed 6 caplets or tablets in 24 hours, unless directed by a doctor. The smallest effective dose should be used. Take with food or milk, if occasional and mild heartburn, upset stomach or stomach pain occurs with use. Consult a doctor if these symptoms are more than mild or if they persist. Children: Do not give this product to children under 12 except under the advice and supervision of a doctor.

Warnings: Do not take for pain for more than 10 days or for fever for more than 3 days unless directed by a doctor. If pain or fever persists or gets worse, if new symptoms occur, or if the painful area is red or swollen, consult a doctor. These could be signs of serious illness. If you are under a doctor's care for any serious condition, consult a doctor before taking this product. As with aspirin and acetaminophen, if you have any condition which requires you to take prescription drugs or if you have had any problems or serious side effects from taking any nonprescription pain reliever, do not take MOTRIN® IB without first discussing it with your doctor. If you experience any symptoms which are unusual or seem unrelated to the condition for which you took ibuprofen, consult a doctor before taking any more of it. Although ibuprofen is indicated for the same conditions as aspirin and acetaminophen, it should not be taken with them except under a doctor's direction. Do not combine this product with any other ibuprofen-containing product. As with any drug, if you are pregnant or nursing a baby, seek the advice of a health professional before using this product. IT IS ESPECIALLY IMPORTANT NOT TO USE IBUPROFEN DURING THE LAST 3 MONTHS OF PREGNANCY UNLESS SPECIFICALLY DIRECTED TO DO SO BY A DOCTOR BECAUSE IT MAY CAUSE PROBLEMS IN THE UNBORN CHILD OR COMPLICATIONS DURING DELIVERY. Keep this and all drugs out of the reach of children. In case of accidental overdose, seek professional assistance or contact a poison control center immediately. **Store at room temperature. Avoid excessive heat 40°C (104°F).**

Active Ingredient: Each caplet or tablet contains ibuprofen 200 mg.

Other Ingredients: Carnauba wax, cornstarch, hydroxypropyl methylcellulose, propylene glycol, silicon dioxide, pregelatinized starch, stearic acid, titanium dioxide.

How Supplied: Bottles of 24, 50, 100, and 165 Caplets or Tablets.

Shown in Product Identification Section, page 434

MYCIGUENT® Antibiotic Ointment

Description: *Myciguent* Ointment (each gram contains 5 mg of neomycin sulfate equivalent to 3.5 mg neomycin) is a non-stinging first aid ointment. Also contains anhydrous lanolin, mineral oil, and white petrolatum.

Indications: First aid ointment to help prevent infection and aid in the healing of minor burns, cuts, nicks, scrapes, scratches and abrasions.

Warnings: For external use only. Do not use in the eyes or apply over large areas of the body. In case of deep or puncture wounds, animal bites, or serious burns, consult a physician. Stop use and consult a physician if the condition persists or gets worse. Do not use longer than 1 week unless directed by a physician. Keep this and all medications out of the reach of children. In case of accidental ingestion, seek professional assistance or contact a poison control center immediately.

Dosage and Administration: For adults and children (all ages): Clean the affected area. Apply a small amount of *Myciguent* (an amount equal to the surface area of the tip of a finger) on the area 1 to 3 times daily. May be covered with a sterile bandage.

How Supplied: Available in ½ oz and 1 oz tubes.

MYCITRACIN® Triple Antibiotic Ointment
MYCITRACIN® Plus Pain Reliever

Active Ingredients: Each gram of *Mycitracin* contains 500 units of bacitracin, neomycin sulfate equivalent to 3.5 mg neomycin and 5000 units of polymyxin B sulfate. Each gram of *Mycitracin* Plus Pain Reliever contains 500 units of bacitracin, neomycin sulfate equivalent to 3.5 mg neomycin, 5000 units of polymyxin B sulfate and 40 mg lidocaine. Also contain butylparaben, cholesterol, methylparaben, microcrystalline wax, mineral oil, and white petrolatum.

Indications: Both formulations are first aid ointment to help prevent infection in minor burns, cuts, nicks, scrapes, scratches and abrasions. *Mycitracin* Plus Pain Reliever also temporarily relieves pain.

How Supplied: Available in ½ oz and 1 oz tubes and (*Mycitracin*) 1/32 oz packets.

Shown in Product Identification Section, page 434

PROGAINE®
Shampoo for Thinning Hair

Description: PROGAINE Shampoo has been scientifically formulated to clean delicate thinning hair without damaging while adding body and manageability. PROGAINE is also an ideal shampoo for the user of thinning hair treatments. The exclusive, patented formula for PROGAINE Shampoo has been dermatologist tested on over 1000 adults in 31 medical clinics and proven safe for delicate thinning hair. PROGAINE Shampoo is different from many other shampoos in that PROGAINE contains none of the commonly used coating ingredients such as oils, waxes, silicones, proteins, quaternary ammonium salts, or cationic polymers which may leave a deposit on hair and scalp. PROGAINE is also hypoallergenic; it contains no harsh detergents or additives such as dyes, added formaldehydes, or parabens, commonly found in other shampoos, which may irritate sensitive scalps. PROGAINE Shampoo is pH balanced, ranging from 5.4 to 5.7, and will not affect the scalp's normal pH.

Ingredients:

Normal-to-Oily formula: Water, TEA lauryl sulfate, sodium laureth sulfate, cocamidopropyl betaine, cocamide DEA, propylene glycol, disodium EDTA, citric acid, methylchloroisothiazolinone, methylisothiazolinone, fragrance, and sodium chloride.

Normal-to-Dry formula: Water, sodium laureth sulfate, TEA lauryl sulfate, cocamidopropyl betaine, cocamide DEA, acetamide MEA, disodium EDTA, citric acid, methylchloroisothiazolinone, methylisothiazolinone, fragrance, sodium chloride.

Directions: PROGAINE Shampoo is gentle enough to use for every shampoo. For best results, wet hair and scalp, apply PROGAINE Shampoo, bring to a lather, then rinse. Repeat if desired.

How Supplied: Both the Normal-to-Oily and Normal-to-Dry formulas are available in 5 oz. and 8 oz. bottles.

SURFAK® Capsules
Stool Softener Laxative

Active Ingredients: Each soft gelatin capsule contains 240 mg docusate calcium.

Inactive Ingredients: Alcohol up to 3% (w/w), corn oil, FD&C Blue #1 and Red #40, gelatin, glycerin, parabens, sorbitol, and other ingredients.

Indications: SURFAK is indicated for the relief of occasional constipation. SURFAK generally produces a bowel movement in 12 to 72 hours. SURFAK is useful when only stool softening (without propulsive action) is required to relieve constipation.

Dosage and Administration: Adults and children 12 years of age and over: one capsule by mouth daily for several days or until bowel movements are normal. For use in children under 12, consult a physician.

Warnings: Do not use laxative products when abdominal pain, nausea, or vomiting are present unless directed by a doctor. If you have noticed a sudden change in bowel habits that persists over a period of 2 weeks, consult a doctor before using a laxative. Laxative products should not be used for a period longer than 1 week unless directed by a doctor. Rectal bleeding or failure to have a bowel movement after use of a laxative may indicate a serious condition. Discontinue use and consult your doctor. Keep this and all drugs out of the reach of children. In case of accidental overdose, seek professional assistance or contact a poison control center immediately. As with any drug, if you are pregnant or nursing a

Continued on next page

Upjohn—Cont.

baby, seek the advice of a health professional before using this product.

How Supplied: Packages of 7, 30, 100 and 500 red soft gelatin capsules and Unit Dose 100s (10 × 10 strips).
Store at controlled room temperature (59–86° F) in a dry place.

Shown in Product Identification Section, page 434

UNICAP® Capsules/Tablets
Multivitamin Supplement
100% RDA of Essential Vitamins in Easy to Swallow Capsule
Sugar and Sodium Free Tablet

Indications: Dietary multivitamin supplement of ten essential vitamins for health-conscious families (adults and children 4 or more years of age).

Each capsule contains:

		% U.S. RDA*
Vitamin A	5000 Int. Units	100
Vitamin D	400 Int. Units	100
Vitamin E	30 Int. Units	100
Vitamin C	60 mg	100
Folic Acid	400 mcg	100
Thiamine	1.5 mg	100
Riboflavin	1.7 mg	100
Niacin	20 mg	100
Vitamin B_6	2 mg	100
Vitamin B_{12}	6 mcg	100

Each tablet has same content except:

Vitamin E	15 Int. Units	50

*Percentage of U.S. Recommended Daily Allowance.

Ingredient List:
Capsules: Gelatin, Ascorbic Acid (Vit. C), Soybean Oil, Glycerin, Vitamin E Acetate, Niacinamide, Yellow Wax, Lecithin, Pyridoxine Hydrochloride (B-6), Thiamine Mononitrate (B-1), Riboflavin (B-2), Vitamin A Palmitate, Titanium Dioxide, Corn Oil, Folic Acid, FD&C Yellow No. 5, Ethyl Vanillin, Vanilla Enhancer, FD&C Yellow No. 6, Cholecaliciferol (Vit. D), Cyanocobalamin (B-12).
Tablets: Calcium Phosphate, Ascorbic Acid (Vit. C), Vitamin E Acetate, Hydroxypropyl Methylcellulose, Niacinamide, Artificial Color, Vitamin A Acetate, Magnesium Stearate, Pyridoxine Hydrochloride (B-6), Riboflavin (B-2), Silica Gel, Thiamine Mononitrate (B-1), FD&C Yellow No. 5, Folic Acid, Artificial Flavor, Cholecalciferol (Vit. D), Carnauba Wax, Cyanocobalamin (B-12).

Recommended Dosage: 1 capsule or tablet daily.

How Supplied: Available in bottles of 120 capsules or tablets.

Shown in Product Identification Section, page 434

UNICAP Jr™ Chewable Tablets
Good-tasting, Orange-flavored Chewable Tablet

Indications: Dietary multivitamin supplement providing up to 100% of the RDA of essential vitamins. For **children** 4 or more years of age.

Each tablet contains:

		% U.S. RDA*
Vitamin A	5000 Int. Units	100
Vitamin D	400 Int. Units	100
Vitamin E	15 Int. Units	50
Vitamin C	60 mg	100
Folic Acid	400 mcg	100
Thiamine	1.5 mg	100
Riboflavin	1.7 mg	100
Niacin	20 mg	100
Vitamin B_6	2 mg	100
Vitamin B_{12}	6 mcg	100

*Percentage of U.S. Recommended Daily Allowance.

Ingredient List: Sucrose, Mannitol, Sodium Ascorbate (Vit C), Lactose, Cornstarch, Niacinamide, Citric Acid, Vitamin E Acetate, Povidone, Artificial Flavor, Dextrins, Silica, Calcium Stearate, Pyridoxine HCl (B-6), Artificial Color, Vitamin A Acetate, Thiamine Mononitrate (B-1), Riboflavin (B-2), Folic Acid, Cyanocobalamin (B-12), Cholecalciferol (Vit D).

Recommended Dosage: 1 tablet daily.

How Supplied: Available in bottles of 120 tablets.

UNICAP M® Tablets
Multivitamins and Minerals
Sugar Free and Sodium Free

Indications: Dietary supplement providing up to 100% of the RDA for essential vitamins and minerals, including vitamin C and B-complex vitamins your body cannot store.

Each tablet contains:

		% U.S. RDA
Vitamin A	5000 Int. Units	100
Vitamin D	400 Int. Units	100
Vitamin E	30 Int. Units	100
Vitamin C	60 mg	100
Folic Acid	400 mcg	100
Thiamine	1.5 mg	100
Riboflavin	1.7 mg	100
Niacin	20 mg	100
Vitamin B_6	2 mg	100
Vitamin B_{12}	6 mcg	100
Pantothenic Acid	10 mg	100
Iodine	150 mcg	100
Iron	18 mg	100
Copper	2 mg	100
Zinc	15 mg	100
Calcium	60 mg	6
Phosphorus	45 mg	5
Manganese	1 mg	+
Potassium	5 mg	+

+Recognized as essential in human nutrition, but no U.S. Recommended Daily Allowance (U.S. RDA) has been established.

Ingredient List: Calcium Phosphate, Ascorbic Acid (Vit C) Vitamin E Acetate, Ferrous Fumarate, Cellulose, Niacinamide, Artificial Color, Zinc Oxide, Calcium Pantothenate, Vitamin A Acetate, Potassium Sulfate, Magnesium Stearate, Cupric Sulfate, Silica Gel, Manganese Sulfate, Pyridoxine Hydrochloride, Riboflavin (B-2), Thiamine Mononitrate (B-1), FD&C Yellow No. 5, Folic Acid, Artificial Flavor, Cholecalciferol (Vit D), Potassium Iodide, Carnauba Wax, Cyanocobalamin (B-12).

Recommended Dosage: 1 tablet daily.

How Supplied: Available in bottles of 120 and 500 tablets.

Shown in Product Identification Section, page 434

UNICAP® Plus Iron Tablets
Multivitamin Supplement With 100% of the U.S. RDA of Essential Vitamins Plus Calcium and Extra Iron
Sugar Free and Sodium Free

Indications: Dietary multivitamin supplement providing essential vitamins. 125% of the RDA of Iron plus Calcium for women 12 or more years of age.

Each tablet contains:

		% U.S. RDA*
Vitamins		
Vitamin A	5000 Int. Units	100
Vitamin D	400 Int. Units	100
Vitamin E	30 Int. Units	100
Vitamin C	60 mg	100
Folic Acid	400 mcg	100
Thiamine	1.5 mg	100
Riboflavin	1.7 mg	100
Niacin	20 mg	100
Vitamin B_6	2 mg	100
Vitamin B_{12}	6 mcg	100
Pantothenic Acid	10 mg	100
Minerals		
Iron	22.5 mg	125
Calcium	100 mg	10

*Percentage of U.S. Recommended Daily Allowance.

Ingredient List: Calcium Phosphate, Cellulose, Ascorbic Acid (Vit C), Ferrous Fumarate, Vitamin E Acetate, Artificial Color, Niacinamide, Vitamin A Acetate, Calcium Pantothenate, Magnesium Stearate, Silica Gel, Pyridoxine HCl (B-6), Riboflavin (B-2), Thiamine Mononitrate (B-1), Folic Acid, Artificial Flavor, Cholecalciferol (Vit D), Carnauba Wax, Cyanocobalamin (B-12).

Recommended Dosage: 1 tablet daily.

How Supplied: Available in bottles of 120 tablets.

UNICAP Sr.® Tablets
Vitamins and Minerals for Adults 50+ Based on the National Academy of Sciences–National Research Council Recommendations
Sugar Free and Sodium Free

Indications: Dietary supplement of essential vitamins and minerals formulated for the nutritional needs of adults 50+.

Each tablet contains:

		% RDDA*
Vitamin A (as Acetate and Beta Carotene)	5000 Int. Units	100
Vitamin D	200 Int. Units	100
Vitamin E	15 Int. Units	50
Vitamin C	60 mg	100
Folic Acid	400 mcg	100
Thiamine	1.2 mg	100
Riboflavin	1.4 mg	100
Niacin	16 mg	100

Vitamin B_6	2.2 mg	100
Vitamin B_{12}	3 mcg	100
Pantothenic Acid	10 mg	100
Iodine	150 mcg	100
Iron	10 mg	100
Copper	2 mg	100
Zinc	15 mg	100
Calcium	100 mg	12
Phosphorus	77 mg	10
Magnesium	30 mg	9
Manganese	1 mg	+
Potassium	5 mg	+

* Percentage of Recommended Daily Dietary Allowance for Adults 51 years and over, National Academy of Sciences–National Research Council.

+ Recognized as essential in human nutrition, but no U.S. Recommended Daily Allowance (U.S. RDA) has been established.

Ingredient List: Calcium Phosphate, Cellulose, Ascorbic Acid (Vit C), Magnesium Oxide, Vitamin E Acetate, Ferrous Fumarate, Artificial Color, Zinc Oxide, Niacinamide, Calcium Pantothenate, Vitamin A Acetate, Magnesium Stearate, Potassium Sulfate, Cupric Sulfate, Silica Gel, Beta-Carotene, Manganese Sulfate, Pyridoxine Hydrochloride (B-6), Riboflavin (B-2), Thiamine Mononitrate (B-1), Folic Acid, Artificial Flavor, Cholecalciferol (Vit D), Potassium Iodide, Carnauba Wax, Cyanocobalamin (B-12).

Recommended Dosage: 1 tablet daily.

How Supplied: Available in bottles of 120 tablets.

Shown in Product Identification Section, page 434

UNICAP T® Tablets
Stress Formula
A More Complete Vitamin and Mineral Supplement
Sugar Free and Sodium Free

Indications: Dietary supplement offering higher levels of vitamin C and B-complex vitamins essential for the return to, and maintenance of good health.

Each tablet contains:		% U.S. RDA
Vitamin A	5000 Int. Units	100
Vitamin D	400 Int. Units	100
Vitamin E	30 Int. Units	100
Vitamin C	500 mg	833
Folic Acid	400 mcg	100
Thiamine	10 mg	667
Riboflavin	10 mg	588
Niacin	100 mg	500
Vitamin B_6	6 mg	300
Vitamin B_{12}	18 mcg	300
Pantothenic Acid	25 mg	250
Iodine	150 mcg	100
Iron	18 mg	100
Copper	2 mg	100
Zinc	15 mg	100
Manganese	1 mg	+
Potassium	5 mg	+
Selenium	10 mcg	+

+ Recognized as essential in human nutrition, but no U.S. Recommended Daily Allowance (U.S. RDA) has been established.

Ingredient List: Ascorbic Acid (Vit C), Niacinamide Ascorbate, Cellulose, Hydroxypropyl Methylcellulose, Vitamin E Acetate, Ferrous Fumarate, Artificial Color, Calcium Pantothenate, Calcium Phosphate, Zinc Oxide, Vitamin A Acetate, Magnesium Stearate, Potassium Sulfate, Thiamine Mononitrate (B-1), Riboflavin (B-2), Selenium Yeast, Pyridoxine Hydrochloride (B-6), Cupric Sulfate, Silica Gel, Manganese Sulfate, FD&C Yellow No. 5, Folic Acid, Artificial Flavor, Cholecalciferol (Vit D), Potassium Iodide, Carnauba Wax, Cyanocobalamin (B-12).

Recommended Dosage: 1 tablet daily.

How Supplied: Available in bottles of 60 tablets.

Shown in Product Identification Section, page 434

Wakunaga of America Co., Ltd.

Subsidiary of Wakunaga Pharmaceutical Co., Ltd.
23501 MADERO
MISSION VIEJO, CA 92691

KYOLIC®
Odor Modified Garlic

Active Ingredient: Aged Garlic Extract.

Indications: Dietary Supplement.

Suggested Use: Average serving, four capsules or tablets a day during or after meals.

How Supplied: Liquid—Kyolic-Aged Garlic Extract Flavor and Odor Modified Enriched with Vitamin B_1 and B_{12} (and empty gelatine capsules) 2 fl oz (62 capsules) and 4 fl oz (124 capsules). Kyolic-Aged Garlic Extract Flavor and Odor Modified Plain (and empty gelatine capsules) 2 fl oz (62 capsules) and 4 fl oz (124 capsules).

Tablets and Capsules—Ingredients per Tablet or Capsule:

Kyolic—Super Formula 100 Tablets: Aged Garlic Extract Powder (300 mg), Whey (168 mg) blended with natural vegetable sources: Cellulose and Algin, bottles of 100 and 200 tablets.

Kyolic—Super Formula 100 Capsules: Aged Garlic Extract Powder (300 mg), Whey (168 mg), bottles of 100 and 200 capsules.

Kyolic—Super Formula 101 Garlic Plus® Tablets: Aged Garlic Extract Powder (270 mg) blended with Brewer's Yeast (27 mg), Kelp (9 mg), bottles of 100 and 200 tablets.

Kyolic—Super Formula 101 Garlic Plus® Capsules: Aged Garlic Extract Powder (270 mg) blended with Brewer's Yeast (27 mg), Kelp (9 mg), bottles of 50, 100 and 200 capsules.

Kyolic—Super Formula 102 Tablets: Aged Garlic Extract Powder (350 mg), "Kyolic Enzyme Complex™" [Amylase, Protease, Cellulase and Lipase] (30 mg), bottles of 100 and 200 tablets.

Kyolic—Super Formula 102 Capsules: Aged Garlic Extract Powder (350 mg), "Kyolic Enzyme Complex™" [Amylase, Protease, Cellulase and Lipase] (30 mg), bottles of 100 and 200 tablets.

Kyolic—Super Formula 103 Capsules: Aged Garlic Extract Powder (220 mg), Ester C® [Calcium Ascorbate] (150 mg), Astragulus membranaceous (100 mg), Calcium lactate (80 mg), bottles of 100 and 200 capsules.

Kyolic—Super Formula 104 Capsules: Aged Garlic Extract Powder (300 mg), Lecithin (200 mg), bottles of 100 and 200 capsules.

Kyolic—Super Formula 105 Capsules: Aged Garlic Extract Powder (250 mg), Beta-Carotene (37.5 mg) *d*-Alpha-Tocopheryl Acid Succinate [Vitamin E] (50 mg) in a base of Alfalfa and Parsley, bottles of 100 capsules.

Kyolic—Super Formula 106 Capsules: Aged Garlic Extract Powder (300 mg), *d*-Alpha Tocopheryl Succinate [Vitamin E] (90 mg), Hawthorn Berry (50 mg), Cayenne Pepper (10 mg), bottles of 50 and 100 capsules.

Professional label "SGP" is available in liquid and Aged Garlic Extract powder forms.

Shown in Product Identification Section, page 435

EDUCATIONAL MATERIAL

From Soil to Shelf
Brochure describing our company, garlic fields, aging tanks and factory, plus our product line.

Walker, Corp & Co., Inc.

P.O. BOX 1320
EASTHAMPTON PL. &
N. COLLINGWOOD AVE.
SYRACUSE, NY 13201

EVAC–U–GEN®
[*e-vak-ū-jen*]

Description: Evac-U-Gen® is available as purple scored tablets, each containing 97.2 mg of yellow phenolphthalein. Also contains anise oil, corn syrup solids, D&C red 7, FD&C blue 1, lactose, magnesium stearate, saccharin sodium and sugar.

Action and Uses: For temporary relief of occasional constipation and to help restore a normal pattern of evacuation. A mild, non-griping, stimulant laxative in chewable, anise-flavored form, Evac-U-Gen provides gentle, overnight relief by softening of the feces through selective action on the intramural nerve plexus of intestinal smooth muscle, and increases the propulsive peristaltic activity of the colon. It is frequently helpful in preparing the bowel for diagnostic procedures.

Indications: Because of its gentle and non-toxic nature, Evac-U-Gen is especially recommended for persons over 55,

Continued on next page

Walker, Corp—Cont.

and in the presence of hemorrhoids. It is also suitable in pregnancy and for children. Safe for nursing mothers, Evac-U-Gen does not affect the infant. It may be useful when straining at the stool is a hazard, as in hernia, cardiac or hypertensive patients.

Contraindications: Contraindicated in patients with a history of sensitivity to phenolphthalein. Evac-U-Gen should not be used when abdominal pain, nausea, vomiting, or other symptoms of appendicitis are present.

Side Effects: If skin rash appears, use of Evac-U-Gen or other preparations containing phenolphthalein should be discontinued. May cause coloration of feces or urine if such are sufficiently alkaline.

Warning: Frequent or prolonged use may result in dependence on laxatives. Keep this and all medication out of reach of children.

Administration and Dosage: Adults: chew one or two tablets night or morning. **Children:** Over 6, chew ½ tablet daily. Intensity of action is proportional to dosage, but individually effective doses vary. Evac-U-Gen is usually active 6 to 8 hours after administration, but residual action may last 3 to 4 days.

How Supplied: Evac-U-Gen is available in bottles of 35, 100, 500, 1000 and 6000 tablets.

Shown in Product Identification Section, page 435

Walker Pharmacal Company

4200 LACLEDE AVENUE
ST. LOUIS, MO 63108

PRID SALVE
(Smile's PRID Salve)
Drawing Salve and Anti-infectant

Active Ingredients: Ichthammol (Ammonium Ichthosulfonate) Phenol (Carbolic Acid) Lead Oleate, Rosin, Bees Wax, Lard.

Description: PRID has a very stiff consistency and is almost black in color.

Indication: PRID is an anti-infective salve, which also serves as a skin protective ointment. As a drawing salve, PRID softens the skin around the foreign body, and assists the natural rejection. PRID also helps to prevent the spread of infection. PRID aids in relieving the discomfort of minor skin irritations, superficial cuts, scratches and wounds. PRID is also helpful in the treatment of boils and carbuncles. PRID has been used with some success in the treatment of acne and furunculosis as well as other skin disorders.

Warning: When applied to fingers or toes, do not use a bandage; use loose gauze so as to not interfere with circulation. Apply according to directions for use and in no case to large areas of the body without a physician's direction. Keep out of eyes.

Caution: If PRID salve is not effective in 10 days, see your physician.

Directions For Use: Wash affected parts thoroughly with hot water; dry and apply PRID at least twice daily on a clean bandage or gauze. After irritation subsides, repeat application once a day for several days. DO NOT irritate by squeezing or pressing skin area.

How Supplied: PRID is packaged in a telescoping orange metal can containing 20 grams of PRID salve.

Wallace Laboratories

P.O. BOX 1001
HALF ACRE ROAD
CRANBURY, NJ 08512

MALTSUPEX®
(malt soup extract)
Powder, Liquid, Tablets

Composition: 'Maltsupex' is a nondiastatic extract from barley malt, which is available in powder, liquid, and tablet form. 'Maltsupex' has a gentle laxative action and promotes soft, easily passed stools. Each **Tablet** contains 750 mg of 'Maltsupex' and approximately 0.15 to 0.25 mEq of potassium. Tablet Ingredients: acetylated monoglycerides, FD&C Yellow #5, FD&C Yellow #6, flavor (artificial), hydroxypropyl methylcellulose, polyethylene glycol, povidone, stearic acid, talc, titanium dioxide. Each tablespoonful (½ fl oz) of **Liquid** and each heaping tablespoonful of **Powder** contains the equivalent of 16 g of Malt Soup Extract Powder and 3.1 to 5.5 mEq of potassium. Other Ingredients: none.

Indications: 'Maltsupex' is indicated for the dietary management and treatment of functional constipation in infants and children. It is also useful in treating constipation in adults, including those with laxative dependence.

Warnings: Do not use when abdominal pain, nausea or vomiting are present. If constipation persists, consult a physician. Keep this and all medications out of the reach of children.
'Maltsupex' Powder and Liquid only—Do not use these products except under the advice and supervision of a physician if you have kidney disease.
As with any drug, if you are pregnant or nursing a baby, seek the advice of a health professional before using this product.

Precautions: In patients with diabetes, allow for carbohydrate content of approximately 14 grams per tablespoonful of **Liquid** (56 calories), 13 grams per tablespoonful of **Powder** (52 calories), and 0.6 grams per Tablet (3 calories). **Tablets only:** This product contains FD&C Yellow No. 5 (tartrazine) which may cause allergic-type reactions (including bronchial asthma) in certain susceptible individuals. Although the overall incidence of FD&C Yellow No. 5 (tartrazine) sensitivity in the general population is low, it is frequently seen in patients who also have aspirin hypersensitivity.

Dosage and Administration: General—The recommended daily dosage of 'Maltsupex' may vary from 6 to 32 grams for infants (2 years or less) and 12 to 64 grams for children and adults, accompanied by adequate fluid intake with each dose. Use the smallest dose that is effective and lower dosage as improvement occurs. Use heaping measures of the **Powder.** 'Maltsupex' **Liquid** mixes more easily if stirred first in one or two ounces of warm water.
Powder and Liquid (Usual Dosage)—**Adults:** 2 tablespoonfuls (32 g) twice daily for 3 or 4 days, or until relief is noted, then 1 to 2 tablespoonfuls at bedtime for maintenance, as needed. Drink a full glass (8 oz) of liquid with each dose. **Children:** 1 or 2 tablespoonfuls in 8 ounces of liquid once or twice daily (with cereal, milk or preferred beverage). **Bottle-Fed Infants (over 1 month):** ½ to 2 tablespoonfuls in the day's total formula, or 1 to 2 teaspoonfuls in a single feeding to correct constipation. To prevent constipation (as when switching to whole milk) add 1 to 2 teaspoonfuls to the day's formula or 1 teaspoonful to every second feeding. **Breast-Fed Infants (over one month):** 1 to 2 teaspoonfuls in 2 to 4 ounces of water or fruit juice once or twice daily.
Tablets—**Adults:** Start with 4 tablets (3 g) four times daily (with meals and bedtime) and adjust dosage according to response. Drink a full glass (8 oz) of liquid with each dose.

How Supplied: 'Maltsupex' is supplied in 8 ounce (NDC 0037-9101-12) and 16 ounce (NDC 0037-9101-08) jars of 'Maltsupex' Powder; 8 fluid ounce (NDC 0037-9001-12) and 1 pint (NDC 0037-9001-08) bottles of 'Maltsupex' Liquid; and in bottles of 100 'Maltsupex' Tablets (NDC 0037-9201-01).
'Maltsupex' **Powder** and **Liquid** are Distributed by

WALLACE LABORATORIES
Division of
CARTER-WALLACE, INC.
Cranbury, New Jersey 08512

'Maltsupex' **Tablets** are Manufactured by

WALLACE LABORATORIES
Division of
CARTER-WALLACE, INC.
Cranbury, New Jersey 08512
Rev. 10/85

Shown in Product Identification Section, page 435

RYNA™
(Liquid)
RYNA-C® Ⓒ
(Liquid)
RYNA-CX® Ⓒ
(Liquid)

Description:
RYNA Liquid—Each 5 mL (one teaspoonful) contains:
Chlorpheniramine maleate.............2 mg
Pseudoephedrine hydrochloride....30 mg
Other ingredients: flavor (artificial), glycerin, malic acid, sodium benzoate, sorbitol, purified water, in a clear, slightly yellow colored, lemon-vanilla flavored demulcent base containing no sugar, dyes, or alcohol.
RYNA-C Liquid—Each 5 mL (one teaspoonful) contains, in addition:
Codeine phosphate..........................10 mg
(WARNING: May be habit-forming)
Other ingredients: flavor (artificial), glycerin, malic acid, purified water, saccharin sodium, sodium benzoate, sorbitol, in a clear, colorless to slightly yellow, cinnamon-flavored, demulcent base containing no sugar, dyes, or alcohol.
RYNA-CX Liquid—Each 5 mL (one teaspoonful) contains:
Codeine phosphate..........................10 mg
(WARNING: May be habit-forming)
Pseudoephedrine hydrochloride....30 mg
Guaifenesin....................................100 mg
Other ingredients: flavors (artificial), glycerin, glycine, malic acid, povidone, propylene glycol, purified water, saccharin sodium, sorbitol, in a clear, colorless, cherry-vanilla-menthol flavored demulcent base containing no sugar, dyes, or alcohol.

Actions:
Chlorpheniramine maleate in RYNA and RYNA-C is an antihistamine that antagonizes the effects of histamine.
Codeine phosphate in RYNA-C and RYNA-CX is a centrally-acting antitussive that relieves cough.
Pseudoephedrine hydrochloride in RYNA, RYNA-C and RYNA-CX is a sympathomimetic nasal decongestant that acts to shrink swollen mucosa of the respiratory tract.
Guaifenesin in RYNA-CX is an expectorant that increases mucus flow to help prevent dryness and relieve irritated respiratory tract membranes.

Indications:
RYNA: For the temporary relief of the concurrent symptoms of nasal congestion, sneezing, itchy and watery eyes, and running nose as occur with the common cold or allergic rhinitis.
RYNA-C: Temporarily relieves cough, nasal congestion, runny nose and sneezing as may occur with the common cold.
RYNA-CX: Temporarily relieves cough and nasal congestion as may occur with the common cold. Relieves irritated membranes in the respiratory passageways by preventing dryness through increased mucus flow.

Warnings:
For RYNA:
Do not give this product to children taking other medication or to children under 6 years except under the advice and supervision of a physician. Do not exceed recommended dosage unless directed by a physician because nervousness, dizziness, or sleeplessness may occur at higher doses. If symptoms do not improve within 3 days or are accompanied by high fever, discontinue use and consult a physician. Do not take this product except under the advice and supervision of a physician if you have any of the following symptoms or conditions: high blood pressure; heart disease; thyroid disease; diabetes; asthma; glaucoma; or difficulty in urination due to enlargement of the prostate.
For RYNA-C and RYNA-CX:
Adults and children who have a chronic pulmonary disease or shortness of breath, or children who are taking other drugs, should not take these products unless directed by a physician. Do not give these products to children under 6 years of age except under the advice and supervision of a physician. A persistent cough may be a sign of a serious condition. If cough persists for more than one week, tends to recur, or is accompanied by fever, rash or persistent headache, consult a physician. Do not take these products for persistent or chronic cough such as occurs with smoking, asthma, emphysema, or if cough is accompanied by excessive phlegm (mucus) unless directed by a physician. Do not take these products if you have glaucoma, asthma, emphysema, difficulty in breathing, difficulty in urination due to enlargement of the prostate gland, heart disease, high blood pressure, thyroid disease, or diabetes, unless directed by a physician. May cause or aggravate constipation.
Do not take these products or give to children for more than 7 days. If symptoms do not improve or are accompanied by fever, consult a physician. Unless directed by a physician, do not exceed recommended dosage because nervousness, dizziness or sleeplessness may occur at higher doses.
For RYNA and RYNA-C:
These products contain an antihistamine which may cause excitability, especially in children, or drowsiness or may impair mental alertness. Combined use with alcohol, sedatives, or other depressants may have an additive effect. Do not drive motor vehicles, operate machinery, or drink alcoholic beverages while taking these products.
As with any drug, if you are pregnant or nursing a baby, seek the advice of a health professional before using these products.

Drug Interaction Precaution: Persons who are presently taking a prescription drug for high blood pressure or depression should not use these products without consulting a physician.

Dosage and Administration:
Adults: 2 teaspoonfuls every 6 hours
Children 6 to under 12 years: 1 teaspoonful every 6 hours.
Children under 6 years: consult a physician.
DO NOT EXCEED 4 DOSES IN 24 HOURS.
Ryna-C and Ryna-CX:
A special measuring device should be used to give an accurate dose of these products to children under 6 years of age. Giving a higher dose than recommended by a physician could result in serious side effects for the child.

How Supplied:
RYNA: bottles of 4 fl oz (NDC 0037-0638-66) and one pint (NDC 0037-0638-68).
RYNA-C: bottles of 4 fl oz (NDC 0037-0522-66) and one pint (NDC 0037-0522-68).
RYNA-CX: bottles of 4 fl oz (NDC 0037-0801-66) and one pint (NDC 0037-0801-68).
TAMPER-RESISTANT BAND ON CAP, PRINTED "WALLACE LABORATORIES". DO NOT USE IF BAND IS MISSING OR BROKEN.

Storage:
RYNA: Store below 30° (86°F).
RYNA-C and RYNA-CX: Store at controlled room temperature. Protect from excessive heat and freezing.
KEEP THESE AND ALL DRUGS OUT OF THE REACH OF CHILDREN. IN CASE OF ACCIDENTAL OVERDOSE, SEEK PROFESSIONAL ASSISTANCE OR CONTACT A POISON CONTROL CENTER IMMEDIATELY.

WALLACE LABORATORIES
Division of
CARTER-WALLACE, Inc.
Cranbury, New Jersey 08512
Rev. 8/88

Shown in Product Identification Section, page 435

SYLLACT®
(Psyllium Hydrophilic Mucilloid for Oral Suspension, U.S.P.)
(Powdered Psyllium Seed Husks)

Description: Each rounded teaspoonful of fruit-flavored **'Syllact'** contains approximately 3.3 g of powdered psyllium seed husks and an equal amount of dextrose as a dispersing agent, and provides about 14 calories. Potassium sorbate, methyl and propylparaben are added as preservatives. Other ingredients: citric acid, dextrose, FD&C Red #40, flavor (artificial), and saccharin sodium.

Actions: The active ingredient in 'Syllact' is hydrophilic mucilloid, non-absorbable dietary fiber derived from the powdered husks of natural psyllium seed, which acts by increasing the water content and bulk volume of stools. It gives 'Syllact' a bland, non-irritating, laxative action and promotes physiologic evacuation of the bowel.

Indications: 'Syllact' is indicated for the treatment of constipation and, when recommended by a physician, in other disorders where the effect of additional bulk and fiber is desired.

Continued on next page

Wallace—Cont.

Warnings: Do not swallow dry. Drink a full glass (8 oz) of water or other liquid with each dose. If constipation persists, consult a physician. Do not use if fecal impaction, intestinal obstruction, or abdominal pain, nausea or vomiting are present. Keep this and all medications out of the reach of children.
As with any drug, if you are pregnant or nursing a baby, seek the advice of a health professional before using this product.

Dosage and Administration: The actual daily dosage depends on the need and response of the patient. Adults may take up to 9 teaspoonfuls daily, in divided doses, for several days to provide optimum benefit when constipation is chronic or severe. Lower the dosage as improvement occurs. Use a dry spoon to measure powder. Tighten lid to keep out moisture.
Usual Adult Dosage—One rounded teaspoonful of 'Syllact' in a full glass (8 oz) of cool water or other beverage taken orally one to three times daily. If desired, an additional glass of liquid may be taken after each dose.
Children's Dosage—6 years and older—Half the adult dosage with the same fluid intake requirement.

How Supplied: 'Syllact' Powder—in 10 oz jars (NDC 0037-9501-13).

Rev. 5/86

WALLACE LABORATORIES
Division of
CARTER-WALLACE, INC.
Cranbury, New Jersey 08512

Shown in Product Identification Section, page 435

Warner-Lambert Company

Consumer Health Products Group
201 TABOR ROAD
MORRIS PLAINS, NJ 07950

PROFESSIONAL STRENGTH EFFERDENT
Denture Cleanser

Cleansing Ingredients: Potassium monopersulfate, sodium perborate, sodium carbonate, sodium tripolyphosphate, EDTA and surfactants.

Other Ingredients: Sodium bicarbonate, citric acid, colors and flavors.

Indications: For effective and convenient daily denture cleaning to remove plaque and stains and to inhibit bacterial growth on dentures and removable orthodontic appliances.

Actions: Efferdent's effervescent cleansing action removes stubborn stains between teeth, whitens and brightens, fights plaque and leaves dentures and removable orthodontic appliances fresh tasting and odor free.

Warnings: Keep out of the reach of children. DO NOT PUT TABLETS IN MOUTH.

Dosage and Administration: For best results, use at least once daily. Dentures may be soaked safely in Efferdent overnight.

How Supplied: Available in boxes of 20, 40, 60, 90, and 120 tablets.

Shown in Product Identification Section, page 435

HALLS® MENTHO-LYPTUS®
Cough Suppressant Tablets

Active Ingredients: Each tablet contains eucalyptus oil and menthol.

Inactive Ingredients: Corn Syrup, Flavoring, Sugar and Artificial Colors.

Indications: For temporary relief of minor throat irritation and coughs due to colds or inhaled irritants. Makes nasal passages feel clearer.

Warning: A persistent cough or sore throat may be a sign of a serious condition. If cough persists for more than 1 week, tends to recur, or is accompanied by fever, rash or persistent headache, or if sore throat is severe, persistent or accompanied by high fever, headache, nausea, and vomiting, consult a doctor. Do not take this product for sore throat lasting more than 2 days or persistent or chronic cough such as occurs with smoking, asthma, emphysema, or if cough is accompanied by excessive phlegm (mucus) unless directed by a doctor. Keep this and all drugs out of the reach of children.

Dosage and Administration: Adults and children 5 years and over: dissolve one tablet slowly in mouth. Repeat every hour as needed or as directed by a doctor. Children under 5 years: consult a doctor.

How Supplied: Halls Mentho-Lyptus Cough Suppressant Tablets are available in single sticks of 9 tablets each, in 3-stick packs, and in bags of 30 tablets. They are available in five flavors: Regular, Cherry, Honey-Lemon, Ice Blue-Peppermint, and Spearmint.

Shown in Product Identification Section, page 435

HALLS® PLUS
Cough Suppressant Tablets

Active Ingredients: Each centerfilled tablet contains eucalyptus oil and menthol.

Inactive Ingredients: Corn Syrup, Flavoring, Glycerin, High Fructose Corn Syrup, Sugar and Artificial Colors

Indications: For temporary relief of minor throat irritation and coughs due to colds or inhaled irritants. Makes nasal passages feel clearer.

Warnings: A persistent cough or sore throat may be a sign of a serious condition. If cough persists for more than 1 week, tends to recur, or is accompanied by fever, rash or persistent headache or if sore throat is severe, persistent or accompanied by high fever, headache, nausea, and vomiting, consult a doctor. Do not take this product for sore throat lasting more than 2 days or persistent or chronic cough such as occurs with smoking, asthma, emphysema, or if cough is accompanied by excessive phlegm (mucus) unless directed by a doctor. Keep this and all drugs out of the reach of children.

Dosage and Administration: Adults and children 5 years and over dissolve one centerfilled tablet slowly in mouth. Repeat every hour as needed or as directed by a doctor. Children under 5 years: consult a doctor.

How Supplied: Halls Plus Cough Suppressant Tablets are available in single sticks of 10 tablets each and in bags of 25 tablets. They are available in three flavors: Regular, Cherry and Honey-Lemon.

Shown in Product Identification Section, page 435

HALLS® Vitamin C Drops

Description: Halls Vitamin C Drops are a delicious way to get 100% of the U.S. Recommended Daily Allowance of Vitamin C. Each drop provides 60 mg. of Vitamin C (100% U.S. RDA).

Ingredients: Sugar, Glucose Syrup, Sodium Ascorbate, Citric Acid, Ascorbic Acid, Natural Flavoring and Artificial Color (Including Yellow 5 and Yellow 6).

Indication: Dietary Supplementation.

How Supplied: Halls Vitamin C Drops are available in single sticks of 9 drops each and in bags of 30 drops. They are available in 2 great-tasting assortments: All-natural citrus flavors (tangerine, lemon, sweet grapefruit, lime and orange) and berry flavors (grape, cherry, strawberry and raspberry).

Shown in Product Identification Section, page 435

LISTERINE® Antiseptic

Active Ingredients: Thymol .06%, Eucalyptol .09%, Methyl Salicylate .06% and Menthol .04%. Also contains: Water, Alcohol 26.9%, Benzoic Acid, Poloxamer 407 and Caramel.

Indications: To help prevent and reduce supragingival plaque and gingivitis; for general oral hygiene and bad breath.

Actions: Listerine Antiseptic has been shown to help prevent and reduce supragingival plaque and gingivitis when used in a conscientiously applied program of daily oral hygiene and regular professional care. Its effect on periodontitis has not been determined. Listerine is the only leading nonprescription mouthrinse that has received the American Dental Association's Council on Dental Therapeutics Seal of Acceptance for helping to prevent and reduce plaque above the gumline and gingivitis.

Directions: Rinse full strength for 30 seconds with ⅔ ounce (4 teaspoonfuls)

morning and night. If bad breath persists, see your dentist.

How Supplied: Listerine Antiseptic is supplied in 3, 6, 12, 18, 24, 32, 48 and 58 fl. oz. bottles.

Shown in Product Identification Section, page 435

LISTERINE ANTISEPTIC THROAT LOZENGES

Active Ingredients: Each lozenge contains: Hexylresorcinol.

Inactive Ingredients: Corn Syrup, Flavors, Glycerin and Sugar.

Indications: For fast temporary relief of minor sore throat pain.

Actions: When allowed to dissolve slowly in the mouth Listerine Lozenges bathes the throat with the soothing pain-relieving action of Hexylresorcinol, a safe and effective topical anesthetic. Listerine Lozenges provide fast temporary relief from minor sore throat pain of colds, smoking and mouth irritations.

Warnings: Severe or persistent sore throat, or sore throat accompanied by high fever, headache, nausea and vomiting, may be serious. Consult physician promptly. Do not use more than 2 days or administer to children under 3 years of age unless directed by a physician. Keep this and all drugs out of the reach of children.

Dosage: 1 lozenge every 2 hours as needed.

Storage: Store at room temperature.

How Supplied: 24 count packages.

Available in: Regular Strength (Hexylresorcinol 2.4 mg.) in Cherry, Lemon-Mint and Regular flavors and Maximum Strength (Hexylresorcinol 4.0 mg.).

Shown in Product Identification Section, page 435

LISTERMINT®
Mouthwash with Fluoride

Active Ingredient: Sodium Fluoride (0.02%). Also contains: Water, SD alcohol 38-B (6.65%), glycerin, poloxamer 407, sodium lauryl sulfate, sodium citrate, flavoring, sodium saccharin, zinc chloride, citric acid, D&C Yellow No. 10, FD&C Green No. 3.

Indications: Aids in prevention of dental cavities and freshens breath.

Directions: Adults and children 6 years of age and older: Use twice a day after brushing teeth with toothpaste. Vigorously swish 10 ml. (2 teaspoonfuls) of rinse between teeth for 1 minute and spit out. Do not swallow the rinse. Do not eat or drink for 30 minutes after rinsing.

Warnings: Children under 12 years of age should be supervised in the use of this product. Consult a dentist or physician for use in children under 6 years of age. Developing teeth of children under 6 years of age may become permanently discolored if excessive amounts of fluoride are repeatedly swallowed. This is not a dentifrice and should not be used as a substitute for regular toothbrushing. Keep this and all drugs out of reach of children.

How Supplied: Listermint with Fluoride is supplied to consumers in 6, 12, 18, 24 and 32 fl. oz. bottles.

Shown in Product Identification Section, page 435

LUBRIDERM® CREAM
Skin Lubricant Moisturizer

Composition:
Scented—Contains Water, Mineral Oil, Petrolatum, Glycerin, Glyceryl Stearate, PEG 100 Stearate, Hydrogenated Polyisobutene, Lanolin, Lanolin Alcohol, Lanolin Oil, Cetyl Alcohol, Sorbitan Laurate, Fragrance, Methylparaben, Butylparaben, Propylparaben, Quaternium-15.
Fragrance Free—Contains Water, Mineral Oil, Petrolatum, Glycerin, Glyceryl Stearate, PEG 100 Stearate, Hydrogenated Polyisobutene, Lanolin, Lanolin Alcohol, Lanolin Oil, Cetyl Alcohol, Sorbitan Laurate, Methylparaben, Butylparaben, Propylparaben, Quaternium-15.

Actions and Uses: Lubriderm Cream is an emollient-rich formula designed for extremely dry skin. Lubriderm Cream relieves the roughness, dryness, and discomfort associated with dry or chapped skin and helps protect the skin from drying.
Lubriderm Cream is particularly effective when applied at nighttime or after bathing to restore and protect the skin's natural suppleness. It smooths on easily and penetrates to help soothe, soften, and moisturize.

Administration and Dosage: Apply as often as needed to extra dry skin areas.

Precautions: For external use only.

How Supplied:
Scented: Available in 2.7 oz. pump container.
Fragrance Free: Available in a 2.7 oz. pump container.

Shown in Product Identification Section, page 436

LUBRIDERM® LOTION
Skin Lubricant Moisturizer

Composition:
Scented—Contains Water, Mineral Oil, Petrolatum, Sorbitol, Lanolin, Lanolin Alcohol, Stearic Acid, Triethanolamine, Cetyl Alcohol, Fragrance, Butylparaben, Methylparaben, Propylparaben, Sodium Chloride.
Fragrance Free—Contains Water, Mineral Oil, Petrolatum, Sorbitol, Lanolin, Lanolin Alcohol, Stearic Acid, Triethanolamine, Cetyl Alcohol, Butylparaben, Methylparaben, Propylparaben, Sodium Chloride.

Actions and Uses: Lubriderm Lotion is an oil-in-water emulsion indicated for use in softening, soothing and moisturizing dry chapped skin. Lubriderm relieves the roughness, tightness and discomfort associated with dry or chapped skin and helps protect the skin from further drying.
Lubriderm's extra-rich formula smoothes easily into skin without leaving a greasy feeling.

Administration and Dosage: Apply as often as needed to hands and body to restore and maintain the skin's natural suppleness.

Precautions: For external use only.

How Supplied:
Scented: Available in 1, 4, 8, 12 and 16 fl. oz. plastic bottles, and a 2.5 ounce tube.
Fragrance Free: Available in 1, 8, 12 and 16 fl. oz. plastic bottles, and a 2.5 ounce tube.

Shown in Product Identification Section, page 436

LUBRIDERM LUBATH®
Skin Conditioning Oil

Composition: Contains Mineral Oil, PPG-15 Stearyl Ether, Oleth-2, Nonoxynol-5, Fragrance, D&C Green No. 6.

Actions and Uses: Lubriderm Skin Conditioning Oil is a lanolin-free, mineral oil–based, bath oil designed for softening and soothing dry skin during the bath. The formula disperses into countless droplets of oil that coat the skin and help lubricate and soften. It is equally effective in hard or soft water and provides an excellent way to moisturize the skin and help counterbalance the drying effects of harsh soaps and hot water.

Administration and Dosage: One to two capfuls in bath, or apply with hand or moistened cloth in shower and rinse. For use as a skin cleanser, rub into wet skin and rinse.

Precautions: Avoid getting in eyes; if this occurs, flush with clear water. When using any bath oil, take precautions against slipping. For external use only.

How Supplied: Available in 8 fl. oz. plastic bottles.

Shown in Product Identification Section, page 436

ROLAIDS®

Active Ingredient: Dihydroxyaluminum Sodium Carbonate 300 mg.

Inactive Ingredients: Corn Starch, Corn Syrup, Flavoring, Magnesium Stearate and Sugar. May also contain pregelatinized starch. Contains 50 mg. sodium per tablet.

Indications: For the relief of heartburn, sour stomach or acid indigestion and upset stomach associated with these symptoms.

Actions: Rolaids® provides rapid neutralization of stomach acid. Each tablet has acid-neutralizing capacity of 75–80 ml. of 0.1N hydrochloric acid and the

Continued on next page

Warner-Lambert—Cont.

ability to maintain the pH of the stomach contents close to 3.5 for a significant period of time.
Due to the relatively low solubility and other physical and chemical properties of dihydroxyaluminum sodium carbonate (DASC), it is for the most part nonabsorbed.
Although sodium is present in DASC, the sodium is available for absorption only when the antacid reacts with stomach acid. When Rolaids are consumed in excess of the amount of acid present in the stomach, this sodium is unavailable for absorption and the active ingredient is passed through the digestive system unchanged, with no sodium released.

Warnings: Keep this and all drugs out of the reach of children. Do not take more than 24 tablets in a 24-hour period, nor use the maximum dosage of this product for more than two weeks, nor use this product if you are on a sodium-restricted diet, except under the advice and supervision of a physician.

Professional Warnings: Prolonged use of aluminum-containing antacids in patients with renal failure may result in or worsen dialysis osteomalacia. Elevated tissue aluminum levels contribute to the development of the dialysis encephalopathy and osteomalacia syndromes. Small amounts of aluminum are absorbed from the gastrointestinal tract and renal excretion of aluminum is impaired in renal failure. Aluminum is not well removed by dialysis because it is bound to albumin and transferrin, which do not cross dialysis membranes. As a result, aluminum is deposited in bone, and dialysis osteomalacia may develop when large amounts of aluminum are ingested orally by patients with impaired renal function. Aluminum forms insoluble complexes with phosphate in the gastrointestinal tract, thus decreasing phosphate absorption. Prolonged use of aluminum-containing antacids by normophosphatemic patients may result in hypophosphatemia if phosphate intake is not adequate. In its more severe forms, hypophosphatemia can lead to anorexia, malaise, muscle weakness, and osteomalacia.

Drug Interaction Precaution: Do not take this product if you are presently taking a prescription antibiotic drug containing any form of tetracycline.

Dosage and Administration: Chew 1 or 2 tablets as symptoms occur. Repeat hourly if symptoms return or as directed by a physician.

How Supplied: Rolaids is available in Regular (Peppermint), Spearmint and Wintergreen Flavors. One roll contains 12 tablets; 3-pack contains three 12-tablet rolls; one bottle contains 75 tablets; one bottle contains 150 tablets.

Shown in Product Identification Section, page 436

CALCIUM RICH/SODIUM FREE ROLAIDS®

Active Ingredient: Calcium Carbonate 550 mg. per tablet.

Inactive Ingredients:
Cherry Flavor: Corn Starch, D&C Red No. 27, Flavoring, Magnesium Stearate, Mannitol, Polyethylene Glycol, Sugar and Titanium Dioxide.
Assorted Fruit Flavors: Colors (D&C Red No. 27, FD&C Blue No. 1, Red 40, Yellow 5 [Tartrazine] and Yellow 6), Corn Starch, Flavoring, Magnesium Stearate, Mannitol, Pregelatinized Starch and Sugar.
Peppermint Flavor: Corn Starch, Flavoring, Magnesium Stearate, Mannitol, Pregelatinized Starch, Sugar and Titanium Dioxide.

Indications: For the relief of heartburn, sour stomach or acid indigestion and upset stomach associated with these symptoms.

Actions: Calcium Rich/Sodium Free Rolaids provides rapid neutralization of stomach acid. Each tablet has an acid neutralizing capacity of 110 ml of 0.1N hydrochloric acid and the ability to maintain the pH of the stomach contents at 3.5 or greater for a significant period of time. Each tablet contains less than 0.4 mg of sodium and provides 22% of the Adult U.S. RDA for calcium.

Warnings: Do not take more than 14 tablets in a 24-hour period or use the maximum dosage of this product for more than 2 weeks except under the advice and supervision of a physician. Keep this and all drugs out of the reach of children.

Dosage and Administration: Chew 1 or 2 tablets as symptoms occur. Repeat hourly if symptoms return or as directed by a physician.

How Supplied: Calcium Rich/Sodium Free Rolaids is available in Peppermint, Cherry and Assorted Fruit Flavors. One roll contains 12 tablets: 3-pack contains three 12-tablet rolls; one bottle contains 75 tablets; one bottle contains 150 tablets.

Shown in Product Identification Section, page 436

EXTRA STRENGTH ROLAIDS®

Active Ingredient: Calcium Carbonate 1000 mg. per tablet.

Inactive Ingredients: Acesulfame Potassium, Colors (FD&C Blue No. 1, FD&C Yellow No. 5 [Tartrazine] and Titanium Dioxide), Corn Syrup, Flavoring, Magnesium Stearate, Pregelantinized Starch and Sugar.

Indications: For the relief of heartburn, sour stomach or acid indigestion and upset stomach associated with these symptoms.

Actions: Extra Strength Rolaids provides rapid neutralization of stomach acid. Each tablet has an acid-neutralizing capacity of 200 ml. of 0.1N hydrochloric acid and the ability to maintain the pH of the stomach contents at 3.5 or greater for a significant period of time. Each tablet contains less than 0.4 mg. of sodium.

Warnings: Do not take more than 8 tablets in a 24-hour period or use the maximum dosage of this product for more than 2 weeks except under the advice and supervision of a physician. Keep this and all drugs out of the reach of children.

Dosage and Administration: Chew 1 or 2 tablets as symptoms occur. Repeat hourly if symptoms return or as directed by a physician.

How Supplied: Extra Strength Rolaids is available in Assorted Mint Flavors. One roll contains 10 tablets: 3-pack contains three 10-tablet rolls; one bottle contains 55 tablets; one bottle contains 110 tablets.

Shown in Product Identification Section, page 436

Westwood-Squibb Pharmaceuticals Inc.
**100 FOREST AVENUE
BUFFALO, NY 14213**

LAC-HYDRIN® FIVE
Fragrance Free—Patented—Softens Even Your Driest Skin

Composition: Water, lactic acid buffered with ammonium hydroxide, glycerin, petrolatum, squalane, steareth-2, POE-21-stearyl ether, propylene glycol dioctanoate, cetyl alcohol, dimethicone, cetyl palmitate, magnesium aluminum silicate, diazolidinyl urea, methylchloroisothiazolinone and methylisothiazolinone.

Action and Uses:
Dry skin care for elbows, knees, feet and hands—LAC-HYDRIN® FIVE is dermatologically tested and guaranteed to soften and smooth even the body's roughest, driest skin.
Elegant enough to use all over, it absorbs quickly without leaving a greasy feel. And it's non-comedogenic—designed not to clog pores and cause acne.
Try LAC-HYDRIN® FIVE, the dry skin product that's unlike any other. With regular use, you'll notice a definite improvement in the appearance of your skin—or your money back.

Administration and Dosage: For best results, apply to dry skin twice a day.

Warnings: Avoid contact with eyes. For external use only.

How Supplied: 8 oz. plastic bottle (NDC 0072-5760-08) and 4 oz. plastic bottle (NDC 0072-5760-04).

Shown in Product Identification Section, page 436

MOISTUREL® CREAM
Skin Lubricant—Moisturizer

Composition: Water, petrolatum, glycerin, PG dioctanoate, cetyl alcohol, steareth-2, dimethicone, PVP/hexadecene copolymer, laureth-23, Mg Al silicate, diazolidinyl urea, carbomer-934, sodium hydroxide, methylchloroisothiazolinone and methylisothiazolinone.

Actions and Uses: A highly effective concentrated formula clinically proven to relieve dry skin and designed not to cause acne or blemishes. Free of lanolins, fragrances, and parabens that can sensitize or irritate skin. Indicated for generalized dry skin.

Administration and Dosage: Apply a small amount as often as needed.

How Supplied: 4 oz. (NDC 0072-9500-04) and 16 oz. (NDC 0072-9500-16) plastic jars.

Shown in Product Identification Section, page 436

MOISTUREL® LOTION
Skin Lubricant—Moisturizer

Composition: Water, petrolatum, glycerin, dimethicone, steareth-2, cetyl alcohol, benzyl alcohol, laureth-23, Mg Al silicate, carbomer-934, sodium hydroxide, quaternium-15.

Action and Uses: MOISTUREL is a non-greasy formula that leaves the skin feeling smooth and soft. Clinically proven to relieve dry skin and designed not to cause acne or blemishes. Free of parabens and fragrances that can sensitize or irritate skin. Indicated for generalized dry skin.

Administration and Dosage: Apply liberally as often as needed.

How Supplied: 8 oz. (NDC 0072-9100-08) and 12 oz. (NDC 0072-9100-12) plastic bottles.

Shown in Product Identification Section, page 436

MOISTUREL®
SENSITIVE SKIN CLEANSER
Pure, Clear and Soap-Free

Composition: Sodium laureth sulfate and laureth-6 carboxylic acid and disodium laureth sulfosuccinate, methyl gluceth-20, cocamidopropyl betaine, water, diazolidinyl urea, and methylchloroisothiazolinone and methylisothiazolinone.

Actions and Uses: Moisturel Sensitive Skin Cleanser is a crystal clear, lathering, soap-free cleanser. It cleans thoroughly without stinging, irritating, or drying. Unlike soaps, Moisturel Sensitive Skin Cleanser rinses refreshingly clean without leaving a film or residue. Its pure and gentle formula makes it ideal for facial use. Its nondrying, noncomedogenic, and fragrance-free formula makes it ideal for cleansing:

- Sensitive skin—even a baby's
- Dry, itchy skin caused by cold and wind, or overexposure to sun
- Skin robbed of moisture by use and removal of cosmetics
- Irritated, allergic skin
- Skin dried by harsh acne medications

Administration and Dosage: With skin wet, gently work Moisturel Sensitive Skin Cleanser into a rich lather by massaging in a circular motion. Rinse thoroughly and pat dry with a soft cloth.

Caution: Avoid contact with eyes. For external use only.

How Supplied: 8.75 oz. (NDC 0072-6420-08) plastic bottle with pump.

Shown in Product Identification Section, page 436

SEBULEX®
Antiseborrheic Treatment Shampoo

Active Ingredients: 2% sulfur and 2% salicylic acid. Also contains: D&C yellow #10, docusate sodium, EDTA, FD&C blue #1, fragrance, PEG-6 lauramide, PEG-14M, sodium dodecyl benzene sulfonate, sodium octoxynol-2 ethane sulfonate and water.

Action and Uses: A penetrating therapeutic shampoo for the temporary relief of itchy scalp and the scaling of dandruff. SEBULEX helps to relieve dandruff and itching, and removes excess oil. It penetrates and softens the crusty, matted layers of scales adhering to the scalp, and leaves the hair soft and manageable.

Administration and Dosage: SEBULEX liquid should be shaken before use. SEBULEX is massaged into wet scalp. Lather should be allowed to remain on scalp for about 5 minutes and then rinsed. Application is repeated, followed by a thorough rinse. Initially, SEBULEX can be used daily, or every other day, or as directed, depending on the condition. Once symptoms are under control, one or two treatments a week usually will maintain control of itching, oiliness and scaling.

Caution: If undue skin irritation develops or increases, discontinue use. For external use only. Contact with eyes should be avoided. In case of contact, flush eyes thoroughly with water. Keep this and all drugs out of reach of children.

How Supplied: SEBULEX in 4 oz. (NDC 0072-2700-04) and 8 oz. (NDC 0072-2700-08) plastic bottles.

Shown in Product Identification Section, page 436

SEBUTONE® and SEBUTONE® CREAM
Antiseborrheic Tar Shampoo

Active Ingredients: Coal tar 0.5%, salicylic acid 2%, sulfur 2%. SEBUTONE also contains: D&C yellow #10, docusate sodium, EDTA, FD&C blue #1, fragrance, lanolin oil, PEG-6 lauramide, PEG-90M, sodium dodecyl benzene sulfonate, sodium octoxynol-2 ethane sulfonate, titanium dioxide, and water. SEBUTONE CREAM also contains: Ceteareth-20, D&C yellow #10, dextrin, docusate sodium, EDTA, FD&C blue #1, fragrance, laureth-4, lanolin oil, magnesium aluminum silicate, PEG-6 lauramide, PEG-14 M, sodium dodecyl benzene sulfonate, sodium octoxynol-2 ethane sulfonate, stearyl alcohol, titanium dioxide and water.

Action and Uses: A surface-active, penetrating therapeutic shampoo for the temporary relief of itchy scalp and the scaling of stubborn dandruff and psoriasis. Provides prompt and prolonged relief of itching, helps control oiliness and rid the scalp of scales and crust. Tar ingredient is chemically and biologically standardized to produce uniform therapeutic activity. Wood's light demonstrates residual microfine particles of tar on the scalp several days after a course of SEBUTONE shampoo. In addition to its antipruritic and antiseborrheic actions, SEBUTONE also helps offset excessive scalp dryness with a special moisturizing emollient.

Administration and Dosage: SEBUTONE liquid should be well shaken before use. A liberal amount of SEBUTONE or SEBUTONE CREAM is massaged into the wet scalp for 5 minutes and the scalp is then rinsed. Application is repeated, followed by a thorough rinse. Use as often as necessary to keep the scalp free from itching and scaling or as directed. No other shampoo or soap washings are required.

Caution: If undue skin irritation develops or increases, discontinue use. In rare instances, temporary discoloration of white, blond, bleached or tinted hair may occur. Contact with the eyes is to be avoided. In case of contact flush eyes with water. For external use only. Keep this and all drugs out of reach of children.

How Supplied: SEBUTONE in 4 oz. (NDC 0072-5000-04) and 8 oz. (NDC 0072-5000-08) plastic bottles.
SEBUTONE CREAM in 4 oz. (NDC 0072-5100-01) tubes.

Shown in Product Identification Section, page 436

Whitehall Laboratories Inc.

Division of American Home Products Corporation
685 THIRD AVENUE
NEW YORK, NY 10017

ADVIL®
[ad 'vĭl]
Ibuprofen Tablets, USP
Ibuprofen Caplets
Pain Reliever/Fever Reducer

Warning: ASPIRIN-SENSITIVE PATIENTS. Do not take this product if you have had a severe allergic reaction to aspirin, e.g.—asthma, swelling, shock or hives, because even though this product contains no aspirin or salicylates, cross-reactions may occur in patients allergic to aspirin.

Continued on next page

Whitehall—Cont.

Active Ingredient: Each tablet contains Ibuprofen 200 mg.

Inactive Ingredients: Acacia, Acetylated Monoglycerides, Beeswax or Carnauba Wax, Calcium Sulfate, Colloidal Silicon Dioxide, Dimethicone, Iron Oxide, Lecithin, Pharmaceutical Glaze, Povidone, Sodium Benzoate, Sodium Carboxymethylcellulose, Starch, Stearic Acid, Sucrose, Titanium Dioxide.

Indications: For the temporary relief of minor aches and pains associated with the common cold, headache, toothache, muscular aches, backache, for the minor pain of arthritis, for the pain of menstrual cramps and for reduction of fever.

Dosage and Administration: Adults: Take one tablet every 4 to 6 hours while symptoms persist. If pain or fever does not respond to one tablet, two tablets may be used but do not exceed six tablets in 24 hours unless directed by a doctor. The smallest effective dose should be used. Take with food or milk if occasional and mild heartburn, upset stomach, or stomach pain occurs with use. Consult a doctor if these symptoms are more than mild or if they persist. Children: Do not give this product to children under 12 except under the advice and supervision of a doctor.

Warnings: Do not take for pain for more than 10 days or for fever for more than 3 days unless directed by a doctor. If pain or fever persists or gets worse, if new symptoms occur, or if the painful area is red or swollen, consult a doctor. These could be signs of serious illness. If you are under a doctor's care for any serious condition, consult a doctor before taking this product. As with aspirin and acetaminophen, if you have any condition which requires you to take prescription drugs or if you have had any problems or serious side effects from taking any nonprescription pain reliever, do not take this product without first discussing it with your doctor. **IF YOU EXPERIENCE ANY SYMPTOMS WHICH ARE UNUSUAL OR SEEM UNRELATED TO THE CONDITION FOR WHICH YOU TOOK IBUPROFEN, CONSULT A DOCTOR BEFORE TAKING ANY MORE OF IT.** Although ibuprofen is indicated for the same conditions as aspirin and acetaminophen, it should not be taken with them except under a doctor's direction. Do not combine this product with any other ibuprofen-containing product. As with any drug, if you are pregnant or nursing a baby, seek the advice of a health professional before using this product. **IT IS ESPECIALLY IMPORTANT NOT TO USE IBUPROFEN DURING THE LAST 3 MONTHS OF PREGNANCY UNLESS SPECIFICALLY DIRECTED TO DO SO BY A DOCTOR BECAUSE IT MAY CAUSE PROBLEMS IN THE UNBORN CHILD OR COMPLICATIONS DURING DELIVERY.** Keep this and all drugs out of the reach of children. In case of accidental overdose, seek professional assistance or contact a poison control center immediately.

Professional Labeling: Same as stated under Indications.

How Supplied: Coated tablets in bottles of 8, 24, 50, 100, 165 and 250. Coated caplets in bottles of 24, 50, 100, 165, and 250.

Storage: Store at room temperature; avoid excessive heat 40°C (104°F).

Shown in Product Identification Section, page 436

ANACIN®

[an 'a-sin]

Coated Analgesic Tablets
Coated Analgesic Caplets

Description: Each tablet or caplet contains: Aspirin 400 mg, Caffeine 32 mg. Anacin® has a special protective coating that makes each tablet or caplet easy to swallow.

Indications and Usage: Anacin provides fast relief from the pain of headache, neuralgia, neuritis, sprains, muscular aches, sinus pressure ... discomforts and fever of colds ... pain caused by tooth extraction and toothache ... menstrual discomfort. Anacin also temporarily relieves the minor aches and pains of arthritis and rheumatism.

Warnings: Children and teenagers should not use this medicine for chicken pox or flu symptoms before a doctor is consulted about Reye Syndrome, a rare but serious illness reported to be associated with aspirin. As with any drug, if you are pregnant or nursing a baby, seek the advice of a health professional before using this product. **IT IS ESPECIALLY IMPORTANT NOT TO USE ASPIRIN DURING THE LAST 3 MONTHS OF PREGNANCY UNLESS SPECIFICALLY DIRECTED TO DO SO BY A DOCTOR BECAUSE IT MAY CAUSE PROBLEMS IN THE UNBORN CHILD OR COMPLICATIONS DURING DELIVERY.** Keep this and all medicines out of children's reach. In case of accidental overdose, contact a physician immediately.

Precautions: If pain persists for more than 10 days, or redness is present, or in arthritic or rheumatic conditions affecting children under 12 years of age, consult a physician immediately.

Dosage and Administration: Adults: 2 Tablets or caplets with water every 4 hours, as needed. Do not exceed 10 tablets or 10 caplets daily. Children 6–12 years of age: half the adult dosage.

Professional Labeling: Same as those outlined under Indications.

Inactive Ingredients: Tablets contain Hydroxypropyl Methylcellulose, Microcrystalline Cellulose, Polyethylene Glycol, Starch, Surfactant.
Caplets contain Hydroxypropyl Methylcellulose, Iron Oxide, Microcrystalline Cellulose, Polyethylene Glycol, Starch, Surfactant.

How Supplied: Tablets: In tins of 12's and bottles of 30's, 50's, 100's, 200's and 300's. Caplets: In bottles of 30's, 50's and 100's.

Shown in Product Identification Section, page 436

MAXIMUM STRENGTH ANACIN®

[an 'a-sin]

Coated Analgesic Tablets

Description: Each tablet contains: Aspirin 500 mg, Caffeine 32 mg. Maximum Strength Anacin has a special protective coating that makes each tablet easy to swallow.

Indications and Usage: See Anacin Tablets.

Warnings: See Anacin Tablets.

Precautions: See Anacin Tablets.

Dosage and Administration: Adults: 2 Tablets with water 3 or 4 times a day. Do not exceed 8 tablets in any 24-hour period. Not recommended for children under 12 years of age.

Inactive Ingredients: Hydroxypropyl Methylcellulose, Microcrystalline Cellulose, Polyethylene Glycol, Starch, Surfactant.

How Supplied: Tablets: Tins of 12's and bottles of 20's, 40's, 75's, and 150's.

Maximum Strength ANACIN-3®

[an 'a-sin thre]

Film Coated Acetaminophen Tablets
Film Coated Acetaminophen Caplets

Regular Strength ANACIN-3®

Film Coated Acetaminophen Tablets

Description: Maximum Strength Tablets and Caplets: Each film coated tablet and caplet contains acetaminophen, 500 mg.
Regular Strength: Each film coated tablet contains acetaminophen, 325 mg.

Indications and Actions: Anacin-3 is a safe and effective 100% aspirin-free analgesic and antipyretic that acts fast to provide temporary relief from pain of headache, colds or "flu," sinusitis, muscle aches, bursitis, sprains, overexertion, backache and menstrual discomfort. Also for temporary relief of minor arthritis pain, toothaches and to reduce fever. Anacin-3 is particularly well suited in the presence of aspirin sensitivity, upper gastrointestinal disorders and anticoagulant therapy. It is usually well tolerated by aspirin-sensitive patients.

Warnings: Keep this and all medicines out of children's reach. In case of accidental overdose, contact a physician immediately. As with any drug, if you are pregnant or nursing a baby, seek the advice of a health professional before using this product.

Precautions: If pain persists for more than 10 days or redness is present or in arthritic or rheumatic conditions affecting children under 12, consult a physician immediately.

Dosage and Administration: Maximum Strength—Adults: Two tablets or caplets 3 or 4 times a day. Do not exceed 8 tablets or caplets in any 24-hour period. Regular Strength—Adults: 2 or 3 tablets every 4 hours not to exceed 12 tablets in any 24-hour period. Children (6–12): ½ to 1 tablet 3 to 4 times daily. Consult a physician for use by children under 6 or for use longer than 10 days.

Overdosage: Acetaminophen in massive overdosage may cause hepatic toxicity in some patients. In all cases of suspected overdose, immediately call your regional poison control center or the Rocky Mountain Poison Control Center for assistance in diagnosis and for directions in the use of *N*-acetylcysteine as an antidote. In adults, hepatic toxicity has rarely been reported with acute overdoses of less than 10 grams and fatalities with less than 15 grams. Importantly, young children seem to be more resistant than adults to the hepatotoxic effect of an acetaminophen overdose. Despite this, the measures outined below should be initiated in any adult or child suspected of having ingested an acetaminophen overdose.
Early symptoms following a potentially hepatoxic overdose may include: nausea, vomiting, diaphoresis and general malaise. Clinical and laboratory evidence of hepatic toxicity may not be apparent until 48 to 72 hours post-ingestion. The stomach should be emptied promptly by lavage or by induction of emesis with syrup of ipecac. Patients' estimates of the quantity of a drug ingested are notoriously unreliable. Therefore, if an acetaminophen overdose is suspected, a serum acetaminophen assay should be obtained as early as possible, but no sooner than four hours following ingestion. Liver function studies should be obtained initially and at 24-hour intervals. The antidote, *N*-acetylcysteine, should be administered as early as possible and within 16 hours of the overdose ingestion for optimal results. Following recovery, there is no residual, structural or functional hepatic abnormalities.

Professional Labeling: Same as those outlined under Indications.

Inactive Ingredients: Maximum and Regular Strength Tablets:
Calcium Stearate, Croscarmellose Sodium, FD&C Blue No. 1 Lake, Hydroxypropyl Methylcellulose, Microcrystalline Cellulose, Polyethylene Glycol, Povidone, Propylene Gylcol, Starch, Stearic Acid and Titanium Dioxide.
Maximum Strength Caplets:
Croscarmellose Sodium, D&C Red No. 7 Lake, FD&C Blue No. 1 Lake, Hydroxypropyl Methylcellulose, Polyethylene Glycol, Povidone, Propylene Glycol, Starch, Stearic Acid and Titanium Dioxide.

How Supplied: Maximum Strength Film Coated—Tablets (colored white, imprinted "A-3" and "500")—tins of 12 and bottles of 30, 60, and 100: Caplets (colored white, imprinted "Anacin-3")—bottles of 30's, 60's and 100's. Regular Strength Film Coated—Tablets (colored white, scored, imprinted "A-3") in bottles of 24, 50, and 100.

Shown in Product Identification Section, page 436

ANBESOL® Liquid and Gel
[an 'ba-sol"]
Antiseptic-Anesthetic

Description: Anbesol is an antiseptic-anesthetic which is available in a Maximum Strength and Regular Strength gel and liquid. Baby Anbesol, available in gel, is an anesthetic only and is alcohol-free.
The Maximum Strength formulations contain Benzocaine 20% and Alcohol 60%.
The Regular Strength formulations contain Benzocaine 6.3%, Alcohol 70%, and Phenol 0.5%.
The Baby Anbesol Gel contains Benzocaine 7.5%.

Indications: Maximum Strength and Regular Strength Anbesol are indicated for the fast temporary relief of pain due to toothache, braces, denture and orthodontic irritation, sore gums, cold and canker sores and fever blisters. Regular Strength Anbesol and Baby Anbesol Gel are also indicated for the fast temporary relief of teething pain.

Actions: Temporarily deadens sensations of nerve endings to provide relief of pain and discomfort; reduces oral bacterial flora temporarily as an aid in oral hygiene (Regular and Maximum Stengths only).

Warnings: Flammable. Keep away from fire or flame. Avoid smoking during application and until product has dried. Do not use near eyes. For persistent or excessive teething pain, consult a physician or dentist. Localized allergic reactions may occur after prolonged or repeated use. KEEP THIS AND ALL MEDICINES OUT OF THE REACH OF CHILDREN.

Precautions: Not for prolonged use. If the condition persists or irritation develops, discontinue use and consult your physician or dentist. NOT FOR USE UNDER DENTURES OR OTHER DENTAL WORK.

Dosage and Administration: Apply topically to the affected area on or around the lips, or within the mouth.

For Denture Irritation: Apply thin layer to affected area and do not reinsert dental work until irritation/pain is relieved. Rinse mouth before reinserting dentures. If irritation/pain persists, contact your physician.

Inactive Ingredients:
Maximum Strength Gel: Carbomer 934P, D&C Yellow #10, FD&C Red #40, Flavor, Polyethylene Glycol, Saccharin.
Maximum Strength Liquid: D&C Yellow #10, FD&C Red #40, Flavor, Polyethylene Glycol, Saccharin.
Regular Liquid: Camphor, Glycerin, Menthol, Potassium Iodide, Povidone Iodine.
Regular Gel: Carbomer 934P, D&C Red #33 and Yellow #10, FD&C Blue #1 and Yellow #6, Flavor, Glycerin.
Baby Gel: Carbomer 934, D& C Red #33, Disodium Edetate, Flavor, Glycerin, Polyethylene Glycol, Saccharin, Water.

How Supplied: Maximum Strength Gel in .25 oz (7.2 g) tube, Maximum Strength Liquid in .31 oz (9 mL) bottle. Regular Liquid in two sizes— .31 fl. oz. (9 mL) and .74 fl. oz. (22 mL) bottles. Gel and Baby Gel in .25 oz. (7.2 g) tubes.

Shown in Product Identification Section, page 436

ARTHRITIS PAIN FORMULA™
[är 'thrīt-is ' pān ' for-mye-la]
By the Makers of Anacin® Analgesic Tablets and Caplets

Description: Each caplet contains 500 mg microfined aspirin and two buffers, 27 mg Aluminum Hydroxide and 100 mg Magnesium Hydroxide.
Arthritis Pain Formula is a buffered analgesic and antipyretic with microfined aspirin, which means the aspirin particles are so fine they dissolve more readily. The buffering agents help provide protection against stomach upset that could be associated with large antiarthritic doses of aspirin.

Indications and Actions: Arthritis Pain Formula provides hours of relief from minor aches and pains of arthritis and rheumatism and low back pain. Also relieves the pain of headache, neuralgia, neuritis, sprains, muscular aches, discomforts and fever of colds, pain caused by tooth extraction and toothache, and menstrual discomfort.

Warnings: Children and teenagers should not use this medicine for chicken pox or flu symptoms before a doctor is consulted about Reye syndrome, a rare but serious illness reported to be associated with aspirin. As with any drug, if you are pregnant or nursing a baby, seek the advice of a health professional before using this product. **IT IS ESPECIALLY IMPORTANT NOT TO USE ASPIRIN DURING THE LAST 3 MONTHS OF PREGNANCY UNLESS SPECIFICALLY DIRECTED TO DO SO BY A DOCTOR BECAUSE IT MAY CAUSE PROBLEMS IN THE UNBORN CHILD OR COMPLICATIONS DURING DELIVERY.** Keep this and all medications out of children's reach. In case of accidental overdose, contact a physician immediately.

Precautions: If pain persists for more than 10 days, or redness is present, or in arthritic or rheumatic conditions affecting children under 12, consult a physician immediately.

Dosage and Administration: Adult Dosage: 2 caplets, 3 or 4 times a day. Do not exceed 8 caplets in any 24-hour pe-

Continued on next page

Whitehall—Cont.

riod. For children under 12, consult a physician.

Inactive Ingredients: Hydrogenated Vegetable Oil, Microcrystalline Cellulose, Starch, Surfactant.

How Supplied: In plastic bottles of 40 (non-child-resistant size), 100 and 175 caplets.

CoADVIL™
Ibuprofen/Pseudoephedrine Caplets*
Pain Reliever/Fever Reducer/Nasal Decongestant

WARNING: ASPIRIN-SENSITIVE PATIENTS. Do not take this product if you have had a severe allergic reaction to aspirin, eg—asthma, swelling, shock or hives—because even though this product contains no aspirin or salicylates, cross-reactions may occur in patients allergic to aspirin.

Indications: For temporary relief of symptoms associated with the common cold, sinusitis or flu, including nasal congestion, headache, fever, body aches, and pains.

Directions: *Adults:* Take 1 caplet every 4 to 6 hours while symptoms persist. If symptoms do not respond to 1 caplet, 2 caplets may be used, but do not exceed 6 caplets in 24 hours unless directed by a doctor. The smallest effective dose should be used.
Take with food or milk if occasional and mild heartburn, upset stomach, or stomach pain occurs with use. Consult a doctor if these symptoms are more than mild or if they persist. *Children:* Do not give this product to children under 12 years of age except under the advice and supervision of a doctor.

Warnings: Do not take for colds for more than 7 days or for fever for more than 3 days unless directed by a doctor. If the cold or fever persists or gets worse, or if new symptoms occur, consult a doctor. These could be signs of serious illness. As with aspirin and acetaminophen, if you have any condition which requires you to take prescription drugs or if you have had any problems or serious side effects from taking any nonprescription pain reliever, do not take this product without first discussing it with your doctor. IF YOU EXPERIENCE ANY SYMPTOMS WHICH ARE UNUSUAL OR SEEM UNRELATED TO THE CONDITION FOR WHICH YOU TOOK THIS PRODUCT, CONSULT A DOCTOR BEFORE TAKING ANY MORE OF IT. If you are under a doctor's care for any serious condition, consult a doctor before taking this product.
Do not exceed recommended dosage because at higher doses nervousness, dizziness or sleeplessness may occur. Do not take this product if you have high blood pressure, heart disease, diabetes, thyroid disease or difficulty in urination due to enlargement of the prostate gland, except under the advice and supervision of a doctor.

Drug Interaction Precaution: Do not take this product if you are presently taking a prescription drug for high blood pressure or depression without first consulting your doctor. Do not combine this product with other nonprescription pain relievers. Do not combine this product with any other ibuprofen-containing product. As with any drug, if you are pregnant or nursing a baby, seek the advice of a health professional before using this product.
IT IS ESPECIALLY IMPORTANT NOT TO USE THIS PRODUCT DURING THE LAST 3 MONTHS OF PREGNANCY UNLESS SPECIFICALLY DIRECTED TO DO SO BY A DOCTOR BECAUSE IT MAY CAUSE PROBLEMS IN THE UNBORN CHILD OR COMPLICATIONS DURING DELIVERY. Keep this and all drugs out of the reach of children. In case of accidental overdose, seek professional assistance or contact a poison control center immediately. Store at room temperature; avoid excessive heat (40°C, 104°F).

Active Ingredients: Each caplet contains Ibuprofen 200 mg and Pseudoephedrine HCl 30 mg.

Inactive Ingredients: Carnauba or Equivalent Wax, Croscarmellose Sodium, Iron Oxides, Methylparaben, Microcrystalline Cellulose, Propylparaben, Silicon Dioxide, Sodium Benzoate, Sodium Lauryl Sulfate, Starch, Stearic Acid, Sucrose, Titanium Dioxide.

How Supplied: CoAdvil is an oval-shaped tan-colored caplet supplied in consumer blister packs of 20 and bottles of 48 and 100.

Shown in Product Identification Section, page 436

*Oval-Shaped tablets

COMPOUND W®
['käm-pound W]
Solution and Gel

Description: Compound W is a Salicylic Acid (17% w/w) preparation available as a solution or gel.

Indication: Compound W is indicated for the removal of common warts. The common wart is easily recognized by the rough "cauliflower-like" appearance of the surface.

Actions: Warts are common benign skin lesions which appear mainly on the back of hands and on fingers, but can also appear on other parts of the body. They are caused by an infectious virus which stimulates mitosis in the basal cell layer of the skin, resulting in the production of elevated epithelial growths. The keratolytic action of salicylic acid in a flexible collodion vehicle causes the cornified epithelium to swell, soften, macerate and then desquamate.

Warnings: For external use only. Do not use this product on irritated skin, on any area that is infected or reddened, if you are a diabetic, or if you have poor blood circulation. If discomfort persists, see your doctor. Do not use on moles, birthmarks, warts with hair growing from them, genital warts, or warts on the face or mucous membranes (inside mouth, nose, anus, genitals, or on lips). Flammable. Keep away from fire or flame. Cap bottle tightly and store at room temperature away from heat. Avoid smoking during application and until product has dried. Do not use near eyes. If product gets into the eye, flush with water to remove film and continue to flush with water for 15 minutes. Do not inhale. Keep this and all medicines out of the reach of children. In case of accidental ingestion, seek the advice of a physician or contact a poison control center immediately.

Precautions: If redness or irritation occurs, discontinue product for 2 days and then reapply. Should stinging or irritation recur, discontinue use. Covering the treated wart with a bandage will increase effectiveness but may also increase the chance of irritation. If a bandage is used, first allow the solution or gel to dry thoroughly.

Dosage and Administration: Wash affected area. May soak in warm water for 5 minutes. Dry area thoroughly. If any tissue has loosened, remove by rubbing with a washcloth or soft brush. Apply one drop at a time sufficiently to cover each wart by using the plastic rod provided with the solution or by squeezing the tube. Let dry. Repeat this procedure once or twice daily as needed (until wart is removed) for up to 12 weeks. If the wart shows no improvement, see your physician.

Professional Labeling: Same as those outlined under Indication.

Inactive Ingredients: Solution: Acetone Collodion, Alcohol 1.83% w/w, Camphor, Castor Oil, Ether 63.5%, Menthol, Polysorbate 80. Gel: Alcohol 67.5% by vol., Camphor, Castor Oil, Collodion, Colloidal Silicon Dioxide, Hydroxypropyl Cellulose, Hypophosphorous Acid, Polysorbate 80.

How Supplied: Compound W is available in .31 fluid oz. clear bottles with plastic applicators. Compound W Gel is available in .25 oz. tubes. Store at room temperature.

DENOREX®
[dĕn 'ō-reks]
Medicated Shampoo
DENOREX®
Mountain Fresh Herbal Scent Medicated Shampoo
DENOREX®
Medicated Shampoo and Conditioner
DENOREX®
Extra Strength Medicated Shampoo
DENOREX®
Extra Strength Medicated Shampoo with Conditioners

Description: The Shampoo (Regular and Mountain Fresh Herbal) and the Shampoo with Conditioner contain Coal Tar Solution 9.0%, Menthol 1.5%. The

Extra Strength Shampoo and the Extra Strength Shampoo with Conditioners contain Coal Tar Solution 12.5% and Menthol 1.5%.

Indications: Relieves scaling, itching, flaking of dandruff, seborrhea and psoriasis. Regular use promotes cleaner, healthier hair and scalp.

Actions: Denorex Shampoo is an antiseborrheic and antipruritic which loosens and softens scales and crusts. Coal tar helps correct abnormalities of keratinization by decreasing epidermal proliferation and dermal infiltration. Denorex also contains the antipruritic agent, menthol.

Warnings: For external use only. Discontinue treatment if irritation develops. Avoid contact with eyes. Keep this and all medicines out of children's reach.

Directions: For best results use regularly, but at least every other day. For severe scalp problems use daily. Wet hair thoroughly and briskly massage until you obtain a rich lather. Rinse thoroughly and repeat. Your scalp may tingle slightly during treatment.

Professional Labeling: Same as stated under Indications.

Inactive Ingredients:
Shampoo: Also contains Chloroxylenol, Lauramide DEA, Stearic Acid, TEA-Lauryl Sulfate, Water (plus Hydroxypropyl Methylcellulose in the Mountain Fresh Herbal scent formula), Alcohol 7.5%.
Shampoo and Conditioner: Chloroxylenol, Citric Acid, Fragrance, Hydroxypropyl Methylcellulose, Lauramide DEA, PEG-27 Lanolin, Polyquaternium-11, TEA-Lauryl Sulfate, Water, Alcohol 7.5%.
Extra Strength: Chloroxylenol, FD&C Red #40, Fragrance, Glycol Distearate, Lauramide DEA, Methylcellulose, TEA-Lauryl Sulfate, Water, Alcohol 10.4%.
Extra Strength With Conditioners: Chloroxylenol, Citric Acid, Cocodimonium Hydrolyzed Protein, Dimethicone, FD&C Red #40, Fragrance, Glycol Distearate, Lauramide DEA, Methylcellulose, PEG-27 Lanolin, Polyquaternium-6, TEA-Lauryl Sulfate, Water, Alcohol 10.4%.

How Supplied:
Lotion: 4 oz., 8 oz. and 12 oz. bottles in Regular Scent, Mountain Fresh Herbal Scent, Shampoo and Conditioner, Extra Strength Shampoo, and Extra Strength Shampoo With Conditioners.

Shown in Product Identification Section, page 437

DERMOPLAST®
[der 'mō-plăst]
Anesthetic Pain Relief Lotion

Description: DERMOPLAST Lotion contains Benzocaine 8% and Menthol 0.5%.

Actions: DERMOPLAST is a topical anesthetic and antipruritic.

Indications: DERMOPLAST is indicated for the fast, temporary relief of skin pain and itching due to sunburn, minor cuts, insect bites, abrasions, minor burns, and minor skin irritations.

Warnings: FOR EXTERNAL USE ONLY.
In case of accidental ingestion, seek professional assistance or contact a Poison Control Center. Avoid contact with eyes. Not for prolonged use. If the condition for which this preparation is used persists or if rash or irritation develops, discontinue use and consult physician. Keep this and all drugs out of the reach of children.

Directions: Apply freely over sunburned or irritated skin. Repeat three or four times daily, as needed.

Inactive Ingredients: Aloe Vera Gel, Carbomer 934P, Ceteth-16, Glycerin, Glyceryl Stearate, Laneth-16, Methylparaben, Oleth-16, Propylparaben, Simethicone, Steareth-16, Triethanolamine, Water.

How Supplied: DERMOPLAST Anesthetic Pain Relief Lotion, in Net Wt 3 fl. oz.

DERMOPLAST®
[der 'mō-plăst]
Anesthetic Pain Relief Spray

Description: DERMOPLAST is an aerosol containing Benzocaine 20% and Menthol 0.5%.

Indications: DERMOPLAST is indicated for the fast, temporary relief of skin pain and itching due to sunburn, minor cuts, insect bites, abrasions, minor burns, and minor skin irritations. May be applied without touching sensitive affected areas. Widely used in hospitals for pain and itch of episiotomy, pruritus vulvae, and postpartum hemorrhoids.

Warnings: FOR EXTERNAL USE ONLY. Avoid spraying in eyes. Contents under pressure. Do not puncture or incinerate. Do not use near open flame. Use only as directed. Intentional misuse by deliberately concentrating and inhaling the contents can be harmful or fatal. Do not take orally. Not for prolonged use. If the condition for which this preparation is used persists, or if a rash or irritation develops, discontinue use and consult physician.

Directions for Use: Hold can in a comfortable position 6–12 inches away from affected area. Point spray nozzle and press button. To apply to face, spray in palm of hand. May be administered three or four times daily, or as directed by physician.

Inactive Ingredients: Acetylated Lanolin Alcohol, *Aloe vera* Oil, Butane, Cetyl Acetate, Hydrofluorocarbon, Methylparaben, PEG-8 Laurate, Polysorbate 85.

How Supplied: DERMOPLAST Anesthetic Pain Relief Spray, in Net Wt 2¾ oz (78 g). Do not expose to heat or temperatures above 120° F.

DRISTAN®
[drĭs 'tăn]
Decongestant/Antihistamine/ Analgesic
Coated Tablets and Coated Caplets

Description: Each Dristan Coated Tablet or Coated Caplet contains: Phenylephrine HCl 5 mg, Chlorpheniramine Maleate 2 mg, Acetaminophen 325 mg.

Actions: Phenylephrine HCl is an oral nasal decongestant (sympathomimetic amine) effective as a vasoconstrictor to help reduce nasal/sinus congestion. Phenylephrine produces little or no central nervous system stimulation.
Chlorpheniramine Maleate is an antihistamine effective in the control of rhinorrhea, sneezing and lacrimation associated with elevated histamine levels in disorders of the respiratory tract.
Acetaminophen is both an analgesic and an antipyretic. Therapeutic doses of acetaminophen will effectively reduce an elevated body temperature. Also, acetaminophen is effective in reducing the discomfort of pain associated with headache.

Indications: Dristan is indicated for effective multi-symptom relief of colds/flu, sinusitis, hay fever, or other upper respiratory allergies: nasal congestion, sneezing, runny nose, fever, headache and minor aches and pains.

Warnings: Avoid alcoholic beverages and driving a motor vehicle or operating heavy machinery while taking this product. May cause drowsiness or excitability, especially in children. Persons with asthma, glaucoma, high blood pressure, diabetes, heart or thyroid disease, difficulty in urination due to enlarged prostate gland, or taking an antidepressant drug, should use only as directed by a physician. Do not exceed recommended dosage because at higher doses nervousness, dizziness, or sleeplessness may occur. If symptoms do not improve within 7 days or are accompanied by high fever, discontinue use and see a physician. As with any drug, if you are pregnant or nursing a baby, seek the advice of a health professional before using this product.
Do not give to children under 6. Keep this and all medication out of children's reach. In case of accidental overdose contact a physician immediately.

Dosage and Administration: Adults: Two tablets or caplets every four hours, not to exceed 12 tablets or caplets in 24 hours. Children 6–12: One tablet or caplet every four hours, not to exceed six tablets or caplets in 24 hours.

Inactive Ingredients: Tablets—Calcium Stearate, Croscarmellose Sodium, D&C Yellow #10 Lake, FD&C Yellow #6 Lake, Hydroxypropyl Methylcellulose, Microcrystalline Cellulose, Polyethylene Glycol, Povidone, Starch, Stearic Acid.
Caplets—Calcium Stearate, Croscarmellose Sodium, D&C Red #7 Lake, D&C

Continued on next page

Whitehall—Cont.

Yellow #10 Lake, FD&C Yellow #6 Lake, Hydroxypropyl Methylcellulose, Microcrystalline Cellulose, Polyethylene Glycol, Povidone, Starch, Stearic Acid, Titanium Dioxide.

How Supplied: Yellow/White coated tablets in tins of 12 and blister packages of 24 and bottles of 48 and 100. Yellow/White coated caplets in blister packages of 20 and bottles of 40.

Shown in Product Identification Section, page 437

DRISTAN®
[*drĭs 'tăn*]
Nasal Spray
Menthol Nasal Spray

Description: Dristan Nasal Spray contains Phenylephrine HCl 0.5%, Pheniramine Maleate 0.2%.

Actions: Phenylephrine HCl is a sympathomimetic agent that constricts the smaller arterioles of the nasal passages producing a gentle and predictable decongesting effect. Pheniramine Maleate is an antihistamine that controls rhinorrhea, sneezing, and lacrimation associated with elevated histamine levels in disorders of the respiratory tract.

Indications: Dristan Nasal Spray provides prompt temporary relief of nasal congestion due to colds, sinusitis, hay fever or other upper respiratory allergies.

Warnings: Do not exceed recommended dosage because symptoms may occur such as burning, stinging, sneezing, or increase of nasal discharge. Do not use this product for more than 3 days. If symptoms persist, consult a physician. The use of the dispenser by more than one person may spread infection. For adult use only. Do not give this product to children under 12 years except under the advice and supervision of a physician. Keep these and all medicines out of children's reach. In case of accidental ingestion, seek professional assistance or contact a Poison Control Center immediately.

Dosage and Administration: Squeeze Bottle—With head upright, insert nozzle in nostril. Spray quickly, firmly and sniff deeply.
Metered Dose Pump—Prime the metered dose pump by depressing pump firmly several times. With head upright, insert nozzle in nostril. Depress pump 2 or 3 times, all the way down, with a firm, even stroke and sniff deeply.
Adults: Spray 2 or 3 times into each nostril. Repeat every 4 hours as needed. Children under 12 years: As directed by a physician.

Professional Labeling: Same as those outlined under Indications.

Inactive Ingredients: Dristan Nasal Spray: Alcohol 0.4%, Benzalkonium Chloride 1:5000 in buffered isotonic aqueous solution, Eucalyptol, Hydroxypropyl Methylcellulose, Menthol, Sodium Chloride, Sodium Phosphate, Thimerosal 0.002%, and Water.
Dristan Menthol Nasal Spray: Benzalkonium Chloride 1:5000 in buffered isotonic aqueous solution, Camphor, Eucalyptol, Hydroxypropyl Methylcellulose, Menthol, Methyl Salicylate, Polysorbate 80, Sodium Chloride, Sodium Phosphate, Thimerosal 0.002%, and Water.

How Supplied: Dristan Nasal Spray: 15 mL and 30 mL plastic squeeze bottles, and 15 mL metered dose pumps.
Dristan Menthol Nasal Spray: 15 mL and 30 mL plastic squeeze bottles.

Shown in Product Identification Section, page 437

DRISTAN®
[*drĭs 'tăn*]
Long Lasting Nasal Spray
Long Lasting Menthol Nasal Spray

Description: Dristan Long Lasting Nasal Spray contains Oxymetazoline HCl 0.05%.

Actions: The sympathomimetic action of Dristan Long Lasting Nasal Spray and Dristan Long Lasting Menthol Nasal Spray constricts the smaller arterioles of the nasal passages, producing a prolonged, up to 12 hours, gentle and predictable decongesting effect.

Indications: Dristan Long Lasting Nasal Spray and Dristan Long Lasting Menthol Nasal Spray provide prompt temporary relief of nasal congestion due to colds, sinusitis, hay fever, or other upper respiratory allergies for up to 12 hours.

Warnings: Do not exceed recommended dosage because symptoms may occur such as burning, stinging, sneezing, or increase of nasal discharge. Do not use this product for more than 3 days. If symptoms persist, consult a physician. The use of the dispenser by more than one person may spread infection. Keep these and all medicines out of the reach of children. In case of accidental ingestion, seek professional assistance or contact a Poison Control Center immediately.

Dosage and Administration: Squeeze Bottle—With head upright, insert nozzle in nostril. Spray quickly, firmly and sniff deeply.
Metered Dose Pump—Prime the metered dose pump by depressing pump firmly several times. With head upright, insert nozzle in nostril. Depress pump 2 or 3 times, all the way down, with a firm even stroke and sniff deeply.
Adults and children 6 years of age and over, spray 2 or 3 times into each nostril. Repeat twice daily—morning and evening. Not recommended for children under six.

Professional Labeling: Same as those outlined under Indications.

Inactive Ingredients: Dristan Long Lasting Nasal Spray—Benzalkonium Chloride 1:5000 in buffered isotonic aqueous solution, Hydroxypropyl Methylcellulose, Potassium Phosphate, Sodium Chloride, Sodium Phosphate, Thimerosal 0.002%, and Water.
Dristan Long Lasting Menthol Nasal Spray—Benzalkonium Chloride 1:5000 in buffered isotonic aqueous solution, Camphor, Eucalyptol, Hydroxypropyl Methylcellulose, Menthol, Potassium Phosphate, Sodium Chloride, Sodium Phosphate, Thimerosal 0.002%, Water, and Alcohol 0.4%.

How Supplied: Dristan Long Lasting Nasal Spray: 15 mL and 30 mL plastic squeeze bottles and 15 mL metered dose pump. Dristan Long Lasting Menthol Nasal Spray: 15 mL plastic squeeze bottle.

Shown in Product Identification Section, page 437

Maximum Strength DRISTAN®
[*drĭs 'tăn*]
Decongestant/Analgesic Coated Caplets

Description: Each Maximum Strength Dristan Coated Caplet contains: Pseudoephedrine HCl 30 mg and Acetaminophen 500 mg.

Actions: Pseudoephedrine HCl is an oral nasal decongestant and is effective in reducing nasal/sinus congestion. Acetaminophen is both an analgesic and an antipyretic. This maximum strength nonaspirin pain reliever effectively reduces headache pain and the pain of a sinus cold. Acetaminophen also reduces an elevated body temperature.

Indications: Maximum Strength Dristan is indicated for effective relief without drowsiness from nasal and sinus congestion, sinus pressure and sinus pain due to colds, sinusitis, and upper respiratory allergies.

Warnings: Do not exceed recommended dosage because at higher doses nervousness, dizziness or sleeplessness may occur. Persons with high blood pressure, heart disease, diabetes, thyroid disease, difficulty in urination due to an enlarged prostate gland, or taking an antidepressant drug should use only as directed by a physician. If symptoms do not improve within 7 days, or are accompanied by high fever, discontinue use and see a physician. Do not give to children under 12. As with any drug, if you are pregnant or nursing a baby, seek the advice of a health professional before using this product. Keep this and all medication out of children's reach. In case of accidental overdose, contact a physician immediately.

Dosage and Administration: Adults and children over 12: Two caplets every 6 hours, not to exceed 8 caplets in any 24-hour period. Children under 12 should use only as directed by a physician.

Inactive Ingredients: Calcium Stearate, Croscarmellose Sodium, D&C Yellow #10 Lake, FD&C Yellow #6 Lake, Hydrogenated Vegetable Oil, Hydroxypropyl Methylcellulose, Microcrystalline Cellulose, Polyethylene Glycol, Povidone, Starch, Stearic Acid, Titanium Dioxide.

How Supplied: Yellow coated caplets in blister packages of 24 and bottles of 48 and 100.

Shown in Product Identification Section, page 437

FREEZONE®
['frēz-ōn]
Solution

Description: Freezone is a solution which contains Salicylic Acid 13.6% w/w in a collodion vehicle.

Indications: Freezone is indicated for removal of corns and calluses. Relieves pain by removing corns and calluses.

Actions: Freezone penetrates corns and calluses painlessly, layer by layer, loosening and softening the corn or callus so that the whole corn or callus can be lifted off or peeled away in just a few days.

Warnings: For external use only. Do not use this product on irritated skin, on area that is infected or reddened, if you are a diabetic, or if you have poor blood circulation. If discomfort persists, see your doctor or podiatrist. Flammable. Keep away from fire or flame. Cap bottle tightly and store at room temperature away from heat. If the product gets into eye, flush with water for 15 minutes. Avoid inhaling vapors. Keep this and all drugs out of reach of children. In case of accidental ingestion, seek the advice of a physician or contact a poison control center immediately.

Dosage and Administration: Wash affected area and dry thoroughly. Apply one drop at a time to sufficiently cover each corn/callus. Let dry. Repeat this procedure once or twice daily as needed for up to 14 days (until corn/callus is removed). May soak corn/callus in warm water for 5 minutes to assist in removal.

Inactive Ingredients: Alcohol (20.5%), Balsam Oregon, Castor Oil, Ether (64.8%), Hypophosphorous Acid and Zinc Chloride.

How Supplied: Available in a .31 fl. oz. glass bottle.
Store at room temperature away from heat.

MOMENTUM®
[mō-mĕn 'tum]
Muscular Backache Formula

Description: Momentum contains Aspirin 500 mg, Phenyltoloxamine Citrate 15 mg, per caplet.

Indications: Momentum is indicated for the relief of pain due to stiffness and tight, inflamed muscles.

Actions: The combination of aspirin and phenyltoloxamine citrate act to relieve the pain of tense, knotted muscles. As pain subsides, muscles loosen and become less stiff, more relaxed and mobility is increased.

Warnings: Children and teenagers should not use this medicine for chicken pox or flu symptoms before a doctor is consulted about Reye Syndrome, a rare but serious illness reported to be associated with aspirin. Do not drive a car or operate machinery while taking this medication as this preparation may cause drowsiness in some persons. As with any drug, if you are pregnant or nursing a baby, seek the advice of a health professional before using this product. **IT IS ESPECIALLY IMPORTANT NOT TO USE ASPIRIN DURING THE LAST 3 MONTHS OF PREGNANCY UNLESS SPECIFICALLY DIRECTED TO DO SO BY A DOCTOR BECAUSE IT MAY CAUSE PROBLEMS IN THE UNBORN CHILD OR COMPLICATIONS DURING DELIVERY.** Keep this and all medicines out of children's reach. In case of accidental overdose, contact a physician immediately.

Precaution: If pain persists for more than 10 days or redness is present as in arthritic or rheumatic conditions affecting children under 12, consult a physician immediately.

Dosage and Administration: Adults: Two caplets upon rising, then two caplets as needed at lunch, dinner, and bedtime. Dosage should not exceed 8 caplets in any 24-hour period. Not recommended for children.

Professional Labeling: Same as those outlined under Indications.

Inactive Ingredients: Alginic Acid, Citric Acid, Colloidal Silicon Dioxide, Hydrogenated Vegetable Oil, Microcrystalline Cellulose, Starch and Surfactant.

How Supplied: Bottles of 24 and 48 white, uncoated caplets.

OUTGRO®
['aut-grō]
Solution

Description: Outgro solution contains Tannic Acid 25%, Chlorobutanol 5%.

Indications: Outgro provides fast, temporary pain relief of ingrown toenails.

Actions: Outgro temporarily relieves pain, reduces swelling and eases inflammation accompanying ingrown toenails. Daily use of Outgro toughens tender skin—allowing the nail to be cut and thus preventing further pain and discomfort. Outgro does not affect the growth, shape or position of the nail.

Warnings: For external use only. Do not use Outgro solution for more than 7 days unless directed by a doctor. Consult a doctor if no improvement is seen after 7 days. IF YOU HAVE DIABETES OR POOR CIRCULATION, SEE A DOCTOR FOR TREATMENT OF INGROWN TOENAIL. DO NOT APPLY THIS PRODUCT TO OPEN SORES. IF REDNESS AND SWELLING OF YOUR TOE INCREASES, OR IF A DISCHARGE IS PRESENT AROUND THE NAIL, STOP USING THIS PRODUCT AND SEE YOUR DOCTOR IMMEDIATELY. Flammable. Keep away from fire or flame. Avoid smoking during use and until product has dried. In case of accidental ingestion, contact a physician or call a Poison Control Center immediately. KEEP THIS AND ALL MEDICINES OUT OF CHILDREN'S REACH.

Directions: Cleanse affected toes thoroughly. Using rod in cap, either apply Outgro Solution in the crevice where the nail is growing into the flesh or place a small piece of cotton in the nail groove (the side of the nail where the pain is) and wet cotton thoroughly with Outgro solution several times daily until nail discomfort is relieved. Change cotton at least once daily. Do not use product for more than 7 days unless directed by a doctor (podiatrist or physician). In some instances, temporary discoloration of the nail and surrounding skin may occur.

Inactive Ingredients: Ethylcellulose, Isopropyl Alcohol 83% (by volume).

How Supplied: Available in .31 fl. oz. glass bottles.

OXIPOR VHC®
['äk-si-pōr VHC]
Lotion for Psoriasis

Description: OXIPOR VHC lotion for psoriasis contains Coal Tar Solution 48.5%, Salicylic Acid 1.0%, Benzocaine 2.0%.

Actions: Coal tar solution helps control cell growth and therefore prevents formation of new scales. Salicylic acid has a keratolytic action which helps peel off and dissolve away scales. Benzocaine is a local anesthetic that gives prompt relief from pain and itching. Alcohol is the solvent vehicle.

Indications: OXIPOR VHC has been clinically proven to relieve itching, redness and help dissolve and clear away the scales and crusts of psoriasis.

Warnings: For external use only. Avoid contact with eyes or mucous membranes. Use caution in exposing skin to sunlight after applying product. It may increase your tendency to sunburn for up to 24 hours after application. DO NOT USE in or around rectum or in genital area or groin except on advice of a doctor. Flammable. Keep away from fire or flame. Avoid smoking during application and until product has dried. Do not chill. Not for prolonged use. If condition persists or if rash or irritation develops, discontinue use and consult physician. Keep out of children's reach.

Dosage and Administration: Shake bottle well before each application. SKIN: Wash affected area before applying to remove loose scales. With a small wad of cotton, apply twice daily. Allow to dry before contact with clothing.
SCALP: Apply to scalp with fingertips making sure to get down to the skin itself. Leave on for as long as possible, even overnight. Shampoo. Then remove all loose scales with a fine comb. This product may temporarily discolor light-col-

Continued on next page

Whitehall—Cont.

ored hair. Discoloration can be prevented by reducing the time the product is left on the scalp. Also be sure to rinse product out of hair thoroughly.

Professional Labeling: Same as those outlined under Indications.

Inactive Ingredients: Alcohol 81% by volume, water.

How Supplied: Available in 1.9 oz. and 4.0 oz. bottles. Store at room temperature.

POSTURE®
[*pos 'tūr*]
600 mg
High Potency Calcium Supplement

Description: Each film-coated tablet of POSTURE® contains Tribasic Calcium Phosphate 1565.2 mg, which provides 600 mg of elemental calcium. POSTURE® is specially formulated not to produce gas.

Two tablets contain:		For Adults— % U.S. RDA*
Elemental Calcium...... (as calcium phosphate)	1200 mg	...120%

*Percentage of U.S. Recommended Daily Allowance

Indication: POSTURE® Tablets provide a daily source of calcium to help maintain healthy bones or to supplement dietary calcium intake when directed by a physician.

Directions for Use: One or two tablets daily, or as recommended by a physician. Keep Out of Reach of Children.

Inactive Ingredients: Croscarmellose Sodium, Ethylcellulose, Magnesium Stearate, Microcrystalline Cellulose, Polyethylene Glycol, Povidone, Sodium Lauryl Sulfate.

How Supplied: In bottles of 60 scored tablets.

Shown in Product Identification Section, page 437

POSTURE®-D
600 mg
High Potency Calcium Supplement with Vitamin D

Description: Each film-coated tablet of POSTURE®-D contains Tribasic Calcium Phosphate 1565.2 mg, which provides 600 mg of elemental calcium and 125 IU of Vitamin D. POSTURE®-D is specially formulated not to produce gas.

Two tablets contain:		For Adults— % U.S. RDA*
Elemental Calcium...... (as calcium phosphate)	1200 mg	...120%
Vitamin D....................	250 IU	.... 63%

*Percentage of U.S. Recommended Daily Allowance.

Indication: POSTURE®-D Tablets provide a daily source of calcium and Vitamin D to help maintain healthy bones or to supplement dietary intake of calcium and Vitamin D when directed by a physician.

Directions for Use: One or two tablets daily, or as recommended by a physician. Keep Out of Reach of Children.

Inactive Ingredients: Croscarmellose Sodium, Ethylcellulose, Magnesium Stearate, Microcrystalline Cellulose, Polyethylene Glycol, Povidone, Sodium Lauryl Sulfate.

How Supplied: In bottles of 60 scored tablets.

Shown in Product Identification Section, page 437

PREPARATION H®
[*prep-e 'rā-shen-āch*]
Hemorrhoidal Ointment and Cream
PREPARATION H®
Hemorrhoidal Suppositories

Description: Preparation H is available in ointment, cream and suppository product forms. The **Ointment** contains Live Yeast Cell Derivative supplying 2,000 units Skin Respiratory Factor per ounce of Ointment, and Shark Liver Oil 3.0% in a specially prepared Rectal Petrolatum Base.
The **Cream** contains Live Yeast Cell Derivative supplying 2,000 units Skin Respiratory Factor per ounce of Cream and Shark Liver Oil 3.0% in a specially prepared Rectal Cream Base containing Petrolatum.
The **Suppositories** contain Live Yeast Cell Derivative, supplying 2,000 units Skin Respiratory Factor per ounce of Cocoa Butter Suppository Base and Shark Liver Oil 3.0%.

Actions: Live Yeast Cell Derivative acts by increasing the oxygen uptake of dermal tissues and facilitating collagen formation. Shark Liver Oil has been incorporated to act as a protectant which softens and soothes the tissues. Preparation H also lubricates inflamed, irritated surfaces to help make bowel movements less painful.

Indications: Preparation H helps shrink swelling of hemorrhoidal tissues caused by inflammation and gives prompt, temporary relief in many cases from pain and itch in tissues.

Precautions: In case of bleeding, or if your condition persists, a physician should be consulted.

Dosage and Administration: Ointment/Cream: Before applying, remove protective cover from applicator. Lubricate applicator before each application and thoroughly cleanse after use. It is recommended that Preparation H Hemorrhoidal ointment/cream be applied freely to the affected rectal area whenever symptoms occur, from three to five times per day, especially at night, in the morning, and after each bowel movement. Frequent application with Preparation H ointment/cream provides continual therapy which leads to more rapid improvement of hemorrhoidal symptoms. **Suppositories:** Whenever symptoms occur, remove wrapper, insert one suppository rectally from three to five times per day, especially at night, in the morning, and after each bowel movement. Frequent application with Preparation H suppositories provides continual therapy which leads to more rapid improvement of hemorrhoidal symptoms.

Professional Labeling: Same as those outlined under Indications.

Inactive Ingredients: Ointment—Beeswax, Glycerin, Lanolin, Lanolin Alcohol, Mineral Oil, Paraffin, Phenylmercuric Nitrate 1:10,000 (as a preservative), Thyme Oil.
Cream—BHA, Cellulose Gum, Cetyl Alcohol, Citric Acid, Disodium EDTA, Glycerin, Glyceryl Stearate, Lanolin, Methylparaben, Phenylmercuric Nitrate, 1:10,000 (as a preservative), Propyl Gallate, Propylene Glycol, Propylparaben, Simethicone, Sodium Lauryl Sulfate, Stearyl Alcohol, Water, Xanthan Gum. May also contain Glyceryl Oleate and/or Polysorbate 80.
Suppositories — Beeswax, Glycerin, Phenylmercuric Nitrate 1:10,000 (as a preservative), Polyethylene Glycol 600 Dilaurate.

How Supplied: Ointment: Net Wt. 1 oz. and 2 oz. **Cream:** Net wt. 0.9 oz. and 1.8 oz. Store at controlled room temperature or in a cool place but not over 80° F. **Suppositories:** 12's, 24's, 36's and 48's. Store at controlled room temperature in cool place but not over 80° F.

Shown in Product Identification Section, page 437

PRIMATENE®
[*prīm 'a-tēn*]
Mist
(Epinephrine Inhalation Aerosol Bronchodilator)

Description: Primatene Mist contains Epinephrine 5.5 mg/mL.

Action: Epinephrine is a sympathomimetic agent which eases breathing for asthma patients by reducing spasms of bronchial muscles.

Indications: Primatene Mist is indicated for temporary relief of shortness of breath, tightness of chest, and wheezing due to bronchial asthma.

Dosage and Administration: Inhalation dosage for adults, children 12 years of age and older, and children 4 to under 12 years of age: Start with one inhalation, then wait at least 1 minute. If not relieved, use once more. Do not use again for at least 3 hours. The use of this product by children should be supervised by an adult. Children under 4 years of age: Consult a physician. Each inhalation delivers 0.22 mg. of epinephrine.

Warnings: Do not use this product unless a diagnosis of asthma has been made by a physician. Do not use this product if you have heart disease, high blood pressure, thyroid disease, diabetes, or difficulty in urination due to enlargement of the prostate gland unless directed by a physician. As with any drug, if you are pregnant or nursing a baby, seek the advice of a health professional before using this product. Do not use this product if you have ever been hospitalized for asthma or if you are taking any prescription drug for asthma unless directed by a physician. Keep this and all drugs out of the reach of children. In case of accidental overdose, seek professional assistance or contact a poison control center immediately. DO NOT CONTINUE TO USE THIS PRODUCT, BUT SEEK MEDICAL ASSISTANCE IMMEDIATELY IF SYMPTOMS ARE NOT RELIEVED WITHIN 20 MINUTES OR BECOME WORSE. DO NOT USE THIS PRODUCT MORE FREQUENTLY OR AT HIGHER DOSES THAN RECOMMENDED UNLESS DIRECTED BY A PHYSICIAN. EXCESSIVE USE MAY CAUSE NERVOUSNESS AND RAPID HEART BEAT AND POSSIBLY, ADVERSE EFFECTS ON THE HEART. DRUG INTERACTION PRECAUTION: Do not use this product if you are presently taking a prescription drug for high blood pressure or depression, without first consulting your physician.

Precautions: Contents under pressure. Do not puncture or throw container into incinerator. Using or storing near open flame or heating above 120° F (49° C) may cause bursting. Store at room temperature 59° F–86° F (15° C–30° C).

Directions For Use of The Mouthpiece:
The Primatene Mist mouthpiece, which is enclosed in the Primatene Mist 15mL size (not the refill size), should be used for inhalation only with Primatene Mist.

1. Take plastic cap off mouthpiece. (For refills, use mouthpiece from previous purchase.)
2. Take plastic mouthpiece off bottle.
3. Place other end of mouthpiece on bottle.
4. Turn bottle upside down. Place thumb on bottom of mouthpiece over circular button and forefinger on top of vial. Empty the lungs as completely as possible by exhaling.
5. Place mouthpiece in mouth with lips closed around opening. Inhale deeply while squeezing mouthpiece and bottle together. Release immediately and remove unit from mouth. Complete taking the deep breath, drawing the medication into your lungs and holding breath as long as comfortable.
6. Then exhale slowly keeping lips nearly closed. This distributes the medication in the lungs.
7. Replace plastic cap on mouthpiece.
8. The Primatene Mist mouthpiece should be washed once daily with soap and hot water, and rinsed thoroughly. Then it should be dried with a clean, lint-free cloth.

Inactive Ingredients: Alcohol 34%, Ascorbic Acid, Fluorocarbons (Propellant), Water. Contains No Sulfites.

How Supplied:
½ Fl. oz. (15mL) With Mouthpiece.
½ Fl. oz. (15mL) Refill
¾ Fl. oz. (22.5mL) Refill

Shown in Product Identification Section, page 437

PRIMATENE®
[*prīm 'a-tēn*]
Mist Suspension
(Epinephrine Bitartrate Inhalation Aerosol Bronchodilator)

Description: Primatene Mist Suspension contains Epinephrine Bitartrate 7.0 mg/mL.

Action: Epinephrine is a sympathomimetic agent which eases breathing for asthma patients by reducing spasms of bronchial muscles.

Indications: Primatene Mist Suspension is indicated for temporary relief of shortness of breath, tightness of chest, and wheezing due to bronchial asthma.

Dosage and Administration: Shake before using. Inhalation dosage for adults, children 12 years of age and older, and children 4 to under 12 years of age: Start with one inhalation, then wait at least 1 minute. If not relieved, use once more. Do not use again for at least 3 hours. The use of this product by children should be supervised by an adult. Children under 4 years of age: Consult a physician. Each inhalation delivers 0.3 mg. Epinephrine Bitartrate equivalent to 0.16 mg. Epinephrine Base.

Warnings: Do not use this product unless a diagnosis of asthma has been made by a physician. Do not use this product if you have heart disease, high blood pressure, thyroid disease, diabetes, or difficulty in urination due to enlargement of the prostate gland unless directed by a physician. As with any drug, if you are pregnant or nursing a baby, seek the advice of a health professional before using this product. Do not use this product if you have ever been hospitalized for asthma or if you are taking any prescription drug for asthma unless directed by a physician. Keep this and all drugs out of the reach of children. In case of accidental overdose, seek professional assistance or contact a poison control center immediately.
DO NOT CONTINUE TO USE THIS PRODUCT, BUT SEEK MEDICAL ASSISTANCE IMMEDIATELY IF SYMPTOMS ARE NOT RELIEVED WITHIN 20 MINUTES OR BECOME WORSE. DO NOT USE THIS PRODUCT MORE FREQUENTLY OR AT HIGHER DOSES THAN RECOMMENDED UNLESS DIRECTED BY A PHYSICIAN. EXCESSIVE USE MAY CAUSE NERVOUSNESS AND RAPID HEART BEAT AND POSSIBLY, ADVERSE EFFECTS ON THE HEART. DRUG INTERACTION PRECAUTION: Do not use this product if you are presently taking a prescription drug for high blood pressure or depression, without first consulting your physician.

Precautions: Contents under pressure. Do not puncture or throw container into incinerator. Using or storing near open flame or heating above 120° F (49° C) may cause bursting. Store at room temperature 59° F–86° F (15° C–30° C).

Directions For Use of The Inhaler:

1. SHAKE BEFORE USING.
2. HOLD INHALER WITH NOZZLE DOWN WHILE USING. Empty the lungs as completely as possible by exhaling.
3. Purse the lips as in saying "O" and hold the nozzle up to the lips keeping the tongue flat. As you start to take a deep breath, squeeze nozzle and can together, releasing one full application. Complete taking a deep breath, drawing medication into your lungs.
4. Hold breath for as long as comfortable. Then exhale slowly, keeping the lips nearly closed. This distributes the medication in the lungs.
5. The Primatene Mist Suspension nozzle should be washed once daily. After removing the nozzle from the vial, wash it with soap and hot water, and rinse thoroughly. Then it should be dried with a clean, lint-free cloth.

Inactive Ingredients: Fluorocarbons (Propellant), Sorbitan Trioleate. Contains No Sulfites.

How Supplied: ⅓ Fl. oz. (10mL) pocket-size aerosol inhaler.

PRIMATENE®
[*prīm 'a-tēn*]
Tablets

Description: Depending upon the state (see How Supplied), Primatene Tablets are available in 3 formulations:
Regular Formula: Theophylline Anhydrous 130 mg, Ephedrine Hydrochloride 24 mg.
P Formula: Theophylline Hydrous 130 mg, Ephedrine Hydrochloride 24 mg, Phenobarbital 8 mg (⅛ gr) per tablet. (Warning: May be habit forming.)
M Formula: Theophylline Anhydrous 130 mg, Ephedrine Hydrochloride 24 mg, Pyrilamine Maleate 16.6 mg per tablet.

Actions: Primatene Tablets contain two bronchodilators, theophylline, a methylxanthine, and ephedrine, a sympathomimetic amine. The pharmacologic action of theophylline may be mediated through inhibition of phosphodiesterase with a resulting increase in intracellular cyclic AMP. The β-adrenergic ephedrine acts by a different mechanism to produce cyclic AMP. Used at the start of an asthma attack, Primatene acts to (1) open bronchial tubes so breathing is natural, (2) relax bronchial muscles, (3) reduce congestion. Primatene helps relieve the asthma spasms, thus permitting sleep at night and freedom from associated anxiety by day.

Indications: Primatene Tablets are indicated for relief and control of attacks of bronchial asthma and associated hay fever.

Warnings: If symptoms persist, consult your physician. Some people are sensitive to ephedrine and, in such cases, temporary sleeplessness and nervous-

Continued on next page

Whitehall—Cont.

ness may occur. These reactions will disappear if the use of the medication is discontinued. Do not exceed recommended dosage.
People who have heart disease, high blood pressure, diabetes or thyroid trouble or difficulty in urination due to enlargement of the prostate gland should take this preparation only on the advice of a physician. Both the "M" and "P" formulae may cause drowsiness. People taking the "M" or "P" formula should not drive or operate machinery.
As with any drug, if you are pregnant or nursing a baby, seek the advice of a health professional before using this product. Keep all medicines out of reach of children.

Dosage and Administration: Adults: 1 or 2 tablets initially and then one every 4 hours, as needed, not to exceed 6 tablets in 24 hours. Children (6–12): One half adult dose. For children under 6, consult a physician.

Inactive Ingredients:
Regular Formula): Croscarmellose Sodium, D&C Yellow No. 10 Lake, FD&C Yellow No. 6 Lake, Magnesium Stearate, Microcrystalline Cellulose, Silica, Starch, Stearic Acid.
P Formula (Phenobarbital): Colloidal Silicon Dioxide, D&C Yellow No. 10, FD&C Yellow No. 6, Magnesium Stearate, Sodium Starch Glycolate, Starch, Surfactant.
M Formula (Pyrilamine Maleate): D&C Yellow No. 10 Lake, FD&C Yellow No. 6 Lake, Hydrogenated Vegetable Oil, Magnesium Stearate, Microcrystalline Cellulose, Sodium Starch Glycolate, Surfactant, Talc.
Contains No Sulfites.

How Supplied: Available in three Primatene Tablet forms, Regular Formula, "M" Formula, and "P" Formula. (Regular) Primatene Tablets are primarily available in the West and Southwest only. "P" Formula, containing phenobarbital, is available in most states. In those states where phenobarbital is Rx only, "M" Formula, containing pyrilamine maleate, is available. Both "M" and "P" formulas are supplied in glass bottles of 24 and 60 tablets. (Regular) Primatene Tablets are supplied in 24 and 60 tablet thermoform blister cartons.

Shown in Product Identification Section, page 437

RIOPAN®
[*rī'opan*]
magaldrate
Antacid

Description: RIOPAN is a buffer antacid containing the unique chemical entity Magaldrate. Each teaspoonful (5 mL) of suspension contains Magaldrate, 540 mg. Each Chew Tablet or Swallow Tablet contains Magaldrate, 480 mg. RIOPAN is considered dietetically sodium-free (containing not more than 0.004 mEq, 0.1 mg sodium per teaspoonful or tablet).

Actions: Magaldrate, the active ingredient in RIOPAN, demonstrates a rapid and uniform buffering action. The acid-neutralizing capacity of RIOPAN is 15.0 mEq/5mL and 13.5 mEq/tablet. RIOPAN does not produce acid rebound or alkalinization.

Indications: Riopan is indicated for the relief of heartburn, sour stomach, and acid indigestion. For symptomatic relief of hyperacidity associated with the diagnosis of peptic ulcer, gastritis, peptic esophagitis, gastric hyperacidity, and hiatal hernia.

Dosage and Administration: RIOPAN (magaldrate) Antacid *Suspension*—Take one or two teaspoonfuls, between meals and at bedtime, or as directed by the physician. RIOPAN Antacid *Chew Tablets*—Chew one or two tablets, between meals and at bedtime, or as directed by the physician. RIOPAN Antacid *Swallow Tablets*—Take one or two tablets, between meals and at bedtime, or as directed by the physician. Take with enough water to swallow promptly.

Warnings: Patients should not take more than 18 teaspoonfuls (or 20 tablets) in a 24-hour period or use the maximum dosage for more than two weeks, or use if they have kidney disease except under the advice and supervision of a physician.

Drug Interaction Precaution: Do not use in patients taking a prescription antibiotic drug containing any form of tetracycline.

Inactive Ingredients: Chew Tablets: Flavor, Magnesium Stearate, Polyethylene Glycol, Sorbitol, Starch, Sucrose, Titanium Dioxide. Swallow Tablets: Flavor, Magnesium Stearate, Menthol, Microcrystalline Cellulose, Polyethylene Glycol, Starch, Talc, Titanium Dioxide. Suspension: Flavor, Glycerin, Potassium Citrate, Saccharin, Sorbitol, Xanthan Gum, Water.

How Supplied: RIOPAN Antacid *Suspension*—in 12 fl oz (355 mL) plastic bottles. Individual Cups, 1 fl oz (30 mL) ea., tray of 10—10 trays per packer. Store at room temperature (approximately 25°C). Avoid freezing. RIOPAN Antacid *Chew Tablets*—in bottles of 60 and 100. Also, single roll-packs of 12 tablets and 3-roll rollpacks of 36 tablets. RIOPAN Antacid *Swallow Tablets*—Boxes of 60 and 100 in individual film strips (6 x 10 and 10 x 10, respectively).

Shown in Product Identification Section, page 437

RIOPAN PLUS®
[*rī'opan*]
magaldrate and simethicone
Antacid plus Anti-Gas

Description: RIOPAN PLUS is a buffer antacid plus anti-gas combination product containing the unique chemical entity Magaldrate. Each teaspoonful (5mL) of suspension contains Magaldrate, 540 mg and Simethicone, 40 mg. Each Chew Tablet contains Magaldrate, 480 mg and Simethicone, 20 mg. RIOPAN PLUS is considered dietetically sodium-free, containing not more than 0.004 mEq (0.1 mg) sodium per tablet or 0.013 mEq (0.3 mg) per teaspoonful.

Actions: Magaldrate, the active antacid ingredient in RIOPAN PLUS, provides a rapid and uniform buffering action. The acid-neutralizing capacity of RIOPAN PLUS is 15.0 mEq/5mL and 13.5 mEq/tablet. RIOPAN PLUS does not produce acid rebound or alkalinization. Simethicone reduces the surface tension of gas bubbles so that the gas is more easily eliminated.

Indications: RIOPAN PLUS is indicated for the relief of heartburn, sour stomach and acid indigestion, accompanied by the symptoms of gas. For symptomatic relief of hyperacidity associated with the diagnosis of peptic ulcer, gastritis, peptic esophagitis, gastric hyperacidity, and hiatal hernia. For postoperative gas pain.

Dosage and Administration: RIOPAN PLUS (magaldrate and simethicone) Antacid plus Anti-Gas *Suspension*—Take one or two teaspoonfuls between meals and at bedtime, or as directed by the physician.
RIOPAN PLUS Antacid plus Anti-Gas *Chew Tablets*—Chew one or two tablets, between meals and at bedtime, or as directed by the physician.

Warnings: Patients should not take more than 12 teaspoonfuls (or 20 tablets) in a 24-hour period, or use the maximum dosage for more than two weeks, or use if they have kidney disease, except under the advice and supervision of a physician.

Drug Interaction Precaution: Do not use in patients taking a prescription antibiotic drug containing any form of tetracycline.

Inactive Ingredients: Chew Tablets: Flavor, Magnesium Stearate, Methylcellulose, Polyethylene Glycol, Silica, Sorbitol, Starch, Sucrose, Titanium Dioxide. Suspension: Flavor, Glycerin, PEG-8 Stearate, Potassium Citrate, Saccharin, Sorbitan Stearate, Sorbitol, Xanthan Gum, Water.

How Supplied: RIOPAN PLUS Antacid plus Anti-Gas *Suspension*—in 12 fl oz (355 mL) plastic bottles. Individual Cups, 1 fl oz (30 mL) ea., tray of 10—10 trays per packer. Store at room temperature (approximately 25°C). Avoid freezing.
RIOPAN PLUS Antacid plus Anti-Gas *Chew Tablets*—in bottles of 60 and 100. Also, single rollpacks of 12 tablets and 3-roll rollpacks of 36 tablets.

Shown in Product Identification Section, page 437

RIOPAN PLUS® 2

[*rī'opan plus 2*]

magaldrate and simethicone
Double Strength
Antacid plus Anti-Gas

Description: RIOPAN PLUS 2 is a double strength buffer antacid plus antigas combination product containing the unique chemical entity Magaldrate. Each teaspoonful (5 mL) of suspension contains Magaldrate, 1080 mg and Simethicone, 40 mg. Each Chew Tablet contains Magaldrate, 1080 mg and Simethicone, 20 mg. RIOPAN PLUS 2 is considered dietetically sodium-free (containing not more than 0.013 mEq, 0.3 mg per teaspoonful or 0.021 mEq, 0.5 mg per tablet).

Actions: Magaldrate, the active antacid ingredient in RIOPAN PLUS 2, provides a rapid and uniform buffering action. The acid-neutralizing capacity of Double Strength RIOPAN PLUS 2 is 30 mEq/5 mL and 30.0 mEq/tablet. RIOPAN PLUS 2 does not produce acid rebound or alkalinization. Simethicone reduces the surface tension of gas bubbles so that the gas is more easily eliminated.

Indications: RIOPAN PLUS 2 is indicated for the relief of heartburn, sour stomach and acid indigestion accompanied by the symptoms of gas. For symptomatic relief of hyperacidity associated with the diagnosis of peptic ulcer, gastritis, peptic esophagitis, gastric hyperacidity, and hiatal hernia. For postoperative gas pain.

Dosage and Administration: RIOPAN PLUS 2 (magaldrate and simethicone) *Suspension*—Take one or two teaspoonfuls between meals and at bedtime, or as directed by the physician.
RIOPAN PLUS 2 Chew Tablets—Chew one or two tablets, between meals and at bedtime, or as directed by the physician.

Warnings: Patients should not take more than 12 teaspoonfuls (or 9 tablets) in a 24-hour period, or use the maximum dosage for more than two weeks, or use if they have kidney disease, except under the advice and supervision of a physician.

Drug Interaction Precaution: Do not use in patients taking a prescription antibiotic drug containing any form of tetracycline.

Inactive Ingredients: Chew Tablets: Flavor, Magnesium Stearate, Methylcellulose, Polyethylene Glycol, Saccharin, Silica, Sorbitol, Starch, Sucrose, Titanium Dioxide. Supension: Flavor, Glycerin, PEG-8 Stearate, Potassium Citrate, Saccharin, Sorbitan Stearate, Sorbitol, Xanthan Gum, Water.

How Supplied: RIOPAN PLUS 2 *Suspension*—in 12 fl oz (355 mL), 6 fl oz plastic bottles. RIOPAN PLUS 2 Chew Tablets—in bottles of 60.

Shown in Product Identification Section, page 437

SEMICID®

[*sĕm 'ē-sĭd*]

Vaginal Contraceptive Inserts

Description: Semicid is a safe and effective, nonsystemic, reversible method of birth control. Each vaginal contraceptive insert contains 100 mg of the spermicide nonoxynol-9. It contains no hormones and is odorless and nonmessy.
When used consistently and according to directions, the effectiveness of Semicid is approximately equal to other vaginal spermicides, but is less than oral contraceptives.

Actions: Semicid dissolves in the vagina and blends with natural vaginal secretions to provide double birth control protection: a physical barrier, plus an effective sperm killing barrier that covers the cervical opening and adjoining vaginal walls.
Semicid requires no applicator and has no unpleasant taste. Unlike foams, creams and jellies, Semicid does not drip or run, and Semicid inserts are easier to use than the diaphragm. Also, Semicid does not effervesce like some inserts, so it is not as likely to cause a burning feeling. Semicid provides effective contraceptive protection when used properly. However, no contraceptive method or product can provide an absolute guarantee against becoming pregnant.

Indication: For the prevention of pregnancy.

Warnings: Do not insert in urinary opening (urethra). Do not take orally. If irritation occurs, discontinue use. If irritation persists, consult your physician. Keep this and all contraceptives out of the reach of children.

Precautions: If douching is desired, one should wait at least six hours after intercourse before douching. If either partner experiences irritation, discontinue use. If irritation persists, consult a physician.
If your doctor has told you that it is dangerous to become pregnant, ask your doctor if you can use Semicid.
If menstrual period is missed, a physician should be consulted.

Dosage and Administration: To use, unwrap one insert and insert it deeply into the vagina. It is essential that Semicid be inserted at least 15 minutes before intercourse; however, Semicid is also effective when inserted up to 1 hour before intercourse. If intercourse is delayed for more than 1 hour after Semicid is inserted, or if intercourse is repeated, then another insert must be inserted. Semicid can be used as frequently as needed.

Inactive Ingredients: Benzethonium Chloride, Citric Acid, D&C Red #21 Lake, D&C Red #33 Lake, Methylparaben, Polyethylene Glycol, Water.

How Supplied: Strip Packaging of 10's and 20's.
Keep Semicid at room temperature (not over 86°F or 30°C).

Shown in Product Identification Section, page 437

SLEEP-EZE 3®

[*slēp-ēz*]

Nighttime Sleep Aid Tablets
Diphenhydramine Hydrochloride

Description: Sleep-eze 3 is a nighttime sleep-aid that contains Diphenhydramine Hydrochloride, 25 mg per tablet.

Indication: Sleep-eze 3 helps to reduce difficulty in falling asleep.

Action: Sleep-eze 3 contains diphenhydramine, an antihistamine with anticholinergic and sedative action.

Warnings: Do not give to children under 12 years of age. Insomnia may be a symptom of serious underlying medical illness. If sleeplessness persists continuously for more than 2 weeks, consult your physician. As with any drug, if you are pregnant or nursing a baby, seek the advice of a health professional before using this product.
Do not take this product if you have asthma, glaucoma, emphysema, chronic pulmonary disease, shortness of breath, difficulty breathing or difficulty in urination due to enlargement of the prostate gland except under the advice and supervision of a physician.
In case of accidental ingestion or overdose, contact a physician or Poison Control Center immediately. Keep this and all medicines out of children's reach.

Drug Interaction: Avoid alcoholic beverages while taking this product. Do not take this product if you are taking sedatives or tranquilizers, without first consulting your doctor.

Precaution: This product contains an antihistamine and will cause drowsiness. It should be used only at bedtime.

Dosage and Administration: Take 2 tablets 20 minutes before going to bed.

Inactive Ingredients: Croscarmellose Sodium, Dicalcium Phosphate, D&C Yellow No. 10, FD&C Yellow No. 6, Magnesium Stearate, Microcrystalline Cellulose, Stearic Acid.

How Supplied: Packages of 12's, 24's, and 48's.

TODAY®

[*tü-dā*]

Vaginal Contraceptive Sponge

Description: Today Vaginal Contraceptive Sponge is a soft polyurethane foam sponge containing nonoxynol-9, a spermicide used by millions of women for over 25 years.
Today Sponge is Effective, Safe, and Convenient. Today Sponge provides 24-hour contraceptive protection without hormones, allowing spontaneity. Today Sponge is easy to use, nonmessy and disposable.

Active Ingredient: Each Today Sponge contains nonoxynol-9, one gram.

Inactive Ingredients: Benzoic acid, citric acid, sodium dihydrogen citrate,

Continued on next page

Whitehall—Cont.

sodium metabisulfite, sorbic acid, water in a polyurethane foam sponge.

Indication: For the prevention of pregnancy.

Actions: Used as directed, Today Vaginal Contraceptive Sponge prevents pregnancy in three ways: 1) the spermicide nonoxynol-9 kills sperm before they can reach the egg; 2) Today Sponge traps and absorbs sperm; 3) Today Sponge blocks the cervix so that sperm cannot enter.
Today Sponge is designed for easy insertion into the vagina. It is positioned against the cervix, and while in place provides protection against pregnancy for 24 hours. The soft polyurethane foam sponge is formulated to feel like normal vaginal tissue and has a specially designed ribbon loop attached to an interior web for maximum strength.
In clinical trials of Today Sponge in over 1,800 women worldwide who completed over 12,000 cycles of use, the method-effectiveness, i.e., the level of effectiveness seen in women who followed the printed instructions exactly and who used Today Sponge every time that they had intercourse, was 89 to 91%.

Instructions: Remove one Today Sponge from airtight inner pack, wet thoroughly with clean tap water, and squeeze gently until it becomes very sudsy. The water activates the spermicide. Fold the sides of Today Sponge upward until it looks long and narrow and then insert it deeply into the vagina with the string loop dangling below. Protection begins immediately and continues for 24 hours. It is not necessary to add creams, jellies, foams, or any other additional spermicide as long as Today Sponge is in place, no matter how many acts of intercourse may occur during a 24-hour period. Always wait 6 hours after your last act of intercourse before removing Today Sponge. If you have intercourse when Today Sponge has been in place for 24 hours, it must be left in place an additional 6 hours after intercourse before removing it.
To remove Today Sponge, place a finger in the vagina and reach up and back to find the string loop. Hook a finger around the loop. Slowly and gently pull the Sponge out. Some women, especially first-time users, may have difficulty removing the Sponge. This situation may be due to tension or unusually strong muscular pressure. Simple relaxation of the vaginal muscles and bearing down should make it possible to remove the Sponge without difficulty. See User Instruction Booklet (Section 7) for details on removing Today Sponge or call the Today TalkLine 1-800-223-2329.

Warnings: Some cases of Toxic Shock Syndrome (TSS) have been reported in women using barrier contraceptives including Today® Sponge. Although the occurrence of TSS is uncommon, some studies indicate that there is an increased risk of non-menstrual TSS with the use of barrier contraceptives, including Today Sponge. Today Sponge should not be left in place for more than 30 hours after insertion. If you experience two or more of the warning signs of TSS including fever, vomiting, diarrhea, muscular pain, dizziness, and rash similar to sunburn, consult your physician or clinic immediately. If you have difficulty removing the sponge from your vagina or you remove only a portion of the sponge, contact the Today Talk Line or consult your physician or clinic immediately. Today Sponge should not be used during the menstrual period. After childbirth, miscarriage or other termination of pregnancy, it is important to consult your physician or clinic before using this product. If you have ever had Toxic Shock Syndrome do not use Today Sponge.
A small number of men and women may be sensitive to the spermicide in this product (nonoxynol-9) and should not use this product if irritation occurs and persists. If you or your partner have ever experienced an allergic reaction to the spermicide used in this product, it is best to consult a physician before using Today Vaginal Contraceptive Sponge. If either you or your partner develops burning or itching in the genital area, stop using this product and contact your physician.
A higher degree of protection against pregnancy will be afforded by using another method of contraception in addition to a spermicidal contraceptive. This is especially true during the first few months, until you become familiar with the method. In our clinical studies, approximately one-half of all accidental pregnancies occurred during the first three months of use. Where avoidance of pregnancy is essential, the choice of contraceptive should be made in consultation with a doctor or a family planning clinic. Any delay in your menstrual period may be an early sign of pregnancy. If this happens, consult your physician or clinic as soon as possible. Keep this and all drugs out of reach of children. In case of accidental ingestion of Today Sponge, call a poison control center, emergency medical facility or doctor. (For most people ingestation of the spermicide alone should not be harmful.) As with any drug, if you are pregnant or nursing a baby, seek professional advice before using this product.

How To Store: Store at normal room temperature.

How Supplied: Packages of 3s, 6s, and 12s.

Shown in Product Indentification Section, page 437

TRENDAR®
Ibuprofen Tablets, USP
Menstrual Pain & Cramp Reliever

Warning: ASPIRIN SENSITIVE PATIENTS. Do not take this product if you have had a severe allergic reaction to aspirin, e.g. asthma, swelling, shock or hives, because even though this product contains no aspirin or salicylates cross-reactions may occur in patients allergic to aspirin.

Indications: For the temporary relief of painful menstrual cramps (dysmenorrhea); also headaches, backaches and muscular aches and pains associated with premenstrual syndrome.

Dosage and Administration: Adults: Take 1 tablet every 4 to 6 hours at the onset of menstrual symptoms and while pain persists. If pain does not respond to 1 tablet, 2 tablets may be used but do not exceed 6 tablets in 24 hours, unless directed by a doctor. The smallest effective dose should be used. Take with food or milk if occasional and mild heartburn, upset stomach, or stomach pain occurs with use. Consult a doctor if these symptoms are more than mild or if they persist. Children: Do not give this product to children under 12 except under the advice or supervision of a doctor.

Warnings: Do not take for pain for more than 10 days unless directed by a doctor. If pain persists or gets worse, or if new symptoms occur, consult a doctor. These could be signs of serious illness. If you are under a doctor's care for any serious condition, consult a doctor before taking this product. As with aspirin and acetaminophen, if you have any condition which requires you to take prescription drugs or if you have had any problems or serious side effects from taking any nonprescription pain reliever, do not take this product without first discussing it with your doctor. If you experience any symptoms which are unusual or seem unrelated to the condition for which you took ibuprofen, consult a doctor before taking any more of it. Although ibuprofen is indicated for the same conditions as aspirin and acetaminophen, it should not be taken with them except under a doctor's direction. Do not combine this product with any other ibuprofen-containing product. As with any drug, if you are pregnant or nursing a baby, seek the advice of a health professional before using this product. IT IS ESPECIALLY IMPORTANT NOT TO USE IBUPROFEN DURING THE LAST 3 MONTHS OF PREGNANCY UNLESS SPECIFICALLY DIRECTED TO DO SO BY A DOCTOR BECAUSE IT MAY CAUSE PROBLEMS IN THE UNBORN CHILD OR COMPLICATIONS DURING DELIVERY. Keep this and all drugs out of the reach of children. In case of accidental overdose, seek professional assistance or contact a poison control center immediately.

Active Ingredient: Each tablet contains Ibuprofen 200 mg.

Inactive Ingredients: Acacia, Acetylated Monoglycerides, Beeswax, Calcium Sulfate, Colloidal Silicon Dioxide, Dimethicone, Iron Oxide, Lecithin, Pharmaceutical Glaze, Povidone, Sodium Benzoate, Sodium Carboxymethylcellulose, Starch, Stearic Acid, Sucrose, Titanium Dioxide.

Professional Labeling: Same as stated under Indications.

How Supplied: Coated tablets in bottles of 20's & 40's.

Storage: Store at room temperature; avoid excessive heat 40°C (104°F).

Winthrop Consumer Products

Division of Sterling Drug Inc.
90 PARK AVENUE
NEW YORK, NY 10016

BRONKAID® Mist
(Epinephrine)

Description: BRONKAID Mist, brand of epinephrine inhalation aerosol. Contains: Epinephrine, USP, 0.5% (w/w) (as nitrate and hydrochloric salts). Also contains: Alcohol 33% (w/w), ascorbic acid dichlorodifluoromethane, dichlorotetrafluroethane, purified water. Each spray delivers 0.25 mg epinephrine. Contains no sulfites.

Indication: For temporary relief of shortness of breath, tightness of chest and wheezing due to bronchial asthma.

Warnings: FOR ORAL INHALATION ONLY. Do not use this product unless a diagnosis of asthma has been made by a doctor, or if you have heart disease, high blood pressure, thyroid disease, diabetes, or difficulty in urination due to enlargement of the prostate gland, if you have ever been hospitalized for asthma or if you are taking any prescription drug for asthma. **Do not use this product more frequently or at higher doses than recommended, unless directed by a doctor.** Keep this and all drugs out of the reach of children. In case of accidental overdose, seek professional assistance or contact a poison control center immediately. As with any drug, if you are pregnant or nursing a baby, seek the advice of a health professional before using this product.
Excessive use may cause nervousness and rapid heart beat, and, possibly, adverse effects on the heart. **Do not continue to use this product, but seek medical assistance immediately if symptoms are not relieved within 20 minutes or become worse.**

Drug Interaction Precaution: Do not use this product if you are presently taking a prescription drug for high blood pressure or depression, without first consulting your doctor.

Warnings: Avoid spraying in eyes. Contents under pressure. Do not break or incinerate. Using or storing near open flame or heating above 120°F may cause bursting.

Dosage: Inhalation dosage for adults and children 4 years of age and older. Start with one inhalation, then wait at least one (1) minute. If not relieved, use once more. Do not use again for at least 3 hours. The use of this product by children should be supervised by an adult. Children under 4 years of age, consult a doctor.

Directions for Use:
1. Remove cap and mouthpiece from bottle.
2. Remove cap from mouthpiece.
3. Turn mouthpiece sideways and fit metal stem of nebulizer into hole in flattened end of mouthpiece.
4. Exhale, as completely as possible. Now, hold bottle **upside down** between thumb and forefinger and close lips loosely around end of mouthpiece.
5. Inhale deeply while pressing down firmly on bottle, once only.
6. Remove mouthpiece and hold your breath a moment to allow for maximum absorption of medication. Then exhale slowly through nearly closed lips.

After use, remove mouthpiece from bottle and replace cap. Slide mouthpiece over bottle for protection. When possible rinse mouthpiece with tap water immediately after use. Soap and water will not hurt it. A clean mouthpiece always works better.

How Supplied:
Bottles of ½ fl oz (15 ml) NDC 0024-4082-15 with actuator. Also available—refills (no mouthpiece) in 15 mL (½ fl oz) NDC 0024-4083-16 and 22.5 mL (¾ fl oz) NDC 0024-4083-22.

Shown in Product Identification Section, page 437

BRONKAID® Mist Suspension
(Epinephrine Bitartrate)

Active Ingredients: Each spray delivers 0.3 mg epinephrine bitartrate equivalent to 0.16 mg epinephrine base. Contains epinephrine bitartrate 7.0 mg per cc. Also contains: Cetylpyridinium chloride, dichlorodifluoromethane, dichlorotetrafluoroethane, sorbitan trioleate, trichloromonofluoromethane. Contains no sulfites.

Indication: Provides temporary relief of shortness of breath, tightness of chest, and wheezing due to bronchial asthma.

Warnings: FOR ORAL INHALATION ONLY. Do not use this product unless a diagnosis of asthma has been made by a doctor, or if you have heart disease, high blood pressure, thyroid disease, diabetes, or difficulty in urination due to enlargement of the prostate gland, if you have ever been hospitalized for asthma or if you are taking any prescription drug for asthma. **Do not use this product more frequently or at higher doses than recommended, unless directed by a doctor.** Keep this and all drugs out of the reach of children. In case of accidental overdose, seek professional assistance or contact a poison control center immediately. As with any drug, if you are pregnant or nursing a baby, seek the advice of a health professional before using this product.
Excessive use may cause nervousness and rapid heart beat, and, possibly, adverse effects on the heart. **Do not continue to use this product, but seek medical assistance immediately if symptoms are not relieved within 20 minutes or become worse.**

Drug Interaction Precaution: Do not use this product if you are presently taking a prescription drug for high blood pressure or depression, without first consulting your doctor.

Warning: Avoid spraying in eyes. Contents under pressure. Do not break or incinerate. Using or storing near open flame or heating above 120°F may cause bursting.

Administration:
1. SHAKE WELL.
2. HOLD INHALER WITH NOZZLE DOWN WHILE USING. Empty the lungs as completely as possible by exhaling.
3. Purse the lips as in saying the letter "O" and hold the nozzle up to the lips, keeping the tongue flat. As you start to take a deep breath, squeeze nozzle and can together, releasing one full application. Complete taking deep breath, drawing medication into your lungs.
4. Hold breath for as long as comfortable. This distributes the medication in the lungs. Then exhale slowly keeping the lips nearly closed.
5. Rinse nozzle daily with soap and hot water after removing from vial. Dry with clean cloth.

Before each use, remove dust cap and inspect mouthpiece for foreign objects. Replace dust cap after each use.

Dosage: Inhalation dosage for adults and children 4 years of age and older. Start with one inhalation, then wait at least one (1) minute. If not relieved, use once more. Do not use again for at least 3 hours. The use of this product by children should be supervised by an adult. Children under 4 years of age; consult a doctor.

Professional Labeling: Same as stated under Indication.

How Supplied:
⅓ fl oz (10 cc) pocketsize aerosol inhaler, NDC 0024-4082-10 with actuator.

BRONKAID® Tablets

Description: Each tablet contains ephedrine sulfate 24 mg, guaifenesin (glyceryl guaiacolate) 100 mg, and theophylline 100 mg. Also contains: magnesium stearate, magnesium trisilicate, microcrystalline cellulose, starch.

Indication: For symptomatic control of bronchial congestion and bronchial asthma. Clears bronchial passages. Helps relieve shortness of breath, plus helps loosen phlegm.

Continued on next page

This product information was effective as of November 1, 1990. Current information may be obtained directly from Winthrop Consumer Products, Division of Sterling Drug Inc., by writing to 90 Park Avenue, New York, NY 10016.

Winthrop Consumer—Cont.

Warnings: Do not use this product unless a diagnosis of asthma has been made by a doctor, or if you have heart disease, diabetes, difficulty in urination due to enlargement of the prostate gland, if you have ever been hospitalized for asthma or if you are taking any prescription drug for asthma unless directed by a doctor. Do not continue to use this product, but seek medical assistance immediately if symptoms are not relieved within an hour or become worse. Some users of this product may experience nervousness, tremor, sleeplessness, nausea, and loss of appetite. If these symptoms persist or become worse, consult your doctor.

Drug Interaction Precaution: Do not use this product if you are presently taking a prescription drug for high blood pressure or depression. Do not exceed recommended dosage unless directed by a physician.

Warnings: As with any drug, if you are pregnant or nursing a baby, seek the advice of a health professional before using this product. Keep this and all drugs out of the reach of children. In case of accidental overdose, seek professional assistance or contact a poison control center immediately.

Dosage and Administration: *Adult Dosage:* 1 tablet every four hours. Do not take more than 5 tablets in a 24-hour period. Swallow tablets whole with water. *Children under 12 years of age:* Consult a doctor. *Morning Dose:* An early dose of 1 tablet (for adults) can relieve the coughing and wheezing caused by the night's accumulation of mucus, and can help you start the day with better breathing capacity. *Before an Attack:* Many persons feel an attack of asthma coming on. One BRONKAID tablet beforehand may stop the attack before it starts. *During the Day:* The precise dose of BRONKAID tablets can be varied to meet your individual needs as you gain experience with this product. It is advisable to take 1 tablet before going to bed, for nighttime relief. However, be sure not to exceed recommended daily dosage.

How Supplied:
Boxes of 24 NDC 0024-4081-02.
Boxes of 60 NDC 0024-4081-06.

Shown in Product Identification Section, page 437

CAMPHO-PHENIQUE®
[*kam 'fo-finēk*]
COLD SORE GEL

Description: Contains phenol 4.7% (w/w) and camphor 10.8% (w/w). Also contains: Colloidal silicon dioxide, eucalyptus oil, glycerin, light mineral oil.
Use at the first sign of cold sore, fever blister and sun blister. Symptoms (tingling, pain, itching).

Indications: For relief of pain and itching due to cold sores, fever blisters and sun blisters. To combat infection from minor injuries and skin lesions.
Also effective for:
Minor skin injuries: abrasions, cuts, scrapes, burns, razor nicks and chafed or irritated skin.
Insect bites: mosquitoes, black flies, sandfleas, chiggers.

Warnings: Not for prolonged use. Not to be used on large areas. In case of deep or puncture wounds, serious burns, or persisting redness, swelling or pain, or if rash or infection develops, discontinue use and consult physician. Do not bandage if applied to fingers or toes.
Avoid using near eyes. If product gets into the eye, flush thoroughly with water and obtain medical attention. Keep this and all drugs out of the reach of children. In case of accidental ingestion, seek professional assistance or contact a poison control center immediately.

Directions for Use: For external use. Apply directly to cold sore, fever blister or injury three or four times a day.

How Supplied: Tubes of 0.23 oz (6.5 g) NDC 0024-0212-01 and 0.50 oz (14 g) NDC 0024-0212-02.

Shown in Product Identification Section, page 437

CAMPHO-PHENIQUE® Liquid
[*kam 'fo-finēk*]

Description: Contains phenol 4.7% (w/w) and camphor 10.8% (w/w). Also contains: Eucalyptus oil, light mineral oil.

Actions: Pain-relieving antiseptic for scrapes, cuts, burns, insect bites, fever blisters, and cold sores.

Indications: For relief of pain and to combat infection from minor injuries and skin lesions.

Warnings: Not for prolonged use. Not to be used on large areas or in or near the eyes. In case of deep or puncture wounds, serious burns, or persisting redness, swelling or pain, or if rash or infection develops, discontinue use and consult physician. Do not bandage if applied to fingers or toes.
Keep this and all drugs out of the reach of children. In case of accidental ingestion, seek professional assistance or contact a poison control center immediately.

Directions for Use: For external use. Apply with cotton three or four times daily.
4 oz size only: Do not use more than ½ the contents of the 4 fl oz bottle in any 24-hour period.

How Supplied:
Bottles of ¾ fl oz (NDC 0024-5150-05)
1 ½ fl oz (NDC 0024-5150-06)
4 fl oz (NDC 0024-5150-04)

Shown in Product Identification Section, page 438

CAMPHO-PHENIQUE™
[*kam 'fo-finēk*]
TRIPLE ANTIBIOTIC OINTMENT PLUS PAIN RELIEVER

Description: Contains bacitracin 500 units, neomycin sulfate 5 mg (equiv to 3.5 mg neomycin base), polymyxin B sulfate 5000 units, lidocaine HCl 40 mg (or diperodon HCl 10 mg) (Pain Reliever). Also contains white petrolatum.

Actions: Pain-relieving triple antibiotic with anesthetic to help prevent infection in minor cuts, scrapes, burns and other minor wounds.

Indications: Helps prevent infections in minor cuts, burns, and other minor wounds. Provides soothing, nonstinging temporary relief of pain and itching associated with these conditions.

Warnings: For external use only. In case of deep or puncture wounds, animal bites or serious burns, consult physician. If redness, irritation, swelling or pain persists or increases, or if infection occurs, discontinue use and consult physician. Do not use in eyes or over large areas. Keep this and all drugs out of the reach of children. In case of accidental ingestion seek professional assistance or contact a poison control center immediately.

Directions: Apply directly to the affected area and cover with a sterile gauze if necessary. May be applied 1 to 3 times daily as the condition indicates.

How Supplied: Tubes of 0.50 oz (NDC 0024-2015-05) and 1.0 oz (NDC 0024-2015-01).

Shown in Product Identification Section, page 438

FERGON® TABLETS
[*fur-gone*]
brand of ferrous gluconate
FERGON® ELIXIR

Composition: FERGON (ferrous gluconate, USP) is stabilized to maintain a minimum of ferric ions. It contains not less than 11.5 percent iron.
Each FERGON tablet contains 320 mg (5 grains) ferrous gluconate equal to approximately 36 mg ferrous iron. Also contains: acacia, carnauba wax, dextrose excipient, FD&C Red No. 40, D&C Yellow No. 10, FD&C Blue No. 1, gelatin, kaolin, magnesium stearate, parabens, povidone, precipitated calcium carbonate, sodium benzoate, starch, sucrose, talc, titanium dioxide, yellow wax. Not USP for dissolution.
FERGON Elixir contains: ferrous gluconate 6%. Also contains: alcohol 7%, flavor, glycerin, liquid glucose, purified water, saccharin sodium. Each teaspoon (5 mL) contains 300 mg (5 grains) ferrous gluconate equivalent to approximately 34 mg ferrous iron.

Action and Uses: FERGON preparations produce rapid hemoglobin regeneration in patients with iron-deficiency anemias. FERGON is better utilized and better tolerated than other forms of iron because of its low ionization constant and

solubility in the entire pH range of the gastrointestinal tract. It does not precipitate proteins or have the astringency of more ionizable forms of iron, does not interfere with proteolytic or diastatic activities of the digestive system, and will not produce nausea, abdominal cramps, constipation or diarrhea in the great majority of patients.
FERGON preparations are for use in the prevention and treatment of iron deficiency. They should be taken when the need for iron supplement therapy has been determined by a physician.

Warnings: Since oral iron products interfere with absorption of oral tetracycline antibiotics, these products should not be taken within two hours of each other. Keep this and all drugs out of the reach of children. As with any drug, if you are pregnant or nursing a baby, seek the advice of a health professional before using this product. In case of accidental overdose, seek professional assistance or contact a poison control center immediately.

Dosage and Administration: *Adults* —One to two FERGON tablets or one to two teaspoonfuls of FERGON Elixir daily. *For children and infants,* as prescribed by physician.

How Supplied: FERGON Tablets of 320 mg (5 grains) bottle of 100 (NDC 0024-1015-10), bottle of 500 (NDC 0024-1015-50). FERGON Elixir, 6% (5 grains per teaspoonful) bottle of 1 pint (NDC 0024-1019-16).

Shown in Product Indentification Section, page 438

NāSal™ Moisturizer AF
Saline (buffered)
0.65% Sodium chloride
Nasal Spray, Spray Pump and Drops

Description: The nasal spray, nasal spray pump and nose drops contain sodium chloride 0.65%. Also contains: benzalkonium chloride and thimerosal 0.001% as preservative, mono- and dibasic sodium phosphates as buffers, purified water.
Contains No Alcohol.

Actions: Immediate relief for dry nose. Formulated to match the pH of normal nasal secretions to help prevent stinging or burning.

Indications: Provides immediate relief for dry, inflamed nasal membranes due to colds, low humidity, allergies, minor nose bleeds, overuse of topical nasal decongestants, and other nasal irritations. As an ideal nasal moisturizer, it can be used in conjunction with oral decongestants.

Adverse Reactions: No associated side effects.

Warnings: Keep this and all drugs out of the reach of children. In case of accidental ingestion seek professional assistance or contact a poison control center immediately. The use of the dispenser by more than one person may spread infection.

Dosage and Administration: *Spray* —For adults and children: with head upright, spray twice in each nostril as needed or as directed by physician. To spray, squeeze bottle quickly and firmly. *Nasal Spray Pump*—For adults and children—spray twice in each nostril as often as needed or as directed by a physician. Hold bottle with thumb at base and nozzle between first and second fingers. With head upright, insert nozzle in nostril. Depress pump two times, all the way down, with a firm even stroke and sniff deeply. Repeat in other nostril. Do not tilt head backward while spraying. *Nose Drops* —For infants and adults: 2 to 6 drops in each nostril as needed or as directed by physician.

How Supplied: Nasal Spray—plastic squeeze bottles of 15 mL (½ fl. oz.) NDC 0024-1316-01.
Nose Drops—MonoDrop® bottles of 15 mL (½ fl. oz.) NDC 0024-1315-01.

Shown in Product Identification Section, page 438

NEO-SYNEPHRINE®
Pediatric Formula, Mild Formula, Regular Strength, and Extra Strength.
phenylephrine hydrochloride

Description: This line of Nasal Sprays, Drops and Spray Pumps contains phenylephrine hydrochloride in strengths ranging from 0.125% (drops only) to 1%. Also contains: benzalkonium chloride and thimerosal 0.001% as preservatives, citric acid, purified water, sodium chloride, sodium citrate.

Action: Rapid-acting nasal decongestant.

Directions: For adults: with head upright, spray 2 or 3 times, or squeeze 2 or 3 drops into each nostril. May be repeated in four hours as needed.

Indications: For temporary relief of nasal congestion due to common cold, hay fever, sinusitis, or other upper respiratory allergies.

Precautions: Some hypersensitive individuals may experience a mild stinging sensation. This is usually transient and often disappears after a few applications. Do not exceed recommended dosage. Do not use this product for more than 3 days. If symptoms persist, consult a doctor. Frequent and continued usage of the higher concentrations (especially the 1% solution) occasionally may cause a rebound congestion of the nose. Therefore, long-term or frequent use of this solution is not recommended without the advice of a physician.
Prolonged exposure to air or strong light will cause oxidation and some loss of potency. Do not use if brown in color or contains a precipitate.

Adverse Reactions: Generally very well tolerated; systemic side effects such as tremor, insomnia, or palpitation rarely occur.

Warnings: Keep these and all drugs out of the reach of children. In case of accidental ingestion seek professional assistance or contact a poison control center immediately. The use of the dispenser by more than one person may spread infection.
Do not use this product if you have heart disease, high blood pressure, thyroid disease, diabetes, or difficulty in urination due to enlargement of the prostate gland unless directed by a doctor.

Dosage and Administration: *Topical* —dropper or spray. The *0.25% solution* is adequate in most cases *(0.125% for children 2 to 6 years).* In resistant cases, or if more powerful decongestion is desired, the *0.5% or 1% solution* should be used. Also used as *0.5% jelly.*

How Supplied: Nasal spray 0.25%—15 ml (for children and for adults who prefer a mild nasal spray)—NDC 0024-1348-03; nasal spray 0.5%—15 ml (for adults)—NDC 0024-1353-01; nasal spray 1%—15 ml (extra strength for adults)—NDC 0024-1352-02; nasal spray pump 0.5%—15 ml bottle (½ fl. oz.) NDC 0024-1353-04; nasal solution 0.125% (for infants and small children), 15 ml bottles—NDC 0024-1345-05; nasal solution 0.25% (for children and adults who prefer a mild solution), 15 ml bottles—NDC 0024-1347-05; nasal solution 0.5% (for adults), 15 ml bottles—NDC 0024-1351-05; nasal solution 1% (extra strength for adults), 15 ml bottles—NDC 0024-1355-05; and water soluble nasal jelly 0.5%, ⅝ oz tubes—NDC 0024-1367-01.

Shown in Product Identification Section, page 438

NEO-SYNEPHRINE®
Maximum Strength 12 Hour
oxymetazoline hydrochloride
Nasal Spray 0.05%

Description: *Adult Strength Nasal Spray* and *Nasal Spray Pump* contain: Oxymetazoline Hydrochloride 0.05%. Also contain: Benzalkonium Chloride and Phenylmercuric Acetate 0.002% as preservatives, Glycine, Purified Water, Sorbitol, may also contain Sodium Chloride.

Action: 12 HOUR Nasal Decongestant.

Indications: Provides temporary relief, for up to 12 HOURS, of nasal congestion due to colds, hay fever, sinusitis, or allergies. NEO-SYNEPHRINE MAXIMUM STRENGTH 12-HOUR Nasal Spray and Pump contain oxymetazoline which provides the longest-lasting relief of nasal congestion available.

Continued on next page

This product information was effective as of November 1, 1990. Current information may be obtained directly from Winthrop Consumer Products, Division of Sterling Drug Inc., by writing to 90 Park Avenue, New York, NY 10016.

Winthrop Consumer—Cont.

Warnings: Do not exceed recommended dosage because symptoms may occur such as burning, stinging, sneezing, or increase of nasal discharge. Do not use these products for more than 3 days. If symptoms persist, consult a physician. The use of the dispenser by more than one person may spread infection.
Do not use this product if you have heart disease, high blood pressure, thyroid disease, diabetes, or difficulty in urination due to enlargement of the prostate gland unless directed by a doctor.
Keep this and all drugs out of the reach of children. In case of accidental ingestion, seek professional assistance or contact a poison control center immediately.

Dosage and Administration: *Adult Strength Nasal Spray*—For adults and children 6 to under 12 years of age (with adult supervision): 2 or 3 sprays in each nostril not more often than every 10 to 12 hours. Do not exceed 2 applications in any 24-hour period. Children under 6 years of age: consult a doctor. To administer, hold head upright, spray 2 or 3 times in each nostril twice daily—morning and evening. To spray, squeeze bottle quickly and firmly.
Nasal Spray Pump—For adults and children 6 to under 12 years of age (with adult supervision): 2 or 3 sprays in each nostril not more often than every 10–12 hours. Do not exceed 2 applications in any 24 hour period. Children under 6 years of age: consult a doctor. Hold bottle with thumb at base and nozzle between first and second fingers. To administer, hold head upright and insert spray nozzle in nostril. Depress pump 2 or 3 times, all the way down, with a firm even stroke and sniff deeply. Repeat in other nostril. Do not tilt head backward while spraying.

How Supplied: *Nasal Spray Adult Strength*—plastic squeeze bottles of 15 ml (½ fl. oz.) NDC 0024-1390-03; *Nasal Spray Pump*—15 ml bottle (½ fl. oz.) NDC 0024-1389-01.

Shown in Product Identification Section, page 438

NTZ®
Long Acting
Oxymetazoline hydrochloride
Nasal Spray 0.05%
Nose Drops 0.05%

Description: Both the nasal spray and nose drops contain Oxymetazoline Hydrochloride 0.05%. Also contain: Benzalkonium Chloride and Phenylmercuric Acetate 0.002% as preservatives, Glycine, Purified Water, Sorbitol, and may also contain Sodium Chloride.

Actions: 12 Hour Nasal Decongestant.

Indications: Provides temporary relief, for up to 12 hours, of nasal congestion due to colds, hay fever, sinusitis, or allergies. Oxymetazoline hydrochloride provides the longest-lasting relief of nasal congestion available. It decongests nasal passages up to 12 hours, reduces swelling of nasal passages, and temporarily restores freer breathing through the nose.

Warnings: Not recommended for children under six. Do not exceed recommended dosage because symptoms may occur such as burning, stinging, sneezing, or increase of nasal discharge. Do not use these products for more than 3 days. If symptoms persist, consult a physician. The use of the dispenser by more than one person may spread infection. Do not use this product if you have heart disease, high blood pressure, thyroid disease, diabetes, or difficulty in urination due to enlargement of the prostate gland unless directed by a doctor. Keep these and all drugs out of the reach of children. In case of accidental ingestion seek professional assistance or contact a poison control center immediately.

Dosage and Administration: Intranasally by spray and dropper. *Nasal Spray*—For adults and children 6 years of age and over: With head upright, spray 2 or 3 times in each nostril twice daily—morning and evening. To spray, squeeze bottle quickly and firmly. *Nose Drops*—For adults and children 6 years of age and over: 2 or 3 drops in each nostril twice daily—morning and evening.

How Supplied: *Nasal Spray*—plastic squeeze bottles of 15 ml (½ fl. oz.) NDC 0024-1312-02. *Nose Drops*—bottles of 15 ml (½ fl. oz.) with dropper NDC 0024-1311-03.

pHisoDerm®
[fi-zo-derm]
Skin Cleanser and Conditioner

Description: pHisoDerm, a nonsoap emollient skin cleanser, is a unique liquid emulsion containing sodium octoxynol-2 ethane sulfonate solution, water, petrolatum, octoxynol-3, mineral oil (with lanolin alcohol and oleyl alcohol), cocamide MEA, imidazolidinyl urea, sodium benzoate, tetrasodium EDTA, and methylcellulose. Adjusted to normal skin pH with hydrochloric acid. Contains no hexachlorophene. pHisoDerm contains no soap, perfumes, or irritating alkali. Its pH value, unlike that of soap, lies within the pH range of normal skin.

Actions: pHisoDerm is well tolerated and can be used frequently by those persons whose skin may be irritated by the use of soap or other alkaline cleansers, or by those who are sensitive to the fatty acids contained in soap. pHisoDerm contains an effective detergent for removing soil and acts as an active emulsifier of all types of oil—animal, vegetable, and mineral.
pHisoDerm produces suds when used with any kind of water—hard or soft, hot or cold (even cold seawater)—at any temperature and under acid, alkaline, or neutral conditions.
pHisoDerm deposits a fine film of lanolin components and petrolatum on the skin during the washing process and, thereby, helps protect against the dryness that soap can cause.

Indications: A sudsing emollient cleanser for use on skin of infants, children, and adults.
Useful for removal of ointments and cosmetics from the skin.

Directions: For external use only.
HANDS. Squeeze a few drops of pHisoDerm into the palm, add a little water, and work up a lather. Rinse thoroughly.
FACE. After washing your hands, squeeze a small amount of pHisoDerm into the palm or onto a small sponge or washcloth, and work up a lather by adding a little water. Massage the suds onto the face for approximately one minute. Rinse thoroughly. Avoid getting suds into the eyes.
BATHING. First wet the body. Work a small amount of pHisoDerm into a lather with hands or a soft wet sponge, gradually adding small amounts of water to make more lather. Rinse thoroughly.

Caution: pHisoDerm suds that get into the eyes accidentally during washing should be rinsed out promptly with a sufficient amount of water.
pHisoDerm is intended for external use only. pHisoDerm should not be poured into measuring cups, medicine bottles, or similar containers since it may be mistaken for baby formula or medications. If swallowed, pHisoDerm may cause gastrointestinal irritation.
pHisoDerm should not be used on persons with sensitivity to any of its components.

How Supplied: pHisoDerm is supplied in three formulations for regular, oily and dry skin. It is packaged in sanitary squeeze bottles of 5 and 16 ounces. The regular formula is also supplied in squeeze bottles of 9 ounces and plastic bottles of 1 gallon.

Shown in Product Identification Section, page 438

pHisoDerm®
Cleansing Bar

Description: pHisoDerm Cleansing Bar, is a unique cleansing bar containing sodium tallowate, coconut oil, water, glycerin, petrolatum, lanolin, sodium chloride, BHT, trisodium HEDTA, and titanium dioxide.

Actions: pHisoDerm Cleansing Bar is formulated to clean thoroughly, removing dirt and oil. Special emollients leave skin feeling soft and smooth, not tight and dry. pHisoDerm Cleansing Bar contains no detergents or harsh ingredients which could irritate delicate skin.

Administration: Use every time you wash. First wet area to be washed. Using hands, sponge or washcloth, mix with water and work up a creamy lather. Massage the suds onto the area to be washed for approximately one minute. Rinse thoroughly. Avoid getting suds into the eyes.

Precautions: pHisoDerm Cleansing Bar suds that get into the eyes accidentally during washing should be rinsed out promptly with a sufficient amount of water. pHisoDerm Cleansing Bar is intended for external use only. It should not be used on persons with sensitivity to any of its components.

How Supplied: pHisoDerm Cleansing Bar is supplied in an Unscented and Lightly Scented formula. It is packaged in specially coated cardboard cartons containing a 3.3 oz. bar.

Shown in Product Identification Section, page 438

pHisoDerm® FOR BABY
[fi 'zo-derm]
Skin Cleanser

Description: pHisoDerm FOR BABY, a nonsoap emollient skin cleanser, is a unique liquid emulsion containing sodium octoxynol-2 ethane sulfonate solution, water, petrolatum, octoxynol-3, mineral oil (with lanolin alcohol and oleyl alcohol), cocamide MEA, fragrance, imidazolidinyl urea, sodium benzoate, tetrasodium EDTA, and methylcellulose. Adjusted to normal skin pH with hydrochloric acid. Contains no hexachlorophene or irritating alkali. Its pH value, unlike that of soap, lies within the pH range of normal skin.

Actions: pHisoDerm FOR BABY gently cleans babies' delicate skin without irritating. Petrolatum and lanolin leave skin soft and smooth and protect against dryness.
pHisoDerm FOR BABY rinses easily without leaving a soapy film. The powder fragrance leaves skin smelling fresh and clean.

Precautions: pHisoDerm FOR BABY suds that get into babies' eyes accidentally during washing should be rinsed out promptly with a sufficient amount of water.
pHisoDerm FOR BABY is intended for external use only. It should not be poured into measuring cups, medicine bottles, or similar containers since it may be mistaken for baby formula or medications. If swallowed, pHisoDerm FOR BABY may cause gastrointestinal irritation.
pHisoDerm FOR BABY should not be used on babies with sensitivity to any of its components.

Administration: First wet the baby's body. Work a small amount of pHisoDerm FOR BABY into a lather with hands or a soft wet sponge, gradually adding small amounts of water to make more lather. Spread the lather over all parts of the baby's body, including the head. Avoid getting suds into the baby's eyes. Wash the diaper area last. Be sure to carefully cleanse all folds and creases. Rinse thoroughly. Pat the baby dry with a soft towel.

How Supplied: pHisoDerm FOR BABY is packaged in soft plastic, sanitary, squeeze bottles of 5 and 9 ounces and can be opened and closed with one hand.

Shown in Product Identification Section, page 438

pHisoPUFF®
[fi-zo-puf]
Nonmedicated Cleansing Sponge

Description: pHisoPUFF is a nonmedicated cleansing sponge with a special dual layer construction combining a white polyester fiber side and a green sponge side.

Actions: pHisoPUFF cleanses two ways: (1) white fiber side for extra thorough cleansing to gently remove the top layer of dead skin cells, free dirt, debris, and oil trapped in this layer and reveal new, fresh skin cells and (2) green sponge side works to cleanse and rinse skin clean. Using this side will help apply your cleanser or soap more evenly. Also good for removing eye makeup.

Precautions: Do not use pHisoPUFF fiber side on skin that is irritated, sunburned, windburned, damaged, broken, or infected. Do not use on skin which is prone to rashes or itching.

Administration: For the green sponge side: Wet pHisoPUFF with warm water, apply pHisoDerm® or another skin cleanser of your choice, and develop a lather. Glide sponge over your face up and down, back and forth, or in a circle; whatever is the easiest for you. Rinse face and dry.
For the white fiber side: Wet pHisoPUFF with warm water, apply pHisoDerm or another skin cleanser of your choice, and develop a lather. Try pHisoPUFF on the back of your hand before using it on your face. Experiment by changing the pressure and speed with which you move it. Now move pHisoPUFF gently and slowly over your face. Use no more than a few seconds on each area. You can move it in any direction, whichever comes natural to you. Rinse face and dry. As you use this fiber side more often, usage and pressure may be increased to best fit your skin sensitivity. Always rinse your pHisoPUFF thoroughly each time you use it. Hold under running water, let it drain, then give it a few quick shakes.

How Supplied: Box of 1 pHisoPUFF.

Shown in Product Identification Section, page 438

WinGel®
[win 'jel]
Liquid and Tablets

Description: Each teaspoon (5 mL) of liquid contains a specially processed, short polymer, hexitol-stabilized aluminum-magnesium hydroxide equivalent to 180 mg of aluminum hydroxide and 160 mg of magnesium hydroxide. Also contains: benzoic acid, flavor, methylcellulose, purified water, red ferric oxide, saccharin sodium, sodium hypochlorite solution, sorbitol solution.
Each tablet contains a specially processed, short polymer, hexitol-stabilized aluminum-magnesium hydroxide equivalent to 180 mg of aluminum hydroxide and 160 mg of magnesium hydroxide. Also contains: D&C Red No. 28, FD&C Red No. 40, flavor, magnesium stearate, mannitol, saccharin sodium, starch. Smooth, easy-to-chew tablets.

Action: Antacid.

Indications: An antacid for the relief of acid indigestion, heartburn, and sour stomach. Nonconstipating. For the symptomatic relief of hyperacidity associated with the diagnosis of peptic ulcer, gastritis, peptic esophagitis, gastric hyperacidity, and hiatal hernia.

Warnings: *Adults and children over 6*—Patients should not take more than eight teaspoonfuls or eight tablets in a 24-hour period or use the maximum dosage of the product for more than 2 weeks, except under the advice and supervision of a physician.
Keep this and all drugs out of the reach of children. In case of accidental overdose, seek professional assistance or contact a poison control center immediately.

Drug Interaction Precautions: Antacids may react with certain prescription drugs. Do not take this product if you are presently taking a prescription antibiotic drug containing any form of tetracycline. If the patient is presently taking a prescription drug, this product should not be taken without checking with the physician.

Dosage and Administration: *Adults and children over 6*—1 to 2 teaspoonfuls or 1 to 2 tablets up to four times daily, or as directed by a physician.
Acid Neutralization: The acid neutralization capacity of WinGel liquid and tablets is not less than 10 mEq/5 ml.

How Supplied:
Liquid—bottles of 6 fl oz (NDC 0024-2247-03) and 12 fl oz (NDC 0024-2247-05).
Tablets—boxes of 50 (NDC 0024-2249-05) and 100 (NDC 0024-2249-06).

Winthrop Pharmaceuticals
90 PARK AVENUE
NEW YORK, NY 10016

BRONKOLIXIR®
Bronchodilator • Decongestant

Description: Each 5 mL teaspoonful contains:

Ephedrine sulfate, USP	12 mg
Guaifenesin, USP	50 mg
Theophylline, USP	15 mg
Phenobarbital, USP	4 mg

(Warning: May be habit forming.)
Also contains: Alcohol 19% (v/v), FD&C Red #40, Flavors, Glycerin, Purified Water, Saccharin Sodium, Sodium Chloride, Sodium Citrate, Sucrose.

Continued on next page

This product information was effective as of September 10, 1990. Current detailed information may be obtained directly from Winthrop Pharmaceuticals, Division of Sterling Drug Inc., by writing to 90 Park Avenue, New York NY, 10016.

Winthrop Pharm.—Cont.

Indications: For symptomatic control of bronchial asthma. BRONKOLIXIR is also helpful in overcoming the nonproductive cough often associated with bronchitis or colds.

Warnings: Frequent or prolonged use may cause nervousness, restlessness, or sleeplessness. Phenobarbital may cause drowsiness. Do not use if high blood pressure, heart disease, diabetes, or thyroid disease is present, unless directed by a physician. Ephedrine may cause urinary retention, especially in the presence of partial obstruction, as in prostatism. Keep this and all drugs out of the reach of children. In case of accidental overdose, seek professional assistance or contact a poison control center immediately. As with any drug, if you are pregnant or nursing a baby, seek the advice of a health professional before using this product.

Dosage: *Adults*—2 teaspoons every three or four hours, not to exceed four times daily. *Children*—**over six**—one half the adult dose; **under six**—as directed by physician.

How Supplied: Bottle of 16 fl oz (NDC 0024-1004-16)

BRONKOTABS®
Bronchodilator • Decongestant

Description: Each tablet contains ephedrine sulfate, USP, 24 mg; guaifenesin, USP, 100 mg; theophylline, USP, 100 mg; phenobarbital, USP, 8 mg. (Warning: May be habit forming.)
Also contains: Magnesium Stearate, Magnesium Trisilicate, Microcrystalline Cellulose, Starch.

Indications: For symptomatic control of bronchial asthma.

Warnings: Frequent or prolonged use may cause nervousness, restlessness, or sleeplessness. Phenobarbital may cause drowsiness. Do not use if high blood pressure, heart disease, diabetes, or thyroid disease is present unless directed by a physician. Ephedrine may cause urinary retention, especially in the presence of partial obstruction, as in prostatism. Keep this and all drugs out of the reach of children. In case of accidental overdose, seek professional assistance or contact a poison control center immediately. As with any drug, if you are pregnant or nursing a baby, seek the advice of a health professional before using this product.

Dosage: *Adults*—1 tablet every three or four hours, four to five times daily. *Children:* **over six**—one half the adult dose; **under six**—as directed by physician.

How Supplied: Bottle of 100 (NDC 0024-1006-10)

DRISDOL®
brand of ergocalciferol oral solution, USP (in propylene glycol)
Vitamin D Supplement

Description: 200 International Units (5 μg) per drop. The dropper supplied delivers 40 drops per mL.

Indication: For the prevention of vitamin D deficiency in infants, children, and adults.

Warnings: Keep this and all drugs out of the reach of children. In case of accidental overdose, seek professional assistance or contact a poison control center immediately.

Dosage: 2 drops daily. This dose provides the US Recommended Daily Allowance for vitamin D for infants, children, and adults.

How Supplied: Bottles of 2 fl oz (NDC 0024-0391-02)

pHisoDerm
(See Winthrop Consumer Products.)

ZEPHIRAN® CHLORIDE
brand of benzalkonium chloride
ANTISEPTIC
AQUEOUS SOLUTION 1:750
TINTED TINCTURE 1:750
SPRAY—TINTED TINCTURE 1:750

Description: ZEPHIRAN Chloride, brand of benzalkonium chloride, NF, a mixture of alkylbenzyldimethylammonium chlorides, is a cationic quaternary ammonium surface-acting agent. It is very soluble in water, alcohol, and acetone. Aqueous solutions of ZEPHIRAN Chloride are neutral to slightly alkaline, generally colorless, and nonstaining. They have a bitter taste, aromatic odor, and foam when shaken. ZEPHIRAN Chloride Tinted Tincture 1:750 contains alcohol 50 percent and acetone 10 percent by volume. ZEPHIRAN Chloride Spray—Tinted Tincture 1:750 contains alcohol 92 percent. The Tinted Tincture and Spray also contain an orange-red coloring agent.

Clinical Pharmacology: ZEPHIRAN Chloride solutions are rapidly acting anti-infective agents with a moderately long duration of action. They are active against bacteria and some viruses, fungi, and protozoa. Bacterial spores are considered to be resistant. Solutions are bacteriostatic or bactericidal according to their concentration. The exact mechanism of bactericidal action is unknown but is thought to be due to enzyme inactivation. Activity generally increases with increasing temperature and pH. Gram-positive bacteria are more susceptible than gram-negative bacteria (TABLE 1). [See table above.]

TABLE 1
Highest Dilution of ZEPHIRAN Chloride Aqueous Solution Destroying the Organism in 10 but not in 5 Minutes

Organisms	20°C
Streptococcus pyogenes	1:75,000
Staphylococcus aureus	1:52,500
Salmonella typhosa	1:37,500
Escherichia coli	1:10,500

Pseudomonas is the most resistant gram-negative genus. Using the AOAC Use-Dilution Confirmation Method, no growth was obtained when *Staphylococcus aureus, Salmonella choleraesuis,* and *Pseudomonas aeruginosa* (strain PRD-10) were exposed for ten minutes at 20°C to ZEPHIRAN Chloride Aqueous Solution 1:750 and Tinted Tincture 1:750.
ZEPHIRAN Chloride Aqueous Solution 1:750 has been shown to retain its bactericidal activity following autoclaving for 30 minutes at 15 lb pressure, freezing, and then thawing.
The tubercle bacillus may be resistant to aqueous ZEPHIRAN Chloride solutions but is susceptible to the 1:750 tincture (AOAC Method, 10 minutes at 20°C).
ZEPHIRAN Chloride solutions also demonstrate deodorant, wetting, detergent, keratolytic, and emulsifying activity.

Indications and Usage: ZEPHIRAN Chloride aqueous solutions in appropriate dilutions (see Recommended Dilutions) are indicated for the antisepsis of skin, mucous membranes, and wounds. They are used for preoperative preparation of the skin, surgeons' hand and arm soaks, treatment of wounds, preservation of ophthalmic solutions, irrigations of the eye, body cavities, bladder, urethra, and vaginal douching.
ZEPHIRAN Chloride Tinted Tincture 1:750 and Spray are indicated for preoperative preparation of the skin and for treatment of minor skin wounds and abrasions.

Contraindication: The use of ZEPHIRAN Chloride solutions in occlusive dressings, casts, and anal or vaginal packs is inadvisable, as they may produce irritation or chemical burns.

Warnings: Sterile Water for Injection, USP, should be used as diluent in preparing diluted aqueous solutions intended for use on deep wounds or for irrigation of body cavities. Otherwise, freshly distilled water should be used. Tap water, containing metallic ions and organic matter, may reduce antibacterial potency. Resin deionized water should not be used since it may contain pathogenic bacteria.
Organic, inorganic, and synthetic materials and surfaces may adsorb sufficient quantities of ZEPHIRAN Chloride to significantly reduce its antibacterial potency in solutions. This has resulted in serious contamination of solutions of ZEPHIRAN Chloride with viable pathogenic bacteria. Solutions should not be stored in bottles stoppered with cork closures, but rather in those equipped with appropriate screw-caps. Cotton, wool, rayon, and other materials should not be stored in ZEPHIRAN Chloride solutions. Gauze sponges and fiber pledgets used to apply solutions of ZEPHIRAN Chloride to the skin should be sterilized and stored in separate containers. Only immedi-

TABLE 2
Correct Use of ZEPHIRAN Chloride

ZEPHIRAN Chloride solutions must be prepared, stored, and used correctly to achieve and maintain their antiseptic action. Serious inactivation and contamination of ZEPHIRAN Chloride solutions may occur with misuse.

CORRECT DILUENTS	INCOMPATIBILITIES	PREFERRED FORM
Sterile Water for Injection is recommended for irrigation of body cavities. *Sterile distilled water* is recommended for irrigating traumatized tissue and in the eye. *Freshly distilled water* is recommended for skin antisepsis. *Resin deionized water* should not be used because the deionizing resins can carry pathogens (especially gram-negative bacteria); they also inactivate quaternary ammonium compounds. *Stored water* is not recommended since it may contain many organisms. *Saline* should not be used since it may decrease the antibacterial potency of ZEPHIRAN Chloride solutions.	Anionic detergents and soaps should be thoroughly rinsed from the skin or other areas prior to use of ZEPHIRAN Chloride solutions because they reduce the antibacterial activity of the solutions. Serum and protein material also decrease the activity of ZEPHIRAN Chloride solutions. Corks should not be used to stopper bottles containing ZEPHIRAN Chloride solutions. Fibers or fabrics when stored in ZEPHIRAN Chloride solutions adsorb ZEPHIRAN from the surrounding liquid. Examples are: Cotton — Gauze sponges Wool — Rayon Rubber materials Applicators or sponges, intended for a skin prep, should be stored separately and dipped in ZEPHIRAN Chloride solutions immediately before use. Under certain circumstances the following commonly encountered substances are incompatible with ZEPHIRAN Chloride solutions: Iodine — Aluminum Silver nitrate — Caramel Fluorescein — Kaolin Nitrates — Pine oil Peroxide — Zinc sulfate Lanolin — Zinc oxide Potassium permanganate — Yellow oxide of mercury	ZEPHIRAN Chloride Tinted Tincture 1:750 is recommended for preoperative skin preparation because it contains alcohol and acetone which enhance its cleansing action and promote rapid drying. ZEPHIRAN Chloride Tinted Tincture 1:750, containing acetone, is recommended when it is desirable to outline the operative site. (Aqueous solutions of ZEPHIRAN Chloride used in skin preparation have a tendency to "run off" the skin.) Caution: Because of the flammable organic solvents in ZEPHIRAN Chloride Tinted Tincture 1:750 and Spray, these products should be kept away from open flame or cautery.

ately prior to application should they be immersed in ZEPHIRAN Chloride solutions.

Since ZEPHIRAN Chloride solutions are inactivated by soaps and anionic detergents, thorough rinsing is necessary if these agents are employed prior to their use.

Antiseptics such as ZEPHIRAN Chloride solutions must not be relied upon to achieve complete sterilization, because they do not destroy bacterial spores and certain viruses, including the etiologic agent of infectious hepatitis, and may not destroy *Mycobacterium tuberculosis* and other rare bacterial strains.

ZEPHIRAN Chloride Tinted Tincture 1:750 and Spray contain flammable organic solvents and should not be used near an open flame or cautery.

If solutions stronger than 1:3000 enter the eyes, irrigate immediately and repeatedly with water. Prompt medical attention should then be obtained. Concentrations greater than 1:5000 should not be used on mucous membranes, with the exception of the vaginal mucosa (see Recommended Dilutions).

Precautions: In preoperative antisepsis of the skin, ZEPHIRAN Chloride solutions should not be permitted to remain in prolonged contact with the patient's skin. Avoid pooling of the solution on the operating table.

ZEPHIRAN Chloride solutions that are used on inflamed or irritated tissues must be more dilute than those used on normal tissues (see Recommended Dilutions). ZEPHIRAN Chloride Tinted Tincture 1:750 and Spray, which contain irritating organic solvents, should be kept away from the eyes or other mucous membranes.

Preoperative periorbital skin or head prep should be performed only before the patient, or eye, is anesthetized.

Adverse Reactions: ZEPHIRAN Chloride solutions in normally used concentrations have low systemic and local toxicity and are generally well tolerated, although a rare individual may exhibit hypersensitivity.

Directions for Use:

General: For most surgical applications, the recommended concentration of ZEPHIRAN Chloride Aqueous Solution or ZEPHIRAN Chloride Tinted Tincture is 1:750 (0.13 percent). Liberal use of the solution is recommended to compensate for any adsorption of ZEPHIRAN Chloride by cotton or other materials.

To use ZEPHIRAN Chloride Spray—Tinted Tincture 1:750, remove protective cap, hold in an UPRIGHT position several inches away from the surgical field or injured area, and apply by spraying freely.

Preoperative preparation of skin: ZEPHIRAN Chloride solutions 1:750 are recommended as an antiseptic for use on unbroken skin in the preoperative preparation of the surgical field. Detergents and soaps should be thoroughly rinsed from the skin before applying ZEPHIRAN Chloride solutions. The detergent action of ZEPHIRAN Chloride solutions, particularly when used alternately with alcohol, leaves the skin

Continued on next page

This product information was effective as of September 10, 1990. Current detailed information may be obtained directly from Winthrop Pharmaceuticals, Division of Sterling Drug Inc., by writing to 90 Park Avenue, New York NY, 10016.

Winthrop Pharm.—Cont.

smooth and clean. When ZEPHIRAN Chloride solutions are applied by friction (using several changes of sponges), dirt, skin fats, desquamating epithelium, and superficial bacteria are effectively removed, thus exposing the underlying skin to the antiseptic activity of the solutions.

The following procedure has been found satisfactory for preparation of the surgical field. On the day prior to surgery, the operative site is shaved and then scrubbed thoroughly with ZEPHIRAN Chloride Aqueous Solution 1:750. Immediately before surgery, ZEPHIRAN Chloride Tinted Tincture 1:750 or Spray is applied to the site in the usual manner (see Precautions). If the red tinted solution turns yellow during the preparation of patient's skin for surgery, it usually indicates the presence of soap (alkali) residue which is incompatible with ZEPHIRAN solutions. Therefore, rinse thoroughly and reapply the antiseptic. Because ZEPHIRAN Chloride Tinted Tincture 1:750 contains alcohol and acetone, its cleansing action on the skin is particularly effective and it dries more rapidly than the aqueous solution. The Tinted Tincture is recommended when it is desirable to outline the operative site.

Recommended Dilutions: For specific directions, see TABLES 2 and 3.

Surgery

Preoperative preparation of skin: Aqueous solution 1:750 and Tinted Tincture 1:750 or Spray

Surgeons' hand and arm soaks: Aqueous solution 1:750

Treatment of minor wounds and lacerations: Tinted Tincture 1:750 or Spray

Irrigation of deep infected wounds: Aqueous solution 1:3000 to 1:20,000

Denuded skin and mucous membranes: Aqueous solution 1:5000 to 1:10,000

Obstetrics and Gynecology

Preoperative preparation of skin: Aqueous solution 1:750 and Tinted Tincture 1:750 or Spray

Vaginal douche and irrigation: Aqueous solution 1:2000 to 1:5000

Postepisiotomy care: Aqueous solution 1:5000 to 1:10,000

Breast and nipple hygiene: Aqueous solution 1:1000 to 1:2000

Urology

Bladder and urethral irrigation: Aqueous solution 1:5000 to 1:20,000

Bladder retention lavage: Aqueous solution 1:20,000 to 1:40,000

Dermatology

Oozing and open infections: Aqueous solution 1:2000 to 1:5000

Wet dressings by irrigation or open dressing (Use in occlusive dressings is inadvisable.): Aqueous solution 1:5000 or less

Ophthalmology

Eye irrigation: Aqueous solution 1:5000 to 1:10,000

Preservation of ophthalmic solutions: Aqueous solution 1:5000 to 1:7500

TABLE 3
Dilutions of ZEPHIRAN Chloride Aqueous Solution 1:750

Final Dilution	ZEPHIRAN Chloride Aqueous Solution 1:750 (parts)	Distilled Water (parts)
1:1000	3	1
1:2000	3	5
1:2500	3	7
1:3000	3	9
1:4000	3	13
1:5000	3	17
1:10,000	3	37
1:20,000	3	77
1:40,000	3	157

Accidental Ingestion: If ZEPHIRAN Chloride solution, particularly a concentrated solution, is ingested, marked local irritation of the gastrointestinal tract, manifested by nausea and vomiting, may occur. Signs of systemic toxicity include restlessness, apprehension, weakness, confusion, dyspnea, cyanosis, collapse, convulsions, and coma. Death occurs as a result of paralysis of the respiratory muscles.

Treatment: Immediate administration of several glasses of a mild soap solution, milk, or egg whites beaten in water is recommended. This may be followed by gastric lavage with a mild soap solution. Alcohol should be avoided as it promotes absorption.

To support respiration, the airway should be clear and oxygen should be administered, employing artificial respiration if necessary. If convulsions occur, a short-acting barbiturate may be given parenterally with caution.

How Supplied:

ZEPHIRAN Chloride Aqueous Solution 1:750

Bottles of 8 fl oz (NDC 0024-2521-04) and 1 gallon (NDC 0024-2521-08)

ZEPHIRAN Chloride Tinted Tincture 1:750 (*flammable*)

Bottles of 1 gallon (NDC 0024-2523-08)

ZEPHIRAN Chloride Spray—Tinted Tincture 1:750 (*flammable*)

Bottles of 1 fl oz (NDC 0024-2527-01) and 6 fl oz (NDC 0024-2527-03)

ZW-83-H

This product information was effective as of September 10, 1990. Current detailed information may be obtained directly from Winthrop Pharmaceuticals, Division of Sterling Drug Inc., by writing to 90 Park Avenue, New York, NY 10016.

Wyeth-Ayerst Laboratories

Division of American Home Products Corporation
P.O. BOX 8299
PHILADELPHIA, PA 19101

Wyeth-Ayerst Tamper-Resistant/Evident Packaging

Statements alerting consumers to the specific type of Tamper-Resistant/Evident Packaging appear on the bottle labels and cartons of all Wyeth-Ayerst over-the-counter products. This includes plastic cap seals on bottles, individually wrapped tablets or suppositories, and sealed cartons. This packaging has been developed to better protect the consumer.

ALUDROX®

[*al'ū-drox*]
Antacid
(alumina and magnesia)
ORAL SUSPENSION

Composition: *Suspension*—each 5 ml teaspoonful contains 307 mg aluminum hydroxide [$Al(OH)_3$] as a gel and 103 mg of magnesium hydroxide. The inactive ingredients present are artificial and natural flavors, benzoic acid, butylparaben, glycerin, hydroxypropyl methylcellulose, methylparaben, propylparaben, saccharin, simethicone, sorbitol solution, and water. Sodium content is 0.10 mEq per 5 ml suspension.

Indications: For temporary relief of heartburn, upset stomach, sour stomach, and/or acid indigestion.

Directions: *Suspension*—Two teaspoonfuls (10 ml) every 4 hours or as directed by a physician. Medication may be followed by a sip of water if desired.

Warnings: Do not take more than 12 teaspoonfuls (60 ml) of suspension in a 24-hour period or use maximum dosage for more than two weeks except under the advice and supervision of a physician. As with any drug, if you are pregnant or nursing a baby, seek the advice of a health professional before using this product.

Drug Interaction Precautions: Do not take this product if you are presently taking a prescription antibiotic drug containing any form of tetracycline.

Keep at Room Temperature, Approx. 77°F (25°C).

Suspension should be kept tightly closed and shaken well before use. Avoid freezing.

Keep this and all drugs out of the reach of children.

How Supplied: *Oral Suspension*—bottles of 12 fluidounces.

Shown in Product Identification Section, page 438

Professional Labeling: Consult *1991 Physicians' Desk Reference.*

AMPHOJEL®
[am 'fo-jel]
Antacid
(aluminum hydroxide gel)
ORAL SUSPENSION • TABLETS

Composition: *Suspension*—Each 5 ml teaspoonful contains 320 mg aluminum hydroxide [$Al(OH)_3$] as a gel, and not more than 0.10 mEq of sodium. The inactive ingredients present are artificial and natural flavors, butylparaben, calcium benzoate, glycerin, hydroxypropyl methylcellulose, methylparaben, propylparaben, saccharin, simethicone, sorbitol solution, and water. *Tablets* are available in 0.3 and 0.6 g strengths. Each contains, respectively, the equivalent of 300 mg and 600 mg aluminum hydroxide as a dried gel. The 0.3 g (5 grain) tablet is equivalent to about 1 teaspoonful of the suspension and the 0.6 g (10 grain) tablet is equivalent to about 2 teaspoonfuls. Each 0.3 g tablet contains 0.08 mEq of sodium and each 0.6 g tablet contains 0.13 mEq of sodium.

Indications: For temporary relief of heartburn, upset stomach, sour stomach, and/or acid indigestion.

Directions: *Suspension*—Two teaspoonfuls (10 ml) to be taken five or six times daily, between meals and at bedtime or as directed by a physician. Medication may be followed by a sip of water if desired. *Tablets*—Two tablets of the 0.3 g strength, or one tablet of the 0.6 g strength, five or six times daily, between meals and at bedtime or as directed by a physician. It is unnecessary to chew the 0.3 g tablet before swallowing.

Warnings: Do not take more than 12 teaspoonfuls (60 ml) of suspension, or more than twelve 0.3 g tablets, or more than six 0.6 g tablets in a 24-hour period or use this maximum dosage for more than two weeks except under the advice and supervision of a physician. May cause constipation. As with any drug, if you are pregnant or nursing a baby, seek the advice of a health professional before using this product.

Drug Interaction Precautions: Do not use this product if you are presently taking a prescription antibiotic containing any form of tetracycline.
Keep tightly closed and store at room temperature, Approx. 77°F (25°C).
Suspension should be shaken well before use. Avoid freezing.
Keep this and all drugs out of the reach of children.

How Supplied: *Suspension*—Peppermint flavored; without flavor—bottles of 12 fluidounces. *Tablets*—a convenient auxiliary dosage form—0.3 g (5 grain) bottles of 100; 0.6 g (10 grain), boxes of 100.
Shown in Product Identification Section, page 438

Professional Labeling: Consult *1991 Physicians' Desk Reference.*

BASALJEL®
[bā 'sel-jel]
(basic aluminum carbonate gel)
ORAL SUSPENSION •CAPSULES •TABLETS

Composition: *Suspension*—each 5 ml teaspoonful contains basic aluminum carbonate gel equivalent to 400 mg aluminum hydroxide [$Al(OH)_3$]. The inactive ingredients present are artificial and natural flavors, butylparaben, calcium benzoate, glycerin, hydroxypropyl methylcellulose, methylparaben, mineral oil, propylparaben, saccharin, simethicone, sorbitol solution, and water. *Capsule* contains dried basic aluminum carbonate gel equivalent to 608 mg of dried aluminum hydroxide gel or 500 mg aluminum hydroxide [$Al(OH)_3$]. The inactive ingredients present are D&C Yellow 10, FD&C Blue 1, FD&C Red 40, FD&C Yellow 6, gelatin, polacrilin potassium, polyethylene glycol, talc, and titanium dioxide. *Tablet* contains dried basic aluminum carbonate gel equivalent to 608 mg of dried aluminum hydroxide gel or 500 mg aluminum hydroxide. The inactive ingredients present are cellulose, hydrogenated vegetable oil, magnesium stearate, polacrilin potassium, starch, and talc.

Indications: For the symptomatic relief of hyperacidity, associated with the diagnosis of peptic ulcer, gastritis, peptic esophagitis, gastric hyperacidity, and hiatal hernia.

Warnings: Do not take more than 24 tablets/capsules/teaspoonfuls of BASALJEL in a 24-hour period, or use this maximum dosage for more than two weeks except under the advice and supervision of a physician. Dosage should be carefully supervised since continued overdosage, in conjunction with restriction of dietary phosphorus and calcium, may produce a persistently lowered serum phosphate and a mildly elevated alkaline phosphatase. A usually transient hypercalciuria of mild degree may be associated with the early weeks of therapy. As with any drug, if you are pregnant or nursing a baby, seek the advice of a health professional before using this product.

Dosage and Administration: *Suspension*—two teaspoonfuls (10 ml) in water or fruit juice taken as often as every two hours up to twelve times daily. Two teaspoonfuls have the capacity to neutralize 23 mEq of acid. *Capsules*—two capsules as often as every two hours up to twelve times daily. Two capsules have the capacity to neutralize 24 mEq of acid. *Tablets*—two tablets as often as every two hours up to twelve times daily. Two tablets have the capacity to neutralize 25 mEq of acid. The sodium content of each dosage form is as follows: 0.13 mEq/5 ml for the suspension, 0.12 mEq per capsule, and 0.12 mEq per tablet.

Precautions: May cause constipation. Adequate fluid intake should be maintained in addition to the specific medical or surgical management indicated by the patient's condition.

Drug Interaction Precautions: Alumina-containing antacids should not be used concomitantly with any form of tetracycline therapy.

How Supplied: Suspension—bottles of 12 fluidounces.
Capsules—bottles of 100 and 500.
Tablets (scored)—bottles of 100.
Shown in Product Identification Section, page 438

Professional Labeling: Consult *1991 Physicians' Desk Reference.*

CEROSE-DM®
[se-ros 'DM]
Cough & Cold Formula
Sugar Free • Non-Narcotic

Description: Each teaspoonful (5 mL) contains 15 mg dextromethorphan hydrobromide, 4 mg chlorpheniramine maleate, and 10 mg phenylephrine hydrochloride. Alcohol 2.4%. The inactive ingredients present are artificial flavors, citric acid, edetate disodium, FD&C Yellow 6, glycerin, saccharin sodium, sodium benzoate, sodium citrate, sodium propionate, and water.

Indications: For the temporary relief of cough due to minor throat and bronchial irritation as may occur with the common cold or with inhaled irritants. Temporarily relieves nasal congestion, runny nose, and sneezing due to the common cold, hay fever, or other upper respiratory allergies.

Directions: Adults and children 12 years of age and over: One teaspoonful every four hours as needed. Children 6 to under 12 years of age: One-half teaspoonful every four hours as needed. Do not exceed six doses in a 24-hour period. For children under 6 years, consult a doctor.

Drug Interaction Precaution: Do not take this product if you are presently taking a prescription drug for high blood pressure or depression without first consulting your doctor.
Each teaspoonful (5 mL) contains 15 mg dextromethorphan hydrobromide, 4 mg chlorpheniramine maleate, and 10 mg phenylephrine hydrochloride. Alcohol 2.4%. The inactive ingredients present are artificial flavors, citric acid, edetate disodium, FD&C Yellow 6, glycerin, saccharin sodium, sodium benzoate, sodium citrate, sodium propionate, and water.
Warnings: May cause marked drowsiness; alcohol may increase the drowsiness effect. Avoid alcoholic beverages while taking this product. Use caution when driving a motor vehicle or operating machinery. Do not take this product if you have heart disease, high blood pressure, thyroid disease, diabetes, asthma, glaucoma, emphysema, chronic pulmonary disease, shortness of breath,

Continued on next page

difficulty in breathing, or difficulty in urination due to enlargement of the prostate gland unless directed by a doctor. This product may cause excitability, especially in children. Do not exceed recommended dosage because at higher doses nervousness, dizziness, or sleeplessness may occur. Do not take this product for more than 7 days. A persistent cough may be a sign of a serious condition. If symptoms persist for more than one week, tend to recur, or are accompanied by fever, rash, or persistent headache, consult a doctor. Do not take this product for persistent or chronic cough such as occurs with smoking, or if cough is accompanied by excessive phlegm (mucus) unless directed by a doctor. As with any drug, if you are pregnant or nursing a baby, seek the advice of a health professional before using this product.
Keep this and all drugs out of the reach of children. In case of accidental overdose, seek professional assistance or contact a Poison Control Center immediately.
Keep tightly closed—below 77° F (25° C).

How Supplied: Cases of 12 bottles of 4 fl. oz.; bottles of 1 pint.

Shown in Product Identification Section, page 438

COLLYRIUM for FRESH EYES

[ko-lir 'e-um]

a neutral borate solution
EYE WASH

Description: Soothing Collyrium Eye Wash for Fresh Eyes is specially formulated to soothe, refresh, and cleanse irritated eyes. Collyrium Eye Wash is a neutral borate solution that contains boric acid, sodium borate, thimerosal (not more than 0.002% as a preservative) and water.

Indications: To cleanse the eye, loosen foreign material, air pollutants or chlorinated water.

Recommended Uses:
Home—For emergency flushing of foreign bodies or whenever a soothing eye rinse is necessary.
Hospitals, dispensaries and clinics—For emergency flushing of chemicals or foreign bodies from the eye.

Directions: Puncture bottle by twisting clear cap fully down onto bottle; then remove clear cap from bottle and discard. Remove the eyecup from plastic bag. Rinse blue eyecup with clear water immediately before and after each use. Avoid contamination of rim and interior surface of cup. Fill blue eyecup one-half full with Collyrium Eye Wash. Apply cup tightly to the affected eye to prevent the escape of the liquid and tilt head backward. Open eyelids wide and rotate eyeballs to thoroughly wash eye. Recap by twisting blue eyecup fully onto bottle for storage and subsequent use.

Warnings: Do not use if solution changes color or becomes cloudy, or with a wetting solution for contact lenses or other eye care products containing polyvinyl alcohol. This product contains thimerosal (not more than 0.002% as a preservative). Do not use this product if you are sensitive to mercury.
To avoid contamination do not touch tip of container to any surface. Replace cap after using. If you experience eye pain, changes in vision, continued redness, irritation of the eye, or if the condition worsens or persists, consult a doctor. Obtain immediate medical treatment for all open wounds in or near the eye.
The Collyrium for Fresh Eyes bottle is sealed for your protection. Prior to first use, remove cap and squeeze bottle. If bottle leaks, do not use.
Keep this and all medication out of the reach of children.
Keep bottle tightly closed at Room Temperature, Approx. 77°F (25°C).

How Supplied: Bottles of 4 fl. oz. (118 ml) with eyecup.

Shown in Product Identification Section, page 438

COLLYRIUM FRESH™

[ko-lir 'e-um]

Sterile Eye Drops
Lubricant
Redness Reliever

Description: Collyrium Fresh is a specially formulated sterile eye drop which can be used, up to 4 times daily, to relieve redness and discomfort due to minor eye irritations caused by dust, smoke, smog, swimming, or sun glare.
The active ingredients are tetrahydrozoline HCl (0.05%) and glycerin (1.0%). Other ingredients include benzalkonium chloride (0.01%) and edetate disodium (0.1%) as preservatives, boric acid, hydrochloric acid and sodium borate.

Indications: For the temporary relief of redness due to minor eye irritations or discomfort due to burning or exposure to wind or sun.

Directions: Tilt head back and squeeze 1 to 2 drops into each eye up to 4 times daily, or as directed by a physician.

Warnings: Do not use if solution changes color or becomes cloudy. Remove contact lenses before using. If you have glaucoma, do not use this product except under the advice and supervision of a physician. Overuse of this product may produce increased redness of the eye. To avoid contamination, do not touch tip of container to any surface. Replace cap after using. If you experience eye pain, changes in vision, continued redness or irritation of the eye, or if the condition worsens or persists for more than 72 hours, discontinue use and consult a physician.
Keep this and all medication out of the reach of children.
Retain carton for complete product information.
Keep bottle tightly closed at Room Temperature, Approx. 77°F (25°C).

How Supplied: Bottles of ½ fl. oz. (15 ml) with built-in eye dropper.

Shown in Product Identification Section, page 438

NURSOY®

[nur-soy]

Soy protein isolate formula
READY–TO–FEED
CONCENTRATED LIQUID
POWDER

Breast milk is preferred feeding for newborns. NURSOY® milk-free formula is intended to meet the nutritional needs of infants and children who are not breastfed and are allergic to cow's milk protein and/or intolerant to lactose. NURSOY Ready-to-Feed and Concentrated Liquid contain sucrose as their carbohydrate. NURSOY Powder contains corn syrup solids and sucrose as its carbohydrate. Professional advice should be followed.

Ingredients (in normal dilution supplying 20 calories per fluidounce): 87% water; 6.7% sucrose; 3.4% oleo, coconut, oleic (safflower) and soybean oils; 2.3% soy protein isolate; 0.10% potassium citrate; 0.09% monobasic sodium phosphate; 0.04% calcium carbonate; 0.04% dibasic calcium phosphate; 0.03% magnesium chloride; 0.03% calcium chloride; 0.03% soy lecithin; 0.03% calcium carrageenan; 0.03% calcium hydroxide; 0.03% L-methionine; 0.01% sodium chloride; 0.01% potassium bicarbonate; taurine; ferrous, zinc, and cupric sulfates; L-carnitine; (68 ppb) potassium iodide; ascorbic acid; choline chloride; alpha-tocopheryl acetate; niacinamide; calcium pantothenate; riboflavin; vitamin A palmitate; thiamine hydrochloride; pyridoxine hydrochloride; beta-carotene; phytonadione; folic acid; biotin; cholecalciferol; cyanocobalamin.
NURSOY Powder contains corn syrup solids and sucrose. NURSOY Ready-to-Feed and Concentrated Liquids contain only sucrose.

PROXIMATE ANALYSIS
at 20 calories per fluidounce
READY-TO-FEED, CONCENTRATED LIQUID, and POWDER

	(W/V)
Protein	2.1 %
Fat	3.6 %
Carbohydrate	6.9 %
Ash	0.35%
Water	87.0 %
Crude fiber	not more than 0.01%
Calories/fl. oz.	20

Vitamins, Minerals: In normal dilution, each liter contains:

A	2,000	IU
D_3	400	IU
E	9.5	IU
K_1	100	mcg
C (ascorbic acid)	55	mg
B_1 (thiamine)	670	mcg

B_2 (riboflavin)	1000	mcg
B_6	420	mcg
B_{12}	2	mcg
Niacin	5000	mcg
Pantothenic acid	3000	mcg
Folic acid (folacin)	50	mcg
Choline	85	mg
Inositol	27	mg
Biotin	35	mcg
Calcium	600	mg
Phosphorus	420	mg
Sodium	200	mg
Potassium	700	mg
Chloride	375	mg
Magnesium	67	mg
Manganese	200	mcg
Iron	12.0	mg
Copper	470	mcg
Zinc	5	mg
Iodine	60	mcg

Preparation: *Ready-to-Feed* (32 fl. oz. cans of 20 calories per fluidounce formula)—shake can, open and pour into previously sterilized nursing bottle; attach nipple and feed. Cover opened can and immediately store in refrigerator. Use contents of can within 48 hours of opening.
Prolonged storage of can at excessive temperatures should be avoided.
Expiration date is on bottom of can.
WARNING: DO NOT USE A MICROWAVE TO PREPARE OR WARM FORMULA. SERIOUS BURNS MAY OCCUR.

Concentrated Liquid —For normal dilution supplying 20 calories per fluidounce, use equal amounts of NURSOY® liquid and cooled, previously boiled water.
Note: Prepared formula should be used within 24 hours.
Prolonged storage of can at excessive temperatures should be avoided.
Expiration date is on bottom of can.
WARNING: DO NOT USE A MICROWAVE TO PREPARE OR WARM FORMULA. SERIOUS BURNS MAY OCCUR.

Powder —For normal dilution supplying 20 calories per fluidounce, add 1 scoop (8.9 grams or 1 standard tablespoonful) of NURSOY POWDER, packed and leveled, to 2 fluidounces of cooled, previously boiled water. For larger amounts of formula, add ¼ standard measuring cup of powder (35.5 grams), packed and leveled, to 8 fluidounces (1 standard measuring cup) of water.
Note: Prepared formula should be used within 24 hours.
Prolonged storage of can at excessive temperatures should be avoided.
Expiration date is on bottom of can.

WARNING: DO NOT USE A MICROWAVE TO PREPARE OR WARM FORMULA. SERIOUS BURNS MAY OCCUR.

How Supplied: *Ready-to-Feed* —presterilized and premixed, 32 fluidounce (1 quart) cans, cases of 6 cans;
Concentrated Liquid —13 fluidounce cans, cases of 12 cans;
Powder —1 pound cans, cases of 6 cans.

Questions or Comments regarding NURSOY: 1-800-99-WYETH.

Shown in Product Identification Section, page 439

SMA®
Iron fortified
Infant formula
READY-TO-FEED
CONCENTRATED LIQUID
POWDER

Breast milk is the preferred feeding for newborns. Infant formula is intended to replace or supplement breast milk when breast feeding is not possible or is insufficient, or when mothers elect not to breast feed.
Good maternal nutrition is important for the preparation and maintenance of breast feeding. Extensive or prolonged use of partial bottle feeding, before breast feeding has been well established, could make breast feeding difficult to maintain. A decision not to breast feed could be difficult to reverse.
Professional advice should be followed on all matters of infant feeding. Infant formula should always be prepared and used as directed. Unnecessary or improper use of infant formula could present a health hazard. Social and financial implications should be considered when selecting the method of infant feeding.
SMA® is unique among prepared formulas for its physiologic fat blend, whey-dominated protein composition, amino acid pattern, mineral content and inclusion of beta-carotene and nucleotides.
SMA, utilizing a hybridized safflower (oleic) oil, became the first infant formula offering fat and calcium absorption equal to that of human milk, with a physiologic level of linoleic acid. Thus, the fat blend in SMA provides a ready source of energy, helps protect infants against neonatal tetany and produces a ratio of vitamin E to polyunsaturated fatty acids (linoleic acid) more than adequate to prevent hemolytic anemia and yields a serum lipid profile comparable to the breast-fed infant.
By combining reduced minerals whey with skimmed cow's milk, SMA reduces the protein content to fall within the range of human milk, adjusts the whey-protein to casein ratio to that of human milk, and subsequently reduces the mineral content to a physiologic level.
The resultant 60:40 whey-protein to casein ratio provides protein nutrition superior to a casein-dominated formula. In addition, the essential amino acids, including cystine, are present in amounts close to those of human milk. So the protein in SMA is of high biologic value.
Five nucleotides found in higher amounts in human milk compared to infant formula have been added to SMA at the levels found in breast milk. Clinical studies have demonstrated that these additions allow for plasma lipid levels and gut bifidobacteria which are similar to human milk-fed infants. Benefits to the immunological system have also been proven.
The physiologic mineral content makes possible a low renal solute load which helps protect the functionally immature infant kidney, increases expendable water reserves and helps protect against dehydration.
Use of lactose as the carbohydrate results in a physiologic stool flora and a low stool pH, decreasing the incidence of perianal dermatitis.

Ingredients: SMA Concentrated Liquid or Ready-to-Feed. Water; nonfat milk; reduced minerals whey; oleo, coconut, oleic (safflower or sunflower), and soybean oils; lactose; soy lecithin; taurine; cytidine-5′-monophosphate; calcium carrageenan; adenosine-5′-monophosphate; disodium uridine-5′-monophosphate; disodium inosine-5′-monophosphate; disodium guanosine-5′-monophosphate; *Minerals:* Potassium bicarbonate and chloride; calcium chloride and citrate; sodium bicarbonate and citrate; ferrous, zinc, cupric, and manganese sulfates. *Vitamins:* ascorbic acid, alpha tocopheryl acetate, niacinamide, vitamin A palmitate, calcium pantothenate, thiamine hydrochloride, riboflavin, pyridoxine hydrochloride, beta-carotene, folic acid, phytonadione, biotin, cholecalciferol, cyanocobalamin.

SMA Powder. Lactose; oleo, coconut, oleic (safflower or sunflower), and soybean oils; nonfat milk; whey protein concentrate; soy lecithin; taurine; cytidine-5′-monophosphate; adenosine-5′-monophosphate; disodium uridine-5′-monophosphate; disodium inosine-5′-monophosphate; disodium guanosine-5′-monophosphate. *Minerals:* Potassium phosphate; calcium hydroxide; magnesium chloride; calcium chloride; sodium bicarbonate; ferrous sulfate; potassium hydroxide; potassium bicarbonate; zinc, cupric, and manganese sulfates; potassium iodine. *Vitamins:* Ascorbic acid, choline chloride, inositol, alpha tocopheryl acetate, niacinamide, calcium pantothenate, vitamin A palmitate, riboflavin, thiamine hydrochloride, pyridoxine hydrochloride, beta-carotene, folic acid, phytonadione, biotin, cholecalciferol, cyanocobalamin.

PROXIMATE ANALYSIS at 20 calories per fluidounce READY-TO-FEED, POWDER, and CONCENTRATED LIQUID:

	(W/V)
Fat	3.6 %
Carbohydrate	7.2 %
Protein	1.5 %
60% Lactalbumin (whey protein)	0.9 %
40% Casein	0.6 %
Ash	0.25%
Crude Fiber	None
Total Solids	12.6 %
Calories/fl. oz.	20

Continued on next page

Wyeth-Ayerst—Cont.

Vitamins, Minerals: In normal dilution, each liter contains:

A	2000	IU
D_3	400	IU
E	9.5	IU
K_1	55	mcg
C (ascorbic acid)	55	mg
B_1 (thiamine)	670	mcg
B_2 (riboflavin)	1000	mcg
B_6 (pyridoxine hydrochloride)	420	mcg
B_{12}	1.3	mcg
Niacin	5000	mcg
Pantothenic Acid	2100	mcg
Folic Acid (folacin)	50	mcg
Choline	100	mg
Biotin	15	mcg
Calcium	420	mg
Phosphorus	280	mg
Sodium	150	mg
Potassium	560	mg
Chloride	375	mg
Magnesium	45	mg
Manganese	100	mcg
Iron	12	mg
Copper	470	mcg
Zinc	5	mg
Iodine	60	mcg

Preparation: *Ready-to-Feed* (8 and 32 fl. oz. cans of 20 calories per fluidounce formula)—shake can, open and pour into previously sterilized nursing bottle; attach nipple and feed immediately. Cover opened can and immediately store in refrigerator. Use contents of can within 48 hours of opening.
Prolonged storage of can at excessive temperatures should be avoided.
Expiration date is on bottom of can.

WARNING: DO NOT USE A MICROWAVE TO PREPARE OR WARM FORMULA. SERIOUS BURNS MAY OCCUR.

Powder—(1 pound can)—For normal dilution supplying 20 calories per fluidounce, use 1 scoop (8.3 grams or 1 standard tablespoonful) of powder, packed and leveled, to 2 fluidounces of cooled, previously boiled water. For larger amount of formula, use ¼ standard measuring cup of powder (33.2 grams), packed and leveled, to 8 fluidounces (1 standard measuring cup) of water. Three of these portions make 26 fluidounces of formula.
Prolonged storage of can of powder at excessive temperatures should be avoided.
Expiration date is on bottom of can.

WARNING: DO NOT USE A MICROWAVE TO PREPARE OR WARM FORMULA. SERIOUS BURNS MAY OCCUR.

Concentrated Liquid—For normal dilution supplying 20 calories per fluidounce, use equal amounts of SMA® liquid and cooled, previously boiled water.
Prolonged storage of can at excessive temperatures should be avoided.
Expiration date is on bottom of can.

WARNING: DO NOT USE A MICROWAVE TO PREPARE OR WARM FORMULA. SERIOUS BURNS MAY OCCUR.
Note: Prepared formula should be used within 24 hours.

How Supplied: *Ready-to-Feed*—presterilized and premixed, 32 fluidounce (1 quart) cans, cases of 6 cans; 8 fluidounce cans, cases of 24 (4 carriers of 6 cans). *Powder*—1 pound cans with measuring scoop, cases of 6 cans. *Concentrated Liquid*—13 fluidounce cans, cases of 24 cans.

Also Available: SMA® lo-iron. For those who appreciate the particular advantages of SMA®, the infant formula closest in composition nutritionally to mother's milk, but who sometimes need or wish to recommend a formula that does not contain a high level of iron, there is SMA® lo-iron with all the benefits of regular SMA® but with a reduced level of iron of 1.4 mg per quart. Infants should receive supplemental dietary iron from an outside source to meet daily requirements.
Concentrated Liquid—13 fl. oz. cans, cases of 24 cans. *Powder*—1 pound cans with measuring scoop, cases of 6 cans. *Ready-to-Feed*—32 fl. oz. cans, cases of 6 cans.
Preparation of the standard 20 calories per fluidounce formula of SMA® lo-iron is the same as SMA® iron fortified given above.

Questions or Comments regarding SMA: 1-800-99-WYETH.

Shown in Product Identification Section, page 439

WYANOIDS® Relief Factor
[*wi'a-noids*]
Hemorrhoidal Suppositories

Description: Active Ingredients: Live Yeast Cell Derivative, Supplying 2,000 units Skin Respiratory Factor Per Ounce of Cocoa Butter Suppository Base and Shark Liver Oil 3%. **Inactive Ingredients:** Beeswax, Glycerin, Phenylmercuric Nitrate 1:10,000 (as a preservative), Polyethylene Glycol 600 Dilaurate.

Indications: To help shrink swelling of hemorrhoidal tissues and provide prompt, temporary relief from pain and itching.

Usual Dosage: Use one suppository up to five times daily, especially in the morning, at night, and after bowel movements, or as directed by a physician.

Directions: Remove wrapper and insert one suppository rectally using gentle pressure. Frequent application and lubrication with Wyanoids® Relief Factor provide continual therapy which will lead to more rapid improvement of rectal conditions.

Caution: In case of bleeding or if the condition persists, the patient should consult a physician. Keep this and all medicines out of the reach of children. Do not store above 80°F.

How Supplied: Boxes of 12 and 24.

Shown in Product Identification Section, page 439

EDUCATIONAL MATERIAL

Audiovisual Programs
The ***Wyeth-Ayerst Audiovisual Catalog,*** listing audiovisual programs available through the Wyeth-Ayerst Audiovisual Library or on loan through the local Wyeth-Ayerst representative, can be obtained by writing Professional Service, Wyeth-Ayerst Laboratories, P.O. Box 8299, Philadelphia, PA 19101.

Zila Pharmaceuticals, Inc.
777 EAST THOMAS ROAD
PHOENIX, AZ 85014-5454

ZILACTIN® Medicated Gel
ZILABRACE™ Oral Analgesic Gel
ZILADENT™ Oral Analgesic Gel
ZILACTOL™ Medicated Liquid

Description: **ZILACTIN** is well recognized by many physicians, dentists and pharmacists as the best treatment available to stop pain and speed healing of canker sores, fever blisters and cold sores. **ZILABRACE** is for cuts and sores caused by braces, retainers and other dental appliances. **ZILADENT** is for sores and irritations common to denture wearers. **ZILABRACE** and **ZILADENT** are specially formulated with a topical anesthetic in varying levels determined to be safe and effective. All three products have the unique ability to form a tenacious, occlusive film which holds the medication in place for hours while it relieves pain. This usually permits pain-free eating and drinking even when challenged by acidic beverages. **ZILACTOL,** a non-film-forming medicated liquid, is specially formulated to treat developing cold sores and fever blisters before they break out.

Active Ingredients: **ZILACTIN**—Tannic Acid (7%); **ZILABRACE**—Benzocaine (10%); **ZILADENT**—Benzocaine (6%); **ZILACTOL**—Tannic Acid (7%)

Application: ZILACTIN, ZILABRACE and **ZILADENT:** Apply four times a day for the first three days and then as needed. Dry the affected area with a gauze pad, tissue or cotton swab. Apply a thin coat of **ZILACTIN, ZILABRACE** or **ZILADENT** and allow 30–60 seconds for the gel to dry into a film. **ZILACTOL:** Apply every one to two hours for the first three days and then as needed. For maximum effectiveness use at first signs of tingling or itching. Moisten a cotton swab with several drops of **ZILACTOL.** Apply directly on the developing cold sore or fever blister and allow to dry for 15 seconds.

Warnings: A mild, temporary stinging sensation may be experienced when applying **ZILACTIN, ZILABRACE, ZILADENT** or **ZILACTOL** to an open cut, sore or blister. DO NOT USE IN OR NEAR EYES. In the event of accidental contact with the eye, flush immediately and continuously for ten minutes. Seek immediate medical attention if pain or irritation persists. As with all medications, keep out of the reach of children.

How Supplied: Zila products are available in a 7.1 gm tube (**ZILACTIN, ZILABRACE, ZILADENT**) and 10 ml bottle (**ZILACTOL**). Each product is also available to doctors directly from Zila in full-size and single-use packages.

*U.S. patent numbers 4,285,934 and 4,381,296

Distributed by:
ZILA Pharmaceuticals, Inc.
Phoenix, AZ 85014–5454

Shown in Product Identification Section, page 439

EDUCATIONAL MATERIAL

Samples and literature are available to physicians and dentists on request.

SECTION 7

Diagnostics Devices and Medical Aids

This section is intended to present product information on Diagnostics, Devices and Medical Aids designed for home use by patients. The information concerning each product has been prepared, edited and approved by the manufacturer.

The Publisher has emphasized to manufacturers the necessity of describing products comprehensively so that all information essential for intelligent and informed use is available. In organizing and presenting the material in this edition the Publisher is providing all the information made available by manufacturers.

In presenting the following material to the medical profession, the Publisher is not necessarily advocating the use of any product.

Lavoptik Company, Inc.
661 WESTERN AVENUE N.
ST. PAUL, MN 55103

LAVOPTIK® Eye Cups

Description: Device—Sterile disposable eye cups.

How Supplied: Individually bagged eye cups are packed 12 per box, NDC 10651-01004.

LifeScan Inc.
a Johnson & Johnson company
1051 S. MILPITAS BOULEVARD
MILPITAS, CA 95035-6314

ONE TOUCH®
BLOOD GLUCOSE MONITORING SYSTEM

Description: The One Touch System provides more accurate blood glucose monitoring results for your patients with diabetes because its simple procedure reduces inaccurate readings. The One Touch System eliminates the need for user timing, wiping or blotting. Simple procedure: insert strip, press power, apply sample. Results in 45 seconds. Memory stores the most recent 250 results. Clinically proven more accurate in the hands of patients, the One Touch System helps patients achieve greater accuracy because test results are virtually technique-independent.[1] "A system such as the One Touch, which eliminates the need for the operator to start and time the test and remove the blood, results in an improvement in precision and accuracy . . . "[2]

How Supplied: One Touch® Blood Glucose System—Complete Kit—Each Complete Kit contains everything your patients need to begin blood glucose monitoring:

One Touch Blood Glucose Meter
—with 250 Test Memory and
—prompts in 7 languages, including Spanish
25 One Touch Test Strips
Carry Case
Penlet™ Blood Sampling Pen
25 Lancets
One Touch Glucose Control Solution
Instructional Audio Cassette
Owner's Booklet
4 N-Cell Batteries

For a One Touch System demonstration and a complete review of clinical data, contact your LifeScan Professional Representative. For the name of your local representative, call toll free:

In the United States: 1 800 227-8862
In Canada: 1 800 663-5521

1. *Diabetes Care,* Vol. 11, No. 10, November-December 1988, pp 791-794.
2. *Ibid.*

Ortho Pharmaceutical Corporation
Advanced Care Products
RARITAN, NJ 08869

ADVANCE®
Pregnancy Test

Active Ingredients: Human Chorionic Gonadotropin (HCG) alpha chain specific monoclonal antibody HCG, beta-chain specific antibody/enzyme conjugate, chromogenic substrate solution, and buffer solution.

Indications: An in-vitro pregnancy test for use in the home that can detect the presence of HCG in the urine as early as one (1) day past last missed period.

Actions: ADVANCE will accurately detect the presence or absence of HCG in urine in just thirty minutes. It is as accurate as pregnancy test methods used in many hospitals.

Dosage and Administration: Perform the test according to instructions. If, after thirty minutes, a blue color appears on the rounded end of the COLORSTICK, the patient can assume she is pregnant. If the rounded end of the COLORSTICK remains white, and no blue color can be seen, no pregnancy hormone has been detected and the patient is probably not pregnant. The test results may be affected by certain health conditions such as an ovarian cyst or ectopic pregnancy and by certain medications such as thiazide diuretics, plurothiazine, hormones, steroids, chemotherapeutics, and thyroid drugs. For additional reassurance, a toll-free telephone number is included in each package insert. This service is staffed by Registered Nurses who can answer any questions the patient may have about her results, or how she performed the test.

How Supplied: Each ADVANCE test contains a plastic COLORSTICK, a plastic vial containing buffer solution, a glass tube containing dried test chemicals, a glass tube containing color developing solution, a test stand with urine collection and instructions for use.

Storage: Store at room temperature (59°–86°F). Do not freeze.

Shown in Product Identification Section, page 420

DAISY 2®
Pregnancy Test

Active Ingredients: Human Chorionic Gonadotropin (HCG) antibody HCG antibody/enzyme conjugate, and chromogenic substrate solution.

Indications: An in-vitro pregnancy test for use in the home that can detect the presence of HCG in the urine as early as the first day of a missed period.

Actions: DAISY 2 will accurately check the presence or absence of HCG in urine in just 5–8 minutes. It is the same pregnancy test method used in many hospitals.

Dosage and Administration: Perform the test according to instructions. If, after 5–8 minutes, a plus (+) sign has formed in the center of the test cube, the patient is probably pregnant. If a minus (−) sign appears, no pregnancy hormone has been detected and the patient is probably not pregnant. In the unlikely event that neither sign appears, the test system has not worked properly and the patient should call the toll free number included in each package insert. This toll free number is staffed by Registered Nurses who can answer any questions the patient may have about her results, or how she performed the test. All home pregnancy test kits recommend a second test if the first test indicates that the patient is not pregnant and her period does not begin within a week. This second test may be needed because the patient may have miscalculated her period, or her body may not have accumulated enough hormone for a true reading. Many women like the reassurance that comes from double-checking the results. DAISY 2 makes this double checking easy and convenient by providing two complete and identical tests in each kit. The test results may be affected by certain health conditions such as a ovarian cyst or ectopic pregnancy and certain medications such as thiazide diuretics, plurothiazine, hormones, steroids, chemotherapeutics, and thyroid drugs.

How Supplied: Each DAISY 2 kit contains everything needed to perform two tests, two plastic test cubes, two glass tubes containing dried test chemicals, two plastic vials containing developing solution, two test stands with urine cup and urine dropper and instructions for use.

Storage: Store at room temperature (59–86°F). Do not Freeze.

Shown in Product Identification Section, page 420

FACT PLUS™
Pregnancy Test

Active Ingredients: Human Chorionic Gonadotropin (HCG) antibody, HCG antibody/colored conjugate.

Indications: An in-vitro pregnancy test for use in the home that can detect the presence of HCG in the urine as early as the first day of a missed period.

Actions: FACT PLUS will accurately detect the presence or absence of HCG in urine in as soon as 5 minutes using urine collected at any time of day. One step FACT PLUS is the same pregnancy test method used in many hospitals.

Dosage and Administration: Using the urine dropper, drop five drops of urine in the Urine Well of the test disk. Wait for red to appear in End of Test Window (may take about 5 minutes). If, after the End of Test Window has turned red, a plus (+) sign has formed in the center of the test disk, the patient is proba-

Continued on next page

Ortho Pharm.—Cont.

bly pregnant. If a minus (−) sign appears, no pregnancy hormone has been detected and the patient is probably not pregnant. In the unlikely event that neither sign appears the test system has not worked properly and the patient should call the toll free number included in the package insert. This toll free number is staffed by Registered Nurses who can answer any questions the patient may have about her results, or how she performed the test. The test results may be affected by various other factors and medications such as thiazide diuretics, plurothiazine, hormones, steroids, chemotherapeutics, and thyroid drugs.

How Supplied: Each FACT PLUS kit contains a plastic test disk, a urine collection cup, a urine dropper, and complete instructions for use.

Storage: Store at room temperature (59–86°F). Do not freeze.

Shown in Product Identification Section, page 420

Parke-Davis

Consumer Health Products Group
Division of Warner-Lambert Company
201 TABOR ROAD
MORRIS PLAINS, NJ 07950

e·p·t® STICK TEST
Early Pregnancy Test

BEFORE YOU BEGIN THE e·p·t TEST:

- CAREFULLY READ THROUGH THIS ENTIRE INSERT.
- YOU CAN USE THIS TEST ANY TIME OF THE DAY, PROVIDED THAT YOU DO NOT DRINK ANY LIQUIDS OR EAT ANY FOOD FOR AT LEAST 3 HOURS BEFORE PERFORMING THE TEST.
- IF YOU HAVE ANY QUESTIONS, CALL TOLL-FREE 1-800-562-0266, OR IN NEW JERSEY CALL 1-800-338-0326.
- REGISTERED NURSES ARE AVAILABLE TO ANSWER YOUR CALLS CONFIDENTIALLY.
- **e·p·t** IS VIRTUALLY 100% ACCURATE IN LABORATORY TESTS.

HOW e·p·t WORKS:
When a woman becomes pregnant, her body produces a special hormone known as hCG (Human Chorionic Gonadotropin), which appears in the urine. **e·p·t** can detect this hormone as early as the first day you miss your period.
If you test positive, you can assume you are pregnant and should see your doctor. A negative result means that no hCG has been detected and you can assume that you are not pregnant.

WHEN TO USE e·p·t:
e·p·t can detect hCG hormone levels in your urine as early as the day your period should have started. **e·p·t** can be used on the day of missed period as well as any day thereafter.

THE e·p·t TEST CONTAINS:

A. A pouch containing the test stick. The test stick has a small round window, a larger oval window, and an opening in the lip which is covered by the cap. (A small paper packet (desiccant), helps keep the test fresh. Throw this away. It is NOT part of the test).
B. A urine collection cap.
C. A tray that holds the test contents, with a built-in holder for the test stick.

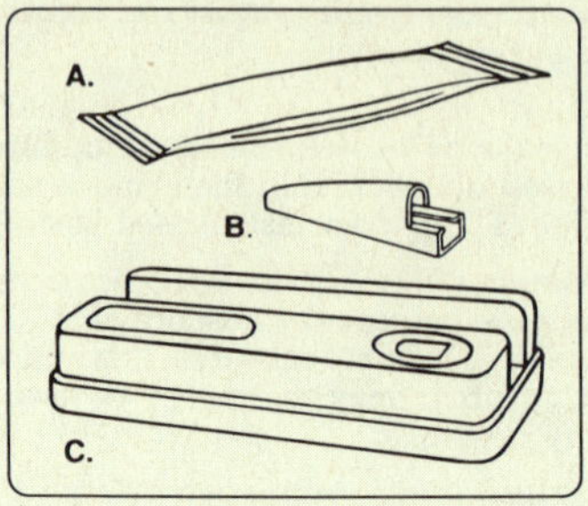

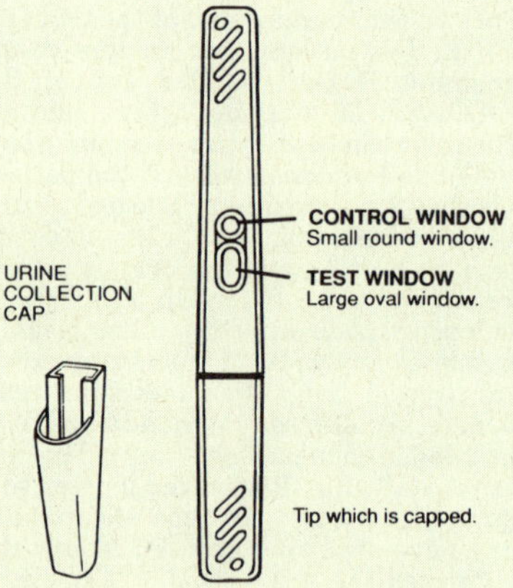

The e·p·t test is easy to perform.
SIMPLY DO THE FOLLOWING:

- **REMOVE THE TEST STICK FROM THE POUCH.**
Tear by the small notch on the end of the pouch.
Take off the cap.
- **SLIDE THE TEST STICK INTO THE URINE COLLECTION CAP.**
Make sure that the opening in the tip faces the cap area (see illustration). The cap should fit easily on the stick. Make sure that the ridges on the cap and the test stick are both on the same side.

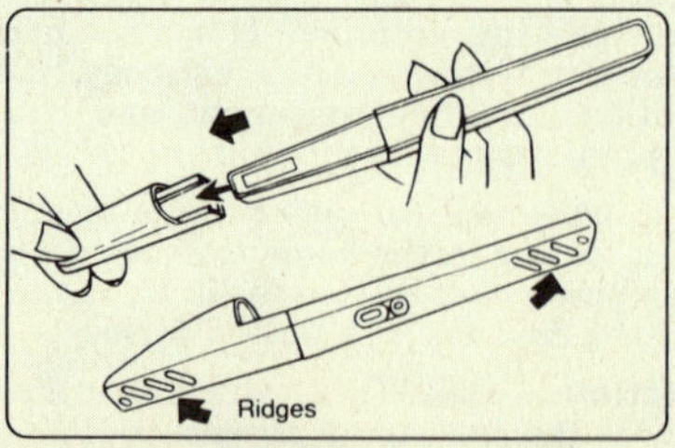

- **COLLECT URINE.**
With the urine collection cap facing you, and pointing in a downward direction, hold the test stick in your urine stream until the cap is filled with urine. The test and control windows should be facing away from you. Do not let urine splash the test and control windows on the test stick.
NOTE: You do not need to use first morning urine. However, do not eat or drink anything for at least 3 hours before you collect your urine.

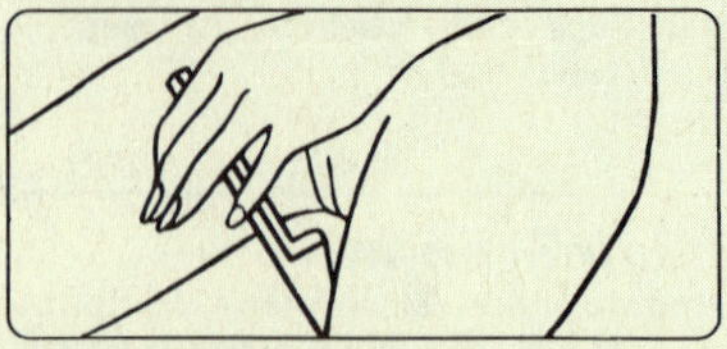

- **PLACE THE TEST STICK INTO THE HOLDER ON THE TRAY.**
(Optional)
The test stick should fit easily into the built-in holder in the tray.

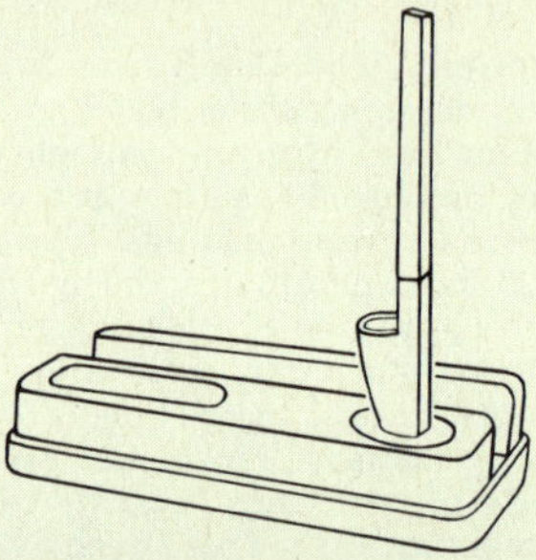

- **WAIT 4 MINUTES.**
DO NOT READ THE TEST RESULTS UNTIL AFTER 4 MINUTES.
(Earlier results may be invalid.)
NOTE: As the urine moves up the test stick, a dark pink or purple color will move across both windows. This color will fade after a few minutes. This is the normal way the test works.

READING THE e·p·t TEST RESULTS:

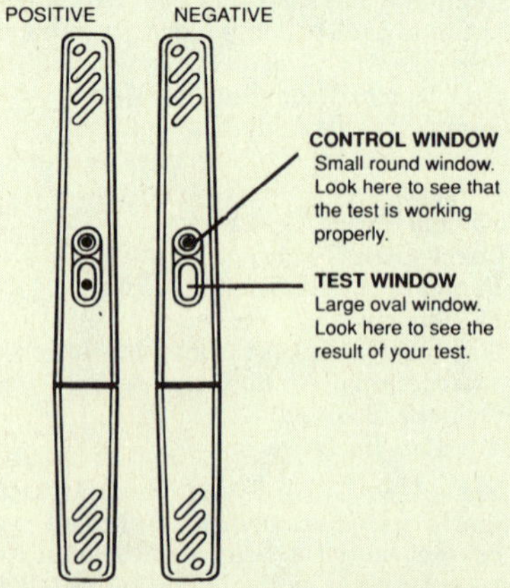

- **READ THE CONTROL WINDOW.**
A pink or purple circle will appear in the Control Window whether you are pregnant or not. This tells you that the **e·p·t** test is working properly. Now you can read your results in the Test Window.

IMPORTANT: If there is no color in the Control Window, call the toll-free number and DO NOT read the result in the Test Window since the result may be incorrect.

- **READ THE TEST WINDOW.**

  POSITIVE—After the test stick has been in the urine for four minutes, you can assume you ARE PREGNANT if a circle of ANY SHADE of pink or purple remains in the Test Window.

  NEGATIVE—You can assume you ARE NOT PREGNANT if after four minutes NO CIRCLE is seen in the Test Window.

NOTE: EVEN IF A VERY FAINT PINK OR PURPLE CIRCLE IS VISIBLE IN THE TEST WINDOW, THE RESULT IS POSITIVE.

(The color of the circle in the Test Window DOES NOT HAVE to match the color of the circle in the Control Window).

Ingredients:
Test stick containing gold sol particles coated with hCG antibodies and anti-hCG antibodies.
*Not to be taken internally.
For in-vitro diagnostic use.
Store at 59°–86°F.

If this is a 2 kit package, save the tray for use with the second test stick.

QUESTIONS YOU MAY HAVE ABOUT e·p·t:

When can I do the test?
e·p·t can detect hCG levels as early as the first day of your missed period. You can perform the test at any time of the day as long as you did not eat or drink anything for at least 3 hours before performing the test.

Can I collect my urine in a cup instead of in the urine collection cap?
Yes. If you collect urine in a cup, place the urine collection cap on the test stick. Then dip the cap side into the cup to fill the cap with urine. Continue the test as instructed.
You can cover and store your urine in the refrigerator. Be sure to do the test the same day the urine was collected and let the urine warm to room temperature before testing.
NOTE: After your urine has been stored for several hours, a sediment may form at the bottom of the container. DO NOT mix or shake the urine. Use only the urine at the top of the container.

What if the test changes color, but the color isn't the same as the picture in the brochure?
If the test is positive, the Test Window will retain a circle of some shade of pink or purple color after the 4 minutes the test stick was in the urine. The color can be ANY SHADE of pink or purple and DOES NOT HAVE TO MATCH the color pictured or the color present in the Control Window.
NOTE: A positive test result in a range of pink or purple shades. **e·p·t** is so sensitive that it can detect pregnancy as early as the day of a missed period. However, during pregnancy, each day after a missed period results in higher levels of hCG (the pregnancy hormone) in the urine. This is why testing a few days or a week after a missed period will result in a darker test result than the first day of a missed period.

What do I do if the test result is positive?
If the test result is positive, you should see a doctor to discuss your pregnancy and next steps. Early prenatal care is important to ensure the health of you and your baby.

What do I do if the test result is negative?
If the test result is negative, no pregnancy hormone (hCG) has been detected and you are probably not pregnant. However, you may have miscalculated when your period was due. If your period does not start within a week, repeat the test. If you still get a negative result after the second test, and your period still has not started, you should see a doctor.

What if I don't wait the full 4 minutes before reading the test result?
If you read the test result before the full 4 minutes have passed, you may not give the test enough time to work, and the results may be inaccurate.

After I perform the test, how long will the result last?
The result of the test is valid for 24 hours after you perform the test. Simply replace the urine collection cap with the original cap to preserve the test results.

What if I don't think the results of the test are correct?
If you follow the instructions carefully, you should not get a false result. Certain drugs and rare medical conditions may give a false result. Analgesics, antibiotics, and birth control pills should not affect the test result. If you repeat the test and continue to get an unexpected result, contact your doctor.

IF YOU HAVE FURTHER QUESTIONS ABOUT **e·p·t** CALL TOLL-FREE 1-800-562-0266 WEEKDAYS 8 AM to 5 PM EST. IN NEW JERSEY, CALL 1-800-338-0326.

Marketed by
PARKE-DAVIS Consumer Health Products Group
©1990 Warner-Lambert Company
Morris Plains, NJ 07950 USA
Shown in Product Identification Section, page 421

Products are indexed by generic and chemical names in the
YELLOW SECTION

Whitehall Laboratories Inc.

Division of American Home Products Corporation
685 THIRD AVENUE
NEW YORK, NY 10017

CLEARBLUE EASY™
Pregnancy Test Kit

Clearblue Easy is the easiest and one of the fastest pregnancy tests available because all you have to do is hold the absorbent tip in your urine stream, replace the cap, and in 3 minutes you'll know the test is complete when a blue line appears in the small window. The large window shows the test result. If there is a blue line in the large window, you are pregnant. If there is no line, you are not pregnant.

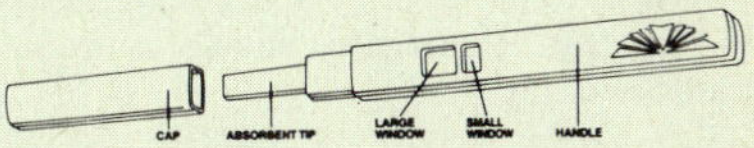

Clearblue Easy is a rapid, one-step pregnancy test for home use which detects tiny amounts of the pregnancy hormone HCG (human chorionic gonadotropin) in the urine. This hormone is produced in increasing amounts during the first part of pregnancy. Clearblue Easy uses sensitive monoclonal antibodies to detect the presence of the hormone from the first day of a missed period.
The pregnancy hormone, HCG, is most concentrated in your first morning urine, so it is recommended that you use this urine, particularly if you test on the day of your missed period.
A negative result means that no pregnancy hormone was detected and you are probably not pregnant. If your period does not start within a week, you may have miscalculated the day your period was due. Repeat the test using another Clearblue Easy test. If the second test still gives a negative result and you still have not menstruated, you should see your doctor.
Clearblue Easy is specially designed for easy use at home. However, if you do have questions about the test or results, give the Clearblue Easy TalkLine a call at 1-800-223-2329. A specially trained staff of advisors is available 24 hours a day to answer your questions.
Produced by Unipath Ltd., Bedford, U.K.
Unipath, Clearblue Easy and the fan device are trademarks.
Distributed by Whitehall Laboratories, New York, NY 10017.
Shown in Product Identification Section, page 436

CLEARPLAN EASY™
One-Step Ovulation Predictor

CLEARPLAN EASY is the easiest home ovulation predictor test to use because of its unique technological design. It consists of just one piece and involves only one step to get the results. To use CLEARPLAN EASY, a woman simply urinates on the absorbent tip (a woman

Continued on next page

Whitehall—Cont.

can test any time of day) for 5 seconds, and after 5 minutes, she can read the results. A blue line will appear in the small window to show her that the test has worked correctly. The large window indicates the presence of luteinizing hormone (LH) in her urine. If there is a line in the large window which is similar to or darker than the line in the small window, she has detected her LH surge.

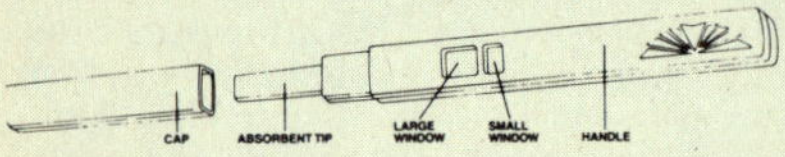

Laboratory tests confirm that CLEARPLAN EASY is over 98% accurate in detecting the LH surge as shown by radioimmunoassay (RIA).

CLEARPLAN EASY employs highly sensitive monoclonal antibody technology to accurately predict the onset of ovulation, and, consequently, the best time each month for a woman to try to become pregnant. The test monitors the amount of LH in a woman's urine. Small amounts of LH are present during most of the menstrual cycle, but the level normally rises sharply about 24 to 36 hours before ovulation (which is when an egg is released from the ovary). CLEARPLAN EASY detects this LH surge which precedes ovulation so that a woman knows 24–36 hours beforehand the time she is most able to become pregnant.

A woman will be most fertile during the 2 to 3 days after an LH surge is detected. Sperm can fertilize an egg for many hours after sexual intercourse. So, if sexual intercourse occurs during the 2–3 days after a similar or darker line appears in the large window, the chances of getting pregnant are maximized.

CLEARPLAN EASY contains 5 days of tests. If, because a woman's cycles are irregular or if for any other reason a woman does not detect her LH surge after 5 days of testing, she should continue testing with a second CLEARPLAN EASY kit. CLEARPLAN EASY offers users the support of a 24-hour TalkLine (1-800-223-2329). This service is operated by trained advisors who are available to answer any questions about using the test or reading the results.

Produced by Unipath Ltd., Bedford, U.K. Unipath, CLEARPLAN EASY and the fan device are trademarks.

Distributed by Whitehall Laboratories, New York, NY 10017.

Shown in Product Identification Section, page 436

Certified Poison Control Centers

The poison control centers in the following list are certified by the American Association of Poison Control Centers. To receive certification, each center must meet certain criteria. It must, for example, serve a large geographic area; it must be open 24 hours a day and provide direct dialing or toll-free access; it must be supervised by a medical director; and it must have registered pharmacists or nurses available to answer questions from the public.

Staff members of these centers are trained to resolve toxicity situations in the home of the caller, but, in some instances, hospital referrals are given.

The centers have a wide variety of toxicology resources, including a computer capability covering some 350,000 substances that are updated quarterly. They also offer a range of educational services to the public as well as to the health-care professional. In some states, these large centers exist side by side with smaller poison control centers that provide more limited information.

AMERICAN ASSOCIATION OF POISON CONTROL CENTERS

ALABAMA

Alabama Poison Control Systems, Inc.
809 University Boulevard East
Tuscaloosa, AL 35401
Emergency Numbers:
(800) 462-0800 (AL only);
(205) 345-0600

Children's Hospital of Alabama - Regional Poison Control Center
1600 Seventh Avenue, South
Birmingham, AL 35233-1711
Emergency Numbers:
(205) 939-9201; (205) 933-4050;
(800) 292-6678

ARIZONA

Arizona Poison & Drug Information Center
Arizona Health Sciences Center,
Room 3204K
University of Arizona
Tucson, AZ 85724
Emergency Numbers:
(602) 626-6016; (800) 362-0101
(AZ only)

Samaritan Regional Poison Center
Good Samaritan Medical Center
1130 East McDowell Road,
Suite A-5
Phoenix, AZ 85006
Emergency Number:
(602) 253-3334

CALIFORNIA

Fresno Regional Poison Control Center of Fresno Community Hospital and Medical Center
P.O. Box 1232
2823 Fresno Street
Fresno, CA 93715
Emergency Numbers:
(209) 445-1222; (800) 346-5922
(CA only)

Los Angeles County Medical Association Regional Poison Control Center
1925 Wilshire Boulevard
Los Angeles, CA 90057
Emergency Numbers:
(213) 484-5151; (800) 77 POISN

San Diego Regional Poison Center
UCSD Medical Center,
225 Dickinson Street
San Diego, CA 92103
Emergency Numbers:
(619) 543-6000; (800) 876-4766

San Francisco Bay Area Regional Poison Control Center
San Francisco General Hospital,
Room 1E86
1001 Potrero Avenue
San Francisco, CA 94110
Emergency Numbers:
(415) 476-6600; (800) 523-2222
(415, 707 only)

UCDMC Regional Poison Control Center
2315 Stockton Boulevard
Sacramento, CA 95817
Emergency Number:
(916) 453-3414

COLORADO

Rocky Mountain Poison and Drug Center
645 Bannock Street
Denver, CO 80204-4507
Emergency Numbers:
(303) 629-1123; (800) 332-3073
(CO only)

D.C.

National Capital Poison Center
Georgetown University Hospital
3800 Reservoir Rd., NW
Washington, DC 20007
Emergency Number:
(202) 625-3333

FLORIDA

Florida Poison Information Center at the Tampa General Hospital
P.O. Box 1289
Tampa, FL 33601
Emergency Numbers:
(813) 253-4444; (800) 282-3171
(FL only)

GEORGIA

Georgia Poison Control Center
Grady Memorial Hospital
Box 26066
80 Butler Street, SE
Atlanta, GA 30335-3801
Emergency Numbers:
(404) 589-4400; (800) 282-5846
(GA only);
(404) 525-3323 (TTY)

KENTUCKY

Kentucky Regional Poison Center of Kosair
Children's Hospital
P.O. Box 35070
Louisville, KY 40232-5070
Emergency Numbers:
(502) 589-8222; (800) 722-5725
(KY only)

MARYLAND

Maryland Poison Center
20 North Pine Street
Baltimore, MD 21201
Emergency Numbers:
(301) 528-7701; (800) 492-2414
(MD only)

MASSACHUSETTS

Massachusetts Poison Control System
300 Longwood Avenue
Boston, MA 02115
Emergency Numbers:
(617) 232-2120; (800) 682-9211
(MA only)

MICHIGAN

Blodgett Regional Poison Center
1840 Wealthy SE
Grand Rapids, MI 49506
Emergency Numbers:
(800) 832-2727 (MI only);
(800) 356-3232 (TTY)

Poison Control Center, Children's Hospital of Michigan
3901 Beaubien Boulevard
Detroit, MI 48201
Emergency Numbers:
(313) 745-5711; (800) 462-6642 (MI only)

MINNESOTA

Hennepin Regional Poison Center
Hennepin County Medical Center
701 Park Avenue
Minneapolis, MN 55415
Emergency Numbers:
(612) 347-3141;
(612) 337-7474 (TTY)

Minnesota Regional Poison Center
St. Paul-Ramsey Medical Center
640 Jackson Street
St. Paul, MN 55101
Emergency Numbers:
(612) 221-2113; (800) 222-1222 (MN only)

MISSOURI

Cardinal Glennon Children's Hospital Regional Poison Center
1465 South Grand Boulevard
St. Louis, MO 63104
Emergency Numbers:
(314) 772-5200; (800) 392-9111 (MO only); (800) 366-8888;
(314) 577-5336 (TTY)

MONTANA

Rocky Mountain Poison and Drug Center
645 Bannock Street
Denver, CO 80204-4507
Emergency Number:
(800) 525-5042 (MT only)

NEBRASKA

Mid-Plains Poison Control Center
8301 Dodge Street
Omaha, NE 68114
Emergency Numbers:
(402) 390-5400; (800) 642-9999 (NE only); (800) 228-9515 (Surrounding states)

NEW JERSEY

New Jersey Poison Information and Education System
201 Lyons Avenue
Newark, NJ 07112
Emergency Numbers:
(201) 923-0764; (800) 962-1253 (NJ only)

NEW MEXICO

New Mexico Poison and Drug Information Center
University of New Mexico
Albuquerque, NM 87131
Emergency Numbers:
(505) 843-2551; (800) 432-6866 (NM only)

NEW YORK

Long Island Regional Poison Control Center
Nassau County Medical Center
2201 Hempstead Turnpike
East Meadow, NY 11554
Emergency Number:
(516) 542-2323

New York City Poison Control Center
455 First Avenue, Room 123
New York, NY 10016
Emergency Numbers:
(212) 340-4494;
(212) POISONS

OHIO

Central Ohio Poison Center
Columbus Children's Hospital
700 Children's Drive
Columbus, OH 43205
Emergency Numbers:
(614) 228-1323; (800) 682-7625 (OH only); (614) 228-2272 (TTY)

Cincinnati Drug and Poison Information Center
231 Bethesda Avenue, M.L. #144
Cincinnati, OH 45267-0144
Emergency Numbers:
(513) 558-5111; (800) 872-5111

OREGON

Oregon Poison Center
Oregon Health Sciences University
3181 SW Sam Jackson Park Road
Portland, OR 97201
Emergency Numbers:
(503) 279-8968 (local);
(800) 452-7165
(OR only)

PENNSYLVANIA

Delaware Valley Regional Poison Control Center
One Children's Center
34th & Civic Center Boulevard
Philadelphia, PA 19104
Emergency Number:
(215) 386-2100

Pittsburgh Poison Center
3705 Fifth Avenue at DeSoto Street
Pittsburgh, PA 15213
Emergency Number:
(412) 681-6669

RHODE ISLAND

Rhode Island Poison Center - Rhode Island Hospital
593 Eddy Street
Providence, RI 02902
Emergency Numbers:
(401) 277-5727

TEXAS

North Texas Poison Center
P.O. Box 35926
Dallas, TX 75235
Emergency Numbers:
(214) 590-5000; (800) 441-0040
(TX only)

Texas State Poison Center
The University of Texas Medical Branch
Galveston, TX 77550-2780
Emergency Numbers:
(409) 765-1420; (713) 654-1701 (Houston); (512) 478-4490 (Austin); (800) 392-8548 (TX only)

UTAH

Intermountain Regional Poison Control Center
50 North Medical Drive, Building 428
Salt Lake City, UT 84132
Emergency Numbers:
(801) 581-2151; (800) 456-7707
(UT only)

WEST VIRGINIA

West Virginia Poison Center
West Virginia University Health Sciences Center/Charleston Division
3110 MacCorkle Avenue, SE
Charleston, WV 25304
Emergency Numbers:
(304) 348-4211; (800) 642-3625
(WV only)

WYOMING

Rocky Mountain Poison and Drug Center
645 Bannock Street
Denver, CO 80204-4507
Emergency Number:
(800) 442-2702 (WY only)